PRESCRIPTION
for
Herbal Healing

SECOND EDITION

PRESCRIPTION

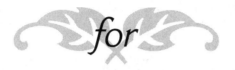

for

Herbal Healing

SECOND EDITION

PHYLLIS A. BALCH, CNC

Revised and Updated by

STACEY BELL, DSC

AVERY

a member of Penguin Group (USA) Inc. · New York

Published by the Penguin Group

Penguin Group (USA) Inc., 375 Hudson Street, New York, New York 10014, USA • Penguin Group (Canada),
90 Eglinton Avenue East, Suite 700, Toronto, Ontario M4P 2Y3, Canada (a division of Pearson Penguin
Canada Inc.) • Penguin Books Ltd, 80 Strand, London WC2R 0RL, England • Penguin Ireland,
25 St Stephen's Green, Dublin 2, Ireland (a division of Penguin Books Ltd) • Penguin Group
(Australia), 250 Camberwell Road, Camberwell, Victoria 3124, Australia (a division of Pearson
Australia Group Pty Ltd) • Penguin Books India Pvt Ltd, 11 Community Centre, Panchsheel Park,
New Delhi–110 017, India • Penguin Group (NZ), 67 Apollo Drive, Rosedale, North Shore 0632,
New Zealand (a division of Pearson New Zealand Ltd) • Penguin Books (South Africa) (Pty) Ltd,
24 Sturdee Avenue, Rosebank, Johannesburg 2196, South Africa

Penguin Books Ltd, Registered Offices: 80 Strand, London WC2R 0RL, England

Most Avery books are available at special quantity discounts for bulk purchase for sales promotions, premiums,
fund-raising, and educational needs. Special books or book excerpts also can be created to fit specific needs.
For details, write Penguin Group (USA) Inc. Special Markets, 375 Hudson Street, New York, NY 10014.

Library of Congress Cataloging-in-Publication Data

Balch, Phyllis A., date.
Prescription for herbal healing : an easy-to-use A-to-Z reference to hundreds of common disorders and
thier herbal remedies / Phyllis A. Balch.—2nd ed.
p.   cm.
Includes bibliographical references and index.
ISBN 978-1-58333-452-2
1. Herbs—Therapeutic use.   I. Title.
RM666.H33B355   2012   2011049379
615.3'21—dc23

Printed in the United States of America
1   3   5   7   9   10   8   6   4   2

Neither the publisher nor the authors are engaged in rendering professional advice or services to the individual
reader. The ideas, procedures, and suggestions contained in this book are not intended as a substitute for
consulting with your physician. All matters regarding your health require medical supervision. Neither the
authors nor the publisher shall be liable or responsible for any loss or damage allegedly arising from any
information or suggestion in this book.

While the authors have made every effort to provide accurate telephone numbers and Internet addresses at the
time of publication, neither the publisher nor the authors assume any responsibility for errors, or for changes
that occur after publication. Further, the publisher does not have any control over and does not assume any
responsibility for author or third-party websites or their content.

CONTENTS

A Note from the Authors,   ix
Acknowledgments,   xi
Preface,   xiii
How to Use This Book,   xv
Targeting Herbal Treatment,   xvii

Part One   Understanding Herbal Healing

Introduction,   3
Principles of Herbal Healing,   5

The Herbs,   14
The Formulas,   159

Part Two   Herbal Prescriptions for Common Health Problems

Introduction,   187
Acne,   188
Alcoholism,   190
Allergies,   191
Alzheimer's Disease,   196
Anemia,   198
Angina,   200
Ankles, Swollen,   202
Anxiety Disorder,   203
Asthma,   205
Atherosclerosis,   209
Athlete's Foot,   211
Attention Deficit Disorder/Attention
    Deficit Hyperactivity Disorder
    (ADD/ADHD),   212
Bed-Wetting,   215
Bell's Palsy,   216
Benign Prostatic Hypertrophy
    (BPH),   217
Bladder Cancer,   219
Bladder Infection (Cystitis),   221
Boil,   223
Bone Cancer,   225
Breast Cancer,   226
Bronchitis and Pneumonia,   230
Bruising,   232
Burns,   233
Bursitis,   234
Cancer,   236
Canker Sores (Aphthous Ulcers),   246
Carpal Tunnel Syndrome,   247
Cataracts,   248
Celiac Disease,   250
Cellulite,   252

Cervical Cancer,   252
Chronic Fatigue Syndrome,   255
Cirrhosis of the Liver,   257
Colic,   259
Colorectal Cancer,   260
Common Cold,   262
Congestive Heart Failure,   264
Constipation,   267
Cough,   269
Crohn's Disease,   271
Cuts, Scrapes, and Abrasions,   274
Dandruff,   275
Depression,   276
Diabetes,   279
Diabetic Retinopathy,   284
Diaper Rash,   285
Diarrhea,   286
Dry Mouth,   288
Ear Infection,   290
Eczema,   292
Emphysema,   295
Endometrial Cancer,   296
Endometriosis,   297
Erectile Dysfunction,   299
Eye Problems,   301
Fibrocystic Breasts,   305
Fibroids, Uterine (Uterine
    Myomas),   307
Fibromyalgia Syndrome,   309
Food Poisoning,   310
Fracture,   313
Gallstones,   314
Gastritis,   316
Glaucoma,   318

Gonorrhea and Chlamydia,   320
Gout,   322
Hair Loss,   323
Halitosis (Bad Breath),   325
Hangover,   326
Headache,   327
Heart Attack (Myocardial
    Infarction),   329
Heat Stress,   332
Hemorrhoids,   333
Hepatitis,   335
Herpesvirus Infection,   338
High Blood Pressure
    (Hypertension),   341
High Cholesterol,   344
HIV/AIDS,   346
Hives,   351
Hodgkin's Lymphoma,   353
Hyperthyroidism,   355
Hypothyroidism,   356
Indigestion,   358
Infertility,   361
Influenza,   364
Insect Bites,   366
Insomnia,   368
Intermittent Claudication,   370
Iron Overload,   371
Irritable Bowel Syndrome,   371
Kidney Cancer (Renal Cell
    Carcinoma),   374
Kidney Disease,   375
Kidney Stones,   377
Laryngitis,   379
Leukemia,   381
Liver Cancer,   383
Lung Cancer,   385
Lupus,   387
Lyme Disease,   389
Lymphedema,   390
Macular Degeneration,   391
Mastitis,   393
Measles,   394
Memory Problems,   395
Ménière's Disease,   397
Menopause-Related
    Problems,   399
Menstrual Problems,   401
Migraine,   403
Mononucleosis,   406
Morning Sickness,   407

Motion Sickness,   407
Multiple Sclerosis,   409
Mumps,   410
Muscles, Sore,   412
Myasthenia Gravis,   412
Nails, Infected,   413
Nausea,   415
Nosebleed,   416
Osteoarthritis,   417
Osteoporosis,   420
Ovarian Cancer,   422
Ovarian Cyst,   424
Overweight,   425
Pain, Chronic,   427
Parasitic Infection,   429
Parkinson's Disease,   432
Pelvic Inflammatory Disease,   433
Peptic Ulcer,   435
Periodontal Disease,   437
Premenstrual Syndrome (PMS),   439
Prostate Cancer,   442
Prostatitis,   445
Psoriasis,   446
Restless Legs Syndrome,   448
Rheumatoid Arthritis,   450
Ringworm,   452
Seizure Disorders,   453
Sex Drive, Diminished,   455
Shin Splints,   457
Sinusitis,   458
Skin Cancer,   460
Sprains and Strains,   463
Stomach Cancer,   464
Strep Throat,   465
Stress,   467
Stroke,   468
Sweating, Excessive,   470
Syphilis,   471
Tendinitis,   472
Tinnitus (Ringing in the Ears),   473
Toothache,   474
Tuberculosis,   476
Vaginosis,   477
Varicose Veins,   478
Vitiligo,   480
Vomiting,   481
Warts,   482
Wrinkles,   484
Yeast Infection
    (Yeast Vaginitis),   485

Part Three   Techniques of Herbal Healing

Introduction,   489
Acupuncture,   489
Aromatherapy,   490
Bowel Retraining,   491
Compresses,   492
Douches,   492
Estrogen-Reducing Diet,   492
Foot Baths,   493
Hand Baths,   493
Kegel Exercises,   493
Massage,   494

Ointments,   494
Plasters,   495
Poultices,   495
Relaxation Techniques,   496
Sitz Baths,   498
Skin Washes,   499
Steam Inhalations,   499
Syrups,   499
Teas,   499
Tinctures,   500

References,   501
Appendix A: Glossary,   613
Appendix B: Resources,   619
Index,   626

A NOTE FROM THE AUTHORS

For each medical condition that appears in Part Two of this book, recommendations of beneficial herbs are listed. We have provided specific precautions for the use of many of the beneficial herbs, so as to alert the reader to proper use. For a more in-depth discussion of the precautions associated with these herbs, please refer to the discussion of the individual herb in Part One.

ACKNOWLEDGMENTS

I wish to acknowledge the following people, who both advised and supported me as I prepared and wrote *Prescription for Herbal Healing*: my daughter, Cheryl Keene; my grandchildren, Ryan and Rachel; my research and editing staff, Christina DiMaio and Debbie Rimer; Theresa Auman, who managed Good Things Naturally; the manufacturers and suppliers who allowed me to test their products before I recommended them to my readers; and my readers, who have remained loyal throughout the years.

PREFACE

Open this herbal encyclopedia before you open your medicine cabinet. This book may help with illnesses from colds and flu to mitigating pain from arthritis. You can easily and quickly look up your ailment or disorder, get a clear explanation of what may have caused it, and find a list of herbal options to use in treating that particular illness or condition. You will get straightforward alternatives so that you can establish when and if you should call a qualified health-care professional. *Prescription for Herbal Healing* is a collection of herbal treatments that are reliable and understood in scientific terms. It offers precise herbal "prescriptions" that can be used to treat an array of health conditions. It lists herbs and formulas that can amplify the benefits of a healthy diet, nutritional supplementation, and natural healing techniques. It presents clear information on the compatibility of herbs with conventional medication in the treatment of health conditions. It points out possibilities for combining herbal healing with conventional treatment with outcomes that neither can achieve alone for various conditions.

It's amazing how far we have come in natural healing, without serious side effects. Herbal treatments are capable of healing all kinds of disorders and all parts of the body. Many countries, especially the European countries and China, are ahead of the United States in using natural products such as herbs, but even in North America, many doctors now blend the best of conventional medicine with alternative healing and have found powerful new treatments that work. In Germany, herbal medicine is prescribed in the same way as regular pharmaceuticals. The major herbs have been evaluated by scholars, and the information compiled into a tome called *The Complete German Commission E Monographs*. Until recently, the book was only available in German, but has since been translated into English. Herbal medicine has come so far in the United States that the *PDR* (*Physicians' Desk Reference*)— a compilation of manufacturer's prescribing information of prescription drugs and the "bible" for all physicians in the United States—now includes an entire book devoted to herbal remedies in its publication series.

Part One of this book defines the principles and materials of herbal healing. Then it lists over 200 of the plants used in traditional herbal healing and the scientific evidence for their use in extending health. It gives the most current scientific explanation of how each herb has been used successfully for centuries as a healing tool. It also provides current clinical information on the herbal formulas of ayurveda, traditional Chinese, Native American, and South American medicine most widely used today, as well as several modern herbal formulas of great healing potential.

Although every herb and formula listed in Part One has been employed by one or more of the great schools of traditional herbal healing for centuries, they also are used in modern medical practice across the globe, including Europe, Egypt, Israel, Japan, and the United States. The herbs and formulas listed in Part One are at least understood in chemical terms and can be used with predictable results with modern medicine—most are considered safe according to *The Complete German Commission E Monographs*. Interestingly, most conventional drugs were originally derived from plant sources. The problem with this is that to make a pharmaceutical drug, the component of the herb believed to be responsible for its activity is extracted and concentrated. In their whole form, herbs are buffered because they contain many different components. Because of this, they may be less likely to cause side effects (which can sometimes be worse than the original problem). However, herbs also may cause side effects. When there are side effects, such effects are noted and explained in detail in this book.

People need to be educated about their treatment options and the potential risks involved. Anything you can do to help yourself, to empower yourself, helps you to get rid of the sense of hopelessness when disease strikes. It's never too late to protect your health. There is no reason you should not know about your body and how it works, even as doctors know these things.

Not every herb recommended in Part One has been confirmed as effective by statistically controlled, randomized, double-blind, clinical studies such as is the norm with conventional medicines. But every herb and formula listed in this book is known to be safe when used as prescribed and has a long history of healing benefits.

Part Two of this book shows how these herbs and formulas can be used to treat over 150 specific conditions. This information is also based on scientific studies. It is included for those who wish to provide themselves with the widest range of possibilities for gaining health. This section reveals how herbs manage disease processes. It discusses the use of herbs with diet and nutritional supplements. It also lists dozens of therapeutic practices for which there is objective evidence. Herbs, nutrition, and personally directed healing therapies are included to give the reader even greater opportunity to take charge of his or her health.

Part Three provides information on making baths, compresses, creams, lotions, ointments, and tinctures. This information is included for those who are most comfortable using herbs as a healing art, as a healing connection to the natural world. Part Three also includes entries that describe healing techniques such as acupuncture and massage therapy, which can be useful complements to any herbal program.

This entire book has been written with an acute and personal awareness of the frequently overwhelming cost of health care. The most economical approach to regaining and maintaining health is a combination of conventional medicine with supplemental approaches. Except for minor conditions, the herbs and formulas in this book are not chosen to replace conventional medicine. Instead, they are intended to work with conventional medicine, to help it work more quickly, effectively, painlessly, and economically.

Of course, for herbs to be useful with conventional medicine, it is essential to pay attention to herb safety. In July 2009, the Food and Drug Administration developed guidelines called GMPs (good manufacturing practices) for preparation of all dietary supplements, including herbs. We have only included herbs produced by manufacturers that follow the new GMPs. These herbs are generally recognized as safe and are processed by known manufacturing practices into safe forms. Special notes on safety for administration to children and during pregnancy and nursing are included where needed. Always read the precautions that are included in this book for each herb before using it. And since the philosophy of this book is that herbs can be used with a doctor's prescribed medication, interactions of herbs and drugs are noted throughout the text. And of course, your doctor should be aware of the *Physicians' Desk Reference (PDR) for Herbal Medicines* to help you make informed choices.

We thank you for choosing to read this book. Its purpose is to make the process of treating disease and returning to health a little easier for you. May this book help you use the best of herbal healing and, when needed, modern medicine to find greater health than you have ever known before.

HOW TO USE THIS BOOK

This book is a comprehensive guide for the layperson seeking to use herbs to enhance health and manage disease. Herbs can be used with other dietary supplements and conventional health treatments to relieve diseases that threaten comfort, health, or life itself. Herbs also can be used to improve athletic performance, enhance sexual response, and complement a healthy diet. This book has been designed to be a user-friendly reference to the most readily available, effective, and reliable herbal remedies.

While not every herbal remedy will work for every person, there are so many herbs available that you'll likely find the right one or mixture to suit you. If you are disease-free, herbs are available to help you stay that way. Disease varies from person to person, and treating only the symptoms and not correcting the cause will not bring about a cure. The key to finding the right remedy is relying on the professional diagnosis of a qualified health practitioner in addition to self-evaluation. When symptoms are understood and conditions requiring urgent medical care are ruled out, then it is possible to choose the right herb or herbs to add to your plans for personal health.

Many herbs have been used successfully for centuries to treat a multitude of health problems. Other herbs offer benefits in the context of conventional, modern medical treatment. Herbs may extend the effects of medication, enabling lower dosages. However, changes in your medications should always be under the supervision of the prescribing doctor. Herbs may also soften conventional medication's side effects. In some cases, herbs may gradually replace manufactured medicine altogether. As herbs and conventional treatments gradually relieve symptoms and their causes, complementary healing techniques may accelerate recovery. Diet, nutritional supplements, massage, meditation, exercise, and other disciplines can round out a treatment plan.

This book has been written to provide the easiest way of choosing the most effective herbal treatments. It is divided into three parts. Part One offers an overview of the principles and materials used in herbal healing, and describes the herbs and herbal formulas recommended in this book. Each entry gives a description of the herb or formula and a brief review of how it is understood in terms of science-based medicine. The entries describe how each herb and formula can be used by itself, and how it can be used with other herbs, nutritional supplements, and prescription medications. Information has been updated to comply with what is presented in *The Complete German Commission E Monographs* and the *Physicians' Desk Reference (PDR) for Herbal Medicines.*

Part Two is an alphabetical listing of the health conditions that can be treated with herbs. Each entry begins with a brief discussion of the condition in mainstream medical terms that physicians use in describing their diagnosis. Then the entry lists A-to-Z options for dealing with the condition. There are *recommendations* for diet, nutritional supplementation, and complementary healing practices that can help herbs and medicine work even better. There are *considerations* for exploring further possibilities for healing, avoiding harmful interactions, and accommodating individual needs in therapy.

Part Three gives information needed for preparing herbs at home. This book also includes appendices listing sources of herbal products and a glossary for easy reference. The author has used some 2,000 technical references documenting the scientific validity of the herbs and formulas described in this book. Searches in medical literature, called Pubmed (www.ncbi.nlm.nih.gov/pubmed), were done to capture the latest high-quality science. This is the same website that your physician will use to seek the best treatment practices for your condition.

This book is designed so that it may be read as a reference manual, by individual herb, disease, and healing techniques. It is also designed to be read from cover to cover by the layperson and health-care practitioners with special commitment to herbal healing in the creation of health. It is designed to give you the information you need for a confident discussion with your health-care providers.

This book is not, however, a manual for self-diagnosis. It is usually simple to match the symptoms of minor complaints of short-term illnesses to the applicable herbal remedy. In these cases, self-assessment can be verified with a doctor. It is always imperative to consult a medical doctor when symptoms persist, cause acute pain, render unbearable disability, or appear to be life-threatening. Readers who find it difficult to locate qualified health-care practitioners knowledgeable in herbal medicine may refer to Appendix B: Resources.

TARGETING HERBAL TREATMENT

Practitioners of herbal medicine have found that certain herbs and herbal preparations tend to benefit specific organs, systems, and functions of the body. In most cases practitioners learn about herbs and their uses from *The Complete German Commission E Monographs* and the *PDR for Herbal Medicines*, where the specific herb for an organ or organ system is defined. This section illustrates the locations of various organs and systems, and lists some of the herbs often used for disorders that affect them. Note that an individual herb listed for a particular organ, system, or function may not benefit every problem that affects it. See the individual entries in Part Two for disorder-specific recommendations. These illustrations are provided for information only.

CARDIOVASCULAR SYSTEM

The cardiovascular organs, structures, and functions depicted here include the blood vessels, circulation, the heart, and the lymph nodes.

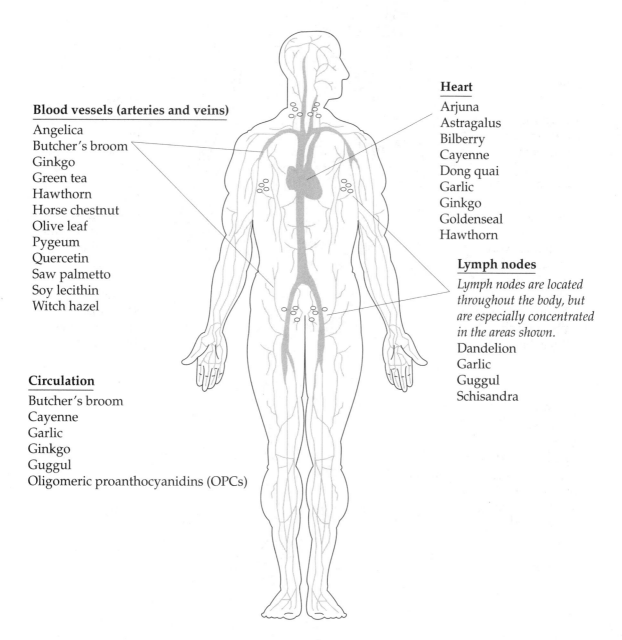

Blood vessels (arteries and veins)
Angelica
Butcher's broom
Ginkgo
Green tea
Hawthorn
Horse chestnut
Olive leaf
Pygeum
Quercetin
Saw palmetto
Soy lecithin
Witch hazel

Circulation
Butcher's broom
Cayenne
Garlic
Ginkgo
Guggul
Oligomeric proanthocyanidins (OPCs)

Heart
Arjuna
Astragalus
Bilberry
Cayenne
Dong quai
Garlic
Ginkgo
Goldenseal
Hawthorn

Lymph nodes
Lymph nodes are located throughout the body, but are especially concentrated in the areas shown.
Dandelion
Garlic
Guggul
Schisandra

STRUCTURAL TISSUES

The structural tissues depicted here are the bones, hair, joints, muscles, and skin.

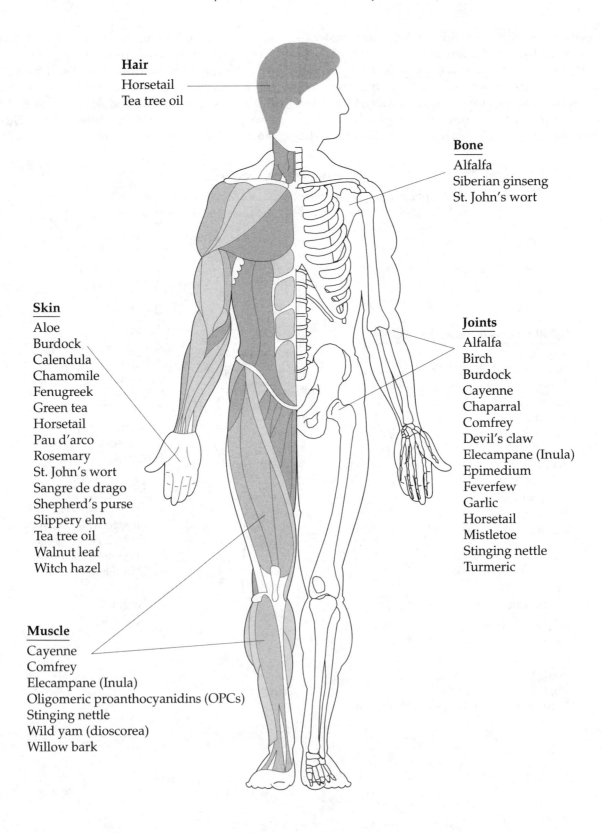

Hair
Horsetail
Tea tree oil

Bone
Alfalfa
Siberian ginseng
St. John's wort

Skin
Aloe
Burdock
Calendula
Chamomile
Fenugreek
Green tea
Horsetail
Pau d'arco
Rosemary
St. John's wort
Sangre de drago
Shepherd's purse
Slippery elm
Tea tree oil
Walnut leaf
Witch hazel

Joints
Alfalfa
Birch
Burdock
Cayenne
Chaparral
Comfrey
Devil's claw
Elecampane (Inula)
Epimedium
Feverfew
Garlic
Horsetail
Mistletoe
Stinging nettle
Turmeric

Muscle
Cayenne
Comfrey
Elecampane (Inula)
Oligomeric proanthocyanidins (OPCs)
Stinging nettle
Wild yam (dioscorea)
Willow bark

ENDOCRINE SYSTEM, NERVOUS SYSTEM, AND URINARY TRACT

The endocrine organs depicted here are the adrenal glands, the thymus, the thyroid, and the pancreas.
Portions of the nervous system represented are the brain and the central nervous system.
The urinary tract organs shown are the kidneys and bladder.

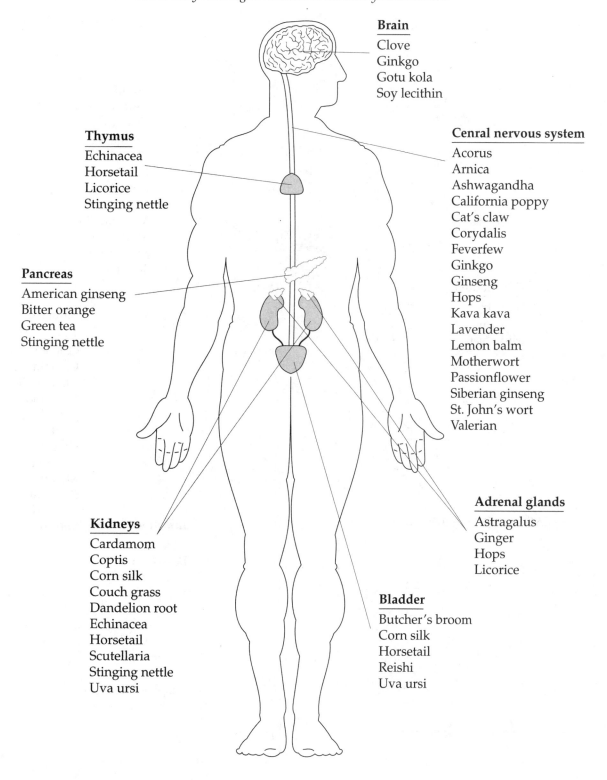

Brain
Clove
Ginkgo
Gotu kola
Soy lecithin

Cenral nervous system
Acorus
Arnica
Ashwagandha
California poppy
Cat's claw
Corydalis
Feverfew
Ginkgo
Ginseng
Hops
Kava kava
Lavender
Lemon balm
Motherwort
Passionflower
Siberian ginseng
St. John's wort
Valerian

Thymus
Echinacea
Horsetail
Licorice
Stinging nettle

Pancreas
American ginseng
Bitter orange
Green tea
Stinging nettle

Adrenal glands
Astragalus
Ginger
Hops
Licorice

Kidneys
Cardamom
Coptis
Corn silk
Couch grass
Dandelion root
Echinacea
Horsetail
Scutellaria
Stinging nettle
Uva ursi

Bladder
Butcher's broom
Corn silk
Horsetail
Reishi
Uva ursi

DIGESTIVE SYSTEM AND RESPIRATORY TRACT

The digestive organs shown here are the gallbladder, intestines, liver, and stomach.
The portion of the respiratory tract depicted is the lungs.

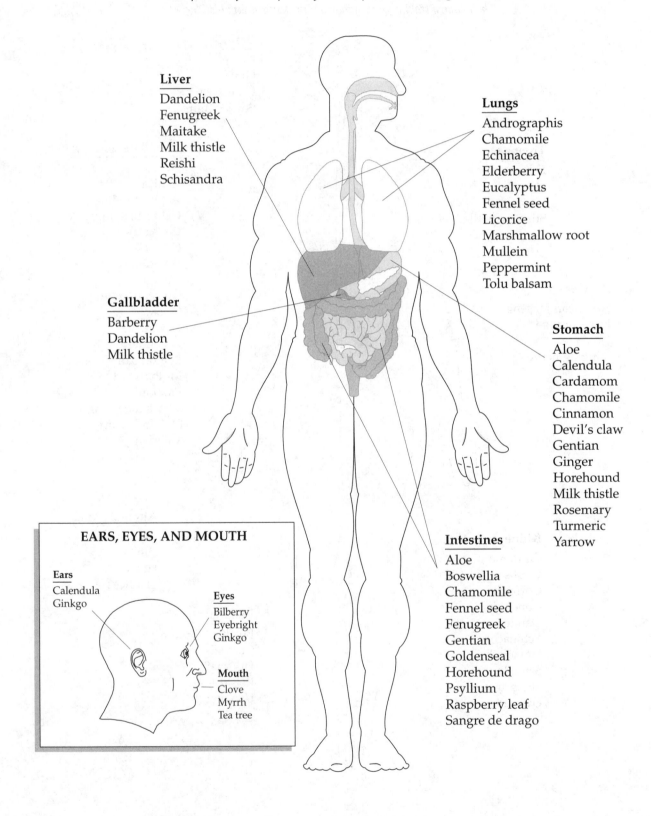

Liver
Dandelion
Fenugreek
Maitake
Milk thistle
Reishi
Schisandra

Gallbladder
Barberry
Dandelion
Milk thistle

Lungs
Andrographis
Chamomile
Echinacea
Elderberry
Eucalyptus
Fennel seed
Licorice
Marshmallow root
Mullein
Peppermint
Tolu balsam

Stomach
Aloe
Calendula
Cardamom
Chamomile
Cinnamon
Devil's claw
Gentian
Ginger
Horehound
Milk thistle
Rosemary
Turmeric
Yarrow

Intestines
Aloe
Boswellia
Chamomile
Fennel seed
Fenugreek
Gentian
Goldenseal
Horehound
Psyllium
Raspberry leaf
Sangre de drago

EARS, EYES, AND MOUTH

Ears
Calendula
Ginkgo

Eyes
Bilberry
Eyebright
Ginkgo

Mouth
Clove
Myrrh
Tea tree

PART ONE

Understanding
Herbal Healing

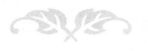

Introduction

At a time when medicine has made some of the greatest advances in its history, something unexpected has begun to happen. Herbs, which have always been the principal form of medicine for the majority of the world's population, have once again become popular throughout the developed world. Striving to stay healthy in the face of chronic stress, pollution, and obesity, more and more people are taking charge of their health with herbs.

Herbal supplement sales were more than $250 million in the United States in 2010 according to Dr. Mark Blumenthal, president of the American Botanical Council. Multi-herb formulations are more common than single herbs and sales of multi-herbs are expected to continue to increase by 9 percent each year in the United States. Women use slightly more herbs than men (60 percent versus 56 percent), and middle-age people are the biggest users of herbs. Some of the top-selling herbs are garlic, echinacea, saw palmetto, ginkgo, soy, cranberry, ginseng, black cohosh, St. John's wort, and milk thistle.

As the use of herbs in the United States has skyrocketed, the U.S. government has become increasingly interested in assessing the safety and effectiveness of herbs. In August 2010, the Office of Dietary Supplements (ODS), which is part of the U.S. Food and Drug Administration (FDA), and the National Center for Complementary and Alternative Medicine (NCCAM), part of the National Institutes of Health (NIH), funded five research centers to study the effectiveness and biological action of botanicals. These studies may provide data that will help develop new ways to reduce the risk of disease.

The "epidemic" of herb use is evident not only in North America and Europe, but also in China, Japan, Korea, and Latin America. Around the world, health-care practitioners are increasingly using herbs and other natural therapies alongside modern forms of treatment, with a renewed understanding of the body's own power to heal.

The healing art of herbalism grew from hundreds of millions of personal healing experiences over centuries before the advent of scientific technology. Herbal remedies that resulted in cures were recognized, remembered, and gradually categorized by the great schools of herbal healing. They were recorded by Egyptian medicine, Indian ayurveda, traditional Chinese medicine, and Japanese Kampo; the teachings of Hippocrates, Dioscorides, Hildegard von Bingen, and Paracelsus; and the native healing systems of Africa, Australia, and the Americas.

The ancient arts of herbal healing used *plants* to relieve carefully defined patterns of symptoms. The traditional herbal healer recognized changes in body and mind. Then he or she used herbs to re-create the healthful conditions of balance that existed in the person before the disease struck. Patterns of symptoms are unique to the individual, so the results of treatment could vary slightly from person to person. As long as both healer and patient stayed within the limits of the craft, the results on the patient were positive. Still, the techniques of treatment could not be applied to all people.

Making medicine available to most everyone was an outcome of the science of chemistry. Basic physiological processes are thought to be the same in all people, and the chemicals that change them can be expected to yield the same results in anyone who takes them. These chemicals then could be mass-produced. In recent years, the chemical techniques that revolutionized the pharmacy have been applied to the understanding of herbs.

The science of herbal healing uses herbs as sources of chemicals that modify known physiological processes that are altered in disease states. Since herb-derived chemicals are understood in terms of these basic physiological processes, they are also expected to yield the same results in anyone who takes them. While most herbs cannot yet be mass-produced, the potential of herbal medicine lies not in staying within limits but in going beyond them—using herbs to soften, support, and reinforce the healing efficacy of other forms of alternative and conventional treatments.

The recent renewal of interest in herbal medicine has been made possible by the same method that once seemed destined to replace it: herbs are not only good medicine, but more and more are being recognized as scientific medicine. Herbs are now subjected to clinical testing in the same way as other medicines are, in scientifically designed double-blind tests. These clinical trials make sure that an herb's effects lie in the herb itself rather than in the wishful thinking (either positive or negative) of the researchers.

Companies also systematically test tens of thousands of plants as sources of compounds from which new drugs might be designed. The natural components of herbs can then be manufactured into medicines. In cell lines, the chemical components of some herbs are angiogenesis inhibitors, which stop the growth of blood vessels that supply tumors. Others are signal transducers, which activate genes to eliminate toxin-damaged cells, or protease inhibitors, which stop the multiplication of viruses. However, just because cell lines respond favorably to a particular herb does not necessarily mean that taking that herb will result in the same outcome. Taking herbal recommendations from a health-care provider specially trained in herbal medicine may increase the likelihood that the herb will offer the maximum benefit.

The renewed confidence in herbal medicine has also been made possible by the efforts of well-intentioned practitioners, manufacturers, and government officials who strive to ensure that the promises made on a label of an herb product are met by the product inside the bottle.

Manufacturers of herbal products are working with groups such as the American Botanical Council, the Herb Research Foundation, and the U.S. Pharmacopeia to develop the scientific techniques needed to verify the quality of herbal products. Moreover, many American manufacturers and distributors of herbal products keep current with scientific research in China, Europe, Japan, and especially Germany, places where herbs are part of mainstream medicine.

Today, the FDA has standards of preparation of all dietary supplements, including herbs. The FDA requires that the ingredients listed on a label are to be found in the product and that it is free of harmful toxins such as pesticides. The FDA does not allow medical claims to be made for any herbal product, even if there is scientifically sound information to support its use. Rather, herbs and dietary supplements can make structure/function claims. These claims refer to supporting a part of the body, such as ginkgo supports brain health. In contrast, drugs can carry claims about disease management, and the FDA also allows the same claims for homeopathic remedies.

Another reason the revitalization of herbal medicine has come about is that while modern drugs have achieved a great deal in disease treatment, they also have contributed to ill health. Every modern drug comes with warnings of side effects. A standard textbook for pharmacists even states, "If a drug is stated to have no side effects, then it is strongly suspected it has no central benefit."

Medication errors cause at least one death every day and injure approximately 1.3 million people annually in the United States. Today, tens of millions of people in the United States depend on prescription and over-the-counter (OTC) medications to sustain their health—as many as 3 billion prescriptions are written annually.

Conventional drugs are also costly. A year's supply of the latest diabetes medication can cost more than $4,000. A year's treatment with an HIV "cocktail" can cost $11,000 to $40,000. The cost of treating chronic disease overwhelms not only individuals, but also their insurance companies. Although herbs cannot replace the essential treatments for chronic disease, in some instances they can shorten a treatment course with the expensive drug, with fewer side effects and lesser expense.

Of course, herbs have side effects as well. Some have such severe side effects that they are not recommended for consumption. In such cases, we have not included these herbs in this edition of our book. In updating our research on herbs for this edition of *Prescription for Herbal Healing*, we relied on two important herbal texts. The first is the *Complete German Commission E Monographs: Therapeutic Guide to Herbal Medicines*. The commission was established in 1978 to help physicians integrate herbs with conventional medicine. Later this tome was translated into English, and it details how to use herbs, proper dosages, contraindications, adverse effects, drug interactions, and how the herbs work. The second book is the *Physicians' Desk Reference for Herbal Medicines*, which provides essential information for intelligent and informed decision-making on herbs and herbal remedies.

None of the drawbacks, however, requires choosing between conventional medicine and an herbal alternative. Many physicians are caring, conscientious, and superbly trained. The physician should always be considered when a problem exists.

But it is also important to receive just the right amount of treatment. Given the staggering expense of modern medicine, every person wants to make sure of maximizing the financial investment in his or her health. People desire assurance that the methods their doctors use allow the body to heal through its own abilities. Although many medical schools in the United States now offer courses in complementary medicine, making sure the best possible treatment is received is a responsibility that must be assumed *with* the doctor. The goal of this book is to provide a solid base of knowledge to help readers share responsibility for the process of healing by making informed—and confident—choices.

The gift that herbal medicine confers is the restoration of control to the individual. Herbs can and should be used with conventional medicine, providing just the right amount of help for the body to regain its balance after an assault by disease. Herbal medicine has an ageless ability to improve the condition of the whole person and can be wisely used to help anyone achieve a better state of health than ever experienced before.

Principles of Herbal Healing

Just a few decades ago, the most widely recognized advertising slogan in America was "Better living through chemistry." Promoting the virtues of plastics, pesticides, and pharmaceuticals, this motto came to be a catchphrase for progress in all of modern life, even medical treatment.

The fact that chemistry brought progress to health-care is incontrovertible. The discovery of new drugs resulted in treatments for conditions that were once invariably fatal, such as certain forms of cancer and most cases of diabetes. Antibiotics made it possible to treat common and equally life-threatening infections contracted by injury, surgery, or epidemic. Pharmacological advances enabled better living with chronic conditions such as lupus, depression, and thyroid problems. It was thought to be only a matter of time before modern, chemically oriented medicine even found a cure for the common cold.

The 1980s and 1990s, however, brought widespread recognition of recurring problems in treating disease with manufactured drugs. Many people judged that the side effects of chemotherapy for cancer outweighed its potential benefits. Novel drugs for diabetes carried the risk of liver failure. New strains of infectious diseases appeared that were resistant to antibiotics. Some people taking treatment for lupus, depression, and thyroid problems abandoned it because they felt the treatments caused worse symptoms than the disease.

By 1999, a small fraction—about 2 percent—of the American public had abandoned chemical medicine altogether and had begun using alternative medicine exclusively. This 2 percent of the public reported using herbs and visiting nontraditional healers. These dedicated followers of natural medicine rejected blood pressure measurements, cholesterol testing, annual physical exams, influenza vaccinations, prostate examinations, breast examinations, mammograms, and Pap tests.

Today, a majority of the American public—about 54 percent, according to polls—still used "chemical" medicines (ones sold by prescription or over-the-counter [OTC]) exclusively. But preliminary survey data indicate that 38 percent of the people in the United States have come to recognize that the best option for treatment today is complementary treatment, using the doctor's prescriptions and herbal options together judiciously.

This section describes the principles of effective herbal treatment. It gives simple *rules* for recognizing when herbal treatment is best and how it works in concert with conventional medical therapies. This section also describes the *materials* of effective herbal treatment. These are the teas, tablets, tinctures, capsules, and extracts used in everyday treatment with herbs. It explains how to recognize the health conditions that benefit from herbal treatment the most, and how the standardization process helps make self-treatment with herbs easy and safe. It also lists the various outlets where healing herbs may be found.

RULES FOR HERBAL TREATMENT

Successful use of herbs for healing requires a few commonsense rules. While these guidelines are self-evident to most people, they are also in complete harmony with the basic principles of modern pharmacology. These principles of herbal treatment apply to all of the herbs and all of the conditions listed in this book.

Rely on Conventional Medicine for Emergency Treatment

When a health condition is an immediate threat to life, treatment administered by a physician is always the best choice. Herbal, nutritional, and complementary treatments are out of place in emergency care. Or, as the distinguished complementary health expert Dr. Dean Ornish frequently comments, "I never tell a patient admitted to the emergency room with a heart attack that she should eat more broccoli."

The following are examples of symptoms that call for prompt medical attention:

- A lump that appears anywhere.
- Chest pains/heart palpitations/pain that radiates down the left arm and chest.
- Coughing with green or yellow mucus.
- Difficulty swallowing.
- Fever over 102°F.
- Known or suspected bone fracture.
- Known or suspected poisoning.
- Known or suspected stroke.
- Loss of consciousness.
- Severe allergic reactions.
- Severe burns.
- Severe high blood pressure.
- Severe infection.
- Severe persistent pain.
- Uncontrolled bleeding.
- Uncontrolled diarrhea.
- Uncontrolled vomiting.

These represent an acute phase of illness. Usually potent medications and medical and surgical procedures will quickly correct the situation and prevent death. Once the emergency phase is over, the body goes into a chronic phase, where long-term convalescence may be needed. This is the time when herbal medicines work best.

Choose the Right Herb for the Diagnosis

The first step in choosing the right herb for the diagnosis is getting the right diagnosis. Self-diagnosis of aches and pains, colds and flu, minor injuries, and predictable fluctuations in chronic conditions is usually valid. Among people who are otherwise healthy, even choosing the wrong herb for these conditions will not interfere with long-term health. Most health conditions, however, require evaluation by someone other than the person experiencing them. Objective evaluation and medical evaluation are usually an important step in choosing the right herb.

The second step in selecting the right herb for the diagnosis is matching the diagnosis with an available herb. With over 5,000 medicinal herbs available worldwide, even the most knowledgeable herb experts do not know them all. Most nations of the world have developed government-approved volumes known as pharmacopeias to provide a comprehensive guide to matching symptoms and signs to specific herbs and herbal formulas. The pharmacopeias of the United States are known as the *United States Pharmacopeia (USP)* and *The National Formulary*. There is also *The American Herbal Pharmacopoeia*, a reference guide that will eventually include summaries of scientific research on over 300 herbs commonly used in the United States. Along with translations of foreign works such as *The Complete German Commission E Monographs,* a tremendous amount of scholarly information is available for the safe use of medicinal herbs. *The Physicians' Desk Reference for Herbal Medicines* is another excellent volume that outlines clearly how doctors can prescribe herbs to patients.

This information is also available through popular publications such as this one. The information in these scholarly works has become required reading for writers of all herb manuals, including this one. And while it is not necessary to read technical works to be able to use an herb with confidence, much of the original scientific research on which the recommendations in responsible herb guides are based may be found on the Internet.

More Is Not Necessarily Better

After choosing the right herb, the next step in effective herbal treatment is taking the right dosage. The dosages of both herbs and prescription drugs are determined according to their most important pharmacological properties, *therapeutic range.*

The therapeutic range of any herbal or conventional medication is the difference between the smallest dose that will do anyone any good and the largest dose that everyone can take without causing harm. Therapeutic range is a measure of the safety of the herb or drug. An herb or drug with a narrow therapeutic range is more dangerous than one with a wider range. Most herbs or drugs with a broad therapeutic range are safe.

Most herbs have a broad therapeutic range. It is very difficult to take a toxic dose of most herbs, but deaths have been reported in the medical literature. The caffeine in green tea (or coffee or any other caffeine-containing beverage), for instance, is theoretically poisonous. It could be fatal if you drank a dose of 50 liters (approximately 12 gallons) of green tea, which contains 10 grams of caffeine.

Green tea is considered nontoxic because it is impossible for anyone to drink 12 gallons of the beverage in a single sitting. Even if it were possible to drink 12 gallons of green tea, the 10 grams of caffeine it contains would still be nontoxic because the caffeine from the first few liters of green tea would break down long before the caffeine from the last liters of green tea could ever reach the bloodstream. However, because green tea is available in capsule form, consuming the equivalent of 12 gallons of tea is possible. Always consult an herbal expert or follow the instructions on the label.

It is possible to take a toxic dose of some other herbs, but extremely unlikely. The bronchitis herb coltsfoot, for example, contains pyrrolizidine alkaloids that can cause liver damage. Moreover, the blossoms of the plant are more toxic than the leaf and root. For this reason, it is important to seek a qualified health-care professional well versed in herbal medicine, and always check the precautions for an herb before using it.

While large doses of herbs are usually safe, they are almost never necessary. Always take the smallest dosage within the therapeutic range of the herbs recommended in this book first. Then gradually increase the dosage to the maximum recommended if symptoms do not improve. If no benefit is derived, seek medical attention from a health-care professional trained in herbal medicine.

Plan for Long-Term Improvement

Herbs usually act gently and slowly. In pharmacological terms, herbs are said to have a long *onset of action.* This term refers to how quickly a drug or herb begins to achieve its desired effect on the body. Herbs usually have both a broad therapeutic range and a slow onset of action. That is, most herbs are generally safe, and taking a little more or a little less is likely to yield the same result. However, their action is slow.

An example of an herb with a long onset of action is one of the most commonly used herbs in the United States, psyllium. This herb is used in dozens of OTC products for the relief of constipation. Using psyllium powder results in immediate relief of constipation by increasing the bulk of stool, but at first it may also cause bloating and gas. This is due to the bacterial breakdown of indigestible fibers in the herb. Only over a period of one to three months do new bacteria establish themselves in the colon to digest

The Origins of Traditional Chinese Medicine

The most widely used system of herbal medicine in the world today, traditional Chinese medicine (TCM), is an example of how herbalism began as a means of demystifying medical practice. In the second century BCE, Chinese scholarship produced perhaps the earliest medical textbook, *The Yellow Emperor's Canon of Internal Medicine*. This book consisted of two parts, a discussion of medical philosophy later known as the *Basic Questions* and a guide to medical practice known as the *Magic Pivot*. The knowledge recorded in this source book included not only the early elements of herbal medicine, but also magic, astrology, and geomancy in a combination that eventually came to be called *fang ji*.

Although *fang ji* was a considerable improvement over no treatment at all, it was not adequate for every medical need. Four centuries after the writing of *The Yellow Emperor's Canon*, the Chinese master herbalist Zhang Zhonjing lived in a time of plague. In about 190 CE, a devastating epidemic killed many members of his family. "My relatives were plenty," he wrote, "the number more than two hundred. However, from the beginning of the Chien An era to now, two-thirds of them have died of infection."

Master Zhang was understandably distraught with the doctors of his day. "They do little but vie for fame and power and delight themselves with improving their physical appearance," he wrote, "and they do not thoroughly study the principles of health before they begin to practice, but merely follow their teachers with no attempt to change their science's outlooks."

In response to his great loss, Zhang Zhongjing sought to replace magic with medicine—herbal medicine. "I pitied those who were ill and could not be cured. So I studied the medicine of the old classics and collected many herbal prescriptions, and compiled them into a book." Zhang's book later became the basics of both traditional Chinese medicine and Japanese kampo medicine. Zhang taught that herbal medicines should conform to people, instead of the other way around. His central idea was that if the disharmonies causing diseases in individuals were carefully studied, then knowledge of the specific combinations of herbs useful in treatment would naturally follow.

Over the centuries, the Chinese refined the notion of person-centered medicine with the development of the principle of Four Examinations. This method consists of examining the patient by sight (especially the tongue), examining the patient by sound and smell, inquiring about symptoms, and touching the patient through a process known as palpation, and, in more modern Oriental medicine, pulse reading. The essence of diagnosis was and is embodied in the charge given every student of TCM: "Listen to your patients; they are telling you their diagnosis."

The Four Examinations yield a diagnosis in terms of the Eight Indicators, cold and heat, deficiency and excess, interior and exterior, and yang and yin. Although there are subtleties in the definition of these indicators, at least the first three pairs of indicators are intuitively clear for most people in Western cultures. Heat is an outside environmental influence, the dominant atmospheric energy of summer. Heat symbolizes the body's normal processes that keep it warm. Heat also can be the body's reaction to an invasion of cold, fever, sweating, and inflammation to repel pathogens in winter. In the metaphor of traditional Oriental medicine, cold is an environmental energy that attacks the surface of the body. When the body is under attack of cold, the body will try to defend successive layers of tissues from cold's attack.

The next pair of indicators is similarly easy to understand. Excess and deficiency measure the person's degree of vitality and ability to withstand disease. People with signs of excess react vigorously to disease, with a state of elevated physiological function. They are susceptible to diseases of excess, such as high blood pressure or insomnia. They are treated with herbs that "drain" the energy imbalance caused by the disease. Persons with signs of deficiency show a week healing response, with a state of diminished physiological functioning. They are susceptible to the opposites of the diseases of excess, such as low blood pressure and drowsiness. They are treated with formulas that energize the body's response to disease.

The last four of the Eight Indicators are used to explain a diagnosis rather than to make a diagnosis. In the theory of ancient Chinese medicine, diseases were thought to first invade the "exterior" defenses of the body and work their way progressively to the "interior" defenses. The body at first employs "yang" energy to fight the disease, and then "yin" energy to preserve itself.

The terminology of the Eight Indicators is used by practitioners of TCM and kampo throughout the world today. Although this manner of describing disease is symbolic and metaphoric, the notions of interior and exterior and yang and yin have led to insights that prompted the recognition of ancient herbal formulas as effective remedies for modern diseases. Modern medicine's understanding of many chronic viral infections illustrates the progression of disease to the "yin" stage. Chronic viral hepatitis, for example, is accompanied by flulike symptoms, with nausea and vomiting as its outset. These are analogous to "yang" symptoms. After the initial signs of infection, however, the hepatitis virus may lie dormant in the liver for weeks, months, or years. The real battle of the body against the disease is one of "yin" energies, or containment. Recognizing the traditionally understood stages of disease in the experience of modern case histories of viral infection led to trials of ancient formulas as treatments. These treatments have proved to be among the most effective of all treatments available for hepatitis and many other chronic viral infections, described in greater detail in The Formulas.

---

fibers without releasing gas. This adjustment of the body (and its symbiotic bacteria) is needed to bring about the full-healing result of the herbal treatment.

Many of the herbs used to treat chronic conditions have a long latent period during which results are not noticed. It may be necessary to use these herbs for several months before they help the body accomplish desired changes. Herbs that have to be taken for several weeks or months before achieving results are identified where they are recommended in this book. There are also many herbs that act more quickly, such as echinacea and goldenseal. In citing published data on herbs, we include the time it took the participants in the study to derive benefit. This will give you a general idea of how long it might take to experience changes in your health.

If You Don't Get Better, Try Something Else

While this rule might seem obvious, it is easy to forget that for an herb or any other treatment to be considered effective, it must produce demonstrable results. In many cases, proving that the herb (or drug) works requires measurement. The only way to know that an herb helps lower high blood pressure is to take blood-pressure readings. The only way to know an herb helps control diabetes is to take blood sugar readings. The only way to know an herb helps weight loss is to step on a scale.

If measurements have been taken and an herb is found not to work, it is important to reconfirm the diagnosis. This is especially true if the herb is being taken on the basis of self-diagnosis. If using ginkgo for several months does not help memory, for example, there is always a possibility of a more serious disorder. Ginkgo has been shown to be most effective in cases of mild cognitive impairment. More advanced states are not shown to benefit from it. A qualified health-care practitioner can help sort out symptoms to make a more refined diagnosis.

Herbs to Avoid

In July 2008, the FDA imposed GMPs (good manufacturing practices) for the preparation of herbal products. You should determine that the herbs you are using are made under GMP. In September 2010, *Consumer Reports* published an article, "Dangerous Supplements." The article identified a dozen supplements that should be avoided because they pose serious health risks. However, if you use these herbs as described in this book, you should avoid these complications. Using herbs from nonreputable sources or taking them without the supervision of a health-care practitioner increases the chances of problems. Every herbal remedy should have the name and address of the manufacturer on the label. If not, do not use it.

The potentially dangerous herbal products include:

Name (also known as)	Possible dangers	Comments
Aconite	Toxicity, nausea, low blood pressure, respiratory paralysis, heart-rhythm disorders, death	Unsafe
Bitter orange	Fainting, heart rhythm disorders, stroke, death	Possibly unsafe; similar to ephedrine, which was banned in 2004
Chaparral	Liver damage, kidney problems	Likely unsafe; the FDA advises against its use
Colloidal silver	Bluish skin, mucous membrane discoloration, neurological problems, kidney damage	Likely unsafe; the FDA advised about the risk of discoloration in 2009
Coltsfoot	Liver damage, cancer	Likely unsafe
Comfrey	Liver damage, cancer	Likely unsafe
Country mallow	Heart attack, heart arrhythmia, stroke, death	Likely unsafe
Germanium	Kidney damage, death	Likely unsafe; in 1993 the FDA warned that it was linked to serious side effects
Greater celandine	Liver damage	Possibly unsafe
Kava kava	Liver damage	Possibly unsafe; in 2002 the FDA issued a warning against its use
Lobelia	Toxicity; overdose can cause fast heartbeat, low blood pressure, coma, and possibly death	Likely unsafe; in 1993 the FDA warned against its use
Yohimbe	Normal doses cause high blood pressure and rapid heart rate; high doses cause low blood pressure, heart problems, and death	Likely unsafe; in 1993 the FDA warned that it was linked to serious adverse events

Herbs Not Recommended for Use by the German Commission E

According to the German Commission E, some herbs should not be taken because they present a possible health risk. However, there are places in this book where we include herbs listed above and below. In some cases, this seeming contradiction is due to the fact that a different part of the plant is being recommended—for example the leaf versus the stem. This is one reason it is very important to be clear about which part of the plant

Herb	Risk
Angelica seed and herb	Photosensitivity
Basil	Cancer causing
Bilberry leaf	High dose may cause intoxication
Bishop's weed fruit	Allergic reactions
Bladderwrack	Hyperthyroidism
Borage	Liver damage
Byronia	Numerous side effects cited
Celery	Allergic skin reactions
Chamomile, Roman	Rare allergic reactions such as rash
Cinnamon flower	Skin allergies
Cocoa	Skin allergies
Colocynth	GI irritation
Coltsfoot	Liver damage
Delphinium flower	Heart problems (low blood pressure)
Elecampane	Skin allergy
Ergot	Allergic reactions
Goat's rue	Hypoglycemia
Hound's tongue	Liver damage
Kelp	Hyperthyroidism
Lemongrass, citronella oil	Toxic to alveoli when oil is inhaled
Liverwort herb	Skin irritation

Herb	Risk
Madder root	Carcinogenic
Male fern	Wide spectrum of adverse reactions
Marjoram	Potential unclear risks
Marsh tea	Overdose may result in poisoning
Monkshood	Serious, varied spectrum of adverse reactions
Mugwort	Fetal abortion
Nutmeg	Thought process changes
Nux vomica	Spastic central nervous system
Oleander leaf	Poisoning
Papain	Increased bleeding
Parsley seed	Large doses of oil produce vascular congestion
Pasque flower	Skin irritations
Periwinkle	Suppression of immune system
Petasites leaf	Liver damage
Rhododendron, rusty-leaved	Poisoning
Rue	Liver and kidney damage
Saffron	Inadvertent abortion
Sarsaparilla root	Gastric irritation
Scotch broom flower	Contraindicated for MAOI therapy and low blood pressure
Senecio herb	Liver damage
Soapwort herb, red	Mucous membrane irritation
Tansy flower and herb	Poisoning
Walnut hull	Cancer causing
Yohimbe bark	Nervousness, sleeplessness, high blood pressure

you are using and why you are using it. It is also possible that the German Commission E scientists just got it wrong. These tables are included as a guide. You be the judge.

The German Commission E also does not recommend the following herbs because there was a lack of scientific documentation to support claims made by the supplement industry. However, since the German Commission E issued its guidelines, new research has shown some of these herbs to be effective in managing certain disorders. Please refer to specific herb entries for a discussion of the herb's uses and cautions.

Ash	Hollyhock flower	Oregano
Alpine lady's mantle	Horse chestnut leaf	Orris root
Blackberry root	Hyssop	Papaya leaf
Burdock root	Jambolan seed	Peony
Calendula herb	Linden charcoal	Pimpinella
Chestnut leaf	Linden flower, silver	Raspberry leaf
Cornflower	Linden leaf	Red sandalwood
Damiana leaf and herb	Loofa	Rose hip and seed
Dill weed	Lungwort	Rupturewort
Echinacea angustifolia herb and root/Pallida herb	Mentzelia	Spinach leaf
Eyebright	Milk thistle herb	Strawberry leaf
Ginkgo biloba leaf	Mountain ash berry	Sweet woodruff
Hawthorn berry	Muira puama	Verbena herb
Hawthorn flower	Night-blooming cereus	Veronica herb
Hawthorn leaf	Oat herb	White dead nettle herb
Heather herb and flower	Olive leaf	Zedoary rhizome
Hibiscus	Olive oil	

TOP REASONS WHY PEOPLE TAKE HERBS

According to the German Commission E, one-third of adults use herbs. Many herbal products are used to treat minor conditions and illnesses (coughs, cold, upset stomach). Herbs can substitute for a conventional OTC medication, but the regulatory mechanisms (FDA and Congress) do not allow the herbs to carry specific claims to these sorts of conditions. Also, herbs are used to support general health. The top health reasons given for using herbs included:

- Boosting energy: 60 percent
- Preventing colds: 56 percent
- Boosting immune system: 54 percent
- Improving sleep: 43 percent
- Helping prostate: 18 percent of the 500 males in the survey

Homeopathy: The Law of Similars

Homeopathy is not covered in this book per se, although there are some homeopathic remedies included where appropriate, because there are many herbs that are used almost strictly in homeopathy. It is important to note that homeopathic remedies are governed by different regulations than herbs and dietary supplements. The term *homeopathy* is derived from the Greek words *homeo* (similar) and *pathos* (suffering or disease). It is the practice of treating syndromes and conditions that constitute disease, with remedies that have produced similar symptoms in healthy subjects. Homeopathy seeks to stimulate the body's ability to heal itself by giving very small doses of highly diluted substances. In this way, homeopathic medicines treat illness by going with rather than against symptoms that are seen as the body's natural defenses. In contrast, conventional medicine acts to suppress symptoms or illness.

Homeopathic medicine uses plants as well as minerals and animal by-products. Most are provided as diluted solutions made from the starting compound. Remedies are taken orally by pill, powder, or drop form or rubbed topically.

The U.S. Food and Drug Administration (FDA) has recognized homeopathic medicines as drugs since 1938. An estimated 3.9 million U.S. adults and approximately 900,000 children use homeopathic remedies. Homeopathic remedies are regulated in the same manner as nonprescription, over-the-counter (OTC) drugs. However, because homeopathic products contain little or no active ingredients, they do not have to undergo the same safety and efficacy testing as prescription and new OTC drugs. The FDA does require that homeopathic remedies meet certain legal standards for strength, purity, and packaging. The labels on the remedies must include at least one major indication (i.e., medical problem to be treated), a list of ingredients, the dilution, and safety instructions. In addition, if a homeopathic remedy claims to treat a serious disease such as cancer, it needs to be sold by prescription. Only products for self-limiting conditions (minor health problems like a cold or headache that go away on their own) can be sold without a prescription. Most remedies are considered safe and not likely to cause adverse reactions when administered under the supervision of trained professionals.

When asked what factors would make them decide to use herbs, people responded:

- Recommended by physicians: 66 percent
- It can't hurt and might help: 41 percent
- Because nothing else has helped: 34 percent
- Heard about it in the news: 26 percent
- Friends using herbs: 15 percent

Only 4 percent said they'd never use herbs.

MATERIALS OF HERBAL TREATMENT

Many, perhaps 50 percent, of all conventional medications are refinements of herbal medicines. The isolation of morphine from opium in 1806 was the first time that chemical methods were used to extract the active chemical constituents of an herb. The chemical processes used to isolate morphine led to the production of codeine, the widely used cough suppressant. Chemical processing of cinchona bark yielded quinine, a malaria treatment that is still important today. The nasal spray cromolyn sodium (sold under the brand names Nasalcrom, Intal), the chemotherapy drug paclitaxel (Taxol), and the heart drug digoxin (Lanoxicaps, Lanoxin) were all developed from chemicals found in herbs. Today, many new drugs are being developed recombinantly, which means that yeast or bacteria are "trained" to make unique compounds shown to be effective at combating a specific disease. Even plants and animals can be genetically modified to make new drugs. If you are taking one of these newer drugs, you need to contact a trained health-care professional to find the best and safest herbs that go with these new drugs.

Synthesizing chemicals that are very similar to the naturally occurring active constituents of an herb allows for the manufacture of potent, fast-acting drugs that can be mass-produced. Of special importance to drug makers is the fact that synthetic chemical compounds can be patented, while herbs cannot. The law grants exclusive rights to the makers of chemical drugs that it does not grant to the manufacturers of herb products. Patent protection allows drug companies to sell chemical drugs at much higher prices, but the effects of the drugs are more likely to be as expected, whereas with herbs, there is a much greater variation in the amount of the active ingredients and therefore the effects are not always as consistent.

In some cases herbs offer some advantages over drugs derived from them; for example, they are often less toxic and less expensive. Of course, if you require conventional medicine for a serious illness whether it is made from herbs or not, you should take it. There are many herbs that work synergistically with certain drugs, so ask your health-care provider before taking any herbs with prescription drugs.

In truly ancient times, the only way to take an herb was to eat the herb raw, whether leaf, root, berry, or bark. The apothecaries of second- and third-century China prescribed finely ground herbs held together with binders, not all of which would be considered foods today: honey, rice porridge, beeswax, clay, pulverized fossils, and even horse manure (used primarily in formulas designed to restore the sense of taste). Ayurvedic herbalists prescribed *churnas*, herbs held together by sugar and myrrh, a method of making medicines still used in ayurveda today.

In modern times, other convenient and healthful forms of herbs are readily available. The most common forms of herbal remedies are listed here. Techniques for making herbal remedies at home are described in Part Three.

Capsules

Capsules consist of a two-part gelatin shell whose halves are fitted together after the herb is placed inside. In addition

Herbal Medicine in Ancient Egypt

The oldest recorded system of medicine originated in Egypt. Its oldest surviving medical text, known as the Ebers Papyrus, dating 1,500 years before recorded Chinese medicine, lists 700 medicinal herbs. Several of these herbs, including aloe vera and senna, have been used continuously for 3,500 years.

The Ebers Papyrus was perhaps the first recorded attempt to separate magic from medicine. It contains 877 herbal recipes concerning a great variety of diseases and symptoms, and only recommended incantations for 12 diseases for which the causes were completely unknown. Although the emphasis in this school of treatment was not mystical, the physician was still presented as a powerful figure above his patients, who always announced the diagnosis with one of three statements:

- "An ailment which I will treat."
- "An ailment with which I will contend."
- "An ailment not to be treated."

Fortunately, the hopeless diagnosis was recommended for only three diseases of the time. The papyri then taught the physician to continue treatment until symptoms resolved in one of three ways:

- "Until he recovers."
- "Until the period of his injury passes by."
- "Until thou knowest that he has reached decisive point."

Although Egyptian medicine was not a magical system, Egyptian physicians were deified. The earliest physician whose name has been recorded, Imhotep, was the wazir of Zoser, founder of the Third Dynasty, in approximately 3000 B.C.E. Imhotep was a learned man, astronomer, physician, and architect. By the time the Ebers Papyrus was recorded, Imhotep was worshiped as a hero, as a blameless physician, and, later still, as the god of medicine.

As an extension of worship, Egyptian medicine was exclusively disease-centered rather than person-centered (except to the extent that it exalted the physician).

---

to gelatin, the capsule shell may contain glycerin or another softening agent and water. Many (but not all) encapsulated formulations of herbal remedies also contain flavoring agents, dyes, and preservatives. It is important to read the label if it is necessary to avoid these artificial ingredients.

Some herbs such as devil's claw and peppermint are deactivated by contact with digestive juices. Other herbs can be so diluted that they become ineffective if they come in contact with food and water in the stomach. Capsules for these herbs are given an enteric coating with a cellulose fiber to delay the release of the herb until the capsule has reached the stomach or intestine.

It is important to take enteric-coated capsules one hour before, rather than during or after, meals. Particles as large as a capsule remain in the stomach until all other food in the stomach is digested. If the enteric-coated capsule is taken with food, or after food, it will be exposed to all the stomach acid released to digest the food and may release the herb prematurely.

Extracts

Extracts are concentrated preparations of herbs. Liquid extracts, more commonly called fluidextracts (written as one word rather than two), combine one part of the herb with one part of water or alcohol (ethanol), or one part of the herb with one part of a mixture of water and alcohol. Solid extracts are made by dissolving the chopped herb in a chemical solvent such as ethanol or another suitable solvent. After the herb is soaked in the solvent, the liquid is filtered out and gently dried at low heat for use in capsules or tablets. Drying the herb removes all of the solvent, leaving only the desired constituents of the herb behind.

The chemical constituents of an herb are much more concentrated in a solid extract than in the raw herb. The most widely sold solid extract in the world, ginkgo biloba extract (GBE), has fifty times the concentration of the biologically active ginkgolides found in ginkgo leaf. This concentration process makes it possible to take several small capsules weighing about one-quarter of a gram (less than one-hundredth of an ounce) for a daily dose of ginkgo instead of 10 to 15 grams (one-third to one-half an ounce) ginkgo leaf in teas.

Granules

Granules consist of powdered herb held together with binders. The binder may be cellulose fiber, gelatin, milk sugar, or table sugar, among other possibilities. The granules may or may not be fashioned into pills or tablets. Granules are most frequently encountered in imported Chinese patent medicines used for the treatment of digestive complaints.

Lozenges

Lozenges, also known as dragées, pastilles, and troches, have a round, oblong, tabletlike appearance but differ from tablets in that they are not made by compression but are molded or cut from pliable mixtures of sugar, acacia gum, gelatin, and a small amount of the herb.

Medicinal Spirits

Medicinal spirits or essences are the volatile oils of herbs preserved in a mixture of water and alcohol (ethanol). The most widely used medicinal spirit, peppermint, is made by dissolving the oil extracted by crushing peppermint leaves in alcohol; other medicinal spirits are made by distillation. To distill an herb, the herb is pulverized and mixed with alcohol. It is allowed to stand until the oil glands in the herb have burst and released their aromatic oils. The essential oil is heated, evaporated, captured in a "still," and preserved in alcohol.

People who have alcohol-related medical problems should avoid medicinal spirits.

Plant Juices

Plant juices are pressed from finely chopped herbs to which water has been added. Commercial preparations of plant juices are pasteurized. Herbs used in OTC plant juices include birch leaf, dandelion, echinacea, garlic, radish, and St. John's wort.

Syrups

Sugar-sweetened syrups were an invention of ancient Arabic healers that reached Europe in the early Middle Ages. The word *syrup* is derived from the Arabic *scherbet*, meaning a sugary juice beverage. The sweet taste of syrup makes it the preferred form of herbs to be given to children.

Syrups usually consist of two-thirds sugar, the high sugar content making it impossible for microbial contaminants to grow. Diluting a syrup invites bacterial growth. Syrups that are made without sugar should be stored in the refrigerator.

Tablets

Tablets are made by compressing granules or powders into a cylindrical mold. Tablets usually contain very small amounts of an extract suspended in a binder with colors, flavors, lubricants, and disintegrating agents. *Coated* tablets are covered with dyes, fat, sugar, and wax to protect the medicinal ingredients inside. Coating tablets protects them against heat, light, moisture, and breakage, and masks any unpleasant taste in the medicinal core.

Teas

Teas can be prepared from single herbs or mixtures of herbs. Teas for acute conditions are almost always brewed with single herbs. Teas for chronic conditions, and the teas used in traditional Chinese medicine, are almost always mixtures of herbs.

Of all the forms in which herbs may be used, teas have the gentlest and slowest effects on the body. The degree to which the active constituents of the herbs used to make the teas will be absorbed is unpredictable. For this reason, the best way to describe the results from taking a tea is "Drink the tea, wait and see."

Despite their unpredictable benefits and their slow onset of action, teas are especially safe. Teas are usually the best way to use herbs to treat young children. (For detailed instructions for making teas, *see* TEAS in Part Three.)

Tinctures

A tincture is a mixture of herb(s), ethanol, and water. Children's "tinctures" usually substitute glycerol for alcohol. Although the main ingredients in any tincture are alcohol, glycerol, and/or water, many tincture labels are printed with separate lists of herbs and the *excipients,* or liquids in which they are dissolved. People who are sensitive to alcohol, or parents buying tinctures for small children, need to read both lists to make sure the liquid with which the tincture is made is not alcohol (ethanol). (For more information on tinctures, *see* TINCTURES in Part Three.)

SHOPPING FOR HERBS

Herbal medicines can be bought through a number of different types of outlets. There are several places to look:

• *Asian markets.* In regions with a large Asian immigrant population, there are food markets that carry Asian specialties and also sell traditional Asian herbal medicines. One caveat: as many of these herbs are imported, it is not possible to guarantee that the herbs are free of toxins such as pesticides.

• *Health food and retail stores.* Many of these stores carry a wide selection of herbs. Labeling laws in the United States do not allow an herb's exact uses to be listed on the package. However, herbs, like all dietary supplements, carry what is called a "structure/function" claim. This means that the herb may be identified for the part of the body that it affects. For example, St. John's wort may carry the claim "supports brain health." Health food stores are arguably the safest places to buy herbs. The bigger stores typically only buy from companies that follow the General Manufacturing Practices (GMP) set forth by the FDA. And these companies often do their own testing as well to verify that the product contains exactly what is stated on the label and that it is free of harmful substances such as pesticides.

• *Herb shops.* Most herb shops carry a wide selection of both packaged and loose herbs, and the proprietor is usually knowledgeable about the products he or she sells.

• *Internet and catalogs.* Like marketers of other alternative health products, many herb distributors operate mail-order and online services offering an equally broad range of herbal products. Buying on the Web is very convenient, especially for hard-to-find herbal formulas. It is important to deal with a reputable company, though, because the product cannot be inspected before purchase. (*See* Appendix B: Resources for the names, addresses, telephone numbers, and websites of a number of recommended mail-order and online sources of herbal and other products.)

• *Compounding pharmacies.* To obtain herbal products for unique individual needs, consult a compounding pharmacy. Compounding pharmacies are local drugstores that prepare custom-made medications of all kinds. Compounding pharmacists are usually "problem-solvers" who can prepare herbs (as well as most prescription medications) to meet specific individual needs that cannot be met by mass production at a factory. A compounding pharmacist can prepare herbs and medications using unique delivery systems, such as lozenges, lollipops, or transdermal gels. For a young patient, a compounding pharmacist might prepare an alcohol-free syrup in vanilla, butternut, cantaloupe, tutti-frutti, or some other unique flavor. For a person who has a difficult time swallowing a capsule, a compounding pharmacist can make a suspension instead.

Compounding pharmacists also can process bulk herbs bought at wholesale prices into economical capsules, pills, and tablets. This is especially economical for individuals with chronic conditions who may use a lot of herbs.

The services of compounding pharmacies are little known to the public because they are prohibited from advertising *specific* compounded products. However, any compounding pharmacy can provide custom-made herbal products. To find a compounding pharmacist in your area, call the International Academy of Compounding Pharmacists. (*See* Appendix B: Resources.)

THE CASE FOR STANDARDIZATION

Herbs are plants. Just as there are very different outcomes of nature and nurture in the characteristics of individual people, there are many differences among individual plants. We all know that there are different kinds of teas and different vintages of wines and that there are low-acid and high-acid kinds of coffee. Similarly, there can be great differences in the concentrations of healing constituents in different herbs of the same species, especially when they are gathered in the wild.

Much of the training of the herbal healer in history was centered on recognizing plants with the greatest healing potential. The Chinese herb fu zi (a kind of aconite), for example, contains pain-relieving mesaconitines when it is grown or gathered from a height of over 2,500 feet (800 meters), but not when it is collected at sea level. Botanists exploring the Amazon rain forest at first ridiculed the local healers' insistence that cat's claw with one size of hooks on its stems could be used to treat illness, while cat's claw with another size of hooks on its stems could not. Decades later, chemical analysis showed that the plants selected by the healers contained healing alkaloids that most of the plants collected by the early botanists did not.

The modern consumer unfortunately lacks access to traditional healers knowledgeable of plants in the wild. In the place of this knowledge, modern technology offers standardized extracts, herbal products chemically tested and confirmed to contain a minimum dosage of all the *known* active constituents of the herb.

The first step of the standardization process is knowing the producer. Commercial buyers rely on growers to apply consistent methods of cultivation and to harvest herbs at the appropriate stage of growth, season, temperature, and time of day. Long-term relationships of mutual trust between growers and buyers are the goal of the herb industry.

The second step in standardization is confirming the identity of the herb purchased. The buyer's experience in how an herb should look, smell, and taste is an essential part of this process. This step also usually entails microscopic examination of a sample of the herb to ensure that it is the species of plant required. In some cases, the buyer may prepare a chemical extract to ascertain that the herb contains minimum amounts of those plant chemicals known to have healing effects. This is called a Certificate of Analysis. In other cases, the medicinal value of the herb will be verified by measurements of ash or water content. Manufacturers also routinely test for the presence of heavy metals, especially arsenic, lead, and mercury, in order to exclude them.

The third step in standardization is sanitary storage. Bacteria, insects, and molds must be excluded from the storage space.

To ensure the quality of the standardized product, the herbs selected for use are processed as extracts (*see* page 11). Not every batch, however, comes out with the same concentration of the important constituents. Extracts must be analyzed by technical means, usually by high-performance liquid chromatography (HPLC), to make sure they contain the needed chemicals.

Once each batch has been analyzed, herb manufacturers blend batches of extract together in a way that ensures a consistent concentration of specific ingredients or groups of compounds. If the therapeutic power of the product is influenced by a single group of compounds, this quality adjustment is accomplished by adding or subtracting binders and fillers from the final mix.

Standardization is critical for making a quality, mass-produced herbal product. Equally effective products are available from professional herbalists who have the knowledge and take the time to collect high-quality herbs from their gardens or from the wild. Their traditional products, however, cannot be mass-produced.

The Herbs

The previous section described the basic principles of herbal treatment. It explained how chemical medicines are measured doses of single ingredients, while herbs are blends of various compounds that work together to rejuvenate the physiological processes that need help. It described the ways in which herbs allow a precise match between an individual's symptoms and treatment, reducing side effects and increasing effectiveness of measures to treat disease and establish health.

This section lists the herbs used widely today. It is a guide to the herbs most frequently recommended in Part Two, which discusses individual disease conditions. Herbs that are used to treat very specific or unique conditions are listed where applicable in the entries in Part Two.

Each entry in this section starts with a description of the plant. Following the plant description is a summary of the evidence for using the herb in the treatment of the conditions for which it is listed in Part Two. Finally, each entry gives Considerations for Use. This tells how to take the herb, how long it takes to work, and how it interacts with prescription medications that people who use the herb usually also take. Since specific dosages vary for different conditions, this information is given in Part Two.

Any herb or medication that is strong enough to heal may be also strong enough to harm when used improperly or for too long. This issue is addressed in each applicable entry, as are situations that would preclude the use of the herb, such as pregnancy or a possibly harmful drug interaction. It is always important to consult a qualified health-care provider if there is *any* question as to whether or not an herbal treatment is appropriate in any specific case.

ACEROLA

Latin name: *Malpighia* species (Malpighiaceae [tropical cherry] family)
Other common names: Antilles cherry, Barbados cherry, cereso

General Description

The acerola is a bushy tree that grows to a height of ten to fifteen feet. It is native to the West Indies and southern Texas southward to northern South America. Acerola is often cultivated as an ornamental shrub, particularly in the southeastern United States. The fleshy red fruits are about the size of a cherry and can be eaten fresh or used to make jams and jellies. They also are an important commercial source of natural vitamin C.

Acerola is one of the richest food sources of vitamin C.

On average, 100 grams (3.5 ounces) of ripe acerola fruits contains 17,000 milligrams of vitamin C. (The vitamin C content varies depending on the season, climate, location, and ripeness of the fruit.) For the sake of comparison, 100 grams of oranges contains only 50 milligrams of vitamin C. Acerola has a carotene content comparable to that of carrots and also supplies a small amount of magnesium, niacin, pantothenic acid, potassium, vitamin B_1 (thiamine), and vitamin B_2 (riboflavin). The vitamin content of acerola is highest before it ripens, while the fruit is still green. As the fruit begins to ripen, it loses much of its vitamin content, which is why it is harvested green.

Evidence of Benefit

Acerola is used primarily for its vitamin C content and free-radical-scavenging abilities, but it also has small amounts of other vitamins and minerals. The acerola fruit also contains other substances, like provitamin A, that intensify the antioxidative (cell-protective) effects of vitamin C.

Vitamin C is an essential nutrient and must be supplied by the diet. It is known to be a natural detoxifier and antioxidant. Vitamin C may indirectly protect the body from the effects of pollution. It is necessary for the formation and maintenance of collagen, which is a primary protein of the skin and connective tissues, and is necessary for a healthy liver and adrenal gland function.

Benefits of acerola and vitamin C for specific health conditions include the following:

• *Aging.* Research on aging has focused on free radicals as one of the causes of oxidative damage to the body leading to a gradual failure of the immune system. Vitamin C is effective at scavenging free radicals, limiting damaging oxidation reactions in the body, and stimulating the immune system, thus possibly slowing the aging process.

• *Angina.* As an exceptionally rich source of vitamin C, acerola may help people who must use nitroglycerin tablets to avoid becoming habituated to the drug.

• *Bronchitis.* Vitamin C has anti-infective activity and helps the immune system to regain balance, enabling it to fight the infection. In studies, hospital patients with bronchitis recovered faster when they took vitamin C supplements.

• *Cancer.* Studies show that people who regularly eat foods high in vitamin C have a lower than average risk of developing various malignancies, especially cancer of the stomach and esophagus. Whether regular supplementation with acerola reduces this risk is unknown.

• *Colds and flu.* Taking 2,000 to 4,000 milligrams of vitamin C with acerola has been found to ease symptoms of colds and flu and to shorten the duration of the infection.

• *Glaucoma.* Glaucoma involves an increase in intraocular pressure (fluid pressure in the eyeball) that develops when the drainage mechanism for this fluid becomes impaired. Many studies show that vitamin C lowers intraocular pressure, but there are no specific human studies indicating that acerola does this.

• *Herpes.* The acids in acerola break down mucus, in which the herpesvirus multiplies. The high concentration of vitamin C provided by the herb interacts with the micronutrient copper to eliminate as many as 99.994 percent of the viruses that would be shed by infected cells, according to laboratory studies. Clinical studies of herpes treatment have found that vitamin C, but not acerola, reduces pain and swelling, and speeds the healing of scabs by several days.

• *Parkinson's disease.* Acerola is an excellent source of antioxidants important for maintaining mental function. Laboratory studies in cells of people with Parkinson's disease suggest that acerola may help maintain levels of available vitamin C in brain tissue when the people also are taking vitamin E.

• *Wrinkles.* Acerola extracts are used in antioxidant skin-care products to fight cellular aging. According to South American herb expert Leslie Taylor, acerola contains mineral salts that promote the remineralization of tired and stressed skin, as well as mucilage and proteins that prevent drying. Acerola has been shown in cell studies to fight fungal infections, but human studies are lacking.

Considerations for Use

The easiest way to use acerola is as a natural vitamin C tablet called "vitamin C USP with acerola." To avoid changes in metabolism that cause the body to require large amounts of vitamin C for normal health, take no more than one to two tablets per day for Parkinson's disease. However, speak to your doctor before you take acerola if you have Parkinson's disease. Use acerola tablets for herpes only when lesions break out. Be sure to drink six to eight glasses of water daily when taking acerola.

Acerola replaces vitamin C that may be depleted during treatment with tetracycline antibiotics, corticosteroids such as prednisone, and oral contraceptives. Avoid acerola for two to three weeks after any surgical procedure for cancer. Acerola should also be avoided during chemotherapy with agents designed to deprive cancer cells of vitamin C, such as melphalan (Alkeran).

People who have hemachromatosis (iron overload disease) should avoid acerola and other vitamin C supplements, since taking over 200 milligrams of vitamin C per day increases iron absorption. People with this disorder who are being treated with deferoxamine (Desferal), however, benefit from taking acerola, since the additional vitamin C helps the drug remove iron from circulation. Do not do this without your doctor's permission.

There is no danger of overdose through the use of acerola skin creams. But before using such a cream, test it on a small area to see if any sign of an allergic reaction develops. If there is no redness or swelling forty-eight hours later, apply the cream as needed.

There is some evidence that vitamin C supports the synthesis of calcium oxalate, which can become concentrated in the urine, a condition known as ascorbate-induced hyperoxaluria. For some people, this may result in the formation of kidney stones. This is a rare situation, however. Such a response to vitamin C may be genetically determined, so if you have a family history of kidney stones, screening for ascorbate-induced hyperoxaluria is recommended.

How much vitamin C is enough? In 1999, the *Journal of the American Medical Association* and the *American Journal of Clinical Nutrition* reported studies that showed that cells cannot absorb more vitamin C than the amount provided by taking 200 milligrams of vitamin C one or two times a day. This would seem to imply that high-potency sources of vitamin C such as acerola provide ascorbic acid that is "wasted" by the body. Still, few clinical studies show that too much vitamin C from acerola is harmful.

Body tolerance is the largest dose of vitamin C a person can take without experiencing gas, loose stools, or diarrhea. You can find your body tolerance by starting with a relatively low dose, perhaps 500 to 1,000 milligrams with each meal, and gradually increasing the dose every day until you notice any of symptoms mentioned above. Then decrease the dose slightly to the largest amount you can tolerate, with continued adjustment as needed. These recommendations are for adults; do not give children these high amounts of vitamin C without consulting a pediatrician.

ACORUS

Latin name: *Acorus gramineus* (Araceae [sweet flag] family)
Other common names: chang pu, gramineus, shi chang pu, sweet flag rhizome

General Description

Acorus is a grasslike, rhizome-forming perennial plant resembling an iris. It inhabits wet areas like the edges of streams and around ponds and lakes. The rhizomes have an aromatic, spicy fragrance, and are used in herbal medicine. Acorus is the Japanese relative of the American herb calamus, also known as sweet flag.

Evidence of Benefit

Acorus is an antioxidant that has special effects on the central nervous system. It is used by the Akha people of

Thailand for stomachache. The Chinese use it for vomiting, diarrhea, abdominal pain, and dysentery. This herb eliminates phlegm and tranquilizes the mind, and has been used to treat amnesia, heart palpitations, insomnia, tinnitus, chronic bronchitis, and bronchial asthma.

Benefits of acorus for specific health conditions include the following:

• *Drug withdrawal.* Acorus affects the brain during withdrawal from cocaine, heroin, and morphine. During the first one to ten days of withdrawal, addicts experience intense drug cravings, nausea, and vomiting. Acorus can blunt gastric upset during the acute phase of drug withdrawal (although it has no effect on the cravings themselves) through its ability to prevent the secretion of the inflammatory chemical histamine.

• *Seizure disorders.* Acorus is used to treat a broad range of brain conditions. It works by protecting brain tissue from toxic free radicals, which are released in the presence of excess oxygen. When the flow of oxygen is restored to previously oxygen-deprived brain cells, these cells are temporarily unable to use all the oxygen available to them. The oxygen escapes the biochemical pathways that usually control it and free-radical damage results. The resulting tissue damage in the brain can lead to memory loss or seizures. Acorus helps prevent the formation of free radicals of oxygen and the resulting brain tissue damage. It is most effective when taken *before* circulation is restored, that is, in the first few days to a month after a head injury or stroke.

Considerations for Use

Acorus is most commonly supplied by practitioners of traditional Chinese medicine (TCM). It is usually sold in the United States as chang pu or shi chang pu, in the form of powders, teas, and tinctures.

The herb's American relative calamus contains the potentially cancer-causing chemical beta-asarone, which has caused it to be banned for use in the United States. Although the form of acorus used in TCM is legal in the United States, it is restricted in Canada. Many other countries ban the use of both acorus and calamus in herbal medicine. Acorus should *never* be used without professional supervision.

AGRIMONY

Latin name: *Agrimonia eupatoria* (Rosaceae [rose] family)
Other common names: church steeples, cocklebur, liverwort, stickwort

General Description

Agrimony has paired leaves, green above and silvery beneath, growing along a three-foot (ninety-centimeter) stem. It is characterized by its spikes that bear rows of tiny yellow flowers known as church steeples. It is grown throughout much of the United States and southern Canada and is harvested in the summer, when it produces its yellow flowers. It prefers full sun and average soils, and tolerates dry weather. All of the aboveground parts of the plant are used in herbal medicine.

Evidence of Benefit

Agrimony is a nontoxic astringent, or binding herb, that is especially safe for children. Traditionally, agrimony is one of the most renowned vulnerary (wound-healing) herbs. The Anglo-Saxons taught that it would heal wounds, snakebite, and warts. In France, it is applied for sprains and bruises. It is still fully appreciated in herbal practice as a mild astringent and tonic, useful for coughs, diarrhea, and relaxed bowels.

Benefits of agrimony for specific health conditions include the following:

• *Bed-wetting, bladder infections.* Agrimony stops irritation of the urinary tract that can increase a child's urge to urinate. It also works in adults who have had a history of cystitis (bladder infection).

• *Bleeding.* Agrimony has been used for thousands of years to stop bleeding and bruising, and encourage clot formation. Agrimony acts by "tanning" skin cells, making them impermeable to bleeding. This action also prevents bacteria from entering the wound.

• *Diabetes.* Experiments in animals indicate that infusions of agrimony can prevent the development of type 1 diabetes, although it is not known whether the herb could have the same effect in humans.

• *Diarrhea.* Agrimony is effective against diarrhea, especially in small children.

• *Jaundice and liver problems.* Agrimony's astringents exhibit tonic and diuretic properties. Agrimony has a reputation for treating jaundice and other complaints.

• *Skin problems.* Agrimony can be applied topically to the skin in places of mild inflammation.

Considerations for Use

Agrimony is used in teas or tinctures. Its low toxicity makes it particularly suitable for children's illnesses. But consult your child's pediatrician first before giving it to a child. It has been approved by the German Commission E for use in diarrhea, inflammation of the skin, and inflammation of the mouth and pharynx. However, the herb has a high tannic acid content and too much could lead to digestive complaints.

While agrimony is an effective treatment for many forms of diarrhea, it can aggravate constipation. The tannins in agrimony cause pectin fibers to cross-link and bind. Blockage can result if you take agrimony at the same time as psyllium powders, such as Metamucil, or if you take it with prunes or prune juice.

Agrimony affects the immune system. It stimulates the body to produce immune bodies known as B cells. These cells produce complex chemicals known as antigens that attack invading microbes. A number of other conditions, however, result from attacks on *healthy* tissues by B cells with defects in their genetic programming. For that reason, people with rheumatoid arthritis, myasthenia gravis, Graves' disease, Hashimoto's thyroiditis, lupus, Sjögren's syndrome, or any other autoimmune disease should avoid agrimony. People who are susceptible to sunlight should not use agrimony, as they may develop skin rashes. Those who are taking anticoagulation or high blood pressure drugs should not take this herb. Pregnant and lactating women should avoid this herb.

ALFALFA

Latin name: *Medicago sativum* (Fabaceae [legume] family)
Other common names: buffalo herb, lucerne, purple medic

General Description

Alfalfa is a perennial herb that grows to a height of three feet (ninety centimeters). It has three-lobed leaves, blue-violet or yellow flowers, and spiraling seed pods. It is cultivated in many regions of the world. It is not picky as to soil, but it does prefer full sun and regular watering. The aerial (aboveground) parts of the plant are used in herbal medicine.

Alfalfa originated in the Middle East. By the sixteenth century, it had been planted in England, and it arrived in 1736 in the thirteen colonies that later formed the United States. English and American herbalists used alfalfa in the same way they used the related plant, clover—to treat stomach upset.

The Arabs called alfalfa the "father of all foods." The leaves of the alfalfa plant contain some minerals, such as calcium, magnesium, and potassium, as well as other nutrients, such as carotene. Alfalfa leaf tablets have protein and vitamins A, D, E, and K. Alfalfa extract is a good source of chlorophyll and carotene. The leaves contain eight essential amino acids.

Evidence of Benefit

Alfalfa has helped many with cardiovascular, nervous, and digestive system issues. Traditionally it was used in treating diabetes in people with a poorly functioning thyroid gland. There is also evidence in animal and cell studies that components in alfalfa may lower cholesterol and have antifungal effects.

Benefits of alfalfa for specific health conditions include the following:

• *Atherosclerosis.* Scientific studies with animals have found that alfalfa leaf extracts lower total cholesterol and the "bad" cholesterol, low-density lipoprotein (LDL) levels, without lowering the "good" cholesterol, high-density

lipoprotein (HDL). In one study people who had high cholesterol levels used 40 to 80 grams of alfalfa seeds for eight weeks and it lowered their total cholesterol and the LDL levels. The typical dose is 40 grams of heat-prepared seeds, three times a day. Alfalfa may also help shrink atherosclerotic plaques. Alfalfa's effect on atherosclerosis is probably due to its effect on the activity of immune cells known as macrophages. Macrophages are drawn to sites of wear and tear in artery linings, where they form a platform on which cholesterol can collect. Alfalfa regulates macrophages in such a way that they are less likely to "lodge" in the linings of arteries and accumulate cholesterol. Alfalfa also slows the progress of atherosclerosis by keeping cholesterol from entering the body from food. The alfalfa saponins, which are soaplike compounds, form an insoluble foam with cholesterol inside the intestine. The resulting foam cannot be absorbed through the walls of the intestine and is excreted in the stool.

• *Cancer.* Alfalfa has important uses in counteracting the effects of cancer chemotherapy. White blood cells, including granulocytes, leukocytes, and T cells, are the body's first line of defense against infection. Alfalfa extracts may increase the production of these white cells by as much as 60 percent. Studies in animals have found that alfalfa completely reverses immune depression caused by treatment with the cancer chemotherapy drug cyclophosphamide (Cytoxan, Neosar). Although alfalfa suppresses the action of macrophages (*see* above), it does not inhibit the activity of any of the immune cells the body needs during the first stages of infection.

• *Endometriosis.* Doctors may prescribe synthetic estrogen, usually in the form of birth control pills, for the treatment of endometriosis. Naturopaths have favored herbs and foods with phytoestrogens, natural plant hormones that are related to estrogen but are less potent than the body's own estrogens. Alfalfa sprouts contain phytoestrogens that also block the body's estrogen receptor sites, thereby reducing the effect of a woman's own hormones.

• *Fungal infections.* The saponins found in alfalfa have well-documented antifungal properties. When applied topically in studies using pigs, alfalfa helped improve skin tone that was damaged by *Trichophyton mentagrophytes*. In addition, an extract of alfalfa was shown to treat cryptococcosis and candidiasis.

• *Menopause-related problems.* Hot flashes and other menopausal symptoms are rare among women who consume a lot of legumes, such as black beans, mung beans, and soybeans, which have mild estrogenic activity. Alfalfa has demonstrable estrogenic activity, too. In addition to acting like estrogen in women whose own sex hormone production has declined, phytoestrogens also appear to reduce the risk of estrogen-linked cancers such as breast cancer. Laboratory experiments show that phytoestrogens are effective in preventing tumors of the breast tissue.

• *Nosebleed.* Alfalfa contains vitamin K, which helps blood clot normally. The level of vitamin K in alfalfa is not so high as to interfere with normal circulation.

• *Osteoporosis.* Clinical studies in Japan have found that vitamin K_2, found in alfalfa and in green leafy vegetables such as kale and spinach, can partially prevent bone loss caused by estrogen deficiency. The vitamin interacts with vitamin D to increase the formation of new bone. The combination is not sufficient, however, to completely compensate for osteoporosis caused by estrogen-depleting medications.

• *Ulcers.* Herbalists have long used alfalfa to treat ulcers, with good results. The bioflavonoids found in alfalfa build capillary strength and reduce inflammation of the stomach lining, while alfalfa's vitamin A helps to maintain the stomach's health. The herb's enzymes aid in food assimilation.

Considerations for Use

Alfalfa is not recommended as *primary* treatment for any condition. Instead, it should be taken in capsules, tablets, or ointment, or eaten as fresh raw sprouts that have been rinsed thoroughly to remove mold. The sprouting process creates an outstanding environment for microorganism propagation, so care must be taken before eating them. Treating alfalfa with chlorine or other disinfectants may not be enough to reduce the pathogen growth. Some have proposed radiation as the best alternative. Alfalfa seeds should never be eaten unless sprouted because they contain high levels of the toxic amino acid canavanine.

Alfalfa is especially useful for replacing vitamin K that is depleted during treatment with a wide variety of drugs. Vitamin K deficiency is common among people being treated with antibiotics such as amoxicillin (Amoxil, Polymox, Trimox), cefaclor (Ceclor), gentamicin (Garamycin), streptomycin, and tetracycline as well as many others. It also may occur during treatment with the cholesterol-lowering drugs cholestyramine (Locholest, Prevalite, Questran) and colestipol (Colestid), any steroid drug taken internally, or the drugs ethotoin (Peganone), mephenytoin (Mesantoin), and phenytoin (Dilantin), which are used to treat seizure disorders. It is important to take alfalfa products certified as grown organically, since the plant concentrates cadmium, copper, lead, nickel, and zinc when it is grown in contaminated soils.

Not everyone can benefit from alfalfa. Alfalfa should be avoided by pregnant women and by people with gout and systemic lupus erythematosus. Alfalfa reduces the effectiveness of immunosuppressive drugs. Patients who have had an organ transplant should avoid alfalfa supplements if taking antirejection drugs such as cyclosporine. Alfalfa also reduces the effectiveness of prednisone. Many patients with lupus use this medication to reduce inflammation. Alfalfa (and alfalfa sprouts) also should be avoided by people taking prescription warfarin (Coumadin) or other anticoagulants.

ALOE

Latin name: *Aloe barbadensis/capensis/vera*

General Description

Aloe, or aloe vera, is a prickly, gray-green succulent native to Africa but cultivated around the world. It is a perennial with leaves that can grow up to two feet (sixty centimeters) long, and it bears spikes of yellow or orange flowers. The leaves contain a clear gel that is applied in skin treatments. A dried yellow sap taken from the leaf base, aloe bitters, is used internally.

Evidence of Benefit

Aloe is an immune stimulant, laxative, and anti-inflammatory agent. In clinical trials aloe has been shown to have a wide range of benefits for the skin and in the treatment of cancer and ulcerative colitis.

Benefits of aloe for specific health conditions include the following:

• *Acne.* Aloe vera has been shown to be an effective treatment for acne when taken orally or applied topically. When combined with *Ocimum gratissimum* oil and given topically, the product performed significantly better than a placebo.

• *Burns and other wounds.* Scientific studies with animals have shown that aloe vera sap activates macrophages, the immune cells that fight bacterial infection. This allows burns to heal cleanly. The sap stimulates the circulation of blood at the body's surface, which accelerates wound healing. Aloe vera juice speeds healing because it increases the amount of oxygen carried by the blood to the cells. Aloe gel is a mild anesthetic that relieves itching, swelling, and pain. Aloe also helps repair damaged cells and prevents burns from scarring. Moreover, aloe contains enzymes, carboxypeptidase and bradykininase, that relieve pain, reduce inflammation, and decrease redness and swelling. Clinical studies have confirmed that burns and cuts treated with aloe vera gel heal as much as six days faster than burns and cuts treated with unmedicated dressings or with chemical antiseptic gels.

• *Cancer.* Alo A, a medically active complex sugar in aloe, stimulates and regulates various components of the immune system. It stops both the processes of inflammation necessary for tumors to gain new blood supplies and the growth of tumors themselves. In a skin cancer study involving animals, aloe gel and vitamin E cream together produced remission approximately 33 percent of the time, compared with 3 percent when no treatment was given. In addition, certain compounds in aloe seem to prevent cancer-causing substances from entering liver tissue. Aloe works best for skin issues—such as skin toxicities—that are a common side effect of radiation therapy to treat cancer. Mixing aloe with a mild soap seemed to reduce skin rash and redness in women who received very high doses of radiation for their breast cancer. Patients with head and neck cancer did not seem to benefit from using aloe after they received radiation therapy.

• *Constipation.* Aloe bitters are a fast and effective remedy for constipation used widely outside the United States. When compared with other herbal stimulant laxatives such as cascara sagrada or senna, aloe draws less fluid into the large intestine from the rest of the body. This makes it less likely than cascara or senna to cause dehydration or electrolyte disturbances. Aloe juices have the same effect as bitters on constipation but are less reliable and offer less relief. Aloe has anthraquinones that directly affect intestinal mucosa by increasing colonic motility, enhancing colonic transit time, and inhibiting water and electrolyte excretion. They also cause less irritation to the bowel compared to other anti-diarrheal agents. Aloe softens the stool, and the onset of action is six to twelve hours after ingestion. In one study, when combined with psyllium and celandine, aloe allowed for softer stools, less laxative dependence, and more frequent bowel movements in a group of patients with chronic constipation compared to a placebo treatment.

• *Hemorrhoids.* Aloe gel helps heal wounds and can be applied topically. India's ayurvedic physicians recommend drinking ½ cup of aloe juice three times a day until hemorrhoid flare-ups are gone.

• *Herpes simplex.* In one study, an extract of the leaf of the aloe made into a cream healed genital sores more quickly than an aloe gel. The gel or cream was applied three times a day and there were no significant side effects. In another study, a leaf extract was effective at treating first lesions of herpes simplex prepared in a cream after five weeks. The patients who received the cream with aloe healed more quickly than the placebo group and showed a 67 percent cure rate—only 13 percent of those who were cured developed herpes again in the next twenty months.

• *Psoriasis.* In one study, an extract of aloe leaf effectively cured or reduced the signs of psoriasis in a group of sixty subjects. The mean Psoriasis Area and Severity Score (a marker of disease) was lower in the aloe group after sixteen weeks compared to the placebo group. Eighty-three percent of the patients in the aloe group saw improvements, compared to only 7 percent of the control group. However, another study found that aloe vera gel did not improve the redness and swelling of skin in patients with psoriasis faster than the placebo after one month.

• *Radiation exposure.* Aloe protects against skin-damaging X-rays. Aloe is an effective antioxidant that absorbs the free radicals caused by radiation. Many studies have been conducted in patients receiving radiation therapy and taking aloe. However, in a systematic review on the subject, aloe was not found to be more effective than a placebo in treating skin lesions and mouth sores. Most patients studied had breast cancer or head and neck cancer.

• *Ulcerative colitis.* Aloe gel is an effective anti-inflammatory for this condition. In one study, patients took aloe for four weeks and had reduced bowel inflammation.

• *Ulcers.* Aloe has been shown to be effective in healing long-term leg ulcers compared to other therapies. In one study, an aloe gel prepared from fresh leaves was applied locally three to five times a day. In addition, pressure ulcers (bed sores) were healed faster with aloe according to a standardized measurement (Pressure Sore Status).

• *UV light damage.* In one study healthy volunteers who had four areas of the skin irradiated with UV light and received topical aloe gel from the plant leaf did not experience less redness or swelling compared to those who received no treatment.

• *Vitamin deficiency.* In one study aloe vera preparations made from the leaf of the plant increased the absorption of vitamins E and C.

Considerations for Use

Use aloe gels for skin problems, aloe bitters for constipation, and aloe juice for other disorders, as directed in individual entries in Part Two.

Aloe gel is available commercially and may also be taken from one's own plants. Leaves up to one foot long may be removed from the plant without causing damage. The best time of day for cutting aloe leaves is midafternoon, when the plant has moved a maximum amount of sap into the leaf.

Be aware that there are many so-called aloe vera products on the market that actually contain very little aloe vera. They are watered-down imitations that are not as beneficial as bona fide aloe vera. Read product labels. Aloe vera should be listed as a primary ingredient—that is, it should be the first- or second-listed ingredient.

Aloe bitters and aloe juice should not be taken *internally* during pregnancy, lactation, or menstruation. Children under twelve years of age should not take it. Aloe is also contraindicated in cases of rectal bleeding, intestinal obstruction, and acutely inflamed intestinal disease. It should not be used for acute surgical abdomen bowel obstruction or fecal impaction, appendicitis, and abdominal pain of unknown origin. Any laxative, herbal or otherwise, affects the rate at which other orally administered drugs are absorbed into the bloodstream. Therefore, prescription medication and aloe laxatives should be taken at different times.

Long-term internal use (more than two weeks) of aloe is not recommended because the fluid drawn into the stool can result in depletion of electrolytes, especially potassium. Loss of potassium is even greater when aloe is taken internally with potassium-wasting diuretic drugs. Depletion of potassium by excessive use of aloe laxatives theoretically could lead to toxic buildup of calcium in the bloodstream and kidney damage in women who take calcium carbonate (such as Caltrate 600) for osteoporosis. Potassium depletion also can cause serious mineral imbalances in persons who take forms of lithium, including Cibalith-S, Eskalith, Lithobid, Lithonate, and Lithotabs, for the treatment of bipolar disorder. The internal use of aloe should likewise be avoided by people who take potassium-depleting drugs for high blood pressure or congestive heart failure, such as hydrochlorothiazide (found in diuretic drugs sold under a wide range of brand names) or furosemide (Lasix).

Scientists have debated whether aloe-emodin, aloe's laxative compound, can damage colon cells. The most recent finding is that, when taken as directed, aloe poses no risk of cancer or genetic damage. Among people who abuse aloe and similar laxative herbs over a period of at least a year, *and* who develop other colon changes, about 3 percent can be expected to develop colorectal cancer within five years. This can be compared with the approximately 4 percent of the population as a whole who will develop colorectal cancer at some point in their lives. Stopping aloe use before twenty weeks have passed gives the body a chance to reverse its effects. Aloe juice does not carry the risks of aloe bitters for colon cancer.

Ayurvedic medicine uses aloe to stimulate fertility in women. Women who take birth control pills should avoid the internal use of aloe, although application of aloe to the skin will not interact with oral contraceptives.

Aloe may increase the risk of low blood sugar when it is used in conjunction with antidiabetic medications. In addition, aloe should not be used with digoxin, as it can cause toxicity.

AMERICAN GINSENG

Latin name: *Panax quinquefolium* (Araliaceae [ginseng] family)

General Description

In appearance, American ginseng is a smaller version of its more famous Asian cousin. (*See* GINSENG.) It is a slow-growing perennial plant with a large, fleshy root and a one- to two-foot-high stem. The leaves are divided into three to seven sharp-toothed, lance-shaped leaflets. The scented yellow-green flowers grow in June and July. The fruits, which follow the blossoms, are two-seeded red berries. American ginseng is found from Maine to Georgia and from Oklahoma to Minnesota. Unfortunately, it is now an endangered species in much of this area. Asians highly value the ginseng grown in Wisconsin. (*See* "Ginseng Among the Native Americans" below.)

The root, coarsely chopped, is the part used in herbal medicine. A good-quality root has first a sweet and then a bitter flavor as it is chewed. For most applications, wildcrafted American ginseng is more effective than field-grown ginseng.

Evidence of Benefit

American ginseng is a "cooler" alternative to Chinese (also known as red or Korean) ginseng (*Panax ginseng*) for persons who have high blood pressure or for treatment during summer months. It is used primarily for increased mental efficiency, stamina, and energy. Ginseng contains components called ginsenosides that stimulate the immune system and fight fatigue and stress. They do this by supporting the adrenal glands and the use of oxygen by exercising muscles.

American ginseng also boosts the immune system and reduces the risk of cancer. It also may promote appetite and is helpful for rheumatism, headaches, colds, coughs,

Ginseng Among the Native Americans

The plant now known as Korean or red ginseng was the most popular herb in China for thousands of years. By the beginning of the sixteenth century, supplies of wild ginseng were growing scarce, so the Chinese were forced to look for other sources. Amazingly, an almost identical plant grew in North America, and Native Americans had also put it to the same medicinal uses.

In 1709, Petrus Jartoux, a Jesuit missionary to China, received four pieces of American ginseng after accompanying a mapping expedition. He found himself so reinvigorated by the herb after his exhausting journey that he published his observations in the *Philosophical Transactions of the Royal Society of London*. Father Jartoux noted that he thought the plant could be found in the cold, damp forests of French Canada, similar to the areas of China where it grew wild. Another Jesuit missionary working among the Mohawk tribe in Quebec, Père Lafitau, read Father Jartoux's account in 1714. Lafitau promptly located the same plant, called *gar-ent-oguen*, or "man plant," by the Iroquois.

This plant turned out to have the same medicinal qualities as

Chinese ginseng. Not only did the Iroquois use the same plant, they used it for the same purposes as the Chinese. By 1748, the Jesuits were selling tons of American ginseng in China for the then-unimaginable price of five dollars a pound.

Ginseng was used throughout North America. The Cherokee of North Carolina called ginseng the "plant of life" and used the root for cramps, dysmenorrhea, and symptoms that we would now identify as premenstrual syndrome. The Potawatomi used ginseng to mask the unpleasant tastes of other medicines. The Alabamans took ginseng for stomach pains and nausea, and used it to pack wounds to stop bleeding. The Creek used ginseng for bronchial disease, cough, croup, and fever. The Menominee used ginseng as the Chinese did, to stimulate mental capacity and as a general tonic.

One of the most unusual uses of ginseng came from the Pawnee, who combined ginseng with two other herbs into a love potion. Possession of this medicine supposedly served to attract all persons to the holder, regardless of animosities. If the hair of a desired woman was added to the mixture, she was said to be incapable of resisting.

bronchitis, constipation, lung problems, cystitis, and symptoms of menopause. Native Americans use a tea made from the herb to treat nausea and vomiting. It has also been used as an ingredient in "love potions."

Benefits of American ginseng for specific health conditions include the following:

• *Attention deficit hyperactivity disorder (ADHD).* One preliminary study showed that American ginseng and ginkgo may help treat this condition, but more studies are needed.

• *Cancer.* American ginseng has been shown to inhibit tumor growth in cell culture studies. One study showed that the growth of colorectal cancer cells was slowed with ginseng.

• *Colds and flu.* Two studies showed that people who took a specific product (Cold-FX) made from American ginseng for four months and who got colds had them for a shorter duration and had fewer of them compared to placebo.

• *Diabetes.* Researchers found that ginseng lowered blood sugar levels in people with diabetes. The effect was seen on both fasting blood glucose and on postprandial (after eating) levels. American ginseng may be a viable alternative to conventional forms of treatment for type 2 diabetes, but more studies are needed.

• *High blood pressure.* American ginseng contains compounds saponins that regulate both the strength of the heartbeat and blood pressure. If the body is deficient in potassium, these saponins slow the *rate* at which heart muscle fibers contract. If there is excess potassium, the saponins increase the *strength* with which heart muscle fibers contract. Maintaining optimal potassium levels also eases high blood pressure. Laboratory tests show that American ginseng also lowers blood pressure by stimulating the conversion of the amino acid arginine to nitric oxide (NO), which causes the walls of blood vessels to relax. This action prevents the release of a protein known as endothelin, which can cause blood vessels to constrict during a heart attack.

• *Infertility.* Various Native American groups used American ginseng in the treatment of infertile women, although no clinical studies have confirmed the usefulness of the herb for this purpose. However, it is known that American ginseng shares compounds with Chinese ginseng that stimulate the pituitary gland to in turn stimulate growth of the uterine lining.

• *Stress.* Like other forms of ginseng, American ginseng traditionally has been applied to restoring health after long periods of illness or prolonged stress. Research suggests that American ginseng aids the body in adapting to different temperatures and stress when taken regularly. These effects are termed adaptogenic. Taken over a course of one to three months, American ginseng regulates the body's production of stress hormones. The next time the individual is exposed to stress, stress reactions are greatly reduced. Although the exact mechanisms of activity are not known, it is likely that American ginseng protects a portion of the brain known as the hippocampus from the effects of stress hormones. This prevents memory problems, a common complaint among people under stress. This mechanism would also explain the usefulness of American ginseng in preventing loss of memory and cognitive ability in people who suffer from bipolar disorder, depression, and a disorder of the adrenal glands known as Cushing's disease.

Considerations for Use

American ginseng is most commonly available in a dried form and added to water or water and alcohol to produce a tincture, although many vendors supply high-quality root for use as a tea. It is also sold in capsules, powders, and tablets. All forms of the herb should be avoided if your stomach does not produce enough acid to digest food properly.

Since American ginseng stimulates fertility, it also should be avoided by women in the first week after starting any new brand of oral contraceptive. This effect is especially pronounced in women who take birth control pills with antibiotics or barbiturates. American ginseng should be avoided by women who take prescription drug treatments for which pregnancy is contraindicated, especially isotretinoin (Accutane), which causes birth defects. Women who are breast-feeding or have a history of breast cancer should not use it. American ginseng should not be used by children except under a doctor's supervision.

Some people report experiencing insomnia when taking American ginseng, especially if they also consume foods or beverages containing caffeine. This adverse effect can be lessened by reducing the dose of American ginseng or by avoiding it later in the day. Other side effects include anxiety, diarrhea, headache, breast pain, and vaginal bleeding. People with high blood pressure should avoid this product, or be under the close supervision of their physician.

Other contraindications include taking ginseng with blood-thinning medications (anticoagulants such as warfarin), as it renders them less effective. Ginseng may also increase the effects of medications like antipsychotic medications used to treat psychiatric disorders such as schizophrenia and bipolar disorder. American ginseng may increase the stimulant effect and side effects of some medications taken for ADHD, including amphetamine and dextroamphetamine (Adderall) and methylphenidate (Ritalin).

There is a condition called ginseng abuse syndrome caused by long-term use of ginseng in an amount over 15 grams per day, which greatly exceeds the normal recommended daily dose. Symptoms of this condition include high blood pressure and nervousness. This should not be a big concern unless you are taking such high doses—in which case you should seek professional help.

Standardized extracts for American ginseng are not available. However, American ginseng can be safely taken in the amount of 1 to 2 grams from the fresh root (not extract) per day in capsule or tablet form or 1 to 2 teaspoons of a 1:5 tincture three times a day.

ANDIROBA

Latin name: *Carapa guianensis* (Meliaceae [mahogany] family)

General Description

Andiroba is a towering rain forest tree, reaching a height of up to 300 feet (90 meters), found in tropical Brazil, Colombia, and Guyana. It produces fragrant flowers and a brown, woody four-cornered nut three to four inches (eight to ten centimeters) across that resembles a chestnut and contains an oil-rich kernel. The oil of the nut, the tree bark, leaves, and seed oil are used medicinally.

Evidence of Benefit

Andiroba oil is an anti-inflammatory due to the presence of compounds known as limonoids. It promotes normal circulation to the skin and relieves pain and swelling. The Northwest Amazons use the bark and leaves for fever-reducing and worm-inhibiting tea, and externally as a wash for skin problems, ulcers, and insect bites, and as an insect repellent. Brazilians use the seed oil as an antiarthritic and anti-inflammatory, while the fruit oil is ingested for coughs.

Tests on cells have shown that the bark is antibacterial, the flowers are antitumor, and the heartwood is antifungal. Gelatin capsules containing the oil have been used for the treatment of some cancers in Brazil.

Benefits of andiroba for specific health conditions include the following:

• *Arthritis and rheumatism.* Hot andiroba oil is rubbed into the skin to relieve arthritis and rheumatism. Andiroba oil contains beneficial omega-3 fatty acids. These essential fatty acids are quickly absorbed through the skin. They offset the production of chemicals that cause inflammation leading to reduced swelling and decreased production of inflammatory chemicals, which reduces pain. However, this has not been shown in human studies.

• *Skin damage from cuts, age spots, and psoriasis.* Andiroba oil may accelerate healing of skin damage by providing myristic acid, one of the chemical building blocks of an enzyme that links together the proteins that form the skin's protective outer layer. One of the fatty acids found in andiroba oil, linolenic acid, was shown in a laboratory study to slow the growth of skin cells in psoriasis and age spots.

Considerations for Use

Andiroba is used as an oil applied to the skin. It is also used as a base for antiwrinkle creams such as Aveda and Oil of Olay. The fats in the oil transport healing alpha-hydroxy acids and other ingredients as they moisturize and protect the skin.

ANDROGRAPHIS

Latin name: *Andrographis paniculata* (Acanthaceae [acanthus] family)
Other common names: chiretta, chuan xin liang, fah tolai, kalmegh, king of bitters, kiryat

General Description

Andrographis is a branched, erect annual plant that grows in forests and wastelands in China, India, Pakistan, and Thailand. Its leaves and stems are harvested in late summer for medicinal use. It is cultivated extensively in China and Thailand, and in the East and West Indies.

Evidence of Benefit

Andrographis is an ancient medicinal herb with an extensive history in Asia. It has immune system effects, so it has been used to treat upper respiratory infections, fever, herpes, sore throat, and a variety of other chronic and infectious diseases. It has also been used for diabetes, gastrointestinal disorders such as diarrhea, indigestion, and weight loss. In Scandinavian countries, it is commonly used to prevent and treat the common cold. There have been some studies in cancer, AIDS, and a variety of bacterial and viral diseases.

Benefits of andrographis for specific health conditions include the following:

• *Atherosclerosis and heart attack.* Clinical studies in China have found that andrographis prevents the formation of blood clots and that use of the herb may prevent *restenosis,* or "reclogging," of arteries after angioplasty. The herb changes the way the linings of blood vessels respond to calcium, helping them to stay open.

• *Cancer.* It has been shown that if a cancer cell can be made to mature (or differentiate), it will not have the ability to grow out of control. Results of a study have demonstrated that andrographis has potent cell-differentiation-inducing activity on leukemia cells. Moreover, extracts from andrographis leaves are cytotoxic (cell-killing) against cancer cells. Japanese researchers have reported that andrographis stops stomach cancer cells from multiplying.

• *Cold, fever, and flu.* Andrographis prevents infections with rhinoviruses, the type of viruses most often responsible for the common cold. Taking 200 milligrams a day of an andrographis preparation (marketed as Kanjang) throughout the cold season was shown to reduce the risk of catching a cold by over 50 percent. Andrographis also relieves runny nose, headache, sore muscles, sore throat, swollen lymph nodes, and fatigue, although a dose of 1,200 milligrams or more a day (up to 6 grams) may be needed for this effect. Andrographis has also been used to reduce fever and pain, and for disorders of the intestinal tract.

• *Diarrhea and other intestinal disorders.* Extracts of andrographis have been shown to have significant effects against the diarrhea associated with *Escherichia coli* (*E. coli*) bacterial infections. In one study, chronic inflammation of the colon was treated with a combination of 60 grams of andrographis and 30 grams of rehmannia (*Rehmannia glutinosa*), with a cure rate of 72 percent. Twenty-six percent experienced symptomatic relief.

• *Hepatitis; liver and gallbladder problems.* The primary active ingredient in andrographis, andrographolide, increases bile flow and the levels of bile salts and bile acids. It was found to be more potent than silymarin (an active ingredient in milk thistle), which is used clinically as a hepatoprotective agent. Also, the andrographolides present in andrographis are potent stimulators of gallbladder function, therefore reducing the probability of gallstone formation.

Considerations for Use

Andrographis should be used in the form of tablets made from a standardized extract. The combination of andrographis with echinacea and zinc has been used to prevent and treat colds, while other standardized preparations of the herb are useful for other applications. Andrographis reduces fertility in both men and women, and should be avoided during pregnancy and nursing.

Formal toxicological studies have confirmed that andrographolide and other andrographis compounds have very low toxicity. In rare cases, some people who use andrographis experience dizziness and heart palpitations. Some may have an allergic reaction ranging from minor skin rash to more serious anaphylaxis. Other side effects include gastric discomfort, vomiting, and loss of appetite.

ANGELICA

Latin name: *Angelica archangelica* (Apiaceae [parsley] family)
Other common names: garden angelica, wild parsnip

General Description

Native to the Middle East, angelica grows one to two feet tall and grows in pots for indoor use. It bears bright green serrated leaves and greenish-yellow flowers. The medicinal parts include the seed, whole herb, and root.

Evidence of Benefit

Angelica is a remedy for colic, gas, sour stomach, and heartburn. It improves appetite and circulation, warms the body, and relieves spasms of the stomach and bowels and feeling of fullness. Angelica may also be a good herb to add to treatments for lung diseases, coughs, colds, and fevers.

Benefits of angelica for specific health conditions include the following:

• *Angina and high blood pressure.* Angelica contains fifteen compounds that act much like calcium channel blockers, a class of drug that is a standard treatment for angina and high blood pressure. However, no human studies currently support its use for heart disease.

Considerations for Use

Folklore indicates that angelica was used for coughs, bronchitis, symptoms related to menstruation, loss of appetite, stomach and intestinal cramps, and liver ailments. It has not been shown to be effective for kidney disease and neuralgic complaints. Angelica should not be taken by pregnant women. People with diabetes should avoid using angelica, and it may increase sensitivity to the sun. It also may increase the risk of bleeding, so those with this problem should not use it, or use it only under the supervision of a medical professional. There are no known hazards when the typical doses are used, which include 4.5 grams in herb, 1.5 to 3 grams in extract (1:1), and 1.5 grams in tincture (1:5).

ANISE

Latin name: *Pimpinella anisum* (Apiaceae [parsley] family)
Other common names: pimpinel seed, sweet cumin

General Description

Anise is a highly aromatic, low-growing plant that produces feathery leaves and small yellow and white flowers on stalks that reach a height of one to two feet (thirty to sixty centimeters). It is native to the Mediterranean coasts of west Asia and is cultivated in Egypt, Spain, and Turkey. The essential oil, distilled from the seeds, is used in medicine. The seeds also are used in the manufacture of flavored liqueurs, such as the French anisette and the Greek ouzo, and in the flavoring of food.

Evidence of Benefit

Anise is a secretagogue, an herb that stimulates the body to secrete fluids to clear out congestion and normalize digestion. It may reduce intestinal spasms and is an antibacterial and antiviral agent. It may even be an effective insect repellent. It has been approved by the German Commission E for the common cold, cough, bronchitis, fever, inflammation of the mouth and pharynx, dyspeptic complaints, and loss of appetite.

Benefits of anise for specific health conditions also may include the following:

• *Bad breath.* The seeds of this licorice-flavored herb have been used for thousands of years to freshen the breath. You can boil a few teaspoons of seeds in a cup of water for a few minutes, strain, and then drink or use as a mouthwash.

• *Colic.* Anise seeds are an ingredient in paregoric, an opium mixture that is used to settle the stomach and was once commonly given to colicky babies. Unlike paregoric, anise seed contains no opiates and has no potentially harmful sedative effect on the central nervous system. Anise also stops spasmodic flatulence and aids digestion.

• *Influenza, sinusitis, and other respiratory ailments.* The essential oil in anise seeds stimulates secretions from the linings of the throat and lungs. Anise seed teas are particularly appropriate in cases of unproductive cough. Used as a cough suppressant, anise is an ingredient in many cough medicines and lozenges. It also gives them a better flavor. The Greeks use teas made from anise and fennel for asthma and other respiratory ailments. They both contain creosol and alpha-pinene, which help to loosen bronchial secretions. As an expectorant, anise helps to loosen and get rid of phlegm in the respiratory tract.

Considerations for Use

When made as a homeopathic remedy, *Pimpinella anisum*, anise is used for shoulder pain and lumbago. Anise may be prepared as an essential oil and applied topically or taken as a tea. The essential oil is employed in aromatherapy, and the whole seeds are used in cooking. Aromatherapy with anise and foods prepared with anise (such as anise cookies) have the same but milder action as anise used as an herb.

You should avoid anise if you are allergic to anise and anethole, or if you have an allergic and/or inflammatory skin condition. Large doses are narcotic and slow down the circulation and may cause difficulty in breathing. Use this herb in moderation only. It should not be used during pregnancy. Anise has been shown to interfere with drugs that clot the blood and it may increase the risk of bleeding if used with them.

ARJUNA

Latin name: *Terminalia arjuna* (Combretaceae [myrobalan] family)

General Description

Native to the Indian subcontinent, arjuna is an evergreen tree with yellow flowers and conical leaves that reaches a towering 100 feet (30 meters). The bark and fruit have been used medicinally since the sixth century BCE.

Evidence of Benefit

Arjuna is among the most frequently prescribed herbs for cardiovascular health and specifically for congestive heart failure and low blood flow. It has been shown to lower blood pressure in animals. The bark of the arjuna tree contains calcium salts, magnesium salts, tannins, and glycosides. In ayurvedic medicine, it is considered to be a stimulant, tonic, and astringent and is used to treat hemorrhages, diarrhea, dysentery, edema, skin problems like ulcers, and fractures. It may be a sedative and may increase the activity of barbiturates. In addition, it has been found to have antibacterial and antimutagenic properties.

Benefits of arjuna for specific health conditions include the following:

• *Acne.* In one study, when combined with other herbs such as aloe, neem, and turmeric, subjects with acne experienced improvements in skin color and quality. The product was given in tablet form and as a cream; both forms needed to be taken for the remedy to be effective.

• *Angina, congestive heart failure, and heart attack.* The primary benefit of arjuna is improvement of cardiac muscle function and improved pumping activity of the heart. It is thought that the saponin glycosides are the reason for the beneficial effects of arjuna. The flavonoids and oligomeric proanthocyanidins (OPCs) it contains help to strengthen blood vessels and have antioxidant activity. Arjuna is used as a heart tonic to treat heart failure and edema, a condition in which fluid accumulates in the ankles and legs because the heart is not circulating blood properly. In a three-month study of angina patients who took arjuna, Indian physicians tracked a number of health indicators, including blood pressure, high-density lipoprotein (HDL, or "good") cholesterol, and frequency of angina attacks. Overall, there was a 50 percent reduction in the frequency of attacks, with lower systolic blood pressure and slightly increased HDL cholesterol levels. The more unstable the angina, however, the less arjuna helped the condition in the first three months of treatment. However, a double-blind study over a period of twenty-four months led to reduced symptoms, increased mobility, and patient reports of increased quality of life. Using arjuna regularly for one year can strengthen the heart to its best condition. In a review of seven articles on the use of arjuna and heart disease, all showed positive effects lowering blood lipids (total and low-density lipoprotein [LDL, or "bad"] cholesterol). Using 500 milligram capsules of arjuna every eight hours, over six weeks, patients with congestive heart failure had fewer signs of poor heart function and improvements in breathing (shortness of breath was diminished) and they were less fatigued. The left injection fraction increased, which is a key indicator of improved heart function. The study continued for twenty-eight months and patients continued to improve. No major safety issues appeared during this time.

Considerations for Use

Arjuna is commonly available in capsule form made from powder, and as a liquid. Ayurvedic formulas containing arjuna usually combine this herb with as many as thirty other cardioprotective herbs. Since arjuna has a powerful effect on heart muscle, it should be taken for angina or congestive heart failure only after consulting a physician. The dose varies by the patient according to ayurvedic medicine, but one study showed benefit at 3.88 grams of powder per day. No health hazards are known if taken in proper doses.

ARNICA

Latin name: *Arnica montana* (Asteraceae [composite] family)

General Description

Arnica is an aromatic perennial that grows to one foot (thirty centimeters) in height. It has downy, egg-shaped leaves and bright yellow daisylike flowers. Arnica grows in the mountains of Europe, Siberia, Canada, and the northern United States. The parts used in herbal medicine include the ethereal oil of the flowers, the dried flowers, the dried leaves (collected before the plant flowers), the fresh roots, and the dried rhizome and roots.

Evidence of Benefit

Arnica is an antibiotic, anti-inflammatory, and pain reliever. It has immune-stimulating, antiseptic, and wound-healing properties. Arnica extracts have been used in both herbal and homeopathic forms to help minimize the effects of tissue trauma and to assist in the healing process. It has been used in Europe for centuries to reduce bruising and swelling and to shorten recovery time after physical trauma. It also is used to treat inflammation of the mouth and throat, inflammation caused by insect bites, and superficial swelling (phlebitis). It has a long history of use among Native Americans as a major healing plant. It is primarily for external usage as a tincture or salve.

Arnica is also one of the most important herbs in homeopathic medicine. It is used in a 3x dilution for motion sickness and in a 10x dilution for seizure disorders, and in dilutions between 3x and 10x for a variety of other conditions. It is approved for use by the German Commission E for fever and colds, inflammation of the skin, bronchitis, inflammation of the mouth and pharynx, rheumatism, blunt injuries, and infection.

Benefits of arnica for specific health conditions include the following:

• *Carpal tunnel syndrome, fractures, and other injuries.* Arnica prevents bruising and swelling after traumatic skin injuries by preventing blood platelets, the cells involved in the clotting process, from gathering at the site of the injury. It stops pain and swelling in tired and painful muscles by reversing the effects of pain-causing prostaglandins. Arnica contains sesquiterpene lactones, helanalin, and dihydrohelanalin, compounds that alleviate pain, reduce inflammation, and fight bacteria. It is useful for joint and rheumatic pain.

Double-blind studies with marathon runners in the 1990 Oslo (Norway) Marathon found that applying arnica to the skin before an athletic event reduced pain and stiffness experienced after the event. Also, recent reports indicate that arnica may be effective in reducing postoperative swelling.

• *Diabetic eye disease (retinopathy).* Homeopathic arnica has been used to treat diabetic eye disease, which can cause severe vision loss or blindness. In one study, arnica produced significant improvement in retinal sensitivity and functional improvement in the retinal area. The patients in this study all had insulin-dependent diabetes and the retinopathy was related to it. There were no side effects from the arnica. In another study, patients experienced improvements in red critical retinal flicker fusion, a marker of vision.

• *Inflammation of the knee joint (gonarthrosis).* In one study, a homeopathic preparation of arnica and other compounds (such as *Sanguinaria canadensis*) was shown to be effective at reducing knee pain in patients with gonarthrosis. Patients received two injections a week and they saw some improvement after five weeks. Pain and joint stiffness improved in 90 percent of the subjects and no adverse side effects were observed. In another study, a homeopathic arnica preparation (30x dilution) was used to mitigate pain after knee surgery. In this randomized study the arnica group, compared to placebo, showed less postoperative swelling. However, the difference was only significant for patients who underwent a specific knee operation (cruciate ligament reconstruction), but not for arthroscopy or artificial knee joint implantation.

• *Muscle pain.* Arnica has been used to treat muscle pain or myalgia, which can be a sign of serious disease. In one study, a combination of arnica and Rhus tox in a 30x dilution reduced delayed onset muscle soreness. However, those patients who received the placebo experienced similar benefits. In another study, a gel preparation of arnica flowers (20 percent tincture) applied to limbs reduced muscle pain compared to a placebo. Moreover, there was better blood flow, less swelling, and reduced feeling of heaviness in the legs.

• *Pain management.* Arnica has been used in various forms for the management of pain. In one study, homeopathic arnica significantly decreased pain score (a validated composite of how painful someone feels) after a tonsillectomy. There were no differences in the use of analgesics or antibiotics, however. In another study, arnica was used as a topical gel, but it did not lessen the pain of osteoarthritis of the hands compared to the placebo gel. An arnica homeopathy preparation also did not reduce postoperative pain or antibiotic use in women following hysterectomy. Similarly, there was no benefit of arnica at reducing pain following oral surgery.

Misunderstood Artemisia

Several herb handbooks warn that artemisia may have intoxicating effects similar to those of marijuana. Whether you consider this to be desirable or undesirable, it is simply not true.

This misunderstanding stems from the use of a form of artemisia known as absinthe, a fashionable drink in the nineteenth century. The herb became associated with the death of the American writer Edgar Allan Poe and the suicide of the painter Vincent Van Gogh. It was immortalized in a painting by Edgar Degas, which shows a haunting portrait of two absinthe drinkers, hollow-eyed and oblivious to all

but the intoxicating beverage. Of course, the absinthe drinkers in the picture were merely models.

Thujone, the intoxicating chemical in artemisia, and tetrahydro-cannabinol (THC), the active ingredient of marijuana, have similar molecules, and both attach to the same receptor sites in the brain. However, the thujone content of alcoholic beverages containing artemisia is less than one-twentieth of the amount needed for intoxication. Any "high" from artemisia comes from the alcohol in which it is dissolved.

Considerations for Use

Arnica is used in cream form. It should not be applied to mucous membranes, eyes, broken skin, or to an open wound, and it should *never* be taken internally except as a homeopathic remedy, where the amount ingested is very small. It is contraindicated in people with a known sensitivity to members of the daisy family such as chamomile, marigold, and yarrow. Eating large quantities of the flower or roots can be poisonous. It should not be used for more than two weeks at a time, and if a rash develops, its use should be discontinued. Arnica contains compounds that act in the same manner as oxytocin (Pitocin), a drug used to induce labor. For this reason, pregnant women should not use arnica in any form. Patients who are prone to excessive bleeding should avoid arnica.

ARTEMISIA

Latin name: *Artemisia capillaris* (Asteraceae [composite] family)
Other common names: capillaris, Chinese wormwood, yen chen hao

General Description

Artemisia, known in literature as wormwood, is a bushy perennial that grows from two to four feet (60 to 120 centimeters) high. It bears tiny yellow-green flowers from July to October. It is native to Japan, Taiwan, and northern China.

Herbalists use broken pieces taken from the top of the softly aromatic plant. Unfortunately, a misunderstanding about wormwood's chemical properties has led some to condemn artemisia as a dangerous drug. (*See* "Misunderstood Artemisia," above.)

Evidence of Benefit

Artemisia has several useful antimicrobial properties. It is also a cholagogue, a substance that stimulates the production of bile in laboratory studies. Benefits of artemisia for specific health conditions include the following:

• *Bladder and parasitic infections.* Artemisia may help eliminate parasites. It has been used to help treat urinary tract infections (UTIs) caused by *Klebsiella* bacteria, but not as

the only treatment. Laboratory studies have shown that artemisine (a compound found in artemesia) may be effective against the organisms that cause river blindness.

• *Constipation and diarrhea.* Artemisia may help with intestinal disturbances by soothing inflamed intestinal tissues and aiding digestion.

• *Liver disorders.* Artemisia in laboratory studies increases the secretion of bile into the gastrointestinal tract, which possibly can support liver function. Used with gardenia (*Gardenia jasminoidis*), it has been shown to increase the rate of liver cell regeneration.

Considerations for Use

Artemisia is used in teas or tinctures. The practitioners of traditional Chinese medicine (TCM) who supply artemisia usually refer to this herb and the products made from it as yen chen hao.

ASAFOETIDA

Latin name: *Ferula asafoetida* (Apiaceae [parsley] family)
Other common names: devil's dung, food of the gods, hing, narthex

General Description

Asafoetida is a perennial plant native to Afghanistan, Iran, and Pakistan. It grows six feet (two meters) tall from a fleshy taproot, and bears composite leaves and umbels of white flowers at its head. Asafoetida produces a gum gathered in summer from the roots of plants at least four years old (if a plant is not a minimum of four years old, its gum is considered worthless). The oldest plants are the most productive. The stems are cut off, and successive slices are made through the roots. The gum wells up and is collected after it has hardened.

Despite its common name devil's dung, asafoetida was the favorite flavoring of ancient Rome. With a pungent aroma that is more persistent than garlic, asafoetida is still used as an ingredient in Worcestershire sauce.

Evidence of Benefit

According to ayurvedic medicine, asafoetida is a valuable spice and remedy for nervous disorders, colic, and bowel spasms. In cell cultures, it has been shown to be a mild anticancer agent and may kill *Salmonella typhimurium*. Asafoetida has been used in Chinese medicine to treat intestinal parasites. In ayurvedic medicine, asafoetida has been used for asthma, whooping cough, flatulence, constipation, disease of the liver and spleen, and epilepsy. Homeopathic asafoetida remedies are used for low acid levels in the stomach, and to control stomach pressure, flatulence, and loose stools. It has not been shown to be of benefit for chronic gastritis, dyspepsia, and irritable colon.

Benefits of asafoetida for specific health conditions include the following:

• *Colic.* Asafoetida is a local stimulant of mucous membranes, especially in the alimentary tract. As a result, it is useful in reducing flatulence and easing colic, and as a laxative medicine.

• *Insect bites.* Due to its pungent smell, asafoetida repels insects from the skin and body.

• *Irritable bowel syndrome (IBS).* Asafoetida oil relieves gas buildup and irritation in IBS. It also calms muscle spasms and digestive disturbances associated with anxiety.

• *Nervous disorders.* Asafoetida was one of the most commonly prescribed herbs throughout the nineteenth century for the treatment of hysteria and for many symptoms associated with mood swings and depression.

Considerations for Use

Asafoetida is used as a powder or tincture. As a tincture, 20 drops is a single dose. The pale yellow or orange-yellow essential oil, occasionally used in aromatherapy in place of garlic, is not a substitute.

The uncooked herb can cause nausea and vomiting. Using asafoetida over long periods may cause lip swelling, throat irritation, gas, diarrhea, and burning urination. It can cause convulsions in susceptible individuals. Genital swelling has been observed following external administration on the abdomen. This herb should be *avoided* during pregnancy.

ASHWAGANDHA

Latin name: *Withania somnifera* (Solanaceae [nightshade] family)
Other common names: Indian ginseng, winter cherry, withania

General Description

Ashwagandha is a plant in the same family as the tomato. It grows as a stout shrub that reaches a height of 5 feet (1.5 meters). Like the tomato, ashwagandha bears yellow flowers and red fruit, though the fruit is berrylike in size and shape. Ashwagandha grows prolifically in India, Pakistan, and Sri Lanka. All parts of the plant are used in herbal medicine.

Ashwagandha is a Hindi name meaning "horse's smell." The term refers not only to the smell of a horse, but also to a horse's strength. Some herbalists refer to ashwagandha as Indian ginseng, since it is used in ayurvedic medicine in the same way that ginseng is used in traditional Chinese medicine (TCM).

Evidence of Benefit

Ashwagandha has been used for more than 2,500 years as a "vitalizer." Today, we would place it in the category of adaptogens. It is rejuvenating, balancing, strengthening, and calming to the nervous system. Ashwagandha is useful for relieving fatigue, nervous exhaustion, and memory loss. This herb also has a reputation as an aphrodisiac and is believed to help prevent sterility in males and sexual ailments. A mild sedative, ashwagandha reduces mental chatter and promotes calm sleep. It also promotes tissue regeneration and slows the aging process.

It is excellent for use in bodybuilding and for any type of physical sport, as it gives an instant charge of long-lasting energy without the use of stimulants. Ashwagandha contains iron and may promote growth in children and improve hemoglobin levels. In addition, ashwagandha has shown promise in treating hypothyroidism (low levels of thyroid hormone in the blood).

Benefits of ashwagandha for specific health conditions include the following:

• *Alzheimer's disease and memory problems.* Ashwagandha helps correct memory loss by modifying the way in which the brain uses acetylcholine, a chemical that transmits messages from nerve cell to nerve cell. If oxygen levels are low, the brain acquires acetylcholine by destroying its own cells. The cell remnants form neurofibrillary tangles, blocking the transmission of nerve signals and resulting in Alzheimer's-like symptoms. Ashwagandha decreases the likelihood that the brain will cannibalize its own cells. This action reduces cognitive deficit and memory loss in diseases such as Alzheimer's disease and dementia.

• *Arthritis and carpal tunnel syndrome.* Animal studies have found that naturally occurring steroids in ashwagandha are more potent than treatment with the synthetic steroid hydrocortisone for controlling inflammation. These natural steroidal compounds also reduce the pain of arthritis as effectively as aspirin and phenylbutazone when given in the same amount, but without the immune-depressing side effects those drugs cause. Patients who have trouble with balance (called cerebral ataxias) gained better balance with ashwagandha. In a clinical study of patients with osteoarthritis, ashwagandha and other herbs reduced pain and disability significantly.

• *Autoimmune disorders.* Ashwagandha increases red and white blood cell counts after treatment with azathioprine (Imuran, Azasan), cyclophosphamide (Cytoxan, Neosar), or prednisone for autoimmune diseases such as lupus.

• *Cancer.* Ashwagandha extracts increase platelet counts, red blood cell counts, and white blood cell counts during cancer chemotherapy treatment with cyclophosphamide (Cytoxan, Neosar). Animal studies in India also have found that ashwagandha sensitizes cancer cells to radiation treatment, making treatments approximately 50 percent more effective. Studies have shown that ashwagandha is helpful in putting cancer tumors of the breast, central nervous system, colon, and lung into regression without killing healthy tissues. The herb may also help prevent chemotherapy-induced neutropenia (low white blood cell count). However, the effectiveness of ashwagandha in the treatment of patients with cancer is not yet determined.

• *Diabetes.* Improvements in high blood sugar levels and insulin sensitivity (how well insulin works) have been detected in the animal studies of type 2 diabetes.

• *Sex drive, diminished.* Ashwagandha is a sexual "grounding" herb that reduces the frequency of premature ejaculation and increases sexual stamina. Ashwagandha's active principles, alkaloids and with anoloids, have longevity-enhancing and sexually stimulating properties.

• *Stress.* Ayurvedic medicine has used ashwagandha as a general tonic for centuries to stimulate long-term endurance. Ashwagandha contains steroidlike compounds that may increase resistance to stress.

Considerations for Use

Ashwagandha is available in capsule form. The product you choose should be standardized for with anolides.

When used to increase sex drive, ashwagandha should not be taken in instances of acute sexual anxiety, as its effects take hold only after about one week of daily use. For the conditions listed above, be sure *not* to use a product called ashwagandha oil. That is a combination of ashwagandha with almond oil and rose water designed to be used as a facial toner. Do not eat ashwagandha berries, as they can cause severe gastrointestinal pain. Taking ashwagandha with tranquilizers may result in drowsiness and loss of coordination. You should avoid this herb if you are taking prescription drugs for anxiety, insomnia, or a seizure disorder. Human toxicity studies for ashwagandha are limited.

ASTRAGALUS

Latin name: *Astragalus membranaceus* (Fabaceae [legume] family)
Other common names: locoweed, milk vetch root

General Description

Astragalus is a bushy member of the legume family with hairy stems that grow to a height of sixteen inches (forty centimeters). Herbal medicine uses long, thin, diagonal sections of astragalus root that show the exterior at each end. The root should be long, thick, and firm, and have a sweet taste.

Evidence of Benefit

Astragalus has an unusual ability to stimulate certain immune functions while depressing others. It is an overall body tonic that is used to strengthen digestion, increase metabolic activity, and stimulate the immune system. It is highly beneficial for anyone who experiences fatigue, low vitality, and frequently recurring infections. It also may normalize the function of the heart and kidneys. It is a potent antioxidant and has been shown to protect lipids from oxidizing in rat heart mitochondria. It also has a diuretic effect. Astragalus is most effective when it is used long term, on a daily basis.

Benefits of astragalus for specific health conditions include the following:

• *Angina, atherosclerosis, congestive heart failure, and heart attack.* Astragalus increases how much blood the heart can pump (which is limited in heart disease) in patients with chest pain. It strengthens the left side of the heart, the part that is usually sluggish in heart disease, and slows heart rate in those whose hearts are beating too fast. In one study, astragalus helped patients who had just had a heart attack. Within thirty-six hours of the attack, the herb improved left-sided ventricular function. There also was reduced lipid peroxidation and increased superoxide dismutase activity on red blood cells, suggesting that astragalus worked as an antioxidant. Astragalus balances the levels of salt and water in the body so that the heart and kidneys function better. In one study, participants with congestive heart failure who had trouble mobilizing fluid benefited from taking astragalus. In another study, combining astragalus with *Angelica sinensis* significantly lowered total cholesterol and low-density lipoprotein (LDL, or "bad") cholesterol, as well as serum triglycerides in rats. In patients with ischemic heart disease (a narrowing of blood vessels), astragalus improved chest pain. When taken with the herbs coptis and scutellaria, astragalus makes the blood more fluid, which helps prevent coronary arteries from becoming clogged by clots. (*See* COPTIS and SCUTELLARIA.) In this regard, it may be used like aspirin, but if you are taking aspirin, ask your physician before stopping it and switching to astragalus. Clinical testing also has shown that astragalus increases the effectiveness of lidocaine, the drug used in emergency rooms to treat the weak, erratic heartbeat of ventricular fibrillation, a common and life-threatening complication of heart attack. The herb also protects heart tissues from damage after blood returns to them after a heart attack or bypass surgery.

Chinese researchers have had good preliminary results using astragalus compounds called astragalosides in treating congestive heart failure. Patients treated by injection regain an average of approximately 20 percent of their heart function in two weeks of treatment. Whether similar benefits can be obtained from orally administered astragalus products is not yet known.

Other Chinese doctors have found that astragalus offers more effective relief than the drug nifedipine (Procardia) for angina pain. More than 80 percent of angina patients improved on astragalus treatment without the dizziness, giddiness, heartburn, or headache that nifedipine can cause.

• *Cancer.* Chinese studies have found that astragalus increases the activity of natural killer (NK) cells and lymphokine-activated killer (LAK) cells, an immune-system component. Synthetic IL-2, used for colorectal cancer, lymphoma, melanoma, and kidney cancer, is extremely toxic when concentrated, but the simultaneous use of IL-2 and astragalus increases the drug's effectiveness. This allows the use of a lower, less toxic dosage of IL-2. In addition, astragalus stops the spread of cancers known to respond to gene p53, a tumor-suppressing gene that acts as a molecular "patrolman" to keep defective cells from multiplying. Astragalus is commonly used in cancer patients to enhance the effectiveness and reduce side effects of chemotherapy.

Chinese studies of the treatment of small cell lung cancer with standard chemotherapy drugs—carmustine (Gliadel, BiCNU), cyclophosphamide (Cytoxan, Neosar), methotrexate (Rheumatrex, Trexall), and vincristine (Oncovin, Vincasar)—combined with astragalus and ginseng produced dramatic increases in longevity. In general, patients had a reduced risk of death after twelve and twenty-four months and shrunken tumor size. For small cell lung cancer patients treated with conventional medicine and astragalus, the response rate has been reported to be as high as 98 percent. In one study, people with lung cancer survived as long as seventeen years on the combination therapy. (*See* GINSENG.)

A mixture of astragalus and ligustrum prevents red-cell depletion during mitomycin (Mutamycin) cancer therapy. Astragalus alone, however, is effective in preventing depletion of white blood cells during chemotherapy. A clinical study involving 115 patients receiving various forms of chemotherapy found that 83 percent had higher white blood cell counts when given astragalus.

A meta-analysis of four studies showed that astragalus and other herbs counteracted the side effects of chemotherapy in 374 patients with colon cancer. The herb appeared to stimulate the immune system.

• *Cochlear damage.* In one study, a combination of astragalus and *Pyrola rotundifolia* protected against cochlear damage caused by gentamicin, a potent antibiotic.

• *Common cold.* Chinese studies have shown that using astragalus during cold season reduces the number of colds caught and shortens the duration of those that are caught. If you tend to get colds and flu often, astragalus can help you build up a natural resistance. It increases the body's production of interferon, which helps to protect against viruses invading the cells. Astragalus also helps the macrophages, immune cells that kill off viruses, to become faster and more efficient.

• *Diabetes.* The traditional use of astragalus as a diabetes treatment has been confirmed by modern research. One study included people with diabetes who had various complications of the disorder, including an eye disease called diabetic retinopathy. Participants in this study were given 2 to 3 grams (approximately a tablespoon) of a mixture of equal parts of astragalus and another herb, rehmannia, three times a day for three months. Improvements in blood flow through the eye were noted in 82 percent of participants. Fasting blood sugar was kept below 150 milligrams per deciliter (mg/dL) for 77 percent of participants, without the use of other medications.

• *Infertility.* In ancient Chinese medicine, astragalus seed was used to treat infertile men. Tests have shown that the herb does increase sperm motility, or the vigorous activity of sperm.

• *Liver and gastrointestinal tract ailments:* The herb strengthens the movement and muscle tone of the intestine to increase movements of food through the GI tract. In one study, liver cells were protected by astragalus after being exposed to carbon tetrachloride. Animals excreted less SGPT (a marker of liver disease) with an ethanol root extract of astragalus and the liver cells appeared to be protected.

Considerations for Use

Astragalus is used in capsules, fluid extracts, teas, and tinctures. Even in large doses, it is nontoxic. Laboratory animals fed astragalus have been able to eat up to 10 percent of their body weight in astragalus without ill effects. Daily doses in humans are 2 to 6 grams of the dried root per day and as a fluid extract of 4 to 12 milliliters. A powdered root capsule (250 to 500 milligrams) can be taken as two capsules, three times a day.

Chinese tradition teaches that astragalus should not be used in people with a known autoimmune disorder and during an acute infection, or for colds and flu, especially if there is fever or a skin infection. The main reason is that deep immune tonics, such as astragalus, are believed to strengthen the chi (energy) of the virus, and a more superficial immune stimulator is needed.

Astragalus helps the body compensate for immune damage induced by many kinds of prescription medications. In addition to the conditions listed in Part Two, astragalus is useful in preventing side effects from Cibalith-S, Eskalith, Lithobid, Lithonate, and Lithotabs, all forms of lithium used in the treatment of bipolar mood disorder. Astragalus is useful for immune damage caused by lithium without inducing release of immune cells known as macrophages, which can damage nerve tissue.

Astragalus is incompatible with prescription medications often given after a heart attack. As much as 2 percent of astragalus root is made up of coumarins, which are chemically similar to the prescription blood-thinning drug warfarin (Coumadin). People who take warfarin should avoid astragalus because of the potential for bleeding. A class of high blood pressure medications known as beta-blockers may be less effective when taken with astragalus. Persons taking beta-blockers, which include atenolol (Tenormin), metoprolol (Lopressor), propranolol (Inderal), and many other medications, should also avoid this herb. Astragalus should be used with caution by anyone who is on immunosuppressive therapy, such as people with autoimmune diseases and those who have received organ transplants. It should be discontinued before surgery, as it may increase the risk of bleeding. Astragalus is rich in selenium and if taken in large amounts could be toxic and result in neurological damage and lead to paralysis.

AVENA

Latin name: *Avena sativa* (Poaceae [haygrass] family)
Other common names: oat extract, wild oats

General Description

Avena is the green tops of the cereal plant oats, harvested just before the plant is in full flower. Oats originated in France, England, Poland, Germany, and Russia. Its use as a medicine preceded its use as a food.

Avena sativa is Latin for "wild oats." The sexual stimulation resulting from the consumption of this herb is said to be the source of the phrase "sowing one's wild oats." Stallions fed wild oats are said to become libidinous, and some studies suggest that "wild oats" have a similar effect on the human male.

Evidence of Benefit

In folk medicine, as well as with current herbalists, avena is used to treat nervous exhaustion, insomnia, and weakness of the nerves. It is an anti-inflammatory and sedative. This herb contains small amounts of calcium, phosphorus, and the B-complex vitamins, as well as other vitamins, minerals, and micronutrients.

Benefits of avena for specific health conditions include the following:

• *Attention deficit disorder (ADD).* Herbalists report that oat top extract reduces symptoms of withdrawal from methylphenidate (Ritalin), and relieves sadness and mild depression in adults with ADD. Do not give avena to your child if he or she has ADD without consulting your child's physician. Avena has pharmacological actions similar to those of opium, which may account for its calming effects.

• *Eczema.* Avena or oatmeal baths may soothe inflamed skin.

• *Nervousness and menopause.* Avena is nerve food. It nourishes the nervous and hormonal systems, and can ease hot flashes and symptoms of premenstrual syndrome (PMS). It should be taken daily for menopausal symptoms, and for two weeks per month for premenopausal problems.

• *Sex drive, diminished.* Avena has been shown to heighten thoughts and pleasure associated with sex by freeing up testosterone, the sex hormone most closely tied to libido, that gets bound to various compounds in the body. As we age, the binding of testosterone increases, and bound testosterone is not as effective as free testosterone. One double-blind study showed that both males and females experienced a dramatic increase in sexual desire, performance, sensation, and sexual activity after taking avena. There is evidence in laboratory studies, however, that avena may act on the hypothalamus and stimulate the release of luteinizing hormone (LH). This action may correct the normal production of testosterone in men, but human studies showing this action are lacking.

Considerations for Use

Avena is used as a bath for eczema and as a tincture, usually in combination with other herbs, for treatment of diminished sex drive.

BARBERRY

Latin name: *Berberis* species, most commonly *Berberis vulgaris* (Berberidaceae [barberry] family)
Other names: berberry, paundice berry, mountain grape, Oregon grape, pipperidge, sow berry

General Description

Barberry is a thorny, deciduous shrub that grows to a height of ten feet (three meters). Protected by thorny stems and tough leaves, it bears small yellow flowers in spring followed by purple berries in autumn. Native to Europe, northern Africa, and central Asia, barberry has been naturalized in North America. The bark of both the stem and root and also the berries are used to make herbal medicines.

Evidence of Benefit

Barberry contains vitamin C, which increases immune function and may prevent scurvy. It has a mild diuretic effect. Homeopathic preparations are used for kidney stones, gout, rheumatism, liver and gallbladder disorders, and dry skin diseases such as psoriasis. Unproven uses include opium withdrawal, jaundice, tuberculosis, piles, renal disease, malaria, and leishmaniasis.

Benefits of barberry for specific health conditions include the following:

• *Cuts, scrapes, and abrasions; infections of the bladder, eyes, nails, reproductive tract, sinuses, skin, throat; and parasitic infection.* In cell studies, berberine (a compound in barberry) kills a vast variety of germs—among them the parasites *Leishmania* and *Plasmodium* (the organism that causes malaria); *Pseudomonas, Salmonella, Shigella, Staphylococcus, Streptococcus,* and *Vibrio* bacteria; and various kinds of fungi—and is very active against a number of others. Some laboratory tests have found that berberine is a more potent antibiotic than the sulfa drugs against some kinds of infections. Berberine also is effective against some bacteria that have become antibiotic-resistant. But human data are unavailable to support its use in such cases.

• *Diarrhea.* One study found that individuals suffering from cholera-induced diarrhea experienced significant relief from acute diarrhea after twenty-four hours with a dosage of 100 milligrams of barberry four times a day.

• *Gallstones, kidney stones, and liver problems.* The stem and root bark of barberry have been used to improve liver function and to treat gallstones. It has been purported to prevent kidney stones in some people, but it is not indicated as a treatment.

• *Gastritis and peptic ulcers.* Berberine kills *Helicobacter pylori,* a bacterium implicated in both ulcers and chronic gastritis. Animal studies have shown that the compounds in barberry can reduce muscle spasms, which might further explain their usefulness in gastrointestinal disorders. Alcohol extracts of barberry may help with heartburn and stomach cramps.

• *Immunity.* Extracts of barberry have been used to fight infections, feverish colds, and urinary tract infections (UTIs), although to date these uses are largely unproven.

Considerations for Use

Barberry is available in capsules, ointments, tablets, and tinctures. The tincture can be used to make compresses. It can be made into a tea as well. The daily dosage of the infusion of tea is 2 grams in 250 milliliters of water, to be sipped. A tincture dose is 20 to 40 drops daily. Homeopathy doses are 5 drops, 1 tablet, or 10 globules every thirty to sixty minutes for an acute illness or one to three times daily for a chronic illness.

Side effects are rare when barberry is used properly. However, dosages of over 4 grams will bring about light stupor, nosebleeds, vomiting, diarrhea, and kidney irritation. Treatment may be required to treat this poisonous state.

Another of the chemical constituents of barberry, palmitine hydroxide, is believed to interfere with the maturation of sperm cells in the testes. Studies indicate that this effect may contribute to sterility in men. Men who are seeking to become fathers should avoid barberry.

Berberine alone has been reported to interfere with normal bilirubin metabolism in infants, raising a concern that it may worsen jaundice. Also, there are reports that it can stimulate the uterine muscles. For these reasons, berberine-containing plants, including barberry and goldenseal, should not be used by pregnant women or nursing mothers. Also, strong extracts may cause stomach upset, so they should be used for no more than two weeks at a time.

BILBERRY

Latin name: *Vaccinium myrtillus* (Ericaceae [blueberry] family)
Other common names: blueberry, huckleberry, trackleberry, whortleberry, wineberry burts

General Description

Bilberry refers to the leaf of the blueberry bush, a shrub that grows to about one foot (thirty centimeters) in height and that produces sweet blue berries. It is found in North America and Europe on damp, acidic soils.

In Elizabethan times, English herbalists referred to bilberries as *wortleberries* and prescribed them for diarrhea and stomach complaints. American herbalists later combined "whortleberries" with gin to make a diuretic.

Evidence of Benefit

Bilberry is said to possess antioxidant and antiseptic properties. It has several pharmacological actions, such as wound healing, anti-ulcer, anti-artery clogging, and vasoprotective (keeps blood flowing). Bilberry extract strengthens capillaries, which not only protects the eye from the hemorrhaging associated with diabetic retinopathy, but also aids in treating other vascular disorders, such as varicose veins. Extracts of the leaves in animals have been shown to kill *Staphylococcus aureus* and *Escherichia coli* (*E. coli*). It is approved by the German Commission E for treatment of diarrhea (taken internally) and inflammation of the mouth and pharynx (used topically).

Benefits of bilberry for specific health conditions include the following:

• *Cataracts.* In one study, bilberry prevented the development of further lens opacity in the eyes of 97 percent of the patients with mild senile cortical cataracts. A bilberry extract of 180 milligrams and 100 milligrams of vitamin E was given twice a day for eight months. After four months, improvements were observed in the treatment group but not the placebo group.

• *Diabetes.* Bilberry's component (anthocyanosides) may help patients with diabetic retinopathy. This is a progressive worsening of vision caused by elevated blood glucose levels. In one study, using 160 milligrams of bilberry anthocyanosides extract (Myrtocyan) twice a day for one month improved the eyes in 77 to 90 percent of the participants. Using a different preparation of the bilberry (Tegens) at the same concentration and dose for one year, improvements were seen in 50 percent of the patients compared to 20 percent in the placebo group. Patients with diabetic retinopathy have an increase in polymeric collagen synthesis in the eye, which leads to eye damage. Using 600 milligrams of bilberry anthocyanosides per day for two months decreased the synthesis of this collagen. Several human studies have shown that bilberry extracts have improved symptoms in patients with retinopathy related to diabetes. Patients experienced changes in their eye tests that revealed the retinas were becoming normal. Retinal hemorrhage decreased or disappeared, less collagen was made, which is seen in retinopathy, and the retinas looked healthier when the doctor used an ophthalmoscope. Patients took an extract of about 160 milligrams of bilberry anthocyanosides twice a day in most studies.

• *Dysmenorrhea (painful menstruation).* Bilberry may help women with painful periods. In one study, taking anthocyanins from bilberry (320 milligrams per day) resulted in fewer women with a history of chronic primary dysmenorrhea having nausea, vomiting, and breast tenderness.

• *Heart disease.* Bilberry extracts serve as antioxidants to reduce the oxidation of the low-density lipoprotein (LDL, or "bad") cholesterol, which reduces the risk of heart disease. It also increases cAMP, which in turn reduces thromboxane A_2 in the platelets, which clot the blood. These actions improve blood flow and reduce the risk of cardiovascular disease. In one study, using 480 milligrams of bilberry anthocyanin along with vitamin C (3 grams daily) resulted in decreased platelet aggregation (stickiness) after thirty to sixty days.

• *Night vision problems.* In addition to stimulating circulation in the eye, bilberry stimulates the regeneration of rhodopsin, the purple pigment that is used by the rods in the eye for night vision. This effect has been confirmed in some but not all clinical observations and controlled tests. The use of 240 milligrams of bilberry anthocyanoside improved night vision the best, two hours after ingestion. The response of the pupil to light was demonstrated by greater contraction, faster movement, and greater acceleration in less time. Improvement to macular recovery as well as night vision was found in subjects after using 60 milligrams of anthocyanosides for one week. Use of bilberry extracts seemed to improve retinal sensitivity even in daylight so that objects were less fuzzy and clearer, and twilight vision also was improved. The participants took 150 milligrams a day of dry hypo alcohol bilberry extract.

• *Peptic ulcer.* In animal studies, cyanidins from bilberry counteract the formation of peptic ulcers caused by alcohol, allergy, nonsteroidal anti-inflammatory agents (NSAIDs), and stress. The bilberry is able to reduce prostaglandin E_2 without affecting stomach acid. This was accomplished by taking 600 milligrams of anthocyanin pigment from bilberry, twice daily for ten days. These changes are important to reduce the risk of stomach ulcers and still allow food to be digested.

• *Venous insufficiency.* In one study, both pregnant women and patients with varicose veins experienced improved blood flow, reduced bruising, less leg swelling and pain, and less of a heavy feeling in their legs. Participants in the study used 240 to 320 milligrams a day of bilberry anthocyanosides.

Considerations for Use

Bilberry is available in tablets and capsules made from bilberry extract and as a dried herb bagged for making teas. Some products combine bilberry with lutein, another supplement useful in maintaining eye health. The active ingredients in bilberry extracts break down rapidly in the body. For this reason, frequent, small doses are preferable to larger, less frequent doses. Bilberry herbal extract in capsules or tablets standardized to provide 36 percent anthocyanosides can be taken in the amount of 60 to 160 milligrams three times per day.

Many of the earliest clinical studies of bilberry (conducted in the 1950s and 1960s) noted that its effects were greater when patients also took beta-carotene. For best results, you should eat dark-green, yellow, and orange vegetables daily while taking bilberry.

You should not use extremely high doses of bilberry teas or take teas of this herb for more than one month at a time. If blood appears in the urine, discontinue use.

Bilberry should not be taken during pregnancy or lactation. If you are taking anticoagulants such as warfarin (Coumadin), or if you have bleeding disorders, check with your doctor before taking bilberry, as the anticoagulant dose may need adjusting.

BIRCH

Latin name: *Betula* species (Betulaceae [birch] family)
Other common names: black birch (American species), silver birch (European species), sweet birch (*Betula lenta*), white birch

General Description

The birch is a slender deciduous tree that grows to a height of 100 feet (30 meters). The leaves are dark green on their upper sides and pale green on their lower sides. While birch bark, flowers, leaves, and sap are all used in herbal medicines, birch leaf is the part used most often. Birch leaf is slightly bitter and faintly aromatic.

Evidence of Benefit

Birch leaf is antibacterial, anti-inflammatory, and antispasmodic. It also helps diseases of the kidney. In Europe, birch is used to relieve the pain and swelling of arthritis and to heal boils and sores. Recent tests in Finland have found that birch leaf extracts kill the bacterium *Staphylococcus aureus*. One component of birch bark is called betulin, which targets a factor that causes genes to tell the body to make cholesterol, fatty acids, and triglycerides. In one study, mice were fed a high-fat diet that mimicked a typical Western diet. The addition of an extract from birch leaf lowered blood lipids and reduced body fat and the animals' insulin was more responsive to glucose. More work is needed to see if these favorable changes occur in humans.

Traditional healers have long considered the leaves of the European white and silver birch effective in remedying skin rashes, hair loss, and rheumatic complaints.

Benefits of birch leaf for specific health conditions include the following:

- *Arthritis, rheumatism, and muscular pain.* Sweet birch is thought to be an analgesic and good for all kinds of muscular pain. For rheumatism and arthritis, it is often used as an adjunct with other therapies.

- *Skin ailments.* Birch tar, used externally, may reduce parasitic infestation on the skin, and help with dry skin (eczema) and psoriasis. It was traditionally used for scabies.

Considerations for Use

It is preferable to use birch leaf as a tea for all conditions except for bladder and kidney infections. The tea can also be used as a douche. (*See* DOUCHES in Part Three.) Women with impaired heart or kidney function can experience adverse side effects from this, however, and should avoid birch leaf douches. Birch tar may cause skin irritations, so it should not be used on sensitive areas of the body. Birch leaves should not be used for swelling or edema where there is reduced heart or kidney function.

BITTER MELON

Latin name: *Momordica charantia* (Cucurbitaceae [gourd] family)
Other common names: balsam pear, bitter cucumber, bitter gourd, cerasee, karela, momordica

General Description

Bitter melon is a climbing vine that reaches a height of six feet (two meters). It has deeply lobed leaves, yellow flowers, and orange-yellow fruit. Native to southern Asia and an important ingredient in Asian cuisine, bitter melon is cultivated in warm-weather regions throughout the world. Although the seeds, leaves, and vines of bitter melon all have been used in herbal medicine, the fruit—which looks like a cucumber with bumps—is the primary part of the plant used medicinally.

Evidence of Benefit

Bitter melon is a useful agent for treating diabetes, as it lowers blood sugar levels. In folk medicine, bitter melon is used to treat colds, flu, and fever. It has traditionally been used to treat parasites, worms, digestive disorders, and skin diseases like psoriasis.

Bitter melon improves the body's ability to use blood sugar and improves glucose tolerance. Also, at least one animal study noted that bitter melon fruit juice may cause a renewal and recovery of the insulin-producing beta cells of the pancreas.

Benefits of bitter melon for specific health conditions include the following:

- *Cancer.* Patients with cancer have compromised immune systems indicated by decreases in white blood cell counts and in natural killer (NK) cells, which directly attack cancer cells. In one study, bitter melon intake seemed to help patients with head and neck cancer who were undergoing radiation therapy. A transporter protein (P-glycoprotein) similar to NK cells was improved compared to a placebo. NK cell numbers did not improve, however.

- *Diabetes.* Bitter melon is widely used in the treatment of type 2 diabetes. In one study, fasting and postprandial blood glucose levels went down after drinking a homogenized suspension of the bitter melon pulp. Eighty-six of the 100 patients with type 2 diabetes responded favorably. In another study, 50 patients received bitter melon or a placebo for four weeks. No changes were observed in fructosamine, which is a marker of insulin levels in the blood.

Considerations for Use

The easiest place to find bitter melon is an Asian food market. Bitter melon can be taken in whole fruit form or as a momordica extract, tincture, or juice. The latter forms are most likely to be available from practitioners of traditional Chinese medicine (TCM). It also is sold as a dried herb powder. The daily dose is 1 gram. You should not use the tincture for diabetes control, since this form does not lower blood sugar levels. For people with diabetes, it is likely that long-term results will be better if bitter melon is combined with the herb gurmar (*Gymnema sylvestre*). If you are taking insulin or medication to reduce blood sugar, bitter melon might amplify the effect, and you may need to reduce your dose of medication. Bitter melon may potentiate cholesterol-lowering drugs, so blood lipids should be monitored when using this herb.

Ingestion of excessive amounts of bitter melon juice can cause abdominal pain and diarrhea. Anyone with hypoglycemia (low blood sugar) should not take bitter melon, because it could worsen the problem. Bitter melon should not be used during pregnancy, as it can stimulate the uterus and was traditionally used for abortions. Women who are lactating should avoid it as well because it is transferred to the baby in the milk. Bitter melon reduces fertility in both males and females.

BITTER ORANGE

Latin name: *Citrus aurantium* (Rutaceae [citrus] family)
Other common names: chih-shih, neroli, orange

General Description

Bitter orange is the whole, unripe fruit of the mandarin orange. Smaller fruits are preferred in herbal medicine. The peel, known as chen-pi, is also used medicinally.

Evidence of Benefit

Bitter orange contains synephrine, which has decongestant effects on the respiratory system and also may help with blood pressure, digestion, constipation, gastritis, and abdominal distention. The herb has been used in Chinese medicine for thousands of years to improve circulation and liver function, stimulate gastrointestinal functions, and treat indigestion and bronchitis. It also has been used for gout, sore throat, and sleeplessness.

Bitter orange is a potent stimulant of certain nerves that control the circulation of blood. It also constricts small arteries in the nose, sinuses, and eustachian tubes to counteract allergic reactions. Chinese formulas containing the herb have been used for coughs, colds, and anorexia to reduce apathy, and for uterine and anal prolapse. The German Commission E has approved this herb for loss of appetite and stomachache.

Benefits of bitter orange for specific health conditions include the following:

• *Indigestion.* Bitter orange has been used to relieve nausea and soothe stomach disturbances such as indigestion, gas, and bloating. Research has shown that it is effective in shrinking a distended stomach.

• *Overweight.* Bitter orange has the ability to bind to a specific subgroup of B cell receptors called B-3 receptors. This binding effect causes an increase in the rate at which fat is released from body stores for energy production, and increases the resting metabolic rate. It has been added to herbal weight-loss formulas as a replacement for epinephrine. However, the effect in weight reduction is still controversial and awaits more clinical assessment.

Considerations for Use

Bitter orange is available from Asian food markets and Chinese pharmacies, but it is also available in weight-loss products at drugstores and mass-market stores. A typical dose in a tea is one cup, a half hour before meals, which is 4 to 6 grams of the herb or 1.2 grams of the extract. It is best used as a tea.

Bitter orange acts on the uterus and the intestines. In small doses, bitter orange inhibits contractions of these organs, while in large doses, it stimulates contractions. Bitter orange should not be used with cocaine, codeine, or other narcotic pain relievers, since the combination can cause irregular heartbeat and high blood pressure. It should be used with caution during pregnancy and in cases of low energy. It has been reported to have a contraceptive effect. Bitter orange can make the skin more sensitive to sunlight, especially for fair-skinned individuals, and may cause skin redness, swelling, blisters, and pigment spots.

BLACK COHOSH

Latin name: *Cimicifuga racemosa* (Ranunculaceae [peony] family)
Other common names: black snakeroot, bugbane, cimicifuga (in traditional Chinese medicine), squawroot

General Description

Black cohosh is a perennial herb that bears a three- to nine-foot (one- to three-meter) spike covered with creamy white flowers. This shade-loving plant is found in the woodlands of the Atlantic seaboard states and eastern Canada. The rhizome and roots of a number of closely related species are used in herbal medicine. Black cohosh is not related to blue cohosh.

Many of the earliest patent medicines contained high concentrations of black cohosh. It was the main ingredient in Lydia Pinkham's Vegetable Compound, an over-the-counter remedy promoted in the early nineteenth century as relieving stress and nervous tension in women. It became the best-selling herb in the world for treatment of menstrual problems such as hot flashes, night sweats, and mood swings.

Evidence of Benefit

Black cohosh balances hormone levels in both men and women. Historically it was used for aches and pains, sore throat, and bronchitis. A tincture was also used as a sedative, and to treat fever and snakebite. The most important use of black cohosh is in maintaining the therapeutic response to estrogen replacement therapy (ERT) as ERT is gradually withdrawn. The herb is also useful in the treatment of stress-related symptoms during menopause and premenstrual syndrome (PMS) if psychoactive medications cause intolerable side effects. Black cohosh also nourishes the respiratory system and soothes sore throat. It has been approved by the German Commission E for female sexual dysfunction and PMS.

Benefits of black cohosh for specific health conditions include the following:

• *Fibroids (uterine myomas).* Black cohosh contains at least three classes of compounds that act to regulate hormone use. These compounds bind to receptor sites in the reproductive tract, the brain, and other organs that otherwise would receive estrogen. This reduces overall estrogen activity when estrogen levels are high. These substances also block the formation of luteinizing hormone (LH), which stimulates a surge of estrogen production in the first fourteen days of the menstrual cycle. This stimulates estrogen production when estrogen levels are low. The dual action of the herb allows it to stabilize the body's estrogen usage.

• *Infertility.* One of the chemical constituents of black cohosh, ferulic acid, increases the motility and viability of sperm cells by protecting their cell walls from oxidation by compounds released from environmental toxins.

• *Menopause-related problems and premenstrual syndrome (PMS).* Black cohosh offsets a decline in estrogen by providing powerful plant compounds called phytoestrogens that mimic the hormone's effects. These phytoestrogens bind to hormone receptors in the uterus, breast, and other parts of the body. As a result, black cohosh is reported to lessen hot flashes, vaginal dryness, headaches, dizziness, depressed mood, and other hormone-related symptoms. This makes the herb useful as a substitute for ERT, especially when compared with synthetic hormone replacement therapies. Black cohosh does not appear to simulate the growth of breast tumors, unlike conventional hormone replacement therapy, which has been linked to a slightly increased risk of breast cancer when taken over the long term. Some researchers even think the phytoestrogens might prevent tumor growth by keeping the body's own estrogen from stimulating breast cells. Black cohosh compounds likewise regulate estrogen production before menopause, and are especially useful for treating blurred vision and migraine associated with PMS. It has antispasmodic properties that may lessen menstrual discomforts. Black cohosh may increase the blood flow to the uterus, reducing the intensity of particularly painful cramps.

Considerations for Use

Black cohosh is available in capsules, fluid extracts, tablets, and tinctures. The dosage is 40 milligrams per day, when made into a 40 percent alcohol solution. The herbs should not be used longer than six months unless advised by a physician. Taking too much may cause vomiting, headaches, dizziness, limb pain, and low blood pressure. About 10 percent of women who use black cohosh experience mild stomach upset for one to two weeks after starting the herb. To reduce the chance of stomach upset, take black cohosh with meals. Allow up to eight weeks to see benefits for menopausal problems. During this time some women have been able to reduce the dosage of ERT. There are no firm data that black cohosh can be substituted for ERT, and its cardioprotective effects are unknown.

Black cohosh should not be taken with immunosuppressive drugs used in patients who have had organ transplants. In particular, it should not be used with azathioprine and cyclosporine. The herb can also potentiate the action of blood pressure–lowering medications, so these should not be used together. Black cohosh may enhance the effectiveness of tamoxifen, and should not be used together without consulting an oncologist. If you are taking iron, don't take black cohosh at the same time because it binds to iron and makes it unable to be absorbed.

Girls who have not reached puberty should not take black cohosh. The herb should be avoided altogether during pregnancy or while nursing, and by anyone who has an estrogen-sensitive cancer. Black cohosh may interfere with the action of hormonal medications (birth control pills or replacement hormones), so you should consult with a physician before combining it with such medications. You should also consult with your doctor before trying black cohosh if you have heart disease. Black cohosh may have a mild sedative effect, so it should not be taken

with tranquilizers. It may also interfere with blood pressure medication.

Some herbal authorities have speculated that the estrogen-like qualities of black cohosh could be hazardous to women with undiagnosed breast cancer. This is particularly true for breast cancers that are sensitive to estrogen.

Be sure not to confuse black cohosh with blue cohosh, which may be toxic.

BOSWELLIA

Latin name: *Boswellia serrata* (Burseraceae [frankincense] family)
Other common names: dhup, frankincense, Indian olibanum, mastic, olibanum, salai gugal

General Description

Boswellia is a large branching tree about twelve feet high found in the dry hilly areas of India. The purified extract of the gummy resin tapped from the tree trunk is used in modern herbal preparations. Along with myrrh, boswellia was traded for centuries in the Middle East, as seen by biblical references to this substance under the name frankincense. Boswellia is aromatic, granular, and translucent.

Evidence of Benefit

Boswellia is one of the most ancient and respected herbs in ayurvedic healing. Traditionally it was used to treat arthritis, colitis, coughs, sores, snakebites, and asthma. Researchers and clinicians are finding that boswellia is a potent anti-inflammatory, antiarthritic for both rheumatoid arthritis and osteoarthritis, and pain reliever without any side effects. The gum and oil also are used in cosmetics, perfumes, and skin-care products.

Benefits of boswellia for specific health conditions include the following:

• *Arthritis.* Laboratory studies have shown that boswellic acids, active components in boswellia, deactivate the hormonal triggers for inflammation and pain in osteoarthritis. These acids effectively shrink inflamed tissue and could stimulate the growth of cartilage, increase blood supply to inflamed joints, and enhance the repair of local blood vessels damaged by inflammation. In one study, patients with knee pain derived benefit from boswellia at 333 milligrams per capsule, taken three times a day for eight weeks. When the patients were receiving the boswellia, they experienced less pain intensity and swelling, and improved knee function.

Clinical studies using boswellia have showed some good results in both osteoarthritis and rheumatoid arthritis. Several studies have reported dramatic improvement within two to four weeks. Experimental and clinical usage of boswellia indicates that it does not produce any side effects, such as irritation, ulcers, and effects on heart rate and blood pressure, which are associated with most anti-inflammatory and antiarthritic drugs.

• *Inflammation.* Boswellia extracts have been shown to inhibit the synthesis of pro-inflammatory mediators including prostaglandins and leukotrienes. This action may help treat diseases like inflammatory bowel disease, asthma, and arthritis. Boswellia seems to work better in treating chronic asthma symptoms rather than acute asthma.

• *Ulcerative colitis and Crohn's disease.* One double-blind study reported that boswellia may be helpful for ulcerative colitis. A recommended dose is 400 milligrams of boswellia, standardized to contain 37.5 percent of gum resins, three times daily. The full effect may take as long as four to eight weeks to develop. Another study used 300 milligrams of gum resin of boswellia, three times a day for six weeks in patients with chronic colitis. Ninety percent of the patients improved with minimal side effects. Another group of patients got the standard drug treatment (sulfasalazine), and only 60 percent improved. Crohn's patients took 800 milligrams of boswellia serrata extract or placebo, three times a day for one year. There were no differences between the two groups in terms of tolerance, days in remission, and time to remission. Thus, boswellia seems to be better for ulcerative colitis patients than for those with Crohn's disease.

Considerations for Use

Boswellia is available as an extract labeled for its content of boswellin. Many product labels include the name *boswellin.* Since boswellin stimulates blood circulation, you should not use any boswellia product during pregnancy.

Few side effects have been reported with boswellia other than an occasional allergic reaction, such as diarrhea, skin rash, or nausea. However, it is not recommended for young children, pregnant or nursing women, or those with severe liver or kidney disease.

BRAHMI

Latin name: *Bacopa monniera* (Scrophulariaceae [snapdragon] family)
Other common names: Indian pennywort, water hyssop

General Description

Brahmi is a perennial creeping herb with crinkled leaves and white flowers related to spinach and snapdragons. It grows floating in the waters of tropical marshes and wetlands in Florida, Central America, and India. The tops of the plant are used in herbal medicine. An important herb in ayurvedic medicine, brahmi is closely related to an herb with similar medicinal properties, gotu kola. (*See* GOTU KOLA.)

Evidence of Benefit

Of all Indian herbal therapies, brahmi has been established as a powerful nerve and brain tonic. It is the main revitalizing herb for the nerves and the brain cells. It has a reputation for increasing intelligence, longevity, and circulation in the brain, improving both short-term and long-term memory, and decreasing senility and aging.

Traditional ayurvedic practitioners used the herb for a number of conditions, including blood cleansing, fevers, inflammations, joint pain, and a variety of skin problems. It also was known to stimulate hair, skin, and nail growth.

Benefits of brahmi for specific health conditions include the following:

• *Alzheimer's disease, attention deficit disorder (ADD), memory problems, and Parkinson's disease.* Brahmi may be useful in treating a variety of conditions that involve impaired mental capacity. Laboratory studies indicate that brahmi improves intellectual function primarily by balancing the chemicals gamma-aminobutyric acid (GABA) and glutamate in the brain. This allows the orderly firing of nerve cells involved in verbal memory and symbol recognition. However, there are few human studies using brahmi for improving mental capacity.

The two main active incredients in brahmi, bacosides A and B, have been shown to increase protein kinase activity and new protein synthesis in regions of the brain associated with long-term memory. Animal studies have found that brahmi produces faster performance times, reduces errors, improves acquisition and retention of learning, decreases forgetfulness, and increases the ability to adapt to new learning.

• *Anxiety disorder and stress.* Brahmi induces a sense of calm and peace. It helps reduce the restlessness and distraction that nervousness causes. Coupled with its unique ability to improve cognitive function, brahmi may be useful for those who spend time in stressful work or study environments.

• *Irritable bowel syndrome (IBS).* A study that evaluated brahmi in the treatment of IBS found the herb to have beneficial effects, especially if diarrhea was the predominant symptom.

Considerations for Use

Brahmi is available as a bacoside extract in tablet form. In ayurvedic medicine, brahmi is used as a rasayana, a traditional formulation that includes spices and honey to make a palatable mixture. The effectiveness of brahmi is increased by simultaneous supplementation with inositol and/or a B-vitamin complex. For best results, adults should take 3,000 milligrams one or twice daily. It may take four weeks to see an improvement. Brahmi is best taken at the beginning of the day and again in mid- to late afternoon, or before doing meditation or yoga.

The herb is often combined with the circulatory boosters ginkgo and lecithin. These herbs have independent modes but work well synergistically to improve cognitive function.

Women with conditions of excess estrogen production (or who take estrogen replacement therapy [ERT] or birth control pills) should avoid brahmi, since an interaction between estrogen and increased GABA can cause temporary hearing loss.

BROMELAIN

Latin name: bromelain is extracted from pineapple, *Ananas comosus* (Bromeliaceae [bromeliad] family)

Description

Bromelain is a proteolytic (protein-digesting) enzyme found in the stem and fruit of the pineapple plant. It is extracted from pineapple juice pulp by the use of chemical solvents such as acetone or methanol, or by filtration. Although both processes result in a safe and effective product, buyers may want to read product literature to ensure purchase of a natural product. In Hawaii, some herb shops sell a pineapple latex, collected directly from the plant, that contains high concentrations of bromelains A and B.

Evidence of Benefit

Bromelain is best known as a digestive aid and for its anti-inflammatory effects after traumatic injuries and surgery. It also helps the digestion of proteins, stops blood clot formation, and has antiviral properties.

Bromelain has been used to treat heart disease, arthritis, upper respiratory tract infection, and Peyronie's disease, which affects the genitourinary tract and can cause sexual dysfunction in men. It is also used to promote healing of wounds caused by burns because it has been shown to debride wounds (remove dead skin). It also may help with other skin conditions. Bromelain may increase the actions of chemotherapy drugs in animals and lengthen their survival from lung and breast cancer and leukemia. It also has been used for arthritis, bruises, burns, cancer prevention, cancer treatment, circulatory disorders, edema, and indigestion.

Benefits of bromelain for specific health conditions include the following:

• *Cancer.* Studies in mice have shown that bromelain has antitumor effects and is protective against getting cancer. Bromelain can be used along with enzymes as an adjuvant to cancer treatments. Survival was increased in animals; however, clinical data in humans are lacking. Bromelain works by slowing tumor growth by stimulating the body to release immunosuppressive compounds.

• *Chronic rhinosinusitis.* Bromelain was shown to provide faster relief when given to children with irritation of the nasal membranes from allergens or infections. With this condition, normal flow of sinus fluid is disrupted and you feel a stuffy nose, blockage in the nose, and swelling in the nose. The bromelain offered relief from these symptoms.

• *Crohn's disease, diabetes, gastric ulcers, and gastric upset.* Bromelain intensifies the digestive process by breaking down proteins. This makes it easier for the stomach to pass food to the intestine. This effect can counteract gastroparesis, a condition caused by long-term diabetic nerve damage in which the stomach is unable to pass food along properly. It relieves the symptoms of gastrointestinal upset, aids in the healing of gastric ulcers, and is used as a digestive enzyme for pancreatic insufficiency. Controlling gastroparesis is of considerable importance in diabetes management, since delays in passing food through the digestive tract make the timing of insulin injections and diabetes medications difficult. By helping to regulate the digestive process, bromelain use makes it possible for people with diabetes to more accurately estimate when to take insulin or other medications. Bromelain's ability to speed protein digestion also makes it useful in treating Crohn's disease.

• *Osteoarthritis.* In one study, bromelain (90 milligrams), along with other enzymes (trypsin and rutoside), was compared to a standard nonsteroidal anti-inflammatory drug (NSAID), diclofenac, in osteoarthritis patients. Both treatments were given twice a day. Standard measurements of pain and mobility were assessed. There were no differences in joint stiffness and physical function. Bromelain with these other compounds may offer a safe and effective alternative to NSAIDs.

• *Premenstrual syndrome (PMS).* Bromelain balances the body's production of prostaglandins, a class of regulatory hormones including a number of substances that cause smooth muscles to contract. As a smooth-muscle relaxant, bromelain may decrease spasms of the cervix accompanying PMS.

• *Rheumatoid arthritis.* Bromelain blocks formation of kinins, compounds that cause swelling. Patients with rheumatoid arthritis (RA) have an overproduction of cytokine-transforming growth factor-beta (TGF-beta), which leads to chronic inflammation. In one study, patients who had elevated levels of TGF-beta at the start of the study with bromelain and other proteolytic enzymes experienced a decrease, so the direct utility of bromelain is unknown. Also, patients had RA and other conditions (osteomyelofibrosis and herpes zoster). All are related to chronic inflammation, which bromelain can fix.

Considerations for Use

Bromelain is available in tablet form. A typical dose is 80 to 320 milligrams daily in two to three doses. When it is used by itself, as much as 50 percent of the medication is passed out of the digestive tract unabsorbed. Many manufacturers combine bromelain with the digestive enzyme papain so that more bromelain actually enters the bloodstream. These formulas are preferable to pure bromelain. For use as a digestive aid, 500 milligrams with each meal is recommended. Generally, you should take bromelain for only eight to ten days, but it may be tolerated for longer periods. Talk to your physician if you want to take it longer.

Taking bromelain with tetracycline will increase the concentration of the antibiotic in the bloodstream. While this increases the ability of the antibiotic to ward off infection, it also increases the risk of allergic reactions. You should not take bromelain if you are taking warfarin (Coumadin) or any other medication to thin the blood.

No serious side effects of bromelain have been reported, but it may cause nausea, vomiting, diarrhea, and excessive menstrual bleeding. People who are allergic to pineapple may experience allergic reactions, including skin reactions and asthma. Check with your health-care provider before taking bromelain if you have a blood-clotting disorder, liver or kidney disease, or hypertension, or if you are pregnant or lactating.

BUPLEURUM

Latin names: *Bupleurum chinense* (northern bupleurum), *Bupleurum scorzoneraefolium* (southern bupleurum) (Apiaceae [parsley] family)
Other common names: chai hu, Chinese thorowax root, hare's ear root, saiko

General Description

Bupleurum is a perennial in the same family as carrots and parsley. It grows up to three feet high, with sickle-shaped leaves and clusters of small yellow flowers at the top of the plant. The root, the part used in herbal medicine, is harvested in the spring and autumn.

Evidence of Benefit

Bupleurum is an important Chinese tonic herb for the liver and circulatory system. It also helps to moderate emotional instability associated with sluggish liver function and may play a supportive role in patients with hepatitis C by possibly stabilizing the liver tissue and preventing toxins from entering it. It has traditionally been very effective for treatment of intermittent fevers, colds, malaria, and gastrointestinal disorders. This herb seems to exert a tonic effect on the heart and the lungs, making it useful for improving kidney function. Patients who are on steroids may get some relief from this herb, as it may allow them to take lower doses of steroids. This has only been shown in animal studies, however. These benefits are mainly derived because bupleurum is an anti-inflammatory and stimulates immune function.

Benefits of bupleurum for specific health conditions include the following:

• *Allergies.* Bupleurum has been shown in animal studies to lessen the symptoms of allergies by acting as an antihistamine.

• *Bone cancer.* Bupleurum enhances the production of interferon, an immune-system chemical used in cancer treatment. (For more detailed information on this effect, *see* MINOR BUPLEURUM DECOCTION *under* The Formulas.) The herb also contains rutin, a bioflavonoid that helps restrain cancer cells from multiplying indefinitely. Whether it works in bone cancer patients is not known. Bupleurum when used with other herbs has been used for liver cancer. The saikosaponins in this herb promote a strong immune system by modulating T-lymphocyte function and promoting IL-2 production. These compounds in the herb also inhibit arachidonic acid metabolism, which leads to improved immune function.

Considerations for Use

Bupleurum is available in the form of saikosaponin extract at Chinese pharmacies, as chai hu from practitioners of traditional Chinese medicine (TCM), and in combination with other herbs such as those in many important Chinese herbal formulas. Some over-the-counter (OTC) formulas available at retail stores combine bupleurum with dong quai or scutellaria. (*See* DONG QUAI and SCUTELLARIA.) Bupleurum also can be used as a tea.

Like many other herbs, bupleurum requires the help of friendly bacteria living in the human intestine to be therapeutically useful. These bacteria transform the compounds in the herb into bodily chemicals that relieve inflammation. Therefore, bupleurum should not be taken at the same time as antibiotics, which often kill off these bacteria. Large doses of bupleurum may cause gastroenteritis, intestinal colic, or diarrhea due to the saponin content.

Bupleurum should not be used during pregnancy or if you are undergoing interferon therapy for hepatitis. There have been reports of adverse drug-herb reactions linked to lung tissue damage. If you are using nonsteroidal anti-inflammatory drugs (NSAIDs), you should consult with your prescribing physician before taking bupleurum. There have been reports of interstitial lung disease occurring with its use.

BURDOCK

Latin name: *Arctium lappa* (Asteraceae [composite] family)
Other common names: bardana, beggar's buttons, hareburr, appa, love leaves

General Description

Burdock, a relative of the sunflower, grows to a height of 5 feet (1.5 meters) and bears reddish-purple flower heads covered with spiny bracts. In summer, the grayish-red seeds are harvested, and the roots of two-year-old plants are dug. Although native to Asia and Europe, this biennial is now widespread throughout the United States. The ripe seed and fresh and dried roots are the most important parts of the plant used for medicinal purposes.

Evidence of Benefit

Although no human data exist, in animals and in vitro studies, burdock has been shown to be an antibacterial, anticancer, antioxidant, antiviral, anti-inflammatory, and liver protectant.

In traditional Chinese medicine (TCM), burdock root is used in combination with other herbs to treat skin redness, ulcers, sore throats, tonsillitis, colds, and measles. It is also used as a diuretic and blood purifier. Externally it is used for dry skin like psoriasis and seborrhea of the scalp.

Benefits of burdock for specific health conditions include the following:

• *Arthritis, gout, and sciatica.* Consistent use of the tea (made from the root or seeds) may ease arthritis, gout, and sciatica by reducing the swelling around joints.

• *Boils, dandruff, and eczema.* Herbal practitioners in Japan and Europe have long used burdock root and seeds in treatments for chronic skin diseases, especially eczema. European herbalists use burdock root, which seems to work by preventing the body's own immune system from attacking the skin. Burdock root oil extract (Bur oil) has traditionally been popular in Europe as a scalp treatment applied to improve hair strength, shine, and body, and to combat hair loss. It has been used to ease dandruff and scalp itching.

• *Cancer.* Cancer researchers have discovered a substance in burdock root capable of reducing cell mutation, in either the absence or the presence of metabolic activation. Japanese researchers named this new property the B-factor. Burdock has gained fame as one of the four potent herbs in Essiac tea, an important alternative cancer remedy. Laboratory studies with animals suggest that the dietary fiber arctiin, found in burdock seed, may slow or stop the growth of breast cancer in the early stages, in which the number of cancer cells increases rapidly. This fiber may have similar benefits against leukemia, and colon and pancreatic cancers.

• *Liver diseases.* In animal studies, burdock has been shown to heal a damaged liver and protect it from further damage. It worked as well as silymarin in maintaining healthy liver blood tests and liver tissue. There are no human data available.

Considerations for Use

Look for burdock-seed cereals, available as gobo or goboshi, in Japanese groceries, and for burdock oil and tincture in health food stores. Burdock root is sometimes labeled as "cut and sifted burdock root" or by its Latin name, *Arctium lappa*. Burdock is also available as a tea.

Traditional herbalists recommend a tea made from 2.5 grams of burdock in 150 milliliters (6 ounces) of hot water and taken twice a day, or 460 to 475 milligrams per day in capsule form. The use of burdock root at these dosage levels is generally safe. However, large quantities of burdock root may stimulate the uterus. This herb should therefore be used with caution during pregnancy, especially during the first trimester. It can safely be combined with other pharmaceutical drugs other than alcohol extract of disulfiram or metronidazole, due to their alcohol content. Burdock may cause a rash on the skin if it comes in contact with the herb.

BUTCHER'S BROOM

Latin name: *Ruscus aculeatis* (Liliaceae [lily] family)
Other names: Jew's myrtle, kneeholm, knee holy, pettigree, sweet broom

General Description

Butcher's broom is an evergreen bush in the lily family. Growing to three feet (one meter) in height, it has leaf-like branches with a terminal spine, greenish-white flowers, and shiny red berries. Until the twentieth century, the dried plant was used as a broom throughout Europe, giving the herb its name. Both the aerial (aboveground) parts and the root of the plant are gathered in summer when the herb is in bloom for use in herbal medicine. Also, the dried rhizome and root are used.

Evidence of Benefit

In animal studies, butcher's broom is known for its cleansing properties, especially with blood vessels. It contains agents that support circulation (especially to the legs). It also reduces urine retention, which may make it useful in treating bladder infections. For humans, it has been approved by the German Commission E for hemorrhoids (itching and burning) and venous conditions such as poor blood flow in the legs that causes pain and heaviness. It is also suitable for cramps in the legs, itching, and swelling.

Benefits of butcher's broom for specific health conditions include the following:

• *Hemorrhoids.* Butcher's broom tightens the dilated blood vessels that form hemorrhoids. The herb is particularly effective for relief of burning and itching hemorrhoids.

• *Swelling.* Placebo-controlled, double-blind clinical trials have shown that butcher's broom extracts, taken over a period of three months, reduce swelling in the upper arm after surgical treatment for breast cancer. The reduction of swelling was proportionally greater in tissues with the thinnest layers of fat.

• *Varicose veins.* One of the chemical constituents of butcher's broom, ruscogenin, is a potent inhibitor of the enzyme elastase, which accelerates the recycling of tissues lining the veins. Unlike some other herbs used for varicose veins, butcher's broom enhances the action of hyalouronidase, an enzyme vital for fertility in women. Due to the presence of steroidal compounds, butcher's broom helps to make veins stronger and less porous. It encourages blood to move up out of the legs, helps to tighten the veins and decrease inflammation, and also helps to reduce pain.

German clinical studies have confirmed that butcher's broom creams reduce the swelling of varicose veins during pregnancy. Researchers found that wearing support stockings plus applying a ruscogenin cream resulted in an average dilation of varicose veins of 2.1 millimeters during pregnancy. Wearing support stockings but not using the cream resulted in an average dilation of 3.4 millimeters. Using neither ruscogenin cream nor support stockings during pregnancy resulted in an average dilation of varicose veins of 4.5 millimeters. In other words, none of the treatments eliminated varicose veins entirely, but butcher's broom cream plus the use of support stockings reduced the "spread" of the veins by half and the amount of blood diverted into them by 90 percent.

Considerations for Use

Butcher's broom is available in ruscogenin tablets, capsules of ruscogenin powder, and in a commercial capsule in which butcher's broom is combined with rosemary oil. When taken internally, butcher's broom is considered to be more effective if taken with vitamin C. Creams are available from compounding pharmacies. Some commercial preparations combine ruscogenin with another plant extract, hesperidin, for treatment of lymphedema.

A dosage of 7 to 11 milligrams of total ruscogenin extract is generally recommended. At this dosage, no side effects have been reported. Large doses of butcher's broom can cause vomiting, purging, weakening heart, lowered nerve strength, and low blood pressure. Large doses have been reported to cause poisoning, and advanced stages of toxicity can cause complete respiratory collapse.

Although no reports of adverse interactions have been noted when taken in normal doses, it is conceivable that butcher's broom may cause stomach complaints and queasiness in rare cases. Do not use during pregnancy unless your obstetrician agrees.

CAJUEIRO

Latin name: *Anacardium occidentale* (Anacardiaceae [sumac or pistachio] family)
Other common names: cashew nut shells, jambu (not to be confused with jambul)

General Description

Cajueiro is a tropical evergreen tree in the same plant family as the mango, poison ivy, and poison oak. Cajueiro is native to Brazil and grows in tropical regions throughout the world. Growing to a height of thirty feet (ten meters), it has large oval leaves and bears pink-striped yellow flowers on long stems. The cajueiro "fruit" is actually a thickened stem. The true fruit is just below the thickened portion of the stem, and contains red or yellow flesh surrounding the cashew nut. The nut, removed from its bark, is used principally as a food. The bark, "fruit," nuts, and resin of the tree are used medicinally.

Evidence of Benefit

Cajueiro contains naturally occurring analogs of the latest diabetes drugs pioglitazone (Actos) and rosiglitazone (Avandia), without their potential for liver damage or weight gain. However, this was shown in animals and not humans. Do not use cajueiro if you have diabetes without consulting your physician. Cajueiro is used in tribal medicine in South America as a contraceptive, snakebite cure, and treatment for parasites and vaginitis.

Benefits of cajueiro for specific health conditions include the following:

• *Diabetes.* Laboratory tests suggest that cajueiro lowers blood sugar in mice by inhibiting the action of an enzyme known as tyrosinase. When tyrosinase is blocked, receptor sites on cells in the intestines become more sensitive to insulin. Insulin "instructs" the cells to absorb more of the amino acids leucine, phenylalanine, tyrosine, and valine. With higher concentrations of these amino acids in the body, the body suffers less protein breakdown and wasting caused by uncontrolled diabetes. This protects against kidney damage. The animal studies show cajueiro to have only a weak antidiabetic effect.

• *Parasitic infection.* In the Bahía region of Brazil, 65 percent of cases of leishmaniasis, an ulcerating skin disease, are successfully treated with cajueiro. In cell studies, cajueiro extracts are over 90 percent effective against the parasites that cause schistosomiasis (bilharzia).

Considerations for Use

Cajueiro is available as a tincture. Check with your doctor if you plan on using this herb. When using cajueiro for diabetes, patience is required, as lower blood sugar may not be observed for three to four weeks. However, blood sugar should be measured as usual to make sure the combination of cajueiro and prescribed insulin and/or other medications does not lower sugars excessively. The oil in the nut shell can cause skin irritation if it is not heated first to render the oil less caustic. Never eat cashews raw. They are not dangerous after being roasted in the shell.

CALENDULA

Latin name: *Calendula officinalis* (Asteraceae [composite] family)
Other common names: gold-bloom, marigold, marybud, pot calendula, pot marigold

General Description

Calendula is an annual or biennial aromatic native to the Mediterranean countries. Its name refers to its tendency to bear flowers by the calendar, once a month in warm climates, usually during the new moon. "Marigold" refers to the Virgin Mary, and marigolds are traditionally used in Catholic celebrations concerning the Virgin Mary.

Calendula bears many-petaled orange or yellow flowering heads two to three inches (four to seven centimeters) in diameter. Grown widely as a garden flower, calendula is cultivated for use in herbal medicine in Eastern Europe and throughout Latin America. The flowers are used in herbal preparations and the petals are a good source of lycopene and lutein.

Evidence of Benefit

Calendula is an antibacterial, anti-inflammatory, antiparasitic, and painkilling agent for minor injuries and topical infections and irritations. It also can help with wound healing. Some of the chemical components of calendula have shown potential in laboratory tests as a reverse transcriptase inhibitor for the treatment of HIV/AIDS. When mixed with other herbs, it may help reduce earache in children with acute otitis media, although some studies do not support its use in this context. Animal and cell studies suggest that calendula can kill cancer cells. Preliminary data support its use topically for prophylaxis of acute dermatitis during radiation therapy in cancer patients.

Benefits of calendula for specific health conditions include the following:

• *Bowel diseases.* Calendula reduces the inflammation that causes pain in these disorders. It reduces the general tension that can promote bowel problems, relaxing the nervous constriction of the digestive muscles to help the bowels.

• *Conjunctivitis.* Calendula washes are useful in treating chronic conjunctivitis. They are antibacterial and stimulate the growth of healthy tissue in the membranes surrounding the eye.

• *Gastritis.* German studies have demonstrated that calendula prevents the hormonal reactions that produce swelling and inflammation in the stomach lining, specifically by acting on the inflammatory prostaglandin E_2 (PGE_2). Calendula has a strong bactericidal effect that may counteract infection with *Helicobacter pylori*, a bacterium associated with both gastritis and peptic ulcers. Calendula and comfrey taken together may have a healing effect on duodenal and peptic ulcers and increase the effectiveness of antacids. (*See* COMFREY.)

• *Inflammation.* In cells, calendula inhibits cyclooxygenase-2 (COX-2), a key enzyme mediating inflammation. Synthetic drugs (such as Vioxx) that act as COX-2 inhibitors and targeted arthritis, Alzheimer's disease, and some cancers have been removed from the market by the FDA. Calendula may help in these conditions, but more human studies are needed.

• *Mucous membrane and skin disorders.* Calendula is widely used as an additive to cosmetic skin creams. Used in these creams, it stimulates the production of collagen, filling in wrinkles. Calendula creams also hydrate winter-dried skin, relieve pain and inflammation caused by conditions such as mastitis and hemorrhoids, and alleviate vaginal itching caused by menopausal tissue changes. In addition, this herb has antibacterial action that allows it to prevent and treat various types of infection. Wound healing studies have only been conducted on animals, but the results are positive.

Calendula creams are used in Europe to prevent skin damage from drying, insect bites, and sunburn. Europeans also make wide use of them for preventing diaper rash and inflammations of the mouth, nose, and throat. Used externally, calendula helps to soothe, heal, and protect a baby's sensitive skin.

Indian researchers report that aerosol sprays of calendula extracts stop bleeding from cuts and scrapes while preventing infection. Calendula washes kill *Staphylococcus aureus*, a common germ that infects abrasions, burns, and cuts. Calendula, used externally, helps injured skin to rejuvenate. In one study, skin pain and redness were reduced with topical calendula when used by women with breast cancer who were receiving radiation therapy to the breast. This study was an open label study, so results are not conclusive and more work is needed. However, this treatment may offer benefit to women who do not respond to other therapies.

Considerations for Use

Calendula is available in creams, eyedrops, teas, and tinctures. As a cream, it is recommended in a 2 to 5 percent ointment, and applied topically three to four times a day. As a tincture, it should be 1:1 in 40 percent alcohol or 1:5 in 90 percent alcohol. These preparations may be further diluted in 1:3 boiled water for compresses. Calendula is also found in toothpaste and mouthwashes, as it has active compounds that are effective against oral bacteria. Combinations of calendula and comfrey may be available from compounding pharmacies.

Because of the cumulative nature of the very mild antibacterial toxins present in the herb, it is advisable to use calendula *teas* for no more than two weeks or until symptoms subside, whichever comes first. Wait six weeks before resuming the tea. Anyone allergic to members of the Aster/Compositae family such as ragweed and marigold should avoid this herb.

When calendula is taken internally, it can increase the sedative effect of medications for anxiety and insomnia.

It also may increase the activity of blood glucose–lowering drugs or insulin and may help decrease blood lipids and triglycerides. Consult your physician if you are taking any of these drugs before using calendula. Use caution while driving or operating machines if taking calendula and such medications at the same time. Insufficient information is available about using calendula in children, so check with your child's pediatrician before giving it to a child. There is little data on the use of calendula during pregnancy and lactation, so its use should be avoided.

CALIFORNIA POPPY

Latin name: *Eschscholzia californica* (Papaveraceae [opium poppy] family)

General Description

This herb, the state flower of California, is a two-foot-high (sixty-centimeter) annual with finely cut leaves and bright orange, pink, red, or yellow flowers. It is widely grown as a garden plant in both the United States and Europe. The aboveground parts of the poppy are used in herbal medicine.

Evidence of Benefit

California poppy is a calming and anti-inflammatory agent. In Native American herbal medicine, it is used to ease toothache. The main active principle in California poppy is californidine, which has a sleep-inducing, sedative effect. California poppy also contains an alkaloid called protopine, which is similar in structure to morphine, but it is not addictive and has different effects on the body. Although unproven, it may help with the following issues: insomnia, aches, nervous agitation, bed-wetting in children, diseases of the bladder and liver, sadness, and nervous system weakness.

Benefits of California poppy for specific health conditions include the following:

• *Anxiety.* California poppy is closely related to the opium poppy, but it has a very different effect on the central nervous system. Unlike the opiates found in the opium poppy, the alkaloid components of California poppy do not cause addiction or disorientation as they induce relaxation (in lower doses) or sleep (in higher doses). In one study, patients with mild or moderate generalized anxiety disorder benefited from a product made from 20 milligrams of dry aqueous extract of California poppy, hawthorn, and magnesium. After three months, there was an improvement in the total anxiety score, somatic score, and self-assessment score. California poppy appears to be an effective and safe alternative treatment for mild to moderate anxiety.

• *Stress.* The California poppy has sleep-inducing and sedative effects that help relieve muscle tension.

Considerations for Use

California poppy may be blended with corydalis in an over-the-counter (OTC) formula. Homeopathy preparations are also available as drops or tablets. They can be taken every thirty to sixty minutes for acute use and one to three times daily for chronic use. It can also be used in teas, which are made using 2 grams of the herb per 150 milliliters (¾ cup) of water. Pregnant women should avoid California poppy, since it may cause uterine contractions. Caution should be taken when giving it to children; it is stronger than other herbs such as chamomile flowers or fennel seed for sedation.

CARDAMOM

Latin name: *Amomum villosum* (Zingiberaceae [ginger] family)
Other common names: cardamon, grains-of-paradise

General Description

Cardamom is a medicinal herb native to tropical China and Vietnam. It is closely related, but not identical, to the cardamom grown in India and Sri Lanka as a spice. Cardamom is a perennial that grows to a height of fifteen feet (five meters), with mauve-streaked white flowers and very long, lance-shaped leaves. The seed pods are used medicinally and oil is extracted from them.

Evidence of Benefit

According to folk medicine, cardamom helps with digestive problems, vomiting and diarrhea, morning sickness, and loss of appetite. In Chinese medicine, it is used for stomachache, nausea, vomiting, and flatulence. Ayurvedic physicians use it to treat ulcers and malaria. The essential oil is antibacterial and antifungal.

Benefits of cardamom for specific health conditions include the following:

• *Dyspepsia.* Cardamom works best on upset stomachs according the German Commission E.

• *Urinary incontinence.* Cardamom is used in ayurvedic medicine to help control urinary incontinence in both men and women.

Considerations for Use

Cardamom is most frequently used as a tincture and liquid extract, which are made from ground seeds. The average daily dose is 1.5 grams of the herb, and you need 1 to 2 grams a day. It also may be used as a tea. The spice cardamom has the same effects as the medicinal herb—provided the spice is fresh. It should not be taken by anyone with gallstones unless a physician is consulted. There are no known other side effects or drug interactions.

Why Cats Love Catnip

Catnip is a favorite herb of felines. The herb is known to induce pleasure behaviors (purring, relaxation) in cats, but it is probably equally attractive to cats for its effects on their objects of prey. Brazilian researchers have found that catnip has a short-term effect on mice similar to that of amphetamines, causing frenzied behavior and seizures. Then, in the long term, it causes mice to become drowsy and then cataleptic. Catnip also causes drowsiness in birds. Catnip need not be fed to cats, but can be used to scent pillows or cloths where the cats stay.

CATNIP

Latin name: *Nepeta cataria* (Lamiaceae [mint] family)
Other common names: catmint, catswort, field balm

General Description

Catnip is a downy aromatic mint that grows to a height of three feet (one meter). The plant has heart-shaped gray-green leaves and whorls of white flowers with purple spots. It is native to Europe and has become naturalized in North America, growing along dry roadsides and in mountainous regions up to altitudes of 5,000 feet (1,500 meters). The tops of the plant are gathered for herbal use in the fall.

Evidence of Benefit

Catnip, best known for its peculiar attractiveness to cats, is a carminative (an agent that helps to expel gas) and gastric stimulant in humans. It is used in folk medicine to treat colds, colic, and fevers. It has also been used in nervous disorders and migraines, since it seems to have a calming effect. In England and France, it was a culinary and medicinal herb and was used as a stimulating drink before black tea became popular. Although catnip is typically used as a calming agent, the tea actually seems to have stimulating properties. Some reports have shown that smoking catnip produces a psychedelic effect. Catnip contains constituents that have local anesthetic effects that could cause central nervous system depression or stimulation when absorbed.

Benefits of catnip for specific health conditions include the following:

• *Influenza.* Catnip teas have long been used in traditional herbal medicine to quell digestive disturbances, especially those accompanying flu or asthma. Catnip stimulates gastric secretions. This aids the movement of food and infection out of the digestive tract, while relaxing tight muscles and generally inducing relaxation. Recent laboratory research has confirmed that catnip is antimicrobial.

• *Insomnia.* Catnip is a potent sleep-inducer for humans. It is often used to help get children to sleep or settle them down. Catnip calms without affecting you the next day.

Considerations for Use

Catnip is usually used as a tea. The bulk herb is available in herb shops and health food stores. The flowers are used for tea and the aerial parts are used for capsules. Tea should be consumed three times a day using about 10 teaspoons in 1 liter of water. Catnip also is available in capsules, which are 380 milligrams per capsule, and are taken as needed. Catnip should not be used during pregnancy. There are no known side effects when used at the correct amounts. Children should only take catnip if they are under the supervision of a pediatrician. There has been a report of a child chewing on a catnip tea bag and developing lethargy and abdominal pain.

CAT'S CLAW

Latin names: *Uncaria guianensis* or *Uncaria tomentosa* (Rubiaceae [madder] family)
Other common names: garbato, paraguaya, tambor hausea, toron, uña de gato

General Description

The cat's claw plant, which comes from the rain forest areas of Central and South America, is a tropical creeping vine that grows up, and sometimes connects, canopy trees, reaching a length of up to 100 feet (30 meters). It is in the same plant family as coffee. The bark is used in herbal medicine.

Evidence of Benefit

Used by native peoples in South America as a contraceptive, cat's claw is an anti-inflammatory agent and immune stimulant. It is also good for all forms of arthritis. It has also been shown to have anticancer, antioxidant, antiviral, and cardiovascular effects. In folk medicine, it has been used for diarrhea and gastritis.

Benefits of cat's claw for specific health conditions include the following:

• *Arthritis.* Cat's claw is a rich source of sterols, which have anti-inflammatory activity. Animal studies have found that the herb reduces swelling by approximately 50 percent.

• *Bowel disorders.* In animal studies, cat's claw was shown to protect the intestine from damage from indomethacin, a nonsteroidal anti-inflammatory drug (NSAID).

• *Cancer.* Austrian researchers have confirmed that cat's claw supports a body affected by cancer by stimulating the immune system. It also inhibits the proliferation of human tumor cells such as for leukemia. Cat's claw also has been shown to directly kill cancer cells in cell line studies. The additional immune-system boost may allow some people to take the full course of chemotherapy needed to prevent recurrence of the disease. As an antioxidant, cat's claw supports the body during chemotherapy and radiation treatments, and removes toxic metabolites. In one study two people—one a smoker and the other a nonsmoker—were given cat's claw. The cat's claw had no effect on the nonsmoker, but the smoker experienced a decrease in the genetic mutation activity that could lead to cancer, specifically lung cancer. The effect continued eight days after the treatment was withdrawn.

• *Colds.* The immune-stimulant effects of cat's claw allow it to support immune function to possibly fight off cold viruses.

• *HIV/AIDS.* The advantage of cat's claw for treating AIDS is that it helps the body produce T cells and other white blood cells in normal numbers. This can prevent excessive immune stimulation that can provoke herpes outbreaks or give HIV opportunities to become drug-resistant. In a study of thirteen HIV-positive patients who took 20 milligrams daily of cat's claw containing 12 milligrams per gram total of pentacyclic oxindole alkaloids for up to five months, the patients showed an increase in absolute lymphocyte count (part of the white blood cells). However, a marker of HIV infection—the T4/T8 ratio—did not change.

Considerations for Use

Cat's claw is available in capsule and tincture forms. The daily dosage is 250 to 1,000 milligrams, and the total alkaloid equivalent is 10 to 30 milligrams. People with limited kidney function should consult their physician, as there is evidence that cat's claw may be associated with renal failure. It should not be used by pregnant women or nursing mothers. Patients with autoimmune diseases or who are on immunosuppressants to prevent rejection of implanted organs, including bone marrow, should not use cat's claw. This herb may increase the risk of bleeding if you are taking anticlotting medications, so the two should not be used together.

The healing alkaloids in cat's claw tinctures are released from tannins by the action of acid in the stomach. If they are absorbed through the tongue, they lose their effect. For this reason, you should always take cat's claw tincture with at least 6 ounces (¾ cup) of water to avoid absorption through the tongue. You can add 1 tablespoon of lemon juice or 1 teaspoon of vinegar to the water to increase the acidity of the solution. This releases even more alkaloids from tannin. Some brands of cat's claw tincture are made with vinegar. If you use one of these brands, you do not need to add lemon juice or vinegar to the water you use to wash down the tincture. If you do not use one of these types of tincture, or if you use pills or tablets, be sure to add lemon juice or vinegar to the water you drink while taking the herb to assure its bioavailability.

CATUABA

Latin name: *Erythroxylum catuaba* (Erythroxylaceae [coca] family)

General Description

Catuaba (pronounced with the accent on the last syllable) is a Brazilian rain forest tree with alternating leaves and trumpet-shaped flowers. It is in the same plant family as coca, the plant from which cocaine is derived, but lacks the narcotic alkaloids found in coca. The bark is used in herbal medicine.

Evidence of Benefit

Catuaba has been used as an aphrodisiac in the treatment of erectile dysfunction (ED) and prostatitis.

Benefits of catuaba for specific health conditions include the following:

• *Erectile dysfunction and prostatitis.* Catuaba is the most famous of the Brazilian aphrodisiac plants, noted for its ability to strengthen erections. The Tupi people, who first discovered the herb's sexually stimulating properties, even recorded its qualities in song. Catuaba's use results in increased erotic dreams and increased sexual interest. In cell studies, the herb also seemed to normalize prostate function.

• *HIV/AIDS.* Scientific studies in Japan have confirmed that catuaba inhibits the ability of HIV to destroy cells, but it has not been shown to be effective in patients. The herb may protect people with AIDS against infection with *Escherichia coli* (*E. coli*) or *Staphylococcus aureus*, but again these are in cell line studies. Catuaba is not recommended as a primary treatment for AIDS, but rather as a defense against opportunistic infection. Check with your doctor if you have HIV infection before using this herb.

Considerations for Use

Catuaba is most commonly available as a tincture. For maximum effect, take the tincture in a small amount of water to which is added 1 teaspoon (4 milliliters) of lemon juice. Acidifying the tincture releases alkaloids and tannins.

CAYENNE

Latin name: *Capsicum* species (Solanaceae [nightshade] family)
Other common names: African pepper, bird pepper, chili, chili pepper, goat's pod, paprika, red pepper, Zanzibar pepper.

General Description

Cayenne is a perennial but frost-sensitive shrub that grows to a height of three feet (one meter). It is covered with scarlet-red, conical fruits that, when fresh, contain plump, white seeds. Native to Mexico and Central America, cayenne was brought to Europe in the seventeenth century by the Spanish. It is a mainstay of the cuisines of much of Latin America and the American Southwest. Although cayenne is a unique species, any of the over 130 species of pepper that contain capsaicin can be used medicinally. The fresh or dried fruits are used medicinally.

Evidence of Benefit

Cayenne is an anti-inflammatory and anti-irritant. It relieves pain, has antimicrobial effects, and may even have an anticancer effect. It can ease aspirin-induced upset stomach, and is a digestive aid. It seems to be a detoxifying agent and specifically protects the stomach. It also may help blood clot more effectively. In folk medicine, cayenne has been used for painful muscle spasms, frostbite, and as a gargle for hoarseness and sore throats. It also was used for preventing seasickness, heart disease, and stroke. In ayurvedic medicine, cayenne is used for gout, arthritis, sciatica, coughs, and hoarseness. It can lower a fever associated with malaria, yellow fever, and scarlet fever. It is also used for cholera and edema. When combined with ginger and rhubarb, it can treat anorexia nervosa. As a homeopathic remedy, cayenne is used for inflammation of the urinary tract, alimentary canal, and mouth, and for middle ear infections.

Benefits of cayenne for specific health conditions include the following:

• *Arthritis, diabetic neuropathy, and sore muscles.* Capsaicin in cayenne acts as a counterirritant, causing temporary pain to the skin that depletes the chemical messengers of pain for the joint. Applied as a cream, capsaicin permeates the skin, enters the nerve, and eliminates substance P, which stops the pain message from reaching the brain. Leaving a concentrated form on the skin for a long period of time may cause skin irritation. However, a review of the medical literature failed to find overwhelming positive benefits over placebo in arthritis patients. In patients with diabetes who had nerve pain, cayenne cream was effective in some patients, but burning was a frequent side effect, and many patients stopped using it. Another group of patients with diabetes and nerve pain experienced significant reduction in pain status (a 45 percent reduction on the pain severity scale) using a 0.75 percent cream applied four times a day. Half of the patients improved or were cured. Cayenne seemed to relieve pain in patients with osteoarthritis rather than those with the rheumatoid form of the disease. In another study, patients with osteoarthritis used a 0.75 percent cream four times a day for four weeks. Afterward, they had less pain and were less tender. According to the German Commission E, cayenne is used for rheumatism and muscular soreness. Cayenne has been shown to reduce postoperative nerve pain after breast surgery, amputation, and thoracotomy.

• *Cough.* In one study, children with cystic fibrosis or asthma seemed to benefit from cayenne.

• *Female sexual dysfunction.* The herb cream improves circulation and may promote female orgasm. It should not be used for more than two days and then should not be used again for two weeks. Longer usage can cause festering dermatitis, blistering, and ulceration.

• *Overweight.* A clinical study conducted by scientists at Laval University in Quebec found that eating cayenne at breakfast decreased appetite and led to lower fat and calorie intake throughout the day. Cayenne helps boost your metabolism and induces the body to burn off more fat instead of storing it in the body. It may also help attenuate postprandial hyperglycemia when taking 30 grams per day of 55 percent cayenne.

• *Stomach ailments.* The inside of the stomach can be protected from extensive aspirin use by taking cayenne in advance of aspirin, as it delays gastric mucosal damage compared to aspirin alone.

Considerations for Use

For external application, use cayenne in the form of capsaicin cream; for internal applications, use cayenne powder, mixed with a starchy food. Do not apply capsaicin cream to broken skin, and avoid contact with the eyes or mouth. If redness occurs, stop using it. It should clear up within seventy-two hours. The daily dose is 10 grams externally in a cream and as a tincture of 1:10 dilution. Homeopathic remedies are 5 drops, 1 tablet, or 10 globules every thirty to sixty minutes for acute problems or one to three times a day for chronic issues.

Both capsaicin and cayenne are difficult to remove from contact lenses. Even cleaning the lenses twice will leave enough capsaicin to cause severe eye irritation. Do not use any lens that may be contaminated with capsaicin or cayenne without seeing an ophthalmologist or optometrist.

Some medical concerns exist. Long-term use in Mexico was associated with an increased risk of gastric cancer. Cayenne may be anticancer at low doses and carcinogenic at high doses. Topical application of more than 1 percent cream may be toxic to nerves. Cayenne may reduce the ability of the blood to clot and some people are allergic to it, experiencing sneezing and runny nose. Chronic exposure to this herb may lead to an increased cough. If you are using an ACE inhibitor (angiotensin-converting enzyme) and experience coughing, discontinue its use. If you are using anticoagulants, do not use cayenne. Concurrent use of barbiturates or aspirin with cayenne may decrease their effectiveness. If you are taking theophylline to help with breathing, the drug may become toxic if combined with cayenne, so they should not be used together.

Taking cayenne powder internally on a regular basis or eating a diet high in hot peppers reduces the ability of the activity of the liver enzyme known by the abbreviation

CYP1A2. The liver requires this enzyme to eliminate a number of common medications, including clomipramine (Anafranil), clozapine (Clozaril), imipramine (Tofranil), olanzapine (Zyprexa), tacrine (Cognex), theophylline (Elixophyllin, Theolair, Theo-Dur, and others), warfarin (Coumadin), and zileuton (Zyflo). It is possible that taking cayenne with any of these medications could increase the medication's side effects.

CHAMOMILE

Latin names: *Chamomilla recutita* or *Matricaria recutita* (Asteraceae [composite] family)
Other common names: Hungarian chamomile, wild chamomile

General Description

Chamomile is a sweetly aromatic annual plant native to Europe. Reaching a height of two feet (sixty centimeters), this herb has finely cut leaves and numerous flower heads with white petals and yellow centers. The flower heads, picked in full bloom in the summer, are preferred in herbal medicine.

Evidence of Benefit

Chamomile has antianxiety, antihistamine, anti-inflammatory, antioxidant, and antispasmodic properties. It also may lower blood sugar and protect against cancer. As an antibacterial herb, chamomile may inhibit the growth of underarm bacteria, which eliminates underarm perspiration odor.

Benefits of chamomile for specific health conditions include the following:

• *Allergies.* If chamomile is steamed or placed in hot water, a substance called chamazulene, which has markedly antiallergenic properties, is formed. Studies have found that chamazulene prevents the formation of inflammatory leukotrienes, thereby inhibiting the generation of toxic free radicals needed to trigger the allergic response. A compound in the herb's essential oil reinforces the effect of chamazulene by blocking the release of histamine. Chamazulene also stops stomach irritation caused by the release of free radicals that activate histamine. This explains chamomile's traditional use in soothing upset stomach.

• *Anxiety, attention deficit disorder (ADD), insomnia, and stress.* Chamomile has traditionally been used as a calmative for persons under stress. Herbalists especially recommend it for sleeplessness in children. Laboratory tests on animals show that inhaling the vapors of essential oil of chamomile reduces the body's production of adrenocorticotropic hormone (ACTH), a stress hormone. Inhaling the essential oil lowers stress and makes other stress-reduction drugs, such as diazepam (Valium), more effective.

• *Cuts, scrapes, and abrasions.* Chamomile creams reduce the "weeping" of fluid from cuts and scrapes and have been used on skin ulcers. A German study of people who had undergone dermabrasion for the removal of tattoos found that chamomile creams reduced both the amount of fluid lost and the size of the wounds. In another study, cancer patients receiving chemotherapy were given a mouthwash of chamomile three times a day for two weeks and their mouth sores did not heal better compared to a control group. However, in a case study on a woman who was receiving methotrexate for rheumatoid arthritis, a chamomile mouthwash was shown to help with mouth sores. The patient was completely healed after four weeks. According to the German Commission E, chamomile is approved for treatment of inflammation of the skin and mucous membranes and diseases of the skin and gums. It may also act as a deodorant.

• *Endometrial cancer.* Chamomile contains apigenin, a chemical that prevents the production of proteins that allow cancer cells from anchoring to new sites in cell lines.

• *Irritable bowel syndrome (IBS) and morning sickness.* Naturopathic physicians in the United States frequently recommend chamomile tea as part of a treatment program for IBS because of its antispasmodic properties, which also makes it useful in treating morning sickness. Chamomile is more effective when used with ginger. (*See* GINGER.)

• *Peptic ulcers.* For over twenty years, medical researchers have recognized the value of chamomile in preventing and treating peptic ulcers. Chamomile's anti-inflammatory and antihistamine actions soothe inflammation throughout the digestive tract. When the discomfort of peptic ulcers is compounded by diarrhea, chamomile hastens recovery, especially if a high-fiber diet is maintained.

• *Premenstrual syndrome (PMS).* Traditional herbal medicine in England used chamomile as one of the five "opening" herbs for the treatment of irregular menstruation. Chamomile contains spiroether, a very strong antispasmodic agent that relaxes aching and tense muscles, and alleviates premenstrual pain.

Considerations for Use

People who are allergic to ragweed or members of the Compositae family (chrysanthemums) should avoid contact with chamomile because it could produce dermatitis or anaphylaxis.

Chamomile is used in teas and tinctures internally, and in creams and compresses externally. (*See* COMPRESSES in Part Three.) More than those of most other herbs, the effects of chamomile are cumulative. Use chamomile for at least three to four weeks before deciding whether or not it is effective.

Choose products made from German chamomile,

Chamomilla recutita, or *Matricaria recutita,* rather than Roman chamomile, *Anthemis cotula.* In a few rare instances, Roman chamomile produces allergic skin reactions, but the allergenic compound in Roman chamomile is not found in German chamomile. It is also important to buy a chamomile product that consists only of flowers, without leaves and stems mixed in. Leaves and stems have much lower content of therapeutic essential oils than flowers.

Chamomile contains the natural blood-thinners known as coumarins. Since these chemicals in the herb are similar to the prescription drug warfarin (Coumadin), avoid chamomile teas when taking warfarin. However, some argue that the risk may not be significant and chamomile may be taken with warfarin. Check with your doctor if you are on blood-thinners before using chamomile. It may also cause drowsiness.

CHANCA PIEDRA

Latin names: *Phyllanthus niruri,* also known as *Phyllanthus amarus* (Euphorbiaceae [spurge] family)
Other common names: phyllanthus (in ayurvedic medicine), quebra pedra

General Description

Chanca piedra is a tropical plant that bears graceful branches of densely packed, alternating leaves growing from a central stem. Although chanca piedra is sometimes called "kidney stone tree," it is not a tree but rather a small herb. The aerial (aboveground) parts of the plant are used in herbal medicine.

Evidence of Benefit

Chanca piedra is used as a "stone breaker" in both human and veterinary herbal medicine. It is a favorite natural treatment for kidney problems in guinea pigs and hamsters. Scientists are investigating several compounds in the herb as antiviral treatments for hepatitis B and HIV.

Benefits of chanca piedra for specific health conditions include the following:

• *Diabetes.* Clinical trials with small numbers of patients in India have found that taking chanca piedra for a week lowers blood sugar levels in people with diabetes. This herb's main value in treating diabetes, though, is in the prevention of long-term complications within the eyes and central nervous system. If blood sugars are out of control for a long period of time, large amounts of glucose flow into tissues that do not need insulin to absorb it, especially the brain, nerve tissues, and the lens of the eye. An enzyme in these tissues, aldose reductase, converts glucose to sorbitol, which is a nerve toxin that destroys nerve tissues in the process of diabetic neuropathy. Japanese researchers have found that chanca piedra contains aldose reductase inhibitors that stop the process of nerve

damage in cell studies. It is not clear that it works this way for patients with diabetes. If you have diabetes, check with your doctor first before using this herb.

• *High blood pressure.* In about 60 percent of people who have primary high blood pressure, raising the amount of sodium (salt) in the blood starts a chain reaction that raises the kidneys' production of the enzyme angiotensin II, which causes the walls of the arteries to constrict, raising blood pressure. Scientists at Japan's Toyama University have isolated a compound from chanca piedra that acts on the kidneys as an angiotensin-converting enzyme (ACE) inhibitor, which reverses this effect. This action could lower blood pressure among people who are salt-sensitive, but there are no human studies to confirm this. The work was done in cell studies only.

• *Kidney stones.* The name of chanca piedra in Portuguese, *quebra pedra,* literally means "stone breaker." Traditionally, this herb has been used throughout tropical South America for the treatment of kidney stones and urinary tract infections (UTIs). A German physician, Wolfram Wiemann, gave chanca piedra to more than 100 people with kidney stones in Germany, and found that 94 percent of these people eliminated the stones within two weeks. He concluded that chanca piedra caused no side effects other than cramping during passage of the stones in a few people. Dr. Wiemann believed the herb provided a permanent cure for kidney stones. Subsequent research in Brazil has confirmed that chemicals in chanca piedra keep calcium crystals, especially crystals of calcium oxalate, from entering kidney cells. This was done in cell lines and not in human studies. If you have kidney stones, check with your doctor before using chanca piedra.

Considerations for Use

Chanca piedra is used in tablet and tincture form. Tablets are most often labeled by the ayurvedic name of the herb, phyllanthus, while tinctures are usually manufactured by companies that import the herb from South America and call it chanca piedra or quebra pedra.

CHAPARRAL

Latin name: *Larrea divaricata* (Zygophyllaceae [guaiac] family)
Other common names: creosote bush, gobernadora, hediondilla, larrea

General Description

The term *chaparral* refers broadly to a thicket of dwarf shrubs. The most common shrub in the chaparrals of the southwestern United States and northern Mexico is a dark-green, olive-scented shrub also known as chaparral. Extracts from this plant are, like creosote, used as a preservative for lumber. The leaves and flowers of the plant are used in herbal medicine.

Evidence of Benefit

Chaparral has potent and long-lasting anti-inflammatory and analgesic effects in the treatment of arthritis. It also has been shown to have anticancer effects. Nordihydroguai-aretic acid (NDGA), a compound found in chaparral, is a powerful antioxidant that may help to prevent the kind of cell damage that can lead to cancer. But this has only been shown in cell lines and animal studies. NDGA was removed from the U.S. Food and Drug Administration's Generally Recognized as Safe (GRAS) ingredient list in 1968 due to reports of liver damage. Chaparral is used for the common cold, menstrual cramps, and snakebites, to promote urination, and to control spasms.

Benefits of chaparral for specific health conditions include the following:

• *Arthritis and carpal tunnel syndrome.* The major traditional use of chaparral in Mexican herbalism is as a bath or liniment to relieve the inflammation and pain of arthritis, sometimes in combination with osha. (*See* OSHA.)

Considerations for Use

Chaparral should be used externally *only,* as a bath and in small amounts. (*See* HAND BATHS in Part Three.) In one seven-year period, there were eighteen reports of toxic liver damage from the internal use of chaparral in the United States. Some people required liver transplantation. Others reported side effects including fatigue, jaundice, cirrhosis, kidney failure, and renal cell carcinoma. Some people developed hepatitis from its use. Mexican toxicological studies have found that internal use of this herb causes serious signs of toxicity and pathological changes, such as a marked reduction of growth, pronounced irritability and aggressiveness, and a marked shrinkage of the testicles. In addition, chaparral contains compounds that can both increase the risk of sunburn and cause skin irritation to parts of the body not exposed to sun. When using chaparral, be sure to avoid sunlight exposure on any treated skin (or use a sunscreen), and do not use the herb more than once in any thirty-day period. Chaparral should not be used if you have kidney, lymph, or liver problems. If you are using MAO inhibitor drugs, excessive doses of chaparral may interfere with their effectiveness.

CHEN-PI

Latin name: *Citrus reticulata* (Rutaceae [citrus] family)
Other common name: bitter orange peel

General Description

Chen-pi is the fresh peel of the mandarin orange, the whole fruit of which is also used in herbal medicine. (*See* BITTER ORANGE.) Chen-pi comes in large pieces, thin-skinned, pliable, red, oily, and aromatic. The first taste of the herb is slightly sweet, but the aftertaste is bitter and then pungent.

Evidence of Benefit

Chen-pi has been used to quell allergic reactions and digestive upsets. In addition, it contains compounds that increase the heart's output and other compounds that act together as a contraceptive for women, but these findings were done in cells rather than people with these problems.

Benefits of chen-pi for specific health conditions include the following:

• *Allergies.* Chen-pi is used in traditional Chinese medicine (TCM) to prevent and treat allergic reactions. The whole fruit also can be used for this purpose.

• *Diarrhea, indigestion, nausea, and peptic ulcer.* Bitter orange peel teas may relax the body's smooth muscles. This may account for the herb's effect on the digestive system, relaxing the muscles that hold food in place in the digestive tract.

Considerations for Use

Bitter orange peel is used as a tea or tincture. TCM urges caution in using this herb when "red" symptoms (such as red tongue, redness in the face with fever and cough, and spitting of blood) are present.

Women who are pregnant or who have menstrual problems should not use this herb. In small doses, bitter orange peel inhibits contractions of the uterus and intestines, but in large doses, bitter orange peel stimulates contractions of the uterus and intestines.

CHINESE SENEGA ROOT

Latin name: *Polygala tenuifolia* (Polygalaceae [senega] family)
Other common names: polygala, polygala tenuifolia root

General Description

Chinese senega root is a low-growing perennial with lance-shaped leaves that have toothed edges. Its flowers are white tinged with mauve or yellow. Herbal medicine uses the white root.

Evidence of Benefit

Chinese senega root has been used for hangover. This herb also stimulates both bronchial secretions and uterine contractions, and kills some kinds of bacteria. However, these observations were made in cell line studies rather than in people.

Benefits of Chinese senega root for specific health conditions include the following:

• *Hangover.* Compounds in Chinese senega root affect the rate at which the body absorbs ethanol, the alcohol in alcoholic beverages. In animal studies, these compounds block as much as 90 percent of the ethanol that otherwise would have been absorbed into the body. Japanese researchers are developing products based on this herb to prevent alcohol intoxication.

• *Seizure disorders.* Physicians in Hong Kong report cases that indicate Chinese senega root reduces the chance that seizures will occur during periods of emotional stress.

Considerations for Use

Chinese senega root is best used as a tincture, but is sometimes prescribed by traditional Chinese medicine (TCM) practitioners as a tea. You should always use this herb under professional supervision, especially if you have a seizure disorder. You should not use Chinese senega root if you have gastritis or ulcers, or during pregnancy.

CHIRETTA

Latin name: *Swertia chirayita* (Gentianaceae [gentian] family)
Other common names: chirayata (Hindi), Indian balmony, Indian gentian, swertia

General Description

Chiretta is a native herb of the foothills of the Himalayas in northern India and Nepal. An annual growing to a height of three feet (one meter), chiretta bears a single stalk covered with pale green, purple-tinged flowers and paired leaves. The aboveground parts of the plant are harvested in summer when the plant is in flower.

Evidence of Benefit

Chiretta is a bitter herb that stimulates digestion, especially of fats, and helps to normalize blood sugars. It has been used for dyspeptic disorders, loss of appetite, and disorders of the GI tract.

Benefits of chiretta for specific health conditions include the following:

• *Diabetes.* Diabetic laboratory animals with high baseline blood sugar levels show reduced blood sugar levels after treatment with chiretta. However, animals do not show this reduction in sugar levels after treatment if they have low levels to start with. This suggests that chiretta may be useful in controlling blood sugar levels without the risk of hypoglycemia from overdose. Other animal studies have found that chiretta is more effective at controlling blood sugars than the common antidiabetic drug tolbutamide (Orinase).

• *Nausea.* The bitter taste of chiretta triggers a reflex reaction that stimulates the production of saliva and gastric juices. This action stops nausea as well as bloating, hiccups, and indigestion. It can help improve appetite.

Considerations for Use

Intensely bitter chiretta is best used as a tincture, although it is also available as a tea. A typical dose is 15 to 20 drops, three times a day before meals, or for nervous disorders, use the same amount between meals. Chiretta is also included in the imported Chinese patent medicine Tian Xian. Chiretta should not be used by people who have gastric or duodenal ulcers because it stimulates gastric juice secretion.

CINNAMON

Latin name: *Cinnamomum cassia* (Lauraceae [laurel] family)
Other common names: cassia, cinnamon bark, cinnamon twig

General Description

Cinnamon, used in cooking throughout the world, comes from a tropical evergreen tree that reaches a height of between thirty and sixty feet (thirty meters). The tree grows in low-lying rain forests in India, Sri Lanka, the Philippines, and the West Indies. Herbal medicine uses its soft reddish-brown bark and young twigs, both of which are cut and allowed to ferment in the field before being gathered for drying. Cinnamon leaf oil is also used.

Evidence of Benefit

Cinnamon is one of the world's most widely used digestive aids. It is also used as a supplement for loss of appetite and dyspeptic complaints, and it has been approved for use for these conditions by the German Commission E. In folk medicine cinnamon has been used for exhaustion and flatulence. Ayurvedic medicine employs it for toothache, nausea and vomiting, and dyspepsia. The cinnamaldehyde in the bark's essential oil is antibacterial and antifungal, and promotes gastric motility. It has a mildly estrogenic effect in animal tests. It may also serve as an insecticide.

Benefits of cinnamon for specific health conditions include the following:

• *Fibroids and menstrual problems.* Before the twentieth century, cinnamon tinctures were the standard remedy for uterine bleeding. Certain forms of cinnamon have been found to inhibit a substance in the blood called thromboxane A_2, which causes platelets in the blood to clump together and form clots. Inhibiting thromboxane leads to less clotting and a more normal blood flow. This action, paradoxically, reduces uterine bleeding by stimulating blood flow *away* from the uterus.

• *Indigestion.* Perhaps the most common medicinal application of cinnamon is in the relief of intestinal gas. Both teas and tinctures are equally effective in quelling flatulence.

• *Liver cancer.* Two chemicals extracted from cinnamon, camphornin and cinnamonin, have been shown in laboratory tests on cell lines to stop the growth of liver cancer and melanoma cells. Compounds in cinnamon are known to deactivate plasmin, a substance that allows cancer cells to infiltrate surrounding tissue. In addition, cinnamon stimulates the body's production of tumor necrosis factor

(TNF), an immune-system chemical that fights cancer. Cinnamon bark can contain the fungus *Antrodia cinnamomea*, producer of a substance that has been shown to kill leukemia cells in animal testing.

• *Peptic ulcer.* A compound found in cinnamon, propanoic acid, stops the formation of stomach ulcers without interfering with the production of gastric acid.

Considerations for Use

Cinnamon can be used as an oil added to water or as a tea, or it can be grated onto food. The daily dosage is 2 to 4 grams of the bark or 0.05 to 0.2 grams of essential oil. Cinnamon oil should not be used during pregnancy. People who are allergic to tolu balsam or any of the many products containing tolu balsam should avoid the medicinal use of cinnamon oils and the use of cinnamon oils in aromatherapy. (*See* TOLU BALSAM.)

CLOVE

Latin name: *Syzygium aromaticum* (Myrtaceae [clove] family)

General Description

The clove is an evergreen tree with pointed leaves that is native to the Molucca Islands and cultivated in Brazil, Madagascar, Indonesia, and Zanzibar (Tanzania). Oil of cloves is extracted from the leaf and/or flowers, and is the principal form of clove used medicinally. The fresh and dried flower buds are also used in herbal formulas in traditional Chinese medicine (TCM).

Evidence of Benefit

Oil of cloves is anti-inflammatory, antimicrobial, analgesic, antiviral, and antifungal. It may protect the liver, reduce inflammation of the mouth and pharynx, and help with dental pain when used as a topical anesthetic. It also may prevent cancer, inhibit platelet aggregation, and protect nerves from toxins. In ayurvedic medicine it is used for halitosis, eye disease, toothache, flatulence, colic, and anorexia.

Benefits of clove oil for specific health conditions include the following:

• *Food poisoning.* Clove oil kills some types of bacteria, including *Pseudomonas aeruginosa*, *Shigella* (all species), *Staphylococcus aureus*, and *Streptococcus pneumoniae*, all of which can be involved in food poisoning. However, it is not known as a food poisoning treatment.

• *Headache.* In one study, clove oil–containing ointment was effective in treating headaches. The ointment was rubbed on the forehead at thirty-minute intervals. Compared to a placebo, the participants had less pain at five minutes and at two hours. Another group got the standard treatment of paracetamol (acetaminophen), but the clove group got faster relief.

• *Herpes.* Clove oil increases the effectiveness of acyclovir (Zovirax), a drug used to treat the viral infections underlying these disorders.

• *Peptic ulcer.* Oil of cloves may reduce the sensation of gas pressure within the stomach that is frequently troubling for people with peptic ulcers. The eugenol in clove oil depresses the transmission of nerve impulses that convey a feeling of bloating and gas, although it does not directly stop the production of gas.

• *Periodontal disease and toothache.* Clove blossoms and clove oil have been used around the world for generations to relieve pain from toothache and dental treatment. Oil of cloves is combined with zinc oxide to make an analgesic paste that is inserted into the region of an extracted tooth to kill bacteria and reduce pain. Clove oil should be avoided, however, in treating pain due to root canal work, as it may cause inflammation.

Considerations for Use

Do not give clove oil to infants or children under the age of six, as it can cause gastric upset or excitement. Clove oil is very strong and can cause irritation if used in its pure form; mild high blood pressure can occur as well as difficult breathing. Diluting it in water or another type of oil, such as olive oil, is recommended. Mouthwashes of 1 to 5 percent of essential oil are used. People using anticoagulants should avoid using clove oil.

CODONOPSIS

Latin name: *Codonopsis pilosula* (Campanulaceae [bluebell or lobelia] family)
Other common name: poor man's ginseng

General Description

Codonopsis is a twining perennial. It reaches a length of 5 feet (1.5 meters) and has oval leaves and purple-veined green flowers. Herbal medicine uses the long, sweet taproot. It is a native of Asia and is now cultivated throughout the world.

Evidence of Benefit

Codonopsis has been used for stomach pain and headache. Codonopsis reduces stress and enhances tolerance to stress. It also boosts stamina.

Benefits of codonopsis for specific health conditions include the following:

• *Headache.* Codonopsis is employed in traditional Chinese medicine (TCM) to treat headaches accompanied by high blood pressure, muscular tension, and indigestion.

• *Lupus.* In cell studies, codonopsis restrains the immune system in lupus, a disease in which the immune system attacks the DNA found in the body's own skin cells. If you have lupus, ask your doctor before using this herb. It has not been shown to be effective in patients.

• *Peptic ulcer.* In animal studies, codonopsis has been found to prevent the formation of peptic ulcers induced by stress. Codonopsis may be useful for ulcers that are compounded by loss of appetite, diarrhea, or vomiting.

• *Vomiting.* Codonopsis has been used for centuries to treat appetite loss, diarrhea, and vomiting. Laboratory studies suggest that codonopsis extracts act by reducing the secretion of pepsin in the stomach and by slowing the rate at which the stomach passes food to the intestines.

Considerations for Use

Codonopsis is available in tablets, teas, and tinctures. It is a relatively inexpensive herb that is often substituted for ginseng in herbal tonics labeled as "ginseng." (*See* GINSENG.) While the substitution makes herbal formulas less expensive for manufacturers to produce, in many cases codonopsis is actually more effective for the intended purpose of the formula than the more expensive ginseng.

If you are interested in using codonopsis in the treatment of ulcers, you should do so under supervision of your doctor.

COIX

Latin name: *Coix lachryma-jobi* (Gramineae [grass] family)
Other common names: coicis, hatomugi, Job's tears

General Description

Coix is an East Asian grain that bears six to fifteen seed heads, similar to wheat's single seed head, on alternating sides of a single stalk. Grown throughout China as a food crop, coix is harvested at the end of autumn when its seeds have ripened. Quality coix seed is full, large, round, and white.

Evidence of Benefit

Coix contains some essential fatty acids that relieve inflammation and has some antiviral effects. However, it has only been tested in cell studies.

Benefits of coix for specific health conditions include the following:

• *Nails, infected.* In cell line studies in Japan, coix has been found to stop viral infections, such as those that cause warts under the nails, by stimulating the immune system to destroy infected cells. A study of seven healthy volunteers who took two capsules of coix three times a day for four weeks found that the herb stimulated production of T-helper cells, immune cells that stimulate other immune

cells to attack the virus. These people did not have nail problems, however.

Considerations for Use

Coix, a food as well as an herb, can be taken on a long-term basis. Coix cereal is available in Japanese groceries as hatomugi. Since coix promotes urination, it should not be used during pregnancy and by people who have urinary incontinence.

COLEUS

Latin names: *Coleus forskohlii,* also known as *Plectranthus barbatus* (Lamiaceae [mint] family)
Other common names: colforsin, makandi

General Description

Coleus is a highly aromatic type of mint that grows on the dry slopes of the Himalayan foothills. It is also found in gardens in warm temperate areas of Kenya, Myanmar (Burma), Nepal, Sri Lanka, and Tanzania, where it is used both medicinally and for flavoring pickles. The root and leaves are harvested at the end of summer or the dry season for medicinal use. In the United States, coleus is most often used as an extract standardized for its principal active constituent, forskolin.

Evidence of Benefit

Coleus is the most potent herbal antihistamine. It has been used for cancer, obesity, glaucoma, asthma, and heart failure. It has also been used for allergies, eczema, insomnia, and high blood pressure.

Benefits of coleus for specific health conditions include the following:

• *Asthma.* Forskolin, the main active ingredient of coleus, stabilizes the mast cells in the lining of the lungs to keep them from releasing massive amounts of histamine in response to irritation. It is able to open up the airways, acting as a bronchodilator. This prevents asthma attacks in response to exposure to dust particles, smoke, and allergens. A clinical study involving sixteen asthma patients in Austria found that forskolin can be more effective in controlling attacks than inhalers. The patients received 10 milligrams of dry forskolin powder and had improved bronchodilation.

• *Eczema.* One of the causes of eczema is believed to be a defect in the central nervous system's ability to activate beta-agonists, chemicals that stop the release of histamines that cause skin inflammation. Forskolin is not only a potent antihistamine in itself, but it also reactivates these chemicals. It also has been useful in treating psoriasis.

• *Glaucoma.* Coleus may reduce intraocular pressure (IOP), which is useful in treating glaucoma. In one study, forskolin in eye drop form was put in one eye and not the other; it was only effective at lowering IOP in the treated eye.

• *Heart disease.* Coleus has been shown to reduce blood pressure when given intravenously. In one study, it also improved left ventricular function, increased heart rate, and reduced arterial pressure. It also may increase cerebral blood flow and be useful after a stroke.

• *High blood pressure.* Coleus lowers blood pressure while slowing the pulse and strengthening the heartbeat, without increasing the heart's need for oxygen. Forskolin also relaxes the smooth muscles surrounding the arteries to lower blood pressure. The chemical accomplishes this by activating "slow" calcium channels, complementing the effect of prescription calcium channel blockers.

• *Overweight.* Forskolin has been shown to be useful for weight loss, as it stimulates fat burning in the fat cells. In one study, overweight women experienced an 8 percent loss of body fat after using coleus for eight weeks. In another study, participants did not lose weight when taking 500 milligrams a day of a coleus extract made up of 10 percent forskolin compared to a placebo. However, the treatment group had higher white blood cell counts, suggesting improved immune response. They also felt fuller but did not eat fewer calories.

Considerations for Use

Coleus should be used in the form of forskolin extract. Coleus products for high blood pressure frequently contain forskolin extract mixed with extracts of hawthorn and/or valerian that may not be listed prominently on the label. (*See* HAWTHORN and VALERIAN.) Coleus products for inflammation are frequently mixed with bupleurum and/or licorice. (*See* BUPLEURUM and LICORICE.) A daily dose is 5 to 10 milligrams of forskolin unless prescribed otherwise.

Because it relaxes and dilates the blood vessels, forskolin reduces the load on the heart. It also enhances the ability of heart muscle to contract, without affecting the heart's consumption of oxygen. Forskolin should not be used with anticoagulants because they inhibit platelet aggregation. People taking warfarin (Coumadin) or other blood-thinning medications should not take coleus or forskolin unless advised to do so by a physician. Forskolin may increase the effectiveness of antihypertensive drugs, so it should be avoided by those who use them. If you have low blood pressure or ulcers, or are pregnant or lactating, you also should not use this herb.

COLTSFOOT

Latin name: *Tussilago farfarae* (Asteraceae [composite] family)
Other common names: assfoot, British tobacco, coughwort, fieldhove, foalswort, horsehoof, tussilago

General Description

Coltsfoot is an herb that looks like the dandelion. Native to Asia and Europe, it has become naturalized in North America, where it is a common sight along roadsides and in open areas. It also has spread to the mountains of northern Africa. Herbal medicine uses the fresh and dried flower buds.

Evidence of Benefit

Coltsfoot relieves congestion. This property makes it useful in treating bronchitis, cough, laryngitis, and pneumonia. Coltsfoot alkaloids are antibacterial and anti-inflammatory. It is used for mild inflammation of the oral and pharyngeal mucosa. It has been used in cigarettes to help cure smoking addiction.

Benefits of coltsfoot for specific health conditions include the following:

• *Bronchitis, cough, laryngitis.* Small doses of coltsfoot open the bronchial passages, although large doses close them. The herb also contains mucilages that coat the throat, relieving irritation.

Considerations for Use

Coltsfoot is traditionally used in tea form, although it also appears in over-the-counter (OTC) formulas for colds and congestion. You should *not* give coltsfoot to a child in cold-remedy form.

Wild coltsfoot contains pyrrolizidine alkaloids, compounds that can induce liver cancer even in very small amounts. However, the amounts of these alkaloids that occur naturally in a standard dose of coltsfoot is less than one-hundredth of the amount that produces toxicity. Moreover, a genetically engineered variety of coltsfoot that contains none of the offending substances is now available. Therefore, you should use only a coltsfoot product that is *certified pyrrolizidine-free.* In particular, do not use tinctures. If other products with these alkaloids are used, you should not consume more than 1 microgram of total pyrrolizidine alkaloids with 1.2 unsaturated necine structure. The product should not be used for more than four to six weeks a year. When made with wild coltsfoot, such tinctures contain ten times the concentration of alkaloids as teas made with the same amount of the herb. In addition, wild coltsfoot tinctures can aggravate high blood pressure. No form of this herb should be used during pregnancy and lactation.

COMFREY

Latin name: *Symphytum officinale* (Boraginaceae [borage] family)
Other common names: ass ear, black root, blackwort, bruisewort, healing herb, knitbone, salsify, slippery root, wallwort

General Description

Comfrey is a European plant that has been naturalized in temperate zones around the world. A compact perennial that bears one or two stalks growing to a height of three feet (one meter), comfrey is distinguished by white, pink, or lavender flowers and arrowlike leaves. The entire plant is used in traditional herbal medicine, although only the dried aerial (aboveground) parts of the plant are reliably nontoxic. In much of central Europe, comfrey leaves make a traditional May Day salad, although the root should never be eaten.

Evidence of Benefit

Comfrey relieves pain and inflammation caused by injuries and degeneration, especially the symptoms of muscular skeletal disorders. Anticancer activity has been demonstrated for comfrey in cell lines. It can also be used for bruises and sprains and to promote bone healing. In folk medicine, the root was used for rheumatism, pleuritis, and as an anti-diarrheal agent.

Benefits of comfrey for specific health conditions include the following:

• *Inflammation.* Comfrey has been studied for use in musculoskeletal disorders. In one study, people with rheumatism were treated with a pyrrolizidine alkaloid–free ointment for four weeks. Not all subjects experienced improvements and it seemed to depend on the specific diagnosis. Comfrey seemed to work best on muscle pain (myalgia) and not as well on osteoarthritis-associated pain. Pain and functional complaints improved for all, but again the muscle pain group saw more improvement. The benefits were noted within four hours, so comfrey should be applied three times a day.

• *Pain.* Comfrey is used a pain reliever. In one study, an extract of comfrey root ointment was applied to the knees of patients with osteoarthritis for three weeks and their pain was significantly reduced during rest and movement. In another study, an ointment was applied to unilateral ankle sprains. The treated group had less swelling and pain, and improved mobility compared to a placebo group. The participants who received the ointment used it four times a day for eight days.

• *Skin problems and injuries.* Comfrey relieves pain and speeds healing of pus-filled wounds, and accelerates tissue healing in cases of insect bite. It treats skin tags and common, flat, and filiform warts. In addition, comfrey stops reddening and irritation of the skin around wrinkles. Comfrey's astringent tannins form a protective surface over wounds that promotes healing. This herb contains allantoin, a compound that helps stimulate the growth of new cells. It aids healing through cell proliferation.

Considerations for Use

The preferred way to use comfrey is as an allantoin cream. It can also be used in poultices. (*See* POULTICES in Part Three.) You should avoid letting the cream come into contact with unaffected skin and wash your skin after application, as allantoin may be irritating.

Comfrey leaf tea can be taken with calendula to alleviate gastritis. (*See* CALENDULA.) Compounding pharmacists can make this combination. Do not use comfrey pepsin tablets, as these are significantly more risky than comfrey tea. Comfrey *root* should *never* be taken internally. Comfrey contains pyrrolizidine alkaloids, which have been linked to liver and lung cancers, among other disorders, but the root is much more toxic than the leaf. Therefore, you should not use comfrey internally if you have liver disease or cancer, or if you regularly consume alcohol. In animal studies, comfrey has been shown to induce liver cancer.

As a further precaution against toxicity, do not use comfrey if you are taking antibiotics, prescription medication for yeast infections, fluoxetine (Prozac), cyclosporine (Neoral, Sandimmune, SangCya), cholesterol-lowering medications, calcium channel blockers for high blood pressure, or steroids in any form. These medications compete for a liver enzyme that is necessary to neutralize any toxic compounds that may be ingested with comfrey. Do not use orally for more than four to six weeks a year.

Applied to the skin as a cream, comfrey is nontoxic. The cream should be 5 to 20 percent of the dried herb. Daily doses should not exceed 100 micrograms of pyrrolizidine alkaloids. Comfrey should not be used on babies or during pregnancy.

COPAIBA

Latin name: *Capifera* species (Fabaceae [legume] family)
Other common names: balsam copaiba, copal, Jesuit's balsam, mal-dos-sete-días

General Description

Copaiba is a giant tropical legume found in the rain forests of Brazil, Colombia, and Venezuela. It grows to sixty to one hundred feet (twenty to thirty meters) in height. The part used medicinally is the resin that accumulates in cavities within the tree trunk. The tree is tapped in much the same manner as a rubber tree. Once its resin is collected, the sap is distilled to concentrate its essential oils.

Evidence of Benefit

Copaiba has been used for skin inflammation and irritation. Copaiba shampoos may relieve dandruff. Copaiba has beneficial effects on mucous membranes.

Benefits of copaiba for specific health conditions include the following:

• *Arthritis, eczema.* Copaiba may relieve the symptoms of a wide range of diseases that cause inflammation of soft tissue or mucous membranes. Laboratory tests show that the resin acts by reducing the permeability of capillary walls to histamine, the chemical responsible for painful swelling in all of these conditions. The volatile oil is antimicrobial and could prevent secondary infections in eczema, but this has not been shown to be true in people.

Considerations for Use

Copaiba is available as an oil and in shampoos for external use, and as a tincture for internal use. Taking very large amounts internally can be toxic. Many topical products combine copaiba with tolu balsam. If you are allergic to tolu balsam, you should make sure to use pure copaiba oil.

COPTIS

Latin name: *Coptis chinensis* (Berberidaceae [barberry] family)
Other common names: Chinese goldthread, coptidis, coptis rhizome

General Description

Coptis, a low-growing relative of the peony, is native to the mountains of China. Herbal medicine uses the root, which is dug up in the autumn and sliced.

Evidence of Benefit

Coptis is an East Asian relative of the American herb goldenseal. The best known of the herb's active constituents is berberine, a chemical coptis shares with barberry, goldenseal, and Oregon grape root. (*See* BARBERRY; GOLDENSEAL; and OREGON GRAPE ROOT.) Berberine has antimicrobial properties against *Escherichia coli* (*E. coli*) and other organisms. Berberine targets bacterial protein used in cell division and *E. coli* is unable to adhere to body tissues.

Benefits of coptis for specific health conditions include the following:

• *Diabetes*. This herb has traditionally been used for diabetes. In one study, patients with type 2 diabetes took 500 milligrams of berberine (the active main component in coptis) three times a day for thirteen weeks. In the group that took the plant extract, glucose regulation was improved to a degree similar to another group who received a glucose-lowering drug, metformin. The herb also lowered triglycerides and cholesterol in the blood, but the drug did not. About one-third of the subjects taking the herb complained of gastrointestinal discomfort, including diarrhea, constipation, flatulence, and abdominal pain. However, when the dose was reduced to 300 milligrams, three times a day, the symptoms went away.

• *Urinary infection*. In rats, berberine completely protected rat bladders from induced hemorrhagic cystitis. In clinical studies, berberine reduced stool *E. coli* content, diarrhea, and risk of urinary tract infection (UTI). It is more effective at preventing UTIs than treating them.

Considerations for Use

Coptis is available in capsules, ointments, powders, and tinctures. It can be used to make compresses and poultices.

When using coptis, it is very important to pay close attention to dosage. Small amounts of coptis stimulate the brain and result in alertness, while the use of large amounts result in drowsiness. Similarly, small doses of coptis increase blood pressure, but large doses lower it.

Coptis has several relatively uncommon side effects. There is some evidence that the berberine in coptis can interfere with the absorption of tetracycline antibiotics. It may also lower blood sugar, so if you have diabetes and have not used this herb before, you should use it with caution. The tannins in coptis tinctures may cause stomach irritation, so tinctures of the herb should be avoided if you have diarrhea or chronic heartburn. People with Raynaud's disease who use relatively high dosages of coptis may find that it aggravates numbness and tingling. This effect is minor and temporary. You should not use this herb if you are pregnant or nursing.

CORDYCEPS

Latin name: *Cordyceps sinensis* (Clavicipitaceae [antler fungus] family)
Other common names: dong chong xia cao, vegetable caterpillar, yarshagumba

General Description

The name *cordyceps* in Chinese literally means "winter bug summer herb." It is an antlered fungus that grows in insect larvae, usually before the insect's cocoon is formed. The short, sticklike fungus has a fat, full, round, yellow-white cross-section. It is gathered in the early summer. Although this fungus is found throughout Japan and in China, as well as on the Atlantic seaboard of the United States, it is very difficult to collect from the wild and so is usually grown in laboratories in tissue cultures.

Medicinal mushroom expert Christopher Hobbs writes that in ancient China, cordyceps was used exclusively in the emperor's palace because it was very scarce. It was prepared by stuffing it into the stomach of a duck, and then slowly roasting the duck over a low flame. Then the cordyceps was removed, and the duck was eaten for eight to ten days.

Evidence of Benefit

Cordyceps relieves conditions that traditional Chinese medicine (TCM) associates with the kidneys, including high cholesterol and ringing in the ears. It was also used for fatigue, sexual dysfunction, cough, and as an immune stimulant. The herb is an aphrodisiac that has been used as a cure for erectile dysfunction (ED). Cordyceps has been shown to increase testosterone in mice. It has also been used in cancer treatment and has antitumor effects in cells. Cordyceps strengthens the immune system of people who have undergone radiation therapy, chemotherapy, or surgery, and helps to strengthen people who have had long-term illnesses or suffer from exhaustion. Cordyceps is known to boost energy levels and increase endurance in athletes.

Benefits of cordyceps for specific health conditions include the following:

• *Cancer.* Cordyceps delays the diffusion of cancer cells and is able to control the division of cancer cells. It also increases the ability of the immune system's T cells and macrophages to engulf and destroy invaders. It therefore may aid in the fight against cancer. However, as yet, few clinical studies are available to support its use in cancer patients.

• *Congestive heart failure, kidney disease, lung cancer (in the elderly).* Cordyceps improves a variety of conditions in elderly patients. Patients with congestive heart failure had improved quality of life with 3 to 4 grams a day. Using 3 to 4.5 grams a day improved respiratory symptoms such as shortness of breath and sleep. Improved renal function was seen in patients with chronic renal disease such as creatinine clearance, blood urea nitrogen, and serum creatinine. More patients who had lung cancer completed radiation and chemotherapy with 2 to 5 grams of cordyceps.

• *Tinnitus.* Cordyceps helps people with tinnitus caused by fluid accumulation in the inner ear. It is not helpful for tinnitus accompanied by a long history of auditory nerve disorder, however. Elderly patients with tinnitus and other ailments such as fatigue, dizziness, and intolerance to cold had improvements with 3 grams a day.

Considerations for Use

Cordyceps is available in tablets and tinctures. You should not use it if you have a hormone-sensitive disorder such as breast cancer (for women) or prostate cancer (for men). Most manufacturers of cordyceps products also caution that the fungus should be used by adults only, and that people who use anticoagulant drugs, asthma inhalers, or immunosuppressant drugs for lupus, myasthenia gravis, psoriasis, rheumatoid arthritis, or Sjögren's syndrome should consult a health-care provider before using the herb.

CORN SILK

Latin name: *Zea mays* (Poaceae [haygrass] family)
Other common names: Indian corn, maidis stigma, maize silk, zea

General Description

Corn silk is a collection of the stigmas of the female flowers of the corn plant. It is gathered in summer immediately after the corn tassels appear but before the flowers are fertilized to produce kernels of corn. Although corn is native to Central America, most of the corn silk used in herbal medicine comes from Albania, Bulgaria, and the former Yugoslavia. The medicinal part is the seed.

Evidence of Benefit

Corn silk is a diuretic and a rich source of potassium. It is used for disorders of the urinary tract and as an aid in kidney and bladder disorders, although these uses are unproven. Traditional Chinese medicine uses it for treatment of the liver. Its active components stimulate the heart, increase blood pressure, and sedate the digestive tract.

Benefits of corn silk for specific health conditions include the following:

• *Carpal tunnel syndrome, high blood pressure, and premenstrual syndrome (PMS).* Corn silk encourages urination, while the potassium in the herb offsets potassium loss caused by increased urination. Compared with other diuretics, this combination in corn silk reduces the likelihood of muscle cramps and irregular heartbeat due to a loss of electrolytes through increased urination.

Considerations for Use

Corn silk is used as a tea. Use 2 teaspoons of the herb per cup of water. Drink one cup every other day. It also comes in a tincture that is prepared by adding 20 grams of the herb to 100 milliliters of 20 percent alcohol. Taken with the blood pressure drug quinapril (Accupril), corn silk can cause excessive potassium levels, leading to heart flutter, muscle twitches, or even atrial fibrillation, a disturbance in heart rhythm in which the heart muscle twitches rapidly and weakly rather than beating strongly and steadily. Taken with the appetite suppressant drug phentermine (Adipex-P, Fastin, Phentercot, Zantryl, and others), however, corn silk helps to conserve potassium and to prevent loss of coordination and fatigue.

CORYDALIS

Latin name: *Corydalis yanhusuo* (Papaveraceae [opium poppy] family); *C. cava*
Other common names: corydalis rhizome, early fumitory, squirrel corn, turkey corn, yan-hu-suo

General Description

Corydalis is a low-growing plant with narrow leaves and pink flowers native to northern China, Japan, and Siberia. This opium-poppy relative survives the harsh conditions of northeast Asia by storing most of its energy reserves in its hard bright yellow tuber. It also is indigenous to southern and central Europe in the *Corydalis cava* form. The root is unearthed in autumn, dried, and then sliced into cross-sections for use in herbal medicine. The active compounds, such as tetrahydropalmatine, which is associated with analgesia and sedation, are found in lesser amounts in the *C. cava* form compared to the Chinese *C. yan-hu-suo* form.

Evidence of Benefit

Corydalis is hypnotic, sleep-inducing, hallucinogenic, sedative, and tranquilizing. It also suppresses the central nervous system, reduces blood pressure, and impedes movement of the small intestine. Folk medicine used it for worm infestation, menstrual disorders, and Parkinson's disease. Externally it was applied to poorly healing wounds and ulcers. Homeopathy corydalis remedies help with inflammation associated with the respiratory tract and eyes, rheumatism, and diarrhea.

Benefits of corydalis for specific health conditions include the following:

• *Anxiety, insomnia, and restless legs syndrome.* The sedative qualities of corydalis make it useful in the treatment of insomnia and anxiety. Its alkaloids increase the sleep-inducing effect of barbiturates and are about 40 percent as effective as morphine in inducing sleep. American herbalists blend corydalis with California poppy to treat nervousness, insomnia, agitation, and anxiety. (*See* CALIFORNIA POPPY.)

• *Cataracts.* Alcohol extracts of corydalis slow the formation of cataracts associated with diabetes.

Considerations for Use

For anxiety, insomnia, and restless legs syndrome, corydalis is best used blended with California poppy. In the treatment of cataracts, corydalis should be used under professional supervision only. Muscle tremors can occur with too high a dose.

Corydalis should not be used during pregnancy. Continuous use of corydalis results in tolerance and may also lead to a cross-tolerance to morphine. Anyone who uses any type of a sleeping aid, especially a barbiturate, should be careful of the additive effects of sleeping pills and corydalis.

COUCH GRASS

Latin names: *Elymus repens, Graminis rhizoma,* or *Agropyron repens* (Poaceae [haygrass] family)
Other common names: dog grass, quackgrass

General Description

Couch grass is an invasive weed found in the Americas, northern Asia, Australia, and Europe. It is similar to, and sometimes misidentified as, Johnson grass. A vigorous perennial growing to a height of three feet (one meter), couch grass has long, creeping rhizomes, slender leaves, and erect flower spikes bearing green flowers in two rows. The rhizome and the seeds are used in herbal medicine.

Evidence of Benefit

Couch grass is a rich source of healing mucilages that soothe and relieve inflamed sore throat. It has been used to treat difficult urination and kidney stones since the time of the Roman Empire.

Benefits of couch grass for specific health conditions include the following:

• *Kidney problems.* Couch grass is useful for inflammatory diseases of the urinary tract and for prevention of kidney stones.

Considerations for Use

Couch grass is used as a tea or used to irrigate the kidneys. When used as an irrigant, it is important to consume copious amounts of water. No irrigations should be done in those with edema due to heart or kidney failure. The bulk herb is available from online retailers and in herb shops. Herb gardeners attempting to grow couch grass should exercise caution, since it easily becomes an uncontrollable weed.

DAMIANA

Latin name: *Turnera diffusa* (Turneraceae [damiana] family)

General Description

Damiana is an aromatic shrub of the hot and humid reaches of Texas, Mexico, Central America, and Namibia. Growing to a height of six feet (two meters), it bears upward-growing stems with pale, smooth, green leaves and small, yellow flowers. The leaves are harvested for medicinal use in summer, when the plant is in flower.

Evidence of Benefit

Few clinical studies have been performed on damiana. Animal studies indicate that the herb has blood sugar–lowering effects and is an anti-inflammatory. It also seems to bind progesterone but not estrogen and may be helpful in menopause formulas and to increase sexual function. Damiana has been associated with improved sexual function for both men and women. It contains elements that directly stimulate the nerves, genitals, blood circulation, and metabolism. It has been reported to give a mild narcotic "high" that lasts for about an hour. Longer use of damiana increases its potency and helps to regulate sex hormones in women.

Damiana along with other herbs is used to treat sexual trauma, lack of sexual desire and pleasure, and erectile dysfunction (ED). However, it must be used consistently for several weeks before an effect is noticed. It may also act to clear the kidneys, help with digestion, relieve constipation, clear coughs, and help control bed-wetting.

Damiana is a stimulating nerve tonic used for debility, depression, and lethargy. It is used in Germany for its tonic action on the hormonal and central nervous systems.

Benefits of damiana for specific health conditions include the following:

• *Depression, nervousness.* Damiana has been used to stimulate people with depression because it is a natural monoamine oxidase (MAO) inhibitor. However, there is as yet no clinical research on its use in treating depression. It may also help to increase the appetite and to reduce. nervousness.

• *Erectile dysfunction, menopause-related problems, and reduced sex drive.* Damiana has been used as an aphrodisiac since the time of the Maya. A clinical study involving 1,000 men in the United States and Europe indicates that the herb can relieve erectile failure in attempts at repeated intercourse after orgasm. A combination of damiana and muira puama is associated with an increased frequency of intercourse, morning erections, and stability of the erection during intercourse. (*See* MUIRA PUAMA.) In women, in addition to anecdotal reports of increased sex drive, damiana helps reduce hot flashes.

Considerations for Use

Damiana is available as a tincture, in capsules, and dried for making teas or smoking. If damiana is taken in large doses, the tannins it contains can interfere with the absorption of iron from food or supplements, and also with the absorption of many common medications. This effect can be avoided by adding a teaspoon of lemon juice to the water in which the tincture is taken. It also can increase the effect of diuretics.

Damiana can lower blood sugar. People with type 1 diabetes should use this herb with caution. It may also cause low blood sugar if it is taken with sulfonylureas, which are used to treat diabetes. This class of drugs includes glipizide (Glucotrol), glyburide (DiaBeta, Glynase, Micronase), tolbutamide (Orinase), and others.

Damiana is on the U.S. Food and Drug Administration's generally recognized as safe (GRAS) list and is widely used as a food flavoring. However, damiana contains low levels of cyanidelike compounds, so excessive doses may be dangerous. There is a report of someone who drank 8 ounces and experienced tetanus-like convulsions. Its safety for young children, pregnant or nursing women, and people with severe liver or kidney disease has not been established. The only common side effect of damiana is occasional mild gastrointestinal distress.

DAN SHEN

Latin name: *Salvia miltiorrhiza* (Lamiaceae [mint] family)
Other common names: cinnabar root, red root sage, tan shen

General Description

Dan shen is a hardy perennial mint cultivated in Mongolia and Manchuria. Growing to a height of thirty-two inches (eighty centimeters), it has toothed oval leaves and clusters of purple flowers. The root harvested from late autumn to early spring is used in herbal medicine. It is coarse and purplish-black inside, with small white spots.

Evidence of Benefit

Dan shen is commonly known as a heart tonic. It has been used to strengthen and tone the heart and helps it to beat in a steady, regular rhythm. It may also help the liver and stimulates the production of bile.

Used in traditional herbal medicine to prevent pain, dan shen also protects nerve cells from free-radical damage in cell studies. Benefits of dan shen for specific health conditions include the following:

• *Fibroids (uterine myomas) and menstrual problems.* Dan shen is useful for short-term treatment of skipped periods or uterine fibroids. Authorities on traditional Chinese medicine (TCM) note that the herb "releases" congealed blood, as shown by dark-red clots during menses, and eases pelvic congestion.

• *Heart disease.* Dan shen extracts relax the smooth muscles that support the coronary arteries and increase circulation to the heart. The herb contains a substance called tanshinone IIA_1, which slows the transmission of nerve impulses within the heart, slowing the pulse while increasing the heart's ejection fraction, or the percentage of available blood that the heart's main pumping chamber pumps into the blood vessels with each beat. This work was done in rabbits, so whether it works in the same way in people is not known. If you have heart disease, check with your physician first before using this herb.

In laboratory tests, dan shen was shown to prevent the formation of clots in the bloodstream and reduce blood cholesterol and triglyceride levels. It enhances the heart-healthy effect of unsaturated fatty acids and protects heart and nerve cells from a kind of free-radical damage known as reperfusion injury, which occurs when blood circulation is restored after heart attack or stroke, by increasing the effectiveness of vitamin E. Clinical researchers in China have reported improvements in people taking dan shen for angina, stroke, and phlebitis. Surgical experiments with animals indicate that dan shen may prevent recurrence of blockages after angioplasty.

• *Hepatitis.* Dan shen may be effective in treating chronic hepatitis. Experimentally, it has been reported to be effective in suppressing fibrosis in the liver. If you have hepatitis, check with your doctor before using this herb.

Considerations for Use

Dan shen is used in tea and tincture forms. For angina and other circulatory problems, you should use this herb only under professional supervision.

Long-term use of dan shen for fibroids or menstrual

problems can be harmful, since the herb stimulates estrogen production. Dan shen should be used for such conditions only under the supervision of a knowledgeable practitioner and for no more than twenty-eight days at a time, followed by a four-week break. You should not use dan shen at all if you have an estrogen-sensitive disorder such as breast cancer. People taking warfarin (Coumadin), aspirin, or nonsteroidal anti-inflammatory drugs (NSAIDs) on a regular basis also should avoid dan shen entirely, because it increases the risk of bleeding. You should inform your physician or dentist prior to any surgical or dental procedure if you are taking this herb.

DANDELION

Latin name: *Taraxacum officinale* (Asteraceae [composite] family)
Other common names: blowball, cankerwort, Irish daisy, lion's tooth, monk's head, priest's crown, swine snout, wild endive, witch's gowan, yellow gowan

General Description

Known best in North America as a weed that pops up in freshly cut lawns, dandelion grows wild in most of the world and is cultivated as an herb in China, France, and Germany. Young leaves are picked in the spring for tonic salads. In the early summer, before the plant blooms, leaves are harvested for the manufacture of medicinal teas and tinctures. The roots of two-year-old plants are dug in the fall, when they have their greatest concentration of the complex carbohydrate inulin, for use in tablets and tinctures.

Evidence of Benefit

Historically, the herb was considered a rich source of beta-carotene and potassium. According to folk medicine, dandelion was used for disturbances in bile flow, inflammatory conditions of the urinary tract, and dyspepsia. It was also used for liver and gallbladder disorders, hemorrhoids, gout, rheumatic disorders, eczema, and other skin conditions. The herb has a diuretic effect and is used for kidney and bladder complaints. Traditional Chinese medicine (TCM) uses it for acute mastitis and urinary disorders. Ayurvedic medicine uses it for chronic ulcers, tuberculosis, flatulence, colic, kidney disease, gout, and liver ailments. The German Commission E has approved it for stomach complaints, infections of the urinary tract, liver and gallbladder complaints, and loss of appetite. However, in a comprehensive review on the topic in humans, dandelion did not reduce inflammation, work as an antioxidant, counter cancer or colitis, treat diabetes, or work as a diuretic. New work has shown that it can suppress the growth of colon cancer cells and mouse melanoma cell lines.

Benefits of dandelion for specific health conditions include the following:

• *Bladder infection and premenstrual syndrome (PMS).* Unlike many conventional diuretics, which cause a loss of potassium, dandelion leaves are rich in potassium. Using the herb as a diuretic results in a net gain of this vital mineral. Because of its diuretic effect, dandelion helps to relieve fluid retention in PMS and counteract urine retention in bladder infections.

• *Constipation, hemorrhoids, and indigestion.* German research has shown that dandelion root is a mild bitter, or appetite stimulant. Bitters of all types activate a reflex that increases the secretion of digestive juices by the lining of the stomach. Dandelion root has a significant cleansing effect on the liver by stimulating the production of bile, which ultimately results in increased transport of a variety of potentially noxious compounds to the stool. Increasing the release of bile also relieves constipation without causing diarrhea and stops spasms of the bile duct.

• *Liver problems and gallstones.* The bitter principles in dandelion increase bile production and bile flow in the liver. This makes it useful for people with sluggish liver function due to alcohol abuse or poor diet. It is restorative to the liver and helps reduce the risk of developing gallstones, but you should avoid it if you already have gallstones, since increasing the flow of bile could increase pressure against the stones.

• *Overweight.* European herbalists frequently prescribe dandelion tinctures as a weight-loss aid. Dandelion reduces water weight through its diuretic effect. Dandelion may increase bile flow to improve fat metabolism in the body. In one laboratory study, animals that were given daily doses of dandelion extract for a month lost up to 30 percent of their body mass.

Considerations for Use

Dandelion can be taken in tablet, tea, or tincture form. Tea can be consumed in the morning and evening. If you use a tincture, 10 to 15 drops should be taken three times a day.

Dandelion may cause increased stomach acidity and ulcer pain. Some people have reported heartburn, stomachache, and mild diarrhea with its use. There have also been rare reports of low blood sugar, contact dermatitis, and allergies. If you have ileus, gallstones, or biliary tract obstructions, you should avoid this herb. Dandelion should not be used as a substitute for pharmaceutical diuretics for hypertension. If you are using potassium supplements, avoid taking dandelion because it may interfere with the absorption of the supplements. Dandelion may increase the risk of bleeding in those who are using anticoagulant drugs. People with known allergies to related plants, such as chamomile and yarrow, should use dandelion with caution.

Dandelion also should be avoided during antibiotic treatment, especially treatment with ciprofloxacin (Cipro), ofloxacin (Floxin), lomefloxacin (Maxaquin), norfloxacin (Noroxin), and enoxacin (Penetrex), since it may keep concentrations of these antibiotics from peaking in the bloodstream, diminishing their ability to fight infection.

DEVIL'S CLAW

Latin name: *Harpagophytum procumbens* (Pedaliaceae [sesame] family)
Other common names: grapple plant, wood spider

General Description

Devil's claw is a trailing perennial vine native to the Transvaal of South Africa. Bearing bright purple flowers with five petals in early spring, the plant grows to a length of 5 feet (1.5 meters). It is especially common along roadsides and on sandy soils from which other vegetation has been cleared. The plant gets its name by virtue of its barbed, fibrous fruit, but the root is the part of the plant used in herbal medicine.

Evidence of Benefit

Devil's claw is an anti-inflammatory and painkilling agent when used in its recommended form. It also inhibits the production of inflammatory compounds that worsen many diseases, such as heart disease and diabetes. In folk medicine, devil's claw has been used in an ointment for skin injuries and disorders. As a dried root, it is used for pain relief, pregnancy discomforts, arthritis, allergies, and disorders of the kidney, bladder, liver, and gallbladder. It has also been used in South Africa as an appetite stimulant. As a homeopathic remedy, it can be used for chronic rheumatism. According to the German Commission E, it is approved for stomach complaints, loss of appetite, and rheumatism. However, there are numerous conflicting reports in clinical studies on its use as an anti-inflammatory agent. It may be that it is more effective when combined with an anti-inflammatory herb, such as willow bark.

Benefits of devil's claw for specific health conditions include the following:

• *Arthritis, carpal tunnel syndrome, gout, and tendinitis.* The use of devil's claw in the treatment of pain required a number of tests before the herb was accepted within the scientific community. Animal tests showed that it relieves inflammation and stops pain, but the first set of tests with healthy human volunteers found no significant anti-inflammatory or analgesic power. Moreover, chemical analysis of the herb found that it did not act in the same way as aspirin and nonseroidal anti-inflammatory drugs (NSAIDs). The resolution of the conflicting findings concerning devil's claw is that the analgesic components of the herb break down the longer they are in contact with the gastric juices of the stomach. Taking devil's claw in an enteric-coated form protects it from digestion in the stomach. This increases its usefulness in controlling pain.

Repeated clinical trials found enteric-coated tablets of the herb effective against pain. Questions about the pharmacology of the herb were clarified when it was discovered that devil's claw contains chemicals, like those in many other pain-relieving herbs, that stimulate circulation and carry inflammatory chemicals away from affected tissues.

Devil's claw has been most extensively tested for relief of lower back pain. In an open label study, seventy-five patients with knee or hip osteoarthritis took 2.4 grams of devil's claw from a product called Doloteffin for twelve weeks. Standardized measurements of pain and disability were reduced by 25 percent and adverse side effects were minor. A randomized, double-blind study in Germany with 183 subjects produced the surprising result that not only was devil's claw effective in relieving lower back pain, it was most effective for people who had the most severe, radiating pain, with numbness in the extremities.

Considerations for Use

To relieve pain, devil's claw has to be taken in the form of an enteric-coated capsule. Enteric-coated capsules should be taken one hour *before* meals. Since the pain-relieving chemicals in the herb are activated by intestinal bacteria, the herb is less effective during and for one to two weeks after antibiotic treatment of any kind. It can also be used in an ointment or a liquid extract. The daily dosage for appetite loss is 1.5 grams of the herb. In homeopathy, devil's claw doses are 5 to 10 drops, 1 tablet, or 5 to 10 globules, one to three times a day. The ointment should be applied one to three times a day.

Devil's claw should not be used in the presence of stomach or duodenal ulcers because it stimulates gastric juices. If you have gallstones, consult a doctor before using this herb. It may interact with and decrease the effectiveness of anticoagulants and cardiac antiarrhythmic drugs. Devil's claw may also interact with antacids, rendering them less effective, and with digoxin by weakening heart muscle contractions. It may slow heart rate in people with congestive heart failure. Occasionally, devil's claw causes mild diarrhea. If this happens, you should take the next dose on an empty stomach. You should not use devil's claw if you are pregnant or nursing.

DIOSCOREA

See WILD YAM.

DONG QUAI

Latin name: *Angelica sinensis* (Apiaceae [parsley] family)
Other common names: Chinese angelica root, dang gui, tang kuei

General Description

Dong quai is the dried and sliced root of Chinese angelica, a plant native to China, Korea, and Japan. When grown under cultivation, this plant is a sturdy perennial that reaches heights of up to six feet (two meters). The herb bears bright green leaves and clusters of white flowers.

Evidence of Benefit

Dong quai has different actions depending on which part of the root is used. The head of the root has anticoagulation properties and the main root serves as a tonic and pain reliever. The tail of the root eliminates blood stasis. Dong quai has antispasmodic effects. It also relieves some, but not all, of the symptoms of menopause and premenstrual syndrome (PMS). It is used in the treatment of arthritis, chronic kidney inflammation, various blood-vessel disorders, pernicious anemia, and neuralgia. In traditional Chinese medicine (TCM), dong quai is used to treat boils that develop at sites of injury to the skin. It is also used in TCM for treating amenorrhea, menopausal symptoms, and fibroid tumors. In addition, it has been used for high blood pressure, rheumatism, ulcers, anemia, allergies, constipation, and to strengthen the uterus before pregnancy. In Japan, dong quai is used as an analgesic, sedative, and nutrient.

Benefits of dong quai for specific health conditions include the following:

• *Atherosclerosis, heart attack, and high blood pressure.* Dong quai teas contain active compounds that prolong the resting period between heartbeats and dilate the coronary blood vessels, increasing coronary blood flow. Together, these actions lower blood pressure. Of additional importance to people at risk for heart attack, dong quai inhibits the release of a chemical in the blood that promotes the formation of clots and starts inflammatory reactions. Experiments with animals have found that dong quai reduces the formation of atherosclerotic plaques on artery walls.

• *Infertility.* One of the chemical components of dong quai, ferulic acid, increases the motility and viability of sperm cells by protecting their membranes from the action of cell-harming free radicals. There is some evidence, however, that ferulic acid *increases* the risk of free-radical damage to sperm cells in men undergoing chemotherapy with bleomycin (Blenoxane), a cancer chemotherapy treatment sometimes chosen for its relatively minor effects on the immune system.

• *Leukemia and other cancers.* Some herb experts have speculated that dong quai has the potential to protect healthy white blood cells during chemotherapy. Dong quai is known to contain compounds that, possibly when activated by exposure to sunlight as white blood cells circulate to the skin, greatly increase the effectiveness of chemotherapy drugs for leukemia, thereby indirectly sparing healthy cells. One study found that a water extract of dong quai was shown to have estrogen activity. Women

at risk for breast cancer should carefully consider the use of this herb, and if you have breast cancer, you should not use it at all.

• *Menopause-related problems, menstrual problems, migraine, ovarian cysts, and premenstrual syndrome (PMS).* One of dong quai's best-known uses is that of a regulator for the female reproductive system. Some of its compounds stimulate the uterus, while others relax the uterus. The compounds that stimulate the uterus are water-soluble and are absorbed into the body from teas or capsules containing freeze-dried herb. The compounds that relax the uterus have a very high boiling point, are soluble in alcohol, and are provided by tinctures.

There is some agreement among herb experts that this herb helps stop cramping and migraine attacks of PMS, and eases the pain of ovarian cysts. There is less agreement over whether it stops hot flashes. In 2004, the North American Menopause Society stated that there is insufficient evidence that dong quai is superior to placebo for reducing menopausal vasomotor symptoms. In a study completed in 2004, 354 women with two or more symptoms were randomized to three groups: black cohosh; multibotanicals with black cohosh and dong quai and eight other herbs; and soy with the same multibotanicals. After one year, none of the three treatments led to meaningful reductions in menopausal symptoms. However, many women have reported that taking the herb for four to six weeks stops hot flashes related to entering menopause. Most women report that the herb is better for intermittent hot flashes than for unremitting heat. It is reportedly more effective for women who enter menopause after surgery. These women tend to have more severe hot flashes than women who enter menopause gradually. A clinical study at San Francisco's Kaiser Permanente Center was unable to confirm a benefit of the herb in treating hot flashes, but the investigation was limited to women who had not had surgery to remove their ovaries. Investigations into dong quai's actions at a chemical level tend to confirm that it can control hot flashes in cell lines but not necessarily in humans. One of the chemicals in the herb stops the production of free radicals of nitric oxide that cause veins to dilate just before a hot flash. In one study, fifty women (ages 44 to 65 years) took dong quai along with other herbs such as milk thistle and red clover and they experienced fewer hot flashes, a reduction in night sweats, and improved sleep quality. However, it is not clear that these actions were attributable to dong quai alone.

Considerations for Use

Dong quai is available in a variety of forms—oral, subcutaneous for use in acupuncture therapy, and an intravenous form that is available in China. In extract or tablet form dong quai is usually taken in amounts of 2 to 3 grams two to three times a day. It is important to remember that the compounds in dong quai that stimulate the uterus are water-soluble, and absorbed into the body from all forms *except* tinctures. The compounds in dong quai that relax the uterus are soluble in alcohol, and are absorbed into the body *only* from tinctures. It is best to avoid all forms of dong quai during pregnancy and breast-feeding. You should not use dong quai tinctures to treat insufficient menstrual flow, as they will further decrease flow. You should avoid dong quai for thirty days after the first symptoms of a herpes infection or recurrence, as this herb inhibits the body's defenses against the virus.

Dong quai is contraindicated for patients with hemorrhagic disease, excess blood loss during menses, chronic diarrhea, abdominal bloating, or acute infections like a cold or flu. Possible side effects from its use include fever, gastrointestinal disturbances, and increased bleeding. There has been one report of serious bleeding in a woman who was taking warfarin (Coumadin) at the same time as dong quai. The woman recovered one month after discontinuing the herb. People who take prescription blood-thinners should avoid this herb.

Avoid exposure to the sun if you are taking dong quai, as it can cause photodermatitis (an abnormal skin reaction to the sunlight, or more specifically, to ultraviolet [UV] rays). While this effect is very rare, persons taking prescription medications that increase risk of sunburn, such as angiotensin-converting enzyme (ACE) inhibitors (including captopril [Capoten], lisinopril [Prinivil, Zestril], and fosinopril [Monopril]) for high blood pressure, should avoid dong quai. Also, patients taking benzodiazepines may experience increased muscle relaxation and sedative effects. For those taking testosterone, watch for increased androgenic effects, such as acne, hirsutism, and behavior changes.

ECHINACEA

Latin name: *Echinacea* species, especially *Echinacea angustifolia* and *Echinacea purpurea* (Asteraceae [composite] family) Other common names: black sampson, hedgehog, purple coneflower, red sunflower, rudbeckia, sampson root

General Description

The echinaceas are a group of North American prairie perennials known for their purple daisylike flowers and leaves covered with coarse hairs. Growing to a height of twenty inches (fifty centimeters), they are native throughout the United States east of the Rockies. They also have been naturalized in Europe. The medicinal parts, depending upon the variety, are the roots, leaves, and whole plant.

Evidence of Benefit

Echinacea is used extensively to boost the immune system, treat colds and flu, fight infection, help speed wound healing, and reduce inflammation. Herbal medicine generally uses two species of echinacea, *E. angustifolia* and

E. purpurea. Since each of the species has slightly different effects, specific disorders are usually best treated with one or the other.

Researchers have found that echinacea's immune-stimulating properties are due to a host of polysaccharides and phytosterols. They help to activate macrophages that are directly involved in the destruction of bacteria, viruses, and other infectious agents. Echinacea also increases production of interferon, an important part of the body's response to viral infections such as colds and flu. It has been specifically shown to activate an important class of white blood cells known as natural killer (NK) cells.

In folk medicine, Native Americans used this herb externally for burns, swelling of the lymph nodes, and insect bites. Internally, it was used for pain associated with headaches and stomachaches, measles, coughs, and gonorrhea. It was also used for rattlesnake bites. Today, the herb is used for prophylaxis and treatment of flu, sepsis, and mild to moderate cold infections. Externally, the herb is used for treatment of poorly healing wounds and inflammatory conditions such as abscesses and leg ulcers. There is no evidence that echinacea is useful for those who are at increased susceptibility to infection due to temporarily lowered resistance, treatment of leucopenia following radiation therapy, or chemotherapy. On the other hand, the German Commission E has approved the *E. purpurea* herb for use for the common cold, coughs and bronchitis, fever and colds, infections of the urinary tract, inflammation of the mouth and pharynx, infections, and wounds and burns.

Benefits of echinacea for specific health conditions include the following:

• *Chronic fatigue syndrome (CFS) and yeast infection. E. purpurea* acts against *Candida albicans,* the microorganism that can cause yeast infections. In German studies, echinacea acted by stimulating the immune-system cells known as macrophages to engulf and consume yeast cells by 30 to 45 percent, but did not increase the numbers of immune cells overall. The advantage of keeping the number of macrophages constant is that it helps to avoid inflammatory reactions that can accompany infection. These studies were on animals and human studies do not exist. Echinacea could be useful for people with CFS because yeast infections may accompany symptoms of this disorder. *E. purpurea* has been shown to stimulate cellular immune function of immune cells in patients with CFS.

• *Colds, cough, influenza, and upper respiratory infections.* Echinacea is one of the most studied herbs in humans; still there is quite a bit of conflicting data on whether it is effective at preventing colds or for shortening their duration once they appear. The major problem is that echinacea preparations differ widely from one clinical trial to another. There are more than 200 different preparations that use various species and parts of the plant (root, herb, or both), as well as many methods of extracting the active ingredient. Adding to the confusion is that some so-called echinacea-containing products contained no herb at all.

In 2006, a Cochrane Collaboration review was conducted that compared the effectiveness of echinacea with a placebo, no treatment, or another treatment. This is a system often used in medicine to compare different studies on the same thing, such as a particular herb or drug. Of the sixteen studies identified, most looked at whether echinacea was effective for preventing and treating a cold. Nine out of the sixteen studies showed that echinacea was beneficial for treating a cold, but not one showed echinacea to be effective at reducing the chances of catching a cold. Because of the lack of standardization of the herb, another comprehensive review of eleven studies found echinacea not to be beneficial for treating the common cold.

Even when a standardized echinacea was used in a well-controlled study, where 437 participants were given a cold virus, there was no difference from the placebo group in length of sickness, the amount of virus measured in the blood, volume of nasal secretions, or nasal-lavage specimen measurement of key immune-system cells. This study used *E. angustifolia* root.

• *Ear infection. E. angustifolia*, especially when used with goldenseal, stops drainage and speeds healing. (*See* GOLD-ENSEAL.) This combination of herbs increases the body's production of immune globulins that attack both bacteria and viruses, such as those that commonly cause ear infection.

• *Herpes.* Treatment with the plant and root extract of *E. purpurea* had no significant benefit in patients with recurrent genital herpes.

Considerations for Use

Since *E. angustifolia* and *E. purpurea* are not completely interchangeable, you should try to use the species of echinacea suited to each specific condition. (The entries for specific disorders in Part Two designate appropriate species, forms, and dosages.) All forms of echinacea are extraordinarily nontoxic. Do not take echinacea for longer than three months. If used over the long term, *E. purpurea* can deplete the body's stores of vitamin E.

Depending upon which form is used, there are different recommended daily doses. For the *E. purpurea* herb, the dose is 6 to 9 milliliters of the juice; for the *E. purpurea* root, it is 30 to 60 drops as a tincture, and for the *E. pallid* herb and root, a daily dose is 900 milligrams. For the *E. angustifolia* herb and root, there is no daily dose because of the lack of efficacy. For external use, at least a 15 percent pressed juice product is desirable.

Side effects of all forms are minimal and rare except when it is provided intravenously or used for longer than the recommended time. With intravenous use, side effects include headache, dizziness, nausea, constipation, skin redness, and some breathing difficulties in persons known to have other allergies.

If you have an autoimmune disease such as rheumatoid arthritis or lupus, or a chronic infection such as HIV/AIDS or tuberculosis, you should not use echinacea. This is especially important for persons with HIV/AIDS. In stimulating immune function, echinacea slightly increases the production of T cells, the immune cells attacked by HIV. When there are more T cells, the virus has both more cells to infect and more opportunities to mutate into a drug-resistant form. People with diabetes and those who tend to get allergies should not get intravenous echinacea.

If you are trying to get pregnant, it is probably best not to take echinacea. Both of the most widely used echinacea species contain a substance that can interfere with the release of unfertilized eggs into the fallopian tube, so they may decrease a woman's fertility. This has only been demonstrated in animals, however.

There are numerous drug interactions with echinacea that pose major and moderate risks. There is preliminary evidence that *E. purpurea* contains chemicals that deactivate CYP3A4, a liver enzyme that breaks down a wide range of medications. These medications could theoretically increase in the blood, causing an overdose state. The medications processed by this enzyme include anabolic steroids and corticosteroids; the chemotherapy drug methotrexate (Rheumatrex, Trexall), used in the treatment of cancer and lupus; astemizole (Hismanal), an antihistamine prescribed for allergies; nifedipine (Adalat, Procardia) and captopril (Capoten), used for high blood pressure; sildenafil (Viagra), prescribed for erectile dysfunction (ED); and many others. In general, *E. purpurea* seems to interact with the same medications that interact with grapefruit juice or quercetin. (*See* QUERCETIN.) While this possible effect of echinacea might help maintain levels of these drugs in the bloodstream and make them more effective, it might also cause them to accumulate to levels at which they produce side effects. If the expected side effects of any of these medications occur while taking echinacea, discontinue the herb.

Echinacea should be used with caution by people who are allergic to ragweed or to plants in the sunflower family. Claims that a combination of echinacea and goldenseal boosts the immune system have been borne out by laboratory experiments with animals that show that the two herbs augment different, but complementary, immune globulins. Before taking an echinacea-and-goldenseal combination, be sure to observe the precautions listed for goldenseal. (*See* GOLDENSEAL.)

Echinacea should be avoided immediately before, during, and after organ transplantation if a drug such as cyclosporine (Neoral, Sandimmune) or tacrolimus (Prograf) is prescribed to prevent rejection of the transplanted organ. Taking basiliximab (Simulect), an immunosuppressant, daclizumab (Zenapax), azathioprine (Imuran), and other drugs to prevent organ rejection with echinacea is not advised because the effectiveness of the drug will be reduced.

ELDERBERRY

Latin name: *Sambucus nigra* (Caprifoliaceae [honeysuckle] family)
Other common names: black-berried alder, boor tree, bounty, elder, elder black, ellanwood, ellkorn

General Description

The elder is a deciduous tree that grows to thirty-five feet (twelve meters) in height, and bears oval leaves and cream-colored flowers followed by purplish-blue berries in autumn. Native to Europe, elder is especially common in England, where is it is a popular hedge tree. The flowering tops and berries of the plant as well as the bark, dried roots, and fresh leaves are used in herbal medicine.

In England, elder was once known as "nature's medicine chest." The Druids believed that elder was inhabited by the Elder Mother, and that cutting the branches of the tree without first repeating a placatory incantation would invite her wrath.

Evidence of Benefit

Elderberry is one of the most effective herbs for preventing and treating colds and upper respiratory infections, eczema and other skin disorders, and to reduce pain and inflammation. It may also be helpful for patients with diabetes, as it fosters increased glucose uptake out of the blood into the tissues. Elderberry stimulates the immune system and has shown some activity in preliminary trials against viruses such as herpes simplex and HIV.

In folk medicine, elder flowers are used internally as a tea for colds and fever. Elder flower also serves as a gargling mixture for respiratory disorders such as coughs and head colds. It has been used by nursing mothers to increase lactation. Elderberry has been used for swelling and inflammation. Homeopathic remedies exist for inflammation of the respiratory tract. Elderberry is approved by the German Commission E for coughs and bronchitis as well as for fevers and colds. It also may be good for hay fever and sinusitis.

Benefits of elderberry for specific health conditions include the following:

• *Asthma, bronchitis, influenza, and sinusitis.* Elderberry contains substances that disarm the neuraminidase enzyme of flu viruses, preventing them from penetrating healthy cells. It has been shown to be effective against eight strains of flu virus; vaccines are usually only effective against one or two types. Once infected, elderberry has been shown to speed recovery by as many as three days. A clinical trial of elderberry syrup (Sambucol) found that it cured 90 percent of flu infections within seventy-two hours. In the same trial, patients receiving a placebo needed six days for recovery. Later these same investigators found that 15 milliliters of the same syrup four to five times a day shortened symptoms by four days. Those using the elderberry also were less likely to use other symptom-relief medications. Elderberry also relieves nasal congestion, fever, and sore throat.

Considerations for Use

Elderberry is best used in the form of Sambucol, a patented herbal medicine from Israel that is active against various strains of viruses. The daily dose is 10 to 15 grams. It also comes as tinctures and is used in teas. It is preferable to use Sambucol rather than unprocessed elderberries. Some reported side effects include dizziness, headache, convulsions, and rapid heartbeat. Large dosages of elderberry juice can also cause uncontrollable diarrhea. Uncooked or unripe berries can cause nausea and vomiting. The stem of the plant should be *avoided* due to its cyanide content.

Elderberry should not be used with patients who have diabetes or low blood iron. The herb seems to form a complex with iron, which may become toxic in the blood.

ELECAMPANE

Latin name: *Inula helenium* (Asteraceae [composite] family)
Other common names: alant, elfdock, horse-elder, inula, scabwort, velvet dock, wild sunflower, yellow starwort

General Description

Elecampane, a flowering perennial in the sunflower family, is related to echinacea. Native to Europe and temperate Asia, it bears asterlike yellow flowers at the top of its ten-foot (three-meter) stems. The root is dug in autumn, washed, cut up, and dried at a high temperature for use in herbal medicines. It has recently been introduced into the United States and China.

The Latin name of elecampane comes from Helen of Troy, who was supposed to have carried the herb with her while being abducted by Paris. The herb was used by the ancient Greeks and Romans to treat indigestion, melancholy, sciatica, cough, bronchitis, and asthma.

Evidence of Benefit

Elecampane is regarded as a long-term treatment for respiratory diseases such as asthma and bronchitis. It is also recommended as a daily supplement to improve digestion. It also is used for menstrual cramps, worm infestation, and headaches. Homeopathic preparations are used for stomach ulcers and chronic cough. It has antibacterial and antifungal effects in cell lines. One of elecampane's active ingredients, alantolactone, has been used to treat intestinal parasites. It also is somewhat effective against yeast infections.

Benefits of elecampane for specific health conditions include the following:

• *Bronchitis and pneumonia.* Elecampane contains inulin, a mucilage-like polysaccharide that may coat the linings of the bronchial passages. The herb's essential oil is antibacterial.

Considerations for Use

Elecampane is available in capsules, tinctures, and teas; as an ayurvedic medicine called a rasayana; and in combination with other ayurvedic herbs in a commercial preparation. The daily dose of elecampane is 1 gram.

Repeated use of elecampane may cause allergic sensitivity. Symptoms of overdose are cramps, diarrhea, vomiting, and signs of paralysis. It also can cause contact dermatitis. In rare cases, it may be necessary to use a stomach pump and treat the poisoning with medication. Animal studies have shown a reduction in blood sugar with small doses of elecampane, and an increase in blood sugar with large doses. Until further testing shows otherwise, people with diabetes should avoid elecampane. It should not be used by pregnant women or nursing mothers.

EPHEDRA

Latin names: *Ephedra sinica, Ephedra equisetina, Ephedra intermedia* (Ephedraceae [ephedra] family)
Other common names: ma huang, Mormon tea

General Description

Ephedra is a shrub with long, narrow, sprawling stems and very small leaves. At a mature height of only twenty inches (fifty centimeters), the herb is well suited to the cold, windy deserts of its native northern China and Mongolia. Ma huang (the Chinese name for ephedra) is on a list of 365 herbs that dates back to the first century and is the basis of the modern Chinese materia medica.

The herb ephedra is banned in the United States though it is still allowed to be sold in dietary supplements sold by licensed practitioners in traditional Chinese medicine (TCM) formulations that are recommended for their TCM uses. For this reason we have included formulas in this book that contain ephedra. However, we do not recommend using this herb. If you are considering using one of the formulas in this book that contains ephedra, seek the advice of a TCM provider.

EPIMEDIUM

Latin name: *Epimedium grandiflorum* (Berberidaceae [barberry] family)

Other common names: goat wort, herba epimedii, horny goatweed, inyokaku, yin yang huo

General Description

Epimedium is a low-growing herb in the same family as coptis. (*See* COPTIS.) Often used in Chinese medicine as a pungent tea, its yellow-green leaves are traditionally steeped in wine before being fashioned into pills. Its Chinese name yin yang huo is literally translated as "herb for the licentious old goat."

Evidence of Benefit

Epimedium is a versatile Chinese herb traditionally used to treat fatigue, erectile dysfunction (ED), infertility, forgetfulness, back pain, and arthritis. Because of epimedium's ability to dilate capillaries and other blood vessels, it is used to facilitate blood circulation to the brain as well as to the sexual organs, while also lowering blood pressure. Epimedium also stimulates the production of male sex hormones and tonifies the liver. The herb is neuroprotective, has anticancer effects, is an immune-modulator, and has been shown to have anti-HIV activity in cell lines. In Asia, it is used in cancer treatment.

Benefits of epimedium for specific health conditions include the following:

• *Osteoporosis.* One form of epimedium, *E. brevicornum,* is rich in phytosterols that may prevent postmenopausal osteoporosis. In one study, a standardized mixture derived from this herb was given to half of a group of approximately eighty-five Chinese women who took four capsules a day; the other half took four placebo pills. Both groups also took calcium. After two years, lumbar spine and bone mineral density were significantly better in the *E. brevicornum* group. The authors concluded that the herb helped inhibit bone reabsorption, favored bone formation, and helped prevent bone loss in postmenopausal women.

• *Sexual dysfunction.* Traditional Chinese medicine employs many different herbs including epimedium for raising sexual energy in both men and women. Cancer patients may experience symptoms of sexual dysfunction that include painful intercourse, loss of libido, and difficulty maintaining arousal. These symptoms may be caused by stress hormonal changes due to nervousness about their condition. It is advisable for patients with hormone-sensitive cancers to avoid epimedium, as it has estrogenic effects.

Considerations for Use

Epimedium tablets should be taken as directed by an herbalist. It is a relatively nontoxic herb, but with prolonged use can cause side effects such as dizziness, vomiting, dry mouth, increased thirst, or nosebleed. It also has been shown to induce hyperactivity, spasms, and cramps. If any of these symptoms appear, discontinue the herb. Extreme overdoses can result in exaggerated reflexes, spasms, and respiratory arrest. People with prostate disorders or high blood pressure should avoid epimedium. In addition, patients with congestive heart failure should avoid this herb, as it causes shortness of breath, chest pain, and new arrhythmias.

ESPINHEIRA SANTA

Latin names: *Maytenus* species, especially *Maytenus chuchuhuasa* and *Maytenus ilicifolia* (Celastraceae [tripterygium] family)
Other common names: cancerosa (Spanish), limaosinho (Portuguese), maytenus (in English-language publications outside the United States)

General Description

Espinheira santa is a South American holly. It has an evergreen, hollylike appearance. Throughout South America, the bark or leaf of the plant is soaked overnight in aguardiente (rum) and used as a household remedy for the relief of arthritis, rheumatism, and back pain.

Evidence of Benefit

Espinheira santa has been used as a pain reliever and a muscle relaxant that is good for back pain, arthritis, and rheumatism. It may also help for nervous disorders and helps to soothe and heal stomach ulcers. It also supports the adrenal glands, which may help to improve energy levels, immune response, and digestion.

Benefits of espinheira santa for specific health conditions include the following:

• *Gastritis*. Espinheira santa regulates the production of hydrochloric acid by the stomach and helps to heal wounds in cell lines in animal studies. This explains why it is used in a traditional Brazilian antacid remedy for ulcers. Animal studies show that the herb does not interfere with normal digestion and, when taken orally, has no sedating side effects. Laboratory studies suggest that it may be as effective as the common prescription drug cimetidine (Tagamet).

Considerations for Use

Espinheira santa is available as a tincture. The herb is also sold as unprocessed leaf for use in teas, but almost all vendors require a minimum purchase of 1 kilogram (2.2 pounds), enough herb to supply one person for several years.

EUCALYPTUS

Latin name: *Eucalyptus globulus* (Myrtaceae [clove] family)
Other common names: blue gum, fever tree, gum tree, red gum, stringy bark tree

General Description

Eucalyptus, used in traditional aboriginal herbal remedies, is a tree native to Australia and Tasmania. It is cultivated in warm climates in southern Europe, Africa, Asia, and the Americas, and is used extensively as an ornamental tree in California. The fresh leaves and branch tips can be harvested at any time of year and distilled for their essential oil. Dried leaves can also be used. A closely related plant, *E. macrorryncha,* is a good source of rutin, a bioflavonoid widely recommended for strengthening blood vessels.

Evidence of Benefit

Eucalyptus contains the chemical eucalyptol, which has decongestant and antiseptic properties. It is most commonly used internally to clear the respiratory tract, and externally for rheumatic complaints. Eucalyptus has been used in folk medicine internally for the treatment of bladder diseases, asthma, fever, flu, whooping cough, liver and gallbladder complaints, loss of appetite, and diabetes. Externally it was used for wounds, acne, poorly healing ulcers, stomatitis, bleeding gums, neuralgia, gonorrhea, and as a gastrointestinal remedy. It can be added to toothpaste and mouthwash because it has antiseptic properties. The German Commission E has approved the use of the oil for cough and bronchitis and rheumatism, and of the leaf for cough and bronchitis. A tea made from eucalyptus has been shown to clear clogged nasal passages and prevent wounds from becoming infected.

Eucalyptus has myriad pharmacological properties, including: antibiotic, antifungal, insecticidal, and anticaries agent. It works on the skin and contaminated clothing. One form of the herb, *E. grandis* leaves, has been shown to inhibit the growth of cancer cells of the skin and lung in mouse studies.

Benefits of eucalyptus for specific health conditions include the following:

• *Allergies, common cold, cough, bronchitis.* Eucalyptol, found in many over-the-counter remedies, loosens phlegm in the chest and helps to open clogged nasal passages. It kills several types of bacteria and viruses, including *Escherichia coli, Klebsiella pneumoniae,* and *Salmonella cholera sui.* Using 100 milligram capsules three times daily of cineole (a component in eucalyptus) allowed patients with a cold (termed non-purulent rhinitis) to feel better at day four and day seven of using the herb. Patients had fewer headaches on bending and less nasal secretion and obstruction.

• *Dental plaque.* When used in a chewing gum, the amount of plaque buildup was significantly reduced.

• *Fungal infections.* People with athlete's foot who were treated with a 1 percent eucalyptus oil ointment for one week were cured of the infection.

• *Headaches.* In one study, using eucalyptus and peppermint oil improved cognition performance and muscle and mental relaxation in people with headaches. No changes occurred in pain sensitivity, however. The preparations were applied to the forehead and temples using a small sponge.

• *Minor cuts, tick and insect bites.* Because of its antiseptic properties, eucalyptus can be used as a topical antiseptic for minor cuts and scrapes. A eucalyptus-based insect repellent known as PMD has been shown to be effective in protecting study volunteers from various types of biting insects, including the *Anopheles* mosquito (the insect that spreads malaria), for up to five hours. A eucalyptus extract (Citriodiol) works on repelling mosquitoes, midges, and stable flies, and also is effective at reducing the number of tick bites. In one study, tick attachments decreased from 1.5 ticks to 0.5 over a two-week period in participants who lived in a tick-infested region. In another study, patients with incurable malodorous neoplastic ulcers of the head and neck were given eucalyptus-based oil that they applied twice daily. The study found that the skin ulcers cleared up and the foul smell that is typical of ulcers disappeared by day four. In addition, the quality of life of these patients improved because the foul smell was gone.

Considerations for Use

Eucalyptus is used in aromatherapy and steam inhalations, and is also available in capsule and tea forms. Daily doses of the leaf are 4 to 6 grams and 0.3 to 0.6 gram from the oil. Side effects are rare and include nausea, vomiting, and diarrhea. In addition, there have been reports of skin redness, rash, and a burning stomach pain.

You should never apply eucalyptus oil directly to the nostrils or take it internally, especially in children who may develop laryngeal spasms. Taken internally, eucalyptus oil is highly poisonous. If eucalyptus oil is accidentally swallowed, seek emergency medical help. Since there is a remote possibility that cineole, a component in eucalyptus, may trigger seizures in children, eucalyptus products should not be used around a child who has had seizures or any child under the age of two. Eucalyptus oil affects liver enzymes and can weaken or shorten the effects of other drugs. It should not be used in those who have hypersensitivity to eucalyptus, inflammatory diseases of the gastrointestinal tract or the bile ducts, and serious liver disease. Eucalyptus may lower blood sugar, so those who are already using drugs to lower blood sugar should carefully monitor their blood sugar levels. Concurrent use with barbiturates is ill advised because the herb decreases the drugs' effectiveness. Liver problems may develop when eucalyptus is used with comfrey, borage, coltsfoot, and hound's tooth.

When using eucalyptus, it is important to follow directions carefully, as overdosing is possible. Overdosing can lead to life-threatening poisonings. Such poisoning in children has been reported in the medical literature; over one twelve-year period, there were reports of 109 children being hospitalized from eucalyptus poisoning in one hospital in Australia.

EYEBRIGHT

Latin name: *Euphrasia officinalis* (Scrophulariaceae [snapdragon] family)
Other common name: euphrasia

General Description

Eyebright is a creeping herb related to the snapdragon. It has small, scallop-edged white flowers with yellow spots and a black center, somewhat resembling a bloodshot eye. Historically, eyebright's use for eye problems was due to the Doctrine of Signatures, a sixteenth-century theory that held that a plant's appearance indicated the conditions it could treat. The aerial (aboveground) parts of the plant are used in herbal preparations.

Evidence of Benefit

Eyebright is, as its name suggests, the most widely recommended herb for eyestrain, eye inflammations, stinging and weeping eyes, and oversensitivity to light. It is also used for coughs and hoarseness and seems to protect the liver against poisoning. Eyebright has anti-inflammatory and astringent properties that make it useful in treating congestive states such as hay fever, sinusitis, and nasal congestion. There is also some evidence that individual chemicals in eyebright may be useful for treating other problems, including hepatitis B and respiratory infections.

Benefits of eyebright for specific health conditions include the following:

• *Conjunctivitis and bloodshot eyes.* Many herb experts have expressed the opinion that eyebright's centuries of use as a remedy for conjunctivitis and bloodshot eyes is insufficient to commend it for modern use. Their rejection of this herb is due to the fact that detailed study of some of the chemicals in eyebright was not completed until 1999. Although there is no specific evidence that eyebright as a whole is particularly useful for eye conditions, there is considerable evidence that compounds in the herb are anti-inflammatory. The eyebright chemicals aucubin, ladroside, and veronicoside have been shown to stop inflammation in laboratory animals. Aucubin also stimulates the production of proteins that are involved in the process of healing. Few clinical studies in humans exist.

Considerations for Use

Eyebright is used in compresses and eyedrops, but it also comes in capsule and tablet form. Commercial preparations are preferable to compresses made from home-brewed eyebright teas because they are less likely to be contaminated by bacteria. Some over-the-counter (OTC) eyebright tablets combine the herb with other nutritional factors useful in maintaining ocular health, including bilberry, rutin, and hesperidin. Eyebright tablets can be used along with eyebright compresses and drops for additional benefit.

FENNEL SEED

Latin name: *Foeniculum vulgare* (Apiaceae [parsley] family)
Other common names: bitter fennel, fenkel, fennel fruit, large fennel, sweet fennel, wild fennel

General Description

Fennel is a vegetable with a bulbous, celery-like stem and feathery leaves. It is believed to have originated in the Mediterranean. Today, it has spread to England, Germany, and Argentina. It is also found in Iran, India, and China. The aromatic yellow-green fennel seed used in herbal medicine dries on the plant and is harvested in autumn when the fruit has ripened. Seeds have 4 to 5 percent essential oil. Fennel seed is a common cooking spice and is used in several cultures to prevent gas and upset stomach. It is one of the most important herb crops in Europe, where it is processed into dragées (lozenges), honeys, juices, syrups, and waters.

Evidence of Benefit

Fennel is an antispasmodic, diuretic, pain-reducer, and fever-reducer. It also promotes gastric motility. In folk medicine, the herb was used for fish tapeworms, skin conditions, and various eye complaints, including conjunctivitis. Fennel is also used to stimulate appetite, to soothe digestion, and to hasten healing of muscle strains and hernia. According to the German Commission E, fennel oil and seed are approved for coughs, bronchitis, and dyspeptic complaints.

Benefits of fennel for specific health conditions include the following:

• *Asthma, bronchitis, coughs.* Fennel also has a calming, antispasmodic effect on coughs and bronchitis. The Greeks use teas made from fennel and anise for asthma and other respiratory ailments. Both of these herbs contain creosol and alpha-pinene, which help to loosen bronchial secretions, although fennel seeds contain as much as 8,800 parts per million (ppm) of alpha-pinene, while anise contains only 360 ppm.

• *Dyspepsia.* Fennel relaxes the smooth muscle lining of the digestive tract to aid in digestion. It also helps in expelling gas and kills some types of bacteria. Both fennel seed tea and *diluted* fennel seed oil reduce intestinal spasms, but *pure* fennel seed oil can cause burning inflammation of the lower gastrointestinal tract.

Considerations for Use

Fennel seed is used as essential oil or tea. The daily dose of oil is 0.1 to 0.6 milliliter after each meal. As a tea the daily dosage is 5 to 7 grams of the seed. The tea can be used to make compresses. The need to use fennel for more than two weeks suggests a misdiagnosis; if the symptoms you are treating do not improve in that time, consult a physician.

Fennel seed oil should not be used during pregnancy or for infants and toddlers. Side effects are rare, but sometimes allergies arise, which affect the skin and respiratory system. People with diabetes should consider the sugar content of fennel syrup and honey preparations before taking them; some have enough sugar to affect blood levels and blood sugar–lowering medications.

FENUGREEK

Latin name: *Trigonella foenum-graecum* (Fabaceae [legume] family)
Other common names: bird's foot, Greek hay seed

General Description

Fenugreek is the hard brown, red, and yellow "bean" (seed) of the fenugreek plant, a member of the legume family. This native of the Mediterranean coast of Europe is cultivated for medicinal use in China, India, Morocco, and Turkey. The plant is an annual that grows to a height of a little less than three feet (one meter), and bears three-part leaves along with yellow-white pealike flowers. Fenugreek has been used both as a medicine and as a food spice in Egypt, India, and the Middle East. Fenugreek's ripe, dry seeds are used in herbal treatments.

Evidence of Benefit

Used for centuries in Arabian, Greek, and Indian medicine (unani, sidha, and ayurveda), fenugreek contains potent antioxidants that have beneficial effects on the chemistry of the liver and pancreas. The herb also is used to ease digestive-tract disorders and to enlarge the breasts. Historically, it was used to lower blood sugar and cholesterol levels and for respiratory ailments, and was applied topically for local inflammation, ulcers, and eczema. Although nursing mothers are sometimes told to take it to increase milk production, there is no indication that it promotes lactation. Chinese medicine uses the herb for treating pain in the lower abdomen, erectile dysfunction (ED), and hernia. Ayurvedic medicine uses it for fever, vomiting, anorexia, coughs, bronchitis, and colitis. It is approved by the German Commission E for loss of appetite (used internally) and inflammation of the skin (used externally as a poultice).

Benefits of fenugreek for specific health conditions include the following:

• *Diabetes.* Compounds in fenugreek may help with blood sugar control. Mucilages (25 to 45 percent of the seeds) released from the herb coat the lining of the intestines and keep the stomach from emptying quickly, with the result that glucose enters the bloodstream more slowly after a meal. In addition, an amino acid present in fenugreek, 4-hydroxyisoleucine, stimulates the pancreas to secrete insulin in diabetic rats that received an intraperitoneal version. In humans, fenugreek increases the number of insulin binding sites, which enhances glucose utilization. Fenugreek also contains compounds that help muscle tissue and the liver respond better to insulin, acting in a manner similar to glimepiride (Amaryl) and the "glitazone" drugs, such as rosiglitazone (Avandia). Clinical studies in India have found that relatively large doses of fenugreek seeds (25 grams, or nearly an ounce per day) as an ingredient in bread for fifteen days resulted in a lower blood glucose response to a glucose tolerance test in people with type 2 diabetes. Overall, blood sugar levels were 11 percent lower when fenugreek was consumed compared to when it wasn't.

Other Indian clinical studies have found that larger doses of fenugreek seeds, 100 grams (nearly 4 ounces) per day, have even more dramatic effects in people with type 1 diabetes. In one study, fenugreek treatment reduced the blood glucose levels in response to a glucose tolerance test and the excretion of glucose via the urine by 54 percent. This study also found that fenugreek lowered levels of low-density lipoprotein, (LDL or "bad") cholesterol without affecting high-density lipoprotein (HDL, or "good") cholesterol.

• *Heart disease.* One study showed that fenugreek lowers levels of LDL, or "bad," cholesterol in patients with type 2 diabetes. Here, the participants consumed 25 grams of fenugreek in a soup for twenty-four weeks. Total blood cholesterol and the "bad," LDL, cholesterol decreased, as did serum triglycerides. It is thought that these favorable changes in blood lipids were a result of the galactomannan fiber and saponin components that reduce gastrointestinal absorption of cholesterol and increase bile acid excretion.

Considerations for Use

Fenugreek is used as ground seeds, capsules, or teas. For internal use, the dose is 6 grams a day and external use is 50 grams of powder mixed in one-quarter liter of water (about one cup). Since fenugreek can interfere with iron absorption, people who have anemia should avoid it. (Unlike herbs that contain tannins, fenugreek contains mucilages that interfere with iron absorption, so taking lemon juice with fenugreek does not compensate for its tendency to bind iron as it does with some other herbs.) This herb also can alter balances of the various forms of thyroid hormones, so you should not use it if you take thyroid hormone. The use of more than 100 grams of

fenugreek seeds daily can cause intestinal upset, flatulence, diarrhea, and nausea. Applying too much to the skin can cause undesirable skin reactions.

Fenugreek extracts have been shown to stimulate uterine contractions in animals. Therefore, pregnant women should not take fenugreek in dosages higher than are commonly used as a spice.

Fenugreek can cause the urine to develop an odor that sometimes has been misdiagnosed as a hereditary condition known as maple syrup urine disease. If this occurs, you should discontinue the medicinal use of the herb and not use it in cooking for two to three days before being tested for this condition.

Studies conducted with laboratory animals in India suggest that fenugreek may be especially useful in helping people with type 1 diabetes use the trace element vanadium. If you are taking insulin or blood sugar–lowering medications for diabetes, fenugreek may enhance the effect of these therapies and lower blood sugar too far. It is advisable to seek your doctor's supervision before combining fenugreek with other treatments for diabetes.

Fenugreek may potentiate the activity of anticoagulants and may interact with a class of drugs called MAOIs and hormonal agents.

FEVERFEW

Latin name: *Tanacetum parthenium* (Asteraceae [composite] family)
Other common names: featherfew, featherfoil, midsummer daisy

General Description

The daisylike feverfew is a native plant of southeastern Europe that is now common throughout Australia, Europe, and North America. A perennial growing two feet (sixty centimeters) tall, its white flowers with yellow centers bloom all summer. The aerial (aboveground) parts of the plant are used in herbal medicine.

Evidence of Benefit

In folk medicine, feverfew is used for migraine prophylaxis, digestion problems, intestinal parasites, and gynecological disorders. It also has been used as a wash for inflammation and wounds, as a tranquilizer, an antiseptic, and following a tooth extraction, as a mouthwash. Feverfew has been used in the treatment of headaches and migraines since the first century. It has also been used for allergies, inflammation, arthritis, tinnitus, vertigo, difficulty in labor, toothache, insect bites, asthma, menstrual discomforts, fever, and other aches and pains.

Feverfew is an anti-inflammatory because it inhibits thromboxane B_2 and leukotriene B_4. It also inhibits prostaglandin synthetase and major pathways of arachidonic acid to reduce inflammation. Feverfew can inhibit human blood aggregation and serotonin secretion by platelets. It has antispasmodic effects and is an antihistamine.

Benefits of feverfew for specific health conditions include the following:

• *Migraine.* Feverfew is thought to influence migraine by blocking compounds that cause pain and reduce blood flow to the brain. The advantage of feverfew over many prescription medications for migraine treatment is that feverfew does not cause constipation or stomach upset.

Several studies have been performed on feverfew and migraines. In a systematic review of all human studies, there was insufficient evidence that feverfew worked for migraines, but that its use was safe and in some cases was effective. One of the studies included in this review found that two 50-milligram capsules of feverfew helped when taken at the time of a migraine. Patients experienced less pain, vomiting, photophobia (intolerance to light), and phonophobia (intolerance to sound). There were no reports of adverse effects. Patients with a history of migraines who took one feverfew capsule each day for four months had a reduction in the number and severity of attacks in each two-month period.

It seems that feverfew works best if taken daily as a prophylaxis remedy. In another review of the published literature, those with migraines who took this herb daily had no increase in frequency and severity of attacks compared to a placebo, suggesting that feverfew taken daily may prevent attacks of migraines. In fact, using 6.25 milligrams three times a day for four months reduced migraine frequency and decreased the number of attacks per month, compared to a placebo group. These differences were significant and not due to chance. Other similar studies did not see such an advantage over placebo.

• *Rheumatoid arthritis.* Laboratory studies have shown that feverfew stops white blood cells from absorbing the amino acid thymidine. This in turn reduces the rate at which they can produce inflammatory chemicals known as leukotrienes. This alteration of the cellular chemistry also reduces the production of fatty acid products known as eicosanoids, which are essential to the production of inflammatory chemicals. While clinical studies report mixed results, many people find that taking feverfew for two to three months reduces the severity and frequency of arthritic pain. The advantage of feverfew over many other forms of treatment is that it does not cause stomach upset, but acts in a manner like that of a class of pain relievers known as cyclooxygenase-2 (COX-2) inhibitors such as celecoxib (Celebrex). One study found that patients with rheumatoid arthritis who took 70 to 86 milligrams of feverfew daily for six weeks derived some benefit. Although no improvements were seen in blood tests, the patients who took the feverfew experienced improved grip strength compared to a placebo group.

Considerations for Use

Feverfew should always be taken in the form of encapsulated freeze-dried herb if taken internally. It can also be used externally applied to the forehead. For migraines, capsules of 200 to 250 milligrams taken daily and standardized for 0.2 percent parthenolide content should be used. Freshly dried powdered feverfew made from one to three leaves (25 to 75 milligrams) can be used once or twice a day.

The herb may cause skin allergy or digestive upset. In addition, there are reports of transient increased heart rate and smooth muscle contractions. Some individuals (about 10 percent) have reported a rebound effect when they stopped using the herb for migraines. They experienced headaches, muscle stiffness, insomnia, joint pain, fatigue, nervousness, and tension.

People who are allergic to ragweed may be allergic to this herb as well. In rare cases, feverfew may cause uterine bleeding, so pregnant women should not use it. Nursing mothers also should avoid this herb, since its active components can be passed through breast milk and may cause allergies in the child. It should not be used in children under two years of age.

You should not use feverfew if you take warfarin (Coumadin) or any other blood-thinning drug, such as antiplatelet agents. No detrimental interaction between feverfew and this class of drugs has yet been reported, but it is theoretically possible. If you regularly use over-the-counter (OTC) painkillers such as nonsteroidal anti-inflammatory drugs (NASIDs), you should consult with a physician before taking feverfew. Migraine-type headaches can be a symptom of more serious disease, so proper diagnosis is essential. Avoid using feverfew for two weeks prior to undergoing elective surgery.

FRITILLARIA

Latin name: *Fritillaria thunbergii* (Liliaceae [lily] family)
Other common name: Thunberg fritillaria bulb

General Description

Fritillaria is an Oriental lily that is gathered in the early summer after the aerial (aboveground) parts of the plant have withered. Herbal medicine uses thick slices of the rhizome.

Using the right species of fritillaria is important. Asian herbalists use a second variety of fritillaria, *F. cirrhosa*, that is toxic without careful processing.

Evidence of Benefit

Fritillaria is a cough suppressant that may offer steroid-like relief of inflammation. Traditional Chinese medicine (TCM) practitioners have used it for treating people with illnesses such as pneumonia or bronchial infections who have difficulty bringing up mucus. It has also been used historically to treat swollen glands, nodular swellings, and abscesses in the lungs or breast.

Benefits of fritillaria for specific health conditions include the following:

• *Cough, influenza, and laryngitis.* Fritillaria dilates the bronchial tubes, relieves cough, and reduces salivation. Scientists have found in cell studies that this herb acts in a manner similar to the drug dexamethasone (Decadron, Dexamethasone Intensol, and others), which is used to treat nasal allergy and inflammation.

Considerations for Use

Unprocessed fritillaria, which may be sold in some Chinese pharmacies, should never be taken internally. Since fritillaria stimulates uterine contractions, it should be avoided during pregnancy. People with high blood pressure should not use this herb.

GARLIC

Latin name: *Allium sativa* (Alliaceae [onion] family)
Other common names: allium, clove garlic, garlic bulb, garlic clove, poor man's treacle, stinking rose

General Description

Garlic is a pungent herb used around the world in cooking and natural medicine. The bulb is used fresh or dried, or it can be made into an oil. It is a bulbous perennial with a single stalk that grows to a height of from one to three feet (thirty to ninety centimeters), with green-white or sometimes pale pink flowers. The plant was originally found in Central Asia, where it is the most important herb in unani, or Persian, traditional herbal medicine.

Evidence of Benefit

In folk medicine, garlic was used for inflammation of the respiratory tract, such as whooping cough and bronchitis. It was also used for gastrointestinal ailments, particularly related to flatulence and gastrointestinal spasms. Other uses include for menstrual pain and treatment of diabetes. Externally, it was used for corns, warts, calluses, otitis, muscle pain, arthritis, and sciatica. Ayurvedic medicine uses it for bronchitis, constipation, joint pain, and fever. Homeopathic remedies exist for inflammation of the upper respiratory tract, digestive complaints, and muscle aches.

Garlic is a popular herb for cardiovascular health. Numerous scientific studies support the use of garlic in lowering cholesterol levels and blood sugar, preventing heart attack and stroke, and treating infections and cancer. Garlic may be able to reduce risk of blood clots and inhibit tumors. The German Commission E approves it for raised cholesterol levels, high blood pressure, and arteriosclerosis.

Benefits of garlic for specific health conditions include the following:

• *Atherosclerosis and high cholesterol.* Garlic can help prevent atherosclerosis by lowering cholesterol and triglyceride levels in the blood, inhibiting platelet stickiness, and increasing fibrinolysis, which results in a slowing of blood coagulation. Garlic preparations have been found to reduce the size of plaque deposits in animals by nearly 50 percent. In a four-year double-blind study of 152 individuals, standardized garlic powder at a dosage of 900 milligrams daily significantly slowed the development of atherosclerosis as measured by ultrasound. Another study, which measured the flexibility of the aorta in 200 individuals, reported that the participants taking garlic had more flexibility, indicating less atherosclerosis. Reviews of double-blind studies in humans have found that garlic lowered cholesterol levels in adults by approximately 6 to 12 percent, low-density lipoprotein (LDL, or "bad") cholesterol by 4 to 15 percent, and triglycerides by 15 percent. The high-density lipoprotein (HDL, or "good") cholesterol rose 0 to 22 percent. The corresponding dosages of garlic were 900 to 1,200 milligrams a day with at least 10 milligrams alliin (or total allicin potential of 4,000 micrograms). However, several more recent double-blind studies have found no benefit. At present, it appears that garlic's effects on cholesterol are modest at best and considered a clinically inefficient way to lower cholesterol. The authors concluded that garlic looked promising for reducing the clumping of platelets, but as for lowering total and LDL cholesterol and blood pressure and reducing oxidative stress, the studies have not been definitive.

Despite the conflicting data, a few studies showed promise for using garlic to improve blood lipids. In one study, patients at high risk for heart disease who used 4 milliliters (1,200 milligrams) of aged garlic extract had significantly less plaque buildup in their arteries compared to a control group. Garlic also appeared to protect blood vessels from toxic homocysteine, which is often elevated in heart disease. It seems that garlic prevents a decrease in bioavailable nitric oxide. Patients with heart disease risk factors or vascular problems took aged garlic extract for six weeks.

In a ten-year study, healthy subjects took Allicor, an *A. sativum* preparation, for twelve months and were followed for heart disease risks. The study found that 13 percent of the men and 7 percent of the women experienced a reduced risk compared to people who don't take garlic for many aspects of heart problems, such as lower high blood cholesterol and higher HDL ("good") cholesterol.

• *Cancer.* There have been hundreds of studies on the impact of garlic on cancer. In one study, the use of garlic (the highest intake was 9 to 10 cloves a week compared to 0 to 1) was associated with lower rates of cancer of the colon (40 percent) and stomach (47 percent) in both men and women. In addition, garlic intake was inversely associated with cancer of the prostate and endometrium. In another study, patients with precancerous lesions of the large intestine benefited from using a large dose (2.4 milliliters per day) of aged garlic extract (AGE). After one year, there were fewer and smaller adenomas (benign tumors) in the AGE group. In patients with advanced cancer, AGE improved natural killer (NK) cell numbers and activity, but the quality of life of the patients did not change.

Garlic contains compounds that prevent tumors from developing their own blood supplies, stop tumor formation after exposure to carcinogenic chemicals, and inhibit the spread of tumors once they have started. Other chemicals in garlic reduce the production of toxic free radicals in liver and lung tissue, and retard the proliferation of hormone-sensitive breast and prostate cancer cells. Garlic has been found to prevent the growth of the bacterium *Helicobacter pylori*, one of the risk factors for stomach cancer. However, epidemiological data do not support the use of garlic as an anticancer agent.

Garlic works well with other anticancer treatments. Garlic powder, usually taken in tablet form, increases the effectiveness of selenium supplements in preventing the growth and spread of breast cancer. Animal studies have found that garlic protects tissues from the effects of whole-body radiation. However, garlic is not appropriate for people undergoing treatment with recombinant tumor necrosis factor (rhTNF), since a combination of chemicals in the herb reduces the activity of rhTNF.

• *Diabetes.* Garlic can lower blood sugar levels in people with diabetes, although the reports have shown mixed results. It seems to tie up chemical receptors that otherwise would deactivate insulin, the hormone that controls sugar usage, and also stimulates the pancreas to secrete insulin. It does this without stimulating weight gain, a common side effect of some diabetes medications.

• *Ear infection.* Garlic oil, applied directly to the ear canal, is a traditional remedy for earaches. Tests have found that garlic treatment stopped the growth of aspergillus and candida, two fungi that could possibly cause ear inflammation.

• *Heart attack.* In one study of 432 individuals who suffered heart attacks, those who took garlic had a lower incidence of second heart attacks and about a 50 percent lower death rate. Garlic stimulates fibrinolysis, a process by which blood clots are dissolved. In another study, patients with high cholesterol levels who took 200 milligrams of dried garlic three times a day over four weeks experienced an increase in fibrinolytic activity. However, other markers of blood clotting, such as prothrombin time and platelet aggregation, did not change.

Ajoene, a compound isolated from garlic, inhibits platelets from forming clots. Ajoene tends to build up if you take garlic in small doses over a period of weeks, so taking a single, large dose of garlic does not affect clotting capacity either beneficially (preventing clots) or detrimentally

(increasing the risk of bleeding). Avoid taking garlic in supplement form with thrombolytic agents, as excessive bleeding may occur. Ajoene acts synergistically with the calcium channel blockers diltiazem (Cardizem), nifedipine (Adalat, Procardia), and verapamil (Calan, Isoptin, Verelan), increasing their ability to control racing pulse and high blood pressure. Avoid taking garlic in supplement form for two weeks before undergoing elective surgery.

• *Infections and fungi.* Garlic helps strengthen the immune system against infection by activating "germ-eating" macrophages, cells that are produced by the immune system. In one study, participants who consumed 600 milligrams of garlic powder every day for three months showed significant increases in the number of macrophages in their bloodstream. Garlic has antifungal and antibacterial effects, but these have not been demonstrated in human studies. Garlic appears to have only 1 percent the strength of penicillin against certain types of bacterial infections. Therefore, it should not be considered a substitute for conventional antibiotics, but it can be used as a support against some bacterial infections. Check with your doctor before using these medications with garlic.

• *Peptic ulcer.* Garlic has been shown to inhibit the growth of *H. pylori*, a bacterium implicated in the formation of ulcers in the digestive system. No human studies have been done, however; it has only been studied in cell lines. Moreover, it was compounds extracted from garlic such as diallyl sulfide—not the garlic itself—that were most effective.

• *Miscellaneous.* Garlic increases the potency of preparations of the herb coleus (forskolin) and helps nonsteroidal anti-inflammatory drugs (NSAIDs) such as indomethacin (Indocin) provide greater pain relief. However, using them together increases the risk of bleeding, and therefore you should ask your doctor before using them together.

Considerations for Use

Garlic can be used as enteric-coated tablets, oil, or raw cloves. The daily dose is 4 grams of fresh garlic or the equivalent as an extract. To make garlic oil for an ear infection, steep 1 part minced garlic in 5 parts olive oil. The oil can be refrigerated for up to two weeks.

Garlic can counteract the effects of *Bifidus* and *Lactobacillus* cultures taken to restore normal digestion. It also has been known to cause upset stomach. Raw garlic especially can cause heartburn and flatulence. Other side effects include myalgia (muscle pain), fatigue, vertigo, and headache. Most side effects are considered minor. However, children who have had prolonged contact with garlic on their skin have developed burns or dermatological issues such as a rash. There have been reports of elevated liver enzymes with high doses of garlic.

While desired changes in blood pressure and cholesterol may occur after taking as little as 600 milligrams of garlic in tablet form daily for several weeks, taking more than 900 milligrams of garlic tablets a day is not likely to offer any additional benefit. If you take a blood-thinning drug such as warfarin (Coumadin), you should avoid using garlic medicinally because the herb adds to the drug's effects. Because garlic decreases the blood's clotting tendency, discuss the use of garlic with your physician before undergoing any type of surgery. Other drugs that may be affected by garlic use include: protease inhibitors and cyclosporine, which may have decreased effectiveness if taken with garlic; indomethacin, which when combined with garlic may result in increased bleeding; and insulin, which may need to be adjusted due to the hypoglycemic effects of garlic. Nursing mothers should not use garlic.

GENTIAN

Latin names: *Gentiana lutea* (in angostura bitters and European formulas); *G. scabra* (in traditional Chinese medicine [TCM] formulas) (Gentianaceae [gentian] family)
Other common names: bitter root, bitterwort, English gentian, field gentian, gentian root, pale gentian, wild gentian, yellow gentian (*G. lutea*); Chinese gentian root, gentiana longdancao (*G. scabra*)

General Description

Gentian, a perennial plant that grows up to three feet (one meter) tall, bears alternating leaves on a single stem that is topped with five-petaled yellow flowers. The dried or fresh root is used in herbal medicine. The herb is widely cultivated in China and is harvested from areas of the wild in Spain and the Balkans where it is not yet endangered. Gentian extracts are widely sold in liquor stores under the name "bitters."

In both Chinese and Korean, the terms for gentian can be translated literally as "dragon gallbladder herb." This attests to gentian's ability to treat fiery inflammations of the gallbladder that cause intense discomfort.

Evidence of Benefit

Gentian is an intensely bitter herb that has been used in different cultures for about 3,000 years to treat digestive disorders and to stimulate the appetite. It contains some of the most bitter substances known, and is used to increase saliva, to improve digestive tone, help prevent indigestion and gas, and stimulate the gallbladder and liver. It has been reported to eliminate hiccups, particularly if they are caused by drinking alcohol. It is used as a tonic and in teas to stimulate bile secretion and alleviate loss of appetite, fullness, and flatulence. In homeopathy, it is used for digestive disorders. Gentian is approved by the German Commission E for dyspeptic complaints, loss of appetite, and flatulence.

Benefits of gentian for specific health conditions include the following:

• *Gallstones and indigestion.* Gentian helps to ease gallbladder problems and indigestion. Taken thirty minutes before eating, it increases the appetite, stimulating the production of digestive juices and pancreatic activity, and boosting the blood supply to the digestive tract and intestines. It is especially helpful for fat and protein digestion. Gentian also stimulates the production of bile. Herbalists frequently recommend ingesting this herb before or with large meals. In Europe, and particularly in Germany, gentian bitters are taken before fatty meals as an aid to digestion.

Considerations for Use

Gentian is available in capsules and as bitters. It can be used in teas and as a tonic. Most people find the neutral taste of capsules preferable to the extremely bitter taste of the drink called angostura bitters, also called gentian bitters. The daily dose is 2 to 4 grams of the root and a tincture of 1 to 3 grams made according to known recipes.

If you are pregnant or have high blood pressure or chronic gastrointestinal problems, you should use gentian only under the direction of a health-care professional. In particular, if you have a stomach or duodenal ulcer, do not use gentian. You should avoid gentian altogether if you have diarrhea caused by poor digestion, indicated by undigested food in the stool, or if you have excess stomach acid. Adults over sixty-five and children should use low-strength preparations. You should not give gentian to a child under two years of age.

GINGER

Latin name: *Zingiber officinale* (Zingiberaceae [ginger] family)
Other common names: African ginger, Jamaica ginger

General Description

Ginger is the most widely available and widely used herbal remedy on the planet. In particular, it is indigenous to southeastern Asia and is cultivated in the United States, India, China, the West Indies, and other tropical regions. Billions of people use ginger daily as food and medicine. Ginger is derived from the tuberous rhizome of the perennial plant *Z. officinale*. This perennial plant grows to a height of two feet (sixty centimeters), has lance-shaped leaves, and bears stalks of white or yellow flowers.

Evidence of Benefit

For 2,500 years, ginger has played an important role in Asian medicine. It has traditionally been used to promote cleansing of the body through perspiration, to calm nausea, and to stimulate the appetite. It also has been used as an expectorant and an astringent. In Indian ayurvedic medicine, it is used for anorexia, dyspeptic conditions, and sore throats. Also, in Persian unani tibb systems of medicine, ginger is commonly used for the treatment of arthritis. Traditional Chinese medicine uses it for treating colds, nausea, vomiting, and shortness of breath. In China, ginger also has been put to the novel use of helping to turn breech babies by giving the mother ginger teas before delivery.

Ginger is an inexpensive, effective, and nearly universally available remedy for inflammation and pain. The German Commission E has approved it for loss of appetite, travel sickness, and dyspeptic complaints.

Benefits of ginger for specific health conditions include the following:

• *Arthritis and pain.* Ginger inhibits the production of immune-system components called cytokines, chemicals that create a long-term tendency toward inflammation. The published human data on using ginger to treat pain in osteoarthritis are equivocal, but there are data to show that it contains compounds that do interfere with the inflammatory cascade of inflammation and pain receptors. One study showed that ginger was not as effective at reducing the pain of osteoarthritis as ibuprofen, which is one of the usual treatment methods. On the other hand, ginger has been shown to be useful in treating a number of disorders marked by swelling and pain, such as arthritis. In a two-and-a-half-year study in patients with osteoarthritis and rheumatoid arthritis, participants experienced improvement with ginger when used at amounts of 1 to 2 grams daily. More than half of the patients in both groups experienced reduced swelling and some reported less pain. The herbal treatment relieved symptoms without the side effects of nonsteroidal anti-inflammatory drugs (NSAIDs) and steroids, which are helpful but can cause serious side effects, especially if used for long periods.

• *Atherosclerosis and high cholesterol.* In a study using rabbits (which are a good marker of human blood lipids), ginger significantly improved serum lipids and reduced the degree of heart disease after four weeks. In clinical studies conducted in India, the consumption of 5 grams of dried ginger per day for seven days reversed increases in triglycerides and low-density lipoprotein (LDL, or "bad") cholesterol induced by adding 100 grams (nearly 4 ounces) of butter a day to the diet. In another study, powdered ginger inhibited platelets from clumping in twenty patients with heart disease. Patients took 10 grams of the powdered ginger. Using lower doses, such as 1.5 grams and 3 grams, did not have an effect. Interestingly, raw ginger had no effect in healthy people with normal platelet function.

• *Indigestion, morning sickness, motion sickness, nausea, and vomiting.* One of ginger's best-known uses is quelling queasy stomach and nausea. It is an age-old remedy for morning sickness. In one study, pregnant women using 1 gram of ginger daily for four days had less severe and fewer episodes of nausea and vomiting. However, the German Commission E and the American Herbal Products Association recommend that pregnant women do not use ginger during pregnancy. Pregnant women should consult their obstetrician before using it.

Sometimes ginger is touted for easing motion sickness and for reducing nausea and vomiting after surgery, but these studies have been unconvincing. Ginger root contains compounds called gingerols and shogaols, which work as anti-emetics, drugs that are effective against vomiting and nausea. The added benefit is that the action of these compounds is local on the stomach and does not affect the central nervous system as may other anti-emetics. Ginger stimulates the flow of saliva, bile, and gastric juices. It suppresses gastric contractions while increasing peristalsis, whereby food is pushed down the intestines.

Using 1 gram of ginger root powder reduced symptoms of seasickness such as nausea, vomiting, vertigo, and cold sweating compared to a placebo in a group of naval cadets unaccustomed to sea travel. However, in contrast, another study found that ginger was no better than six other commonly used nonherbal drugs to treat motion sickness. The dose used was 500 milligrams of ginger root.

Controlled clinical studies have not always found ginger to be more effective in relieving nausea than dimenhydrinate (Dramamine), the popular over-the-counter (OTC) remedy for motion sickness.

Ginger may be useful in preventing nausea and vomiting after surgery, especially when combined with the prescription antinausea drug metoclopramide (Octamide, Reglan). Even with metoclopramide, ginger does not completely eliminate postoperative nausea and vomiting, but these disagreeable symptoms could be reduced. However, in a well-controlled study, adding ginger to orally administered metoclopramide in patients who were receiving the chemotherapeutic drug cisplatin, participants experienced less nausea and vomiting. One study found that ginger also eases nausea caused by treatment with methoxsalen (8-MOP, Oxsoralen-Ultra), a drug taken by people undergoing photopheresis, a form of light-activated chemotherapy for treating T-cell lymphoma. A dose of 1,500 milligrams, or three 500-milligram capsules of ginger, was used in the study confirming this use.

• *Parasitic infection.* Ginger contains a chemical called zingibain, which dissolves parasites and their eggs. In Japan, ginger's antiparasitic effect is put to use in the preparation of sushi, which is traditionally eaten with pickled ginger. In the laboratory, ginger extracts have been shown to kill the anisakid worm, a parasite sometimes carried in raw fish, within sixteen hours, about the length of time the parasite would have to establish itself in the digestive tract after consumption of contaminated fish. In addition, ginger tea is useful as a supplement in treating schistoso-miasis, a parasitic disease increasingly prevalent among tourists returning to the United States.

Considerations for Use

Ginger is available in capsules, pickles, tablets, and teas, and as hexanol extracts. Ginger teas can be made into compresses. (*See* COMPRESSES in Part Three.) The daily dosage for pills is 2 to 4 grams of ginger root. Ginger may cause stomach irritation, so no more than 6 grams should be consumed on an empty stomach.

Although there are warnings in Chinese medicine about the use of ginger during pregnancy, used in mod-eration (the equivalent of 2 teaspoons, or 1 gram, two to three times per day) will likely pose no risk to the health of the mother or developing baby. Recent studies indicate that eating as much as 2 to 3 tablespoons of raw ginger or 5 to 8 tablespoons of cooked ginger (15 or 40 grams, respectively) daily will not stimulate uterine contractions. However, do not use ginger without checking with your obstetrician first.

Ginger should not be taken if you have gallstones or are at risk of hemorrhage. Too much ginger can cause skin irritation, central nervous system depression, and cardiac arrhythmias. Ginger can increase the potency of prescrip-tion medications used to prevent blood clots, such as aspi-rin, clopidogrel (Plavix), ticlopidine (Ticlid), or warfarin (Coumadin). Combining ginger with these medications could result in unexpected bleeding. Be sure to discuss the use of ginger with your physician before taking the herb to control nausea after surgery. If bleeding is a major risk, ginger should be avoided.

Ginger can prolong the sleeping time induced by bar-biturates. Ginger has no detectable effects on the central nervous system itself, but probably increases the absorp-tion of barbiturates in the digestive tract. If you are taking any kind of medication to induce sleep, you should use ginger with caution.

The daily consumption of ginger root may interfere with the absorption of dietary iron and fat-soluble vita-mins. Avoid taking ginger for two weeks prior to undergo-ing elective surgery.

GINKGO BILOBA

Latin name: *Ginkgo biloba* (Ginkgoaceae [ginkgo] family)
Other common name: ginkgo, maidenhair-tree

General Description

Ginkgo extract is taken from ginkgo leaf, the fan-shaped leaf of the ginkgo tree. *Ginkgo biloba* is one of the oldest living tree species, dating back to over 300 million years. Individual trees can live for 1,000 years. Ginkgo trees are very resistant to viruses, fungi, insects, pollution, and even radiation. It is indigenous to China, Japan, and Korea, and is also found in Europe and the United States. The medicinal use of ginkgo dates back almost 5,000 years in Chinese herbal medicine. It was used for respiratory tract ailments and for memory loss in older adults.

Evidence of Benefit

Ginkgo is the world's most-used treatment for memory loss and degenerative diseases of the brain and central nervous system. It also aids treatment of a variety of con-ditions ranging from erectile dysfunction (ED) to ringing in the ears.

Ginkgo works in the brain to reduce the progression of dementia probably by reducing white blood cell infil-tration in the brain, curbing lipid peroxidation (prevent-ing fat from going rancid), and increasing blood flow by antagonizing platelet-activating factor (PAF). In one study, by boosting glucose levels using ginkgo, rats had increased mental capacity. Traditional Chinese medicine uses ginkgo for asthma, tinnitus, and angina. Homeopathic remedies include those for tonsillitis and headaches. The German Commission E has approved a limited number of spe-cific standard extracts of ginkgo for symptomatic organic brain dysfunction, intermittent claudication, vertigo, and tinnitus.

Ginkgo also has powerful antioxidant properties in the brain, the retina of the eye, and the cardiovascular system. This activity may help prevent free-radical damage and age-related declines in brain function.

Benefits of ginkgo for specific health conditions include the following:

• *Alzheimer's disease, impaired cognition, memory loss, and Parkinson's disease.* Ginkgo's most exciting application may be in the treatment of impaired cognitive function. This disorder is at least partly related to an inadequate sup-ply of glucose, or blood sugar, to the brain, which may alter functions of brain cells and their supporting struc-tures. Ginkgo can both speed up the process by which the brain uses glucose and increase blood flow to the brain. The herb may also improve the brain's use of a chemi-cal called acetylcholine. (*See* "Ginkgo: The Memory Herb and Alzheimer's Disease" *under* ALZHEIMER'S DISEASE in Part Two.) In one study, healthy elderly persons took 120 milligrams of ginkgo for twelve weeks and memory and learning tasks were assessed by standardized tests. The participants felt better but no improvements were seen in memory or learning. In another study, postmenopausal women who took a standardized ginkgo extract (120 milligrams daily) experienced an improvement in men-tal flexibility after six weeks. In particular, women with an average age of sixty-one years made fewer errors and needed less time to complete mental tasks compared to those in a younger cohort (average age fifty-five years) who did not get these same benefits. In another study, ginkgo also was useful to elderly persons with normal cognitive function in that it prevented or delayed impair-ment of memory. Ginkgo has not been shown to be of help to young people, however. In a group of young people with an average age of twenty years, using two 60-milligram tablets of ginkgo (BioGinkgo) daily, there was no effect on a series of memory tests.

Oral doses of 120 and 240 milligrams of ginkgo extract taken by healthy volunteers have been found to increase the activity of alpha waves and to decrease the activity of theta waves (two types of brain waves). These brain-wave changes indicate that ginkgo is capable of improving cognitive function that can be demonstrated in increased mental sharpness, concentration, and memory. Numerous European studies have indicated that ginkgo improves short-term and long-term memory in people with age-associated memory impairment or mild cognitive impairment.

Researchers also have studied the use of ginkgo to treat older adults with either Alzheimer's disease or mental debility caused by vascular dementia. Several studies have been published on using ginkgo for Alzheimer's disease. Unfortunately, many included inconsistent formulas of ginkgo and mixed the ginkgo with other herbs, making interpretation of the results problematic. One high-purity formula, ginkgo extract (EGb 761), had better and more consistent results. European investigators studying patients with Alzheimer's disease and vascular dementia found that using EGb 761 resulted in improvements in tests of dementia compared to placebo and drug treatments. Improvements were seen in attention, memory, and performance on cognition studies. Using this same extract (EGb 761), patients with uncomplicated, mild to moderate Alzheimer's disease or dementia had improvement in cognitive performance and social functioning. Thus, a standardized ginkgo extract seems to be able to reverse deterioration associated with Alzheimer's disease and dementia.

However, not all studies on the use of ginkgo for Alzheimer's disease, mixed dementia, or vascular-related dementia have produced positive results. Nevertheless, it seems prudent to try ginkgo for impaired cognition, as the studies have all shown the herb to be safe.

Doctors in Germany have recognized for over thirty years that ginkgo may reverse brain damage caused by exposure to toxic chemicals. This makes the herb potentially useful in the treatment of Parkinson's disease. Electroencephalograph (EEG) measurements done on research volunteers who have Parkinson's disease show that ginkgo has a long-lasting positive effect on the metabolism of glucose and oxygen in the brain, but clinical improvements have not been seen.

• *Cancer.* In one study, ginkgo improved the efficacy and tolerability of chemotherapy in patients with advanced colon cancer. Patients were treated with 350 milligrams of ginkgo extract (EGb 761) as an infusion. There also was some evidence that the ginkgo actually slowed the progression of the cancer. In another study, patients who suffered radiation exposure as a result of the Chernobyl accident also experienced a reduced risk of cancer from taking ginkgo. The dosage of ginkgo (EGb 761) used in this study was 40 milligrams three times a day. Additionally, in studies using cell lines, ginkgo *teas* (not extract tablets) that contain quercetin have shown some promise and may accelerate the death of leukemia and Burkitt's lymphoma cells; slow the growth of colon, lung, and liver cancers; and inhibit the growth of estrogen-activated cancers, including bladder cancer, breast cancer, and, when used together with the chemotherapy drug cisplatin (Platinol), ovarian cancer.

• *Cataracts, glaucoma, and macular degeneration.* Macular degeneration is associated with an overgrowth of capillaries in the macula—the part of the retina responsible for fine vision. These tiny blood vessels are often weak and leak into the surrounding tissues, damaging them. Ginkgo can stop this process by deactivating PAF, which is essential for the growth of new capillaries. The extract increases circulation within the eye, which supplies more oxygen to the retina. Ginkgo increases circulation to the lens and acts as a free-radical scavenger, slowing the process of cataract formation. The herb works by reducing retinal edema and cellular lesions in the retina. Thus, ginkgo may be helpful for people with eye conditions, although clinical data are lacking.

• *Erectile dysfunction and diminished sexual desire.* One clinical study found that the use of 240 milligrams of ginkgo extract per day for six months resulted in recovery of potency lost after treatment with drugs for depression. Ginkgo contains compounds that can cause the blood vessels to relax, resulting in a greater blood supply to the penis and stronger erections. An open clinical study (one conducted without use of placebos) found that 76 percent of men who experienced sexual problems caused by taking antidepressant drugs such as fluoxetine (Prozac), sertraline (Zoloft), or phenelzine (Nardil) recovered sexual function after four to six weeks of taking ginkgo. However, another study found no effect on sexual function in men and women who were using antidepressants when they were given 240 milligrams of ginkgo for twelve weeks. Still, ginkgo may have a beneficial effect in enhancing desire, excitement, orgasm, and afterglow in women who experience sexual difficulties as a result of taking antidepressants.

• *Intermittent claudication, heart attack, and stroke.* Heart attack, stroke, and intermittent claudication (poor circulation that causes pain in the legs) all respond to treatment with ginkgo. The underlying factor in all of these conditions is atherosclerosis. When a blood vessel is damaged, PAF causes a leak-sealing clot to develop in the vessel wall and stimulates the production of fibrous tissues that cover the injury site. This provides a platform on which cholesterol may accumulate into a vessel-narrowing plaque. By deactivating PAF, ginkgo reduces the rate at which fibrous tissues are produced. The herb also helps to keep cholesterol-laden macrophages produced by the immune system from pumping even more cholesterol onto the arterial wall. In Germany, where ginkgo is prescribed for intermittent claudication, treatment usually brings relief in six weeks. In one study, most patients who took ginkgo in dosages that ranged from 120 to 160 milligrams for twenty-four weeks were able to walk for longer periods of time pain-free compared to patients who received placebos.

Strokes can happen when a blood clot becomes stuck in a narrowed blood vessel in the brain. By inhibiting plaque development, ginkgo can protect against stroke. The herb also is helpful after a stroke. Much of the damage done by a stroke is caused by the formation of toxic free radicals when oxygen levels increase after circulation is restored. Brain cells cannot process all of the oxygen available to them, and some oxygen "escapes" its normal biochemical pathways. Ginkgo increases the production of scavengers that collect the oxygen free radicals before they can attack the linings of cells. Although these actions have been shown to happen in cell lines and animal studies, studies on stroke patients have not showed that taking ginkgo promotes recovery following an acute ischemic stroke in physical performance or on a brain scan.

• *Multiple sclerosis.* In one study, ginkgo extract EGb 761 (20 milligrams daily) helped patients with multiple sclerosis. After four weeks, patients experienced improvements in fatigue, severity of symptoms, and functionality. Several studies support the use of ginkgo in preventing relapses of multiple sclerosis. These studies indicate that ginkgo is more helpful when used long-term to prevent relapses than in treatment of acute relapse symptoms.

• *Schizophrenia.* Patients with schizophrenia seemed to derive benefit from taking ginkgo. Using *G. biloba* extract (EGb 761), patients showed an improvement in T lymphocytes (immune cells) and superoxide dismutase (an antioxidant). The researchers concluded that these are desirable effects for patients with this condition. Taking ginkgo along with a medication (haloperidol) for schizophrenia enhanced the effectiveness of the drug.

• *Seasonal affective disorder (SAD) and depression.* Ginkgo can be used to treat depression in general by increasing the flow of oxygen to the brain. This is particularly true for older adults if the herb is combined with *appropriate* prescription drugs, but you need to check with your doctor before combining this herb with any prescription drug. Other experiments show that the combination of ginkgo and ginger can reduce anxiety. Research suggests that ginkgo may be useful for elderly people with depression who are not responding to standard antidepressant drugs. One double-blind study found that older adults who had both depression and mild dementia, and who were not responding to antidepressant medications, responded well to ginkgo supplementation. Another study found that ginkgo had no effect on SAD in patients who were not taking other medications. Patients took two tablets of a ginkgo extract containing 24 milligrams of flavones glycosides and 6 milligrams of terpene lactones per tablet.

• *Tinnitus, sudden deafness.* Ginkgo is frequently effective against tinnitus, or the sensation of constant ringing or buzzing noises in the ears, if treatment begins within six to eight weeks of onset. A mini-review of five controlled studies showed favorable results. Doses of ginkgo were typically 120 to 160 milligrams a day. However, other studies conducted more recently did not find any benefit over placebo in cases of tinnitus. It also has been used in clinical trials to treat sudden hearing loss. In one study, up to 40 percent of the subjects regained their hearing after ten days of ginkgo treatment, and it was as effective as pentoxifylline, a drug that is typically used to treat hearing loss. The use of ginkgo or any other herb, however, does not substitute for immediate medical evaluation of tinnitus or hearing loss, since certain conditions cannot be treated with herbs or supplements, and are medically treatable only if promptly diagnosed.

Considerations for Use

Ginkgo is available in extract tablets, liquids, and liposome capsules. Depending upon the indication of use, doses range from 120 to 240 milligrams two to three times a day. The duration of use also varies. For memory, ginkgo should be used for eight to twelve weeks. At that time, you should discuss with your health-care provider if you should continue. For pain-free walking and tinnitus, six to eight weeks usually is enough time to get a benefit. It is possible to use ginkgo teas, but these are useful primarily for conditions that do not involve memory or intellectual ability. This is because the ginkgo compounds that affect the central nervous system are especially concentrated in extracts. (*See* "Principles of Herbal Healing" for a discussion of extracts.)

Mild headaches lasting a day or two and mild upset stomach have been reported in a very small percentage of people using ginkgo. Some people who take extremely large doses experience diarrhea, nausea, vomiting, dizziness, and/or restlessness. If this should occur, you should reduce the dosage. If side effects are severe, discontinue it. In addition, excess bleeding can occur. Most reports of serious reactions are related to eating the fruit and whole leaves, which contain a neurotoxin that can cause coma, convulsion, and death. Extracts made from the leaves do not contain sufficient amounts of the toxins to produce ill effects. A part of the ginkgo contains ginkgolic acids, which are harmful. The German Commission E defines strict ways that ginkgo is to be prepared to avoid toxicity.

Finnish doctors report that a few persons taking ginkgo

experienced orthostatic hypotension, a sudden loss of blood pressure when moving from a seated to a standing position, after using ginkgo for a few days. Again, if this happens, you should lower the dosage or stop taking it. If you have a history of seizure disorders or are taking antiseizure medications, you should avoid this herb. The American Herbal Products Association warns that ginkgo may interact with a class of antidepressants known as monoamine oxidase (MAO) inhibitors in such a way as to increase the risk of seizures. Although there is only a very slight (less than 0.1 percent) probability that taking both ginkgo and one of these drugs would cause seizures, it is important to avoid taking ginkgo if you take amitriptyline (Elavil), bupropion (Wellbutrin, Zyban), or maprotiline (Ludiomil), or if you have used any of these drugs within the past six weeks.

Skin irritations have been known to occur in some cases. It is a good idea to take a six-week "vacation" from ginkgo every six months.

Several other drugs should not be used in conjunction with ginkgo. You should avoid ginkgo if you take blood-thinning medications, and discuss its use with your doctor before having any type of surgery or if you regularly take over-the-counter (OTC) painkillers such as nonsteroidal anti-inflammatory drugs (NSAIDs). Use of sedation medication and ginkgo is not advised. It is possible that ginkgo may alter blood glucose levels, so if you are using insulin, you should monitor blood glucose levels frequently and look for signs of low or high blood glucose levels. Speak to your health-care provider before combining ginkgo with antihypertensive drugs or thiazide diuretics. It is possible that using ginkgo and St. John's wort may result in mental changes. In addition, taking ginkgo and selective serotonin reuptake inhibitors (SSRIs) for depression may result in a hypomanic episode. Speak to your doctor before starting ginkgo if you are using antidepressants.

GINSENG

Latin name: *Panax ginseng* (Araliaceae [ginseng] family)
Other common names: American ginseng, Chinese ginseng, five-fingers, ginseng root, Korean ginseng, Oriental ginseng, red berry, red ginseng

General Description

Ginseng is a low-growing perennial plant native to the cool-summer regions of China; it is also cultivated in Korea, Japan, and Russia. Very seldom found in the wild, it is a labor-intensive crop that takes at least four years to mature. The root of the plant is dug in the fall, washed, steamed, and dried for use in herbal medicine.

Evidence of Benefit

Ginseng has been a part of Chinese medicine for over 2,000 years and has been used for blood disorders, gastric disturbances, vomiting, loss of appetite, cachexia, erectile dysfunction (ED) and sterility, insomnia, and neuralgia. It also was traditionally used to curb emotions, stop agitation, brighten the eyes, enlighten the mind, and increase wisdom. It was believed that continuous use leads to longevity and was commonly used by elderly people to improve mental and physical vitality.

Ginseng is an aphrodisiac, painkiller, and general stimulant. Ginseng helps the liver detoxify the blood, while protecting itself from damage. In some—but not all—studies, it lowers serum triglycerides and cholesterol. Homeopathic remedies exist for rheumatism and debility.

Ginseng is an adaptogen—that is, it increases the body's ability to tolerate stressful situations of all types. It is commonly taken to increase energy, enhance physical performance, prolong life, and increase sexual potency. The German Commission E has approved it for use as a tonic for fatigue and debility, and inability to get out of bed or concentrate during convalescence.

Benefits of ginseng for specific health conditions include the following:

• *Anxiety.* Ginseng therapy may prevent the onset of nervous unrest during treatment with morphine. It has been shown to be slightly more effective than a placebo at improving sleep and mood and lessening fatigue.

• *Cancer.* A study performed in South Korea followed 4,587 men and women aged thirty-nine years and older from 1987 to 1991. Individuals who consumed ginseng regularly were compared with similar individuals who did not. It was reported that in that time, those who used ginseng had a 50 percent lower incidence of death from cancer, especially lung and stomach cancer.

Experiments in China found that when ginseng therapy was combined with traditional radiation and chemotherapy for small cell lung cancer, longevity was extended by three to seventeen years. (The researchers in the study abandoned the controls in their research design when they began getting astonishing results from the treatment, so technically, their results should be regarded as potential rather than proven.) A Korean study found that ginseng destroys lung cancer cells that are resistant to the standard chemotherapy drug cisplatin (Platinol) in cell line studies. Although ginseng therapy does not shrink melanoma tumors, it does appear to keep them from developing a blood supply for further growth. In animal studies, a compound called ginsan, found in ginseng, retarded the growth of melanoma at dosages far lower than those that might cause a toxic reaction.

Polyacetylinic alcohol, another compound found in ginseng, retards cell reproduction in tumors and increases the effectiveness of the drug mitomycin (Mutamycin) in the treatment of stomach cancer. Ginsenosides have been found to induce cell differentiation, a prelude to natural cell death, in human leukemia cells. Clinical studies have found that ginseng protects cells in the digestive tract from injury during radiation therapy. A study of 1,987 people concluded that regular ginseng use lowers the risk of developing many types of cancer.

• *Chronic fatigue and stamina.* Ginseng has been shown to increase natural killer (NK) cells in those with chronic fatigue or AIDS. In terms of stamina during exercise, one study found that participants who took 200 milligrams of a standardized 7 percent *P. ginseng* for three weeks experienced an increase in their heart rate and they were able to sustain aerobic exercise for a longer period of time. Although the results were not significant, ginseng may offer some benefit to those with fatigue or who engage in regular exercise.

• *Cognitive ability.* In one study, conducted over a period of eight to nine weeks, a group of individuals treated with 400 milligrams of *P. ginseng* daily showed significant improvement in abstract thinking. Other studies have found that treatment with ginseng improved the ability to complete a detail-oriented editing task and to perform mental arithmetic, and improved memory, attention, concentration, and the general ability to cope. In one study, young healthy college students who took 100 milligrams of ginseng experienced an improvement in rapid visual information processing and the speed at which they were able to subtract numbers. In another study, using 200 milligrams a day of ginseng also improved subtraction performance and reduced mental fatigue in young adults. In another study, participants (aged around forty years) took 400 milligrams of ginseng for eight weeks and had slightly improved abstract thinking and faster simple reaction times. Compared to a placebo group, there was no benefit of ginseng on concentration and memory in this study.

• *Diabetes.* People with type 2 diabetes often find that after two weeks of taking ginseng tea, their blood sugar levels go down by between 40 and 50 milligrams per deciliter (mg/dL). Studies also have found that taking 100 or 200 milligrams of ginseng in a capsule elevated mood and reduced fasting blood glucose levels in people with type 2 diabetes. Ginseng may reduce insulin requirements and prolong the effect of injected insulin. If you have diabetes, you should take ginseng only under a physician's supervision.

• *Hangover.* Ginseng enhances the breakdown of alcohol in the body. In combination with other herbs, it can help reverse alcohol-induced damage to brain cells in laboratory tests.

• *Erectile dysfunction, infertility, and diminished sex drive.* Ginseng's traditional and best-known use as an aphrodisiac for men has been confirmed by research. Chemicals in ginseng stimulate the part of the brain known as the hypothalamus to direct the production of hormones that stimulate cell growth and healing in the sex organs. Ginseng also promotes better blood circulation within the penis.

A Korean study found that ginseng increases blood flow, and therefore erectile strength, by an average of about 30 percent. The amount needed to achieve this is 1,000 milligrams three times a day. Ginseng also can be used to treat infertility in men. An Italian study of sixty men found that ginseng use increased testosterone levels, as well as the number and motility of sperm cells.

• *High blood pressure.* Ginseng compounds relax the linings of blood vessels, lowering blood pressure. One study found that patients with high blood pressure who took 300 milligrams of red ginseng three times a day experienced improved blood flow over twenty-four months. Blood pressure lowering was thought to be a result of increasing the synthesis of nitric oxide. In some cases, blood pressure may be increased in response to ginseng. People with high blood pressure should not take ginseng without first consulting a doctor.

• *Menopause-related problems.* Ginseng reduces hot flashes, fatigue, insomnia, and depression associated with postmenopausal symptoms. In one study, women received 6 grams of ginseng over thirty days. Laboratory studies indicate that it increases ovarian estrogen production in early menopause. This means that it does not help women who have had their ovaries removed, and that its benefits for menopausal complaints decrease with the affected woman's age.

• *Stress.* Depending upon the part of the ginseng plant that is used, the stress response varies. In some cases, stress will be reduced and heartbeat will slow and palms will be dry; in others, stress will be increased, heart rate will rise, and palms will be sweaty. Some forms of ginseng (non-ginsenoside Rg2 and Rg3) decrease the release of catecholamines (fight or flight hormones), which are usually released during stress. In laboratory experiments, the herb has been found to increase the learning ability of animals under stress and to reduce nicotine-induced hyperactivity. It also reduces digestive upset caused by emotional stress and inhibits ulcer formation. Ginseng compounds may reduce the stress of *anticipated* pain.

Considerations for Use

Ginseng is taken in teas, tinctures, or capsules. You should always make sure that any product you use contains real ginseng (the so-called ginseng drinks in convenience stores almost always do not). One widely available ginseng product that is standardized to contain the important ginsenosides is Ginsana (sold as G115 outside North America), but other ethical preparations of ginseng are available also. The dose is usually 1 to 2 grams a day for three months, with a repeated course if necessary.

In teas, the type of ginseng used makes a difference. The most potent herb is called wild mountain root, imported from Jilin province in China. This grade is also called *jilin root* or *ji lin shen.* It is expensive, but worth the cost if you are treating any serious ailment. *Ginseng whiskers* is a term used for a less expensive form of the herb that is recommended over a compound called *sugar root*, an even less expensive ginseng-flavored rock candy. Field-grown ginseng is thought to be less potent than ginseng gathered in the wild. If you decide to use a tincture, be aware that strengths vary greatly from one manufacturer to another, and that some formulations include the less expensive codonopsis, coptis, or Siberian ginseng. (*See* CODONOPSIS; COPTIS; and SIBERIAN GINSENG.) According to tradition, it is wise to avoid drinking green tea when using ginseng, since it may reduce ginseng's efficacy.

Occasionally, women report menstrual abnormalities and breast tenderness when they take ginseng. However, a large double-blind study found no estrogenic effects that would explain these anecdotal reports. Other studies have found that ginseng has an estrogenic effect, so it should not be used by anyone who is told to avoid estrogen-containing drugs, such as women with estrogen-positive breast cancer. Consumption of extremely large amounts of tincture, 100 milliliters or more, may result in headache. This is an early sign of overdose and means that the dose should be reduced. Gross overdoses—40 to 100 times the normally prescribed amount—of ginseng extract can cause rash and itching all over the body, as well as diarrhea, dizziness, fever, headache, and hemorrhage. Best results usually can be obtained by taking small amounts of ginseng on a regular basis.

Herb users in the warmer climates of the southern United States, particularly those in the Gulf Coast states, may find ginseng that is not used as part of a balanced formula to be excessively warming during the hottest summer weather. Using ginseng during times of extreme heat may result in mild fever or sleeplessness. American ginseng is a "cooler" alternative. (*See* AMERICAN GINSENG. *Also see* "Ginseng Among the Native Americans" *under* AMERICAN GINSENG.)

There have been specific reports of interactions between ginseng and monoamine oxidase (MAO) inhibitor drugs, digitalis, warfarin (Coumadin), diuretics, and high doses of prescription steroids. If you are using ginseng, inform your doctor of this if he or she prescribes any of these drugs. Pregnant women and nursing mothers should not use ginseng. Avoid taking American ginseng (*P. quinquefolium*) and Asian ginseng (*P. ginseng*) for two weeks prior to undergoing elective surgery. Caution should be taken in patients with heart disease or diabetes. Ginseng has the ability to lower blood glucose levels, leading to insomnia, headaches, nervousness, and vomiting in those with and without diabetes. Ginseng has been reported to both lower and raise blood pressure.

GOLDENSEAL

Latin name: *Hydrastis canadensis* (Ranunculaceae [peony] family)

Other common names: eye balm, eye root, ground raspberry, Indian plant, jaundice root, wild curcuma, yellow puccoon, yellow root

General Description

Goldenseal is a North American woodland plant, but it is cultivated elsewhere as well. Growing to a height of one foot (thirty centimeters), goldenseal has a thick yellow root and a single erect stem. The stem supports large overlapping three-lobed leaves and a flower that produces a single red inedible fruit. The roots, used in herbal medicine, are dug from three-year-old plants and dried in the open air before processing.

Evidence of Benefit

Goldenseal is an immensely popular herb sold as an immune booster and antibiotic to be taken at the onset of a cold. However, goldenseal is not an effective systemic antibiotic, because the blood levels of berberine produced by the use of oral goldenseal are far too low to be effective. But the herb does exert an antibiotic effect when used topically and has a long history of being used for infections of the skin. It also may be beneficial in treating sore throats and diseases of the digestive tract because it makes direct contact with the affected areas when used for those problems. Homeopathic uses include the treatment of irregular menstruation, digestive problems, and bronchitis.

The best known of the herb's active constituents is berberine, which possesses strong activity against a wide variety of bacteria and fungi. It also seems to have a soothing effect on inflamed mucous membranes. Goldenseal has been shown to reduce the severity of diarrhea and may help patients who receive an organ transplant to use less of the toxic antirejection drug.

Benefits of goldenseal for specific health conditions include the following:

• *Cancer.* Goldenseal can help increase white blood cells, which become dangerously depressed during chemotherapy and radiation therapy. In one study, 50 percent of the participants had increased white blood cells with goldenseal. Berberine, a component of goldenseal, has strong antitumor activity. In brain cancer studies conducted on cell lines and on rats, goldenseal has been shown to kill cancer cells. In fact, goldenseal was as effective as the usual chemotherapeutic drug. These were not studies done on humans, however.

• *Heartburn.* Goldenseal, like coptis, is a bitter herb that is useful in treating heartburn associated with emotional tension.

• *Heart disease.* In one study, berberine from goldenseal lowered cholesterol levels by 29 percent, low-density lipoprotein (LDL, or "bad") cholesterol by 25 percent, and triglycerides by 35 percent in people with high levels of these. Participants took 500 milligrams twice daily for three months. The goldenseal appeared to work in a different way from statin medications, suggesting that the two could be used together to reduce heart disease risk.

• *Periodontal disease.* Goldenseal destroys the bacteria that cause periodontal disease, whether taken in capsule or tablet form or swished around in the mouth in the form of alcohol-free extract. For quick relief of inflamed gums, the extract can be placed on a piece of gauze or pure cotton and placed on the affected area, and packed up tightly between the lips and the gum.

Considerations for Use

Goldenseal can be used in capsule, ointment, powder, tablet, and tincture forms. It may also be used as a compress. (*See* COMPRESSES in Part Three.) A daily dose is 250 to 500 milligrams of a standardized extract (5 percent hydrastine) three times a day. Goldenseal should be used for a limited amount of time and if symptoms of gastrointestinal distress occur, you should stop taking the herb. Overuse of the herb can create digestive disorders, mucous membrane irritation, constipation, hallucinations, and occasionally deliria. Goldenseal reportedly limits the effectiveness of the anticoagulants heparin and warfarin (Coumadin). You should not take goldenseal if you use these medications. Nor should you take it if you are pregnant or nursing. It also should not be used as a douche.

There is some evidence that the berberine in goldenseal can interfere with drugs that work via the cytochrome P450 3A4–metabolzing system and can make some barbiturates more powerful. Some studies have shown that it decreases the absorption of B vitamins. It may lower blood sugars, so it should be used with caution by people with diabetes who have not used this herb before. If you have heart disease you should not take goldenseal. The tannins in goldenseal tinctures may cause stomach irritation, so you should avoid taking the herb in tincture form if you have diarrhea or chronic heartburn. People with Raynaud's disease who use relatively high dosages of goldenseal may find that it aggravates numbness and tingling, although this effect is minor and temporary.

GOTU KOLA

Latin name: *Centella asiatica* (Apiaceae [parsley] family)
Other common names: centella, hydrocotyle, Indian pennywort, thick-leaved pennywort, white rot

General Description

Gotu kola is a low-growing creeping vine reaching a length of up to twenty inches (fifty centimeters). Native to both India and the southeastern United States, the herb has distinctive fan-shaped leaves that impart a bitter, acrid taste. In India and in Indian cuisines, it is sometimes served as a salad or a cooked vegetable. It also is found in Asia, Sri Lanka, parts of China, western South Sea Islands, Madagascar, South Africa, Mexico, Venezuela, Colombia, and eastern South America. The medicinal parts are aboveground fresh and dried leaves and stems.

Evidence of Benefit

Gotu kola has been used for thousands of years in ayurvedic medicine to revitalize the nerves and brain cells and to treat leprosy, skin ulcers, and other skin problems. Research shows that it has anti-inflammatory effects that help with rheumatism, and it improves the flow of blood throughout the body by strengthening the veins and capillaries. One of its active ingredients, asiaticoside, works to stimulate skin repair and to strengthen skin, hair, nails, and connective tissue. Chinese medicine uses gotu kola for dysentery, diarrhea, vomiting, jaundice, kidney stones, and scabies. Homeopathic remedies include those for skin diseases associated with itching and swelling and for uterine inflammation.

Benefits of gotu kola for specific health conditions include the following:

• *Cognition.* Gotu kola may help with general mental ability. It is likely that the herb protects the blood vessels supplying oxygen to the brain, which normalizes the brain's use of oxygen. Gotu kola also has a reputation for improving memory and concentration. A study conducted in 1992 recorded that memory retention in rats treated with gotu kola was three to sixty times better than that in control animals. Preliminary results in one clinical trial with developmentally disabled children showed that treatment with gotu kola increased scores on tests of intellectual achievement. In one study, children with educable mental retardation showed improvement after six months in several tests of intelligence.

• *Swollen ankles and varicose veins.* Asiaticoside, a component of gotu kola, stabilizes the connective tissue that surrounds the veins of the legs. One study showed that people who just had a vein irritation (post-phlebitis) and were taking gotu kola had improved blood flow and reduced their chance of developing severe vascular disease. While gotu kola significantly improved symptoms of varicose veins, particularly the discomfort, tiredness, and swelling, it did not reduce the unsightliness of veins that were already badly damaged.

• *Wounds, scarring, and periodontal disease.* Many herbal practitioners and physicians report that gotu kola stimulates the regeneration of skin cells and underlying connective tissue. Asiaticoside, in gotu kola, has a beneficial effect on collagen and inhibits its excessive production in scar formation. Studies have reported that gotu kola accelerates the healing of burns and skin grafts and minimizes scarring. Gotu kola cream helps relieve the painful scaly red welts of psoriasis. In one study, when gotu kola was combined with *Punica granatum* (pomegranate), participants' periodontal disease was significantly improved—less bleeding and less gingival disease—after three months.

Considerations for Use

Gotu kola is available in liposome tablets or tinctures, as well as in topical creams. Although gotu kola causes changes on a cellular level in forty-eight to seventy-two hours, clinical studies show that the body does not accumulate a maximum level of asiatic acid, the chief active ingredient, until the herb has been taken for at least three weeks.

Gotu kola should be avoided by women who are pregnant or who are trying to become pregnant, as well as by nursing mothers. It may interfere with oral medications for diabetes such as glipizide (Glucotrol) and tolbutamide (Orinase). Since it may raise cholesterol levels, it should be avoided by people with "borderline" high cholesterol and by anyone taking cholesterol-lowering medications or niacin. You should not use it if you take tranquilizers or sedatives, since it may have a narcotic effect. It should not be given to a child under the age of two. Taken orally in recommended doses, gotu kola appears to be nontoxic. It seldom causes any side effects other than an occasional allergic skin rash. However, there are some concerns that it may be carcinogenic if applied topically to the skin.

GREEN TEA

Latin name: *Camellia sinensis* (Theaceae [tea] family)

General Description

A native of the rainy forests of Southeast Asia, the tea plant is cultivated in Burma, China, India, Japan, Turkey, Pakistan, Malawi, Argentina, Georgia, Sri Lanka, and Africa. The evergreen leaves are limp and downy when young, thick and rounded when mature. In the wild, this small tree grows many small branches. Cultivated tea plants are regularly pruned and kept to a height of about 5 feet (1.5 meters) to make harvesting easy. Only the leaf buds and young leaves are harvested, by hand, to make tea.

Green tea and black tea (the more familiar beverage type of tea) come from the same plant, but green tea is less processed so more of the original plant substances survive in this herb. Green tea contains high levels of substances called polyphenols, which are known to have strong antioxidant, anticarcinogenic, antitumorigenic, antibiotic, and cardioprotective properties.

Evidence of Benefit

Green tea is both a stimulant and an antioxidant with a diversity of healing applications. The polyphenols in green tea are potent antioxidants. Researchers have found that one of the polyphenols, designated epigallocatechin gallate (EGCG), is over 200 times more powerful than the renowned antioxidant vitamin E in neutralizing free radicals. Also, green tea increases energy, which may make it useful as part of a weight-loss program. Green tea may help prevent cancer as well as cavities. Originally it was used for stomach disorders, migraine, symptoms of fatigue, vomiting, and diarrhea. Ayurvedic medicine uses it as a tea for loss of appetite, diarrhea, migraine, heartburn, fever, and fatigue. The Chinese also use it in tea for the same conditions, but also for malaria. Homeopathic remedies are available for cardiac issues (circulation), headaches, states of agitation or depression, and stomach complaints.

Benefits of green tea for specific health conditions include the following:

• *Asthma.* Theophylline, a chemical found in both green and black tea, is extracted from the leaf of the tea plant. Theophylline relaxes the smooth muscles supporting the bronchial tubes, reducing the severity of asthma and bronchitis. Drinking either green or black tea provides theophylline in small doses (0.02 to 0.04 percent), which may not be large enough to affect asthma.

• *Atherosclerosis and high cholesterol.* Green tea lowers blood total cholesterol and low-density lipoprotein (LDL, or "bad") cholesterol without side effects. Clinical studies have shown that green tea slows the oxidation of LDL cholesterol into forms that can cause atherosclerotic plaques, although researchers describe this effect as mild. Black tea has a similar effect. In one study, people who drank five or more cups of green tea compared to those who drank one or fewer had a 42 percent less chance of death due to stroke. Even those who drank one cup a day got some benefit, and the benefit increased according to the number of cups consumed.

• *Breast cancer, endometriosis, fibrocystic breasts.* The polyphenols in green tea occupy many of the sites on the exteriors of cells that otherwise would receive estrogen. This keeps the cells from receiving estrogen, reducing the effects of estrogen on the body. This stops estrogen from stimulating growth of cells in breast, ovarian, and uterine cancer. In one study, women in Japan who had long-term high intakes (five cups a day) of green tea had improved prognosis if they developed breast cancer.

• *Cancer.* A number of animal studies have shown that the polyphenols in green tea may offer significant protection against cancers of the pancreas, prostate, urinary tract, head and neck, colon, stomach, lung, and small intestine.

• *Colorectal cancer and food poisoning.* Green tea catechins kill many types of foodborne bacteria, especially *Clostridium* bacteria, which are associated with colon cancer. Laboratory studies with animals have found that regular consumption of green tea catechins prevents the growth of colorectal tumors.

• *Diabetes.* A couple of human studies have shown that those who consume three cups or more of green tea a day have a 33 percent reduced risk of type 2 diabetes compared to those who drink less than one per day. Even green tea extracts containing 544 milligrams of polyphenols a day lowered insulin levels in patients with borderline diabetes or diabetes over two months. Other parameters such as blood sugar, inflammatory markers, and insulin resistance did not change.

• *Genital warts.* In two studies involving 1,000 people, green tea was applied as an ointment three times a day and 54 percent of the people had their warts cleared by week sixteen compared to only 35 percent in the placebo group.

• *Liver disease and gout.* Researchers have found that components in green tea are able to protect liver cells in rats when they are exposed to hepatotoxic agents. These compounds help to protect the linings of liver cells from damage from oxygen free radicals released by toxins. In addition, green tea may be helpful for gout, as its polyphenols inhibit the enzyme xanthine oxidase, which is responsible for the buildup of uric acid in the blood. This is how the typical treatment, allopurinol, works.

• *Periodontal disease.* Green tea catechins prevent *Streptococcus mutans* from forming dental plaque. (This may explain why early Asians cleaned their teeth with whisks of green tea leaves—before the invention of toothpaste.)

• *Weight loss.* Green tea has a fat-burning capability that promotes fat loss and weight loss and prevents or limits weight regain. In one study, subjects took 90 milligrams of green tea polyphenols and 50 milligrams of caffeine three times a day and fat burning increased by 41 percent, and the amount of calories burned by the body increased as well. These benefits were not seen with caffeine alone, so there is something else in green tea that promotes fat burning and hypermetabolism.

• *Wrinkles.* Green tea may protect the skin from the effects of harmful free radicals that can lead to wrinkling. In one study, women who used a 10 percent green tea cream and 300 milligrams of an extract twice a day for eight weeks had improvement in the elasticity of the skin, but so did the women in the placebo group.

Considerations for Use

Studies suggest that 3 cups (an amount containing the equivalent of 240 to 320 milligrams of polyphenols) of green tea daily provide protection against cancer. However, other research suggests that as much as 10 cups per day is necessary to obtain noticeable benefits. Tablets and capsules containing standardized extracts of polyphenols, particularly EGCG, some providing 97 percent polyphenol content (equivalent to drinking 4 cups of tea), are available. Green tea also can be used in cream form or made into compresses. (*See* COMPRESSES in Part Three.)

Mild side effects have been described, such as stomachache and reduced appetite, when taken internally. Care should be taken in those with a weak heart or renal system, thyroid hyperfunction, or who are susceptible to spasms. Infants may develop anemia from taking too much, so young children should not be given green tea. Pregnant women should avoid green tea as well due to its caffeine content (10 to 50 milligrams per cup depending upon the variety and method of brewing). Caffeine passes to an infant in the milk and may cause a baby to sleep poorly, so it should be avoided if you are nursing. You should not take green tea within one hour of taking herbal teas or patent (over-the-counter [OTC]) medicines. This avoids diluting the decoction in the stomach or interfering with the medication. This is especially important if you are taking codeine, colchicine, or ephedrine, which may become insoluble in the presence of tannins from green or black tea. Finally, you should not drink green tea if you are using ginseng regularly. Green tea can reduce the effectiveness of ginseng. Black tea is not known to have this effect.

People who are taking monoamine oxidase (MAO) inhibitors or the blood-thinner warfarin (Coumadin) should not use green tea medicinally. Green tea contains vitamin K, which directly counteracts the blood-thinning action of warfarin. Certain prescription medications increase the stimulant effects of caffeine found in green tea. These include the ulcer drug cimetidine (Tagamet) and antibiotics such as ciprofloxacin (Cipro), enoxacin (Penetrex), and norfloxacin (Noroxin). Combining green tea (or any other beverage that contains caffeine) with these medications could result in overstimulation and insomnia.

GUGGUL

Latin name: *Commiphora mukkul* (Burseraceae [frankincense] family)
Other common names: guggal, gum guggal, gum guggulu, Indian bedellium

General Description

The mukkul myrrh tree is a medium-sized, thorny tree found throughout India. Guggul and gum guggulu are the names of the yellowish resin exuding from its trunk. This resin is the source of the modern extracts of guggul.

Evidence of Benefit

Guggul has been used to lower serum cholesterol and triglyceride levels, and to treat arthritis and obesity. It is used in ayurvedic medicine to increase circulation, stimulating healthy circulation to the skin, and for hemorrhoids.

Benefits of guggul for specific health conditions include the following:

• *Acne.* A small-scale clinical test found that treating nodulocystic acne with guggulsterones, compounds found in guggul, for three months was as effective as using tetracycline, and produced a 50 percent lower rate of recurrence. Guggulsterones were especially effective in treating this painful form of acne in people with oily skin. This effect is striking because guggulsterones act only by limiting inflammation, and allow the body's own immune processes to do the work of fighting the infection.

• *Congestive heart failure and high cholesterol.* Guggul extracts lower blood cholesterol levels by stimulating the incorporation of cholesterol into the linings of cells, where it is beneficial, and by increasing the excretion of excess cholesterol into the bile to be removed with intestinal wastes. Clinical tests in India have found that about 75 percent of people who used guggulsterones for three months saw their total blood-cholesterol and triglyceride levels go down by 20 to 25 percent. About half the people who used the herb for three months saw higher high-density lipoprotein (HDL, or "good") cholesterol levels. In studies, there have been cases where guggul, when taken by non-Indian people, increased low-density lipoprotein (LDL, or "bad") cholesterol levels compared to a placebo; this was not seen in Indian patients with heart disease. It may be the diet of the Indian population or their genetic makeup that explains the favorable effects.

Considerations for Use

Guggul is taken in the form of guggulsterones, an extract of the resin that has been refined to prevent abdominal discomfort and diarrhea. A common dose is 25 milligrams of guggulsterones three times daily. This herb is also available as an ayurvedic preparation called a rasayana. In addition, guggul is available in tinctures, and in combinations with other "heart-healthy" substances, such as hawthorn, ionositol, and/or niacin.

You should *not* use crude guggulu, which can cause nausea, diarrhea, loss of appetite, and skin rashes. Guggul has been shown to cause headaches, eructation, hiccups, and loose stool. Guggul should be used with caution by people who have Crohn's disease or irritable bowel syndrome (IBS). It also should be avoided by people taking beta-blockers, especially propranolol (Inderal, Innopran), or calcium channel blockers, especially diltiazem (Cardizem), for high blood pressure, since it can make these drugs less available to the body. If you are taking anticoagulants, you should not use guggul because it potentiates the action of the drugs. Guggul should be used with caution by pregnant women and by anyone with liver disease or inflammatory bowel disease and diarrhea.

HAWTHORN

Latin names: *Crataegus* species (Rosaceae [rose] family), *Crataegus laevigata*
Other common names: crataegus, mayflower, quickthorn, whitehorn

General Description

The hawthorn, a member of the rose family, is a thorny deciduous tree that grows to a height of twenty-five feet (eight meters). It bears small white five-petaled blossoms in the late spring that give way to red berries in the late summer. There is considerable debate among researchers as to which parts of the plant have the greatest medicinal value. Fresh and dried berries, fresh and dried flowering tops, dried flowers, dried leaves, and dried flowers and leaves combined are all used beneficially, but the leaves and flowers are the most useful for heart conditions.

Many species of hawthorn are used in herbal medicine. *C. laevigata, C. oxyacantha,* and *C. monogyna* are commonly used in Europe and the United States. Practitioners of traditional Chinese medicine (TCM) employ *C. sinaica,* also known as Japanese hawthorn.

Evidence of Benefit

Hawthorn contains compounds that support the heart and circulatory system. It is most often used to protect against the beginning stages of heart disease, for mild heart muscle weakness, for pressure and tightness of the chest, and for mild arrhythmia. It is also an excellent herb to use to speed recovery from a heart attack. In folk medicine, hawthorn has been used to decrease joint inflammation and decrease fragility of capillaries. TCM uses it for reducing bloating and blood stasis. Homeopathic remedies include those for cardiac insufficiency, uneven rhythm of the heart, and chest pain. The German Commission E approves hawthorn for decreasing cardiac output in class II of the New York Heart Association (NYHA) functional classification system.

Benefits of hawthorn for specific health conditions include the following:

• *Alzheimer's disease and memory loss.* Eastern medicine has long used hawthorn to treat age-related forms of memory problems, and scientific research has identified two ways in which the herb works. One is through its effect on cholesterol (*see* page 84), since fewer and smaller plaques in the arteries supplying the brain means that more blood reaches the brain's tissues. The other way is through its high content of both vitamin C and substances that assist vitamin C, known as cofactors. These substances strengthen tiny capillaries in the brain, especially when these vessels are under stress from high blood pressure or microscopic blood clots. Open capillaries result in more nutrients and oxygen for the brain.

• *Angina, cardiac arrhythmia, and congestive heart failure.* Studies show that substances found in hawthorn interact with key enzymes in the heart to increase the pumping force of the heart muscle and to eliminate arrhythmias. Hawthorn also works to dilate the blood vessels, especially the coronary blood vessels. This enables more oxygen-rich blood to get to the heart and thus to reduce the risk that the heart will be deprived of oxygen, which causes the painful sensations of chest pressure and tightness commonly known as angina pectoris. German studies have confirmed that hawthorn is beneficial for people with angina when taken for at least eight weeks. Hawthorn's action is not immediate, but develops very slowly.

• *Atherosclerosis, congestive heart failure, heart attack, high blood pressure, high cholesterol, and stroke.* A large body of scientific research has shown that the fruit, leaves, and flowers of various hawthorn species dilate the blood vessels, lower blood pressure, and dissolve cholesterol deposits. Hawthorn fights atherosclerosis, in which cholesterol forms plaques on blood-vessel walls. It increases the rate at which low-density lipoprotein (LDL) cholesterol—the "bad," artery-clogging kind of cholesterol—is cleared from the body. Hawthorn also fights atherosclerosis by providing antioxidants, which prevent plaque formation. In one study, using a standardized extract of Crataegus berries (Crataegisan), patients with NYHA class II heart failure were able to better tolerate exercise. These patients took 30 drops of a standardized extract (Crataegisan) three times a day and thirty minutes prior to meals for eight weeks. In another study, patients with heart disease took 600 milligrams a day of hawthorn and did better on a bicycle exercise test.

• *Attention deficit disorder (ADD) and anxiety.* Hawthorn extracts may relieve restlessness, acting out, and anxiety in children; however, it is contraindicated for children twelve years of age and under. The herb not only increases circulation to the brain, but also stops inflammatory responses caused by allergies. Allergies give the brain of a person with an attention deficit problem more information than it can process efficiently. Extracts of *C. laevigata* have a sedative effect on the central nervous system. In one study, patients with anxiety disorders showed improvement in their symptoms using a hawthorn mixture compared to a placebo. Hawthorn was taken with *Eschscholzia californica* (California poppy) in a product called Sympathyl, and they took two tablets twice daily for three months.

• *Diabetic retinopathy.* Laboratory studies indicate that hawthorn has beneficial effects on blood sugar levels and blood viscosity, or stickiness, both of which are implicated in diabetic retinopathy. Few clinical studies exist to support this contention.

Considerations for Use

Hawthorn is available in capsules, tablets, and tinctures. Many people find teas made from hawthorn berries to have a laxative effect.

When buying hawthorn extracts for treatment of anxiety, you should make sure the label states that the source plant is *C. laevigata* or *C. oxyacantha.* The best formulations of hawthorn for supplemental treatment of heart conditions are those containing a standardized extract made from hawthorn leaves and flowers, such as Nature's Way HeartCare Hawthorn Extract. You should use hawthorn as a heart tonic only. It is not a substitute for conventional medical treatment. If you have been diagnosed with angina, cardiac arrhythmias, or congestive heart failure, use this herb only in consultation with a physician.

Side effects from hawthorn include heart palpitations, dizziness, headache, vertigo, hot flashes, and gastrointestinal complaints. In particular, attention should be paid to heart rate and blood pressure. In the case of swelling legs or other problematic symptoms, medical management may be needed. A medical diagnosis is absolutely necessary when pains occur in the heart area, upper abdomen, or area around the neck, or in cases of respiratory distress. Taking large amounts of hawthorn may result in sedation or a dramatic drop in blood pressure, which in turn may cause you to feel faint. Children twelve and under and pregnant or nursing women should use hawthorn only under the direction of a licensed health-care professional. It is not to be used when taking anticlotting or antiarrhythmic drugs. For central nervous system depressants, hawthorn may make the drugs have stronger effects.

HO SHE WU

Latin name: *Polygonum multiflorum* (Polygonaceae [cornbind] family)
Other common names: fo-ti, ho shou wu

General Description

Polygonum is a long vine with tiny leaves on dozens of alternating small branches. It is native to China and grows extensively in Japan and Taiwan. It is also found in the wild in North Carolina. The unprocessed root, known in Chinese medicine as fo-ti, is sometimes used. However, once it has been boiled in a special liquid made from black beans, it is rendered into a better medicine. The processed root is called red fo-ti. Ho she wu has been used to treat infertility, premature aging, weakness, vaginal discharges, numerous infectious diseases, angina pectoris, and erectile dysfunction (ED).

Evidence of Benefit

Ho she wu is a traditional calming herb from Chinese medicine that has been shown to lower cholesterol and triglyceride levels in cells and animal studies. Herbalists also recommend it as a tonic to maintain youthful vigor, increase energy, tone the kidneys and liver, and purify the blood. It is said to have the effects of darkening prematurely gray hair.

Benefits of ho she wu for specific health conditions include the following:

• *High cholesterol.* Ho she wu contains a natural form of lecithin, which could be helpful to reduce arterial plaque and blood pressure. In laboratory tests, it reduces blood levels of cholesterol and triglycerides. One chemical found in this herb has been found to prevent cholesterol from forming blood-vessel plaques in test animals fed large amounts of dietary cholesterol.

• *Nightmares.* Ho she wu is employed in traditional Chinese medicine (TCM) to treat repeated nightmares.

Considerations for Use

Ho she wu is available in capsules and tablets. The unprocessed root, which can cause diarrhea and skin rashes, should not be used. This herb should not be confused with fo-ti tieng, a Chinese herbal medicine made from gotu kola.

HOELEN

Latin name: Poria cocos (Polyporaceae [polypore mushroom] family)
Other common names: China-root, fu-ling, poria, tuckahoe

General Description

Hoelen is a mushroom that grows underground on the roots of pines and other trees around the world. In many parts of the world, hoelen is used as a food rather than as a medicine. This was true in the nineteenth century, when hoelen was known as tuckahoe in the eastern and southern United States. A single mushroom could grow to weigh between fifteen and twenty pounds (seven to nine kilograms). Since large mushrooms could be ground into bread flour, the herb became better known as tuckahoe bread.

Evidence of Benefit

Hoelen is a healing mushroom and a source of potassium. It is also an effective diuretic and has antibacterial properties in cell and animal studies. It is used in both Native American medicine and traditional Chinese medicine (TCM) to treat kidney ailments. Hoelen has also been used in TCM for lowering blood sugar and controlling stomach acids.

Benefits of hoelen for specific health conditions include the following:

• *Kidney disease.* In animal studies, hoelen relieves the chronic kidney inflammation of glomerulonephritis. This is an autoimmune condition that results when the body produces antibodies that attack its own tissues. Sometimes, these antibodies accumulate in the kidney, which becomes clogged and loses its ability to retain essential products. Proteins begin to leak out into the urine, a process that can quickly progress to kidney failure. One of hoelen's main constituents, pachyman, may halt this process by preventing the accumulation of antibodies.

Considerations for Use

Dried or fresh hoelen can be taken daily in food, or it can be brewed into tea. Improvement in chronic conditions may take three to four months of consistent use. Only one case of side effects caused by hoelen, in which an allergic reaction resulted in hives and stomach upset, appears in the medical literature.

Since hoelen benefits people with autoimmune kidney disease through several different mechanisms, eating the unprocessed mushroom is preferable to taking extracts.

HOPS

Latin name: *Humulus lupulus* (Cannabaceae [marijuana] family)

General Description

Hops is a perennial climbing vine found in the wild in Europe, and cultivated in the temperate zones of Asia and the United States for use in making beer. Male and female flowers are borne on different plants. The conelike flowers of the female hops plants are picked for use in brewing beer and in herbal medicine.

Evidence of Benefit

Hops has been used to treat anxiety and insomnia for more than a thousand years. A pillow filled with hops has been used to encourage sleep. According to herbal folklore, elderly women who worked as hops pickers experienced a return of their menstrual cycles and other youthful attributes. This led to the use of hops as a hormonal balancer and general restorative during and after menopause. Folk medicine has used it for stimulating the appetite and increasing the secretion of stomach juices. It also has been used for nerve pain, tension headaches, and intestinal inflammation, and externally for ulcers and skin abrasions. Homeopathic remedies exist for treating nervousness and insomnia. The German Commission E has approved its use for mood disturbances such as restlessness and anxiety and sleep issues.

Benefits of hops for specific health conditions include the following:

• *Indigestion.* Hops contain bitter substances that activate a reflex reaction in the central nervous system. This reflex stimulates the stomach to secrete digestive juices, relieving the feeling of fullness by helping the stomach digest food. The reaction also stimulates the flow of bile. This may help with nervous stomach, colitis, and irritable bowel syndrome (IBS), and also may be a preventative treatment for those prone to ulcers in the GI tract.

• *Insomnia.* Hops, like the beers that are made from it, is a well-known sleep aid. Aging hops for up to two years allows two of the herb's chemical compounds, humulone and lupulone, to create a substance that is chemically similar to chlordiazepoxide (Librium) and diazepam (Valium). In one study, combining hops with another herb, valerian, improved sleep and quality of life in individuals who had mild insomnia. In another study, when these herbs were combined with other herbs such as motherwort and balm leaf, sleep quality was improved in a group of alcohol-dependent patients. They also experienced reduced

UNDERSTANDING HERBAL HEALING | Part One

sleepiness the next day and fewer bad dreams, and sleep-walked less frequently.

• *Menopausal symptoms.* Many studies have been conducted using hops for menopausal symptoms, but the results are conflicting. Much of the problem lies in the lack of standardization of the hops. One group of investigators standardized hops to 8-prenylnaringenin (8-PN). Two doses were administered to two different groups of post-menopausal women—100 micrograms or 250 micrograms of 8-PN. The dose amount had no effect on the results; both groups had reduced menopausal-related discomforts and complaints, especially fewer hot flashes.

Considerations for Use

Hops is available in capsules, powders, and tinctures, and also is taken as a tea. Many commercial formulas combine hops with valerian for their synergistic effect in inducing sleep. (*See* VALERIAN.) For most people 0.5 gram is considered the daily dose.

Hops contains the most potent of all the plant estrogens, prenylnaringenin. For this reason, children of either sex who have not reached puberty should not be given hops. Pregnant women, women with estrogen-sensitive disorders, especially estrogen-dependent breast cancer, and men who have gynecomastia (enlargement of the breasts) or erectile dysfunction (ED) also should avoid this herb. This phytoestrogen can be detected in beer, but the levels in beer are low and should not pose any cause for concern, although the phytoestrogens in hops can cause fat to be deposited into the classic "beer-belly" pattern. Dieters seeking to reduce the waistline should avoid both beer and medicinal application of hops.

The excessive use of hops may cause side effects such as dizziness, cognitive changes, and mild jaundice if used in conjunction with central nervous system depressants, antipsychotics, or alcohol. When used during menses, hops can produce nervousness, dermatitis, and respiratory allergies. Chronic consumption of hops may increase the potency of anesthetics used in surgery. It is wise to avoid using hops for at least two weeks before any type of surgery requiring general anesthesia, and to inform your doctor that you have been using hops before undergoing an operation. Hops should not be taken if you suffer from depression.

You should not take hops during the day if you will be driving or operating heavy machinery, or if you are depressed, as this herb may aggravate that condition. Do not take hops with medications for insomnia or anxiety except under a physician's supervision.

HOREHOUND

Latin name: *Marrubium vulgare* (Lamiaceae [mint] family)
Other common names: houndsbane, marrubio (Spanish), marvel, white horehound

General Description

Horehound is a medicinal mint that is native to Morocco but was carried to Europe and North America long ago by traders and settlers. Horehound flourishes in Britain, where it is cultivated on the corners of cottage gardens and is used to make teas and candy to treat coughs and colds.

Growing to a height of one to two feet (thirty to sixty centimeters), horehound bears densely packed green leaves with white edges on a single stalk. Small white flowers appear at the nodes between leaves and the stem. All the aerial (aboveground) parts of the plant are used in herbal medicine.

Evidence of Benefit

Horehound has been a popular cough and cold remedy since ancient Roman times. It is also a gentle expectorant and digestive aid. Laboratory tests have found that its best-known chemical constituent, marrubiin, is more potent than some well-known pain relief medications. In folk medicine, it has been used for bronchitis, whooping cough, asthma, tuberculosis, diarrhea, jaundice, and painful menstruation. Externally, it was used for skin damage, ulcers, wounds, and as a gargle for mouth and throat irritations. Homeopathic remedies exist for inflammation of the respiratory tract. It is approved by the German Commission E for dyspeptic complaints and loss of appetite as a result of flatulence and bloating.

Benefits of horehound for specific health conditions include the following:

• *Bronchitis, colds, and sinusitis.* The compound marrubiin (sometimes spelled marubin) in horehound stimulates the central nervous system. This results in the secretion of fluids into the bronchial passageways, softening phlegm and making expectoration easier. It also combines the action of relaxing the smooth muscle of the bronchi while promoting mucus production and expectoration.

• *Indigestion.* Marrubiin's stimulation of the central nervous system in turn stimulates the stomach to secrete digestive juices. This relieves feelings of fullness by helping the stomach digest food. The reaction also stimulates the flow of bile, which eases flatulence by changing the chemical composition of the contents of the large intestine. Marrubiin is responsible for horehound's distinctive bitter taste. Horehound also stops high and low blood sugar reactions after eating high-carbohydrate meals and snacks.

Considerations for Use

Horehound is available as a juice, lozenge, or tea. It is also included in the alcohol-free cough syrup Herbs for Kids Horehound Blend. The average dose is 4.5 grams of the herb or 30 to 60 milliliters of the juice.

For treatment of gastrointestinal upset, it is important to take the tea thirty minutes before eating. Horehound should not be used by pregnant women, nursing mothers, children under the age of eighteen, or adults over the age of sixty-five. This herb can mildly increase menstrual flow, so you should not use it if you have menstrual problems. It is a mild laxative if taken in large quantities. If you have heart problems or stomach ulcers, consult with your health-care practitioner before taking horehound.

HORSE CHESTNUT

Latin name: *Aesculus hippocastanum* (Hippocastanaceae [horse chestnut] family)
Other common names: buckeye, common horse chestnut, conqueror tree, Spanish chestnut

General Description

The horse chestnut is a sturdy, domed tree that grows to a height of eighty feet (twenty-five meters). It bears leaves composed of five to seven leaflets, clusters of pink and white flowers, and a spiny green fruit that contains up to three shiny brown seeds as much as two inches (four centimeters) in width. Although the bark, leaves, and seeds are all used in herbal medicine, the most effective form of the herb is an extract of its active constituent, aescin. The herb is indigenous to the mountains of Greece, Bulgaria, the Caucasus, northern Iran, and the Himalayas. It is cultivated in northern Europe, including the British Isles, Denmark, and Russia.

Evidence of Benefit

Horse chestnut leaves have been used as a cough remedy and fever-reducer. They were also used to reduce the pain and inflammation of arthritis and rheumatism. However, horse chestnut is mainly used to tone the walls of veins, helping to prevent these blood vessels from becoming slack or swollen and turning into varicose veins or hemorrhoids. Horse chestnut also reduces fluid retention by normalizing the permeability of blood vessel walls. It can also help ease nighttime leg cramps. It also has been used for eczema, hemorrhoids, and pain before menstruation. Horse chestnut was approved by the German Commission E for pathological conditions of the veins of the legs (chronic venous insufficiency), for example, pains and heaviness in the legs, cramps in the calves during the night, and leg swelling. However, if a physician has already prescribed noninvasive therapies such as leg compresses or supportive stockings, you must be under close supervision if you wish to take horse chestnut.

Benefits of horse chestnut for specific health conditions include the following:

• *Bruises.* Aescin (a compound in horse chestnut) stabilizes fragile capillaries damaged by blunt trauma. Stabilizing the capillaries reduces bleeding and fluid accumulation into bruised soft tissues.

• *Chronic venous insufficiency and ulceration.* From a meta-analysis of the use of horse chestnut for chronic venous insufficiency, the herb improved signs and symptoms such as leg pain and swelling. In a study of patients with leg ulcers from venous ulceration, horse chestnut improved the ulcers compared to a placebo. In another study, pregnant women with leg swelling experienced relief and less swelling from Venostasin, a supplement containing 50 milligrams of aescin, taken twice daily.

• *Hemorrhoids, lymphedema, swollen ankles, and varicose veins.* Studies show that aescin reduces the number and diameter of tiny pores in the capillaries. This inhibits fluid from passing through the capillary membranes, which reduces swelling in the surrounding tissues. This normalizes vessel walls that are abnormally permeable and susceptible to edema. Aescin also "firms up" varicose veins (including hemorrhoids) by increasing the tone of the muscle layers underlying them. In one study, patients using 40 milligrams of aescin extract three times a day for two months had less pain and the size of hemorrhoids was reduced. Improvements were identified after only two weeks using horse chestnut.

Considerations for Use

For internal use, choose horse chestnut tablets standardized to deliver at least 10 milligrams of aescin. Doses start at 10 milligrams of aescin and gradually increase to around 100 milligrams. One hundred milligrams of aescin corresponds to 250 to 312.5 milligrams of extract, which can be administered twice a day in a delayed release form (encapsulated) for postoperative traumatic edema, hemorrhoids, or varicose veins. Most horse chestnut tablets combine aescin extract with citrus bioflavonoids, which also increase venous strength. For external use, use aescin cream, most easily obtained from a compounding pharmacist.

The seeds of the horse chestnut tree are poisonous. If the compound aesculin (not to be confused with aescin, which is beneficial) is not properly removed, the herb can cause vomiting, diarrhea, and paralysis that can become life-threatening, particularly for children. Purified horse chestnut extracts standardized for aescin at the doses listed above are generally safe, although there have been isolated reports of kidney damage in people who consumed very large amounts of aescin. Children are particularly susceptible to high doses of horse chestnut.

Horse chestnut products should not be taken *internally* by women who are pregnant, who are trying to become pregnant, or who are nursing. This herb should be avoided by anyone with liver or kidney disease. If you are taking blood-thinning medication, you should not use horse chestnut unless you do so under the supervision of a physician.

HORSETAIL

Latin name: *Equisetum arvense* (Equisetaceae [horsetail] family)

Other common names: bottle-brush, corn horsetail, horse-tail rush, horse willow, paddock-pipes, queue de cheval, scouring rush, shave grass, toadpipe

General Description

Horsetail is a descendant of giant fernlike plants that covered the earth some 200 million years ago. It has two distinctive types of stems. One variety of stem grows early in spring and looks like asparagus. The mature form of the herb has branched, feathery stems that look like a horse's tail. The other variety sends up hollow, jointed, leafless bamboolike stalks that reach six feet (two meters) in length. At the top, there are spore-bearing structures that resemble horsetails. This plant is widely distributed throughout the northern hemisphere including Europe, but grows in Asia and as far south as Turkey and Iran. The plant is also found in the Himalayas, central and northern China, and Japan. The aerial (aboveground) parts of the nonfruiting stems are used in herbal medicine and can be eaten as a vegetable; they can be used dried or fresh.

Evidence of Benefit

Horsetail was originally recommended by Galen, one of the first renowned physicians of ancient times. Since then, several cultures have used this herb for kidney and bladder problems, arthritis, bleeding ulcers, and tuberculosis. The topical use of horsetail is said to stop the bleeding of wounds and promote rapid healing. Unproven folk medicine uses include treating tuberculosis, heavy menstrual flow, brittle fingernails, loss of hair, gout, and frostbite. Homeopathic remedies exist for urinary tract and kidney disorders. The German Commission E recommends that horsetail be used internally for post-traumatic and static edema, irrigation of a bacterial infection, and inflammation of the lower urinary tract and kidney stones. Externally it is used for treating poorly healing wounds.

Horsetail is rich in silica, which strengthens connective tissue and combats arthritis. Silicon is a vital component for bone and cartilage formation.

Benefits of horsetail for specific health conditions include the following:

• *Bronchitis and emphysema.* The silica in horsetail promotes tissue repair and healing for people with breathing difficulties such as bronchitis and emphysema.

Considerations for Use

Horsetail is available as fluidextract, tea, or tincture. Tinctures and fluidextracts—preparations of the herb subjected to high temperatures during manufacturing—are preferred for medicinal use. The processing neutralizes a harmful enzyme that destroys the vitamin B_1 (thiamine). The average daily intake of the herb is 6 grams.

You should not use horsetail if you are pregnant or nursing. The herb's high selenium content can cause birth defects. Adults over sixty-five and children between two and twelve years old should use low-dose formulas. You should not give horsetail to a child under two years of age, and you should not let a child put the stalks in his or her mouth. The plant contains small amounts of nicotine and other alkaloids that may cause a toxic reaction.

People with cardiac disease or high blood pressure should use horsetail only under a physician's care. Do not take horsetail internally for an extended period of time and do not exceed the recommended dosage. Extended use may cause kidney or heart damage. Do not use horsetail for irrigation therapy if you suffer from edema due to poor kidney or heart function. Notify a doctor if you use the herb as a bath additive and you develop skin lesions, fever, or heart problems.

INULA

See ELECAMPANE.

IPORURU

Latin name: *Alchornea* species (Euphorbiaceae [spurge] family)
Other common names: iporoni, macochihua, niando

General Description

Iporuru is a shrub native to the Amazon and parts of Africa. It grows on low-lying plains that become swamps during the rainy season. It is harvested only during the dry season, when its medically active constituents are present. The bark is used in herbal medicine. Iporuru remedies and products are sold in local markets and herbal pharmacies in Peru.

Evidence of Benefit

Iporuru has been used for respiratory and urinary tract infections and gastrointestinal tract problems. Iporuru bark steeped in aguardiente (rum) is a traditional South American remedy for arthritis, colds, and muscle pains after a long day of fishing or hunting. In Peru, health-care practitioners prescribe iporuru to treat rheumatism and erectile dysfunction (ED), and to reduce blood sugar in people with diabetes. Indigenous peoples of Peru use it to relieve symptoms of osteoarthritis. In Africa, it was frequently used as an aphrodisiac and hallucinogen.

Benefits of iporuru for specific health conditions include the following:

• *Erectile dysfunction and infertility.* Iporuru is a unique traditional treatment for infertility in men in that it is taken by the woman rather than by the man. A plausible explanation for this effect is that the herb increases the receptivity of the cervix to sperm cells. French scientists have proposed that men taking iporuru would have stronger erections, greater penetration, and more viable sperm through the action of yohimbine, a compound found in both iporuru and yohimbe. (*See* YOHIMBE.)

Considerations for Use

Iporuru is available as a tincture. Some commercial formulas combine iporuru with smilax as an aphrodisiac or with cat's claw to relieve inflammation. Overdoses can occur if iporuru is used excessively. Follow dosage directions carefully, as this herb is considered severely toxic. High doses in animal studies cause the animals to become severely agitated. Cases of death in humans have occurred from exhaustion due to overstimulation and hallucinations.

JAMBUL

Latin name: *Eugenia jambolana* (Myrtaceae [clove] family)
Other common names: black plum, jambolan flowers, jamul, java plum, rose apple, syzygium cumini (jambul seeds)

General Description

Jambul is an evergreen tree that can reach up to one hundred feet (thirty meters) in height. It is a common tree throughout Asia and Australia. Jambul is a species of clove used in ayurvedic medicine. Ayurveda uses jambul's fruit and seeds, rather than flowers, as with other kinds of cloves. The ripe fruit has a scent and taste similar to the apricot. Recently, this tree has gained interest because the seeds, leaves, and bark have been shown to lower blood sugar in animal models.

Evidence of Benefit

Jambul tightens and tones tissues, may help to expel gas, and is a general regulator of digestive function. It also may be useful for diarrhea. Researchers in India are investigating its potential as a male contraceptive.

Benefits of jambul for specific health conditions include the following:

• *Cancer.* In cell studies, jambul and the form of clove used in South American folk medicine (Surinam cherry, or *E. uniflora*) contain oleanolic acid, which reduces damage to the heart and liver caused by cancer chemotherapy with doxorubicin (Adriamycin, Rubex). Both jambul and the species of clove more commonly used in cooking (*E. caryophyllata*) contain compounds that activate the detoxifying enzyme glutathione S-transferase in the liver. In laboratory studies with animals, increasing the production of glutathione S-transferase lowered the probability of developing stomach cancer by nearly 80 percent.

• *Diabetes and diabetic retinopathy.* Practitioners of ayurvedic medicine report that jambul fruit pulp lowers blood sugar levels in approximately thirty minutes, while jambul seed lowers blood sugar levels in about twenty-four hours. Speak to your doctor first before using this

herb if you have diabetes. Animal studies suggest that jambul can prevent the formation of cataracts caused by diabetes. Jambul also has been shown in cell studies to short-circuit the chemical reactions that make toxic free radicals. Without these free radicals, macrophages—the immune system's cleanup cells—do not accumulate at injured spots on artery walls, where they can form an artery-clogging foam.

Considerations for Use

Add jambul seeds to cooking daily. Ayurvedic medicine teaches that jambul is synergistic with okra; when okra and jambul are eaten together, jambul's blood sugar–lowering action is intensified.

KAVA KAVA

Latin name: *Piper methysticum* (Piperaceae [black pepper] family)
Other common names: ava, ava pepper, intoxicating pepper, kava, kava pepper, kawa-kawa, tonga

General Description

Kava kava is an evergreen shrub native to the Polynesian islands of the South Pacific. It is commercially cultivated in Australia and Hawaii. The kava kava plant grows to a height of ten feet (three meters), and has fleshy stems and heart-shaped leaves. The dried root is aromatic, bitter, and pungent, leaving the mouth feeling slightly numbed, and is used in herbal medicine.

South Pacific islanders have used kava kava for over 3,000 years. A kava kava root cocktail played an important part in social and ceremonial life. It was especially important during meetings involving conflicts, because kava kava induces a state of relaxation and goodwill among parties trying to reconcile differences. It was also noted for enhancing mental acuity, memory, and sensory perception. The medicinal parts are the peeled, dried cut rhizome, which normally has been freed from the roots, and the fresh rhizome with the roots.

Evidence of Benefit

Kava kava is analgesic, sedative, and mildly euphoriant. It is used mostly for its sedative properties, which do not seem to impair the user's mental alertness. Kava kava also is believed to be an antiseptic and anti-inflammatory agent in the urinary tract, making it suitable for treating urinary tract infections (UTIs) such as cystitis and inflammation of the prostate gland. It is also good for headaches. Folk medicine used the herb as a sleeping agent and sedative, for asthma, rheumatism, gastric symptoms, chronic cystitis, syphilis, gonorrhea, and weight loss. In homeopathic medicine, it is used for excitement and exhaustion. It was also used for gastritis and pain of the urethra. Kava kava is approved by the German Commission E for nervous anxiety, stress, and restlessness.

Benefits of kava kava for specific health conditions include the following:

• *Anxiety, depression, stress, and diminished sex drive.* Several controlled studies have shown that symptoms of generalized anxiety disorder, including agoraphobia, social phobia, and anxiety disorder, were significantly reduced in people who took kava kava as compared with those who took a placebo or benzodiazepines, the standard treatment. Several of the chemical constituents of kava kava interact with the brain's benzodiazepine receptors. These are the same sites that are activated by the tranquilizers chlordiazepoxide (Librium) and diazepam (Valium). These tranquilizers can be addictive, impair memory, and worsen depression, while kava kava improves mental functioning and mood and is not addictive.

Kava kava also contains compounds that relax tension in the skeletal muscles. This effect is achieved by kava kava because it has an ability to inhibit sodium ion currents. Sodium ions have a voltage charge, and reducing the movement of sodium ions leads to muscle relaxation.

• *Insomnia.* One extract of kava kava, WS 1490, has been found to help people who have anxiety-related sleep disorders. In one study, participants who used 200 milligrams a day of kava kava slept better and felt rested after sleeping. This product was used successfully in other studies and produced no side effects or post-study withdrawal symptoms.

Considerations for Use

Kava kava should be taken in the form of tablets standardized to contain 70 percent kavalactones. The dosage used in most clinical studies for anxiety is three 100-milligram tablets daily. Others have suggested that the daily dose of the root extract should be 150 to 300 milligrams twice daily with 50 to 240 milligrams of kava kava pyrones, or 60 to 120 milligrams of kava kava pyrones. You should not take kava kava on a daily basis for longer than three months. You should not take kava kava after consuming alcohol or if you are taking pharmaceutical antidepressants, benzodiazepine tranquilizers, or sleeping pills. It should not be used with anticoagulants, muscle relaxants, monoamine oxidase (MAO) inhibitors, or dopamine agonists. There is one report of an individual becoming disoriented and lethargic after combining alprazolam (Xanax) and kava kava, requiring brief hospitalization. Care should be taken when driving or operating machinery.

Kava kava is contraindicated in patients with endogenous depression because it increases the chance of suicide. Kava kava can cause dyskinesia (an impairment of voluntary movement similar to a tic or spasm), so it should be avoided by those with neurological disorders such as Parkinson's disease. The U.S. Food and Drug Administration (FDA) has advised consumers of the potential risk of severe liver injury associated with kava kava consumption. You should not take kava kava with any other drug or herb that has a potential for hepatic toxicity. Some examples of herbs to avoid when using kava kava include chaparral, Russian comfrey, germander, pennyroyal, and petasites. Most authorities on medicinal herbalism recommend that pregnant women and nursing mothers avoid kava kava. Avoid taking kava kava for two weeks prior to undergoing elective surgery. This herb is not recommended for people with generalized anxiety disorders without checking with their physician.

Chronic overconsumption of kava kava can produce dry skin, labored breathing, and alteration of red and white blood cell counts, but this generally happens only with extremely large doses. People have reported mild and reversible gastrointestinal complaints, and central nervous system problems such as dizziness and headaches and uncoordinated eye movements. Constant, long-term large doses of kava kava have been associated with damage to the liver, skin, eyes, and spinal cord.

KELP

Latin names: Various genera, including *Fucus, Laminaria, Macrocystis, Nerocystis* (Sargassum [kelp] family)
Other common names: bladderwrack (*Fucus vesiculosus*), brown kelp seaweed, marine oak, sea wrack

General Description

The term *kelp* is used to describe a number of brownish-green seaweed species. The brown alga known as bladderwrack is a particularly common source of kelp. Seaweeds used as kelp may grow from a few feet to over one hundred feet (thirty meters) in length, but those most commonly used in herbal medicine are harvested when they are three feet (one meter) long. The entire plant is used. Kelp is harvested year-round in the North Atlantic and Mediterranean, and off the coasts of Japan.

Kelp is an important part of the diet in Japan, Norway, and Scotland. For vegans (vegetarians who eat no animal products at all), it supplies vitamin B_{12}, otherwise found almost exclusively in animal products.

Evidence of Benefit

Kelp is a laxative and contains considerable amounts of iodine. Given its iodine content, it has been used to regulate low thyroid function due to a lack of iodine in the diet (hypothyroidism). However, kelp is no longer recommended for this condition. Kelp also has been proposed as a weight-loss agent. Herbalists rely on kelp's active ingredient, sodium alginate, to treat heavy-metal toxins such as barium and cadmium, and to prevent the body from absorbing strontium-90, a radioactive substance created in nuclear power plants.

Besides iodine, kelp has an enormous supply of essential nutrients, including protein, essential fatty acids, fiber, sodium and potassium salts, and a variety of other substances. The trace mineral content of kelp is among the highest of any single known source.

Benefits of kelp for specific health conditions include the following:

• *Cancer and menstrual symptoms.* Kelp has been demonstrated to have anti-estrogenic effects. It is believed to be responsible for the reduced risk of estrogen-related cancers in Asian populations. It also may lower estradiol levels, thereby altering menstrual cycle patterns. In a study using rats, kelp acted as a competitive inhibitor of estradiol, thereby lengthening the estrous cycles of the rats.

• *Cellulite and skin elasticity.* When applied topically, kelp acts as an anti-collagenase and antioxidant, which improve the skin's elasticity and keeps it supple, and may address cellulite.

• *Constipation.* Kelp is a gentle laxative. Up to 25 percent of its weight consists of algin, a complex carbohydrate that swells in water. Algin forms a gel within the intestines that coats and soothes the intestinal lining and softens the stool.

Considerations for Use

Kelp can be eaten as an occasional dietary item in any quantity desired. It should not be eaten every day, though, to prevent consuming too much iodine. It has been reported that the average kelp-based supplement contains 1,000 micrograms of iodine per dose. The recommended dietary intake of iodine for adults in the United States is 150 micrograms per day, with intakes above 2,000 micrograms per day considered potentially harmful. You should therefore limit consumption of kelp to once a week unless otherwise directed. Make sure that the kelp is harvested from non-polluted waters. Kelp has been known to contain heavy metals such as arsenic, cadmium, and mercury, which can cause kidney disease.

Since iodine is a critical element in many thyroid hormones, it has long been thought that increasing available iodine with kelp would stimulate thyroid hormone production. However, scientists have since learned that too much iodine can actually inhibit thyroid activity. Studies of Japanese coastal cities in which large amounts of kelp are eaten show that this type of diet is associated with very high rates of low-level hypothyroidism, or low thyroid activity. It is as if constant consumption of kelp first stimulates and then depletes thyroid function. For this reason, kelp is no longer recommended for hypothyroidism. You should not take kelp if you suffer from hyperthyroidism, have heart problems, or are pregnant or nursing. Kelp should not be used by patients who have hormone-sensitive cancers. It may have an increased effect when taken with cholesterol-lowering and antihypertensive medications.

KHELLA

Latin name: *Ammi visnaga* (Apiaceae [parsley] family)
Other common names: ammi visnaga, bishop's weed fruit

General Description

Khella is a bitter yet aromatic member of the same plant family as carrots and parsley. The plant grows erect to a height of three feet (one meter), bearing wispy leaves and clusters of small white flowers. In late summer, it produces tiny fruits, which are picked before they have ripened for use in herbal preparations. Native to North Africa, khella appeared in Egyptian medicine as much as 4,000 years ago in formulas to treat kidney stones.

Evidence of Benefit

Khella has been purported to combat spasms in the smooth muscles that line the walls of blood vessels, bronchial airways, and other tubes and ducts, making it useful in the treatment of angina, asthma, atherosclerosis, and kidney stones. It has also been suggested that it may improve circulation in the heart muscle and gives a mild boost to the heart's pumping action.

Benefits of khella for specific health conditions include the following:

• *Angina and atherosclerosis.* Khella may help increase circulation to the heart without reducing blood pressure. European researchers have found that one of the chemical constituents of khella, visnagin, also acts as a calcium channel blocker. In cells and in humans, khella may prevent blood-vessel constriction that would result in raised blood pressure. Two other compounds in khella, khellin and visnadin, keep blood vessels from constricting in response to epinephrine, the hormone pumped into the bloodstream by the adrenal glands during stress. This has only been achieved in cell lines, so the effect on humans is unknown. Khella has been shown to increase the ratio of high-density lipoprotein (HDL, or "good") cholesterol to low-density lipoprotein (LDL, or "bad") cholesterol.

• *Asthma.* Khellin and visnagin have been shown to have antispasmodic action on the muscles lining the bronchial passages in cell studies. Talk to your doctor before using this for an asthma attack.

• *Kidney stones.* The most ancient application of khella is in the treatment of kidney stones. *The Complete German Commission E Monographs* recommends khella for its ability to help the urinary passages heal after the trauma of passing kidney stones.

• *Vitiligo.* Vitiligo is a disorder in which the skin loses its pigment-bearing melanocytes. Some researchers have found that a combination of oral khellin and natural sun exposure caused repigmentation. Khellin, the active constituent of khella, appears to work like psoralen drugs:

It increases the sensitivity of remaining melanocytes (pigment-forming cells) to sunlight, which stimulates re-pigmentation of the skin.

Considerations for Use

Khella is available in tablets (khellin) and tinctures. It can also be taken as a tea and is sometimes applied in prescription creams for vitiligo. Using khella does *not* substitute for emergency treatment of severe asthmatic attacks.

In the treatment of vitiligo, absorption of khellin dramatically increases when the cream is left in contact with the skin for more than thirty minutes. Khella contains a number of compounds that may make skin especially sensitive to ultraviolet light. When taking khella for conditions other than vitiligo, you should avoid tanning lamps and use a sunblock when outdoors. If exposure to strong sunlight is unavoidable, stop using khella. Because khella also contains natural blood-thinning agents, using this herb with prescription blood-thinning medications may create an unacceptable risk of bleeding. People taking such drugs should avoid khella. You should consult your health-care provider before taking this herb if you are pregnant or nursing.

Long-term use of khella can bring on queasiness, dizziness, loss of appetite, headache, and sleep disorders. Regular ingestion of high dosages of khellin (100 milligrams or more) can lead to liver problems.

KUDZU

Latin name: *Pueraria lobata* (Fabaceae [legume] family)
Other common names: ge gen, Japanese arrowroot, kudsu, pueraria, puerariae, pueraria root, radix

General Description

The creeping kudzu vine is native to Japan but now has spread throughout the southeastern United States, Southeast Asia, and potentially throughout tropical and subtropical regions around the world. Under ideal conditions, kudzu can grow one foot (thirty centimeters) per day and up to one hundred feet (thirty meters) in a single growing season. The root is used in herbal medicine.

Kudzu is used in Japan as both food and medicine. The common term *kudzu* in English corresponds to the Japanese term for kudzu starch, used in thickening soups and making noodles. The stems yield a fiber called kokemp that is useful in making cloth and paper.

Evidence of Benefit

Kudzu has been used in traditional Chinese medicine (TCM) since at least the year 100 for the treatment of headache and stiff neck with pain due to high blood pressure. Kudzu has also been used for allergic rhinitis, diarrhea, gastroenteritis, migraines, psoriasis, trauma, and osteoporosis. It is used in modern Chinese medicine as a treatment for angina pectoris. It is also TCM's principal herb for the treatment of alcoholism, diabetes, neck pain, and the common cold. Kudzu has application in the treatment of cancer and is helpful in treating the early stages of deafness and various neurological conditions.

Benefits of kudzu for specific health conditions include the following:

- *Alcoholism.* Chinese physicians have used kudzu as a cure for alcoholism for over 2,000 years. The tea that is used is called *xing-jiu-ling*, which is literally translated as "sober up." A biochemist at Harvard Medical School, Wing Ming Keung, compiled studies of over 300 cases in Hong Kong. In all of the cases he reviewed, kudzu tonics were considered effective for controlling and suppressing the appetite for alcohol, without side effects. In clinical studies, kudzu has been shown to significantly reduce the amount that heavy drinkers drink, increase the number of sips and the time taken to consume each drink, with a decrease in volume of each sip. Participants showed no urge to drink more. No side effects were reported. Kudzu appeared to suppress alcohol intake and reduce withdrawal symptoms.

Researchers at Indiana University have discovered two compounds in kudzu that alter the enzymes that break down alcohol in the liver. As a result, an alcohol by-product called acetaldehyde builds up. When this happens, nausea, facial redness, and general discomfort usually ensue. These compounds work in the same way as the prescription drug disulfiram (Antabuse). Kudzu compounds, however, do not induce nausea to as great an extent as disulfiram, although both treatments increase the discomfort of intoxication.

However, a one-month double-blind study of thirty-eight individuals with alcoholism found no improvement in the participants given kudzu as compared with those given a placebo. One reason for the discrepancy in the results among studies may be that the compound daidzin in kudzu becomes less effective when purified during processing. Kudzu may be more effective if used in its natural state, such as in kudzu tea. It is possible that persons of East Asian ancestry have the greatest response to kudzu as a treatment for alcohol abuse. In East Asia, especially in Korea, as much as 80 percent of the population lacks the enzyme that processes acetaldehyde. Since alcohol tolerance is genetically lower among such persons, kudzu may have a more dramatic effect on them.

- *Cancer.* Kudzu has purported effects on cancer treatment because it prevents the cancer cells from multiplying and has anti-inflammatory properties. Tectorigenin is an isoflavone from kudzu, and it has been shown to have antiproliferative activity against human cancer cells.

Many kinds of cancer, including breast cancer and some forms of melanoma, are stimulated by the hormone estrogen. Kudzu, contains several chemicals that are very similar to estrogen. One of these chemicals, formononetin, has no effect on the body by itself, but is changed by the friendly bacteria in the digestive tract into an estrogen-like compound called daidzein. Daidzein binds to cells that ordinarily would be activated by estrogen, locking out estrogen from activator sites on breast cancer cells, but without stimulating the cancer cells to reproduce. Studies in Japan, the United States, and Finland have shown that the isoflavones, the chemical family that includes for-mononetin, are clearly associated with reduced rates of breast and uterine cancer. However, because kudzu has been shown to have estrogenic effects, it should not be used by individuals with hormone-sensitive cancers and those taking tamoxifen should avoid it.

• *Heart disease.* Flavonoid-like substances in kudzu help improve microcirculation and blood flow through the coronary arteries. Kudzu reduces the heart's need for oxygen and improves coronary circulation. Substances in the herb relax the muscles lining the left coronary vessel and lower the heart rate. One kudzu compound is a beta-blocker, which reduces a racing pulse induced by stress. In addition to being used to lower blood pressure, beta-blockers help to reduce swelling within the eye in people with glaucoma. Peurarin, the beta-blocker in kudzu, can perform the same function. In one study, patients with coronary heart disease who received an intravenous form of kudzu (500 milligrams of puerarin) experienced improvements in insulin resistance, blood lipids, and blood clotting. All of these changes are desirable for such patients.

• *Menopause.* The isoflavones in kudzu may be involved with alleviating symptoms such as hot flashes and night sweats in perimenopausal women. In one study, post-menopausal women who used the equivalent of 100 milligrams of isoflavones from kudzu a day for three months experienced better cognitive function compared to a group of women who received hormone replacement therapy (HRT). Other parameters such as blood lipids or hormone levels did not change with kudzu but did in the HRT group. However, many women are advised against using HRT, and kudzu may offer benefit in terms of cognition for these women.

Considerations for Use

Kudzu is most easily used in tablet form, but also comes in a powder and tea. The tablets are usually standardized so that 10 milligrams of extract is equivalent to 5 grams of the herb. This is an extraordinarily nontoxic herb; taking as much as 3 ounces (about 100 grams) in a single dose has no reported side effects. The oral dose for menopausal symptoms is 100 milligrams isoflavones (standardized from kudzu) and for alcoholism, 2.4 grams of kudzu root extract.

Kudzu should not be used by those who are hypersensitive to it and patients with estrogen receptor–positive types of breast cancer. Too much kudzu can impair liver function. Interactions can occur with certain drugs such

as tamoxifen, antidiabetic drugs, and those that work via the cytochrome P450, 2D6, and 1A2 pathways. It is important to remember that kudzu's estrogen-like effects do not occur until the friendly intestinal bacteria process the herb. For this reason, antibiotic use nullifies the effect of using kudzu, whether by itself or in herbal formulas that contain it, as these drugs may harm the intestinal bacteria.

LAVENDER

Latin names: *Lavandula angustifolia* or *Lavandula officinalis*, *Lavandula vera* (Lamiaceae [mint] family)
Other common names: aspic, English lavender, lavandin, spike lavender

General Description

Lavender is a species of mint native to the Mediterranean region. It is grown there on a large scale, especially in Provence, France. Lavender is a low-growing shrub with multiple stems topped with spikes of purple flowers. The flowers are used in herbal medicine and perfumery.

Lavender was one of the most popular herbs in England during the Victorian era. Women of refinement carried hand-sized aromatic "swooning pillows" filled with lavender and camphor, so that they could be readily revived from a faint. Bed pillows stuffed with lavender (without camphor) were used to induce sleep.

A compound tincture of lavender, known as Palsy Drops, was officially recognized by the British Pharmacopoeia for over 200 years. It was used to relieve muscle spasms, nervousness, and headaches.

Evidence of Benefit

For centuries, lavender has been used as a general tonic, sedative, antispasmodic, diuretic, digestive aid, and gas remedy. Lavender tea and essential oil are prescribed to treat common minor ailments such as insomnia, nervousness, fatigue, headaches, nausea, and gas. Its aroma helps to stimulate mental processes to help patients with dementia and alleviate mild to moderate depression. The essential oil has antiseptic qualities that may kill several types of disease-causing bacteria. It is used to treat skin ailments such as fungus, burns, wounds, eczema, and acne. It also has been used for hair loss called alopecia.

Benefits of lavender for specific health conditions include the following:

• *Acne, headache.* Lavender stops pain caused by headaches and various skin conditions, such as acne, through the action of two compounds found in the essential oil, linalool and linalyl aldehyde. Linalool increases the threshold of pain, meaning that a stronger stimulus is required before pain is felt. In addition to stopping the perception of pain, lavender also inhibits the hormonal reactions that create inflammation and pain. It also contains an essential oil called 1,8-cineole or eucalyptol, which is also found in eucalyptus. This compound has analgesic and anti-inflammatory effects as well.

• *Anxiety, depression, and insomnia.* The use of lavender oil in aromatherapy for sleep problems was verified by investigators in a six-week study involving nursing home residents. Researchers found that when they perfumed the sleeping ward with lavender and lavender oil for two weeks, the residents slept as long as and more soundly than they did during a different two-week interval in which they took sleep-inducing drugs. Lavender baths are considered valuable for soothing and strengthening the nervous system. In one study, patients with severe dementia and agitation benefited from an aroma stream of lavender oil. In another study, for patients with mild to moderate depression, a tincture of lavender oil (60 drops a day) and a medication (imipramine) helped treatment better than either alone. In a study using lavender oil in aromatherapy, patients with dementia and agitation experienced major improvements in agitation, aggressive behavior, and irritability. However, in one study of patients with advanced cancer, there was no benefit from weekly massages of lavender oil in terms of reduced pain or anxiety.

• *Burns.* Lavender's effectiveness against burns was first discovered by chemist René-Maurice Gattefossé, who is considered the father of modern aromatherapy. Gattefossé plunged a hand he had burned in a laboratory accident into the nearest liquid, a container of lavender oil, and noticed that the pain subsided quickly and that his hand healed rapidly, without scarring. Lavender acts to heal burns by stopping the action of hormonelike substances called prostaglandins, which cause swelling and provoke painful constriction in the area of a burn. Lavender oil also protects burned skin from bacterial and fungal infection.

• *Digestive discomfort and gas.* Lavender soothes stomach upset, reduces excess gas, and encourages the flow of blood. Health officials in Germany have endorsed the use of lavender tea for disturbances of the upper abdomen, such as nervous irritable stomach.

Considerations for Use

Lavender oil can be used as is, or used in aromatherapy, baths, compresses, or teas. You should never take lavender oil internally. Using it on the skin can lead to allergic dermatitis. People with gallstones or obstructions of the biliary tract should avoid lavender, because it can stimulate the secretion of bile that cannot be released through the bile duct. Lavender should not be used by those who take sleeping pills, as lavender potentiates the effect of the drug.

Not all species of lavender are tranquilizing; Spanish lavender, for example, has a stimulant effect. Before using any type of lavender oil on a regular basis, try it out to make sure that it has a calming effect. Lavender oil should not be used by pregnant women or nursing mothers.

LEMON BALM

Latin name: *Melissa officinalis* (Lamiaceae [mint] family)
Other common names: balm, bee balm, cure-all, dropsy plant, garden balm, honey plant, melissa, sweet balm

General Description

Lemon balm is indigenous to the east Mediterranean region and West Africa, and is a member of the mint family. Now, it is most widely cultivated in central Europe (Germany), although English gardeners have considered lemon balm a valuable plant since at least the Elizabethan era. As its name suggests, the herb smells strongly of lemon, although this effect is sometimes only noticeable after rubbing the leaves, and can be totally lost when the herb is stored for several months. This low-growing, twenty-inch (seventy-centimeter) perennial bears pairs of mintlike leaves on opposite sides of a square stem. Its small, white flowers appear in summer atop its central stem. The medicinal parts are oils extracted from the dried leaf, fresh leaves, and the whole plant.

Evidence of Benefit

Research has found that lemon balm has a mild sedative effect, antibacterial and antiviral properties, and an ability to relieve cramps and gas. It is used to heal wounds, ease indigestion, relieve menstrual cramps, fight cold sores, relax nerves, soothe and prevent insect stings, and prevent insomnia. It has also been used for hysteria, melancholia, headaches, and high blood pressure. The tea is also recommended for inducing perspiration and relieving fever due to colds and flu. Externally, lemon balm has been used for rheumatism, nerve pains, as an insect repellent, and for stiff neck. Homeopathic remedies use lemon balm for menstrual irregularities. It is approved by the German Commission E for nervousness and insomnia. This herb is gentle enough for babies and children.

Benefits of lemon balm for specific health conditions include the following:

• *Alzheimer's disease.* In one study, lemon balm was used in patients with mild to moderate Alzheimer's disease and participants showed improved cognitive function after sixteen weeks of treatment.

• *Anxiety and stress.* Lemon balm teas have been used for generations to relieve anxiety and sleeplessness. In one study where healthy volunteers were stressed under controlled laboratory conditions, a mixture of lemon balm and valerian soothed them and made them less anxious. Each participant took increasing doses of both herbs and was measured serially. The best combination for alleviating anxiety and inducing calmness was at 600 milligrams of a tablet that had 120 milligrams of valerian with 80 milligrams of lemon balm. Other studies have found that when used with valerian, lemon balm hastens sleep and relaxes muscle tension in persons with attention deficit disorder (ADD), without daytime drowsiness. (*See* VALERIAN.)

• *Herpesvirus infection.* Treatment of herpes infections is complicated by the fact that the virus can become resistant to drug treatment. Lemon balm expands the possibilities of treatment and is useful when prescription treatments fail. It kills off the virus in the test tube in as little as three hours. In one double-blind study, 116 people with herpes received either a placebo or extracts of lemon balm at a concentration of 1 percent in a cream base. The group receiving the active cream experienced significantly greater improvement in symptoms on day two compared to the group receiving the placebo cream. (Herpes outbreaks are usually most painful on the second day after the outbreak.) By day five of the study, 50 percent more individuals in the lemon balm group were symptom-free than in the placebo group. People using lemon balm also experienced less scarring than those using the placebo. This indicates that people who used lemon balm suffered less damage to skin cells. Almost identical results were found in a second clinical study. In addition to shortening the healing period, treatment with lemon balm prevented spread of the infection and quickly relieved the itching, burning, tingling, swelling, stabbing, and redness of a herpes outbreak. Lemon balm has an advantage over other treatments in that it does not induce drug resistance in the virus over time. (*See* HERPESVIRUS INFECTION in Part Two.) In addition, a chemical constituent of lemon balm, rosmarinic acid, acts against viruses, yeasts, and bacteria in the laboratory.

• *Insomnia.* Combined extracts of lemon balm and valerian have been studied as a treatment for insomnia. A double-blind study of twenty people with insomnia compared the benefits of 0.125 milligram of the sedative triazolam (Halcion) against placebo and a combination of valerian and lemon balm. The herbal combination was found to be as effective as the drug.

• *Irritable bowel syndrome (IBS).* Lemon balm stops spasms and relieves pain caused by IBS. The form of the herb that had this antispasmodic action is the essential oil, which may be strong enough to break up spasms but not so strong as to cause constipation. However, no human data are available.

Considerations for Use

Lemon balm is available in creams for application to the skin and in tablets and teas to be taken internally. Lemon balm tablets are usually taken for insomnia or stress and frequently combine lemon balm with valerian.

Animal studies indicate that lemon balm can increase the sedative effect of barbiturates. You should therefore avoid lemon balm tinctures and teas if you take barbiturates for anxiety or insomnia. Lemon balm *creams* do not interact with barbiturate drugs.

People with glaucoma should not use essential oil of lemon balm until more studies are conducted. Studies in laboratory animals suggest that it may raise pressure in the eye.

LENTINAN

See SHIITAKE.

LICORICE

Latin names: *Glycyrrhiza glabra, Glycyrrhiza lepidota, Glycyrrhiza uralensis* (Fabaceae [legume] family)
Other common names: sweet root, sweet wort

General Description

Next to ginger, licorice is the world's most widely used herbal remedy. The licorice plant is a woody-stemmed perennial that grows to a height of six feet (two meters). It bears clusters of creamy white flowers similar in appearance to those of its relative, the lupine. In the autumn, roots of three- to four-year-old plants are dug for medicinal use. The medicinal parts of the herb are the unpeeled dried roots and runners, the peeled dried roots, and the rhizome with the roots.

Evidence of Benefit

Licorice in general has been used for ailments of the gastrointestinal and respiratory tracts. Licorice has been used in traditional Chinese medicine (TCM) for over 3,000 years as a tonic to rejuvenate the heart and spleen and as a treatment for ulcers, cold symptoms, and skin disorders. In ayurvedic medicine, it is used internally for gastric ulcers, headaches, bronchitis, eye disease, and sore throat. Externally, it has been used for wounds and cuts. Folk medicine uses include for appendicitis and constipation, and to increase milk production. It has also been used for epilepsy. Modern herbalists commonly use licorice to treat adrenal insufficiencies such as hypoglycemia, to counteract stress, and to purify the liver and blood. This herb is also used to counteract serious allergic reactions and to treat rheumatoid arthritis. It is approved by the German Commission E for coughs and bronchitis and ulcers of the stomach and duodenum.

Benefits of licorice for specific health conditions include the following:

• *Cancer.* Licorice contains a flavonoid, licochalcone-A, which has been shown to kill cancer cells of acute leukemia and of the breast and prostate. This compound works by lowering the level of bcl-2, a protein that causes resistance to anticancer drugs. More work is needed to see if licorice can be used with anticancer drugs to make them more effective. This flavonoid also may be protective against developing cancer. The most useful forms of treatment for cancer using licorice, however, are Chinese herbal formulas containing licorice and other herbs. (*See* AUGMENTED RAMBLING POWDER; BUPLEURUM AND CINNAMON TWIG DECOCTION; GINSENG DECOCTION TO NOURISH THE NUTRITIVE CHI; HOCHU-EKKI-TO; HOXSEY FORMULA; MINOR BUPLEURUM DECOCTION; PEONY AND LICORICE DECOCTION; PINELLIA DECOCTION TO DRAIN THE EPIGASTRIUM; and SHIH QUA DA BU TANG *under* The Formulas.)

• *Chronic fatigue syndrome (CFS).* Epidemiologists have noted that some people who have CFS also have low blood pressure and other blood-pressure anomalies. This condition stems from adrenal-hormone deficiencies that cause the body to lose both sodium and water, resulting in drops in both blood volume and blood pressure. Licorice can reverse this process. Glycyrrhizinic acid, a chemical related to glycyrrhizin, blocks the activity of an enzyme that destroys the adrenal hormone cortisol. Higher cortisol levels in the bloodstream cause the kidneys to retain more sodium, and with it more water. This leads to higher blood pressure.

• *Diaper rash, skin irritations.* Licorice contains glycyrrhizin, glycyrrhizic acid, and liquiritin, which have anti-inflammatory effects. Therefore, it is possible that licorice can ease inflammatory skin conditions to speed healing and relieve pain.

• *Gastritis and peptic ulcer.* Licorice is useful for a number of digestive disorders. It soothes inflammation and protects the stomach and intestines from the effects of stomach acid. Unlike many ulcer drugs, glycyrrhizinic acid does not reduce acid production in the stomach, which would result in incomplete digestion. Instead, it increases the stomach's defense mechanisms by fortifying the stomach's protective mucous coating. Glycyrrhizinic acid also increases circulation to the cells lining the intestinal wall, boosting their supply of nutrients and oxygen.

Pure glycyrrhizinic acid can cause the retention of sodium and water. Deglycyrrhizinated licorice (DGL), which has no known side effects, is now available as well. DGL inhibits gastric-juice secretion and protects the lining of the stomach from aspirin-induced damage. Two controlled studies suggest that regular use of DGL, in the form of a product that also contains antacids, can heal ulcers as effectively as drugs in the ranitidine (Zantac) family. In one study, another compound in licorice, carbenoxolone, was administered as 300 milligrams daily for one week followed by half that amount for five more weeks. Compared to an anti-ulcer medicine called pirenzepine, both healed ulcers in about 50 percent of the patients. However, newer drugs called H2 blockers have higher success rates. In another study, participants with dyspepsia (upset stomach) who were given licorice root as the major ingredient along with other herbs such as peppermint leaves and caraway over twelve weeks showed improved symptoms by 43 percent compared to only 3 percent in the placebo group. Medical treatments try to prevent the recurrence of ulcers permanently by killing *Helicobacter pylori* bacteria. According to laboratory research, flavonoids in licorice appear to inhibit *H. pylori,* although this has not been shown in human studies to be effective. One study reported fewer recurrences of ulcers among people taking DGL as compared with those taking the drug cimetidine (Tagamet).

• *Hepatitis.* One component of licorice, glycyrrhizin, stimulates interferon gamma produced by immune cells, which acts against viral infections. In particular, it suppresses the secretion of the hepatitis B virus surface antigens in patients with hepatitis B. The licorice compound is thought to bind to liver cells to inhibit the proliferation of the virus. Minor Bupleurum Decoction, a Chinese formula that uses licorice, is also effective against hepatitis B, particularly in children. (*See* MINOR BUPLEURUM DECOCTION *under* The Formulas.) Glycyrrhizin has been used in the treatment of hepatitis C. Using an intravenous preparation of glycyrrhizin and other compounds such as Stronger Neo-Minophagen C (NMC) was shown to improve the liver function of patients with hepatitis C and alcoholic cirrhosis. However, when treatment was stopped, the virus came back.

• *HIV/AIDS, cytomegalovirus, severe acute respiratory syndrome (SARS).* In one study, when the licorice compound glycyrrhizin was given intravenously to people with AIDS, HIV became undetectable after three treatments. There is some question as to the sensitivity of the antigen tests the researchers used to test for the presence of HIV. However, the researchers thought that licorice acted by keeping HIV from multiplying. In another study, forty-two HIV-positive people with hemophilia took glycyrrhizin along with two amino acids. The viral load in these individuals did not drop into the undetectable range, but they did experience relief from oral yeast infections, swollen lymph nodes, and rashes. Their immune and liver function also improved. Some Japanese physicians have experimented with licorice as a means of keeping HIV infection from progressing to full-blown AIDS, but there is not enough research to date to support its use for this purpose. Today, the proper use of drugs can reduce viral loads effectively in most patients. In infants with cytomegalovirus (CMV) who were administered an intravenous preparation of glycyrrhizin from licorice, the virus was eradicated from the blood and liver tests were normalized. In a cell line studies, glycyrrhizin had potent antiviral effects against SARS. No human data are available for licorice and SARS, however.

• *Respiratory ailments.* Glycyrrhizin stops the production of toxic free radicals by acting as an antioxidant. Other components in licorice, such as licoricidin and glabridin, act as anti-inflammatories. These substances reduce swelling of the bronchial passageways to help with bronchitis and possibly asthma. The herb also stimulates the secretion of mucus in the windpipe, which relieves dry cough. Licorice also increases the effectiveness of steroid drugs, which effectively treat a variety of inflammatory conditions but also produce a number of side effects. Clinical studies have shown that glycyrrhizin supplements prednisolone therapy, used in both asthma and lupus, allowing affected individuals to use smaller doses of prednisolone with fewer side effects. Similarly, licorice extends the useful life of cortisone creams used to treat vitiligo, a disorder that causes the skin to lose its pigmentation.

Considerations for Use

There are two types of licorice commonly available: standard licorice and DGL. Each type is best used for certain conditions. For respiratory infections, CFS, or topical use for herpesvirus infections, standard licorice containing glycyrrhizin should be used. Most people can take 4 to 8 grams of ordinary licorice per day, but it should not be taken internally for more than four to six weeks at a time unless under the supervision of a health-care provider.

DGL is used for potential safety problems and is used for conditions of the digestive tract, such as ulcers. Generally, one 300-milligram tablet is chewed three times per day before meals and before bed for the best results. For mouth ulcers, 200 milligrams of DGL powder can be mixed with 200 milliliters of warm water and swished in the mouth for three minutes and then spit out.

Licorice is contraindicated for people with chronic hepatitis, cholestatic diseases of the liver, cirrhosis of the liver, severe kidney insufficiency, diabetes mellitus, hypotonic neuromuscular disorders, arrhythmias, hypertension, and low blood potassium. It should not be used during pregnancy and lactation. Due to its aldosterone-like effects, licorice can cause fluid retention, high blood pressure, and potassium loss and should be avoided by anyone who would be affected by these problems, such as patients with high blood pressure, heart disease, stroke, diabetes, glaucoma, or kidney disease. While taking licorice, it is important to include potassium-rich fruits and vegetables such as bananas and apricots in your diet. Weight gain has been reported in people who took 150 milligrams of glycyrrhetinic acid daily.

People with estrogen-sensitive disorders such as fibrocystic breasts, breast cancer, or uterine cancer, and anyone using estrogen as part of hormone replacement therapy (HRT) should avoid licorice. Also, licorice reduces testosterone levels in men and low libido has been reported. Do not use licorice if you are taking testosterone, as it will decrease the effectiveness of this hormone. For this reason, men who have erectile dysfunction (ED) or who are infertile should avoid this herb. People with hypothyroidism should avoid licorice, since it further reduces the thyroid's production of thyroid hormone or may necessitate larger doses of levothyroxine (Levoxyl, Levothroid, Synthroid).

You should not take licorice internally if you are using corticosteroids. Licorice may increase both its negative and positive effects. Women who are pregnant or nursing should use this herb with caution.

If you are taking a thiazide or other type of diuretic for high blood pressure or congestive heart failure, the use of licorice might lead to excessive potassium loss. Potassium depletion can also cause serious mineral imbalances in people who take any form of lithium for the treatment of bipolar disorder. Do not use licorice if you are taking antidiabetic drugs, insulin, or monoamine oxidase (MAO) inhibitors.

Licorice is a primary ingredient in smokeless, or chewing, tobacco. Excessive use of smokeless tobacco can have all the effects of excessive licorice use, especially high blood pressure.

Finally, consumption of large amounts of licorice *candy* (one-quarter to two pounds or 250 to 1,000 grams) can result in temporary visual disturbances. Temporary loss of visual acuity after consuming large amounts of licorice is due to spasms in the blood vessels supplying the eyes. In all the cases of this problem reported in the medical literature, normal vision returned after several days, although medical treatment was required.

MAITAKE

Latin name: *Grifola frondosa* (Basidiomycetes [button mushroom] family)
Other common names: cloud mushroom, dancing mushroom, hen of the woods, king of mushrooms

General Description

Maitake is a very large mushroom that grows deep in the mountains of northeastern Japan. The word *maitake* is literally translated from Japanese as "dancing mushroom." According to herbal folklore, it was so named because in ancient times people who found maitake could exchange it for its weight in silver, leading to their dancing in celebration. Maitake is recognized by its small, overlapping tongue- or fan-shaped caps, usually fused together at the base of tree stumps or on tree roots. Only recently have Japanese farmers succeeded in producing high-quality organic maitake mushrooms, making this herbal product more widely available.

Evidence of Benefit

Herbalists classify maitake as an adaptogen—an herb that helps the body to adapt to stress and resist infection. Maitake and its extracts have been shown to significantly boost the immune system and build immune reserves. It also contains a number of polysaccharides that have been shown to fight the formation and growth of tumors. Other research has found that maitake has potent liver-protectant properties and can lower blood pressure and blood glucose levels.

Benefits of maitake for specific health conditions include the following:

• *Cancer.* Maitake has been shown to fight some forms of cancer cells. In laboratory tests, powdered maitake increased the activity of three types of immune cells—macrophages, natural killer (NK) cells, and T cells—by 140, 186, and 160 percent, respectively. It reduced tumor formation by 86 percent in mice that were given maitake as compared with mice in a control group. A Chinese clinical study established that maitake treatment reduces the rate of recurrence of bladder cancer after surgery from 65 to 33 percent. Researchers have found that when combined with the standard chemotherapy drug mitomycin (Mutamicyn), maitake inhibits the growth of breast cancer cells—even after tumors are well formed—and prevents the spread of such cells to the liver.

The anticancer compound in maitake, sold commercially as the maitake D-fraction, has shown positive results in American studies on breast and colorectal cancer. Chinese doctors have reported positive results in sixty-three patients who had liver, lung, or stomach cancer, or leukemia. Japanese studies have shown that the response was best in cancers of the breast, liver, and lung; poor response rates were seen with leukemia, stomach, and bone cancers. The best results were seen in all forms of cancer when the maitake D-fraction was taken along with chemotherapy. Maitake also shows some promise for prostate cancer. The beta-glucan found in the mushrooms seems to improve the effectiveness of carmustine, a chemotherapeutic drug for prostate cancer.

• *HIV/AIDS.* Studies have shown that maitake extract kills HIV and enhances activity of T cells. A sulfated version of maitake extract prevents HIV-induced destruction of T cells by as much as 97 percent in vitro (outside the body). Maitake extracts also keep ordinary cells from converting to fat-storage cells under laboratory conditions, and so may help prevent the development of fatty deposits under the skin that can occur as a result of treatment with so-called AIDS cocktails. It is touted for patients with AIDS, but no clinical studies are available.

Considerations for Use

Maitake as well as its fraction, maitake D-fraction, are used medicinally. It is available in capsules or tablets containing the whole fruiting body of maitake, which is higher in polysaccharides. Maitake supplements can be used in the amount of 3 to 7 grams per day. A liquid product with a higher concentration of polysaccharides is available. Maitake is also available fresh or dried for use in food or tea.

This herb should be used as a complementary therapy for chronic conditions such as cancer and HIV/AIDS. It should not be considered a substitute for standard treatments.

Maitake has been used by people with multiple sclerosis (MS) to increase the production of a family of immune-system chemicals called interferons, some of which have been shown to stabilize MS. However, one form of interferon stimulated by maitake, gamma-interferon, can promote destruction of nerve tissue, so people with MS should avoid maitake until this remedy has been more thoroughly tested. Those who are using blood sugar–lowering medications and blood-thinners should not use maitake.

MARSHMALLOW ROOT

Latin name: *Althaea officinalis* (Malvaceae [mallow] family) Other common names: althaea root, cheeses, mallards, Moorish mallow, sweet weed, white mallow, wymote

General Description

Marshmallow is an erect perennial plant that bears hibiscus-like blossoms and grows in wet, marshy areas. The use of marshmallow originated in traditional Greek medicine and spread to Arabian and ayurvedic medicine. Marshmallow is cultivated for medicinal use in Europe and Asia and is naturalized in gardens around the world. Its roots are a rich source of healing mucilages used in herbal medicine, but also used are the mallow flowers, leaves, and syrup. In the nineteenth century, some doctors whipped up a foamy meringue from marshmallow root juices, egg whites, and sugar that later hardened, creating a medicinal candy used to soothe children's sore throats.

Evidence of Benefit

Marshmallow root relieves various forms of irritation and inflammation, especially irritation of mucous membranes. It aids the body in expelling excess fluid and mucus. It strengthens the digestive system and improves the functioning of the immune system. Marshmallow root is an ingredient in many lung preparations and cough syrups, as well as preparations for urinary tract problems, stomach ailments, and wound healing. The German Commission E has approved the leaf for irritations of the mouth and throat, mucus control, and associated dry coughs. The root is used for the same ailments as the leaf as well as for mild inflammation of the gastrointestinal tract.

Benefits of marshmallow root for specific health conditions include the following:

• *Cough and laryngitis.* Approximately 35 percent of the weight of the marshmallow root comes from mucilage, which coats irritated linings of the mouth and throat. Since this mucilage acts in the same way as natural mucus, it prevents cough rather than stimulating the release of mucus. Therefore, marshmallow root is appropriate for dry, hacking coughs rather than for relieving congestion. In addition, the herb is known to stimulate phagocytosis, the immune process in which cells called macrophages engulf and digest infectious microorganisms.

• *Stomach ailments.* Teas of marshmallow root contain complex polysaccharides that form a protective layer on the stomach lining. These polysaccharides swell to twelve to fifteen times their original volume when they meet the fluids of the stomach, completely coating its lining.

Considerations for Use

Marshmallow root is available in fluid extracts, powders, and tinctures for internal use, and as a cream for external use. The usual dose is 6 grams a day. When using the marshmallow syrup, be aware of it sugar content; some have very high amounts of sugar and should be avoided by patients with diabetes.

Marshmallow can impair the absorption of many drugs. Therefore, allow a two-hour period between using this herb and other orally administered drugs. Japanese researchers have learned that the mucilages in marshmallow root can lower blood sugars when *injected* into laboratory animals. For this reason, the official guidelines for the use of medicinal herbs in the European Union counsel caution in the use of the herb by people with diabetes. There is no evidence, however, that marshmallow products taken orally or externally can cause hypoglycemia or otherwise interfere with diabetes treatment.

MATÉ

Latin name: *Ilex paraguariensis* (Aquifoliaceae [holly] family) Other common names: Jesuit's Brazil tea, Jesuit tea, Paraguay tea, yerba maté

General Description

Maté is an evergreen shrub native throughout northern Argentina, southern Brazil, Paraguay, and Uruguay, and naturalized to portions of Texas. First brought under cultivation by Jesuit missionaries, maté has become so popular in South America that commercial maté farming has displaced vast areas of rain forest canopy trees, depriving the animals that lived in them of habitat.

The maté plant sometimes reaches a height of twenty feet (six meters), much lower than the rain forest canopy it replaces in cultivation. It bears large leaves, white flowers, and red fruit. The leaves are made into a tea that is the beverage of choice in much of South America.

Maté was introduced to the United States in the 1970s as a caffeine-free coffee substitute. This wasn't quite true. Maté does contain caffeine, although in lesser amounts than coffee (approximately 50 milligrams per 6-ounce cup versus 100 to 150 milligrams per cup of brewed coffee).

Evidence of Benefit

Maté is a stimulant and a source of trace minerals. Its stimulant effects reinforce the effects of other stimulant herbs. It is a general tonic, invigorating to the body and mentally stimulating. Depending upon the tannin amount of maté,

it can act as a diuretic and can help relieve the fluid retention associated with premenstrual syndrome (PMS).

Benefits of maté for specific health conditions include the following:

• *Weight loss.* Maté may delay gastric emptying to keep you feeling full longer. But it is not yet clear if this is why maté produces weight loss. The primary weight-loss component of maté is caffeine. Caffeine stimulates weight loss by short-circuiting the feedback mechanisms that keep the body from producing more adrenaline when stimulated by herbs such as ephedrine. (*See* EPHEDRINE.) Caffeine does not affect weight loss when used by itself.

Considerations for Use

Despite practices to the contrary in South America, maté tea is most beneficial when drunk only once a day. Maté contains high concentrations of carcinogenic compounds such as polycyclic aromatic hydrocarbons. In addition, the high temperature of the water used to make the tea is thought to facilitate the absorption of carcinogenic substances.

The medical literature has studies showing a relationship between excessive maté use and the risk of many cancers. The investigators in these studies corrected for tobacco use and still found a significant increase in the chance of developing cancers with increased use of maté. There have been studies in Brazil, Uruguay, and Paraguay that linked esophageal, mouth, larynx, lung, and bladder cancer with heavy and prolonged maté drinking. The increased risk is 50 percent for many of these cancers. However, the U.S. Food and Drug Administration (FDA) classifies maté as generally recognized as safe (GRAS) for use as a food additive.

Side effects include insomnia, restlessness, agitation, nausea, vomiting, and headache. Due to its antioxidant activity, maté may interfere with some chemotherapy drugs. Patients with high blood pressure, or women who are pregnant or lactating, should not use maté. Do not use maté when taking aspirin, acetaminophen, theophylline, diuretics, beta-adrenergic agonists, or during chemotherapy.

MILK THISTLE

Latin names: *Carduus marianus*, also known as *Silybum marianum* (Asteraceae [composite] family)
Other common names: Marian thistle, Mary thistle, Mediterranean milk thistle

General Description

Milk thistle is a common weed with a distinctive white marking on its leaves. In European tradition, these markings were believed to be splashes of the Virgin Mary's milk. This spiny perennial grows throughout Europe but is naturalized to Australia and California. Reaching a height of 5 feet (1.5 meters), the plant puts out distinctive purple flowering heads, which may be eaten fresh as a vegetable similar to the artichoke. The seeds are collected and dried for use in herbal medicine.

In Europe, during the Middle Ages, and in later French folk medicine, as well as in traditional Chinese medicine (TCM), the liver was regarded as the seat of the emotions. Depression and emotional distraught were thought to arise from malfunctions of the liver. Milk thistle, available in early spring, served as a spring tonic to relieve winter depression by releasing the pent-up emotions or energies housed in the liver.

Evidence of Benefit

Milk thistle is extraordinarily useful in the treatment of liver diseases such as alcoholic hepatitis, cirrhosis, liver poisoning, and viral hepatitis. Milk thistle is one of the few herbs that have no real pharmaceutical equivalent. It reduces inflammation and is an antioxidant. Traditionally used for functional disorders of the liver and gallbladder such as jaundice, it was also used to treat malaria. Today it is used for dyspepsia, toxic liver, and hepatic cirrhosis. The German Commission E has approved milk thistle for dyspeptic, liver, and gallbladder complaints. According to the German Commission E, milk thistle works in two ways: It alters the structure of the outer cell membrane of the liver cells to prevent toxins such as from food poisoning to get inside the liver cells, and second, it stimulates the action of nucleolar polymerase A, which stimulates the regeneration of new, healthy liver cells.

Benefits of milk thistle for specific health conditions include the following:

• *Alcoholism, cirrhosis, and hepatitis.* Silymarin, an extract of milk thistle, acts on the membranes of the liver cells, preventing the entry of virus toxins and other toxic compounds and thus preventing damage to the cells. It also dramatically improves liver regeneration in hepatitis, cirrhosis, mushroom poisoning, and other diseases of the liver. One study, conducted by a German pharmaceutical firm, looked at 2,637 people who had used milk thistle for various liver disorders, including cirrhosis of the liver, fatty liver, and hepatitis. After eight weeks of taking standardized milk thistle capsules daily, 63 percent of the study participants said their symptoms—including abdominal distention, fatigue, lack of appetite, and nausea—had disappeared. The average improvement in levels of alanine aminotransferase (ALT) and aspartate aminotransferase (AST), enzymes that are markers for liver cell impairment, was 46 percent, and over 73 percent of enlarged livers shrank in size. Only 1 percent of the study participants were forced to discontinue milk thistle because of side effects, such as mild diarrhea, nausea, and stomach upset.

Other studies focused on specific disorders also have shown positive results. In a well-documented double-blind study of 116 individuals who had alcoholic cirrhosis of the liver, German researchers found that milk thistle exerted a profound curative action in as little as two weeks. And in a later study, twenty-nine people with advanced alcoholic liver disease reported relief from nausea and restored appetite after two months' treatment with the milk thistle extract silymarin. In cases of hepatitis B and hepatitis C, a flavonoid complex in silymarin stimulates liver protein creation, enabling the organ to produce new liver cells to replace the old ones damaged by hepatitis infection. This action prevents the replacement of virus-infected liver cells with fibrous tissues or fat.

In one study, patients with alcoholic cirrhosis and those with Child's A group classification of portal hypertension taking 40 milligrams of silymarin three times a day for four years showed an improvement in symptoms and blood tests. Patients without alcoholic cirrhosis but who had Child's B and C group hypertension did not show improvement. However, the survival rate of all subjects taking silymarin was better than those who didn't take it (58 percent versus 39 percent).

• *Cancer.* There are no clinical data on cancer and milk thistle. However, milk thistle was shown to reduce liver toxicity associated with chemotherapy for children with acute lymphoblastic leukemia. Some breast cancers (as well as other forms of cancer) are stimulated by the hormone estrogen. Laboratory studies find that silybin, a chemical found in milk thistle, competes for the receptor sites that would receive estrogen in these kinds of cancer cells. Scientists at Case Western Reserve University in Cleveland, Ohio, have found that silymarin stops the growth of breast cancer cells, both within tumors and, more important, before anchoring themselves in other organs of the body.

Rats given the milk thistle compound silibinin in a very large dosage (equivalent to 30 grams, or approximately 1 ounce, for a 110-pound [55-kilogram] adult) had reduced kidney damage during treatment with the cancer chemotherapy agent cisplatin (Platinol). Another study found that, in addition to protecting the kidneys from damage by either cisplatin or doxorubicin (Adriamycin), silybin increased the cancer-fighting effectiveness of the two drugs. Tests also indicate that silibinin protects against the toxic effects of cisplatin and ifosfamide (Ifex) therapy without diminishing these drugs' effects on testicular cancers.

Milk thistle acts against liver cancer by protecting specialized immune cells in the liver known as Kuppfer cells. These cells engulf bacteria, toxins, and other foreign matter coming into the liver, and also play a role in destroying cancer cells that have entered blood circulation as a first step in spreading to other parts of the body. The silibinin in milk thistle protects the Kuppfer cells from inflammatory reactions without interfering with the action of an immune-system chemical called tumor necrosis factor alpha, which accelerates the destruction of cancer cells by the immune system. Silibinin reduces PSA (prostate-specific antigen), which is released in prostate cancer. It also inhibits the G1 cycle of the cell cycle progression in prostate cancers that do not respond to any other chemotherapy. In stopping the G1 cycle, the cancer growth is arrested as well.

• *Diabetes.* Insulin resistance is very difficult to treat and may be found in patients with cirrhosis of the liver caused by alcohol. In a double-blind study of sixty patients who had both alcoholic cirrhosis of the liver and diabetes, twelve months of treatment with 600 milligrams of silymarin daily resulted in significantly lower fasting blood-glucose levels, less glucose spillover into the urine, and lower proportions of glycosylated hemoglobin, which is a measurement of long-term elevated blood sugars.

Milk thistle may fight diabetes in other ways. Insulin not only transports glucose into muscle cells, but also transports fatty acids into fat cells. Silymarin stimulates the liver so that it can take excessive amounts of insulin out of the bloodstream in people with type 2 diabetes or diabetes arising from alcoholic damage to the liver. By regulating the amount of insulin in circulation, silymarin treatment may prevent weight gain, which usually accompanies excessive amounts of insulin in the bloodstream. In addition, animal studies indicate that milk thistle extract can reduce ketoacidosis, a complication of prolonged, uncontrolled diabetes in which the body is forced to use fats rather than glucose for fuel, producing potentially toxic effects on the central nervous system.

• *Psoriasis.* Naturopathic physicians report that milk thistle reduces the frequency of psoriasis outbreaks. This effect is probably due to its antioxidants and anti-inflammatory compounds.

Considerations for Use

Milk thistle is best used as silymarin gelcaps. The best formulation of silymarin is known as silipide. This is a chemical combination of silybin, the main active ingredient in silymarin, with phosphatidylcholine, the principal active ingredient in soy lecithin. The soy lecithin component of silipide helps the digestive tract absorb silymarin, and then delivers 97 percent of silymarin directly to the tissues where it is needed. This product can be recognized on the shelf by its labeling as a *phytosome*. Milk thistle is less effective when used as seeds, teas, and tinctures, all of which can cause mild diarrhea, severe sweating, abdominal cramping, nausea, vomiting, and weakness. However, many of these side effects were related to a substance found in a commercial product in Australia that was other than silybin. Daily doses are usually 12 to 15 grams of the milk thistle herb, which is the equivalent of 200 to 400 milligrams of silymarin.

Since milk thistle tinctures are made with alcohol, they are not recommended for treatment of liver disease. People who have been diagnosed with a chronic liver disease should have regular blood tests to monitor liver function, and should curb or eliminate alcohol consumption. People with diabetes should monitor blood sugar levels carefully while taking milk thistle.

Milk thistle extract has virtually no side effects and can be used by most people, including women who are pregnant or nursing. However, women who are taking birth control pills should be aware that milk thistle may reduce their effectiveness. Since silymarin stimulates liver and gallbladder activity, it may have a mild laxative effect in some individuals. This usually lasts only two to three days. However, people using metronidazole and butyrophenones or phenothiazines should not use milk thistle. It should not be used with the herb yohimbe.

MISTLETOE

Latin names: *Viscum coloratum, Viscum album* (Loranthaceae [mistletoe] family)
Other common names: all-heal, birdline, devil's fuge, European mistletoe, loranthus, mulberry, mystyldene

General Description

The mulberry mistletoe is a parasitic evergreen shrub that forms bunches as much as ten feet (three meters) across on the limbs of host firs, oaks, and pines. The stem, also called loranthus, is used in herbal medicine. Mistletoe is found mostly in Europe and Iran. It is cultivated in China and Europe but not found in America or Australia.

Mulberry mistletoe is not the same herb as American mistletoe, which is traditionally used in Christmas decorations. (American mistletoe is toxic.) Loranthus has feathery leaves, yellow flowers in clusters of three, and round, sticky white berries. The medicinal parts are the leaves and twigs, collected before berries form. Also used are fresh leaf twigs from fruit collected in autumn, leaves, and berries.

Evidence of Benefit

The lectins, polypeptides, and mucilages in mistletoe have shown immune-stimulating activity in humans when extracts are given by injection. Numerous clinical trials have found that injections of mistletoe extract are beneficial for treating cancer of various organs. There is no evidence that giving mistletoe orally would benefit those with cancer. Depending upon the part of the plant, historical uses vary. The fruits were used for treatment of internal bleeding, epilepsy, heart disease, cramps, and gout. The stems were used to produce a calming effect, treat mental and physical exhaustion, and as an antianxiety agent. It is approved by the German Commission E for degenerative inflammation of the joints and as a palliative therapy for malignant tumors. The tea version may be used for high blood pressure, whooping cough, asthma, amenorrhea, diarrhea, nervous tachycardia, and nervousness.

Benefits of mistletoe for specific health conditions include the following:

• *Cancer.* Mistletoe was introduced into the treatment of cancer in 1917. Today, extracts from the plant, usually given as an injection, are widely used as a supplemental treatment in cancer therapy in Europe. The herb's most important active agents are the lectins, which poison cancer cells and stimulate the immune system.

One meta-analysis combining ten studies on mistletoe and cancer failed to show that it was beneficial as palliative treatment. However, more recent reports suggest that mistletoe is helpful, especially for quality of life. When Iscador, a subcutaneously administered mistletoe extract, was randomly assigned to patients with different forms of cancer, those who got the mistletoe extract lived significantly longer (6 months to 1.7 years) than a group that did not get the treatment. All patients were receiving their usual chemotherapy regimen at the same time. A Swiss study of fourteen breast cancer patients showed that Iscador increased the rate at which breast cells were able to repair their DNA. Repairing DNA prevents mutations that can result in the formation of cancerous cells. At the beginning of the study, the rate at which cancer patients' cells repaired DNA damage was only 16 percent of that in healthy individuals. After just nine days of treatment, the rate increased to nearly 50 percent.

In one study, another drug made from mistletoe extract, Eurixor, did not help patients with head and neck cancer. However, when this same drug was used for patients with advanced breast cancer, there was evidence of increased natural killer (NK) cell activity. Patients with other forms of cancer—such as bladder and colorectal—seem also to benefit from extracts of mistletoe. In animal studies, mistletoe extracts prevent the spread of melanoma to lung tissue by approximately 80 percent. However, the extract must be used *before* the cancer spreads to the lung. Studies in animals have confirmed that mistletoe lectins reduce the risk of leukopenia, or white blood cell deficiency, during chemotherapy with cyclophosphamide (Cytoxan, Neosar). Mistletoe also prolongs survival time and reduces risk of leukopenia after exposure to or treatment with radiation.

Considerations for Use

The U.S. Food and Drug Administration (FDA) lists this plant as "unsafe." Mistletoe should be used only under professional medical supervision as part of an overall treatment plan. At least three standardized injectable extracts have been studied in Europe: Iscador, Helixor, and Eurixor. These products are not designed for self-treatment and are not commercially available in the United States, although they can be bought online. Iscador is the only fermented extract of the three. Each is standardized in a different way. People interested in other injectable forms of mistletoe should consult with a physician.

Commercial mistletoe extracts, which are generally given by injection, have minimal side effects. In rare cases, however, allergic symptoms, including reactions leading to shock, have been reported. An injection usually produces an increase in body temperature and flulike symptoms that indicate the herb is taking effect. The injection site can become inflamed, and abdominal pain with nausea may occur. For both the injectable form and the herb, other side effects include chills, fever, headache, chest pain, low blood pressure, diarrhea, and vomiting. In addition, long-term use of mistletoe extracts may reduce immune cell function in cancer patients. People who take monoamine oxidase (MAO) inhibitors for depression or Parkinson's disease should not receive lectin injections. In addition, those who use blood pressure–lowering medications, digoxin, or heart medicine to control arrhythmias should avoid the extracts as well. Patients with chronic progressive infections like tuberculosis should avoid mistletoe. Pregnant women should not use mistletoe, as it stimulates uterine contractions. Those who are lactating should avoid it as well. Mistletoe can form a complex with iron and create a toxin in the blood, so if you are taking both, allow two hours between each.

MORINDA

Latin names: *Morinda citrifolia, Morinda officinalis* (Rubiaceae [madder] family)
Other common names: ba ji tian, mengkudu, noni

General Description

There are two species of morinda. *M. citrifolia* is native to Malaysia, Australia, and Polynesia. *M. officinalis* grows in India, the Philippines, and throughout Southeast Asia. Morinda is a deciduous creeping vine with twining stems and white flowers. Growers harvest its large, thick, intertwined purple roots in the spring and fall for use in herbal medicine. When boiled to make a tea, the roots yield a characteristic yellow pigment. Both species are used to make noni juice. The medicinal parts of the plant are the leaf, fruit, and root.

Evidence of Benefit

Morinda has been used for hundreds of years to support the entire body and to treat a wide range of symptoms, including poor digestion, fever, high blood pressure, respiratory problems, and immune deficiency. Morinda also is useful for treating menstrual problems. This herb increases energy, stamina, and endurance.

Working at the cellular level, morinda solves problems within the body ranging from cancer to digestive distress. It was historically used for diabetes as a blood purifier.

Benefits of morinda for specific health conditions include the following:

• *Cancer.* There is a lot of interest in morinda and cancer. This herb improved survival in animal studies when combined with low-dose chemotherapy. It also reduces cancer risk by blocking carcinogen-DNA binding. Advanced cancer patients used capsules containing 500 milligrams of ripe morinda, taking a maximum of twenty capsules per day. Patients experienced less pain and increased energy levels and physical function. In one study of 847 patients with cancer who drank noni juice (which is made from morinda fruit), 67 percent showed improvements in their symptoms, 91 percent felt an increase in energy levels, 72 percent lost weight if they were overweight, 87 percent had reduced blood pressure, and 90 percent had a decrease in chronic pain.

• *Menstrual problems.* Morinda also helps smooth out irregular menstrual periods. The scientific reasons for this action are not clear, although traditional Chinese medicine (TCM) practitioners have prescribed morinda for almost 2,000 years in such cases. They most commonly prescribe the herb to women who also have either cold or pain in the back or pelvic region, along with frequent urination or urinary incontinence.

Considerations for Use

Morinda is available in juice, capsule, and tea forms. For capsules, the recommendation is to take morinda with meals three times daily. Morinda works slowly. It must be taken consistently for a period of six to eight weeks before results can be seen. TCM practitioners warn that the herb should be avoided if there is dribbling or difficult urination or with renal failure. Patients with diabetes should monitor their blood sugar levels closely when taking morinda. This herb interacts with chemotherapy and warfarin (Coumadin) by decreasing their effectiveness. Do not take morinda with angiotensin-converting enzyme (ACE) inhibitor drugs.

Several adverse reports have been documented in persons using morinda, including cases of liver toxicity, high blood potassium, and high blood sugar levels in patients with diabetes who used a sugary juice version. The first case report on liver toxicity was in 2005 in Austria, where a man was admitted to the hospital with elevated liver function tests and a diagnosis of acute herbal toxicity from drinking a lot of morinda juice.

MOTHERWORT

Latin names: *Leonurus cardiaca, Leonurus heterophyllus* (Lamiaceae [mint] family)
Other common names: leonurus, lion's ear, lion's tail, throw-wort

General Description

Motherwort is a member of the mint family native to Central Asia, central Europe, Scandinavia, and Russia. It is now naturalized to North Africa. The plant bears toothed, palm-shaped leaves and pink, lipped flowers.

Motherwort is also cultivated as a garden plant. The fresh aerial (aboveground) parts collected during flowering season are used in herbal medicine.

The *L. cardiaca* species of motherwort is used primarily to treat heart conditions. The ancient Greeks and Romans employed this species to treat heart palpitations as well as depression. Centuries later, Europeans considered the herb to have stimulating effects on the uterus.

These uses of motherwort correspond to those in traditional Chinese medicine (TCM), which uses the Asian variety to treat menstrual disorders and to promote recovery of the uterus after childbirth.

Evidence of Benefit

In folk medicine, motherwort is used for asthma, to balance hormones affecting the menstrual cycle in women, and for amenorrhea. Homeopathic remedies exist for heart complaints, flatulence, and hyperthyroidism. The German Commission E has approved it for irregular heartbeats in people with thyroid disorders.

Benefits of motherwort for specific health conditions include the following:

• *Congestive heart failure and hyperthyroidism.* The Latin name for motherwort, "lion heart," belies its centuries of use as a remedy for a weak heart. Motherwort strengthens the heartbeat but does not increase pulse rate. Instead, it sedates and relaxes the coronary arteries, resulting in increased circulation to the heart. *The Complete German Commission E Monographs* prescribes motherwort for irregularities of the heart caused by adrenal overstimulation and overactive thyroid (hyperthyroidism). Alkaloids in the herb, such as lionurine and stachydrine, have been reported to lower blood pressure and depress the central nervous system in laboratory animals.

• *Premenstrual syndrome.* Test-tube studies have shown that low concentrations of lionurine, a compound found in motherwort, induced uterine contractions, but that higher concentrations inhibited contractions. The opposing effects may explain how motherwort can induce both labor and menstruation, and relax the uterus after childbirth. However, it should not be used during pregnancy. It is mildly hypnotic and acts as a sedative, so it may relieve symptoms associated with premenstrual syndrome (PMS).

Considerations for Use

Motherwort is available in fluid extracts and teas. You should use solid (capsule or tablet) forms of the herb with caution, if at all; a dose of 3,000 milligrams of solid extract per day, taken in capsule or tablet form, is likely to cause diarrhea, stomach irritation, or uterine bleeding.

Because of the herb's traditional use for uterine stimulation, motherwort should not be used by pregnant women. If you suffer from a heart disorder or take any medicine for a heart condition, consult with your health-care provider before taking this herb.

MUIRA PUAMA

Latin name: *Ptychopetalum ovata* (Oleaceae [olive] family)
Other common names: marapuama, potency wood, potenzholz

General Description

Muira puama is a tree native to the Amazon rain forest, where it reaches a height of fifty feet (fifteen meters). It has a gray trunk, dark brown leaves, white flowers, and orange to orange-yellow fruits. The bark, root, and wood of the tree are used in herbal medicine. Many traditional remedies require the bark and wood of young plants.

Evidence of Benefit

Muira puama has long been used as an aphrodisiac and a tonic for the nervous system. It is soothing and may be helpful for nervous exhaustion, stress, and trauma. It is also used in formulations designed to treat male pattern baldness.

Benefits of muira puama for specific health conditions include the following:

• *Erectile dysfunction (ED) and diminished sex drive.* Muira puama is a good addition to or replacement for treatment with yohimbe. (*See* YOHIMBE.) Clinical studies of muira puama in France have found that using the herb as a sole treatment restores sex drive and erectile function in 51 to 62 percent of cases. From the preliminary information, it appears that the herb works by enhancing both psychological and physical aspects of sexual function.

Considerations for Use

Muira puama is available as a tincture. It is included in many blends of South American herbs that are marketed for treatment of male pattern baldness and ED. Muira puama is typically combined with catuaba, iporuru, and other rain forest herbs. (*See* CATUABA and IPORURU.)

MULLEIN

Latin names: *Verbascum densiflorum*, also known as *Verbascum thapsus* (Scrophulariaceae [spinach] family)
Other common names: Aaron's rod, blanket-leaf, Cuddy's lungs, duffle, golden rod, Jacob's staff, large-flowered mullein, orange mullein, torches, velvet plant, wild ice leaf

General Description

Mullein is native to regions bordering the Mediterranean Sea and to Ethiopia. It has naturalized in moister areas of Europe and North America, where it is a roadside weed. Like spinach, to which it is related, mullein grows oval leaves close to the ground and puts up a flower spike in early spring. Unlike spinach, mullein's flower spike can extend as high as six feet (two meters). Mullein has slightly hairy, gray-green sulfurous-smelling leaves, along with bright yellow flowers. The herb (at the beginning of the flowering seasons), the root, and the flowers are used in herbal medicine.

Evidence of Benefit

Mullein has been popular as a remedy for respiratory problems such as cough, bronchitis, and asthma. It is also used to soothe throat irritation and clear congestion, control diarrhea, and increase urine production. Mullein has been used for bladder and kidney conditions. Externally, it is used to treat wounds, earaches, middle ear infections, and insect bites, calm the pain and inflammation of hemorrhoids, and soften the skin. It is approved by the German Commission E for support of the respiratory tract in ailments such as cough or bronchitis.

Benefits of mullein for specific health conditions include the following:

• *Bronchitis, cough, influenza, and sore throat.* Mullein relieves upper respiratory congestion in two ways. First, its mucilage soothes injured areas of the mouth and throat. Second, it contains compounds that act on the central nervous system to move phlegm out of the body. Mullein stimulates the cough reflex, but not the fine hairs lining the respiratory passages. This herb tones the mucous membranes of the respiratory system and reduces inflammation while promoting expectoration. These actions are useful in treating chronic bronchitis if there is a hard cough with soreness.

• *Cuts and scrapes, diarrhea, ear infection, and hemorrhoids.* In Germany, mullein flowers are steeped in olive oil and then strained to make a remedy for ear infections. Mullein contains mucilages that coat and soothe areas of the epithelium lining the ear canal that have been injured by infection. Mullein contains tannins, substances that constrict tissue and reduce bleeding. Wounds and hemorrhoids respond favorably when mullein is used externally. The presence of tannins also helps to treat diarrhea by reducing inflammation in the intestines.

Considerations for Use

In the United States, the mullein products that are easiest to find are cold-extracted "oils" in which chopped mullein leaf is steeped in glycerin rather than alcohol. The absence of alcohol makes the liquid safe for treating coughs in children. Mullein also is used in oils and teas, and mullein teas can be made into compresses. While the herb can be used by itself, it is frequently combined with anise, coltsfoot, licorice, and/or marshmallow in commercially prepared teas for the relief of coughs and congestion. (*See* ANISE, COLTSFOOT, LICORICE, and/or MARSHMALLOW ROOT.)

If you have a history of cancer, you should consult your doctor before taking this herb internally, since the tannin found in mullein is thought to have both cancer-promoting and cancer-fighting actions. You should not take mullein if you are pregnant or nursing. Mullein *seeds* should be avoided altogether, as they are toxic and may cause poisoning.

MYRRH

Latin name: *Commiphora myrrha* (Burseraceae [frankincense] family)
Other common names: didin, didthin, guggul gum, guggul resin, mukkul

General Description

Myrrh is a resin harvested from the bark of the myrrh tree, grown in East Africa and the Arabian peninsula, and in the Indian states of Gujarat and Rajasthan. It is also indigenous to eastern Mediterranean countries, Somalia, Ethiopia, Eritrea, and Yemen. Myrrh is aromatic and has a reddish-brown color.

Myrrh was the most widely used analgesic in the ancient Middle East. The renowned Greek physician Hippocrates (460–377 B.C.E.) praised myrrh as a balm for sores, the Romans used it to treat infections of the eye and mouth, and the Hebrews used it as a painkiller. In the Vulgate translation of the Gospel of Mark, the writer records that Jesus was offered "vinum murratum"—a mixture of wine and myrrh—just before the crucifixion, and myrrh is mentioned in the holy scriptures of both Judaism and Islam.

Evidence of Benefit

Myrrh has been used for centuries in Western cultures as an antiseptic for sores and gingivitis, and as an expectorant for congestion. It is a gentle anti-inflammatory for the mouth and throat. Chinese healers valued myrrh for treating bleeding, pain, swelling, and wounds. In ayurvedic medicine, myrrh is used for menstrual disorders, stomach complaints, wounds, ulcers, and skin and mouth inflammation. In folk medicine, it is used to stimulate the appetite and the flow of digestive juices. Myrrh is approved by the German Commission E as a topical treatment for mild inflammation of the oral and pharyngeal mucosa.

Benefits of myrrh for specific health conditions include the following:

• *Canker sores, cuts and scrapes, gingivitis, and strep throat.* European herbalists use tincture of myrrh as an antiseptic gargle and rinse. Unlike other mouthwashes that coagulate the cells lining the mouth and throat to form a protective barrier against bacteria, myrrh acts only to prevent soreness and inflammation, and leaves the linings of the mouth and throat intact. Myrrh stimulates the production of infection-fighting white blood cells and also has a direct antimicrobial effect of its own. It is used to treat infections in the mouth such as mouth ulcers, gingivitis, and pyorrhea. Myrrh is a common ingredient in European toothpastes. It is added to fight the bacteria that cause tooth decay. Herbalists rate myrrh particularly high as a topical antiseptic for wounds, hemorrhoids, and bedsores.

• *Congestion.* Myrrh contains many volatile oils that make it suitable for promoting free breathing during congestive colds, and for clearing mucus-clogged passages. It increases circulation and restores tone and normal secretion.

• *Hyperlipidemia.* In one study, myrrh seemed to act as a mild agent in lowering low-density lipoprotein (LDL, or "bad") cholesterol. However, it did not lower total cholesterol or increase high-density lipoprotein (HDL or "good") cholesterol. But other studies have found that myrrh does lower total cholesterol and triglycerides and that the effects were comparable to those of typical lipid-lowering drugs.

Considerations for Use

In the United States, myrrh is most commonly used as an essential oil or tincture, although it is also included in toothpastes and incense sticks. Dosages are imprecise. As few as 5 drops of essential oil is useful in making a gargle or mouthwash, but more than 30 drops is likely to leave a strong aftertaste. The tincture should always be diluted before use, as undiluted forms may irritate the mouth or cause a burning sensation.

Myrrh is used in traditional Chinese medicine (TCM) and in Tibetan medicine to relieve scanty menstruation. For this reason, women who tend to have heavy periods should avoid it, and it should not be used during pregnancy. Myrrh also should not be used during lactation. Large amounts may have a violent laxative action, and can cause vomiting and an accelerated heartbeat. If bleeding gums or pain persists for longer than two weeks, consult a dentist. Myrrh may lower blood glucose levels, so patients with diabetes should ask their health-care professional before using it. Blood glucose needs to be monitored carefully in patients with diabetes if they use this herb. People with sensitive skin should avoid using myrrh topically.

NONI

See MORINDA.

OLIGOMERIC PROANTHOCYANIDINS (OPCs)

Latin name: *Pinus maritime*
Other common names: grapeseed extract, pine-bark extract

General Description

Oligomeric proanthocyanidins, better known by the abbreviation OPCs, are classified as flavonols and are usually derived from grapeseeds or pine bark. They are also present in red wine, hops, and various flowers, leaves, fruits, berries, nuts, and beans, usually with high concentrations in skins, barks, and seeds. The way in which these versatile healing compounds are distinct from flavonoids is their simple chemical structure, which allows them to be readily absorbed into the bloodstream.

Evidence of Benefit

OPCs are very powerful antioxidants. Vitamin E defends against fat-soluble oxidants, and vitamin C neutralizes water-soluble ones, but OPCs are active against both types. They also help stabilize the walls of blood vessels, reduce inflammation, and generally support tissues containing collagen and elastin, proteins found in cartilage, tendons, blood vessels, skin, and muscle.

Of all the herbs and herbal supplements, OPCs are the most useful in supporting vascular health. They maintain the health of capillaries, which are the channels through which the blood delivers nutrients to individual cells and carries away waste products. Capillaries must be permeable enough to allow nutrients and oxygen to seep through them, but strong enough to prevent too much fluid from flowing out and causing edema. OPCs are popular for preventing heart disease and cancer, revitalizing aging skin, and treating attention deficit hyperactivity disorder (ADHD) and high blood pressure.

Benefits of OPCs for specific health conditions include the following:

• *Allergies.* OPCs stop swelling and inflammation in animal and cell studies. Their antioxidant action prevents the activation of enzymes known as oxygenases, which cause the release of inflammatory chemicals in response to histamine. OPCs increase intracellular glutathione, a powerful antioxidant. Allergy sufferers may find that OPCs eliminate some symptoms of allergy, even in the middle of the allergy season. OPCs do not inhibit the production of antibodies to allergens, and so do not interfere with desensitization treatments (allergy shots).

• *Alzheimer's disease.* Cell studies have shown that Pycnogenol, a patented form of pine-bark extract, can inhibit the accumulation of beta-amyloid, a peptide (protein) that accumulates in the form of plaques in the central nervous system and is toxic to nerve cells, causing a breakdown of cell membranes. These plaques are a characteristic feature of Alzheimer's disease, but human data are lacking. In one study, however, a group of elderly patients with impaired cognitive function benefitted from 150 milligrams a day of Pycnogenol. The patients' working memory was believed to be enhanced in part by its antioxidant activity.

• *Attention deficit disorder (ADD).* Dr. Marion Sigurdson, a psychologist in Tulsa, Oklahoma, reports that OPCs extracted from a mix of grapeseeds and pine bark are as effective as methylphenidate (Ritalin) in the treatment of both adult and childhood ADD. However, others were not able to confirm that OPCs were effective in treating ADHD. The manner in which OPCs affect ADD is not precisely understood, but laboratory studies suggest that OPCs help the brain to regulate its use of two excitatory neurotransmitters, dopamine and norepinephrine. OPCs are also known to be potent antioxidants. If blood circulation to the brain of a person with ADD is impeded by allergy, high blood pressure, or muscular tension, the brain's oxygen supply is reduced. Once circulation is restored, toxic free radicals released by oxidation can flood brain tissue, destroying the linings of cells. OPCs interrupt the formation of oxygen free radicals and prevent damage to cell membranes.

• *Cancer and heart disease.* Medical studies have demonstrated the antioxidant effects of OPCs in persons with cancer and heart disease. They have the ability to inhibit the initiation, promotion, and progression of cancer. Scientists at the University of Arizona found that Pycnogenol helps build resistance to cancer by as much as 40 to 50 percent by boosting the body's first line of cancer defense, the immune system's natural killer (NK) cells. OPCs also work as antioxidants by increasing glutathione, a powerful antioxidant that is good for the heart and fights cancer. OPCs increase nitric oxide, which allows for better blood flow. Finally, it blocks compounds that create an inflammatory state. French researchers have found that grapeseed OPCs increase capillary resistance by 25 percent in people with diabetes and/or high blood pressure. German studies have found that damage from stroke is much lower in laboratory animals first treated with OPCs.

• *Diabetic retinopathy and macular degeneration.* Professor Denham Harman of the University of Nebraska believes that OPCs may be the ideal medicine for macular degeneration. Proanthocyanidins concentrate in the linings of microscopic blood vessels in the eye. These delicate conduits for blood are easily blocked by cellular debris or inflammation. They are also sensitive to injury from high blood pressure or diabetes. As long as the right level of permeability is maintained, however, no damage occurs to the retina. OPCs keep the capillaries permeable enough to deliver nutrients and remove waste products. They prevent excessive permeability that would cause swelling in the nerve tissue itself.

Harman believes that the antioxidant action of proanthocyanidins also helps to protect eye tissue from damage caused by inconsistent levels of oxygen. Two unpublished studies of 100 subjects found that taking 200 milligrams of grapeseed OPCs for five weeks produced improvements in night vision and glare recovery.

• *Swollen ankles, cuts and scrapes, lymphedema, nosebleed, tendinitis, and varicose veins.* When the walls of small blood vessels weaken, the fluids they transport leak out, causing swelling. OPCs strengthen capillary walls by blocking the degradation of the two proteins that give them strength and elasticity, collagen and elastin. This action stops edema and swelling.

The ability of OPCs to strengthen capillary walls has been scientifically verified. A double-blind Italian study of fifty people with varicose veins found that grapeseed OPCs worked faster and longer than the most commonly used prescription drug. The OPCs relieved both the burning and tingling sensations caused by varicose veins and swelling in the lower extremities. All symptoms improved in just thirty days. A French study found that 300 milligrams of grapeseed OPCs taken daily for four weeks reduced the reported incidence of pain, nighttime leg cramps, swelling, and tingling by 50 percent. Although OPCs can relieve the pain and swelling of venous insufficiency, they cannot make visible varicose veins disappear. But regular use might help prevent new ones from developing.

There is some evidence that OPCs can be useful for swelling following an injury or surgery. A double-blind controlled study found that postoperative breast cancer patients who took 600 milligrams of OPCs daily for six months experienced a significant reduction in swelling, pain, and sensations known as paresthesias. Another double-blind controlled study found that OPCs improved the rate at which swelling disappeared following sports injuries.

Considerations for Use

The two principal sources of OPCs are a pine-bark extract called Pycnogenol and a number of products based on grapeseed extract. Both kinds of products supply the active ingredients that are important to vascular health and circulation. Products made from cranberries, hazelnut tree leaves, and lemon tree bark that have been standardized for proanthocyanidins may also be used.

Many nutritionally oriented physicians report best results when Pycnogenol is taken in a dosage of 1 milligram per day for each pound of body weight (or 2 milligrams for each kilogram). For a 150-pound (70-kilogram) person, this would be a dose of approximately 150 milligrams of Pycnogenol daily. If progress is not satisfactory after thirty days, you can double the dosage. However, if you experience congestion, fever, rash, diarrhea, headaches, irritability, or fatigue, you should increase the dosage more slowly. There have been reports of irritability and decreased energy levels, especially when grapeseed is used for ADD and ADHD. For other sources of OPCs, follow the dosage and administration directions on the product label.

Grapeseed extracts are high in tannin and may interfere with iron absorption. You should not take these if you have anemia. If you are taking blood-thinning medication, including aspirin, heparin, pentoxifylline (Trental), or warfarin (Coumadin), high doses of OPCs may pose a risk of excessive bleeding. Do not use grapeseed with immunosuppressive drugs. Due to the high antioxidant content, do not use this herb if you are taking chemotherapy drugs or receiving radiation therapy, as it interferes with the action of these treatments.

Flavonoids: The Missing Link in Vitamin Therapy

No vitamin supplement is more universally accepted than vitamin C. Its discoverer, the Hungarian-American scientist Albert Szent-Györgyi (1893–1986), was awarded the Nobel Prize in Physiology or Medicine for his explanation of the biological oxidation process the vitamin controls. Szent-Györgyi became known as a founder of modern biochemistry. His research, however, found that vitamin C is only a part of a system of cofactors needed for health.

While Szent-Györgyi was still trying to make a purified form of vitamin C, he was approached by a colleague who had a patient with scurvy. In this patient, the vitamin-deficiency disease had caused weak gums and purple blotches on the skin, both due to broken capillaries. The scientist gave the doctor an impure preparation that contained vitamin C plus other compounds. The patient quickly recovered.

Later, Szent-Györgyi and the doctor tried a preparation of pure vitamin C on another patient who had similar symptoms, expecting quicker results. To their surprise, pure vitamin C was of no benefit at all, so they went back to the impure solution. Treated with the mixture of unknown compounds and vitamin C, the second patient also recovered.

In 1935, Szent-Györgyi and a colleague isolated a factor from lemon juice that served as the essential cofactor for vitamin C. This compound increased the resistance and decreased the permeability, or "leakiness," of the capillary wall. Since the decreased permeability was the element in the healing process that was not accomplished by administration of pure vitamin C, the two scientists called the new compound vitamin P.

Szent-Györgyi studied this compound for another forty years. When electron microscopes became available, he observed that the structural proteins in healthy cells were "the color of a good Swiss chocolate." This was due to the presence of an electron transfer system in which vitamin C and its cofactors regulate the transfer of free radicals of oxygen. In cancer cells, however, these same proteins were colorless, indicating that their electron acceptors were missing or had been damaged. When either vitamin C or its cofactors was missing, the free radicals of oxygen produced in the normal process of respiration escaped, and the proteins became free radicals themselves.

By this time, the name vitamin P had been dropped from the literature in the United States, although it still is used in articles published in Russia. Discovering its healing properties had taken over forty years. "Vitamin P" compounds appear in so many foods that it is difficult to experience a deficiency, and American scientists had assumed it had no value.

Flavonoids and oligomeric proanthocyanidins are now known to be essential for promoting good health. The flavonoids and oligomeric proanthocyanidins interact with vitamin C to protect each other from free radicals. Together with vitamin C, they promote vascular health. Their promotion of vascular health may help improve heart disease, some cancers, and degenerative conditions of the eyes.

OLIVE LEAF

Latin name: *Olea europa* (Oleaceae [olive] family)
Other common name: lucca

General Description

Olive is a small evergreen tree native to Mediterranean regions as far as Iran and beyond the Caucasus. Throughout history, the use of its fruit and oil is well documented. Hippocrates, the Greek physician known as the "father of medicine," prescribed olive oil for ulcers, cholera, and muscular pains some 2,500 years ago. Over the ages, numerous folk medicine applications for olive oil have been described. The leaves of the olive have been used for arteriosclerosis, rheumatism, gout, diabetes, and fever. More modern uses include the management of high cholesterol levels, HIV infection, high blood pressure, and infections, as well as promoting urination and treating viral infections.

In the early 1900s, a bitter compound from the leaf, called oleuropein, was isolated and determined to be part of the olive tree's powerful disease-fighting properties. In 1962, researchers found that oleuropein could lower blood pressure and increase blood flow in the coronary arteries, relieve arrhythmias, and prevent intestinal muscle spasms. In the late 1960s, researchers showed that elenolic acid, another component in olive leaf, could kill many kinds of viruses, bacteria, and parasitic protozoans. However, when it was ingested, this compound rapidly became bound to proteins in blood serum, rendering it ineffective. Several years ago, scientific research solved the protein-binding problem. Olive leaf extract is now made from oleuropein and a selected blend of olive leaf extracts, including flavonoids.

Evidence of Benefit

Research and clinical experience suggest that olive leaf extract is beneficial in treating conditions caused by viruses, retroviruses, bacteria, or protozoa. The olive leaf appears to have limited antiviral activity. It has the ability to interfere with critical amino acid production for viruses; it can contain viral infection by inactivating viruses through preventing virus budding or assembly; and it has the ability to penetrate infected cells and stop viral replication there. Olive leaf extract is also effective against bacteria, yeast strains, and fungi that produce conditoxin and other microtoxins that may contribute to chronic fatigue and immune dysfunction syndromes. It is also effective against parasites, both protozoa and worms.

Benefits of olive leaf extract for specific health conditions include the following:

• *Heart disease and high blood pressure.* The powerful antioxidant properties of the olive leaf help protect the heart and circulatory system from free-radical damage. A 1994 experiment found that oleuropein inhibited the oxidation of low-density lipoprotein (LDL, or "bad") cholesterol, which has been connected to various heart problems. Other findings have verified that olive leaf extract can significantly decrease blood pressure. One study found that patients with high blood pressure who took 1.6 grams a day of olive leaf experienced significant decreases in blood pressure, whether they were taking antihypertensive drugs or not. The patients' blood sugar levels decreased as well.

• *HIV infection.* In cell line studies, Olive leaf has been shown to have anti-HIV properties. Its components affect signaling proteins that slow the growth of HIV.

• *Yeast infection.* Candida are single-celled fungi that live in the bloodstream, releasing powerful poisons and toxins as they multiply. By the time we reach adulthood, virtually all of us play host to *Candida albicans*. If the immune system becomes suppressed, a yeast overgrowth may result in a deep-seated infection. Symptoms of this can include fatigue, headaches, muscle aches, constipation, diarrhea, gas, itching, vaginal discharge, premenstrual syndrome (PMS), insomnia, eczema, psoriasis, allergies, sinus problems, recurrent colds and flu, indigestion, respiratory problems, asthma, and weight problems. A sixty-day double-blind, placebo-controlled study of thirty subjects found that such symptoms were reduced by more than 50 percent in all of the subjects who took the olive leaf extract, with no apparent side effects.

Considerations for Use

Olive leaf extract is available in capsule form. Dosages recommended by health professionals include one or two capsules, totaling 250 to 500 milligrams, daily for preventive purposes. For treating symptoms, the recommended dosage varies with the severity of disease. Some individuals have reported rapid relief from acute infections after taking three or more 500-milligram tablets every six hours. Use of olive leaf can trigger colic among gallstone sufferers, so it should not be used by those who have gallstones. Do not put the herb near the eyes, as it may irritate the surface of the eye. Patients with biliary stones also should avoid this herb. There also have been some reports of runny nose and asthma after taking olive leaf.

OREGON GRAPE ROOT

Latin names: *Mahonia aquifolium, Mahonia nervosa, Mahonia repens* (Berberidaceae [barberry] family)
Other common names: alegrita, California barberry, japonica, mahonia, mountain grape, mountain holly, pepperidge, sourberry, sowberry, yellow root

General Description

There are three species of Oregon grape: the small creeping *M. repens*, found in dry places such as Ponderosa pine ecosystems; *M. nervosa,* one to two feet (thirty to sixty centimeters) tall with holly, found in lower elevations in coastal forests and interior cedar-hemlock ecosystems; and *M. aquifolium,* known as tall Oregon grape, which is three to 5 feet (1–1.5 meters) tall. They are used interchangeably for medicinal purposes. All have bright yellow flowers and green berries that ripen to a blue-purple color. The name *Oregon grape* comes from its use as a medicine and food along the Oregon Trail. Its popularity as a food and medicine nearly led to its extinction in the late nineteenth century. Both the leaves and root bark are used medicinally.

Evidence of Benefit

Oregon grape root has bacterial infection fighting properties, and has been used both internally and externally, to heal the skin and soothe mucous membranes. It may help to purify the blood and liver of wastes, and may stimulate the functioning of the gallbladder and liver. As a bitter, it stimulates and improves digestive function.

The best known of the herb's active constituents is berberine, a chemical that Oregon grape root shares with barberry, coptis, and goldenseal. (For additional information about the actions of berberine, *see* BARBERRY.)

Benefits of Oregon grape root for specific health conditions include the following:

• *Diarrhea and gastritis.* Berberine has been shown to help manage diarrhea in patients infected with *E. coli.* In cell studies, it is thought to work by inhibiting the ability of bacteria to attach to human cells, which helps prevent infections, particularly in the intestines and urinary tract.

• *Psoriasis, liver ailments.* Oregon grape root has been tested as a treatment for psoriasis in cell studies, and has been found to reduce psoriatic lesions. Laboratory research suggests that Oregon grape root has some effects at the cellular level that might be helpful in the treatment of psoriasis, such as slowing abnormal cell growth and reducing inflammation. Also, part of its action is to help the liver function to metabolize wastes and toxins. This was only shown in cell studies, and it is not known how it works in people with liver disorders. Skin problems can be treated both internally and externally.

Considerations for Use

Oregon grape root is available in capsules, ointments, tablets, and tinctures. To treat skin problems, topical creams or ointments containing 10 percent Oregon grape extract are generally applied three times daily to the affected skin areas. Oregon grape root can also be used in compresses. (*See* COMPRESSES in Part Three.)

More than other herbs containing berberine, Oregon grape root is mildly sedating. You should use it with caution if you take an antianxiety drug, such as alprazolam (Xanax) or lorazepam (Ativan).

Oregon grape root has several other relatively uncommon side effects. There is some evidence that the berberine in Oregon grape root can interfere with the absorption of tetracyline antibiotics. It may also lower blood sugar, so you should use it with caution if you have diabetes and have not used the herb before. The tannins in Oregon grape root tinctures may cause stomach irritation, so tinctures of the herb should be avoided in treating diarrhea and by people who have chronic heartburn. People with Raynaud's disease who use relatively high dosages of Oregon grape root may find that it aggravates numbness and tingling. This effect is minor and temporary.

Oregon grape root has been reported to cause uterine contractions and to increase levels of bilirubin, so oral preparations of Oregon grape root should be avoided during pregnancy. Oregon grape root is not recommended for long-term use (three weeks or more at a time).

OSHA

Latin name: *Ligusticum porteri* (Apiaceae [parsley] family)
Other common names: chuchupate, Colorado cough root, life root

General Description

As echinacea is the antibacterial herb from the American Great Plains, osha is considered to be the antibacterial herb of the American Rocky Mountains. Osha is a perennial herb bearing glossy, toothed compound leaves and greenish yellow flowers. It has a camphorlike scent due to its essential oil, which is responsible for much of its healing properties. The root of the plant is the part used in herbal medicine.

Evidence of Benefit

Osha has shown antibacterial and anti-inflammatory properties in cell studies. It has been used for viral infections of the sinuses, throat, and upper and lower respiratory systems. It may help bring up respiratory secretions and relax smooth muscle, possibly making it useful for coughs and stuffy noses (colds).

Benefits of osha for specific health conditions include the following:

• *Arthritis.* Osha is a traditional remedy in Native American medicine and home remedies of the American West for providing long-term relief of inflammation.

• *Bronchitis, colds, influenza, and sinusitis.* One of the active constituents of osha is Z-ligustilide, which acts gently against bacterial and yeast infections in cell studies. In the minute quantities provided by the herb, this chemical stops the multiplication of bacteria and yeast cells while relaxing the muscles lining the respiratory passages. The proper dose for this herb is not known, as these studies were only done in cell lines.

Considerations for Use

Osha is available as a tincture and can be made into a hand bath. Most over-the-counter (OTC) osha formulas for colds and flu combine osha with echinacea and goldenseal in an alcohol-based tincture; be sure to read labels carefully if you are sensitive to either herb. (*See* ECHINACEA and GOLDENSEAL.)

It you take this herb on its own for extended periods of time, take a weeklong break every couple of months. Osha should not be used during pregnancy, as large amounts may cause uterine contractions.

PAPAIN

Latin name: Papain is extracted from papaya, *Carica papaya* (Caricaceae [papaya] family)
Other common names: mamaeire, melon tree, papaw

General Description

Papain is a proteolytic (protein-dissolving) enzyme extracted from the milky white latex of unripe papaya fruit. Green papaya, used in Southeast Asia as a salad vegetable, is an excellent source of papain. It is also found in papaya fruit and papaya leaf.

Papayas are indigenous to tropical America and are cultivated in tropical regions all over the world. Worldwide, most papayas are eaten green. In many countries in South Asia and Southeast Asia, green papaya is used to make a tart and tasty salad to accompany yams or rice. Green papaya is a richer source of the therapeutically active papain than is the ripe fruit.

Evidence of Benefit

Papain is a digestive aid for those who have trouble digesting proteins. It is also useful for pain relief. It aids digestion and heartburn, stimulates appetite, and helps to prevent ulcers. Papain also helps bruises and other injuries to heal faster. In ayurvedic medicine, it is used for worm infestation, kidney problems, hemorrhoids, coughs, and bronchitis.

Benefits of papain for specific health conditions include the following:

• *Benign prostatic hypertrophy (BPH)*. Papain relieves acute prostate inflammation. A clinical study involving 399 patients in Russia found that papain treatment reversed rectal lesions induced by extreme prostate enlargement in 97 percent of the men treated.

• *Bruises, sore muscles, sprains and strains, and recovery from surgery.* Several double-blind controlled studies have found that treating individuals with ankle injuries, mild athletic injuries, and finger fractures with proteolytic enzymes resulted in significantly improved healing time. Other double-blind studies have found that treatment with proteolytic enzymes after knee surgery, oral surgery, and nasal surgery improved the speed of recovery.

• *Cancer*. There is some evidence that papain may moderate the immune system. It may work by causing an increase in reactive oxygen atoms or by increasing production of cytokines, which kill cancer cells. In one study, oral enzymes including papain and others (trypsin and chymotrypsin) improved symptoms in patients with breast cancer. The women in the study experienced fewer infections, skin disorders, tumor pain, headache, and muscle wasting. Similarly, those with head and neck cancer who used these same enzymes experienced a reduction in symptoms. On the other hand, enzymes including papain did not lengthen life or improve quality of life in patients with inoperable pancreatic cancer compared to gemcitabine-based chemotherapy.

• *Herpesvirus infection and shingles*. A scientifically controlled study conducted in Germany found that the application of papain creams to skin affected by herpes outbreaks produced pain relief equivalent to that of acyclovir (Zovirax), although the papain took longer than acyclovir to control redness. Overall, acyclovir and papain were judged equally effective in the treatment of shingles (herpes zoster). Although both treatments afforded similar pain relief, people treated with papain experienced fewer side effects.

Considerations for Use

Papain is available in the form of Linked-Papain cream for external use, and as a single-herb capsule and a combined bromelain/papain tablet for internal use. (*See* BROMELAIN.)

Pregnant women should not use papain or eat the unripe papaya fruit, as both could have harmful effects on the fetus and could induce abortion. Allergic reactions such as asthma attack are possible. There is some concern that proteolytic enzymes may cause additional damage to exposed tissue in ulcers. People with malabsorption disorders may want to avoid proteolytic enzymes.

A serious condition called fibrosing colonopathy, which involves damage to the large intestines, has been linked to the use of pancreatic enzymes by children with cystic fibrosis. Until more is known, children with cystic fibrosis who need to take pancreatic enzymes should do so only under the careful supervision of a health-care professional.

Papain may increase the blood-thinning effects of warfarin (Coumadin) and other anticoagulants. If you take anticoagulant medication, you should use papain in moderation only.

PASSIONFLOWER

Latin names: *Passiflora caerulea, Passiflora incarnata* (Passifloraceae [passionflower] family)

Other common names: apricot vine, blue passionflower (*Passiflora caerulea*), maypop

General Description

Passionflower is a climbing vine native to North and Central America, and parts of South America such as Argentina and Brazil. Growing to a length of up to thirty feet (ten meters), passionflower bears three-lobed leaves, purple flowers, and egg-shaped fruit. Passionflower's name comes from an analogy drawn between the appearance of the plant's ornate flowers to elements of the crucifixion of Jesus: three styles for the three nails used to affix him to the cross; five stamens for the five wounds he suffered; and white and purple-blue colors believed to symbolize heaven and purity. The medicinal parts are the whole or cut dried herb and fresh aerial (aboveground) parts. The yellow pulp from the berries is edible.

Evidence of Benefit

The use of passionflower to tranquilize and settle edgy nerves has been documented for over 200 years. This herb relieves muscle tension and helps calm extreme anxiety. It has a depressant effect on the central nervous system and lowers blood pressure. Passionflower is especially good for nervous insomnia.

A wide range of potential therapeutic applications of passionflower are currently being investigated. It relaxes the linings of artery walls; reduces blood pressure; stops chemical reactions that cause nausea and vomiting as a result of withdrawal from cocaine, heroin, or opiate painkillers; and, in laboratory tests, stops the growth of certain kinds of thyroid cancer. It has been approved by the German Commission E for nervousness, restlessness, and insomnia.

Benefits of passionflower for specific health conditions include the following:

• *Anxiety and addiction.* Laboratory studies in France concluded that passionflower reduces anxiety and increases the effectiveness of prescription sleep aids. Compounds in passionflower occupy the same receptor sites in the brain as benzodiazepine drugs, such as chlordiazepoxide (Librium) and diazepam (Valium), but produce less drowsiness. The alkaloids harmane and harmaline, found in passionflower, have been found to act somewhat like monoamine oxidase (MAO) inhibitors, a category of drugs sometimes prescribed for depression and other disorders. One product called Passipay is made from passionflower extract and has been shown to have the same benefit as the drug oxazepam in reducing anxiety in patients with generalized anxiety disorder. Passionflower is sometimes substituted for prescription sedatives for people who are addicted to drugs or alcohol. In one study, men who were addicted to opium benefited during withdrawal from passionflower, according to the Short Opiate Withdrawal Scale. In another study, using passionflower before surgery seemed to reduce the anxiety associated with the upcoming surgery.

Considerations for Use

Passionflower is available as a tea or tincture for the treatment of anxiety and insomnia. Sometimes external forms are available as are homeopathic remedies, which help with sleep, convulsions, and agitation. Do not use passionflower if you are taking anticoagulants. Passionflower may cause symptoms including dizziness, ataxia, nausea, vomiting, constipation, electrocardiogram (ECG) changes, and impaired cognitive function.

You should not use passionflower if you take an MAO inhibitor. Nor should you take passionflower during pregnancy, because it may stimulate the uterine muscles. Women seeking to become pregnant also should not take it. Adults over the age of sixty-five and children between the ages of two and twelve should take only low-strength preparations, and you should not give this herb in any form to a child under two years of age.

Many herbalists recommend using only professionally prepared remedies. *P. caerulea* contains cyanide, and there is some fear that this may accidentally be substituted if you purchase the unprocessed herb.

PAU D'ARCO

Latin name: *Tabebuia* species (Bignoniaceae [pau d'arco] family)
Other common names: ipe-roxo, lapacho, purple lapacho, trumpet bush

General Description

Pau d'arco is a tropical tree that grows to a height of one hundred feet (thirty meters). Although it is an evergreen in the Amazonian rain forest, it is deciduous at higher and colder locations. Plants in the *Tabebuia* genus that include the various species of pau d'arco can flower in a number of colors, but the *roxa* (red-, magenta-, crimson-, and violet-flowering) varieties are used the most in herbal medicine. Medicinal preparations are made from the tree's dried inner bark, sustainably harvested from trees in the wild.

Evidence of Benefit

Pau d'arco extract is an immune stimulant and is effective against bacterial, fungal, viral, parasitic, and yeast infections. It also is considered to be an anti-inflammatory agent.

The inner lining of the bark of either the red or the purple pau d'arco tree has been used for centuries as a treatment for cancer, lupus, infectious diseases, wounds, and many other health conditions. Over the past twenty years, numerous reports from doctors and patients in various publications have spoken of pau d'arco tea's beneficial effects on disorders as varied as arthritis, athlete's foot, the common cold, leukemia, pain, and yeast and other fungal infections. The herb is currently being investigated for effects on cancer and candida. Traditional herbalists agree that it strengthens and balances the immune system.

Benefits of pau d'arco for specific health conditions include the following:

• *Cancer.* One of pau d'arco's main components, lapachol, possesses antitumor properties, and for a time was under active investigation as a possible chemotherapy drug. Unfortunately, when given in high enough dosages to kill cancer cells, lapachol causes numerous serious side effects. It also was shown to have no effect in patients with non-leukemic tumors or chronic myelocytic leukemia. However, herbalists believe that the whole herb may be able to produce benefits equivalent to standard chemotherapy drugs with fewer side effects. It has been reported that drinking a tea made from red or purple pau d'arco may help to combat infection, build up immunity, strengthen cells, and reduce pain and inflammation, but not in place of conventional antibiotics. Some people have reported that the tea appeared to increase effectiveness of chemotherapy while decreasing negative side effects of the chemotherapy treatments. Human studies are lacking, but two have been conducted using an extract of the compound furonaphthoquinone from pau d'arco. One study found that tumor size shrank and some patients with cancer went into remission. The other study had to be stopped prematurely because the patients in this study with leukemia had abnormal bleeding tests, nausea, and vomiting. And there was no evidence of an anticancer effect.

• *Parasitic infection.* Pau d'arco acts against Chagas' disease, a tropical infection that has spread to the United States, especially to southern Texas. Chagas' disease is caused by a protozoan known as *Trypanosoma cruzi*, which attacks muscle tissue in the heart and gastrointestinal tract, as well as skeletal muscles and bone. Pau d'arco may offer protection against the parasite without the side effects associated with the drug nifurtimox, which is the standard conventional treatment for Chagas' disease. These effects can include dermatitis, sterility, nausea and vomiting, nerve damage, and a life-threatening reaction called anaphylactic shock.

The drug-resistant strain of malaria, *Plasmodium falciparum,* has become increasingly common, even in such unlikely locales as San Francisco and the borough of Queens in New York City. Conventional treatments offer no protection against this disease. Laboratory tests, however, have shown that a group of chemicals in pau d'arco known as naphthoquinones stop the multiplication of the malaria parasite even if it is resistant to the standard antimalaria medications, chloroquine (Aralen) and quinine. In addition, pau d'arco prevents the progression of schistosomiasis, a parasitic infection that causes a condition better known as river blindness. However, determining the correct human dose can be problematic, as too much of the herb suppresses immune function and is toxic to cells, while small amounts stimulate immune function. For now, pau d'arco should not be the only treatment used for any of these conditions.

• *Yeast infection.* Pau d'arco stimulates the immune system to produce macrophages, immune cells that engulf and digest bacteria and yeasts. One of the active compounds in pau d'arco, lapachol, may be as effective against yeast infections as the prescription drug ketoconazole (Nizoral).

Considerations for Use

Pau d'arco is available in ointments or lotions for external use, and as capsules or tinctures for internal use. Pau d'arco products frequently combine the herb with other herbs used to treat infection and/or inflammation, such as garlic and goldenseal. Be sure to read labels carefully if you are sensitive to these herbs.

High dosages of lapachol can cause uncontrolled bleeding, nausea, and vomiting. It is much safer to use the whole bark than to take isolated lapachol. Unfortunately, inferior products containing only the outer bark and the wood are sometimes misrepresented as genuine inner bark pau d'arco. Because the pau d'arco constituent lapachol is somewhat toxic, the herb is not recommended for women who are pregnant or nursing. Do not use it with anticoagulants. In a study using male rats, short-term use of the herb caused reproductive toxicity or the inability to procreate.

As of yet, there is no good evidence that pau d'arco is an effective cancer treatment, and it may interfere with the action of prescription anticancer drugs. You should not add it to a conventional chemotherapy regimen without consulting with your physician.

PEPPERMINT

Latin name: *Mentha piperita* (Lamiaceae [mint] family)
Other common names: brandy mint, lamb mint

General Description

Peppermint is a hybrid of watermint and spearmint that was first cultivated near London in 1750. It grows almost everywhere. It is a square-stemmed annual that yields the popular flavoring agent. It grows from 32 to 36 inches (85 to 100 centimeters) high and has aromatic serrated leaves. The two main cultivated forms are the black mint, which has violet-colored leaves and stems and a relatively high essential oil content, and the white mint, which has pure green leaves and a milder taste. The finest-quality peppermint is grown in the northwestern United States and Europe.

Peppermint teas are used around the world to calm queasy stomachs and to quell indigestion. Peppermint leaves contain a volatile (essential) oil that is 50 to 75 percent menthol. This oil is the basis of most medicinal preparations of peppermint. The oil is extracted from the aerial parts (aboveground) of the flowering plant, the dried leaves, flowering branch tips, and the whole plant.

Evidence of Benefit

Peppermint is a general stimulant. A strong cup of peppermint tea circulates quickly and acts more powerfully than any liquor stimulant. This herb has a long history as a digestive aid and as a treatment for the symptoms of cough, colds, and fever. It kills microorganisms that can cause food poisoning, relieves the pain of sprains and strains, and helps freshen lingering bad breath. It also is good for nausea and vomiting. The leaves and oil are approved for different uses by the German Commission E. The peppermint leaves are approved for spastic complaints of the gastrointestinal tract as well as for the gallbladder and bile ducts. It is also helpful for symptoms related to digestion problems such as dyspepsia, flatulence, gastritis, and enteritis. The oil is approved for internal use for spastic discomfort of the upper gastrointestinal system and bile ducts, irritable colon, breathing difficulties, and inflammation of the mouth tissue. Externally, it is approved for muscle pain and neuralgia. Homeopathic remedies include one for colds.

Peppermint oil is effective at protecting food from spoiling, as shown by its amazing ability to stop the growth of *Salmonella* bacteria. Japanese experiments with a number of foods stored at 86°F (30°C) for two days showed that peppermint oil stopped the growth of *Salmonella* and slowed the growth of *Listeria*, another harmful type of microbe.

Benefits of peppermint for specific health conditions include the following:

• *Dyspepsia (upset stomach or indigestion).* If queasiness, nausea, a feeling of fullness, or severe vomiting is a problem, a single cup of peppermint tea will often bring relief. Because of the herb's antispasmodic effects, it eases gas pain and heartburn. In one study, 42 percent of patients with nonulcerative dyspepsia who used a combination of peppermint and caraway oils became pain free after two weeks; after four weeks, 90 percent were pain free.

• *Gallstones.* During an acute attack, peppermint relieves mild spasms of the bile duct. It also helps to dissolve gallstones and increase bile flow. In one study, 73 percent of patients with common bile duct stones who used a peppermint product (Rowachol) passed their stones after eighteen months.

• *Headache and stress.* When it is applied topically, peppermint oil can relieve headache. Researchers at Christian-Albrechts University in Germany found that peppermint oil, applied to the forehead, has the same pain-relieving effect as 1,000 milligrams of acetaminophen. In most subjects, regardless of age or sex or the duration of the headache, peppermint was just as effective at relieving pain as acetaminophen. However, another study showed that peppermint offered only a 10 percent reduction in headaches after fifteen minutes. Applying peppermint oil to the temples can also relax your muscles and decrease tension.

• *Irritable bowel syndrome (IBS).* IBS is a condition in which the intestines pass food through to the colon before it is fully digested, causing cramping and diarrhea. Peppermint oil blocks the contractions of the smooth muscles lining the intestines, reversing some of the symptoms of IBS. In one study, patients with IBS using enteric-coated peppermint oil capsules experienced improvement in symptoms such as abdominal pain, bloating, constipation, diarrhea, and passage of gas or mucus. After one month, 75 percent of the patients had a 50 percent or greater improvement in symptoms. Peppermint oil also worked for children who had IBS or recurrent abdominal pain. For children, the effective dose was 180 to 200 milligrams a day.

Considerations for Use

Peppermint is available in menthol lozenges, peppermint oil, enteric-coated peppermint-oil capsules, and teas. Peppermint oil can be used in aromatherapy. (*See* AROMATHERAPY in Part Three.)

You should never ingest pure menthol, and use leaves with caution and only under the care of a doctor, because they contain substances that can be toxic. Ingestion of leaves should especially be avoided by those with a history of gallstones, as there have been reports of colic or liver pain occurring. Pure peppermint may cause cardiac arrhythmias, and even small doses of pure menthol can be life-threatening. Peppermint leaves are not recommended for use during pregnancy. If you drink peppermint tea on a regular basis, take a few days' break after a week or two.

Peppermint oil is not to be used by anyone with biliary duct problems, gallbladder inflammation, or severe liver damage. When using peppermint oil, it is important not to exceed the recommended dosage. It is not recommended for people with esophageal reflux, as it can lead to gastric complaints. Larger doses may cause burning, gastrointestinal upset, and even seizures. Some people have developed skin rashes, abdominal pain, heartburn, and perianal burning. Do not apply to open wounds or areas such as the eyes. The oil should never be applied to the face of infants and small children, particularly around the nose. There have been some reports of severe asthma-like symptoms. However, rubbing 5 to 15 drops of peppermint oil to the chest and back is safe.

Peppermint can cause depletion of or interference with the heartburn drug cisapride (Propulsid). It is ill-advised to use peppermint with calcium channel blockers, as the drug's effectiveness may be reduced. Drugs that are metabolized by the cytochrome P450 system should not be used with peppermint. If you are using peppermint for gallstone relief, be sure to follow the directions under GALLSTONES in Part Two. You should avoid it altogether if you have any other type of gallbladder disorder.

POLLEN

General Description

Pollen consists of the dustlike, air- or insect-borne male reproductive cells of flowering plants. Pollen is collected by, rather than made by, bees. The pollen used in herbal medicine is collected from various species by hand (without the help of bees). Pollen may be used raw or micronized into separate grains.

While pollen is a plant product, it is not technically an herb, but it has been called the miracle food. It contains vitamins (including the B vitamins and vitamins A, C, E, and K), minerals (including calcium, copper, iron, magnesium, phosphorus, potassium, silicon, zinc, and other trace elements), carbohydrates, fats, proteins, and fatty acids. However, their contribution to the overall nutrient needs of the human body is small.

Evidence of Benefit

Pollen both protects the prostate gland and has some beneficial effects in radiation therapy. It has been suggested that pollen has positive effects in treating disorders of the liver, gallbladder, stomach, and intestines. It may also be beneficial for people with hay fever. The German Commission E has only approved its use, however, for restoring feebleness and loss of appetite.

Many studies in cell lines have shown that pollen contains antibiotic substances that act against bacteria.

Benefits of pollen for specific health conditions include the following:

• *Allergies and hay fever.* Pollen extracts, taken orally, have been used to desensitize people to plants to which they are allergic. In one double-blind study, people with allergies to grass pollen were asked to place drops of liquid grass pollen extract under their tongues daily for three weeks, using a gradually increasing concentration. After three weeks, they took pollen twice a week at a maintenance level. During the next allergy season, they had significantly fewer severe hay fever symptoms than those experienced by a group given placebo drops.

• *Benign prostatic hypertrophy (BPH) and prostatitis.* In controlled studies, approximately 40 percent of men with benign prostatic hyperplasia uncomplicated by prostate stones or narrowing of the urethra found complete relief after one month's treatment with micronized pollen. Another 40 percent found partial relief. Pollen seems to act by reducing the production of enzymes needed for the inflammatory process. It does not affect the body's production or use of testosterone.

An extract of several species of rye pollens has been shown to have anti-inflammatory properties, to relax the muscles that surround the urethra, and to inhibit growth of prostate cells. Rye pollen extract has been reported to improve symptoms of chronic prostatitis in a number of studies, including a trial in which three tablets daily significantly reduced symptoms in 78 percent of those with uncomplicated prostatitis, compared with only one of eighteen with complications such as scar tissue and calcifications.

Considerations for Use

Raw pollen is given in doses approximately ten times larger than micronized pollen, so micronized pollen is the easiest form to use. Raw pollen daily doses are 30 to 40 grams, and for micronized pollen it is 3 to 4 grams. Pine pollen, thought to stimulate testosterone production, is available in micronized form for the treatment of reduced sex drive.

Many people have allergies to inhaled pollens, and reactions to ingested pollen have been reported. Serious reactions such as asthma, hives, and anaphylactic shock, some of them life-threatening, have been reported. If you have severe hay fever or other respiratory allergies, you should use pollen with caution, and only under the supervision of a knowledgeable health-care professional. Other side effects include discomforts of the gastrointestinal tract. Although people with pollen allergies do use pollen to gain relief, the German Commission E does not recommend that people with pollen allergies use pollen.

POLYSACCHARIDE KUREHA (PSK)

Latin name: PSK is extracted from the kawaratake mushroom, *Coriolus versicolor* (Basidiomycetes [button mushroom] family)

General Description

Polysaccharide kureha (PSK), also known as krestin, is an extract from the kawaratake mushroom. In Japanese, *kawaratake* means "mushroom on the riverbank." This mushroom is common in the woods of Japan, China, and the United States. It sports a fan-shaped fruiting body that resembles a turkey tail, which gave it the English common name *turkey-tail mushroom.* The fruiting body can be any of a variety of shades of blue, brown, gray, or white. In Japan, PSK is the most widely sold health food in the country.

Evidence of Benefit

PSK is an antioxidant and immune stimulant. It contains complex polysaccharides that have demonstrated to have some anticancer activity in over twenty years of clinical use in Japan. It works best with other conventional cancer therapies and is most effective in people with cancer of the stomach, esophagus, colon, breast, and lungs. There have been over fifty scientific studies involving PSK. It is virtually nontoxic and readily bioavailable when taken orally.

The same active component in PSK can be purchased as coriolus extract. Studies have shown that healthy individuals who took a onetime dose of 1 gram of this extract had a significant improvement in cellular immune function within twelve hours. Coriolus is effective against hepatitis and is being tested as a treatment for hepatitis C, but PSK is not typically used in this way.

Benefits of PSK for specific health conditions include the following:

• *Atherosclerosis.* Because it is an antioxidant, PSK may protect the linings of artery walls from the action of harmful free radicals. This could arrest the immune cells from attracting low-density lipoprotein (LDL, or "bad") cholesterol that gathers into artery-clogging plaques.

• *Cancer.* PSK's effectiveness against cancer is so widely recognized in Japan that in one year, purchases of PSK accounted for over 25 percent of the nation's entire expenditures for cancer treatment. It is especially beneficial when used together with standard chemotherapy or radiation therapy. PSK slows the spread of tumors by disabling enzymes that allow tumor cells to break out of the matrix that holds healthy cells in their proper places. This is especially useful in increasing the effectiveness of radiation therapy for endometrial cancer. In a study of patients at the National Cancer Center Hospital in Tokyo with fairly advanced endometrial and cervical cancer, some took 3 to 6 grams of PSK every day in conjunction with radiation therapy, while others received radiation alone. After the radiation treatment was completed, 36 percent of the patients who took PSK had no observable cancer cells, while that was true of only 11 percent of those who did not take PSK. The two-year survival rate was 94 percent for patients who took PSK and 74 percent for those who did not. The five-year survival rates were 79 percent and 48 percent, respectively.

Doctors have seen an increase in survival rates when PSK is used with either radiation therapy or chemotherapy for lung cancer. In one study of 185 patients with advanced (stage III) lung cancer, the five-year survival rate for people who received both radiation therapy and PSK exceeded that of those who received radiation alone by 400 percent. In another study involving 169 patients, PSK extended longevity in patients who received chemotherapy by an average of seven weeks.

PSK also helps people with colorectal cancer. It checked the progress of the disease and increased survival rates in one trial involving 124 patients, all of whom were also treated with mitomycin (Mutamycin). PSK reduced the depth to which the cancer invaded the intestinal wall and curtailed the cancer's spread to both lymph nodes and blood vessels. In laboratory studies, PSK has been found to increase the effectiveness of the chemotherapy agent 5-fluorouracil (5-FU). In cell line studies, it reduces the rate of cancer growth in the cecum, the place where the large intestine begins, and reduces the rate at which cancer

enters the lymphatic system. PSK increases the effectiveness of immune-system components called T cells against colorectal tumors, and has also been found to prevent the spread of colon cancer to the liver. In one eighteen-year study, PSK reduced the spread of colon cancer to the peritoneum (the membrane lining the intestinal cavity) and the lungs in 60 percent of the people who took it.

PSK is useful in treating several other cancers. In leukemia, it stops invasion of normal tissues by leukemia cells, and it reduces the likelihood of relapse in childhood acute lymphocytic leukemia after chemotherapy is discontinued. In melanoma, it reduces the rate at which cancer cells spread to the lungs and increases the effectiveness of chemotherapy treatment with cyclophosphamide (Cytoxan, Neosar) and interleukin-2 (IL-2), an immune-system chemical. In ovarian cancer, it helps maintain the body's production of IL-2. In prostate cancer, it reduces the rate of spread in those types of prostate cancer that can spread to the lungs.

Considerations for Use

PSK is available in tablet form. It should be used only under professional supervision. If your health-care provider is unable to find PSK locally, contact JHS Natural Products in Eugene, Oregon. (*See* Appendix B: Resources.)

PRICKLY ASH

Latin names: *Xanthoxylum americanum* and *Xanthoxylum bungeanum* (Rutaceae [citrus] family)
Other common names: angelica tree, xanthoxylum

General Description

Prickly ash is a shrub grown throughout China, especially in Szechuan province. The "Chinese" prickly ash is also found in the southeastern United States. The shiny red fruits are gathered in the late summer and fall for culinary and medicinal use.

Evidence of Benefit

The bark of the prickly ash tree is a tonic and circulatory stimulant. It stimulates the lymphatic system and encourages immune function. Prickly ash has antimicrobial and pain-relieving properties. It has a relaxing effect on the upper digestive tract and could be helpful for cramping, stomach upset, and vomiting.

Benefits of prickly ash for specific health conditions include the following:

• *Circulatory disorders and gallstones.* Prickly ash increases pain-free walking distance, and relieves coldness in the feet and toes. People with sickle cell anemia, which causes circulation problems, who use prickly ash report that it reduces pain. Prickly ash also provides temporary relief from abdominal pain caused by a number of disorders, including ulcers, gallbladder disease, and intestinal spasms. Users of this herb may also see improvement in problems such as hemorrhoids and varicose veins with continued use. Prickly ash also may be helpful in healing other injuries involving swelling or wounds that are slow to heal.

• *Parasitic infection.* The chemical constituents of prickly ash that give it its heat also kill foodborne bacteria and parasites in cell studies. Prickly ash is especially effective against roundworms. Prickly ash in sesame oil arrests pain from roundworms within thirty minutes, although it is not effective in long-standing cases. Powdered prickly ash enemas have been used to treat pinworms in children, and powdered prickly ash in capsules has been used for schistosomiasis, a waterborne infection common in tropical areas, because it increases appetite and lessens tissue destruction. Prickly ash extracts have also been used externally to treat scabies, a parasitic skin condition.

Considerations for Use

Prickly ash can be used as a tea or a plaster, or as an enema.

Oral consumption of prickly ash should be avoided during pregnancy. It may stimulate immune processes in the mother that may be detrimental to the developing child. Do not use in a child without first asking a pediatrician.

PRUNELLA

Latin name: *Prunella vulgaris* (Lamiaceae [mint] family)
Other common names: all-heal, brunella, carpenter's weed, heal-all, heart of the earth, self-heal, sicklewort, xia ku cao

General Description

Prunella is a creeping perennial in the mint family. Native to Asia and Europe, prunella grows in meadows and along roadsides, thriving in sunny areas. When imported to North America and Australia, it quickly became naturalized. The plant bears pointed oval leaves and blue or pink flowers. The aerial (aboveground) parts of the plant are harvested in summer, when the plant is in bloom.

Evidence of Benefit

Prunella is an herbal antiviral agent. It aids in the healing of wounds and bruises, and helps to reduce scarring. Prunella's gentle astringency helps to decrease bleeding. It also reduces lymphatic congestion and eases irritated eyes, mouth, throat, swollen glands, and inflammation. It has been used as a remedy for diarrhea, hemorrhage, and gynecological disorders.

Traditional Chinese medicine (TCM) considers prunella a liver and gallbladder stimulant, and uses it to treat symptoms associated with an unbalanced liver, such as hypertension and conjunctivitis.

Benefits of prunella for specific health conditions include the following:

• *Herpesvirus infection.* A study of 472 Chinese medicinal plants found that prunella was among the ten most effective in the treatment of herpes simplex. Researchers believe that prunella works in two ways: by stopping the virus from growing within cells and by preventing it from binding to cells. It works differently from other antiviral drugs such as acyclovir, so it is possible the two could work together for synergistic effect. In seventy-eight cases of herpetic keratitis, an eye problem caused by herpesviruses, thirty-eight patients treated with prunella eyedrops were cured and thirty-seven improved. Only three did not benefit from the herb.

• *HIV/AIDS.* A study of 204 Japanese medicinal plants found that prunella made one of the strongest showings in terms of anti-HIV properties. At a dosage of 16 micrograms per milliliter, prunella extracts completely eradicated HIV under laboratory conditions in cells. Canadian scientists have confirmed that prunella extracts block cell-to-cell transmission of the virus and interfere with the virus's ability to bind with T cells, immune cells that are destroyed by HIV infection. Scientists at the University of California–Davis have identified the complex sugar in the herb that accounts for its actions against HIV. No human data yet support the use of prunella for patients with HIV, however.

Considerations for Use

Prunella is best taken as a tea or as a gargle solution. Do not use this herb if you have diarrhea, nausea, stomachache, or vomiting. Prunella is easier to obtain from traditional TCM practitioners than in retail shops in most of the United States. However, it can be purchased online. This herb could potentially interfere with the actions of prescription blood-thinners such as clopidogrel (Plavix), dipyridamole (Persantine), heparin, and warfarin (Coumadin).

PSORALEA

Latin name: *Psoralea corylifolia* (Fabaceae [legume] family)
Other common names: babchi seeds, bu gu zhi, psoralea fruit, scurfy pea

General Description

Psoralea is a climbing bean found throughout China. Psoralea seeds, which are harvested in the fall when they have ripened, should be large, solid, and black. Unlike garden beans, psoralea seeds are pungent and bitter.

Evidence of Benefit

Psoralea is one of the main herbs in traditional Chinese and Japanese herbal medicine for the treatment of skin conditions. It has been used in the treatment of eczema and hair loss. In addition, in cell studies it acts against staph infections and may help stimulate the heart. The Chinese name of this herb, *bu gu zhi*, means "tonify bone resin." Psoralea is used to promote bone calcification, making it useful in combination with conventional therapies for osteoporosis and bone fractures. Psoralens, components in psoralea, are active principles for inducing pigmentation of the skin. They cause residual pigmentation when applied on hypopigmented skin, together with increased blood flow and melanin-producing activity in the affected area.

Benefits of psoralea for specific health conditions include the following:

• *Psoriasis.* Psoralea is a natural source of psoralens, a group of chemicals that includes the active ingredient of a conventional psoriasis medication called methoxsalen (8-MOP, Oxsoralen-Ultra). Psoralens make ultraviolet-light therapy for this disorder more effective.

• *Vitiligo.* Psoralea helps with vitiligo, a disorder in which patches of skin lose their pigmentation. In one study, forty-nine patients underwent six months of psoralea treatment. Of these patients, 14 percent were cured and another 19 percent regained pigmentation on at least two-thirds of the affected skin.

Considerations for Use

Psoralea is available in capsules under the names *psoralea seed capsule, scurfy pea,* and *bu gu zhi.* Psoralea is unusual in that it can sensitize the skin to both healing and harmful ultraviolet rays from the sun. Unless this herb is being used to treat a light-sensitive disorder, use sunscreen or avoid sun exposure when taking it. If mild stomach upset occurs when using psoralea, take a ginger tea. (*See* GINGER.)

You should not take psoralea with licorice root. In a few cases, local application may irritate the skin and cause blistering.

PSYLLIUM

Latin names: *Plantago afra, Plantago isaghula, Plantago ovata* (Plantaginaceae [plantain] family)
Other common names: blond psyllium husk, flea seed, Indian psyllium husk, ispaghula, plantago, plantain, sand plantain, spogel

General Description

Psyllium is a low-growing annual that has been cultivated for thousands of years in Asia, Europe, and North Africa. It was one of the first medicinal plants brought to the Americas from Europe. The plant grows in India, Afghanistan, Iran, Israel, Northern Africa, Spain, and the Canary Islands. Psyllium seeds are cultivated in Spain, central Europe, Israel, Russia, India, Pakistan, Japan, Cuba, and southern Brazil. Reaching a height of only sixteen inches (forty centimeters), psyllium bears narrow leaves and clusters of minute off-white flowers. Herbal medicine uses whole seeds and ground plantain seeds, gathered in summer and autumn when the seeds have ripened.

Evidence of Benefit

For centuries, traditional Chinese and ayurvedic physicians have used psyllium to treat diarrhea, constipation, hemorrhoids, and urinary problems. Psyllium is a source of soothing mucilages for the digestive tract. Folk medicine has used psyllium husk and seeds for internal inflammation of the mucous membranes in the urogenital tract, and for dysentery. Externally, psyllium is used for gout and rheumatism, and as an analgesic.

The psyllium mucins are laxative and antidiarrheal. Psyllium is known as one of the gentlest laxatives. It is a bulk-forming laxative that is safe for long-term use.

This herb can lower blood levels of glucose and cholesterol by keeping these substances from being absorbed through the intestines. The U.S. Food and Drug Administration (FDA) approved a health claim for foods and dietary supplements that soluable fiber from psyllium may reduce the risk of heart disease by lowering cholesterol when included as part of a low-fat diet. The German Commission E has approved the use of psyllium according to whether you are using seed husk, blond seed, or black seed. The husk and blond seeds are approved for use to ease bowel movements in cases of chronic constipation disorders when a loose stool is desirable, such as for pregnancy or hemorrhoids, or following rectal surgery. These parts of the psyllium plant also are approved as a secondary medication in the treatment of various kinds of diarrhea and in the treatment of irritable bowel disease (IBS). The black seeds are recommended for chronic constipation and IBS.

Benefits of psyllium for specific health conditions include the following:

• *Constipation, diarrhea, hemorrhoids, irritable bowel syndrome, and ulcerative colitis.* Psyllium is the main ingredient of dozens of over-the-counter (OTC) bulk-forming laxatives. This is because psyllium fibers can absorb many times their bulk in water to form a gelatinous mass and keep the feces hydrated and soft. The resulting bulk stimulates a reflex contraction of the walls of the bowel, followed by emptying. The retention of water by the fibers also stops diarrhea. Unlike stimulant laxatives, psyllium does not cause cramps and has been shown to be superior to docusate sodium in people with idiopathic constipation. In one study, more than 50 percent of patients with this ailment became symptom-free or improved using 15 to 30 grams a day of psyllium seeds. In another study, patients who took 3.26 grams of psyllium with Laxomucil (a dietary fiber supplement) twice daily after surgery to remove hemorrhoids had shorter hospital stays and less pain after a bowel movement compared to another group who took glycerin oil. In one study, bleeding episodes related to hemorrhoids were reduced by half (three down from six episodes over thirty days) when patients used psyllium. Other patients with IBS benefited from psyllium husk in that they had fewer bowel movements and felt better, compared to a control group. There were no differences between the groups in abdominal pain or bloating.

• *Heart disease and type 2 diabetes.* Patients with or at risk for heart disease may benefit from psyllium because it improves blood lipids. In one study, subjects with elevated total and low-density lipoprotein (LDL, or "bad") cholesterol who took 15 grams of psyllium and one-half of their regular statin drug (10 milligrams) experienced a greater reduction in LDL cholesterol than a group taking twice as much statin medication (20 milligrams). Other studies have found that using 5.1 grams of psyllium husk for twenty-six weeks lowers both total cholesterol by 5 percent and LDL cholesterol by 7 percent in people with elevated blood lipids but no organic heart disease. Psyllium was also shown to be useful for patients with type 2 diabetes who had both elevated blood lipids and glucose levels. Patients took between 10 and 15 grams of psyllium husk a day.

Considerations for Use

Psyllium is available as cereal, ground seeds, and powders. Patients who have a narrowing in the gastrointestinal tract, intestinal obstruction, or a threat of either of these conditions should not use psyllium. Also, those with fecal impaction, difficulty swallowing, or difficulty regulating blood sugar levels due to diabetes should consult with their physician before using psyllium. Side effects include distention, flatulence, loss of appetite, and allergic conditions such as sneezing and chest congestion. Psyllium contains substances that can evoke an asthma attack. Psyllium also can inhibit the action of pancreatic enzymes that break down fat, so those with pancreatic issues related to enzymes should avoid psyllium.

To avoid problems with the absorption of prescription drugs, do not use psyllium seed within one hour of taking such medications. Lithium should be taken at least two hours before or after you take psyllium. Avoid using psyllium with licorice and with laxatives, as there is an increased risk of low blood potassium levels. If you are using psyllium for diarrhea, and it lasts more than four days, consult your physician. Also, if you have diabetes, using large quantities of psyllium products may cause your absorbed-sugar levels to go down to the point that you may need to reduce your insulin dosage.

Psyllium tea is a milder alternative to psyllium powders, which should be avoided by people who have tendency to low blood sugar (due to psyllium's delaying action on the absorption of sugar from food) and by people who take oral medications several times a day.

Pregnant women should avoid psyllium and all laxatives, because they stimulate the lower pelvis. People with chronic constipation should seek the advice of a health-care professional. Do not use psyllium to treat ulcers or colitis without consulting your doctor.

When taking psyllium as a laxative, you must drink eight to ten glasses of water throughout the day to prevent blockage of the intestines. Others recommend ¾ cup of water for every 5 grams of psyllium. Start using this herb gradually, so the body can adjust to the increased level of fiber.

PYGEUM

Latin name: *Prunus africanum* (Rosaceae [rose] family)
Other common names: African plum tree, konde-konde, lemalan migambo, ligambo, mfila, natal tree, nuwehout, tenduet, twendet

General Description

Pygeum is an evergreen tree that grows to a height of 120 feet (35 meters). Native to tropical and subtropical Africa, it has oblong leaves, white flowers, and red berries. Wild pygeum trees are classified as environmentally threatened. Some effort is being made to grow pygeum on plantations, but not all herbal products companies are careful in choosing a sustainable supplier. The dried bark is the part used in herbal medicine.

Evidence of Benefit

Pygeum is an anti-inflammatory for the prostate gland. It also improves bladder function. It has a number of unproven uses, such as for fever, erectile dysfunction (ED), kidney disease, malaria, male baldness, prostatic adenoma, and stomach upset. Traditional African medicine has used it for treating chest pain, malaria, and fever.

Benefits of pygeum for specific health conditions include the following:

• *Benign prostate hypertrophy (BPH) and prostate cancer.* Pygeum has been shown in double-blind studies to help men with BPH by diminishing symptoms such as night-time urination, urinary frequency, and residual urine volume. After two months, nocturia (awakening at night to pass urine) was reduced by 19 percent, residual urine decreased by 24 percent, and the total amount of urine expelled at one time increased by 23 percent. Using 75 to 200 milligrams of pygeum a day improved overall symptoms in men with BPH. Pygeum extracts also lower the concentrations of luteinizing hormone (LH) and testosterone circulating through the bloodstream. It is possible that pygeum has 5 alpha-reductase inhibition properties, anti-inflammatory properties, and estrogenic effects. Pygeum may inhibit dihydrotestosterone (DHT)-induced prostate hyperplasia. This keeps swollen prostate tissue from absorbing DHT, which stimulates cell division and growth of prostate tissue. Pygeum extracts also prevent the action of prostaglandins, inflammatory agents produced by the immune system;

reduce levels of the hormone prolactin; and block cholesterol in the prostate.

Considerations for Use

Pygeum is available in capsule form, usually formulated with saw palmetto. (*See* SAW PALMETTO.) However, caution is advised, as adverse events may occur when pygeum is taken with 5 alpha-reductase medications or the herb saw palmetto. Ask your doctor before using pygeum with either of these. The usual recommended dose is 50 to 100 milligrams taken twice daily.

This herb should be used under the supervision of a health-care professional. Frequent monitoring of prostate health is essential during treatment of prostate disorders with pygeum or any other herb. Pygeum should not be used during pregnancy or breast-feeding. There are not sufficient data to warrant giving pygeum to children. In theory, pygeum may inhibit human prostatic 5 alpha-reductase. This could reduce PSA (prostate-specific antigen) levels in the blood, masking otherwise elevated levels. Pygeum may also interact with estrogen and other hormones as well as with herbs and supplements that have estrogen-like constituents.

QUERCETIN

General Description

Quercetin is a bioflavonoid, a type of plant pigment found in almost all herbs and plant foods. It is especially abundant in black tea, blue-green algae, broccoli, onions, buckwheat, red apples, and red wine.

Evidence of Benefit

Quercetin is an antioxidant that has been found to block destructive structural changes in cells, which helps to prevent abnormal cell growth. It also inhibits the synthesis of enzymes that can cause allergic reactions. It is an anti-inflammatory and inhibits the enzymes lipoxygenase and cyclooxygenase, resulting in a reduced number of inflammatory mediators such as leukotrienes and histamine, which results in less swelling, less pain, and stronger immune and cardiac systems. Quercetin has been shown in cell lines to have antiviral activity against HIV, herpes simplex, the polio virus, and the respiratory syncytial virus.

Benefits of quercetin for specific health conditions include the following:

• *Allergies, asthma, emphysema, and hives.* Quercetin quells allergic reactions by preventing the multiplication of cells that secrete histamine, a chemical that causes inflammation and swelling. Quercetin is unlike many other allergy medications in that it acts on the cells that produce histamine rather than on the nerves that stimulate those cells.

As a result, it does not cause drowsiness as common antihistamines do. Its antihistaminic action could increase the ability of the lungs to deal with dust and particle pollution, which in turn helps ease emphysema.

• *Atherosclerosis.* When a blood vessel is injured by disease or high blood pressure, specialized cleanup cells called macrophages accumulate at the site of the injury. Macrophages contain large amounts of cholesterol, which can accumulate and eventually form *foam cells,* which can harden into plaques. Quercetin slows a series of chemical reactions that cause large numbers of macrophages to cluster on artery walls, reducing the risk of plaque formation. Although this has been shown in cell lines and animal studies, there are few human studies to support a role for quercetin in heart disease. However, one study showed that quercetin lowers blood pressure in people with hypertension. After one month, patients who had stage 1 hypertension, according to the American Heart Association, and took 730 milligrams a day of quercetin, experienced a six-point drop in each blood pressure reading (systolic and diastolic).

• *Cancer.* Quercetin has considerable cell line data to support its role as an anticancer agent. However, few human studies exist to support its use. Quercetin is thought to fight cancer in several different ways, each assuring the rapid growth of cancer cells is stopped. Quercetin deactivates enzymes that trigger the multiplication of bladder, breast, colorectal, and ovarian cancer cells, especially those that are stimulated by estrogen. Quercetin binds to estrogen receptor sites more completely than the anti-estrogen drug tamoxifen (Nolvadex), which is often prescribed to prevent the recurrence of estrogen-sensitive breast cancers. By occupying estrogen receptor sites, quercetin keeps cancer-stimulating estrogen in the bloodstream from finding a way to act on cells. Quercetin also could be useful in preventing colon cancer because foods that contain quercetin or quercetin extracts bring the nutrient into direct contact with the cells lining the colon. Laboratory studies have found that quercetin from grapefruit and orange juice reduces the rate of growth of breast cancer cells by 50 percent. The extract also stops chemical processes that give ovarian cancer cells a growth advantage over healthy cells, and increases the tumor-killing capacity of the cancer drug cisplatin (Platinol), while reducing its side effects.

Quercetin plays a special role in the supplemental treatment of multidrug resistance. Cancer cells eventually become resistant to chemotherapy drugs. Quercetin may counteract the chemical processes that lead to resistance, forcing cancer cells to remain responsive to many of the chemotherapy drugs, especially doxorubicin (Adriamycin, Rubex), used for breast cancer, and cyclophosphamide (Cytoxan), used for colon cancer. However, there are no clinical studies that have shown the combination of quercetin and such chemotherapy drugs to be effective.

• *Canker sores.* Quercetin may be effective in the treatment of canker sores. It relieves pain and increases the number of ulcer-free days. Some canker-sore sufferers report similar benefits from quercetin.

• *Cataracts, diabetic retinopathy, and macular degeneration.* Diseases that disturb the circulation of blood in the microscopic capillaries serving the back of the eye can result in retinopathy and macular degeneration, disorders that lead to the loss of sight. In both diabetic retinopathy and macular degeneration, capillaries fail and retina cells die. Quercetin does not correct the blood-vessel defects that cause these disorders, but it does protect the cells of the retina and the eye's lens from the effects of low oxygen levels and neurological toxins. Although this has been shown in cell lines, there are no human studies available.

• *Eczema and wrinkles.* Quercetin eases inflammation of the skin. It increases the production of collagen, a protein that is a major constituent of skin and connective tissue, and of fibronectin, which is responsible for knitting skin cells together into a continuous cover. Russian and Ukrainian studies have found that quercetin helps repair damage to nerve tissues underlying the skin in various kinds of skin wounds. A study conducted at the National Institute of Public Health in the Netherlands concluded that quercetin protects the ability of the skin to block out noxious chemicals after damage by sunburn or exposure to ultraviolet (UV) rays. It has also been shown to inhibit the signs of aging by preventing the breakdown of the collagen matrix in connective tissue, which leads to wrinkles.

• *Prostatitis.* Prostatitis is inflammation and infection of the prostate gland that causes chronic pain and difficulty with urination. Conventional treatment for this condition is often unsatisfactory. A one-month double-blind controlled trial of thirty men with chronic pelvic pain found that taking quercetin at a dose of 500 milligrams twice daily was helpful. In another study of patients with prostatitis, 67 percent of those who took quercetin showed an improvement, compared to only 20 percent of the participants in the placebo group.

Considerations for Use

Quercetin comes in tablet form and now is found in functional foods and beverages for increasing athletic performance. One problem with the supplements is that they are not well absorbed by the body. A special form called *quercetin chaconne* appears to be better absorbed. Many experts recommend taking quercetin with bromelain, which increases the absorption of quercetin and many other medications. (*See* BROMELAIN.) Many naturopathic physicians recommend taking both quercetin and bromelain with vitamin C.

Quercetin interacts with many prescription medications, usually by prolonging the time they remain in circulation in the blood. While this effect is frequently ben-

eficial, it can increase the risk of side effects. Note that these side effects come *from the medication* rather than from quercetin itself. However, because of this interaction, it is important not to take quercetin with certain drugs, including cyclosporine (Neoral, Sandimmune) or nifedipine (Adalat, Procardia). It is also important not to combine quercetin with quinolone antibiotics such as ciprofloxacin (Cipro), levofloxacin (Levaquin), norfloxacin (Noroxin), ofloxacin (Floxin), or trovafloxacin (Trovan), since it may interfere with the action of this class of antibiotic.

RASPBERRY LEAF

Latin name: *Rubus idaeus* (Rosaceae [rose] family)
Other common name: red raspberry

General Description

The raspberry is a deciduous shrub that grows as high as six feet (two meters). It has woody stems with thorns, pale green leaves, white flowers, and edible red berries. The leaves are the part of the plant used in herbal medicine. They are a source of vitamin C and contain lesser amounts of manganese, iron, and niacin. The plant is indigenous to Europe and Asia and is cultivated in temperate climates.

Evidence of Benefit

Raspberry leaf has been used in folk medicine for hundreds of years. It has astringent and stimulant properties and is a popular remedy for many ailments. The most common use of raspberry leaves is as a uterine tonic. It has the ability to relax tight uterine muscles and tighten relaxed uterine muscles. This has led to its use as a stimulant at the beginning of labor to make labor easier. Raspberry leaf also has been used for disorders of the gastrointestinal tract, the respiratory tract, the cardiovascular system, the mouth and throat, and for skin rashes and inflammation. It also has been used for influenza, fever, menstrual problems, diabetes, vitamin deficiencies, as a diuretic, and to purify the skin and blood. However, raspberry leaf is on the German Commission E unapproved list because these purported uses have not been documented.

Benefits of raspberry leaf for specific health conditions include the following:

• *Burns.* Raspberry leaf contains tannins, which may stop burns from oozing. The tannins cause proteins in healing skin to cross-link and form an impermeable barrier. However, human data are lacking for the use of raspberry leaf to treat burns.

• *Diarrhea.* The tannins in raspberry leaf prevent the flow of fluids into the intestines, which makes the stool more solid. Used as a tea, in doses of one to two cups, raspberry leaf helps to relieve diarrhea without stimulating contractions.

• *Premenstrual syndrome (PMS).* Raspberry leaf contains tannins and flavonoids, which help the uterus relax to relieve menstrual cramps. At the same time as it relaxes the uterus itself, it stimulates the muscles that support the uterus. This may allow easier menstrual flow.

• *Sore throat.* Its astringent properties justify using raspberry leaf tea as a mouthwash and gargle for mouth or throat inflammation.

Considerations for Use

Raspberry leaf is used as a tea. It is available as a bottled beverage in many health food stores. (Do not confuse raspberry *leaf* teas with sweetened, raspberry-flavored drinks.) Raspberry leaf can produce a more consistent rhythm of uterine contractions during labor; it has been used by women in late stages of pregnancy. However, it should not be used by pregnant women because there are not enough sound scientific and safety data. It should not be used during breast-feeding. Raspberry leaf may produce changes in blood pressure (both high and low), and if used chronically may be carcinogenic due to its high tannin content.

RED WINE CATECHINS

Latin names: *Vitis vinifera, Vitis labrusca* (Vitaceae [grape] family)
Other common name: resveratrol

General Description

Red wine catechins are extracted from the skin of red wine grapes. The most active red wine catechin is resveratrol, a compound the grape plant manufactures in the skin of the fruit to deter gray mold. Although red wine catechins are found in purple grape juice and red wine, resveratrol is most abundant in immature grapes (which are more susceptible to mold) and in grapes grown in damp climates, especially on Long Island in New York.

Evidence of Benefit

Resveratrol has been studied extensively in cancer cells of leukemia, oral squamous carcinoma cells, neuroblastoma cells, and skin, breast, and prostate cancer cells. Because resveratrol is an anti-inflammatory compound, it may be effective for preventing cancer in the three stages of cancer development. It has been shown to slow the development of atherosclerotic plaques and to protect the heart.

Benefits of red wine catechins for specific health conditions include the following:

• *Bladder cancer, breast cancer, leukemia, and prostate cancer.* Scientists at the University of Illinois at Chicago reported in the prestigious journal *Science* that resveratrol stops not one but three major stages of cancer development. It stops cancer initiation, the stage in which the antioxidant defenses of the body are overwhelmed by cancer-causing chemicals. It stops cancer promotion, the stage in which

the tumor secretes inflammatory chemicals essential for it to establish its own nutrient supplies and spread via the bloodstream. And in leukemia, it promotes differentiation, a process by which the unrestrained multiplication of cancer cells is stopped and white blood cells are returned to their normal life cycle.

Since this announcement, more than 1,300 scientific studies have attributed other cancer-fighting effects to resveratrol. Scientists at the Chungang University in Seoul, Korea, found that it deactivates some forms of the liver enzyme p450. This enzyme is necessary to transform many chemicals into a carcinogenic form. This enzyme system is related to hormone-sensitive cancers such as estrogen receptor–positive breast cancer and prostate cancer. As such, resveratrol should be avoided because it may stimulate the proliferation of tumor cells. However, others have found that resveratrol reduces cell migration and invasion in breast cancer cells. It is clear that more work is needed before it can be recommended for patients with, or at risk, for breast cancer.

Scientists at National Taiwan University discovered that resveratrol acts as an anti-inflammatory agent to lessen the inflamed tissues surrounding a tumor and is essential for leukemia viruses to activate leukemia. Resveratrol inhibits cyclooxygenase (COX) activity by releasing cytokines from macarophages in people with chronic obstructive pulmonary disease (COPD). And a research team at the New York Medical College observed that resveratrol triggered apoptosis, or "cellular suicide," in prostate cancer cells. Men who drink a glass of red wine a day may cut their chances of prostate cancer in half. Men who drink four or more 4-ounce glasses of wine per week have a 60 percent lower incidence of more aggressive types of prostate cancer. Resveratrol also has been shown to inhibit the enzymes CYP1A1, CYP1A2, and CYP1B1 in tumor cells. This may be one of the mechanisms by which resveratrol affects cancer cells.

• *Coronary artery disease (CAD).* Resveratrol has been shown to slow the development of atherosclerotic plaques, thus reducing the risk of CAD. Recently, resveratrol has been shown to inhibit the oxidation of human low-density lipoprotein (LDL, or "bad") cholesterol. Another study has shown that resveratrol, as well as some flavonoids, inhibits platelet aggregation, thus helping to forestall the formation of clots in the blood vessels.

Considerations for Use

Resveratrol is usually taken in tablet form. Unless dietary restrictions prohibit the consumption of sugar, drinking 12 to 14 fluid ounces (450 to 500 milliliters) of purple grape juice or one glass of red wine daily will have similar benefits.

Some studies have reported that the flavonoids in red wine can be absorbed from the intestine more efficiently than those in red grape juice. However, other research has found that there is no significant difference in the levels of catechins between alcoholic and nonalcoholic red wine. In fact, concentrations of catechins in plasma dropped more swiftly if alcohol was consumed. Resveratrol should be avoided by those with hormone-sensitive cancers because this compound activates estrogen and androgen receptors, which leads to stimulation of cancer cells that are hormone sensitive. Resveratrol should not be used in conjunction with antiplatelet drugs.

REISHI

Latin name: *Ganoderma lucidum* (Basidiomycetes [button mushroom] family)
Other common names: ling chi, ling zhi, mushroom of immortality

General Description

In Japan, reishi is known as the "phantom mushroom" because of the difficulty in finding it. Although over 99 percent of all wild reishi mushrooms are found growing on old Japanese plum trees, fewer than ten mushrooms will be found on 100,000 trees. The art of growing reishi indoors was perfected by Shigeaki Mori, who developed an elaborate, two-year-long method of culturing wild reishi spores on plum-tree sawdust. The fruiting body (cap and stem) of the mushroom is employed medicinally.

Reishi grows in six different colors, but the red variety is the most commonly used. It is now cultivated commercially in North America, China, Taiwan, Japan, and Korea. In China, it is known as ling zhi.

Evidence of Benefit

Reishi has been used in traditional Chinese medicine (TCM) for at least 2,000 years and is regarded as the "elixir of life." It still ranks as one of the premier Chinese tonics and has been reported to boost energy, help the body resist disease and stress, and promote longevity.

Contemporary Western herbalists regard reishi as an adaptogen and recommend it as an immune stimulant that activates several different phases of immune defense. It is used to treat allergies and altitude sickness, and it is effective against leukemia cells in cell line studies. It has also shown an ability to fight age-related symptoms such as memory problems.

Benefits of reishi for specific health conditions include the following:

• *Alcoholism and cirrhosis of the liver.* Reishi, when fed to rats, helps protect liver cells from damage induced by carbon tetrachloride poisoning. It may be beneficial for people in earlier stages of alcoholic liver disease who have not yet experienced severe loss of liver function.

• *Bronchitis.* Reishi stimulates the maturation of immune cells known as macrophages, which engulf and digest infectious bacteria. This may prevent secondary infections from developing into cases of chronic bronchitis.

• *Cancer.* Reishi may be a useful agent to fight cancer. The most important components of reishi are its triterpenes and polysaccharides, which inhibit tumor invasion by limiting metastases. Reishi can increase plasma antioxidant capacity and enhance immune response in advanced-stage cancer patients. In one study, patients with advanced cancer in different tissues who took 1,800 milligrams of oral Ganopoly (an extract of reishi) three times a day experienced an increase in T cells and of natural killer (NK) cells. Reishi may counteract the suppression of red and white blood cells that can result from cyclophosphamide (Cytoxan, Neosar) treatment by stimulating the creation of protein in the bone marrow. However, more work is needed to determine whether reishi should be used for patients with cancer.

• *High blood pressure.* There is evidence that reishi can lower both blood pressure and blood cholesterol levels. Scientists at Oklahoma's Oral Roberts University found that compounds in reishi reduce the flow of nerve impulses through the sympathetic nervous system, the portion of the nervous system activated by emotional stress. Russian scientists screening mushrooms as potential cholesterol-lowering drugs have found that reishi extracts stop the accumulation of cholesterol in the arteries of laboratory animals. Two controlled clinical studies have investigated the effects of reishi on high blood pressure in humans. Both found it could lower pressure significantly as compared with a placebo. The subjects with high blood pressure in the second study had not previously responded to medications.

• *Stress.* Eastern physicians have recognized for centuries that reishi can reduce emotional outbursts during long-term stress. Exactly how reishi does this has not been studied, but it is likely due to the herb's effects on the central nervous system. Additionally, doctors at the Hijitaki Clinic in Tokyo have found that reishi helped to decrease physical pain dramatically in two people with neuralgia and two other people with shingles (herpes zoster).

Considerations for Use

Reishi is probably the most widely available medicinal mushroom in the world. It is available not only as a foodstuff, but also in teas, syrups, tablets, and tinctures. Do not use *raw* pulverized reishi. It is best to boil the mushrooms to kill any bacteria that may have been growing on them while they were being cultivated.

Although side effects of reishi are extremely rare, they are not unknown. High doses are potentially toxic. Three to six months of *continuous* use may result in dryness of the mouth, throat, and nasal passages; chronic itch; stomach upset; or nosebleed. These complications occur so seldom that their exact causes are not known, but they may be manifestations of an allergy to the mushroom.

Reishi should be avoided by people who have known allergies to other mushrooms or molds. It should not be used continuously for more than three months at a time. If you take reishi on an ongoing basis, you should take a one-month break every three months, and then resume. If you are taking blood-thinning medications such as heparin or warfarin (Coumadin), you should use reishi only under a doctor's supervision. Do not use reishi with immunosuppressant drugs, antihypertensives, or chemotherapy.

ROOIBOS

Latin name: *Aspalathus linearis* (Fabaceae [legume] family)
Other common names: rooibos tea (English), rotbusch

General Description

Rooibos tea is made from the leaves of the rooibostee, a shrub of 6 feet (1.5 to 2 meters) in height with bright green needle-shaped leaves. It is native to the mountains near Capetown, South Africa. Traditionally, its stems and leaves are bruised with hammers, then left to ferment in the sun. The resulting tea has a characteristic sweet flavor. South Africans have drunk rooibos tea for at least 300 years, and it became widely used in South Africa during World War II, when black tea was unavailable. It is one of the few indigenous plants that have become an important commercial crop. Rooibos tea should be not be confused with honeybush tea.

Rooibos contains at least thirty-seven natural antioxidants, minerals, zinc, and alpha-hydroxy acids. It does not contain caffeine, and it has a very low tannin content.

Evidence of Benefit

Rooibos is an antiviral, antianxiety, and antiallergy agent. Rooibos is used in the treatment of syphilis to stop generalized inflammation and pain, although it is not a treatment for the disease itself. It has a beneficial effect on age-related mental decline. Rooibos is also used as a milk substitute for infants who are prone to colic.

This herb is considered to have considerable antispasmodic activity. There is growing evidence that it contributes to a reduction in heart disease and other ailments associated with aging.

Benefits of rooibos for specific health conditions include the following:

- *HIV/AIDS.* Two Japanese studies have shown that rooibos has activity against HIV. Compounds called complex polysaccharides, found in rooibos, prevent HIV from binding to its target cells. However, in this case, the polysaccharide had to be chemically extracted from the leaves and is not found in tea made by steeping the leaves in water. There is no evidence that rooibos tea fights the HIV virus.

- *Insomnia.* Rooibos tea is a bedtime favorite among South African herbalists, consumers, and even physicians.

It is likely that rooibos helps to induce sleep both directly, by affecting the metabolism of acetylcholine in the brain and preventing excessive firing of the neurons that cause wakefulness, and indirectly, by blocking hormonal reactions that cause inflammation and pain.

Considerations for Use

Rooibos is available as a tea. Like black tea, it inhibits the absorption of iron from food, although rooibos has a lesser effect on iron absorption than does black tea. People with iron-deficiency conditions should avoid both beverages. In one study, rooibos leaves as a tea demonstrated estrogenic activity, so patients with hormone-sensitive cancers should use caution before using it. Some reports of liver toxicity have been reported, so speak to your doctor before using rooibos if you have hepatic issues. Rooibos may interfere with many chemotherapy drugs. There is no information available on the use of rooibos during pregnancy.

ROSEMARY

Latin name: *Rosmarinus officinalis* (Lamiaceae [mint] family)

General Description

Rosemary is an aromatic evergreen shrub that grows to a height of three feet (one meter). It bears thick, narrow, parallel green leaves and pale blue to blue-violet flowers. The leaves and the essential oil distilled from the leaves are used in herbal medicine. Rosemary is also used in food preparation as an antioxidant and preservative, particularly for meats, and in the preparation of liqueurs such as Benedictine and Danziger Goldwasser. It is indigenous to the Mediterranean region and Portugal, and is cultivated there as well as in Central Asia, India, Southeast Asia, South Africa, Australia, and the United States.

Evidence of Benefit

Rosemary is a potent antioxidant, antiseptic, and antispasmodic. In European folk medicine, it was used both internally and externally. Rosemary was ingested for digestive disorders, headaches, menstrual ailments, exhaustion, dizziness, and poor memory. Externally, it has been used for myalgia (muscle pain), neuralgia (nerve pain), and sciatica. There are homeopathic remedies for gastrointestinal disorders. The German Commission E has approved it for oral use for dyspeptic disorders and externally as a supportive therapy for rheumatic disease and circulatory problems. In addition, it has been used for dandruff, greasy scalp, and hair growth. More recently, it has been investigated as a cancer therapy.

Benefits of rosemary for specific health conditions include the following:

- *Alzheimer's disease, memory problems.* Rosemary has had a long history of use for enhancing memory. In one study, participants who received rosemary aromatherapy for three minutes showed decreases in alpha and beta power, which suggests increased alertness. They also had reduced anxiety and exhibited better performance on memory testing. Rosemary is suitable for patients with Alzheimer's disease because it is an antioxidant, anti-inflammatory, and cyclooxygenase-2 (COX-2) inhibitor. COX-2 inhibitors have been proposed for use as drugs for Alzheimer's disease. Rosemary contains natural compounds that inhibit COX-2 (apigenin, carvacrol, eugenol, etc.). It also has ferulic acid, which when fed to mice injected with beta-amyloid (the major constituent of brain plaque) had better cognition compared to a control group. Human studies, however, are lacking.

• *Cancer.* Research shows that rosemary has strong antioxidant effects. Several animal studies indicate that rosemary can prevent cancer-causing chemicals from binding to and causing mutations in cellular DNA. This was later reconfirmed in human cells. Rosemary has been shown to inhibit the carcinogen aflatoxin from binding to liver cells and to prevent benzopyrene from binding to bronchial cells. These results show that its potential protective abilities go beyond one carcinogen and one type of tissue. Other research has found that whole rosemary extract can stimulate liver enzymes that defuse carcinogens and reduce those enzymes that can enhance carcinogens. No human studies are available as this is a new area of research.

• *Circulatory problems, eczema, rheumatic disorders, and sore muscles.* In European folk medicine, rosemary baths were used to prevent bacterial infection complicating eczema. Rosemary baths also stimulate blood circulation to the skin. This action helps the body to circulate the immune cells that cause eczema away from the skin and to circulate antibodies and other immune cells that fight infection to the skin. Rosemary contains camphor, which increases the blood supply to the skin. Because of this property, using rosemary in the bath helps to reduce pain in rheumatic muscles and joints. Rosemary baths also help to improve disorders characterized by chronic circulatory weakness, such as low blood pressure, varicose veins, bruises, and sprains.

• *Indigestion and menstrual cramps.* Rosemary helps to relax muscles, including the muscles of the digestive tract and the uterus.

• *Irritable bowel syndrome (IBS).* Rosemary relieves intestinal cramps and spasms. It also eases bloated feelings and stops flatulence. The bitter substances in rosemary stimulate the release of bile, aiding the digestion of dietary fat and lowering cholesterol levels.

Considerations for Use

Rosemary is available as enteric-coated oil capsules, oils (which can be used for aromatherapy), and teas (which can be used as skin washes). Daily doses are 4 to 6 grams of the herb or 10 to 20 drops of the essential oil externally. However, smaller quantities are probably sufficient and safer (for example, 2 drops). Externally, the typical amount is 50 grams of the herb per one bath or 6 to 10 percent essential oil in a semisolid and liquid preparation. Continuous *medicinal* use of rosemary should be avoided by women who have heavy menstrual flow. Since this herb is a uterine stimulant, it should not be used medically during pregnancy. Rosemary leaves taken in large quantities have been used for the purpose of abortion and can result in deep coma, spasm, vomiting, gastroenteritis, uterine bleeding, kidney irritation, and death. The small amounts of rosemary used in cooking do not pose a risk of any side effects. You should *never* ingest the essential oil. It can irritate the stomach and intestines, and cause kidney damage.

SANGRE DE DRAGO

Latin name: *Croton lechleri* (Euphorbiaceae [spurge] family)
Other common names: drago, dragon's blood, sangue de drago

General Description

The sangre de drago tree grows thirty to one hundred feet (ten to thirty meters) high in the Amazon rain forest, sometimes reaching the canopy. When the trunk of the tree is cut or wounded, a resinous sap oozes out, as if the tree were bleeding. This explains the name; sangre de drago is Spanish for "blood of the dragon." The red resin, or "blood," of sangre de drago has been used for hundreds of years as a healing resource both by native peoples of the Amazon basin and by African and European immigrants to the Amazon.

Evidence of Benefit

Sangre de drago fights bacterial, fungal, and viral infections. Tinctures of the herb help to stop bleeding due to peptic ulcers. It is one of the most common traditional medicines in Latin America for adults and children. It has been used for coughs, flu, lung problems, diarrhea, herpes, and stomach ulcers. Topically it has been used for healing wounds, itching, insect bites, and sores.

Benefits of sangre de drago for specific health conditions include the following:

• *Cuts and scrapes, abrasions, eczema, and insect bites.* Sangre de drago resin is applied topically to broken skin and eczema. Within seconds of application, the resin dries to form a protective "second skin." This protective layer allows the underlying skin to regenerate itself without additional risk of abrasion or infection. Sangre de drago contains a latex resin containing an alkaloid called taspine that helps to speed wound healing. It also stops bleeding. Sangre de drago has been confirmed in laboratory studies as an effective treatment for eczema. The crude resin stimulates the contraction of wounds. It also helps the formation of a crust at the wound site, helps skin to regenerate more rapidly, and assists in the formation of new collagen, the main protein found in skin. Some studies have found that the unprocessed herb is four times as effective in treating skin wounds as a chemical extract of the herb. One study found that a topical preparation of taspine increased healing activity and increased the strength of the top of the wound's barrier within five to seven days after application.

• *Diarrhea.* An active compound extracted from sangre de drago, identified as SP-303, has been shown to be beneficial for stopping diarrhea. It acts by inhibiting excess water flow into the intestines. In one study, patients with diarrhea related to AIDS used 500 milligrams of SP-303 four times a day for four days, and there was a significant reduction in stool weight and frequency. In another study, travelers to Jamaica and Mexico who experienced diarrhea were successfully treated with SP-303 at doses ranging from 125 milligrams to 500 milligrams, taken four times a day. The diarrhea was cured 21 percent faster compared to a placebo group. This treatment also has been successfully used for children who develop diarrhea from rotavirus.

• *Vaginitis.* Traditional Peruvian medicine uses sangre de drago as an antiseptic vaginal douche. Bacteria and yeasts need to "root" in the lining of the vagina to take hold and create infection. Sangre de drago makes the lining of the vagina impervious to these microorganisms, which reduces infection. Traditionally, the herb also is used as a vaginal bath for fevers, pyorrhea, draining infections before childbirth, and hemorrhaging after childbirth. There are no modern-day studies to suggest that sangre de drago is effective for these kinds of ailments.

Considerations for Use

Sangre de drago is available in ointments and tinctures. Some importers sell pure liquid resin, which should be taken in doses of no more than 2 to 3 drops in a cup of warm water. Some people have reported that it causes a localized burning sensation upon topical application.

SARSAPARILLA

Latin names: *Smilax* species, especially *Smilax aristolochiae-folia, Smilax febrifuga, Smilax ornata, Smilax regelii* (Smilacaceae [smilax] family)

Other common names: brown sarsaparilla; Costa Rican sarsaparilla; Ecuadorian sarsaparilla; gray sarsaparilla; Guayaquil sarsaparilla (*S. febrifuga*); Honduras sarsaparilla (*S. regelii*); Jamaican sarsaparilla; Mexico sarsaparilla; red sarsaparilla (*S. ornata*); Vera Cruz sarsaparilla (*S. aristolochiaefolia*)

General Description

Sarsaparilla is a woody climbing vine found in rain forests around the world and also in temperate zones in Australia and China. Sarsaparilla has broad, oval-shaped leaves, tendrils, and green flowers. The fragrance of the root is considered pleasant, with a spicy sweet taste. The root is dug year-round and dried for use in herbal preparations.

Evidence of Benefit

Since the 1500s, sarsaparilla has been used throughout the world to treat syphilis and other sexually transmitted diseases. It has a reputation as a blood purifier and general tonic. Sarsaparilla is a sexual stimulant and wound healer. It is also used as a diuretic.

The natural steroidal glycosides found in sarsaparilla have made the herb popular with bodybuilders as an alternative to anabolic steroids for increasing muscle mass. Sarsaparilla also promotes good circulation, balances the glandular system, and stimulates the production of natural hormones. It has also been used for skin diseases, psoriasis, and rheumatic complaints. Homeopathic remedies are available for itching, skin rashes, rheumatism, and inflammation of the urinary organs. It has not been approved by the German Commission E because there is a lack of clinical efficacy documented. In addition, there are significant risks associated with its use, such as gastric irritation and temporary kidney impairment. The claims for rheumatism and gout for sarsaparilla have not been substantiated. However, other experts in herbal medicine disagree and believe that sarsaparilla is safe and does not cause gastric irritation.

Benefits of sarsaparilla for specific health conditions include the following:

• *Eczema and psoriasis.* Conventional medicine has recognized sarsaparilla's worth in treating skin conditions since the 1940s, when *The New England Journal of Medicine* published an article praising the usefulness of sarsaparilla in treating psoriasis. Although no research has been done to ascertain exactly how the herb works, there are numerous reports of its usefulness in treating eczema, psoriasis, and leprosy. Well-done clinical studies are lacking in these areas, however, and the German Commission E specifically states not to use sarsaparilla for psoriasis due to its side effects.

• *Urinary problems.* Historically, sarsaparilla has been used for kidney problems. There is some evidence that it may work as a diuretic, reduce the incidence of urinary tract infections (UTIs), and improve kidney function in patients with diabetic nephropathy. In a study of rats with kidney disease as a result of diabetes, those that received a substance from sarsaparilla called astilbin had improved urine flow.

Considerations for Use

Sarsaparilla is available in capsules and fluid extracts. *Tinctures* of sarsaparilla are ineffective since the active chemical constituents of the herb are soluble in water but not in alcohol. It is also available as a tea.

Large doses of the saponins in sarsaparilla may cause gastrointestinal irritation. If this occurs, you should reduce the dosage or stop taking it.

The German Commission E advises that prescription drugs taken simultaneously with sarsaparilla may be absorbed or excreted more rapidly than when they are taken by themselves. For example, sarsaparilla increases the rate at which the body absorbs digitalis compounds such as digoxin (Lanoxicaps, Lanoxin) and increases the rate at which the body excretes tranquilizers such as the benzodiazepines, a class of medications that includes chlordiazepoxide (Librium) and diazepam (Valium). In general, people who take any prescription drugs regularly should avoid sarsaparilla. Because sarsaparilla may stimulate the production of testosterone, men with prostate disorders should avoid it as well. This herb should not be used by women who are pregnant or nursing.

SAW PALMETTO

Latin name: *Serenoa repens* (Arecaceae [palm] family)
Other common names: American dwarf palm tree, cabbage palm, sabal, serenoa

General Description

Saw palmetto is a low-growing North American palm. It grows wild mainly as isolated plants in the coastal regions of the Carolinas, the Gulf Coast states, and California, and in saw palmetto thickets in Texas. The part of the plant used in medicine is the berry, which has a nutty vanilla-like flavor. The berry can be used partially dried, ripe fresh, and ripe dried.

Evidence of Benefit

Folk medicine has used saw palmetto for inflammation of the urinary tract, bladder, testicles, and mammary glands. It has also been used for bed-wetting, persistent cough, eczema, and improvement of the libido. Homeopathy remedies are used for urination problems and inflammation of the urinary tract. American physicians recognized the usefulness of saw palmetto in hormonal regulation as early as 1856. Doctors prescribed teas of whole dried palmetto berries for breast enlargement, muscle building, and prostate problems.

Saw palmetto has since gained widespread use by doctors and alternative health practitioners as a safe treatment for prostate disorders. In fact, the German Commission E has approved its use for urination problems associated with benign prostatic disease stage I and II. Stage I is characterized by an increase in the frequency of urination, nighttime urination, and weak urinary stream. Stage II is the beginning of decompensation of bladder function accompanied by formation of residual urine and urge to urinate. Saw palmetto also acts as an anti-inflammatory agent.

Benefits of saw palmetto for specific health conditions include the following:

• *Benign prostatic hypertrophy (BPH) and prostate cancer.* Herbalist Andrew Chevallier has called saw palmetto the "plant catheter" for its ability to strengthen the neck of the bladder and to reduce enlargement of the prostate, allowing for the free passage of urine. Saw palmetto's action in this regard has been demonstrated by research. In a double-blind study of thirty men, Italian investigators found that one month's treatment with saw palmetto extract increased urine flow 1,700 percent more than placebo. A study of 110 men by British researchers found that 320 milligrams of saw palmetto extract daily was five times more effective than placebo in improving bladder emptying. In addition, the men did not have as much difficulty, discomfort, or pain in urinating as they had before taking the herb, and reported that they did not have to get up at night to urinate as often. The value of saw palmetto in treating prostate enlargement is so widely recognized in Germany that over 90 percent of German men with prostate enlargement are treated with saw palmetto, often in combination with other herbs.

However, not all studies have shown saw palmetto to be effective in BPH. In one study where men took 160 milligrams of saw palmetto twice a day, there were not significant differences in maximum urinary flow rate, residual volume after voiding, and prostate size compared to placebo. In another study, an extract of saw palmetto, Permixon, did not consistently afford any greater benefit compared to a drug, tamsulosin, except there seemed to be improvement in the amount of "peak urinary flow" symptoms. Two large studies capturing the totality of the evidence also did not support saw palmetto for BPH. However, combining saw palmetto with other herbs seemed to offer benefit to men with chronic prostatitis when the herb was combined with urtica dioica, curcumin, and quercetin. Similarly, adding saw palmetto to vitamin E, cernitin, and beta sitosterol improved subjective symptoms but not objective measurement in patients with BPH. Subjects reported 242 percent improvement in daytime urinary frequency and 258 percent improvement in nighttime urination. In another study, pretreatment with saw palmetto reduced complications during and after surgery for transurethral resection of the prostate and open prostatectomy.

Saw palmetto eases prostate swelling by regulating hormones. If there is an excess of dihydrotestosterone, which stimulates the growth of new cells in the prostate, the prostate can thicken and squeeze the urethra, making urination difficult. Saw palmetto extracts reduce prostate enlargement by reducing the availability of dihydrotestosterone to prostate tissue. Deprived of its hormonal stimulus, cell division in prostate tissue slows. Although saw palmetto prevents the prostate from absorbing dihydrotestosterone, it does not reduce the body's production of testosterone, which would cause changes in sex drive and sexual performance. Saw palmetto extracts also reduce prostate enlargement by short-circuiting the pathways by which inflammation-causing hormones are produced. This action reduces swelling caused by the accumulation of fluid in prostate tissue. It may also account for the fact that saw palmetto extracts offer relief much sooner than their prescription alternatives.

Considerations for Use

Saw palmetto is available as a tablet or saw palmetto liposomes. For prostate conditions, it is often combined with pygeum. (See PYGEUM.) A few locally produced saw palmetto teas are still on the market today. These are *not* recommended for the indications listed here. Most commercial saw palmetto products, however, are made from concentrated extracts of the berries' naturally occurring fat-soluble steroids.

There is some disagreement among experts as to whether saw palmetto berries offer the same benefits as saw palmetto extract. The German Commission E states that the daily dose is 1 to 2 grams of saw palmetto berry, which is equal to 320 milligrams. Saw palmetto berries frequently cause diarrhea, and in rare cases saw palmetto extract can cause stomach upset. Whichever form of the herb is used, it may take four to six weeks to determine if the herb is helping.

Patients with hormone-dependent cancers should be cautious about taking saw palmetto and speak to their doctor first. Saw palmetto is both antiestrogenic and estrogenic, and antiandrogenic. It is not recommended during pregnancy and lactation due to its hormonal effects. Drug-interaction experts Joe and Teresa Graedon suggest that women who are pregnant or may become pregnant should not handle saw palmetto tablets, just as they should avoid contact with finasteride (a synthetic antiandrogen). Additionally, since saw palmetto berries have both estrogenic and antiestrogenic activity, the Graedons suggest that women taking birth control pills or hormone replacement therapy should also avoid saw palmetto products.

You should not use saw palmetto to treat urinary problems without first seeking medical evaluation. Similar symptoms can be caused by more serious conditions, such as prostate cancer, that require medical treatment. Men taking the drugs finasteride (Propecia, Proscar) should inform their doctors if they are also taking saw palmetto, as dosages may have to be adjusted. Saw palmetto should not be used in conjunction with blood-thinners such as warfarin (Coumadin), as there is an increased risk of bleeding. Saw palmetto binds iron, so patients taking supplemental iron should allow two hours between ingestion of saw palmetto and iron.

SCHISANDRA

Latin name: *Schisandra chinensis* (Schisandraceae [schisandra] family)
Other common names: Chinese mock-barberry, five flavor berry, fructus schisandra, gomishi, lemonwood, magnolia vine, omicha, schisandra fruit, wu-wei-zi

General Description

Schisandra is an aromatic woody vine native to northeastern China, Korea, Japan, and the eastern United States. Reaching a length of up to twenty-five feet (eight meters), it bears oval leaves, pink flowers, and spikes of red berries. The berries are dried for use in herbal medicine.

Evidence of Benefit

Schisandra is now a recognized adaptogen—a substance capable of increasing the body's resistance to disease and stress. Chinese medicine uses it for digestion issues such as intestinal inflammation, insomnia, urinary frequency, cough, chronic diarrhea, profuse sweating, and hepatitis. It is said to balance body functions, improve mental function, increase stamina and physical performance, and energize RNA and DNA molecules to rebuild cells. Some reports show that it may lower blood pressure and cholesterol levels, but schisandra is not typically used for these purposes.

Schisandra is also one of the most useful herbs from the herbal traditions of Asia for the treatment of liver diseases. Because it stimulates the central nervous system to maintain breathing, schisandra has been used as an antidote to morphine overdose. It also increases visual acuity and field of vision, as well as tactile sensitivity.

Benefits of schisandra for specific health conditions include the following:

- *Cancer.* Schisandra protects the heart muscle during cancer chemotherapy treatment with doxorubicin (Adriamycin, Rubex), but it does not interfere with doxorubicin's action on cancer cells. A subfraction (or bioactive chemical) of schisandra, gomisin A, was shown to have anticarcinogenic effects in rat livers. Some researchers have suggested that gomisin A has inhibitory effects on liver cancer in animals and may be useful for liver cancer in humans someday. In one study, women being treated with chemotherapy for ovarian cancer experienced improved immunity from a product that contained schisandra (AdMax).

- *Diseases of the liver and hepatitis.* Schisandra protects the liver from chemical damage, particularly damage from chemicals that have to be activated by the liver to become poisonous, such as carbon tetrachloride. Laboratory studies show that schisandra extracts increase the liver's ability to make the enzyme glutathione peroxidase, which deactivates several kinds of toxic free radicals that attack the outer membranes of liver cells. Glutathione peroxidase also helps offset damage done to the liver by chronic viral hepatitis and HIV/AIDS. Schisandra contains lignin compounds that lower high levels of serum glutamic pyruvic transaminase (SGPT) in the blood, which is an indication of hepatitis.

Schisandra's chemical constituent gomisin A blocks the production of the fatty acid arachidonic acid, which is a building block of inflammation-inducing leukotrienes. By blocking the production of arachidonic acid, gomisin A prevents liver inflammation and tissue destruction, and does so without severely compromising the immune system's capacity to respond to the underlying infection. Gomisin A also stimulates liver regeneration. Animal studies show that it stimulates the growth of healthy liver tissue by increasing the production of ornithine decarboxylase, an enzyme critical to protein synthesis in the early stages of tissue recovery. Gomisin A makes schisandra useful in hastening recovery from liver surgery.

• *Cardiomyopathy.* Schisandra has been shown to improve cardiac function when facing cardiomyopathy when used with digoxin. In one study, symptoms of the disease were lessened and there were no side effects when participants used digoxin plus schisandra in a product called Sheng Mei.

• *Insomnia, restless legs syndrome, stress, depression, fatigue, and excessive sweating.* Schizandrin, gamma-schizandrin, deoxyschizandrin, and schizandra are active compounds in schisandra that help to relieve emotional and physical depression and reverse depression of the central nervous system. Animal studies have found that schisandra increases sleeping time when used with the sleep-inducing drug phenobarbital. Schisandra also increases the effectiveness of benzodiazepine tranquilizers, such as chlordiazepoxide (Librium) and diazepam (Valium), allowing patients to take lower doses of these potentially addictive drugs. The herb can be used by itself to treat insomnia, dizziness, excessive sweating, headache, fatigue, and heart palpitations associated with emotional stress. In one study, athletes who took extracts of schisandra and bryonia alba experienced increased physical performance. Both mental and physical fatigue are reduced with schisandra.

• *Skin cancer.* A few animal studies have found that schisandra contains compounds that prevent the development of skin cancer after chemical injury. However, human data are lacking and it was not used historically for this condition.

Considerations for Use

Schisandra is available as capsules and tinctures, and in combination with other herbs, especially hoelen. (*See* HOELEN.) Practitioners of traditional Chinese medicine (TCM) dispense it for use as a tea.

Schisandra should not be used by people with epilepsy,

severe high blood pressure, or intracranial pressure. Some reports of heartburn, peptic ulcer, central nervous system depression, hives, loss of appetite, and stomach upset have been reported. Schisandra may increase the flow of bile. People who have gallstones or blockages of the bile ducts therefore should not use this herb. Schisandra also stimulates the uterus and induces labor, so it should be avoided during pregnancy. It also should not be used during lactation.

SCHIZONEPETA

Latin name: *Schizonepeta tenuifolia* (Lamiaceae [mint] family)
Other common names: Japanese catnip, Japanese mint, jing jie, tenuifolia

General Description

Schizonepeta is native to China and Japan, and is widely cultivated in the Far East. It is a pleasantly aromatic herb with highly dissected foliage and small, clustered lavender blooms that grow in spikes above the foliage. Schizonepeta belongs to the same family as catnip, but it is an annual with a sweet, pinelike aroma. The whole plant is used in herbal medicine.

Evidence of Benefit

Schizonepeta is the principal herb of traditional Japanese medicine for skin infections. The Chinese use the herb to treat symptoms of the common cold: chills, sore throat, and headaches. It may help to lower fever and has an antibacterial action.

Benefits of schizonepeta for specific health conditions include the following:

• *Boils and mastitis.* In laboratory studies, schizonepeta has been shown to heal skin infections by stimulating circulation within the skin and by inducing perspiration. It also has antimicrobial and antiviral effects in cell studies. It may promote healing of skin lesions and eruptions.

Considerations for Use

Schizonepeta is available as a cream from compounding pharmacies for external use. It is dispensed by traditional Chinese medicine (TCM) practitioners as a tea for internal use. You should not use schizonepeta creams on open sores.

SCUTELLARIA

Latin names: *Scutellaria baicalensis, Scutellaria lateriflora, Scutellaria barata,* and more than 350 other species (Lamiaceae [mint] family)
Other common names: baikal skullcap, ban zhi lian, barbat skullcap, blue pimpernel, Chinese scullcap, hoodwort, helmet flower, mad-dog, scute, skullcap, Virginian skullcap

General Description

Scutellaria is a perennial herb native both to the region of Lake Baikal in eastern Siberia and to northern China. It also is indigenous to North America and is cultivated in Europe. It thrives on open grasslands at elevations below 2,000 feet (650 meters) in the wild, and is cultivated both as a medicinal herb and as an ornamental plant. Scutellaria grows to a height of between one and four feet (30 to 120 centimeters), and bears lance-shaped leaves and purple flowers. The root is used medicinally.

Scutellaria has held a central place in Asian medicine for at least 2,000 years. When a tomb built in northwestern China in the second century was excavated, workers found ninety-two wooden tablets containing herbal formulas, many of which listed scutellaria.

Evidence of Benefit

Scutellaria kills bacteria and viruses, and also relieves allergies, asthma, anxiety, and atherosclerosis, and is used as a diuretic. It is used in traditional Chinese medicine (TCM) formulas for the treatment of HIV/AIDS. TCM practitioners also use it for fevers, colds, diphtheria, hepatitis, high blood pressure, and shingles. It is also used in cancer treatments.

Benefits of scutellaria for specific health conditions include the following:

• *Allergies, hay fever, and other respiratory ailments.* Scutellaria contains chemicals that may prevent histamine from provoking hay fever attacks, in a manner similar to that of the prescription drug cromolyn sodium (Intal, Nasalcrom). One of the compounds most prominent in scutellaria, baicalin, interferes with a complex set of hormonal reactions that constrict the bronchial tubes to cause asthma attacks. Equally important, laboratory studies show that scutellaria prevents DNA damage from dexamethasone (Decadron, Intensol), a prescription drug widely used to treat asthma.

Experimental data from China show that scutellaria root inhibits several pneumonia-causing fungi. Chinese physicians sometimes inject a mixture of scutellaria, goldthread, and amur cork tree extracts to treat pneumonia and other respiratory infections.

• *Anxiety, headache, and stress.* The pituitary gland, located at the base of the brain, responds to the perception of stress by releasing adrenocorticotropic hormone (ACTH). This is the hormone that starts the profound changes in body chemistry that make up the stress response. Scutellaria has been reported to stop the overproduction of ACTH in laboratory studies. In one study, scutellaria was shown to reduce anxiety, increase energy levels, and improve cognition.

• *Atherosclerosis, diabetes, heart attack, high blood pressure, and high cholesterol.* In laboratory studies, scutellaria lowers blood cholesterol levels in animals fed a high-fat diet, and stimulates the gallbladder to release bile. Bile flushes cholesterol out of the liver and into the intestines, where it may be excreted. The scutellaria compound baicalin inhibits the process of inflammation on the linings of arteries after injury by bacterial infection (commonly linked to atherosclerosis). This makes it less likely that inflammation will lead to a cascade of immune responses that result in the formation of atherosclerotic plaques. Scutellaria also dilates blood vessels and acts as a diuretic to lower blood pressure. However, there are no clinical studies on scutellaria for any of the conditions discussed here and historically it was not used for them.

• *Attention deficit hyperactivity disorder (ADHD).* A Chinese study looked at the use of a multiple-herb combination that contains scutellaria as an alternative to methylphenidate (Ritalin) treatment in what the Chinese label "minimal brain dysfunction in children," known in North America as attention deficit hyperactivity disorder (ADHD). This treatment was slightly less effective than methylphenidate, but children in the herbal treatment group showed fewer incidents of bed-wetting, plus gains of between four and ten points on intelligence tests.

• *Cancer.* One type of scutellaria, *S. barbata*, has been shown to contain flavonoids that possess anticancer activity. Cell line studies have shown that *S. barbata* exerts anticancer effects by causing the cancer cells to die prematurely, called apoptosis. This same herb also turns off manufacturing of a protein called Bcl-2 protein, which increases white cells' ability to get rid of cancer cells, that is needed by cancer cells to divide. In addition, it seemed to increase immune cell function to kill off cancer naturally. *S. baicalensis* has been shown to reduce prostaglandin E_2 synthesis production by the cancer cells, which reduces cell multiplication. Animal studies have shown that scutellaria exerts anticancer activity against cancers of the breast, liver, prostate, and pancreas. It was most effective in breast and prostate cell lines.

Russian clinics have had success in using scutellaria to increase the effectiveness of the chemotherapy agents 5-fluorouracil (5-FU) and cyclophosphamide (Cytoxan, Neosar) in people with lymphosarcoma. For many years, Chinese medicine has relied on scutellaria for the treatment of liver, lung, and colorectal tumors. Chinese physicians consider this herb to be particularly effective against the cancer-causing effects of fungal toxins, such as aflatoxin, that form in food. Additionally, baicalin reduces the risk of liver cancer caused by iron overload. (*See* IRON OVERLOAD in Part Two.)

• *Gonorrhea and infected nails.* Scutellaria interferes with the growth and reproduction of infectious *Staphylococcus aureus, Streptococcus pneumoniae, Pseudomonas aeruginosa, Corynebacterium diphtheriae* (which causes diphtheria), and *Neisseria meningitidis* (which causes gonorrhea). In one study, penicillin-resistant *Staphylococcus* infections remained sensitive to scutellaria. Tinctures of this herb may be effective against fungal infections of the skin and tongue, but no data exist to support its use for these conditions.

• *Hangover.* In animal studies, scutellaria prevented short-term memory loss due to alcohol intoxication. The herb prevents the inflammation of brain cells by histamine, released when blood-alcohol levels rise. It also protects the lecithin linings of cells in the liver, blood, and immune system.

• *Influenza, viral infection, and vomiting.* Scutellaria shuts down the replication process in influenza viruses A and B, as long as it is administered between eighteen and fifty-four hours before infection. Scutellaria acts against a number of other viruses as well. It does not stimulate the immune system, but instead acts against the viruses themselves. The herb also helps control vomiting, a common complication of viral infection.

• *Periodontal disease.* Laboratory tests have shown that extracts of scutellaria stimulate the growth of collagen in the gums. This action may help to reverse gingivitis. While laboratory tests in themselves do not prove that scutellaria is useful for treating periodontal disease, they do indicate that use of scutellaria formulas for other conditions may have the beneficial side effect of improving periodontal disease.

Considerations for Use

Scutellaria is available in a wide variety of forms. Brand names frequently refer to the herb as *skullcap*. This herb should not be confused with American skullcap (*S. lateriflora*). The two herbs are not interchangeable. Scutellaria, the Asian form of skullcap, may be harder to find, but should be obtainable in Chinese herb stores or via the Internet.

Cases of liver damage have been reported in association with excessive intake of scutellaria. It appears that some scutellaria products also contain germander, an herb known to cause liver damage. You should not use scutellaria if you have diarrhea.

SHEPHERD'S PURSE

Latin name: *Capsella bursa-pastoris* (Brassicaceae [cabbage or crucifer] family)
Other common names: blindweed, case-weed, cocowort, lady's purse, mother's heart, St. James' weed, shepherd's bag, witches' pouches

General Description

Shepherd's purse is a weed in the same plant family as broccoli, cabbage, and mustard. It is a biennial with an erect stem, a rosette of basal leaves, four-petaled white flowers, and heart-shaped seed pods. Its name derives from the appearance of the seed pods, which resemble small purses. All of the aerial (aboveground) parts of the plant are used fresh and dried in herbal medicine.

Before World War I, shepherd's purse was used in mainstream medical practice in Britain and the United States as a remedy for uterine bleeding. During that war, when many herbs became unavailable in Britain, shepherd's purse was used as a substitute for ergot and goldenseal, herbs more commonly used for stopping the flow of blood.

Evidence of Benefit

Shepherd's purse is considered by herbalists to be one of the best herbs for stopping bleeding of all kinds, both external and internal, from superficial cuts and scrapes to internal bleeding of the stomach, the lungs, and, especially, the kidneys and urinary tract. It is prescribed mostly for slowing or stopping excessive menstrual bleeding and other uterine problems. Homeopathic remedies exist for uterine and mucous membrane bleeding.

Studies have shown that shepherd's purse has anti-inflammatory, diuretic, and anti-ulcer properties. It both decreases and increases blood pressure in laboratory tests. Traditional Chinese medicine (TCM) uses shepherd's purse to "brighten vision." Shepherd's purse contains some potassium and vitamin C, nutrients critical to the maintenance of vascular health in the retina. The German Commission E has approved it for symptomatic treatment of mild bleeding such as nosebleeds, menstruation, and wounds and burns. It is also approved for premenstrual syndrome (PMS).

Benefits of shepherd's purse for specific health conditions include the following:

• *Menstrual problems and nosebleed.* Shepherd's purse stops bleeding by the action of a plant protein that acts in the body in the same way as the hormone oxytocin. Oxytocin stimulates the constriction of the smooth muscles that surround blood vessels, especially those in the uterus. Chemical analysis has determined that its effects on slowing and stopping bleeding may also have to do with an ability to accelerate blood coagulation. Studies have also found a uterine-contracting property in shepherd's purse. It also tones the uterus, which explains why women have long taken it after childbirth to help the womb return to normal size.

Considerations for Use

Shepherd's purse is used as tincture or tea, as well as in poultices. A typical dose is 10 to 15 grams of the herb or topically 3 to 5 grams per ¾ cup of water or tea. Shepherd's purse should not be used during pregnancy or breastfeeding. Possible side effects include enlarged pupils, neck swelling, trouble walking, and unusual drowsiness. The herb can also cause low blood pressure, respiratory paralysis, and underactive thyroid. Do not use it if you are taking digoxin, blood pressure–lowering drugs, beta blockers, or sedatives. People with heart or lung disease should use this herb with caution.

SHIITAKE

Latin name: *Lentinus edodes* (Basidiomycetes [button mushroom] family)
Other common names: forest mushroom, hua gu, Japanese mushroom, lentinula

General Description

Wild shiitake mushrooms are native to Japan, China, and other Asian countries, where they typically grow on fallen broadleaf trees. Shiitake is now widely cultivated throughout the world, including the United States. Used as a food for thousands of years in East Asia, shiitake has become popular in the United States as a tasty alternative to the blander mushroom varieties more commonly sold in supermarkets. The fruiting body—fresh and dried—is the part of the plant used medicinally.

According to herbal lore, around the year 200, the Japanese emperor Chuai was offered the shiitake by the Kyusuyu, an aboriginal people of Japan. Shiitake was used even earlier in China, where it was known as *hoang-mo.*

Shiitake is the basis of several extracts, including lentinan. Chemically, the sugars in lentinan form a part of DNA called nucleic acids and are thought to account for lentinan's healing properties. The extract is water-soluble and is not destroyed by exposure to heat, acids, or alkalis. Lentinan possesses immune-enhancing properties, is antiviral and antimicrobial, and has cholesterol-lowering effects.

Evidence of Benefit

Shiitake is good for preventing high blood pressure and heart disease, controlling cholesterol levels, building resistance to viruses and other causes of infections, and fighting diseases such as cancer.

Research indicates that lentinan extracted from shiitake may help some people with hepatitis. Case reports from Japan suggest that lentinan also may be helpful in treating people with HIV/AIDS. Lentinan is generally administered by injection and has been used as an agent to prolong the survival of people receiving conventional cancer therapy. It is an approved drug in Japan to prolong survival in patients with cancer who are undergoing conventional therapies. It is also used to prevent the increase in chromosomal damage induced by anticancer drugs.

Benefits of shiitake for specific health conditions include the following:

• *Cancer.* Japanese physicians have long used lentinan's immune-stimulating capabilities in cancer treatment. Lentinan does not attack cancer cells directly. Instead, it activates the immune system's lymphokine-activated killer (LAK) and natural killer (NK) cells to combat various types of cancers, including carcinoma, hepatoma, and sarcoma. Lentinan also counteracts the formation of prostaglandins that cause inflammation and keep the immune system's T cells from reaching maturity. In addition, specific to colon cancer cells, lentinan can suppress cytochrome 450 1A enzymes, which are known to metabolize pro-carcinogens to active forms and stop cancer cells from forming.

Japanese physicians have found that lentinan stimulates the capacity of specialized blood cells to produce immune-system chemicals, mainly interleukin-1 and tumor necrosis factor (TNF), that prevent the growth and spread of cancer. Lentinan may be useful when surgery is not feasible.

Stomach cancer is unusually difficult to treat because the early symptoms are often so vague that the cancer is usually quite advanced by the time it is detected. Japanese physicians have found that when surgery for advanced stomach cancer is feasible, treatment with a combination of lentinan and chemotherapy improves the quality of life. In one case, a patient whose stomach cancer had spread to the liver and lymph nodes was still alive five years after surgery. The tumors in his liver disappeared after seventeen months of combined treatment with lentinan and the chemotherapy preparation uracil plus ftorafur (UFT).

Japanese physicians also use lentinan to treat breast cancer in women who have had mastectomies without follow-up radiation therapy. When chemotherapy is used, lentinan may help prevent immune-system damage if given before treatment begins. In addition, Japanese studies in animals have shown that lentinan increases the effectiveness of cancer treatment with a specific type of interleukin-2 (IL-2). When used together, the two treatments help prevent the spread of breast cancers to the lung.

Even if cancer has spread to the lung, lentinan can increase survival time. In a group of sixteen people with advanced cancer, Japanese medical researchers injected lentinan directly into malignant areas. All of the patients eventually died, but the average survival time of patients who responded to the treatment was 129 days, compared with 49 days for those who did not respond to the treatment. In another study, patients with pancreatic cancer survived longer when taking 0.14 milligram of lentinan per gram of the shiitake plant. The patients experienced an increase in killer T lymphocytes and a decrease in interleukin-6 and prostaglandin E_2; these changes were thought to boost the immune system and fight the cancer.

On the other hand, patients with prostate cancer who took shiitake mushroom extract for six months had no improvement in prostate-specific antigen (PSA) level (it should have decreased by 50 percent). In fact, in half of the patients, the disease progressed.

• *Chronic fatigue syndrome* (CFS). Japanese physicians report that lentinan is useful for low natural killer cell syndrome (LNKS), a disease that causes disabling fatigue. This disease causes symptoms that are similar to those of

CFS as it is diagnosed in the West. Injected lentinan treatment dosage is 2 milligrams, or 5 milligrams daily taken orally, and has been successful in reversing symptoms, including remittent fever, persistent fatigue, and low NK cell activity.

• *High cholesterol.* Shiitake is beneficial in lowering levels of both total cholesterol and low-density lipoprotein (LDL, or "bad") cholesterol. In animal studies using eritadenine, a chemical found in shiitake, total cholesterol levels were reduced by 25 percent in one week. This effect was more pronounced in subjects who ate high-fat diets than in those on low-fat diets. In another study, subjects consumed ten dried medium-sized mushrooms a day and the reduction in total cholesterol levels ranged from 36 to 45 percent. In animals, shiitake seems to lower blood pressure as well.

• *HIV infection.* Lentin, the protein component of shiitake, has strong antifungal properties and suppresses HIV-1 reverse transcriptase, thereby slowing HIV replication. When administered intravenously to patients with HIV infection, there was a statistical increase in CD4 cells and other white blood counts. However, some side effects occurred, such as breathing difficulty and GI upset. In one study, another part of shiitake, LEM, a carbohydrate xylose-rich extract, was given to HIV patients. Patients used 6 to 9 grams of LEM daily for three to twenty-five months, and symptoms improved in every patient. It seems to work in part by preventing HIV from infiltrating the important immune cells, T lymphocytes.

Considerations for Use

Shiitake can be eaten in food. It is also available in tablets, syrups, and tinctures. People with bladder cancer should not use *raw* shiitake, as it contains a chemical known to cause this disease.

Shiitake has a good record of safety, but may cause temporary diarrhea and abdominal bloating when used in high dosages. Allergic reactions to shiitake are very rare, but when they do occur, they produce a characteristic whorl, similar to hives, on skin exposed to sunlight. There have been reports of patients with lung cancer experiencing decreased lung function from prolonged exposure to shiitake spores. Other reports of side effects include dermatitis, photosensitivity, and food allergy to the shiitake itself. Chronic use may increase eosinophil count, which is indicative of an allergic reaction.

The therapeutic actions of lentinan are highly dose-dependent. Given by injection twice a week, 1 milligram of lentinan is enough to have a therapeutic effect, while doses of more than 10 milligrams of lentinan per week can suppress the immune system. This type of lentinan therapy requires that the health-care provider pay careful attention to the individual's condition and circumstances. Lentinan is also available in powder form. (For sources of powdered lentinan, *see* Appendix B: Resources.)

SIBERIAN GINSENG

Latin name: *Eleutherococcus senticosus* (Araliaceae [ginseng] family)
Other common names: ci wu ju, devil's shrub, eleuthero, eleutherococcus, gum Benjamin siam, touch-me-not

General Description

As its name suggests, Siberian ginseng is a hardy shrub native to the southeastern part of Siberia, just north of China's Amur River. Siberian ginseng also grows in China, Japan, and Korea, and is well adapted to the Pacific Northwest of the United States and British Columbia. A deciduous plant, Siberian ginseng grows to a height of ten feet (three meters) and bears three- to seven-toothed leaflets on each stem. The dried root is used in herbal medicine. Siberian ginseng is in the same family as, but is not identical to, Korean, or red, ginseng. (*See* GINSENG.)

The use of Siberian ginseng dates back about 2,000 years. However, it was "rediscovered" in Siberia in 1855, mistaken for ginseng, and used with good results as a substitute for *Panax ginseng.* Thus, it was named Siberian ginseng.

Evidence of Benefit

Siberian ginseng is considered an adaptogen in that it normalizes body functions. It has been used as a tonic to invigorate and fortify the body against fatigue. It was often used during convalescence from disease to increase work capacity and concentration. Traditional Chinese medicine uses it for kidney pain, urine retention, erectile dysfunction (ED), sleep disturbances, loss of appetite, pain and hip weakness, rheumatoid arthritis, and boosting the immune system. It is an immune stimulant that is especially useful for preventing infection during times of intense physical activity and prolonged periods of stress. In addition, it is a versatile training aid for athletes. (*See* "Siberian Ginseng Goes to the Gym" on page 134.)

Siberian ginseng supports the body by helping the liver detoxify harmful toxins, including chemotherapeutic agents and products of radiation exposure. Preliminary studies in Russia have confirmed the use of the herb for people undergoing chemotherapy and radiation therapy for cancer, to help alleviate side effects, and to help bone marrow recover more quickly.

Benefits of Siberian ginseng for specific health conditions include the following:

• *Cancer and mumps.* Siberian ginseng was found to have a pronounced effect on T cells, mostly T-helper cells, but also cytotoxic and natural killer (NK) cells. It also reduces nitric oxide production, possibly by inhibiting NF-kappa B activity. Siberian ginseng extract was shown to inhibit reactive oxygen species production, which prevents oxygen particles from being released and damaging tissues. Siberian ginseng increases the production of interferon, an immune-system chemical. All of these factors make

Siberian ginseng appealing for further research in treating cancer.

• *Chronic fatigue syndrome (CFS) and viral infections.* Siberian ginseng has a proven ability to prevent upper respiratory infections. Russian studies involving tens of thousands of participants found that taking Siberian ginseng for eight to ten weeks *before* the beginning of the cold and flu season reduces the incidence of these diseases by more than 95 percent. This herb stimulates the activity of several immune-system components: B and T cells, which direct the immune response to infection; macrophages, "germ-eating" cells that attack bacteria; and interferons, which "interfere" with every stage of viral infection.

Research suggests that Siberian ginseng improves stamina. Patients with chronic fatigue who used this herb for six months reported less fatigue. Although the results did not differ from placebo, they were encouraging. The participants took four 500-milligram capsules per day for a total of 2.24 milligrams of eleutherosides, which are one of the active ingredients in Siberian ginseng.

Recent evidence suggests that Siberian ginseng may prove valuable in the long-term management of various diseases of the immune system, including HIV/AIDS, CFS, and autoimmune illnesses such as lupus.

• *Heart disease.* Siberian ginseng supplementation has been shown to reduce LDL-cholesterol ("bad" cholesterol) levels as well as improve the LDL/HDL ("bad"/"good") ratio in postmenopausal women after six months. Other studies have reported that Siberian ginseng is protective of the heart against free-radical damage, reducing platelet aggregation, and lowering blood pressure. These benefits are mainly attributable to the fraction, one of the compounds in the herb called eleutherococcus. In one study, individuals sixty-five years of age and older who had high blood pressure and felt run-down took 300 milligrams of Siberian ginseng (per day) or placebo for eight weeks. After four weeks, those assigned to the herb group had significantly better mental health and social functioning compared to the placebo group. At eight weeks, the groups' results were the same, however.

Considerations for Use

Siberian ginseng is available as eleuthero extracts, tablets, and teas. It is also available in bottled ginseng tonics, but you need to make sure that any such product actually contains *real* Siberian ginseng (*E. senticosus*), and not other herbs that may be falsely labeled as "ginseng."

Using Siberian ginseng may cause insomnia if you take it too close to bedtime, and it has been reported to cause mild, temporary diarrhea in a few users. It has also caused nervousness, tachycardia (fast heartbeat), headache, and low blood sugar. People who have myasthenia gravis, rheumatoid arthritis, or related diseases, such as lupus, psoriatic arthritis, and Sjögren's syndrome, should avoid Siberian ginseng. This herb stimulates the immune system to produce B cells, which in turn release tissue-destructive antibodies, aggravating these conditions. Since Siberian ginseng contains compounds that stimulate testosterone production, men who have prostate disorders should not use it. You should not use Siberian ginseng if you have uncontrolled high blood pressure. It can be used during pregnancy or nursing; however, pregnant or nursing women using this herb should avoid products that also contain *Panax ginseng*. Check with your doctor before taking it to make sure it is safe for you. One woman experienced a hemorrhage when using a product that contained Siberian ginseng with other herbs such as red clover for hot flashes. The problem corrected itself when she stopped using the product. Anyone who takes digoxin (Lanoxicaps, Lanoxin) should seek the advice of a health-care professional before taking Siberian ginseng. This herb-drug combination has been reported to cause dangerously high serum digoxin levels. Animal research has shown that Siberian ginseng can increase the sleep-inducing effects of barbiturates. Persons taking barbiturates for anxiety or insomnia may become more sedated than usual when taking Siberian ginseng.

SLIPPERY ELM

Latin name: *Ulmus rubra* (Ulmaceae [elm] family)
Other common names: Indian elm, moose elm, red elm, sweet elm

General Description

Slippery elm is a large deciduous tree that is native to North America and can now be found planted along streets and growing in forests from Quebec to Florida, from the Dakotas to Texas. It thrives on well-drained soils on high ground, and frequently reaches a height of sixty feet (twenty meters). The inner bark of the trunk and branches is collected in the spring for medicinal use. Slippery elm bark added to hot water has a slippery consistency, explaining its name.

English settlers in North America noticed its widespread use by Native Americans, who soaked the inner bark in water and applied it to wounds. The slippery elm bark would then dry into a natural bandage. Native Americans also wrapped slippery elm around pieces of meat to prevent spoilage. It was mixed with water to make a soothing gruel for children and for sick people of any age.

Evidence of Benefit

Slippery elm has a soothing and healing effect on any part of the body it comes into contact with. It is used in the treatment of sore throats, indigestion, digestive irritation, and stomach ulcers. It is able to neutralize excess acids in the stomach and intestines. It can also be used externally to heal wounds and burns, and can relieve irritated, inflamed, or itchy skin. The mucilage in slippery elm bark is an excellent remedy for irritation and inflammation of

Siberian Ginseng Goes to the Gym

Athletes around the world have adopted Siberian ginseng as a training aid. Athletes use it to increase performance, bolster the immune system against the demands made on it during exercise, reduce fatigue after workouts, and reduce the effects of stress.

The Russians were the first to use Siberian ginseng as a training aid. A Russian scientist named I. I. Brekhman conducted years of painstaking studies on dozens of native Russian plants, trying to find a replacement for red ginseng as a cold- and flu-fighter. Brekhman wanted an herb that would increase resistance to stress and normalize physical function, and do so without causing side effects. All of these qualities are present in Siberian ginseng, which Brekhman and his colleagues found to have an impressive range of benefits.

In time, the herb was investigated as a legal stimulant for the Soviet Union's international athletes. The Soviet (and later, Russian) Olympic team has publicly acknowledged its use of Siberian ginseng since the Munich Olympics of 1972, and the herb was credited by team nutrition and pharmacology adviser Sergei Portugalov for Russia's unexpected capture of eleven gold medals at the Lillehammer Winter Olympics in 1994. Chess players, cosmonauts, musicians, and high-level Russian military officers started using Siberian ginseng, while its use in athletics went global. Basketball player Charles Barkley, for instance, was reported to drink thirty bottles of Siberian ginseng tonic a week.

Unfortunately, scientific studies of Siberian ginseng's usefulness in athletic performance have yielded results that are difficult to interpret. For instance, in a study conducted at Old Dominion University in Virginia, athletes who were given Siberian ginseng had consistently higher maximum heart rates and higher rates of oxygen consumption than athletes who were given a placebo. Athletes taking the herb also did not become exhausted as quickly. Runners had higher concentrations of lactic acid in their muscles after their races, an indication of greater muscular activity. These complicated measurements could be conducted on only sixteen athletes, however, so the study failed to capture statistically significant differences in performance. Other studies have shown positive but not statistically significant benefits from Siberian ginseng.

If the effects of Siberian ginseng are not direct, could they be indirect? The answer seems to be that Siberian ginseng keeps athletes from getting sick and prevents them from becoming run-down through heavy training. It also speeds their return to physiological normalcy following strenuous workouts. Siberian ginseng can, when used over the long term, improve an athlete's overall training program, promote more consistent training, and quicken reflexes and lower race times.

Followers of competitive sports know that simple respiratory infections can dash the competitive hopes of even the most superbly trained athletes. Athletes are easy prey for germs. Intense or prolonged endurance exercise—sometimes even a single workout or race—causes large increases in hormones that can decrease the activity of the immune system, specifically the activity of T and natural killer (NK) cells. The NK cells form an important line of defense against infectious agents, especially against viruses and bacteria that attack the upper respiratory system. Data show that Siberian ginseng, when taken preventively, can reduce athletes' rates of infection by 35 percent. Siberian ginseng spurs the bone marrow and the immune system to greater activity. Some researchers believe that Siberian ginseng increases the synthesis of interferon, a powerful chemical that boosts immune-system activity. Other researchers believe that the herb stimulates the activity of germ-eating macrophages in cell studies. Unfortunately, the effectiveness of Siberian ginseng's infection-fighting components fades fairly quickly, so it must be taken continuously for best results.

Siberian ginseng also reduces fatigue after workouts. It reduces the "burn" after workouts, reducing muscle soreness without the side effects of aspirin and other painkillers. By raising the amount of energy available to the muscles very quickly, Siberian ginseng allows athletes to train consistently and to perform several hard workouts in a short time.

Finally, Siberian ginseng's stress-lowering effect is important to athletes because it moderates the production of cortisol. Overtrained athletes often have high levels of cortisol, which is a catabolic (protein-destroying) stress hormone. Siberian ginseng was shown in cell studies to deactivate cortisol before the hormone could cause tissue damage.

---

the reproductive and respiratory systems, as well as the urinary tract. It has been used for rheumatism, gout, and swollen glands. Different components of the herb act in different ways. The mucilage loosens up congestion such as in the lungs. Insoluble polysaccharides in the mucilage form a viscous material following oral ingestion or when used topically to reduce gastrointestinal transit time, acting as a bulk laxative, and absorbing toxins. Other components are thought to be antitumor and astringent. No human or animal studies have been conducted to support any of these wide-ranging claims, however. It appears to be safe for coughs and minor gastrointestinal complaints, but should not be used for cancer or bronchitis.

Benefits of slippery elm for specific health conditions include the following:

• *Cancer.* Slippery elm is included as part of an antineoplastic remedy called Essiac. From a survey of cancer patients, 16 percent said they had used Essiac, and most of them had gastrointestinal cancers. One-third thought they had benefited psychologically and physically. However, another study found that Essiac does not stop the progression of cancer, does not cure cancer, and is not palliative.

• *Crohn's disease, food poisoning, and irritable bowel syndrome (IBS).* Slippery elm bark may be used for irritation caused by colitis, chronic diarrhea, esophagitis, gastritis, and duodenal and peptic ulcers. The bark consists of an abundance of mucilage, composed of easily digested, nontoxic complex carbohydrates. This mucilage soothes inflammation and stops irritation of the mucous membranes lining the stomach and intestines. Some scientists believe that taking slippery elm by mouth induces a reflex reaction that causes the stomach to secrete more mucus. No clinical data exist to support this belief, however.

Considerations for Use

Slippery elm can be used as a tea, a powder mixed into cold water, or a poultice. Since slippery elm is also a food product, there is no upper limit on dosage, but taking 2 teaspoons dissolved in 1 cup of water is the minimum amount that works, and 5 teaspoons is the maximum that will dissolve in 1 cup of water.

Slippery elm is regarded as safe. However, because of the high mucilage content, it may interfere with the absorption of medications taken at the same time. Contact dermatitis has been reported with topical use. Slippery elm should not be used during pregnancy, as spontaneous abortions have occurred. No data exist on its safety during lactation, so it should be avoided. Slippery elm blocks the absorption of iron, so if you are taking iron supplements, you should separate the two compounds by one to two hours.

SNOW FUNGUS

Latin name: *Tremella fuciformis* (Basidiomycetes [button mushroom] family)

Other common names: bai mu erh, shirokikurage, silver tree-ear fungus, white jelly-leaf, white muer, white tree-ear, wood ear fungus

General Description

Snow fungus is a white, nearly translucent, "trembling" fungus that grows on a great variety of trees throughout Asia and in warmer climates worldwide. The fungus gets the common name of *wood ear* for the way it looks on the decaying logs on which it grows. Good-quality snow fungus has a pale, yellowish-white color and a mucilagelike texture. Chinese and Japanese herbalists have used snow fungus for more than 2,000 years, primarily to increase fluids in the body, for dry coughs, and for palpitations. It has been used as a tonic herb and as a beauty enhancer to improve the complexion.

Evidence of Benefit

Snow fungus is an immune stimulant that may help fight infection as seen in cell studies. Laboratory studies have found that it also demonstrates antitumor activity, lowers levels of low-density lipoprotein (LDL, or "bad") cholesterol, protects the liver, and fights inflammation, and that it may slow the aging process. Supposedly, if snow fungus is eaten regularly, facial freckles will disappear, although this has not been tested in any scientific fashion.

Benefits of snow fungus for specific health conditions include the following:

• *Atherosclerosis and high cholesterol.* In Japan, snow fungus is used to prevent atherosclerosis, in which cholesterol gathers into plaques within the arteries. It does this by lowering total blood cholesterol levels. To date, however, only one preliminary clinical study has confirmed the value of snow fungus for this purpose. However, research on snow fungus polysaccharides as infection-fighters has confirmed that they help maintain cholesterol levels within the linings of cells, where cholesterol is needed, possibly helping to draw it out of the bloodstream.

• *Cancer.* Scientific studies in cells and animals have found that the mucilage-like polysaccharides found in snow fungus fit like keys into receptor sites on certain immune cells. This increases the production of interferon and interleukin-2 (IL-2), two important immune-system chemicals, and stimulates the production of germ-eating macrophages. Snow fungus also increases the activity of natural killer (NK) cells and enhances the effectiveness of antibodies. In addition, snow fungus reduces the rate at which cancers spread in a laboratory setting. In order to grow and spread, tumors have to establish their own blood vessel systems. Snow fungus compounds counteract a blood chemical called platelet-activating factor (PAF), which makes the blood less likely to clot and spin a fibrin "net" on which blood vessels to serve the tumor can form. None of these actions have been confirmed in humans.

Laboratory tests have demonstrated that snow fungus extracts kill cervical cancer cells, as well as those taken from other types of tumors. Snow fungus is known to sensitize the cervix and uterus to radiation treatment, making that treatment more effective. One medical use of snow fungus is to increase white blood cell counts in people undergoing chemotherapy or radiation treatment for cancer. This is a serious condition, however, so do not use snow fungus in this case without first consulting a physician.

Considerations for Use

Snow fungus is available as an extract and in an over-the-counter (OTC) patent medicine called Yin Mi Pian. Like all other so-called jelly fungi, snow fungus has no known toxicity and also can be eaten as a food.

SOY ISOFLAVONE CONCENTRATE

Latin name: Soy isoflavone concentrate is taken from the beans of the soy plant, *Glycine max* (Fabaceae [legume] family)

General Description

The soybean contains several medicinally useful chemicals, including isoflavones and lecithin. (*See* SOY LECITHIN.) The isoflavones most recognized as beneficial are daidzein and genistein, and the closely related compounds daidzin and genistin. These substances have been well researched for their antioxidant and phytoestrogenic properties.

Evidence of Benefit

Soy isoflavones are used medicinally for a variety of indications. In Chinese medicine, they are used for night sweats, confusion, and joint pain. They can be used for blood lipid management in less severe cases and for liver and gallbladder complaints, anemia, nerve conditions, and general debility. The German Commission E has approved their use for elevated serum cholesterol levels.

Benefits of soy isoflavones for specific health conditions include the following:

• *Alzheimer's disease, cognition, and quality of life.* In one study, postmenopausal women who supplemented their diets with soy isoflavones had improved memory but no changes in other measures of cognition. However, in another study, postmenopausal women who used soy protein for one year did not have any improvement on cognition. In a study of young adults who took supplements with soy isoflavones, participants had improvement in memory as well as in mental flexibility, but other aspects of memory did not show improvement. In another study looking at quality-of-life issues in postmenopausal women, women using soy protein with 100 milligrams of soy isoflavones did not benefit after one year. Estrogen is believed to slow the production of amyloid plaques in the brain and help preserve memory, two problems closely associated with Alzheimer's disease. Thus, soy isoflavones may help slow the progress of Alzheimer's disease, although no studies exist to show if this is true.

• *Atherosclerosis and high blood pressure.* Soy isoflavones are protective for the heart. The exact mechanism by which they work is unknown, but it is thought to be related to an isoflavone (phytoestrogen)-induced hyperthyroid state and increased bile acid secretion, which may enhance removal of low-density lipoprotein (LDL, or "bad") cholesterol from the blood. Soy isoflavones may also inhibit oxidation of LDL cholesterol and may alter liver metabolism to enhance removal of LDL by liver cells. In 1995, a review of thirty-eight controlled studies on soy and heart disease concluded that soy isoflavones lower both total cholesterol and LDL cholesterol, the cholesterol that forms fatty plaques in the arteries, and triglycerides, usually without affecting high-density lipoprotein (HDL, or "good") cholesterol. However, in one study, postmenopausal women who consumed soy powder with either low or high soy isoflavone content (1.30 milligrams per gram of soy protein or 2.25 milligrams per gram of soy protein) had an increase in HDL cholesterol and a decrease in total LDL cholesterol.

Total cholesterol typically goes down a small amount— about 6 to 7 percent—with isoflavone supplementation and with soy protein containing isoflavones. However, another study found that men and women with elevated cholesterol levels experienced no benefit on blood lipid levels with 240 milligrams of soy isoflavones.

In one study, people with high blood pressure who took soy protein containing 117 milligrams of soy isoflavones for six months experienced no change in blood pressure. In contrast, patients with mild or moderate high blood pressure who consumed soy milk that provided 143 milligrams of soy isoflavones a day had a mean blood pressure reduction of 17 mmHg (millimeters of mercury). In another study, postmenopausal women with high blood pressure who took 200 milligrams of soy isoflavones did not experience lower blood pressure.

• *Cancer.* Soy may reduce the risk of prostate, lung, and endometrial cancers, but can increase the risk of bladder cancer and endometrial hyperplasia. Conflicting data surround the ability of soy to reduce the risk of breast cancer. Animal data suggest that soy may increase metastasis, and

that one soy isoflavone, genistein, blocks the effects of the breast cancer drug tamoxifen. Epidemiological data from China show that the more soy foods a person consumes, the lower the chance of dying from breast cancer and the lower the chance of recurrence (these women were not taking tamoxifen). But human data show that soy consumption reduces mortality and recurrence in breast cancer patients regardless of tamoxifen use. The strongest evidence in support of soy isoflavones was shown in a study of patients at risk for lung cancer where high intake of soy isoflavones reduced the risk of lung cancer by 72 percent in men and 44 percent in women. Soy isoflavone supplementation may also reduce the adverse effects associated with chemotherapy and radiotherapy. If you have cancer, you should consult your physician before using soy-containing products or soy isoflavones. The similarity of soy isoflavones to the human hormone estrogen allows isoflavones to attach to estrogen receptors in human cells. This blocks actual human estrogen from doing the same. The isoflavones are just different enough from estrogen, however, that they do not always stimulate cells as estrogen does. If you have an estrogen-sensitive form of cancer, check with your doctor before taking soy isoflavones.

Daidzein is one such estrogen-blocking isoflavone. It locks out estrogen from breast-cancer cells without stimulating the cells to reproduce. It also fights cancer by causing immature tumor cells to differentiate, or mature into forms that have normal life spans and are then replaced. Daidzein has been shown to be very potent in forcing differentiation of human leukemia cells and of melanoma cells, even when absorbed in very low concentrations.

Finnish researchers conducted decades of exacting studies to explain why the people of Japan enjoy lower rates of breast, ovarian, prostate, and other cancers. They identified genistein as the common denominator; this is considered to be a stronger anticancer agent than daidzein. Genistein may be valuable in reversing cancer risk associated with certain kinds of obesity in women. Women who are physically inactive and have a genetic tendency toward diabetes often develop insulin resistance, a condition in which the body is forced to produce more and more insulin to transport glucose to the cells where it is needed. In addition to regulating blood sugar, insulin facilitates the transport of fat into fat cells, and fatty tissue produces estrogen. Thus, insulin indirectly activates estrogen and progesterone receptors, an action that stimulates the growth of cells, including estrogen-activated cancer cells. Since genistein blocks estrogen from its receptors on cells, it helps fight the cancer-promoting effects of excess estrogen production.

Genistein counteracts cancer development on several levels. It deactivates a harmful protein called tyrosine protein kinase, a key player in stimulating cell growth. This keeps cancer cells from multiplying. Genistein also affects other key enzymes involved in the cancer-formation process. Like daidzein, genistein causes cancer cells to differentiate, stopping wild multiplication. In addition, genistein stops the process by which tumors develop their own systems of blood vessels. This action deprives cancer cells of nutrients and oxygen, keeping them small. There is also evidence, at least in the case of certain kinds of lung cancer, that genistein complements the action of the gene p53, a "patrol gene" that deactivates cancer cells. Genistein has anticancer effects in breast cancer cell lines (estrogen receptor–positive and estrogen dependent–negative), prostate cancer (androgen-dependent and androgen-independent), neuroblastoma, sarcoma, and retinoblastoma cells. Genistein may act as an antiestrogen by competing for receptor binding, possibly resulting in reduced estrogen-induced stimulation of breast cell proliferation and breast tumor formation. Soy isoflavones reduce breast cancer by decreasing endogenous ovarian steroid levels. Soy isoflavones were found to reduce the risk of endometrial and lung cancer. In prostate cancer, soy protein extracts appear to reduce the progression of disease and they reduce androgen receptor expression in prostate tumors. Genistein may further reduce prostate cancer risk by directly inhibiting the growth of prostate cancer cells and if they occur, causing them to die early (termed *apoptosis*).

• *Menopause-related problems and osteoporosis.* Through their estrogenic action, soy isoflavones help move calcium from the bloodstream into the bones, strengthening their resistance to fracture. Less calcium is lost in the urine than when no soy is consumed. The mild estrogenic activity of soy isoflavones may ease menopause symptoms for some women, without creating estrogen-related problems, as well as having a positive effect in the prevention of osteoporosis. Data on the use of soy isoflavones to treat hot flashes have not been consistent. In one study, using 90 milligrams of soy isoflavones a day for four months in postmenopausal women with breast cancer did not help reduce hot flashes. This was the typical amount of soy isoflavones used in studies with women suffering from hot flashes. A systematic review and meta-analysis of all high-quality studies also found no benefit for using soy isoflavones for hot flashes. However, many women have reported relief from hot flashes using soy isoflavones. The weak estrogenic effect of soy isoflavones could potentially mediate hot flashes triggered by estrogen deficiency, but this action could also cause adverse effects. This dual action could explain the conflicting data on hot flash management using soy isoflavones.

A series of clinical trials around the world has established that soy isoflavones are a useful and safe alternative to estrogen therapy in treating low bone mass or osteoporosis in women who have passed menopause. Animal data suggest that genistein and daidzein have the ability to prevent or reduce bone loss in a manner similar to synthetic estrogen. However, newer data in human studies have produced conflicting results. Some studies showed that soy slowed bone density loss, while others have observed

no effect. In one study, postmenopausal Japanese women who received 100 milligrams of soy isoflavones a day for twenty-four weeks had a significant improvement in bone mineral density.

Considerations for Use

The easiest way to get soy isoflavones is by taking soy isoflavone concentrate. Soy germ also can be used (preferably added to cereals or smoothies), as can cooked soybeans, miso, or tofu (soybean curd). Soy isoflavones are also found in the herb kudzu. (*See* KUDZU.) Of readily available soy foods, roasted soybeans have the highest isoflavone content, about 167 milligrams for a 3.5-ounce serving. Tempeh is next, with 60 milligrams, followed by soy flour, with 44 milligrams. Processed soy products such as soy protein and soymilk contain about 20 milligrams per serving. Although the optimum dosage of isoflavones obtained from food is not known, one study found that ingesting 62 milligrams of isoflavones daily is sufficient to reduce cholesterol. Further, we know that Japanese women eat up to 200 milligrams of isoflavones from soy foods daily.

Although it is not a purely herbal product, ipriflavone, a chemically altered form of soy isoflavones, may be a better choice for preventing and treating osteoporosis, and for preventing bone fractures in weight lifters and participants in contact sports. Clinical testing in Japan has found that treatment with ipriflavone, even without supplemental calcium, prevents bone loss better than calcium supplementation alone. Brands that provide ipriflavone in a corn-oil base may be better absorbed.

Some minor side effects of soy isoflavones include stomach pain, loose stool, and diarrhea. Longer menstrual cycles have been reported. There is a link between fermented soy products and stomach cancer in Asian populations. In Japan, consumption of higher amounts of tofu during middle age resulted in poor cognition and low brain weight. Soy isoflavones were thought to inhibit tyrosine kinase, an enzyme that is involved with neuronal plasticity. In China, there is a twofold increase in bladder cancer in persons with the highest intake of soy. Because isoflavones work somewhat like estrogen, there are concerns that they may not be safe for women who already have breast cancer. Preliminary studies and reports have raised concerns that intensive use of soy products by a pregnant woman could exert a hormonal effect that has an impact on the developing fetus. Soy isoflavones could theoretically interfere with the action of oral contraceptives, although studies have not confirmed this. In each of these cases—breast cancer, pregnancy, oral contraceptives—check with your doctor before taking soy isoflavones or using soy protein. In any regard, do not use tamoxifen and soy products including isoflavones together, because soy decreases the effectiveness of the drug.

Soy products may impair thyroid function or reduce absorption of thyroid medication. People with impaired thyroid function should use soy in moderation or under medical supervision. Do not use soy isoflavones with blood-thinners. There is a minor risk of soy reducing the absorption of iron; to be safe, take them two hours apart.

SOY LECITHIN

Latin name: Soy lecithin is taken from the beans of the soy plant, *Glycine max* (Fabaceae [legume] family)

General Description

Soy lecithin, like soy isoflavone concentrate, is an extract of the soybean. It contains a substance called phosphatidylcholine (PC), which is responsible for its medicinal effects. PC is a major part of the membranes surrounding the cells. But when it is consumed, it is broken down into the nutrient choline rather than being carried directly to cell membranes. Choline is used to make acetylcholine, a nerve chemical essential for proper brain function.

Evidence of Benefit

Soy lecithin provides the building blocks of healthy cell membranes, preventing damage especially to blood and liver cells by oxidation, free radicals, and toxins. More recently, lecithin has been proposed as a remedy for various psychological and neurological diseases, including Tourette's syndrome, Alzheimer's disease, and bipolar mood disorder. Lecithin is approved by the German Commission E for moderate disturbances in fat metabolism, most notably for persons who have high cholesterol levels and cannot reduce them with dietary manipulation alone. In 2001, the U.S. Food and Drug Administration (FDA) approved a nutrient content claim for choline (a nutrient found in lecithin) allowing food labels to say: "Foods that contain over 110 milligrams of choline per serving may claim that they are an excellent source of choline, and those with 55 milligrams per serving may claim that they offer a good source of choline."

Benefits of soy lecithin for specific health conditions include the following:

• *Alcoholism and cirrhosis of the liver.* Numerous clinical and laboratory studies have shown that soy lecithin can protect the liver from damage caused by alcohol, tetrachlorides found in cleaning solvents, the prescription drug paracetamol, and galactosamine, a protein that can irritate the liver. In laboratory studies of chronic hepatitis, soy lecithin has shown an ability to protect the liver against fatty deposits and fibrosis, the development of nonfunctional fibrous tissue. Soy lecithin works on liver cell membranes, and due to its high phospholipid content offers unique protection. Without lecithin every cell in the body would harden and nutrients would be unable to move in and out of the cells. Human data are lacking, however, and soy lecithin is not a treatment for alcoholism at present.

• *Alzheimer's disease and memory problems.* Soy lecithin is a source of phosphatidylcholine (PC), an essential element in the lining of brain cells. Providing additional phosphatidylcholine has a modest effect on Alzheimer's disease, but this supplement is especially beneficial when used with the prescription drug tacrine (Cognex), which helps the brain conserve phosphatidylcholine. Soy lecithin not only provides phosphatidylcholine, but helps to transport tacrine to the brain. Soy lecithin also allows the body to make acetylcholine, an important brain chemical that is low in people with Alzheimer's disease. It is possible that the brain may make more acetylcholine when the person consumes soy lecithin. However, human data are inconclusive at this point in patients with Alzheimer's disease. Soy lecithin also reduces memory loss in smokers and people with high blood pressure, conditions in which large numbers of free radicals that damage brain tissue are generated.

• *Atherosclerosis, gallstones, and high cholesterol.* Soy lecithin can reduce blood cholesterol levels. This occurs through a complex process in which partially digested lecithin is chemically reassembled in the intestinal wall into a form that attracts cholesterol. The lecithin then "steers" larger particles of low-density lipoprotein (LDL, or "bad") cholesterol to the liver, where it is disposed of. People who use niacin to lower their blood cholesterol should consider using lecithin as well because niacin depletes the body of choline. Soy lecithin may reduce cholesterol production and help to prevent the formation of gallstones because most gallstones are composed mostly of cholesterol.

Considerations for Use

Soy lecithin is available in capsules. Other encapsulated soy phospholipids may be identified individually on product labels as 3-sn-phosphatidylcholine, phosphatidylethanolamine, and phosphatidylinositic acid, or as "total phospholipids." Soy lecithin is also available in an over-the-counter (OTC) preparation called Leci-PS.

Soy lecithin may cause mild diarrhea when first used. Although soy lecithin may help reverse alcoholic cirrhosis of the liver, it is important to stop, or at least sharply reduce, alcohol intake when using lecithin.

Ordinary lecithin contains about 10 to 20 percent phosphatidylcholine. However, European research has tended to use soy lecithin products concentrated to contain 90 percent phosphatidylcholine. The following dosages are based on the more concentrated product. For psychological and neurological conditions, researchers have used doses of up to 5 to 10 grams (5,000 to 10,000 milligrams) three times daily. Average daily doses recommended by the German Commission E for lowering cholesterol are 3.5 grams per day. For liver disease, typical doses have been 350 to 500 milligrams taken three times daily. For high cholesterol, doses of 500 to 900 milligrams taken three times daily are common. Most people don't experience side effects when taking between 10 to 30 grams a day of lecithin supplements. However, taking more can cause gastrointestinal problems, diarrhea, weight gain, rash, headache, nausea, vomiting, and dizziness, and produce a "fishy" body odor. If you are taking higher doses of lecithin, you should do so under a doctor's supervision.

The amounts of soy lecithin needed to produce results for people with Alzheimer's disease are relatively expensive, and can cause stomach upset. If you wish to try this type of therapy, take the recommended dosage for three weeks, then continue only if there are noticeable results with no unmanageable side effects.

ST. JOHN'S WORT

Latin name: *Hypericum perforatum* (Hypericaceae [St. John's wort] family)
Other common names: amber, goatweed, hardhay, hypericum, klamath weed, tipton weed

General Description

St. John's wort is a perennial plant native to Great Britain, especially Wales, and to northern Europe, western Asia, and northern Africa. European settlers brought it to the United States in the 1700s. Growing to a height of thirty-two inches (eighty centimeters), it bears bright yellow petals in flowering tops. It was also introduced to eastern Asia, Australia, and New Zealand, and is cultivated in Poland and Serbia. Traditionally, its petals were gathered in midsummer for use in herbal medicine. Today, the entire plant is used. Oils and tinctures made from St. John's wort have a dark red color imparted by hypericin, one of the medicinally active components of the herb.

In Middle English, the term *wort* referred to any plant or vegetable that was used medicinally. St. John's wort got its name because it bloomed on or near June 24, which was known as St. John's Day in the Church calendar. In medieval England, St. John's wort was used to treat attacks of insanity attributed to the work of evil spirits or the devil.

Evidence of Benefit

St. John's wort has antibacterial, antidepressant, anti-inflammatory, antiviral, and pain-relieving properties. This herb's ability to fight depression also makes it useful in treating fatigue, and its ability to relieve pain makes it helpful for treating vocal pain and laryngitis associated with fibromyalgia. Historically it was used for worm infestation, bronchitis, asthma, gallbladder disease, gastritis, bed-wetting, gout, and rheumatism. Oily versions of St. John's wort were prepared for ingestion to treat dyspepsia, and used externally to treat muscle soreness. Chinese medicine used it in a gargle solution for tonsillitis and in a lotion for skin irritations. Homeopathic remedies include those for nervous system issues, depression, and asthma. The German Commission E has approved St. John's wort for internal use for anxiety and depressive moods, and in

an oily mixture for stomach complaints. For external use, it has been approved, when used as an oily mixture, for blunt injuries, skin problems, muscle soreness, and first-degree burns.

Hypericin, a flavonoid component of St. John's wort, is thought to be responsible for the bioactive activities of the herb.

Benefits of St. John's wort for specific health conditions include the following:

• *Burns and skin disorders.* Studies in rats have shown that St. John's wort is more effective for wound healing than placebo or calendula. Clinical studies have found that an ointment prepared by mixing fresh St. John's wort flowers with olive oil greatly accelerates the healing of burns. St. John's wort lotions prevent skin infection with *Staphylococcus aureus* (staph infection). In one study, patients with subacute atopic dermatitis applied a topical cream made from hypericin extract for four weeks and their eczema healed better than the placebo group's eczema. Hypericin-containing extracts may prove useful for the treatment of psoriasis, warts, and certain forms of skin cancer (*see below*).

• *Cancer.* St. John's wort increases sensitivity to light. Photodynamic therapy is a type of treatment based on the ability of cancer cells to selectively take up a specific compound that makes the cancer cells more sensitive to specific wavelengths of light, so that irradiation kills only the cancer cells. In experiments using mice, hypericin was shown to accumulate specifically in tumor tissue. When the hypericin-treated mice were irradiated, tumor growth was inhibited. Similar results have been found in human tumor cells. These results suggest that hypericin can be used as a photodynamic therapy in the treatment of cancer. The use of extracts containing hypericin may prove beneficial for certain types of skin cancer, such as cutaneous T-cell lymphoma, melanoma, and Kaposi's sarcoma. Other studies were done in cell lines of human colon cancer, leukemia, and gastrointestinal tumor cells, and hypericin showed the ability to kill cancer cells, but more work is needed before it can be recommended as a treatment for any type of cancer.

• *Carpal tunnel syndrome.* St. John's wort is anecdotally reported to relieve pain of carpal tunnel syndrome. This is probably due to its ability to improve transmission over the median nerve, the nerve that runs through the carpal tunnel in the wrist. However, there is no historical use of this herb for similar complaints.

• *Crohn's disease, hemorrhoids, and irritable bowel syndrome (IBS).* St. John's wort oil has been used clinically for a variety of digestive ailments. It regulates serotonin, a neurotransmitter that causes digestive irritation, and reduces inflammation and swelling. The tannins in the oil (which are not present in pure hypericin extract) prevent fluids from flowing into the intestines, thereby relieving diarrhea.

For IBS, European doctors usually prescribe St. John's wort oil as an overnight retention enema.

• *Cuts, scrapes, and abrasions.* St. John's wort may keep open wounds from becoming infected. One component in St. John's wort, hyperforin, has antibacterial properties. In laboratory experiments, it shows greater antibiotic activity than sulfa drugs.

• *Depression.* The most common use of St. John's wort is in the treatment of depression. Although the exact way in which the herb works is not yet known, St. John's wort is often described as a "natural Prozac." Hypericin (or, more likely, a group of chemicals in this plant including hypericin) does in fact prevent the reuptake of serotonin by brain tissue, allowing this mood-controlling brain chemical to fight depression. However, St. John's wort has also been described as a natural monoamine oxidase (MAO) inhibitor, acting in the same way as the antidepressant drugs commonly used before fluoxetine (Prozac). The whole herb does not seem to have this effect because it is not concentrated enough. There is also another possible explanation of how St. John's wort works to counteract depression. Scientists at Humboldt University in Berlin have found that hypericin stops the production of cytokines, hormonal messengers that transmit sensations of pain and irritation. Small changes in cytokine balance apparently can make huge differences in brain function, affecting not only depression but also partial seizure disorders. In one study, blood samples were taken from a group of depressed patients and a group of healthy volunteers. Cells were bathed in an extract of hypericum. In both groups there was a reduction in cytokines. It is thought that St. John's wort lowered the number of cytokines, which leads to a decrease in corticotrophin releasing hormone, which triggers depressive moods.

However St. John's wort acts against depression, its effects have been demonstrated in large-scale clinical tests against placebos and other antidepressant medications. A statistical review of twenty-three studies involving 1,757 outpatients with mild to moderate depression found that St. John's wort was better than placebo and had an effect comparable to such antidepressants as amitriptyline (Elavil), maprotiline (Ludiomil), and imipramine (Tofranil). Typical doses of St. John's wort ranged from 350 to 1,800 milligrams a day. Other double-blind studies found that St. John's wort was more effective than fluoxetine (Prozac) and sertraline (Zoloft), and that it caused fewer and less severe side effects. In a meta-analysis of several studies, St. John's wort was shown to be more effective than placebo and as effective as tricyclic antidepressants in treating moderate depression. In one study, 65 percent of the participants who took the herb got better. The participants took 300 milligrams of St. John's wort three times a day to total 900 milligrams daily. Another study of this herb discounted its effects against depression, but that study did not discriminate between mild to moderate depression and severe depression. Other studies of St. John's wort have focused on mild to moderate depression and have found the herb effective. In another study, using an extract of hypericum WS 5570, patients with acute episodes of moderate depression got better and had fewer depressive symptoms, according to the Hamilton Rating Scale for Depression, and also had fewer relapses than a placebo group. The German Commission E has approved the use of St. John's wort for mild to moderate depression. In all probability, the herb does not have usefulness in treating severe depression. And if it is used in cases of severe depression, it should be used in combination with other therapies. In one study of patients with severe depression, hypericum WS 5570 was as effective as a commonly used selective serontonin reuptake inhibitor (SSRI) drug. However, the authors cautioned about using St. John's wort in this way because it has numerous interactions with other medications. The focus has now shifted from efficacy to the potential harmful aspects of the herb.

• *Diabetic neuropathy.* Sometimes, successful treatment of diabetes that has gone uncontrolled for a long time can result in severe nerve pain. This happens because lowering blood sugar leads to restored nerve function, but the "pain fibers" in the nerves are disproportionately stimulated. St. John's wort is an alternative to the tricyclic antidepressant usually prescribed for the condition, amitriptyline (Elavil). Unlike amitriptyline, St. John's wort does not cause secondary effects such as drowsiness, orthostatic hypotension (a sudden drop in blood pressure when you move from a seated to a standing position), or urine retention.

• *Ear infection and herpesvirus infection.* A reduction in ear pain has been reported with use of naturopathic herbal extract eardrops containing hypericum and other herbs. In studies, the product Otikon Otic Solution performed as well as a topical anesthetic and worked without antibiotics. Relief occurred within two to three days, which is also the amount of time it usually takes without any treatment. Hypericin and pseudohypericin, two of the primary active compounds in St. John's wort, inhibit the herpes simplex 1 virus, the type of herpesvirus best known for causing cold sores (fever blisters). Hypericin and pseudohypericin act against a variety of other herpesviruses as well, including cytomegalovirus (CMV). The antiviral process triggered by St. John's wort is enhanced when the user is exposed to sunlight, but no human studies are available to confirm its use for these conditions in humans; all studies were done on cell lines.

• *Headache.* St. John's wort is known to interrupt some of the metabolic pathways activated during tension headaches. The herb may work through its bioflavonoids, which contain a compound that relaxes blood vessels and increases blood circulation.

• *HIV/AIDS.* Hypericin and pseudohypericin have been reported to have activity against some retroviruses, including HIV. Scientists are currently investigating the use of these compounds in fighting HIV.

• *Insomnia and anxiety.* When used by itself, St. John's wort does not increase the time in rapid-eye-movement (REM) sleep (a deep sleep), but does increase the slow-wave sleep. In one study, women took a product called Jarsin, a hypericum extract that supplies 300 milligrams of St. John's wort, three times a day for four weeks. The increase in slow-wave sleep (sleep stages 3 and 4) is postulated to be a significant contributor to the antidepressant effect of St. John's wort. In another study, patients with generalized anxiety disorder experienced symptom relief from 900 milligrams of St. John's wort twice a day. Although the study was only in three patients, the positive effects on the patients' sleep and coping abilities persisted with use of the herb for one year. Laboratory studies show that when animals are given St. John's wort in combination with sleep-inducing medications, it increases total time spent in sleep.

Considerations for Use

St. John's wort is available in a variety of forms. In some people, this herb may cause stomach upset, restlessness, increased urination, headaches, mild allergic reactions, or fatigue. There have been reports of mania, anxiety, and schizophrenia relapse.

No medication, including St. John's wort, is adequate treatment for people who experience a preoccupation with or repeated thoughts of death or suicide. If you do experience such thoughts, you should immediately seek professional help. For other people with depression, St. John's wort should be taken for no less than ten days to two weeks to determine if there is any improvement. If not, and especially if there is no benefit in four to six weeks, the herb should be discontinued. If the herb is helpful, however, there is no limitation on the length of time it can be taken. A dose of hypericin for depression can range from 200 to 1,000 milligrams a day, but as the actual amount of hypericin in St. John's wort varies from product to product, care should be taken in determining the correct dosage for you. For general use, the herb is used at 2 to 4 grams per day.

Many science writers caution that hypericin can sensitize the skin to sunlight, causing a tendency to sunburn. To put this problem in perspective, over 60 million doses of St. John's wort are dispensed every year in Germany alone, and only fewer than a dozen photosensitization reactions have ever been reported. As a caution, though, you should avoid the use of tanning beds or lamps while taking St. John's wort for depression.

If you are taking St. John's wort as an antiviral aid, or to treat cancer or vitiligo, you *need* to expose your skin to sunlight to activate the herb's active constituents, so the preceding caution does not apply. However, you should note that over 85 percent of people with AIDS who take the herb for as long as six months experience at least one episode of severe sunburn. Also, people taking prescription medications that increase risk of sunburn, such as angiotensin-converting enzyme (ACE) inhibitors, commonly prescribed for high blood pressure, should also avoid St. John's wort.

Since the antiviral effect of St. John's wort against HIV has not yet been verified and is still undergoing scientific study, people with AIDS should use this herb only under the supervision of a knowledgeable health-care provider.

Some scientific articles maintain that St. John's wort contains MAO inhibitors, which can cause sudden attacks of severe high blood pressure when combined with the protein tyramine, which is found in aged cheeses, chocolate, and red wine, among many other foods. The studies reporting to find MAO inhibitors in St. John's wort have not been replicated, though, and there are no reports of people taking St. John's wort having symptoms of this kind of drug interaction. However, if you are taking antidepressant drugs, whether MAO inhibitors, tricyclic antidepressants, or SSRIs such as fluoxetine (Prozac); or the painkiller tramadol (Ultram); or the migraine medication sumatriptan (Imitrex), you should *not* take St. John's wort at the same time. Doing so can cause serotonin syndrome, which can be life-threatening. It is characterized by high blood pressure, dizziness, weakness, and agitation that only goes away with discontinuation of the herb. If you are interested in switching from a prescription drug to St. John's wort, you need to let the medication flush out of your system for several weeks (depending on the drug) before you start using the herb. Do not do this without speaking to your doctor.

Other drugs also pose a risk of undesirable interactions. If you are taking digoxin (Lanoxicaps, Lanoxin), cyclosporine (Neoral, Sandimmune), protease inhibitors and non-nucleoside reverse transcriptase inhibitors for HIV infection, birth control pills, amitriptyline (Elavil), warfarin (Coumadin), theophylline (Aerolate, Elixophyllin, Slo-Phyllin, and others), chemotherapy drugs, or antipsychotic medications, St. John's wort might cause these drugs to be less effective. Numerous other prescription drugs pose moderate to major risk to those who use them with St. John's wort. It is best if you are using any prescription drug, even if you think it is benign, such as a contraceptive medication, to contact your doctor first. Of all of the herbs described in this book, St. John's wort interacts with the greatest number of drugs.

If you are taking medications that cause sun sensitivity, such as sulfa drugs, the anti-inflammatory medication piroxicam (Feldene), omeprazole (Prilosec), or lansoprazole (Prevacid), keep in mind that St. John's wort might increase that effect. Similarly, you should not take it if you are planning to undergo any type of surgical procedure. This herb can intensify the effects of anesthesia, resulting in oversedation. Some reports from patients show that St. John's wort increases thyroid-stimulating hormone. If you have thyroid problems, speak to your doctor before using this herb. Use of St. John's wort is contraindicated during pregnancy because it damages reproductive cells. Some people have reported problems with caffeine in combination with St. John's wort. If you experience any unusual symptoms, discontinue one of the two (caffeine or the herb). Others have reported sexual dysfunction when taking St. John's wort. Others have experienced symptoms of withdrawal, such as nausea, anorexia, dry retching, dizziness, thirst, cold, and extreme fatigue, after discontinuing its use.

STINGING NETTLE

Latin name: *Urtica dioica* (Urticaceae [stinging nettle] family)
Other common names: common nettle, greater nettle, nettle

General Description

Stinging nettle is found in temperate climates around the world. A perennial plant growing to a height of 5 feet (1.5 meters), it bears lance-shaped leaves and green flowers with yellow stamens. If you come into contact with fine hairs on the leaves and stem, you may develop a burning pain that lasts for hours. Both the fresh and dried leaves and the roots are used in herbal medicine, but they have very different uses.

Evidence of Benefit

From ancient Greece to the present, nettle has been used for treating coughs, tuberculosis, and arthritis, and as a hair tonic. Stinging nettle leaf is an anti-inflammatory, especially for allergic reactions of the skin, as well as a diuretic. It has been used to relieve symptoms of hay fever and allergies such as runny nose and congestion. It is used to treat urinary tract infections (UTIs), and European folk medicine uses it to treat seborrhea of the scalp and overly greasy hair. The root was also specifically used in folk medicine for edema, rheumatism, gout, and prostatitis.

Taken as a health treatment, stinging nettle root takes the "sting," or inflammation, out of allergic reactions, arthritis, and benign prostatic hypertrophy (BPH). In a study on lupus using mice, stinging nettle seemed to protect the animals from symptoms such as kidney ailments. It also prevents conversion of androgens to estrogens, which may be of benefit to patients with BPH. The German Commission E has approved the use of stinging nettle flowering plant for rheumatism, kidney stones, and infections of the urinary tract. The stinging nettle root has been approved for difficulties in urination related to BPH.

Benefits of stinging nettle for specific health conditions include the following:

• *Allergies (hay fever).* In low doses, stinging nettle root extracts increase the production of T cells, immune cells that act as a controlling mechanism on other immune cells that cause allergic reactions. Stinging nettle root extracts increase the production of interleukin-2 (IL-2), which increases the production of new T cells and sensitizes existing T cells to respond to IL-2. A clinical study with sixty-nine participants at the National College of Naturopathic Medicine in Portland, Oregon, found that stinging nettle was more effective than placebo in treating allergic rhinitis. Nettle leaf has become a popular treatment for allergies. This is probably due to its anti-inflammatory properties. Taken before a meal, nettle leaf has been used for people with certain food sensitivities, but check with your doctor first if you have known food allergies.

• *Arthritis.* Stinging nettle contains extracts that ease arthritic pain. In clinical studies using a leaf extract for rheumatoid arthritis and osteoarthritis, patients had less pain while resting and less pain during movement, and better symptom scores. The herb worked alone or in combination with NSAIDs (nonsteroidal anti-inflammatory drugs).

• *Benign prostatic hypertrophy (BPH).* Stinging nettle root extracts decrease the rate of cell division in the prostate gland. Compounds in stinging nettle bind to receptor sites on prostate cells that otherwise would receive growth hormones such as sex hormone-binding globulin (SHBG). They also interfere with enzymes that are necessary for prostate cell growth. As the growth of prostate cells is slowed, there is less pressure on the urethra and an easier flow of urine. In one clinical study, more than 80 percent of men with BPH experienced improvement in symptoms of the lower urinary tract using stinging nettle. In another study, the root of the stinging nettle improved the International Prostate Symptom Score, which is used by doctors to assess disease impact and improvement in patients. The root is typically used in Germany for patients with BPH to reduce residual urine levels and prostate size. One preparation—a methanol root extract called Bazoton Uno—seemed to be particularly effective using 300 to 600 milligrams a day.

• *Diminished sex drive.* Stinging nettle root keeps testosterone, which contributes to sexual desire in both men and women, in an active (or free) form. Alcohol-soluble components of stinging nettle root known as lignans interact with SHBG to keep it from binding testosterone and taking it out of circulation. For men, the advantage of stinging nettle root over many other treatments for diminished sex drive is that, while it maintains testosterone in a form that energizes the libido, it prevents benign prostate enlargement.

• *Hives and skin irritations.* Stinging nettle leaf may help speed healing of rashes, but this has not been fully explored in human studies. It inhibits this kind of inflammation through its content of scopoletin, beta-sitosterol, and caffeoylmalic acid, which stop a series of chemical steps that leads to a reduction in inflammation and produces an analgesic effect. Caffeoylmalic acid is particularly important to block the arachidonic cascade that triggers inflammation.

Considerations for Use

Stinging nettle leaf is available in capsule and juice forms. It can also be used as a tea. Stinging nettle leaf has a long history of use as a food, and is regarded as safe. The daily dose of the leaf is 8 to 12 grams and of the root is 4 to 6 grams per day. Typically stinging nettle is used as an alcohol-based extract, and in this form the dose is lower. In rare cases, some people develop an allergic reaction, such as a rash, after taking stinging nettle *leaf*. If such a reaction occurs, use of the herb should be discontinued. Others have reported gastrointestinal upset, gingival effects, and increased urination.

Stinging nettle products made from either the leaf or the root of the plant should not be used by people with fluid retention due to congestive heart failure or kidney disease. Men should not use stinging nettle to treat urinary problems without medical examination. Similar symptoms can be caused by a more serious condition, such as prostate cancer, that requires medical treatment. Because stinging nettle leaf reduces the body's production of an immune chemical known as interleukin-6 (IL-6), it should be avoided by people who have or who think they may be coming down with the flu. The root and leaf of the stinging nettle should not be used during pregnancy.

There are concerns that nettle may interact with prescription medications used for diabetes, high blood pressure, and inflammation, as well as sedative medications. Stinging nettle interacts with diclofenac (Voltaren, for arthritis), diuretics, and drugs that work through p450 enzymes. Speak to your doctor if you are taking any of these medications before using stinging nettle. There have not been any reports of actual problems occurring, but if you are taking such medications, you should use nettle with caution. In addition, you should not use uncooked stinging nettles. They may cause kidney damage and other symptoms of poisoning. Stinging nettle is a diuretic and may remove potassium from the body. If nettle is used regularly, you should eat foods high in potassium, such as bananas and fresh vegetables, or take a potassium supplement daily.

TEA TREE

Latin name: *Melaleuca alternifolia* (Myrtaceae [clove] family) Other common names: cajeput oil, melaleuca oil (from Australia)

General Description

The tea tree, which reaches a height of twenty to twenty-five feet (six to eight meters), produces layers of paperlike bark and bears pointed leaves and spikes of white flowers. Native to Australia, the tea tree flourishes in the wet, swampy ground of northern New South Wales and Queensland. The leaves and small branches are picked year-round for distillation into essential oil.

For centuries before Europeans arrived, native Australians used the leaves of this tree as an antiseptic. Named the "tea tree" by Captain Cook, this tree rapidly became a valued remedy used by the European settlers to treat cuts, burns, and insect bites. Tea tree soon became widely recognized as a powerful disinfectant. Some unproven uses include treatment of conditions of the respiratory tract and skin. In folk medicine, it has been used for tonsillitis, pharyngitis, colitis, and sinusitis. Externally, tea tree oil is used for ulcers of the oral mucous membrane, gingivitis, root canal treatments, skin and nail infections, burns, and insect bites.

Evidence of Benefit

Tea tree oil is an antiseptic that is active against many bacteria and fungi. There is promising new evidence in cell studies suggesting that methicillin-resistant *Staphylococcus aureus* is killed by tea tree oil, but whether this can translate into a clinical setting is unknown. However, it is not as effective as oral antibiotics for some conditions. Used as a gargle, it eases sore throats associated with colds. It should not be swallowed.

Australian dentists frequently use tea tree oil mouthwash prior to dental procedures and as a daily preventive measure against periodontal disease. Tea tree oil has deodorant properties, most likely because it suppresses odor-causing bacteria. It controls foot odor and sweetens bad breath.

Benefits of tea tree oil for specific health conditions include the following:

- *Acne.* A clinical study of 124 acne patients found that 5 percent tea tree oil gel was as effective as 5 percent benzoyl peroxide in the treatment of acne. Tea tree oil had fewer side effects than the prescription treatment. A later study found that for mild to moderate acne, a 5 percent topical tea tree oil gel was three to five times more effective than a placebo product, with no side effects.

- *Athlete's foot, ringworm, and yeast infection.* Preliminary double-blind studies have found tea tree oil to be an effective treatment for athlete's foot and other fungal infections of the skin and nails. Tea tree oil also treats ringworm, an infection caused by the same fungus, tinea. Although tea tree oil stops burning and itching, it does not affect the underlying fungal infection causing the disease. Tea tree oil has been proved effective in controlling thirty-two different strains of *Candida albicans,* the microorganism that causes many yeast infections. A concentration of 2 to 4 percent is effective against all yeasts and other fungal pathogens that have been tested. Tea tree oil has been suggested as a treatment for thrush (oral

Candida infection) in people with HIV infection. In one study, a 100 percent solution of tea tree oil was shown to be effective in treating onychomycosis (toenail fungus). The solution was applied twice daily for six months and the results were compared to another therapy—1 percent clotrimazole solution (Lotrimin, Mycelex). In both groups, the fungus was cleared up—in 60 percent of patients, and they remained fungus free for another three months with no treatment.

• *Boils, insect bites, and mastitis.* Even in concentrations as low as 0.5 percent (1 part in 200), tea tree oil kills over 90 percent of *Eshcherichia coli* (*E. coli*) and *Staphylococcus aureus* on human skin. Human studies on these conditions are lacking, however. Some skin irritations are caused by histamine. In a human experimental model where histamine was injected into the participants' forearms, tea tree oil applied topically reduced the swelling.

• *Dandruff.* Tea tree oil shampoos may stop dandruff. Although the exact mechanism by which tea tree oil accomplishes this effect is not known, scientists speculate that the oil stops dandruff by eliminating fungal damage to the skin. This has only been observed in cell line studies.

• *Vaginosis and yeast infection.* An alcohol-free extract of tea tree oil, diluted with water to a 1 percent concentration, may be effective against candidiasis and trichomoniasis if the oil is applied with daily douches combined with weekly application of tea tree oil–soaked tampons. No side effects have been reported from this form of administration.

Considerations for Use

Tea tree oil is used externally in a variety of forms, but it is not taken internally, as it may cause nerve damage and other problems if ingested. The best tea tree products contain oil from the species *M. alternifolia* only, standardized to contain not more than 10 percent cineole (an irritant) and at least 30 percent terpinen-4-ol.

People who are allergic to celery or thyme should not use tea tree oil, since tea tree shares a potential allergen, d-limonene, with these plants. Tea tree oil can be applied to minor cuts, but you should use caution in applying it to more extensive areas of broken skin or rashes not due to fungus. There have been reports of disorientation and dermatitis, as well as changes in hormonal balance, as tea tree oil has weak estrogenic effects.

THYME

Latin name: *Thymus vulgaris* (Lamiaceae [mint] family)
Other common names: creeping thyme, French thyme, garden thyme, mountain thyme, rubbed thyme

General Description

Thyme is an aromatic garden herb in the mint family. Growing to a height of fifteen inches (forty centimeters), it bears small leaves and pink flowers on woody stems. The leaf is used in herbal medicine. This herb is not the same plant species as wild thyme or mother of thyme.

Thyme's common name was probably derived from the Greek word *thumos,* or courage. In medieval times, knights supposedly wore sprigs of thyme as a symbol of courage. Thyme was also used to preserve meat. It is indigenous to the Mediterranean region and neighboring countries, northern Africa, and parts of Asia. It is extensively cultivated.

Evidence of Benefit

Thyme is an antibacterial, antifungal, antiviral, and antioxidant, and has bronchial anti-spasmatic effects. It is used externally for infected wounds and internally for respiratory and digestive infections. Oil of thyme (thymol) is used in commercial mouthwashes (it is the main ingredient in Listerine) and toothpastes. It is not effective against nail fungus despite the fact that components in thyme, thymol, and thyme essential oil have antifungal properties.

Thyme baths are thought to be helpful for neurasthenia, rheumatic problems, bruises, swellings, and sprains. However, avoid whole-body baths except with a doctor's permission in cases involving large skin injuries, acute skin illnesses, severe fever or infectious disease, or cardiac insufficiency. Aromatherapists consider the essential oil a powerful mood-enhancing herb for low spirits, fatigue, mental stress, and premenstrual tension. According to the German Commission E, thyme is approved for bronchitis and coughs.

Benefits of thyme for specific health conditions include the following:

• *Allergies, respiratory; asthma; and cough.* The essential oil of thyme encourages expectoration of phlegm and quells spasms of the bronchial passages. It acts by stimulating the cilia, or hairs, lining the bronchial passages. The cilia push congested mucus outward. Inhaling the steam from thyme placed in hot water is said to give the same antispasmodic and bronchial-clearing effects as the essential oil.

Considerations for Use

Thyme is available as an essential oil, both as a liquid and in enteric-coated capsules. A tea can be made using 1 to 2 grams of dried thyme herb steeped in 1 cup of hot water.

European authorities caution that thyme can cause abdominal contractions. Using thyme oil in bath preparations has, in rare cases, caused severe inflammation and hyperemia (an unusual flood of blood to a particular part of the body). Added to toothpastes, it can cause cracks in the corners of the mouth and a swollen tongue.

You should not use thyme if you have a duodenal ulcer or if you are pregnant. Thyme oil should be used topically only. Taken internally, it can cause vomiting and dizziness, convulsions, coma, and cardiac and respiratory arrest.

If you have any kind of thyroid condition, you should

talk to a health-care professional before taking medicinal doses of thyme. Studies indicate that the herb suppresses normal thyroid activity. It can be used in normal amounts as a food seasoning, however.

TILDEN FLOWER

Latin name: *Tilia cordifolia* (Tiliaceae [tilden] family)
Other common names: basswood, lime tree flower, linden flower

General Description

The tilden tree is an ornamental plant usually seen along the avenues of Europe. It is also found in the United States and in Canada from Quebec to North Dakota and south to North Carolina and Oklahoma. Growing as high as one hundred feet (thirty meters), it has a smooth gray bark, heart-shaped deciduous leaves, and clusters of pale yellow flowers with winglike bracts. The flowers make an excellent honey and an aromatic, pleasant-tasting medicinal tea. Use of the tilden flower began in medieval Europe to promote sweating and to treat feverish colds, flu, and other conditions associated with chilling.

Evidence of Benefit

Tilden flower is used as a home remedy for colds, flu, coughs, fever, headaches, indigestion, and sore throats.

Benefits of tilden flower for specific health conditions include the following:

• *Colds and influenza.* Tilden flowers, especially the bracts at the base of the flower, to which the petals are attached, are rich in a coating, soothing mucilage that relieves a scratchy throat. Several studies indicate that the flowers may enhance a person's resistance to certain kinds of infection, including a type of bacteria commonly associated with mouth infections. Children with flulike symptoms who were treated with tilden flowers developed fewer middle ear infections and other complications than children given conventional antibiotics, and also recovered more quickly. Do not use without consulting your child's pediatrician.

• *Headache and migraine.* The essential oil of tilden flowers contains farnesol, an antispasmodic and muscle relaxant. In laboratory tests on animals, the essential oil dilated blood vessels, lowering blood pressure and relaxing arterial walls. Although this effect is not strong enough to justify the use of tilden flowers in the treatment of high blood pressure in humans, it may be strong enough to counter the constriction of blood vessels that occurs during migraines and other types of headaches.

Considerations for Use

Tilden flower is available as a fluidextract or tea. Product labels sometimes refer to tilden flower as *linden flower.*

Tilden flower teas frequently combine the herb with bitter orange peel, chamomile, meadowsweet, and/or willow bark for maximum analgesic effect. Be sure to read the label if you are sensitive to any of these herbs. This herb should not be used on a daily basis for long periods of time, as long-term use poses a risk of heart damage.

TOLU BALSAM

Latin names: *Myroxylon balsamum, Myroxylon pereirae* (Fabaceae [legume] family)
Other common names: balsam of Peru, balsam of tolu myroxylon, Peru balsam

General Description

Tolu balsam is a resin taken from either of two species of the balsam tree. *M. balsamum,* which provides tolu balsam, is native to Colombia, Jamaica, Peru, Sri Lanka, and Venezuela. *M. pereirae,* which provides Peru balsam, is found not in Peru but in Central America. The name Peru balsam arose from the fact that it was originally shipped to Europe from Peru. Both species of balsam are tall jungle trees that are tapped like rubber trees to yield the vanilla-scented resin.

Evidence of Benefit

Tolu balsam is an antiseptic that fights bacteria and fungi, promotes wound healing, and kills parasites. When taken internally, it helps to loosen phlegm. It also is used in aromatherapy. It has been used in the United States since 1820 for bronchitis, laryngitis, and diarrhea, and as the basis of cough mixtures. It is approved by the German Commission E to treat inflammation of the mucous membranes of the respiratory tract. Folklore states that it was used externally for wound healing. Today, it also may be used in topical preparations for treatment of wounds, ulcers, and scabies, and can be found in hair tonics and antidandruff preparations, and as a natural fragrance in soaps, detergents, creams, lotions, and perfumes.

Benefits of tolu balsam for specific health conditions include the following:

• *Cough and cold.* Tolu balsam works as an expectorant to reduce nasal congestion. It reduces inflammation of the respiratory system to enhance breathing.

Considerations for Use

There are no major side effects for tolu balsam. Used externally, Peru balsam often causes skin reactions such as eruptions, ulcers, swelling, and red patches. Allergic reactions are also possible from internal use. It also may increase your sensitivity to sunlight. Tolu balsam is applied as a cream. Before using it for the first time, apply a dab of the cream to a very small area of unbroken skin and then wait for twenty-four hours to make sure there are no contact allergies.

Tolu balsam is used to provide scent to aperitifs, baby powders, baked goods, calamine lotions, chewing gums, fragrances (such as Opium), hair conditioners, hemorrhoid creams, insect repellents, lip balms, and sunscreens. It also comes in a syrup that is used to make a tincture of 200 grams of tolu balsam and 92.3 percent ethanol. The average daily dose is 0.6 gram of the herb.

TURMERIC

Latin name: *Curcuma longa* (Zingiberaceae [ginger] family) Other common names: curcuma, curcumin, gauri, haldi, Indian saffron, jiang huang, you jin

General Description

Turmeric is a perennial plant found in India and throughout southern and eastern Asia, and it is likely indigenous to India. It grows to a height of three feet (one meter) and bears pairs of lance-shaped leaves on alternate sides of the stem, which sprouts from a knobbed rhizome. The root of the plant is used both as a spice and as a medicine. Turmeric is an essential flavoring spice of Indian curries and other cuisine.

Turmeric is a very important herb in ayurvedic medicine. A symbol of prosperity, it was considered a cleansing herb for the whole body. Specifically, it has been used for treatment of inflammation, wounds, and skin ulcers, itching, stomachache, flatulence, constipation, ringworm infestation, and colic. Practitioners of traditional Chinese medicine (TCM) use turmeric to treat liver and gallbladder problems, stop bleeding, and ease chest congestion and menstrual discomforts. It is also used for chest pain, nosebleeds, and heatstroke.

Evidence of Benefit

Turmeric is the primary anti-inflammatory herb of ayurvedic medicine. Its principal chemical component, curcumin, has anticancer effects in cell lines, and is useful for arthritis through its potent antioxidant action. Curcumin also protects the liver, stimulates the gallbladder, and scavenges free radicals.

Curcumin is an excellent herbal remedy for situations in which high concentrations of antioxidants and anti-inflammatory agents are required.

Benefits of turmeric for specific health conditions include the following:

• *Arthritis and postoperative inflammation.* Clinical studies have confirmed that the volatile oil in turmeric can ease acute pain caused by a number of mechanisms. Its effectiveness is equal to that of steroid preparations such as hydrocortisone and phenylbutazone, but without their side effects. Test-tube and laboratory studies have confirmed that curcumin has anti-inflammatory and antiarthritic activity. This accounts for the long-standing tradition in India of using turmeric to prevent and treat inflammatory conditions such as arthritis. It has been shown to be effective in reducing pain in patients with osteoarthritis of the knee. In one study, an extract of turmeric, Meriva, when used at the equivalent of 200 milligrams of curcumin per day, allowed patients with osteoarthritis to use 63 percent less NSAID (nonsteroidal anti-inflammatory drug) medications and still obtain relief from pain.

• *Atherosclerosis.* Curcumin fights atherosclerosis by deactivating platelet-activating factor (PAF) in cell line studies. This component of the blood seals leaks in blood vessels, in part by stimulating the production of fibrous tissue. This tissue can serve as a platform on which cholesterol can accumulate into plaques. In one study using human subjects, curcumin appeared to increase, rather than decrease, cholesterol levels in the blood. However, in a study on patients with osteoarthritis, turmeric was effective at lowering C-reactive protein, an inflammatory marker that predicts who will get heart disease, by sixteen-fold. More work is needed before turmeric can be recommended for patients with elevated blood cholesterol levels.

• *Cancer.* Curcumin causes the death of cancer cells arising from several different types of tissue. In the laboratory, this compound kills cultures of human leukemia cells. Most of the studies in cell lines were done on pancreatic, breast, and colon cancers. Clinical testing has shown that curcumin increases survival rates in melanoma. It inhibits the spread of melanoma to the lungs. By curtailing the activity of PAF, which is necessary for the formation of the new blood vessels that tumors need to grow, curcumin can keep tumors from spreading throughout the body.

Curcumin can aid recovery from cancer by stimulating the immune system. It stimulates the production of B cells, which are usually depleted in people with chronic leukemia, multiple myeloma, and ovarian cancer. It stimulates the production of T cells, which are depleted in Hodgkin's lymphoma, Kaposi's sarcoma, and any form of carcinoma that has spread from the original site. Curcumin also works well with some cancer treatments, preventing lung damage caused by the chemotherapy drug cyclophosphamide (Cytoxan, Neosar) and by whole-body radiation.

Curcumin is also a powerful cancer preventive. It inhibits the action of p450, a liver enzyme that causes environmental toxins to be processed in ways that make them carcinogenic. It is a strong anti-inflammatory agent and a strong antioxidant. Curcumin also is a potent inhibitor of protein kinase C, which can lead to tumor suppression by blocking signal transduction pathways in the target cells. Thus, some have proposed that curcumin could be a potential third-generation cancer chemopreventive agent. Curcumin is especially useful in the prevention and treatment of colorectal cancer. It works in the same manner as NSAIDs, by suppressing the genes necessary for both the start and the spread of cancer. Curcumin suppresses two genes necessary for the development of colorectal cancer. It prevents damage caused by aflatoxin, a poison produced during improper storage of grains and peanuts. In rodents, curcumin significantly suppressed the promotion/ progression stage of colon cancer cells as well as preventing the invasive adenocarcinomas from spreading. In another rodent study of colon cancer, curcumin was added to the rats' diet and suppressed tumor volume by 57 percent compared to a control diet without added curcumin.

Curcumin may also be helpful for women with breast cancer. Curcumin stopped cancer cells from spreading in several breast tumor cell lines including hormone-dependent and hormone-independent lines. Curcumin also induced cell death in breast cancer cells. These results are promising, but those who are undergoing chemotherapy for breast cancer should limit their intake of turmeric because the herb may limit the effectiveness of the drug treatment cyclophosphamide.

• *Cataracts.* Curcumin quenches cell-damaging free radicals more actively than vitamin E, a noted free-radical scavenger. This prevents cross-linking of proteins in the lens that leads, over a period of many years, to the formation of cataracts. However, there are no clinical data to support the use of curcumin for cataracts.

• *Halitosis and periodontal disease.* Turmeric acts against gum inflammation by halting the action of a gene that creates gum-irritating chemicals. This robs bacteria of a site for growth, and helps prevent both bad breath and periodontal disease. If relying on dietary turmeric to prevent bad breath, it is important to avoid use of curries combining turmeric with the herbs that cause bad breath, such as garlic.

• *HIV/AIDS.* Curcumin may help prevent HIV infection from progressing to full-blown AIDS. Curcumin also counteracts integrase, an enzyme HIV needs to attach itself to human DNA, and reduces some of the tissue destruction seen in HIV/AIDS by selectively deactivating tumor necrosis factor (TNF). However, in an eight-week clinical study, thirty-eight patients with HIV infection had no decrease in viral load taking two different doses of turmeric—one higher and one lower. On the other hand, those in the higher dose group had an increase in CD4 cell count, while those taking the smaller dose had a consistent decrease in these cells. One marker of HIV progression is low CD4 counts, so anything that lowers them should be avoided. Even though these changes in CD4 were not significant, more work is needed before turmeric can be recommended for this population.

• *Ulcerative colitis.* Turmeric has been used for thousands of years for gastrointestinal discomforts. A Japanese study found that 2 grams of curcumin a day was superior to usual treatments such as sulfasalazine or mesalamine. It was particularly good at preventing relapse of the disease, but the herb also improved the clinical score for the disease. No side effects were reported with the herb, but there were numerous side effects with conventional medications, including headache, fever, rash, and kidney inflammation.

Considerations for Use

Turmeric is available as a powder and a tincture. It also can be made into a poultice. Curcumin, the antioxidant component of turmeric, is available in capsules and tablets. Be sure to note whether turmeric or curcumin is the form recommended for your condition. Typically, about 60 to 65 percent of curcumin is absorbed by the body, but in one study when coupled with another product from black pepper, piperine, absorption was increased in animals. Curcumin is also sold in combination with bromelain to enhance absorption. Bromelain has some anti-inflammatory benefits of its own that may add to those of curcumin.

People with congestive heart disease whose cause remains unidentified should avoid curcumin. There is evidence that heart disease can result from the overactivity of a gene called p53 that identifies and eliminates weakened cells in the heart. Curcumin protects gene p53 and therefore may indirectly contribute to the destruction of healthy heart tissue. It also should not be used by people with gallstones or bile duct obstruction. Anyone undergoing chemotherapy should limit their intake of turmeric.

Turmeric should not be used for long periods of time, because it can cause stomach distress. It is not recommended for people with hyperactivity, gastrointestinal ulcers, acute bilious colic, or extremely toxic liver disorders.

If you are pregnant, consult your health-care practitioner before using turmeric. One study in laboratory animals indicated that the use of turmeric reduced fertility. If you are trying to conceive or if you have a history of fertility problems, consult your doctor before using turmeric.

Turmeric is thought to inhibit blood-clotting effect. If you have a blood-clotting disorder, you should consult with your doctor before using this herb.

UVA URSI

Latin name: *Arctostaphylos uva-ursi* (Ericaceae [blueberry] family)
Other common names: bearberry, hogberry, kinnikinnick, mealberry, mountain box, red bearberry, rockberry, upland cranberry

General Description

Uva ursi is a low-lying evergreen shrub in the same family as the blueberry and the upland cranberry. Native to Europe, it is naturalized throughout the temperate zones of the Northern Hemisphere northward to the Arctic Circle. It thrives in sunny yet damp conditions in grasslands, heaths, and thickets. Uva ursi has long, trailing stems bearing dark green leaves that are dull on the lower side. Its bell-shaped pink flowers produce small, glossy red berries in late summer. The berries and dried and fresh leaves are used in herbal medicines.

The name *uva ursi* means "bear's grape" in Latin, and comes from the fact that bears are fond of the fruit. According to British herbalist David Chevallier, the medicinal use of the plant was documented as early as the thirteenth century in the Welsh herbal *The Physicians of Myddfai*.

Evidence of Benefit

Uva ursi leaves have been used for centuries as a mild diuretic and in the treatment of bladder and kidney infections. The leaves also have anesthetic properties that help to numb urinary-tract pain. It has been used for liver ailments. Herbalists also recommend the herb as a diuretic for fluid retention, bloating, and swelling. Homeopathic remedies are for inflammation of the urinary tract. The German Commission E has approved uva ursi for infections of the urinary tract. The tannins in uva ursi act as an astringent, and the phenol glucosides have antibacterial effects. The antimicrobial effect is associated with a substance released from arbutin (an extract of the herb). This makes this herb a urine-sterilizing agent, and some practitioners recommend its use internally and externally for inflammatory conditions such as dermatitis, edema, arthritis, and hyperpigmentation disorders.

Benefits of uva ursi for specific health conditions include the following:

• *Bladder infection and cystitis.* Arbutin is the active ingredient in uva ursi. It is an antiseptic for the urinary tract that is particularly effective against *E. coli* infection. It is also effective against *Proteus* infections, provided steps are taken to ensure alkalization of the urine. The sugar portion of arbutin, and its attached small molecule (hydroquinone), must be broken apart for arbutin to be effective, and the urine must be alkaline for this to happen. This herb prevents bleeding in mild kidney disease and urinary tract infection (UTI). In one study, patients with chronic cystitis benefited from a standardized extract of uva ursi and dandelion root. The benefits can't only be attributed to uva ursi, however, as the other herb was included in the product. It seems that uva ursi should not be used to treat acute cystitis, but it reduced recurrent UTIs by 23 percent in this study. In rats, uva ursi has shown diuretic effects, and it seems worth exploring whether it works in humans.

Considerations for Use

Uva ursi is available in the form of capsules or tablets, preferably standardized for arbutin. It also may be taken as a tea. Daily dose is about 3 grams of the uva ursi, which is equal to 100 to 210 milligrams of water-free arbutin.

Uva ursi is effective against the full range of UTIs only if the urine is alkaline. To achieve this effect, you should avoid consuming acidic agents such as meat, vitamin C, and fruit juice, and you also should take ¼ teaspoon (0.5 gram) of baking soda in ¼ cup (50 milliliters) of water with every dose of herb.

Most authorities caution that uva ursi should be avoided by people with chronic kidney disease, including acidic urine, peptic ulcers, or duodenal ulcers. Uva ursi may aggravate gastroesophageal reflux disease.

Herb expert James Duke reports that uva ursi *sometimes* aggravates tinnitus (ringing in the ears). If this effect occurs, it will be noticed after using the herb for two or three days. Ringing in the ears caused by uva ursi should wear off two or three days after the herb is discontinued. Nausea and vomiting may occur in sensitive adults and children. The herb may temporarily turn the urine green. This is a harmless effect. However, liver damage could occur if the herb is used too long, particularly in children.

This herb should not be used by pregnant or nursing women, or by children under twelve. Avoid taking uva ursi for longer than a week. Take all kidney and bladder infections seriously; they can cause complications if not treated promptly. If symptoms of a UTI persist for more than forty-eight hours, you should always seek medical attention. If you develop symptoms such as high fever, chills, nausea, vomiting, diarrhea, or severe back pain, get medical assistance immediately.

Iron can form harmful complexes when used at the same time as uva ursi; separate the two by one to two hours. Do not use uva ursi if you take thiazide and loop diuretics because the purpose of these drugs is to rid the body of sodium, and uva ursi will cause the body to retain it.

VALERIAN

Latin name: *Valeriana officinalis* (Valerianaceae [valerian] family)
Other common names: all-heal, amantilla, capon's tail, setewale, vandal root, wetwall

General Description

Valerian is a perennial plant native to Europe and northern Asia. It is mainly cultivated in central Europe, England, France, Eastern Europe, Japan, and the United States. It grows four feet (120 centimeters) tall, and bears pinnate leaves and pink flower heads. The root is the part of the plant used in herbal medicine. Valerian root must be carefully dried at temperatures below 105°F (40°C) before use. The taste is both sweet and spicy, and somewhat bitter, but the odor is unpleasant.

Valerian has been used medicinally at least since the time of Hippocrates (460–377 B.C.E.). Ancient medical texts refer to the unpleasant odor of the herb by naming it *phu*.

Evidence of Benefit

Valerian is a tranquilizer and calmative useful for disorders such as restlessness, nervousness, insomnia, hysteria, menstrual problems, headaches, and nervous stomach. It has also been used for menstrual states of agitation, menopause, neuralgia, fainting, and colic uterine spasticity, but many of these uses are unproven. Valerian alkaloids have been known to lower blood pressure. The German Commission E has approved valerian for restlessness and sleeping disorders based on nervous conditions.

Benefits of valerian for specific health conditions include the following:

• *Anxiety, depression, insomnia, and menopause-related problems.* In a large-scale review of human studies on valerian for anxiety, only one seemed to show promise. One of the most common side effects of anxiety and depression is sleep disorders. In one study, people with depression, anxiety, and sleeping issues benefited from a combination of St. John's wort and valerian. The optimal combination for reducing anxiety and improving sleep was 600 milligrams of St. John's wort and 1,000 milligrams of valerian, and the effects took about ten days to manifest.

Most large-scale scientific studies have confirmed valerian's ability to improve the quality of sleep and relieve insomnia, especially the insomnia that sometimes accompanies menopause. These effects occurred without numerous side effects. Dozens of over-the-counter (OTC) sleep aids contain valerian. A double-blind study with 128 participants showed that taking a water-based extract of valerian both improved subjective ratings of sleep quality and reduced sleep latency, the time required to fall asleep. Valerian relieved insomnia without causing grogginess or "hangover" the next morning.

A follow-up study found that valerian was as effective in inducing sleep as barbiturates such as pentobarbital and benzodiazepines such as chlordiazepoxide (Librium). These drugs cause morning sleepiness. Valerian, in contrast, reduced morning sleepiness. The difference, apparently, was that valerian appeared to be nonaddictive and its effects seemed to be milder.

Valerian has a much more pronounced effect when used by people with chronic insomnia than when used by people whose sleeping difficulties are temporary. It is especially suitable for older adults who fall asleep relatively easily but have difficulty staying asleep throughout the night. In addition, this herb relieves panic attacks that occur at night. One clinical study found that using valerian together with St. John's wort was an effective alternative to diazepam (Valium). Some studies in animals have confirmed that valerian does not show overt sedative or tranquilizing effects as compared to diazepam (Valium). Researchers say that a combination of hops and valerian may be as effective as benzodiazepine medications (the group of drugs that includes Valium) for nonchronic and nonpsychiatric sleep disorders.

Valerian has been used safely and effectively in children aged five to fourteen years with sleep difficulties. In one well-controlled trial, where exact measurements of valerian were used daily, children who were intellectually and neurologically deficient (IQ under 70) and their parents slept better and for a longer time period. Do not give valerian to your child without speaking to a pediatrician.

• *Indigestion.* Valerian relaxes the muscles of the digestive tract when under stress. It soothes the digestive system and relieves some types of indigestion, constipation, and stomach cramps, especially when these problems are due to nervous tension.

• *Irritable bowel syndrome (IBS).* Naturopathic physicians sometimes prescribe valerian as one of a combination of herbs useful for the treatment of IBS. One of the chemicals produced when valerian is processed, valerenic acid, not only encourages sleep but also reduces muscle spasms. Although valerenic acid makes sleeping easier, as noted above, it does not force sleep by inducing drowsiness.

Considerations for Use

Valerian is available in the form of valepotriate tablets and as tinctures. The herb can also be made into tea, and it can be used in bathwater. Typical amounts are ½ to 1 teaspoon of the tincture, 2 to 3 grams of the herb, and 100 grams for a bath.

In its natural state, valerian contains a compound known to aid sleep, its essential oil. For this reason, valerian preparations used for insomnia usually state their essential oil content. However, if valerian is combined with herbs such as hops and lemon balm (melissa), a different set of chemicals is responsible for the promotion of sleep. In these compounds, the content of essential oil is not important.

People who use valerian for several months may experience withdrawal symptoms (agitation, headache, insomnia, and racing heart) if they *abruptly* stop using the herb. Used by itself, valerian is almost always free of side effects, although it can increase side effects of barbiturates and tranquilizers such as alprazolam (Xanax), chlordiazepoxide (Librium), diazepam (Valium), or lorazepam (Ativan).

Do not use valerian if you have liver disease, as there have been reports of liver toxicity. Some people complain of gastrointestinal side effects. Symptoms of overdose may include paralysis, weakening of the heartbeat, giddiness, lightheadedness, blurred vision, restlessness, nausea, and, possibly, liver toxicity. Valerian should not be used with prescription medications such as diazepam (Valium) or amitriptyline (Elavil), or with sedative or antidepressant drugs, before consulting with a physician. You should not continue taking valerian if you experience heart palpitations or nervousness after taking it. This herb should not be given to children under the age of fourteen years. It should not be taken with alcohol, nor should it be used by pregnant women or nursing mothers. If you are taking iron, allow one to two hours between taking the iron and the valerian.

Research indicates that valerian does not impair one's ability to drive a car or operate machinery. However, there does appear to be some impairment of attention for a couple of hours after taking valerian. For this reason, it is not a good idea to drive immediately after taking it.

VARUNA

Latin name: *Crataeva nurvula* (Capparaceae [caper] family)
Other common names: barun (in ayurvedic medicine), crataeva, three-leaved caper

General Description

The varuna is a large, deciduous tree frequently cultivated in the vicinity of temples in Bangladesh and India. Growing to a height of fifty feet (fifteen meters), it bears pale yellow flowers and a smooth brown bark. The leaves are harvested in spring and the bark is cut year-round for use in herbal medicine.

Evidence of Benefit

Varuna is the primary ayurvedic herb for kidney and prostate problems. It also has been used to fight urinary tract infections (UTIs).

Benefits of varuna for specific health conditions include the following:

• *Benign prostatic hypertrophy (BPH).* Ayurvedic medicine has traditionally used varuna to relieve difficulty in urination caused by enlargement of the prostate. This effect is probably due to the herb's content of lupeol, a chemical that deactivates enzymes needed to manufacture inflammation-inducing leukotrienes.

• *Kidney stones.* Ayurvedic medicine has used varuna bark to treat kidney stones for over 3,000 years. Scientific research has confirmed that varuna deactivates the enzyme glycolate oxidase. This reduces the body's production of oxalates, which combine with calcium to form kidney stones. One of the other chemical components of varuna, lupeol, reduces the levels of various laboratory markers of kidney damage.

Considerations for Use

Varuna can be taken as a tea or as a tincture. Since this herb is most readily available from practitioners of ayurveda, it should be taken according to the directions given by the herbalist or physician recommending it.

VITEX

Latin name: *Vitex agnus castus* (Verbenaceae [verbena] family)
Other common names: chaste berry, chaste tree fruit, monk's pepper, vitex agnus-castus

General Description

Vitex is an aromatic deciduous tree native to Greece and Italy, and other places in the Mediterranean region and as far as western Asia. It grows to a height of twenty-one feet (seven meters) and bears palm-shaped leaves and small, lilaclike flowers. The ripe yellow-red berries have been harvested in the fall for use in herbal medicine for thousands of years in both Europe and China. In Europe, herbalists also use the leaves and flower tops.

The Greeks knew of vitex in the time of Homer, more than 1,000 years before it was used in China. Homer's seventh century B.C.E. epic the *Iliad* mentions vitex as a symbol of chastity capable of protecting people against evil. According to the first-century Roman historian Pliny, chaste berries strewn on the beds of soldiers' wives was a testimony of the wives' faithfulness while their husbands were in battle. As the common name of the plant, chaste tree, suggests, vitex was thought to reduce the libido. Vitex berries were chewed by monks to stop unwanted sexual desire.

Evidence of Benefit

Vitex has the effect of stimulating and normalizing pituitary gland function. It normalizes the activity of female sex hormones, and is indicated for dysmenorrhea, premenstrual syndrome (PMS), menopausal symptoms, mastalgia (breast pain), and other disorders related to hormone imbalance. Unlike other herbs used for this purpose, vitex does not contain plant estrogens. Instead, it contains at least two forms of testosterone, as well as the growth-stimulant hormones androstenedione and progesterone. Vitex also seems to lower production of the hormone prolactin. Unproven uses for vitex include increasing milk production during lactation, controlling libido, reducing flatulence, suppressing appetite, and inducing sleep. It has also been used for treatment of erectile dysfunction (ED), prostatitis, swelling of the testes, and uterine pain. Homeopathic remedies are available for male sexual disturbances, disturbances of milk flow, and nervous depression. The German Commission E has approved it for irregularities in menstrual cycle, premenstrual complaints, and breast pain. However, the commission cautions that for swelling in the breast or disturbances in menstruation, a physician should be consulted.

Benefits of vitex for specific health conditions include the following:

• *Acne, breast pain, menopause-related problems, menstrual problems, and PMS.* Symptoms related to the menstrual cycle, including cramps, breast pain, and acne flare-ups, among a host of others, are often caused by hormonal imbalances during the luteal phase of the menstrual cycle, the phase that occurs after an egg is released from the ovary. Sometimes, the corpus luteum, the yellowish ovarian scar that forms after the egg is released, produces inadequate amounts of estrogen and progesterone or excessive amounts of testosterone. Vitex restores progesterone concentration by acting on the pituitary-hypothalamic axis rather than directly on the ovaries. A German study found that vitex can reestablish the luteal phase of the period in women whose periods are abnormally short. One particular product, Agnolyt, which contained 9 grams of vitex berry tincture per 100 grams of product, was used in the German study. In addition to balancing hormones, vitex may reduce pain. The analgesic effect of the herb may be due to its content of agnoside.

The most important use of vitex in England is in treating menopausal symptoms. For relieving symptoms such as hot flashes, positive results should be noticed after three months of taking vitex daily. In one study, women took 20 milligrams of a standardized vitex preparation three times a day. Compared to a placebo group, those in the herb group had improved mood, less irritability and anger, and less breast tenderness. Half of the women who got vitex responded favorably. Another study found that 40 milligrams of vitex extract was sufficient to reduce the side effects of PMS in patients with mild to moderate PMS. In another study, two groups of women with breast pain (mastalgia) associated with menstrual cycles were compared; the first group took vitex and the second group a placebo. Half as many women reported to be breast-pain-free in the herb group compared to the placebo group (15 percent versus 8 percent).

Several studies indicate that vitex can help control acne in teenagers, both male and female. It usually starts working after ten days; however, it may take six months or longer to see its full benefit. One side effect of vitex is acne, so caution should be used when taking this herb for this condition.

• *Endometriosis and infertility.* German and Austrian physicians take advantage of vitex's ability to increase the production of progesterone in treating endometriosis, a condition in which the endometrial tissue normally found within the uterus escapes into the abdominal cavity, causing pain and menstrual difficulties. Because it stimulates growth of the uterine lining, vitex is thought to help reverse infertility. However, in one study, a homeopathic remedy containing vitex did not show benefit for female sterility. Further trials are warranted.

• *Prostate cancer.* Theoretically, there are grounds for believing that vitex could be useful in treating prostate cancer, and the herb is frequently recommended for this purpose. At least in laboratory studies, vitex reduces the production of prolactin, a hormone responsible for converting testosterone to dihydrotestosterone, which in turn stimulates the growth of prostate cancer cells. Reducing the production of prolactin theoretically should slow the growth of prostate cancer cells. Whether this effect takes place in the human body, however, is not yet known. Since vitex contains both compounds that stop the conversion of testosterone and the testosterone compounds themselves, it is probably too risky to use this herb as a treatment for prostate cancer. It is not advised to use vitex if you have any hormone-sensitive cancer, such as prostate cancer.

Considerations for Use

Vitex is available in capsules, tablets, and tinctures. In using this herb, it is important to remember that for long-term relief, it is necessary to continue taking the herb for three to six months after symptoms disappear. Vitex should be taken in the morning.

In very rare cases, using vitex can result in a longer period or heavier menstruation. Women of reproductive age must use vitex with caution, since it has been known to stimulate the release of multiple eggs from the ovary, potentially resulting in multiple births. Pregnant women should not take vitex. Despite the herb's traditional use to stimulate lactation, nursing mothers should avoid it because it suppresses the hormone prolactin, which is essential for breast-milk production. Men seeking to become fathers should not take vitex. Animal studies indicate that the seeds can completely halt sperm production, reduce testosterone production, and cause the testicles to atrophy.

Vitex should not be combined with estrogen replacement therapy (ERT) or with birth control pills. Women with estrogen-sensitive cancers originating in the breast, cervix, or uterus should avoid vitex. Animal experiments indicate that medications to regulate dopamine in the brain may be affected in unpredictable ways by this herb. These medications include the psychoactive medication haloperidol (Haldol), prescribed for psychosis, and buproprion (Zyban), prescribed to help smokers who want to quit. Vitex should be used with caution by those who are weak or anemic. Minor gastrointestinal upset and a mild skin rash with itching have been reported in less than 2 percent of the women monitored while taking vitex. Others have reported itching, nausea, vomiting, dry mouth, dizziness, confusion, drowsiness, and agitation while taking vitex.

WALNUT LEAF

Latin names: *Juglans nigra, Juglans regia* (Juglandaceae [walnut] family)
Other common names: black walnut, Caucasian walnut, Circassian walnut, white walnut

General Description

Walnut trees are native to the dry temperate zones of western Asia, China, India, and the southwestern United States. The tree most often used in herbal medicine, the species native to western Asia, also is cultivated for commercial walnut production in Europe and the United States. The leaves are gathered in spring and summer and dried for medicinal purposes.

Walnut leaves have been used in herbal medicine for thousands of years. The Roman naturalist Pliny the Elder reported the cultivation of walnut trees in the first century, the trees having reached Rome from the Middle East. The

Latin name of the tree is derived from reference to the god Jupiter; *Juglans* is derived from combining the name *Jupiter* with *glans* (acorn), meaning "Jupiter's nuts." The famed seventeenth-century English herbalist Nicholas Culpepper combined walnut leaf with honey, onion, and salt to draw out venom from the bites of snakes and spiders.

Evidence of Benefit

During the last century, walnut leaf has been known as one of the "most mild and efficacious laxatives" available. Chinese medicine uses it to treat asthma, beriberi, erectile dysfunction (ED), and constipation. Ayurvedic medicine uses it for rheumatic complaints. The oil of the seeds was used for tapeworm but was reported to have aphrodisiac effects as well as to be useful for dysentery and colic. It has been used as a blood purifier. White walnut also is used in homeopathy as a treatment for liver disorders and intestinal sickness.

Another species of walnut, the black walnut (*J. nigra*), has been used to treat athlete's foot and parasitic infections. Black walnut bark helps relieve constipation and is useful against fungal and parasitic infections. It is used to expel, rather than kill, worms during the normal course of laxative-induced cleansing of the body. Used externally, black walnut is beneficial for eczema, herpes, psoriasis, and skin parasites. It has been shown to exhibit anticancer properties due to the acids and alkaloids it contains. However, other substances such as juglone (a chemical) found in the walnut hulls have been shown to have mutagenic action, and topical use of the hulls has been linked to cancer of the lips and tongue.

The German Commission E has approved walnut leaf for mild, superficial inflammation of the skin and excessive perspiration, especially of the hands and feet.

Benefits of walnut leaf for specific health conditions include the following:

• *Acne and eczema.* Walnut leaves contain astringent tannins. These tannins cross-link skin cells, making them less impermeable to infectious microorganisms, especially fungi. Walnut leaves contain two antibacterial agents, walnut essential oil and juglone, which act directly on infectious microorganisms.

• *Excessive sweating.* Walnut leaf washes "shrink" the sweat glands, possibly reducing perspiration. The herb's tannins cause proteins in the cells lining the sweat glands to cross-link, effectively forming a barrier to the excretion of sweat.

Considerations for Use

Walnut leaf teas can be made into baths, compresses, and skin washes. This herb product is more likely to be obtained from herb shops and other herb suppliers. There are many products that are made with walnut *hulls* combined with other herbs in tinctures for use as a harsh laxative. You should not use walnut hulls instead of walnut leaf for the conditions discussed above.

WILD ANGELICA

Latin name: *Angelica archangelica* (Apiaceae [parsley] family) Other common names: angel's wort, bai zhi, Chinese angelica root, European angelica, garden angelica

General Description

Wild angelica is a sturdy three- to seven-foot (one- to two-meter) shrub topped with flowers similar to those found on Queen Anne's lace. It has a hollow stem and bears three-branched leaves. The herb is harvested between summer and autumn, when the leaves turn yellow. The root is cut lengthwise into thin slices for use in teas. Wild angelica is considered a warm herb, with a spicy flavor. It is found wild on the coasts of the North and Baltic Seas, America, Europe, and China; each cultivates a different species of the plant.

Evidence of Benefit

In laboratory studies, wild angelica inhibits bacteria and viruses, reduces fever, and stimulates respiration. It acts as a disinfectant against a number of infectious microorganisms, including *E. coli,* a cause of diarrhea sometimes from foods. In laboratory studies, it helps to open the coronary blood vessels and increase circulation to the heart. This herb has not been shown to work in people, however.

Benefits of wild angelica for specific health conditions include the following:

• *Diabetes and overweight.* Wild angelica may be useful to fight weight gain, one of the more troubling side effects of oral medications for diabetes. Most of the older medications for type 2 diabetes act by stimulating the pancreas to make insulin. Insulin not only transports glucose into all the cells of the body, but also transports fat into fat cells. In laboratory tests, chemicals in wild angelica cause insulin to move sugar into muscle cells, thus potentially helping to prevent weight gain.

• *Fracture.* Wild angelica could be helpful to reduce the risk of bone fracture in female athletes with irregular menstrual cycles. It also can be helpful to reduce the risk of fracture among people taking steroid treatment. It accomplishes this by inhibiting the release of histamine, but clinical studies are lacking to show that it works.

Considerations for Use

Wild angelica is used in capsules and teas. The easiest way to get the herb is from practitioners of traditional Chinese medicine (TCM). The Chinese term for the herb is *bai zhi.* This herb should not be used during pregnancy. Wild angelica should not be put on open sores.

WILD YAM

Latin name: *Dioscorea opposita* (Dioscoreaceae [yam] family). In the United States, it is often referred to as *Dioscorea villosa.*

Other common names: China root, Chinese yam, colic root, devil's bones, dioscorea, medicinal yam, Mexican yam, tokoro, yuma

General Description

Wild yam is native to moist tropical zones around the world, but it is indigenous to the southern United States and Canada. In the tropics, wild yam vines can climb to a height of twenty feet (six meters), bearing heart-shaped leaves and tiny green flowers. Herbal formulas call for thick, diagonal slices of peeled rhizome. Powdered wild yam serves as a thickening agent for many foods.

Evidence of Benefit

Wild yam has antispasmodic, analgesic, antiarthritic, antiasthmatic, antidiabetic, antitussive, and expectorant effects. It is used for rheumatism, dysmenorrhea, cramps, colic, irritable bowel syndrome (IBS), kidney stones, and neuralgia. In animals, it has been shown to decrease inflammation of the intestine which was induced by indomethacin (a nonsteroidal anti-inflammatory drug [NSAID]) use. In rats it increased bile flow. In an ovariectomized mouse model, wild yam showed estrogen effects and supported mammary development. The root is used as a precursor for manufacturing progesterone and estrogen. It is touted as a natural progesterone, but it has no progesterone-like effects.

Benefits of wild yam for specific health conditions include the following:

• *Female reproductive-tract disorders.* In North and Central America, wild yam is a traditional relaxing remedy for painful and irregular menstruation and ovarian pain. The herb's action is not related to estrogen balance, but rather to its anti-inflammatory action. Diosgenin, a saponin found in wild yam, was shown to have estrogenic and progestogenic effects in mice. It is thought that diosgenin can be converted by the human body into progesterone and other steroid hormones via dehydroepiandrosterone. No scientific evidence supports this idea, however.

• *Heart disease in older people.* In a small group of subjects over the age of sixty-five years, a product with 90 percent wild yam and other herbs such as kola nut and country mallow (EMPRISE) did not significantly affect dehydroepiandrosterone (DHEA) levels. However, reductions in serum triglycerides and phospholipids occurred when wild yam and DHEA were taken together. High-density lipoprotein (HDL, or "good") cholesterol increased as well, but total cholesterol did not change.

• *Menopause.* In a randomized study of fifty women with menopausal symptoms, a wild yam cream was not more effective than a placebo. One teaspoon of the cream was applied twice daily for three months. There were no significant differences in blood pressure, weight, and biochemical and hormonal parameters associated with menopause. There were no side effects.

Considerations for Use

Wild yam is most conveniently used as a tincture, although capsules, creams, and teas may be slightly more effective for the relief of pain. Wild yam is effective even in very low doses and has virtually no toxicity. There is some evidence that wild yam may decrease the anti-inflammatory effect of indomethacin (a NSAID). It may also have an additive estrogenic effect when administered with estrogen-containing drugs. Patients with hormone-sensitive cancers should avoid wild yam.

Some over-the-counter (OTC) medicines sold as wild yam creams contain synthetic progesterone, the same compound used in birth control pills. Almost always, this progesterone is not listed on the label. Be sure to verify that any product you purchase is made solely from herbal ingredients. You should not use wild yam if you are pregnant or nursing.

WILLOW BARK

Latin name: *Salix* species (Salicaceae [willow] family)
Other common names: bay willow, black willow, European willow, pussy willow, white willow bark (*Salicacea alba*)

General Description

Native to Europe, North America, northern Asia, and much of Africa, the willow is usually a low-growing deciduous tree. Under optimum growing conditions, however, it grows to a height of eighty feet (twenty-five meters), bearing green, tapering leaves and catkins in spring. Bark is stripped from two- to five-year-old trees in spring for medicinal use.

Almost 2,000 years ago, the Greek physician Dioscorides recommended "willow leaves, mashed with a little pepper and drunk with wine" to treat lower back pain. During the Middle Ages, willow bark was used in Europe to reduce fever and relieve pain. In 1899, the Bayer Company in Germany introduced a drug composed of a synthetic chemical compound similar to the active compound found in willow bark. Originally used as a brand name, Bayer's term for its product later became one of the best-known generic medicine names—aspirin.

Evidence of Benefit

Like aspirin, willow bark is a proven painkiller, but without many of aspirin's side effects. The analgesic actions of willow are typically slower acting but last longer than standard aspirin products. As with aspirin, uses for willow bark include fever, colds, minor infections, acute and chronic rheumatic disorders, mild headaches, and pain caused by inflammation. Willow bark is also high in tannins, suggesting that it may be of some use in gastrointestinal disorders. The German Commission E has approved its use for disease accompanied by pain, fever, rheumatic ailments, and headaches.

Benefits of willow bark for specific health conditions include the following:

• *Arthritis.* Aspirin has an advantage over its herbal parent in that it is more sure-acting, as willow bark depends on the presence of "friendly" intestinal bacteria to properly digest its components into painkilling compounds. On the other hand, the analgesic compounds from willow bark remain in circulation longer than those from aspirin. The amount of pain-relieving compounds available from willow bark remains at stable levels in the bloodstream for several hours. Unlike aspirin, the salicylates from willow bark have no effect on blood platelets and do not increase bleeding. Clinical testing of willow bark has been conducted in England. Researchers at the Centre for Complementary Health Studies at the University of Exeter gave eighty-two participants with chronic arthritic pain either Reumalex, an herbal drug containing willow bark, or a placebo. After two months of use, the willow bark medication was found to be superior to the placebo pill.

• *Dry mouth.* A clinical study involving ten patients who had had radiation treatment found that Salix SST, a saliva-stimulating lozenge containing the active principles of willow bark, relieved symptoms of dry mouth and improved sleep and speech.

• *Lower back pain and osteoporosis.* Studies have shown that willow bark has pain-relieving effects on people with chronic lower back and osteoporotic pain within a month. One study found that a combination herbal product containing 120 milligrams of salicin from white willow bark reduced knee pain and improved functioning in people with osteoarthritis.

Considerations for Use

Willow bark is available as capsules and salicin tablets, and in various formulations designed specifically for migraines. The typical dose is 60 to 120 milligrams of salicin, which is about 6 to 12 grams of the herb. In Native American medicine, willow bark is used to reduce sexual desire. Chronic use of willow bark may result in diminished sexual interest, although it does not affect physical aspects of sexual performance in either men or women.

If you have had any type of allergic reaction to aspirin or other salicylates, you should not use willow bark. Do not use it if you are pregnant or nursing. Do not take it in combination with aspirin. Long-term use of willow bark is not advisable. Do not give willow bark to a child under sixteen years of age who has symptoms of flu, chickenpox, or any other type of viral infection. As with aspirin, there may be a risk of developing a rare but serious ailment called Reye's syndrome. Do not use willow bark if you have active gastric or duodenal ulcer, hemophilia, asthma, or diabetes. If you are taking blood-thinners or nonsteroidal anti-inflammatory drugs (NSAIDs) avoid white willow–containing products. Limit your intake of alcohol and barbiturates when using this herb, as they may mask symptoms of salicylate overdose and may enhance the toxicity of the salicin from white willow.

WINTERGREEN

Latin name: *Gaultheria procumbens* (Ericaceae [blueberry] family)
Other common names: boxberry, Canada tea, checkerberry, partridge berry, spiceberry, teaberry, wax cluster

General Description

Wintergreen is an aromatic, creeping shrub native to the eastern and northern United States and Canada. It has leathery, oval leaves, small pink or white bell-shaped flowers, and bright red fruit. The berries are used medicinally, and an essential oil is distilled from the herb's glossy green leaves. The oil was once popular as a flavoring in candies, toothpastes, and food, and as an aromatic agent in perfumes.

Native Americans brewed a tea from the leaves to alleviate rheumatic symptoms, headache, fever, sore throat, and various aches and pains. During the American Revolution, wintergreen leaves were used as a substitute for tea, which was then scarce.

Evidence of Benefit

Wintergreen has pain-relieving properties similar to those of aspirin, as well as a refreshing taste. It is good for headaches, arthritis, and muscle and back pain. Regularly applied to painfully swollen, inflamed, or sore muscles and joints, especially if caused by injuries or rheumatic ailments, the essential oil helps to relieve pain. In folk medicine, it has been used for asthma and as an antiseptic.

Benefits of wintergreen for specific health conditions include the following:

• *Carpal tunnel syndrome, sore muscles and joints, and toothache.* Wintergreen oil contains almost 98 percent methyl salicylate. Salicylate is the principal component in aspirin. Wintergreen oil relieves pain through the same mechanism as aspirin, stopping the hormonal reactions that cause inflammation and pain.

Wintergreen also contains small amounts of astringent compounds, called tannins, and a soothing and softening substance called mucilage. They help indirectly to alleviate soreness in muscles and joints, and explain why this herb was traditionally used as a gargle for sore throats.

Considerations for Use

Wintergreen is available as a mouthwash and as an essential oil. The essential oil should be used for external use *only.* It can be used as part of an aromatherapy blend to increase mucus output and clear airways. Wintergreen oil can be harmful if taken internally. If pure wintergreen oil is ingested by a child, 1 teaspoon can be fatal.

Externally, essential oil of wintergreen should be used only for acute pain, since it can be absorbed through the skin and can become toxic to the kidneys and liver. You should not apply the oil to your skin for more than three days out of any month, and you should not use wintergreen oil if you have any degree of chronic kidney or liver disease. You should not apply the oil to the skin of a child under the age of twelve unless directed to do so by a medical professional.

Formulations containing concentrations of 10 to 60 percent methyl salicylate can be applied externally up to four times daily. They should not be used after strenuous exercise or in conjunction with a heating pad, however. Follow package instructions and avoid applying these products after vigorous exercise or in hot weather. Doing so can result in dangerous amounts of certain compounds being absorbed through your skin and into your system.

If you take warfarin (Coumadin) or any other prescription blood-thinning medication, do not use wintergreen, as bleeding problems and other adverse reactions may occur. People taking blood-thinning medication should avoid using any products that contain methyl salicylate.

WITCH HAZEL

Latin name: *Hamamelis virginiana* (Hamamelidaceae [witch hazel] family)
Other common names: hamamelis, hazel nut, snapping hazel, spotted alder winterbloom

General Description

Witch hazel is a leathery-leafed shrub native to the Atlantic seaboard of the United States. The upward-facing surface of its leaves are shiny green, but the bottoms of the leaves are dull gray. Witch hazel trees stand out in the forest in the autumn because as other trees are losing their leaves, the witch hazel is covered with golden-yellow, thread-like flowers, thus making it appealing to landscapers as a desirable ornamental plant. Both the bark and the leaves of the plant are used medicinally.

Native Americans introduced witch hazel to early European settlers. The Native Americans applied a strained decoction of the leaves and twigs to small wounds, insect bites, sore muscles, and joints. They also sipped witch hazel tea to treat bleeding, inflammation, and hemorrhoids. In the nineteenth century, an alcoholic extract of witch hazel was one of the most popular herbs in the United States.

Evidence of Benefit

Witch hazel is a valuable cooling topical astringent for various ailments, including varicose veins, hemorrhoids, abrasions, bruises, and other skin irritations. It is also good for clearing up the redness produced by eczema and for smoothing wrinkles. Witch hazel is used in pads to help soothe discomfort from rectal and vaginal surgery and stitches. The bark decoction also is useful as a gargle in relieving sore throat. There are homeopathic remedies for hemorrhoids, varicose veins, skin inflammation, and bleeding of the mucous membranes. The German Commission E has approved its use for minor injuries of the skin (burns and wounds), local inflammation of the skin and mucous membranes (mouth and pharynx), hemorrhoids, and varicose veins.

Benefits of witch hazel for specific health conditions include the following:

• *Cuts and scrapes, insect bites and stings, and sunburn.* Witch hazel helps to relieve the itching of poison ivy and helps to dry out cold sores. It relieves the itching and burning of insect stings. A tannin found in witch hazel, hamamelitannin (5 percent), has been shown to constrict blood vessels and stem bleeding from abrasions due to shaving nicks. Other tannins in witch hazel help to keep wounds clean, prevent swelling, and combat infection. Witch hazel can cool sunburn and other minor burns. A commercial witch hazel lotion marketed as Eucerin has an anti-inflammatory effect on sunburn. In one clinical study, Eucerin helped reduce sunburn inflammation by 20 percent after seven hours and by 27 percent after forty-eight hours, as compared with 11 to 15 percent, respectively, for other lotions.

• *Diarrhea.* Both witch hazel bark and witch hazel leaf teas are effective against diarrhea, but the gentler witch hazel bark teas are better for use in treating diarrhea (and stomach upset) in children. Check with a pediatrician before giving this tea to a child.

• *Eczema.* A double-blind placebo-controlled clinical test found that witch hazel cream was not as effective as hydrocortisone, but offered a mild yet unmistakable anti-inflammatory effect for eczema, without the side effects of prednisone.

• *Hemorrhoids and varicose veins.* Laboratory experiments have confirmed that witch hazel leaf tinctures (at least if they are injected) increase the tone of the veins. The compounds that perform this function are not found in witch hazel teas or steam-processed witch hazel "water," but rather in alcohol tinctures of the herb. Witch hazel poultices prevent bleeding and weeping from external hemorrhoids. Witch hazel is used in several commercial over-the-counter (OTC) preparations for hemorrhoids, including Tucks and Preparation H. Other commercial products for these conditions frequently combine witch hazel with horse chestnut. (*See* HORSE CHESTNUT.)

• *Periodontal disease.* Witch hazel leaf gargles and mouthwashes form a protective lining over the mucous membranes of the gums and mouth. These products may be useful for sore gums that are accompanied by sore throat.

Considerations for Use

Witch hazel is available as creams, teas, and tinctures; it can also be made into poultices. Do not use the commonly available witch hazel water. While witch hazel water has been approved by the U.S. Food and Drug Administration (FDA), its healing benefits derive from the alcohol rather than the witch hazel itself.

Witch hazel bark teas are intended for treatment of acute rather than chronic diarrhea. If diarrhea persists longer than three days, consult a physician. Always be sure to replace fluids lost during diarrhea by drinking adequate amounts of water.

Witch hazel may cause stomach upset, nausea, vomiting, or constipation, and in rare cases the bark may cause liver damage if too much is absorbed. The volatile oil contains a known carcinogen (safrole), but in small amounts it is unlikely to pose any risk. Due to its high tannin content, witch hazel should not be used over long periods of time. Do not use the commercially prepared witch hazel water internally.

YARROW

Latin name: *Achillea millefolium* (Asteraceae [composite] family)
Other common names: band man's plaything, bloodwort, devil's nettle, milfoil, old man's pepper, soldier's woundwort, thousand weed

General Description

Yarrow is a creeping perennial plant. Growing three feet (one meter) tall, it has white or, occasionally, rose-colored flower heads with yellow centers. Its species name *millefolium* refers to its "thousand leaves." Finely divided, crowded leaves grow on alternate sides of its erect central stems. The leaves, stems, and flowers are used medicinally.

Yarrow appears to have been used as a healing agent virtually since the dawn of the human race. Excavation of a 40,000- to 60,000-year-old Neanderthal grave yielded yarrow (as well as the herbs althea, centauria, ephedra, and senecio). Yarrow's scientific name, *Achillea*, refers to the Greek legend of its use in ointments in the Trojan War. According to legend, Achilles used yarrow to stop bleeding in his soldiers.

Traditional herbalists in Europe, China, and India have used yarrow to stop minor bleeding and to treat wounds and inflammation, especially in the intestinal and female reproductive tracts. It also has traditionally been used as a mild sedative.

Evidence of Benefit

Yarrow is an anti-inflammatory herb useful in the treatment of diarrhea, flatulence, gastrointestinal inflammation, and stomach cramps. This herb can reduce smooth-muscle spasms, which makes it useful for certain gastrointestinal conditions. Yarrow is also a traditional stomach tonic and digestive aid. Unproven uses include as an external palliative treatment for liver disorders and for healing wounds. In folk medicine, it is used for bleeding hemorrhoids, and as a bath to remove perspiration. Homeopathic remedies are for varicose veins, arterial bleeding, and convulsions. Ayurvedic medicine uses a combination of yarrow (*A. millefolium*) with other herbs for patients with liver cirrhosis. Yarrow has anti-inflammatory, antioxidative, immuno-stimulating, and diuretic actions; all of these help patients with cirrhosis by reducing liver blood test values and improving liver test scores (called Child-Pugh).

Yarrow tea has long been used to induce sweating and lower fever. This herb has mild sedative properties that may prevent insomnia. Herbalists prescribe yarrow to relieve cramps and other menstrual pain. It has been approved by the German Commission E internally for loss of appetite and dyspeptic ailments such as mild spastic discomforts of the gastrointestinal tract. Externally it has been used in a sitz bath for painful, cramp-like conditions of psychosomatic origin (in the lower part of the female pelvis).

Benefits of yarrow for specific health conditions include the following:

- *Bruises and pain.* Modern research has confirmed the historical use of yarrow to relieve pain caused by a broad range of conditions. Yarrow teas and tinctures contain salicylate-like derivatives such as stigmasterol and beta-sitosterol that reduce the inflammatory processes, which may accelerate healing. These compounds stop the formation of enzymes necessary for a series of chemical reactions that cause inflammation and pain. Yarrow also contains compounds designated sesquiterpene lactones, which reduce the action of pain-provoking hormones, the prostaglandins. Besides stopping pain, yarrow teas and tinctures kill many kinds of bacteria, some of which, such as *Staphylococcus aureus,* are found on human skin, thus indirectly preventing pain by halting potentially painful infection. In animal studies, a chloroform extract of yarrow (*A. millefolium*) when applied topically had anti-inflammatory effects.

- *Common cold and influenza.* Essential oil of yarrow is used in aromatherapy to relieve colds and flu. The compounds chamazulene and prochamazulene, which are found in the essential oil, are known to act as anti-inflammatory agents. Yarrow is also combined with echinacea, elder flower, ginger, and peppermint leaf in over-the-counter (OTC) extracts used for cold and flu relief.

- *Heart disease and high blood pressure.* In one study, 15 to 20 drops twice a day of a 70 percent ethanol extract of yarrow (*A. wilhelmsii*) lowered low-density lipoprotein (LDL, or "bad") cholesterol in participants after four months, and it continued to go down at month six. There was no change in cholesterol levels in the placebo group. At six months, triglycerides were significantly reduced and high-density lipoprotein (HDL, or "good") cholesterol increased. In another study, using the same yarrow extract product and the same dose, significant decreases in systolic and diastolic blood pressure occurred in patients with stage I hypertension after six months.

Considerations for Use

Yarrow is used in teas (which can be made into poultices) and aromatherapy oils. The herb is most easily purchased in bulk from herb shops. Topical application and/or long-term use can cause skin irritation and/or allergic reactions. If this occurs, stop using the herb. Yarrow may also increase the skin's sensitivity to sunlight.

If you are using yarrow to treat any type of wound, be sure to clean the affected area carefully before applying yarrow because this herb can stop blood flow so quickly that it may seal in dirt or other contaminants. Yarrow should not be used to treat large, deep, or infected wounds. This type of injury requires medical attention.

Yarrow is a uterine stimulant. Although miscarriage is not likely from use of therapeutic doses, the herb nevertheless should not be used during pregnancy and lactation. Women who experience heavy periods or who have pelvic inflammatory disease (PID) also should avoid use of yarrow.

Yarrow is also a biliary stimulant, increasing the production of bile. This action may intensify the pain of gallstones. If you have gallstones, this herb certainly should be avoided during an acute attack. Allow one to two hours between using iron and yarrow, as one can cause the other to be unabsorbable.

Alcohol extracts of yarrow stop sperm production in laboratory mice. Men seeking to become fathers should avoid this herb.

Yarrow is an unusual plant in that it adapts itself to new surroundings easily, and its chemical composition changes readily in response to changes in the environment. For this reason, it is important to use yarrow from the same source every time to get reliable results.

YOHIMBE

Latin name: *Pausinystalia yohimba* (Rubiaceae [madder] family)

General Description

Yohimbe is an evergreen tree native to Cameroon, Congo, and Gabon in central Africa. Growing to a height of one hundred feet (thirty meters) and spanning as much as fifty feet (sixteen meters) across, it has reddish-brown bark, elliptical leaves, and clusters of small, yellow flowers. The bark is the part used in herbal medicine.

Yohimbe is the original source of the chemical yohimbine, which is used in drugs used to treat erectile dysfunction (ED), sold under a number of different brand names, including Aphrodyne, Yocon, Yohimex, Yoman, and others. Yohimbine is also found in the South American herb quebracho.

Evidence of Benefit

Yohimbe is a remedy for ED as well as an aphrodisiac for use by people of both sexes. In traditional African medicine, yohimbe is used both as an aphrodisiac and as a treatment for many skin conditions. It has also been used for debility and exhaustion, although one clinical study found no increase in lean body mass (muscle) or performance in a group of athletes who played top-level soccer and used 20 milligrams a day of yohimbine for three weeks. It is on the Unapproved List in the *German Commission E Monographs*. There is insufficient proof that it is effective and, thus, it is impossible to weigh the risks against the benefits.

Benefits of yohimbe for specific health conditions include the following:

- *Erectile dysfunction and diminished sex drive.* For hundreds of years, people in West Africa and the West Indies have used teas of yohimbe bark as a sexual stimulant for men. There have been a number of studies of yohimbine, the active constituent in yohimbe. This compound inhibits a very specific set of nerve cells, known as the alpha-2-adrenergic system, preventing the flow of blood *out of* the penis. While preventing the flow of blood out of the penis, yohimbine simultaneously stimulates another group of nerve cells known as cholinergic receptors. These nerves regulate the flow of blood *into* the penis. The combined effect increases the strength and duration of erections.

Since yohimbine does not increase testosterone levels, it does not contribute to overgrowth of prostate tissue, male pattern baldness, growth of body hair, aggressive behavior, or other problems associated with excessive amounts of testosterone. Yohimbine is more effective in correcting ED of psychogenic origin than physical origin. Some but not all studies show yohimbe to be beneficial for sexual dysfunction. A meta-analysis of seven high-quality studies using yohimbe for sexual dysfunction found that it had a positive effect compared to placebo with few adverse side effects reported. On the other hand, one study found that a high dose of yohimbine (36 milligrams per day) was no better than placebo for improving sexual performance in patients with mixed-type erectile dysfunction (having ED for more than one reason).

Yohimbine is particularly effective for relieving sexual dysfunction caused by treatment with antidepressant drugs known as selective serotonin reuptake inhibitors (SSRIs). These drugs, including fluoxetine (Prozac), sertraline (Zoloft), and especially paroxetine (Paxil), frequently produce sexual problems in men. In one study, eight of nine men experiencing sexual difficulties after beginning treatment with fluoxetine reported better sexual function after treatment with yohimbine. However, yohimbe is not for use in psychiatric patients, so consult a physician before using it with antipsychotic medications. In another study, all the participants taking yohimbine as prescribed experienced an improvement in sexual performance even after treatment with SSRIs. Yohimbine may also correct sexually depressive side effects of the high blood pressure drug clonidine (Catapres), but yohimbe raises blood pressure so you need to speak to your doctor before using it.

Considerations for Use

Yohimbe is best used as a tincture. The physician may recommend a prescription form of the active chemicals in this herb, such as Yohimbex (yohimbine hydrochloride). Avoid "yohimbe" tablets—these often do not contain actual yohimbe. In fact, many products labeled to contain yohimbe extract contain less than is stated on the label or none at all. At least one study suggests that yohimbe is more likely to be effective if you are fasting or eating a low-fat diet.

Anxiety, dizziness, heart palpitations, and changes in blood pressure are rare side effects, but they can result from even a single dose of either yohimbe or yohimbine. Men receiving medical treatment for anxiety, depression, high blood pressure, migraine, or seizure disorders should consult with their physician before taking this herb. Do not use yohimbe if you have kidney or liver disease, angina pectoris (chest pain), or heart disease, or are pregnant or breast-feeding. Children under twelve should not use yohimbe. Do not use it if you have chronic inflammation of the sexual organs or prostate gland or a history of gastric or duodenal ulcers.

Because the chemical yohimbine is a possible monoamine oxidase (MAO) inhibitor, you should avoid the following substances when using this herb: foods that contain tyramine (chocolate, most French cheeses, liver, organ meats, red wine), nasal decongestants, and weight-loss aids containing phenylpropanolamine. Also avoid high doses of yohimbe, which can result in priapism, a disorder characterized by painful erections that requires surgery.

Yohimbine interacts with an exceptionally large number of over-the-counter (OTC) health remedies and prescription drugs. *It is especially important not to use yohimbe or yohimbine with sildenafil (Viagra), since this herb has the potential to magnify sildenafil's effects on the heart.* Yohimbe, like Viagra, should be avoided by men who use or carry nitroglycerin tablets for angina or chest pain.

Relatively small doses of yohimbine (less than 10 milligrams) can induce mania in people who have bipolar depression. A slightly higher dose (15 to 20 milligrams) can provoke severe high blood pressure in people taking an MAO inhibitor for depression. People with a history of psychosis also should avoid yohimbe, as it has been known to trigger new episodes of psychotic reaction. It can also cause anxiety. Do not use yohimbe with alcohol, as it increases the intoxication potential.

Studies show that the alkaloid yohimbine in yohimbe can have a positive effect in people who are taking fluvoxamine (Luvox), an antidepressant. People who do not respond to fluvoxamine alone may try it in combination with yohimbine, which may greatly increase its effectiveness. Yohimbine may cause side effects, so it should be taken with fluvoxamine under medical supervision. Caution should be used if you are using drugs for high blood pressure, heart disease, or depression, or if you are taking methamphetamines or morphine-based drugs.

The FDA has ruled yohimbine unsafe and ineffective for OTC use, but both yohimbe and yohimbine can be found in health food stores. Regardless of where you live, you should take yohimbe only under medical supervision and only the recommended amounts. Dosages that provide more than 40 milligrams a day of yohimbine can cause a severe drop in blood pressure, abdominal pain, fatigue, hallucinations, and paralysis. Forty milligrams is not very far above the typical recommended dose. If you are taking antidepressants, blood-pressure drugs, or central nervous system stimulants, do not use yohimbine.

The Formulas

The previous section explained how individual herbs work in terms of the chemical principles of modern pharmacy. This section offers an overview of the combinations of herbs into formulas that ancient herbalists—and modern herbalists—have devised to treat complex patterns of symptoms in disease.

Formulas are devised to use herbs in harmony. Over the centuries, practitioners of ayurveda, traditional Chinese medicine (TCM), and the herbal traditions of the Arabic-speaking world and Europe have learned how to match combinations of herbs to combinations of symptoms. Since this involves selecting formulas that match individual people, rather than a disease, the same formula may be applied to different disease conditions as they are understood in conventional medicine. Conversely, two people with the same disease may benefit from different combinations of herbs.

This understanding of how herbal formulas work is not inconsistent with modern medicine. Herbal formulas can be explained as a single "drug" with multiple targets. Each formula is composed of multiple herbs, which in turn contain multiple chemical components. When combined, these chemical components repeatedly interact with multiple sites and targets of a disease. The result is a synergy of responses to very mild treatments that together help correct a disease.

Combinations of herbs in formulas also can act synergistically in other ways. One example of this principle is the chemistry of licorice, which is used in many herbal formulas to treat inflammation. Scientific research has found that the active ingredient in licorice that has the greatest influence on inflammation is glycyrrhetic acid. If used without other herbs, licorice releases only a small amount of glycyrrhetic acid, and this form of the chemical breaks down slowly in the body, offering slow pain relief. If licorice is combined with the optimum amount of peony, however, it releases more of the acid, offering greater pain relief. The acid is bound in a different way so that it breaks down quickly, offering faster pain relief.

Changing the proportions of the herbs, however, alters this balance. Adding too much of an herb can be less effective than not using the herb at all. For this reason, only tried-and-true combinations of the great herbal traditions and the most innovative modern herbalists are recommended in this book.

Herbal formulas are available as teas, tinctures, powders, capsules, and tablets. Most formulas are available in several different forms. Most herbal experts say that Chinese and Japanese herbal formulas are most effective when taken as teas, while ayurvedic formulas are traditionally taken as powders. Most people, however, find the traditional way of taking formulas too time-consuming, and turn to over-the-counter (OTC) extracts and tablets.

Labels are sometimes confusing to first-time users of herbal formulas since they give a range of dosages, such as "take two to three pills daily," rather than an exact dosage. What "two to three pills daily" means in practical terms is that two pills is the minimum anyone can take to improve symptoms, but taking more than three pills provides no additional benefit. In pharmacological terms, formulas have a defined therapeutic range. The lower dosage is about the bottom of the therapeutic range, while the higher dosage is about the top of the therapeutic range.

If a formula doesn't work, the problem is usually in the way the herbs are taken. Formulas should be taken on an empty stomach, with a small amount (½ cup, or 125 milliliters) of warm water. Taking the medication with water assures that it will arrive in the digestive tract. Taking the medication on an empty stomach ensures that it does not chemically react to food.

Just as with conventional medicines, it is possible to get the wrong herbal formula. If a mistake has been made in the choice of formula, taking a small amount of the formula will produce only insignificant side effects. Taking a large amount of any new herbal formula carries the risk of more serious side effects. To stay on the side of safety, use the lowest dosage recommended on the label for at least three days. Then, if there are no problems, increase the amount. (This principle does not apply to herbal formulas prepared by a professional practitioner of ayurveda, kampo, or TCM for a specific patient, only to OTC herbal products. Take professionally prescribed formulas as directed.) As an additional safeguard against side effects caused by taking the wrong herbs, the lowest recommended dosage is best for:

• People who are allergy-prone or who have digestive problems.
• Children, older adults, and people with low body weight.
• People who have chronic disease in addition to the symptoms treated by the formula.

As with any form of medicine, always consult a healthcare practitioner if you have any question about dosage or whether a specific formula is appropriate for your specific case, and especially if you are giving them to your children or taking prescription drugs.

ARREST WHEEZING DECOCTION

This traditional Chinese herbal formula contains apricot seed, coltsfoot, ephedra, ginkgo nut, licorice, mulberry root, perilla seed, pinellia, and scutellaria. This formula contains ephedra. Ephedra is banned in the United States, though it is still allowed to be sold in dietary supplements sold by licensed practitioners in traditional Chinese medicine (TCM) formulations that are recommended for their TCM uses.

The combination is designed for treating asthma, especially if breathing is accompanied by difficult expectoration of thick, yellow sputum. Do not stop your regular medications and speak with your doctor before using this herbal blend. In laboratory studies, the expectorant action of the formula is due to coltsfoot and ephedra. Coltsfoot acts on the nerves that control smooth muscles lining the bronchi to open breathing passageways. In cells, it also reduces the synthesis of nitric oxide, which activates macrophages that in turn increase the volume of phlegm. Used as a tea, coltsfoot supplies mucilages that soothe sore throat.

Ephedra supplies ephedrine, a chemical capable of entering nerve tissue, and increases the activity of the brain centers that control breathing and the constriction of blood vessels in laboratory studies. Ephedrine may cause greater activity of the skeletal muscles that power the diaphragm, making inhalation and exhalation possibly better. Pinellia contains very small doses of nicotine, which also stimulates breathing in cell studies. The other herbs in the formula buffer these stimulant herbs and prevent the agitation, nervousness, or insomnia that might occur if ephedra were used in large doses by itself.

It is possible to take overdoses of this formula. Prolonged overuse of Arrest Wheezing Decoction in tea form can cause skin disorders and shedding of mucous membranes, although this complication is unlikely unless the formula is used for at least six months. Short-term overdoses can cause headache, tremors, irritability, or shortness of breath. If any of these symptoms occur, you should stop taking the formula.

Arrest Wheezing Decoction should not be given to a child under the age of three unless directed by a medical doctor who is familiar with the use of herbs. Reversible liver damage has been known to occur in infants given similar formulas over a period of months. There also has been one case in which taking an ephedra-based formula with the drug furosemide (Lasix), usually prescribed for congestive heart failure, resulted in myocarditis, an inflammation of the heart muscle, from which the patient recovered. Use of this formula should be avoided entirely if you are experiencing diarrhea. Use it with caution if you have a fever, and stop taking it if an existing fever worsens.

ASTRAGALUS DECOCTION TO CONSTRUCT THE MIDDLE

This traditional Chinese herbal formula consists of its namesake astragalus, with cinnamon, ginger, licorice, jujube fruit, malt sugar, and peony root. The Chinese term *construct the middle* refers to the formula's use in stopping spasms and soreness in the middle of the body, that is, the abdomen and stomach.

Japanese scientists have found that the herbs in this formula release chemicals that enter the bloodstream within minutes to cause the brain to release three proteins that control digestion and motion in the intestines: gastrin, motilin, and somatostatin. The secretion of gastrin ensures the normal production of stomach acids needed to digest food. Gastrin can react with the irritant chemical histamine to cause the stomach to churn out large and irritating quantities of acid, but the licorice in the formula limits histamine release. This stops the production of quantities of stomach acid large enough to aggravate or cause ulcers. The somatostatin that the body releases in response to the formula also puts a brake on excessive acid production. Higher levels of motilin ensure that the digested food passes out of the stomach quickly, further ensuring that the stomach produces a minimal amount of acid.

In addition to helping stop production of excess acid in the stomach, this formula promotes the smooth transit of digested food through the intestine. Astragalus may also help to maintain healthy bacteria in the intestine, but this was accomplished in an animal model—not in humans.

The traditional use of this formula in treating vitiligo has not been investigated, but it is known that the formula causes the immune systems of animals to produce more of an immune factor known as interleukin-2 (IL-2), which is sometimes used in the medical treatment of vitiligo.

Traditional Chinese medicine (TCM) recommends this formula as gentle and effective, especially appropriate for children's use. There are no reports of toxicity associated with this formula.

AUGMENTED RAMBLING POWDER

This widely used formula from traditional Chinese medicine (TCM) contains white atractylodis, bupleurum, dong quai, gardenia, hoelen, licorice, moutan, and white peony. *Rambling* refers to a free spirit, and an *augmented* powder was especially effective. This combination of herbs was devised by ancient Chinese herbalists who believed that the combination could free the user from the effects of trapped vital energies of emotion stored in the liver.

In the theory of TCM, when emotions build up beyond the liver's capacity to contain them, they cause the body and mind to "shake." This effect is especially felt on the energy channel supplied by the liver—that is, the external genitalia, the breasts, the centers of the eyes, the spleen, and the crown of the head. The herbs in the formula were thought to redirect emotional energy to the heart and to restore the normal circulation of other energies.

Modern research has found that Augmented Rambling Powder lowers estrogen levels. This makes it effective against disorders affected by estrogen, such as breast cancer, and other disorders of the breast and female reproductive tract. As a complementary treatment for cancer, the formula is used to increase the effectiveness of estrogen-binding drugs, such as tamoxifen (Nolvadex). Do not use this formula if you have breast cancer or are at risk for it before checking with your physician. Augmented Rambling Powder is used to treat symptoms related to imbalances in estrogen, including tenderness in the breasts and lower abdomen, irritability, water retention, headache, and digestive disturbances before and at the beginning of the menstrual period. It has also been used for acne and hepatitis, as it is considered to be a blood nourisher.

For several generations, Chinese doctors have used this formula to treat macular degeneration and an atrophy of the optic nerve that is described in Chinese-language medical journals as resulting from "toxin accumulation." Recent Japanese research has found that the formula acts against macular degeneration by reducing the tendency of the tiny blood vessels serving the retina to secrete collagen, a protein that indirectly clouds the field of vision.

The conditions most commonly treated with this formula include bloodshot eyes, breast and uterine cancer, melanoma, endometriosis, fibrocystic breast disease, fibroids, menstrual problems and symptoms of menopause, ovarian cysts, premenstrual syndrome (PMS), and macular degeneration. It is also used for poor or irregular appetite, epigastric fullness, flushed face, and general fatigue.

Because gardenia contains a compound that can cause early-term miscarriage, women who are trying to become pregnant should not take this formula.

BIOTA SEED PILL TO NOURISH THE HEART

This traditional Chinese herbal formula contains acorus, biota seed, dong quai, hoelen, licorice, lycium, ophiopogon, rehmannia, and scrophularia. The heart to which its name refers is the seat of the emotions and memory in Asian medicine.

Although there have been no clinical investigations of the formula as a whole in the treatment of Alzheimer's disease, attention deficit disorder (ADD), or depression, at least two of the herbs in the formula are known to have effects on the neurological system. The herb for which the formula is named, biota, inhibits the production of platelet-activating factor (PAF) in cell line studies. This factor causes red blood cells to form microscopic clots that can interfere with the supply of oxygen to the brain. The specific way in which biota preserves normal circulation in the brain is by inhibiting the activation of

PAF by serotonin, a chemical that must be conserved to avoid depression. And while biota prevents the formation of blood clots that impede circulation, it does not cause bleeding. The herb is well known in Chinese medicine as an anti-hemorrhage agent. Tests of biota show that, at least for laboratory animals, the herb can offset learning and memory problems caused by damage to brain tissue of mice.

While biota ensures an adequate oxygen supply for brain tissue, acorus protects brain tissue from toxic free radicals that are released from excess oxygen. Especially when the flow of oxygen is restored to previously oxygen-deprived cells, these cells are temporarily unable to use all the oxygen available to them, and free-radical damage results. Tissue damage in the brain can lead to memory loss or seizures. This formula calms the mind while nourishing the heart and tonifying the kidneys.

Thousands of years of experience in using this formula in traditional Chinese herbal medicine indicate that it is best suited for older people. Classics of Chinese herbal medicine describe the use of this formula in recovering the "uniqueness" of the person that may be lost with impairments to memory. The physical symptoms of people who will benefit most from this formula include a tendency toward agitation or aggression, a relatively high energy level, and "dry" symptoms, including constipation, dryness of the mouth, and dry skin. It is also used for anxiety, palpitations, disturbing dreams, insomnia, and night sweating.

BUPLEURUM AND CINNAMON TWIG DECOCTION

Bupleurum and Cinnamon Twig Decoction is a combination of bupleurum, cinnamon, ginger, ginseng, jujube, licorice, peony, pinellia, and scutellaria.

Although this formula has not been put through clinical testing, the properties of several of its principal herbs may explain its usefulness in treating premenstrual syndrome (PMS). Saikosides and other chemical constituents in bupleurum stimulate the pituitary gland to direct the adrenal glands to produce glucocorticoids, which reduce inflammation. Cinnamon, which is also used to control uterine bleeding, helps establish normal circulation to the uterus. Certain forms of cinnamon have been found to inhibit a substance in the blood called thromboxane A_2. Thromboxane causes platelets in the blood to clump together into clots, so inhibiting this chemical leads to less clotting and a more normal blood flow. Ginger has been found to inhibit the production of immune-system compounds called cytokines, an action that reduces inflammation and stimulates blood circulation; this was a cell study, so what happens in humans is unknown. This action could make ginger useful in treating a number of disorders marked by swelling and pain. Ginger also eases indigestion and nausea.

Ginseng stimulates a part of the brain called the

hypothalamus to secrete substances that stimulate cell growth and healing in the sex organs, and licorice is yet another anti-inflammatory. Muscle relaxants are found in both peony and scutellaria, while pinellia helps the nervous system maintain muscle control. Scutellaria additionally stimulates metabolism within brain cells.

This formula counteracts both digestive disturbances and muscle pain in PMS. You should use it with caution if you have a fever, and discontinue use if an existing fever worsens. Since several of the herbs in the formula stimulate estrogen production, Bupleurum and Cinnamon Twig Decoction should not be used for more than two weeks in any month by women who have estrogen-sensitive disorders, such as some forms of breast cancer, uterine fibroids, endometriosis, or fibrocystic breast disease. Ginseng, licorice, or peony used long-term by itself can increase estrogen production, and licorice can increase fluid retention, but neither effect results from short-term use of this formula.

This formula has also been used for joint pain, flatulence, muscular tension, painful muscles, pale tongue, and irregular pulse.

BUPLEURUM PLUS DRAGON BONE AND OYSTER SHELL DECOCTION

This traditional Chinese herbal formula combines a number of herbs and natural products including bupleurum, cinnamon bark, dragon bone (pulverized fossils), ginger, ginseng, hoelen, jujube, pinellia, rhubarb, and scutellaria. Traditionally, the formula also included minium (lead oxide), but this toxic ingredient is no longer used outside of China in making this formula. It was originally used for mental disorders such as epilepsy, schizophrenia, and severe depression.

Ancient Chinese and Japanese herbalists used this formula to treat anxiety, insomnia, palpitations, and other manifestations of nervous tension in people of robust constitution. Modern practitioners have found that it is especially useful for treating hardening of the arteries with the same symptoms. The formula has been shown to increase the ratio of high-density lipoprotein (HDL, or "good") cholesterol to low-density lipoprotein (LDL, or "bad") while reducing nervous tension that may contribute to high blood pressure.

In Japan, this formula is used to treat migraines caused by environmental stresses, such as weather changes, noise, allergens, and drafts. It is commonly used for stimulation of hair growth in bald people, with treatments lasting from two to six months. Japanese physicians have used the formula successfully in treating many other conditions, including depression, risk of heart attack, hyperthyroidism, memory loss, Ménière's disease, migraine, and seizure disorders. Elsewhere, it has purportedly been used for hyperthyroidism, epilepsy, constipation, gastritis, menopausal symptoms, inhibited urination, and rapid pulse. It is also used for withdrawal from nicotine, valium, caffeine, and other substances.

When this formula is used as a bagged tea provided by a traditional Chinese medicine (TCM) or other herbal practitioner, the dragon bone and oyster shell (usually in separate bags) should be boiled for thirty to forty-five minutes before the other ingredients are added. Use this formula with caution if you have a fever, and stop taking it if an existing fever worsens.

CALM THE STOMACH POWDER

This traditional Chinese herbal formula contains atractylodis, chen-pi, licorice, and magnolia bark. It has been used in Chinese herbal medicine since the eleventh century to treat a pattern of symptoms including acid reflux, belching, distention and fullness in the abdomen, heavy sensation in the limbs, increased desire to sleep, loose stools or diarrhea, loss of appetite, loss of sense of taste, nausea, and vomiting.

All four herbs in the formula act directly on these symptoms. Atractylodis stimulates urination. The dosages used in traditional Chinese medicine (TCM) temporarily (for two to three hours) increase urination five- to sevenfold. This reduces the amount of fluid available to cause diarrhea. Bitter orange peel stops a wide variety of allergic reactions, including food allergies. It also stops spasms of the muscles that propel digested food through the intestines.

Licorice soothes inflammation and protects the stomach and intestines from the effects of stomach acid. One of its components, glycyrrhizinic acid, was the first compound proven to promote the healing of ulcers. Unlike many ulcer drugs, glycyrrhizinic acid does not reduce acid production in the stomach, which would result in incomplete digestion. Instead, it increases the stomach's defense mechanisms by fortifying the stomach's protective mucous coating. Glycyrrhizinic acid also increases circulation to the cells lining the intestinal wall, boosting their supply of nutrients and oxygen.

Finally, magnolia bark contains alkaloids that relax tense skeletal muscles, including the muscles that control the anal sphincter. This prevents painful passage of stool. Magnolia bark also has antibiotic effects against streptococcal infections, staph infections, shigella, viral hepatitis, and amoebic infections, but these effects have only been found in cell line studies and may not be applicable to humans.

This formula is traditionally used to induce labor, but home administration for the purpose of inducing labor offers unpredictable results. It should be avoided during pregnancy.

CINNAMON TWIG AND PORIA PILL

This traditional Chinese formula contains cinnamon twig, hoelen (also known as poria), moutan, peach seed, and peony. Chinese herbalists of the fourth century felt that this combination of herbs was so useful that they included it in a book of formulas known as *Essentials from the Golden Cabinet*.

This combination of herbs was designed to treat a pattern of symptoms in women including mild but persistent bleeding of purple or dark blood during pregnancy, accompanied by abdominal pain that increases with pressure. It was also used to treat abdominal spasms, immobile masses in the lower abdomen, and menstrual irregularity.

Cinnamon Twig and Poria Pill is an unusual treatment for these problems in that it stops uterine bleeding by increasing, rather than decreasing, blood circulation. The idea was that if blood was obstructed from its normal pathways, it could have two undesirable effects. It could become "static," causing abdominal tension, amenorrhea, dysmenorrhea, and uterine masses. Or it could "leak," causing uterine bleeding.

Modern Japanese physicians use this formula to treat a collection of symptoms they call "blood effusion," marked by acne and feelings of blood rushing to the head, redness in the face, or coughing with copious phlegm. They use the formula to treat acne in both men and women, but especially women's acne accompanying irregular menstruation. The formula is also used in Japan to treat "blood effusive chills," colds in which there is a feeling of blood rushing to the head.

Research has confirmed the traditional use of this formula for treatment of disorders of the female reproductive tract. Laboratory studies have found that it reduces bloodstream estrogen levels by inhibiting the production of DNA in the ovaries. It therefore does not affect estrogen production in women who have had their ovaries removed. Inhibiting estrogen production reduces the rate of growth of estrogen-receptor positive breast cancers, and may make tamoxifen (Nolvadex) treatment more effective. However, do not use this formula without consulting your physician first if you have breast cancer. Inhibiting the production of estrogen may have an effect on some forms of melanoma and uterine cancer. In endometriosis, a disorder in which the tissue that lines the uterus settles elsewhere in the body, reducing levels of estrogen in the bloodstream slows the rate at which this tissue grows. It similarly slows the development of ovarian cysts and uterine fibroids. This formula has been found in laboratory studies to stop the growth of uterine fibroids without interfering with the menstrual cycle or causing weight gain.

Cinnamon Twig and Poria Pill is also useful in treating reproductive problems in men, especially those caused by variocele, or varicose veins that constrict the spermatic cord. The formula improves circulation in the lower abdomen. In clinical studies in Japan, use of the formula induces a remission from variocele in about 80 percent of cases, and also increases sperm count and motility. Traditionally, the formula is given to men who are "warm-natured," that is, men who prefer cold temperatures to warm temperatures, and who have a tendency to muscle strain. These men are subject to variocele. It is also used for prostatitis.

Cinnamon Twig and Poria Pill shows promise in treating the skin disorder scleroderma. Japanese scientists have found that the formula stops collagen formation in scleroderma-affected cells but not in healthy skin cells. The formula also prevents free-radical damage to brain tissue while circulation is being restored after a stroke. Historically, this formula has not been used for scleroderma or stroke.

Cinnamon Twig and Poria Pill is used by practitioners of traditional Chinese medicine (TCM) in the treatment of acne, breast cancer, fibrocystic breasts, ovarian cysts, endometriosis, menstrual problems, and infertility in both men and women. It should be avoided by women who use birth control pills for contraception.

COPTIS DECOCTION TO RELIEVE TOXICITY

This traditional Chinese herbal formula contains coptis, gardenia, phellodendron, and scutellaria. Widely used in modern Japanese medicine, this formula was originally created to treat a combination of symptoms including dark urine, high fever, dry mouth, and irritability. Today Japanese physicians use Coptis Decoction to Relieve Toxicity to treat insomnia in people with "blood effusive" symptoms: redness in the face, a feeling of blood rushing to the head, high blood pressure. It is used today in Western medicine for septicemia (blood poisoning), dysentery, pneumonia, acute urinary tract infections (UTIs), and skin lesions.

Japanese physicians note that Coptis Decoction to Relieve Toxicity is more effective than conventional antibiotics in treating the bacterial infections that cause acne. By sequestering free radicals from certain chemical processes in the brain, it may protect brain tissue and memory from the effects of restoring oxygen supply after stroke, and may help some people with Alzheimer's disease and depression. However, it was not traditionally used for these applications. It has been shown to protect the lining of the stomach and kill *Helicobacter pylori,* a bacterium that causes peptic ulcers. This formula may be helpful in treating yeast infections aggravated by diabetes, especially thrush and esophageal infections causing heartburn. It is also useful in the treatment of conjunctivitis and inflamed gums.

While this formula is extremely versatile, it must be used with the same precautions that apply to the use of barberry, coptis, goldenseal, and Oregon grape root. Do not use this formula, or any herb or formula containing berberine, during pregnancy, and do not use it daily for a period of longer than two weeks. Do not use it with vitamin B_6 or with protein supplements containing the amino acid histidine, since these supplements counteract the antibacterial effect of berberine. Avoid the formula entirely if you have gallstones.

DONG QUAI AND PEONY POWDER

Also known by its Japanese name, *toki-shakuyaku-san*, this formula combines dong quai and peony with alisma, atractylodis, hoelen, and ligusticum. It has been used in traditional Chinese medicine (TCM) for centuries to treat continuous mild cramping in the lower abdomen during pregnancy. However, if you are pregnant, do not use this formula without consulting your obstretrican. Dong quai, peony, and ligusticum restore the circulation of blood to its normal channels and release the energies of pent-up emotions from the "liver." The other herbs in the formula encourage urination.

In modern Japanese medicine, Dong Quai and Peony Powder is applied to a wide range of conditions that benefit from reduced estrogen production. It is used to treat acne occurring in the first fourteen days of the menstrual cycle, and to stop cyclical growth in endometriosis, fibrocystic breast disease, ovarian cysts, and uterine fibroids. This has only been shown in laboratory studies and not in humans. Unlike some treatments, this formula does not have a "masculinizing" effect because it decreases estrogen production by the ovaries without reducing the ratio of estrogen to testosterone in circulation. In the case of endometriosis, Dong Quai and Peony Powder reduces the formation of inflammatory compounds in endometrial tissue.

An unrelated application of the formula is the treatment of summer colds that cause nasal congestion and chills throughout the body. It is also appropriate for "air-conditioning stress," nasal congestion caused by too many changes from natural to air-conditioned environments in the summer.

Dong Quai and Peony Powder also has been applied to treatment of cognitive disorders of old age. The Japanese herbal product manufacturer Tsumura has sponsored studies of the basic science of the formula, which determined that the formula works by acting on movement of sodium, potassium, and calcium across cell membranes in the brain. These changes in ion balance lessen the production of cell-damaging, oxidative free radicals, but how this translates to human benefit is unknown.

European laboratory studies of Dong Quai and Peony Powder indicate that the formula slows excessive free-radical production in the cardiovascular system, helping slow the process of atherosclerosis. Dong Quai and Peony Powder helps eliminate proteins damaged by free radicals from the stomach, and may increase the production of the protein-digesting hormone trypsin in the stomach, but this was shown in cell studies and not in people.

TCM practitioners also use this formula to treat beriberi, chronic nephritis, pelvic inflammatory disease (PID), and recurrent miscarriage. Since the formula modifies the metabolism of estrogen and progesterone, it should not be used by women who use oral contraceptives.

EIGHT-INGREDIENT PILL WITH REHMANNIA

This traditional Chinese herbal formula contains alisma, astragalus, cornelian cherry, hoelen, moutan peony, rehmannia, schisandra, and wild yam. It was formulated by the Chinese herbalist Fu Qing-Zhu to treat symptoms such as dizziness, lightheadedness, ringing in the ears, diminished hearing, soreness and weakness in the lower back, and profuse perspiration, especially at night. It has also been used for spleen and kidney problems. Newer Western uses include for eye problems, tuberculosis, high blood pressure, urinary tract infections (UTIs), deafness, hyperthyproidism, and retarded growth in children.

Research has shown that this formula has applications far beyond the symptom pattern for which it was designed. Eight-Ingredient Pill with Rehmannia (also known as Rehmannia-Eight Combination) has become one of the most popular herbal treatments for diabetes in Japan. The formula has been shown to lower blood sugar, aid insulin regulation, and slow the progress of diabetic neuropathy in people with type 1 diabetes. It is useful for both type 1 and type 2 diabetes, for people who must take insulin and for those who do not. The primary benefit of Rehmannia-Eight Combination for those who take insulin is a "smoothing out" of insulin's effects. Rehmannia-Eight Combination will not reduce the amount of insulin necessary, but it can give tighter control of blood sugar levels. This helps to prevent eye problems and problems in circulation. This action of the formula also helps keep sugar levels stable in people with diabetes who do not have to take insulin. In Chinese medicine, it is not used as much for diabetes or related conditions.

Japanese scientists have long recognized the ability of the formula to prevent the formation of diabetic cataracts by inhibiting the enzyme aldose reductase. (This is described in greater detail under CATARACTS in Part Two.) The formula also acts by helping maintain the balance of sodium, potassium, and calcium in the lens, which is important in maintaining its transparency. Laboratory tests with the formula suggest that it can delay the development of cataracts by ten to fifteen years.

The formula has been confirmed in laboratory studies as a potential treatment for osteoporosis. In these studies, Eight-Ingredient Pill with Rehmannia prevented the erosion and pocketing of bone in animals deprived of estrogen. Japanese scientists believe that this formula may potentially be as effective as estrogen replacement for preventing osteoporosis. It is often used for low back pain and leg numbness.

Its diuretic herbs—alisma, cornelian cherry, hoelen, and rehmannia—stimulate urination, effectively flushing bacteria out of the genitourinary tract in gonorrhea and pelvic inflammatory disease (PID). In the treatment of high blood pressure, its constituent herb alisma provides extra potassium and increases excretion of sodium, chloride, and urea, which lowers both blood pressure and blood sugar. Laboratory tests indicate that the formula also reduces salt sensitivity and protects against kidney damage. It stops the continuous sweating that can be caused by the form of hyperthyroidism known as Graves' disease. It is a traditional remedy in traditional Chinese medicine (TCM) for problems of menopause including sensitivity to cold in the hands and feet, dry and itchy skin, impaired vision and hearing, and/or abnormalities in urination.

Finally, Eight-Ingredient Pill with Rehmannia eases urination in men with prostate problems. Laboratory studies indicate that it may benefit prostate conditions by altering an enzyme pathway so that the amount of testosterone in circulation to the brain to stimulate sex drive increases, but the detrimental effect of testosterone on prostate tissue decreases. Japanese use it for difficulty with urination, a common problem with prostatic disease.

EPHEDRA DECOCTION

This traditional Chinese herbal formula contains apricot seed, cinnamon bark, ephedra, and licorice. It is also known as Four Emperors Decoction. In ancient Chinese culture, it was common to refer to four important things that were harmonious as a group and not given to extremes as *four gentlemen* or *four emperors*. This phrase was also a Confucian term for a person who exhibits ideal behavior. This formula contains ephedra. Ephedra is banned in the United States, though it is still allowed to be sold in dietary supplements sold by licensed practitioners in traditional Chinese medicine (TCM) formulations that are recommended for their TCM uses.

The symptoms treated by this formula include fever and chills, generalized body aches, headache, and wheezing, all of which can occur with asthma, bronchitis, colds, and flu. Ephedrine, a chemical found in ephedra, rapidly enters nerve tissue, and increases the activity of the brain centers that control breathing and blood-vessel contraction. This may allow the formula to relieve symptoms associated with respiratory disorders. The other herbs in the formula minimize side effects, especially overstimulation, that could be caused by an accidental overdose of ephedra taken by itself.

Research based on laboratory studies shows that Ephedra Decoction not only helps treat the symptoms of colds but may prevent the spread of colds when used at the earliest stages of infection. It may also be useful in treating body aches caused by rheumatoid arthritis. Application of this formula is not limited to treating aches and pains or respiratory problems. Modern clinical research has found that the formula may limit damage to skin from ultraviolet radiation, but this was from an animal study and human benefits are not known.

Because of the buffering herbs in this formula, it is not likely to cause the side effects that might occur from taking ephedra by itself. It should not be used for more than two weeks at a time, however, and it is important to drink eight glasses of water a day while taking this formula to avoid dehydration.

EPHEDRA, ASIASARUM, AND PREPARED ACONITE DECOCTION

This traditional Chinese herbal formula contains asiasarum, ephedra, and aconite that has been steam-processed to remove potential toxins. Ancient Chinese herbalists formulated this combination of herbs to treat a symptom pattern including exhaustion, fever without sweating, and a sensation of severe cold. This formula contains ephedra. Ephedra is banned in the United States, though it is still allowed to be sold in dietary supplements sold by licensed practitioners in traditional Chinese medicine (TCM) formulations that are recommended for their TCM uses.

The pharmacological properties of the herbs in this formula have been extensively researched. Aconite contains an analgesic agent, mesaconitine, which may raise the threshold of pain and help the body attune to both relaxation and stress. In laboratory studies, mesaconitine manipulates the brain's production of norepinephrine, one of the chemicals that "excites" the nervous system. During relaxation, mesaconitine decreases the brain's production of norepinephrine, and during stress, mesaconitine increases the brain's production of norepinephrine.

Asiasarum, known as wild ginger, is also an analgesic. Ephedrine, a chemical found in ephedra, rapidly enters nerve tissue, and increases the activity of the brain centers that control blood-vessel contraction. As blood vessels tighten, less heat is radiated through the skin, and a feeling of warmth results. Ephedrine also stimulates the centers of the brain that control breathing, and may make taking deep breaths easier for people with asthma.

The medical condition most commonly treated with this formula is allergy, particularly allergy to cedar pollen. The formula is most effective when used at the beginning and end of the allergy season. It cannot overcome the effect of direct exposure to massive amounts of cedar pollen. Still, for millions of sufferers of cedar-pollen allergies in Japan and the United States, this formula promises allergy relief without the side effect of drowsiness and without prescription drug interactions.

ESSIAC TEA

Essiac tea was the invention of a Canadian nurse named Rene M. Caisse, who used her last name spelled backward to name the formula. Still the most popular herbal mixture used for treating cancer in North America, one version of the formula, manufactured by the Resperin Corporation, contains just four herbs: burdock root, sheep sorrel, slippery elm bark, and rhubarb root. Another version of the formula, marketed as Flor-Essence, adds four more herbs: blessed thistle, kelp, red clover, and watercress. Both manufacturers claim to manufacture the authentic Caisse formula, but Rene Caisse never authenticated either formula before her death at the age of ninety in 1978. One website, www.essiacinfo.org, claims to be an authorative body on Essiac tea, and says that Rene Caisse's original tea contained four herbs—burdock, slippery elm inner bark, sheep sorrel, and Indian rhubarb root. On this site, they say that "no extensive clinical studies have been performed." If you have cancer and are considering using this formula, speak to your doctor.

Caisse's career as a cancer healer was marked by continuous controversy with Canadian health authorities. Some evaluations critical of the use of her formula were clearly dishonest. Findings in support of the formula are questionable because of the limitations of diagnostic technique in the 1930s, '40s, and '50s—that is, it is possible some patients diagnosed as having cancer and then pronounced cured never actually had the disease. The cases that Canadian health officials acknowledged as cured all involved conventional treatment as well as the use of Essiac tea. Nonetheless, there is a steady stream of well-documented cases of remission from various kinds of cancer after Essiac treatment throughout the 1990s. There have been cases of prostate cancer, advanced bladder cancer, and advanced breast cancer that have gone into remission after use of the formula.

Essiac's efficacy against cancer can be explained in part by the cancer-fighting characteristics of herbs in the formula. Two chemicals in rhubarb, emodin and rhein, may stop the growth of melanoma, breast cancers, and hepatic carcinoma in cell line studies. One of these chemicals, emodin, has been found in the laboratory to greatly enhance the effectiveness of conventional chemotherapies. It makes breast cancer cells more sensitive to paclitaxel (Taxol) and makes certain types of lung cancer cells more sensitive to cisplatin (Platinol) and doxorubicin (Adriamycin, Rubex). Check with your doctor if you have breast cancer and are using these drugs before taking Essiac tea. A closely related chemical, aloe emodin, found in sheep sorrel, has significant activity against leukemia cells. Burdock root increases the rate at which estrogen is excreted into the stool, and red clover blocks estrogen from stimulating breast cancer cells in cell studies.

Taken together, these findings support—but do not prove—the use of Essiac as a treatment to make standard chemotherapy more effective. Essiac is available at almost every health food outlet and can be brewed at home for about five cents a day. The tea has a mild and pleasant taste, and there are no reports of side effects (although injecting Essiac can be fatal). Since rhubarb root and sheep sorrel contain high concentrations of oxalic acid, this formula should be avoided by people who have a history of kidney stones. Rhubarb, a stimulant laxative, is present only in moderate amounts, but should be avoided by people with any kind of intestinal obstruction. Do not use this formula during pregnancy or if you have brain cancer, as the tea may cause swelling.

FIVE-ACCUMULATION POWDER

This traditional Chinese herbal formula contains atractylodis, bitter orange peel, bitter orange slices, cinnamon, ephedra, ginger, hoelen, licorice, ligusticum, magnolia bark, peony, pinellia, platycodon, and wild angelica. The five accumulations to which its name refers are from traditional Chinese medicine (TCM), which attributed many chronic conditions to accumulations of blood, cold, dampness, chi (energy), and phlegm. Imbalances of these five qualities can result in abdominal pain, aversion to food, body aches, diarrhea with rumbling noises, a feeling of fullness in the abdomen and chest, fever and chills without sweating, headache, stiffness in the back and neck, and vomiting. This formula contains ephedra. Ephedra is banned in the United States, though it is still allowed to be sold in dietary supplements sold by licensed practitioners in TCM formulations that are recommended for their TCM uses.

Two of the more active, or chief, herbs in the formula, ephedra and wild angelica, were chosen for their ability to help the body fight the early stages of infection. Ephedra may help relieve respiratory disorders. Wild angelica is a bactericide. In laboratory studies, wild angelica acts against a number of infectious microorganisms, including E. coli, a common cause of diarrhea. It also helps open the coronary vessels and increases circulation to the heart.

The other two chief herbs, cinnamon and ginger, lessen symptoms associated with food poisoning. Cinnamon relieves gas and prevents flatulence. It works by preventing the buildup of inflammatory chemicals in the digestive tract, as shown in cell studies but not in people. A compound found in cinnamon, propanoic acid, may help against the formation of stomach ulcers without interfering with the production of gastric acid. This is important because a lack of gastric acid can lead to indigestion. Ginger has been found in cell studies to inhibit the production of immune-system compounds called cytokines. This action reduces inflammation, stimulates blood circulation, and makes the herb useful in treating disorders marked by swelling and pain. Ginger also eases indigestion and nausea.

Other herbs in the formula complement the effects of the four chief herbs, or change the chemical composition of the tea so that their active ingredients are available in a higher concentration.

The most common application of this formula is the treatment of diarrhea. TCM practitioners also use it to treat mild gastritis and upper respiratory tract infection. It is important to drink eight or more glasses of water a day while taking this formula or any other medication for diarrhea to avoid dehydration.

FIVE-INGREDIENT POWDER WITH PORIA

This traditional Chinese herbal formula contains alisma, atractylodis, cinnamon bark, hoelen, and polyporus, also sometimes called poria. The venerated Chinese herbalist Zhang Zhongjing developed it to treat three overlapping patterns of symptoms:

- Cough, shortness of breath, vertigo, and vomiting of frothy saliva;
- Diarrhea, edema, a generalized sensation of heaviness throughout the body, and vomiting; or
- Fever, headache, irritability, and strong thirst but with vomiting immediately after drinking, and difficulty in urination.

Today, Five-Ingredient Powder with Poria is used for water buildup in the bladder, water buildup in the spleen that relates to diarrhea and acute gastroenteritis, and retention of congested fluids, such as for treating coughs, breathlessness, and dizziness.

The herbal formulation addresses general areas of the kidneys, lungs, spleen, heart, bladder, and stomach. In cell studies, this application can be understood in terms of the herbs making up the formula. Alisma contains complex sugars that stimulate lymph cells to "eat" the pathogenic bacteria and yeasts that can infect the digestive and urinary tracts. Atractylodis, the herb sold in Chinese herb stores as bai zhi, stimulates urination. It encourages the excretion of sodium and relieves fluid retention. In laboratory tests, this effect lasts six to seven hours. Cinnamon relieves gas and prevents flatulence. A compound found in cinnamon, propanoic acid, stops the formation of stomach ulcers without interfering with the production of gastric acid in cell studies. This is important because a lack of gastric acid can lead to indigestion. Hoelen also stimulates urination, but contains a complex carbohydrate known as pachyman, which could prevent inflammation of the kidneys. Polyporus both protects the liver and stimulates the excretion of bile, which stabilizes fats in the digestive tract and reduces diarrhea.

Japanese scientists have found that this formula as a whole acts by decreasing the number of adhesion cells in the kidneys in cell studies. This stimulates urination and reduces the amount of fluid that has to be eliminated through the intestines. Modern Chinese physicians use Five-Ingredient Powder with Poria to treat glaucoma. In a Chinese study of fifty-five glaucoma patients, the formula resulted in lowered intraocular pressures in 63 percent of patients within the first month of use. Chinese physicians report that the formula also relieves Ménière's disease caused by trauma or fever.

Five-Ingredient Powder with Poria is nontoxic. Although it encourages urination, it does not cause loss of potassium or trace minerals. It can be used to treat chronic diarrhea on a long-term basis, but should not be used to treat acute diarrhea for more than a week unless a doctor has ruled out serious underlying disease. Long-term use can lead to loss of appetite, dizziness, vertigo, and a bland taste in the mouth.

FOUR-GENTLEMEN DECOCTION

This traditional Chinese herbal formula contains the four "gentlemen" of traditional chinese medicine (TCM): atractylodis, ginseng, hoelen, and licorice. In Chinese culture, it was common to refer to four important things, in this case, four important herbs, that were harmonious as a group and not given to extremes as *four gentlemen* or *four emperors*. This title was modeled after the Confucian term for a person who exhibits ideal behavior. Chinese herbalists used the four herbs together to remedy a "deficient" constitution, diagnosed from a pale complexion, loose stools, low and soft voice, reduced appetite, and weakness in the limbs.

In this formula, atractylodis may stimulate urination and relieves the body of excess fluid. Ginseng reduces digestive upsets caused by emotional stress and inhibits ulcer formation. Ginseng compounds may even reduce *anticipated* stress.

Studies have found that injected ginseng compounds increase the body's production of adrenocorticotropic hormone (ACTH) and certain steroid hormones, such as adrenaline. This stimulates the natural function of the body's stress-response system, which keeps the adrenal glands from burning out during prolonged periods of stress. However, these observations were made in animals, and whether these things happen in humans is not known.

Hoelen also stimulates urination and helps to protect the kidneys against stress from the breakdown of proteins. It contains poriatin, which in cell line studies stops the production of cytokines, chemical messengers that immune cells use to coordinate attacks on kidney tissues. Poriatin also stops the activity of related chemical messengers of tissue destruction, such as the interleukins and tumor necrosis factor (TNF).

Licorice is useful for a number of digestive disorders. It soothes inflammation and protects the stomach and intestines from the effects of stomach acid. One of the chemical components of licorice, glycyrrhizinic acid, was the first compound proven to promote the healing of ulcers. Unlike many ulcer drugs, glycyrrhizinic acid does not reduce acid production in the stomach, which would result in incomplete digestion. Instead, it increases the stomach's defense mechanisms by fortifying the stomach's protective mucous coating. Glycyrrhizinic acid also increases circulation to the cells lining the intestinal wall, boosting their supply of nutrients and oxygen in cell studies.

Four-Gentlemen Decoction appears as part of many other formulas. These formulas are used to treat diabetes, chronic gastritis, peptic ulcer, irritable bowel syndrome

(IBS), neurasthenia, periodic paralysis, and uterine fibroids, and to stimulate recovery from gastric surgery. Since the herbs in this formula may increase estrogen production, women who have estrogen-sensitive breast cancer or endometriosis, uterine fibroids, or fibrocystic breast disease should not use Four-Gentlemen Decoction. In addition, do not use when facing excess heat, irritability, thirst, and constipation. The formula may cause irritability and dry mouth when used for a prolonged period of time.

FOUR-SUBSTANCE DECOCTION

As its name suggests, this traditional Chinese herbal formula contains four substances—namely, the herbs dong quai, ligusticum, peony, and rehmannia. The masters of Chinese herbalism designed this formula for a pattern of symptoms including blurred vision, dizziness, lusterless nails, pallid complexion, pain around the navel and in the abdomen, and, in women, irregular menstruation with little flow or amenorrhea. The formula is also used in China to treat hard abdominal masses or tumors.

Two of the herbs in this formula, peony and rehmannia, were traditionally known as "blood of the blood" herbs—that is, herbs that help the body create blood. To keep that blood from accumulating as a hard mass when the menstrual period was missed, two herbs to stimulate blood circulation, ligusticum and dong quai, were added to the combination.

Although there has been little or no scientific research on the formula as a whole, its use is supported by what is known about dong quai. There is general agreement among herb experts that this herb helps stop cramping and headaches during the premenstrual period. Investigations into the herb's actions at a chemical level tend to confirm that it stops certain chemical reactions that induce pain by stopping production of free radicals of nitrous oxide, which cause veins to dilate.

Dong quai teas may lower blood pressure and prolong the resting period between heartbeats. They can dilate the coronary blood vessels to increase blood flow to the heart. Dong quai inhibits the release of chemicals into the blood that promote the formation of clots and start inflammatory reactions in cell line studies. This action helps keep microscopic blood vessels in the eye from leaking, helping to protect against macular degeneration, diabetic retinopathy, and the formation of floaters. Dong quai is a traditional treatment for a variety of skin conditions. It does not stimulate the growth of healthy skin cells. Actually, in overdose, it may kill healthy cells. Rather, dong quai compounds called coumarins stimulate circulation to the skin, while other compounds in the herb block the production of inflammation-generating substances called prostaglandins that would normally be transported to the skin by this increased circulation. Dong quai also inhibits the formation of tissue-destructive antibodies at the very beginning of the inflammatory process. That is, dong quai stops the destruction of skin by antibodies, provided it is taken as soon as symptoms are noticed. These studies were done in cells and animals. For humans, the Four-Substance Decoction is used for dull complexion, dry and brittle nails, and pale complexion.

Modern herbalists and naturopathic physicians use this formula to treat a wide range of conditions, including anemia, eye disorders, fibroids, menstrual problems, neurological headaches, and stress. Since the formula may alter the body's metabolism of estrogen and its by-products, it should be avoided by women who take conjugated estrogens (such as Premarin) or oral contraceptives. Do not use this formula when you have diarrhea, poor appetite, or indigestion. It is not to be used if you have a chronic condition, acute blood loss, or labored breathing.

FRIGID EXTREMITIES DECOCTION

This traditional Chinese herbal formula contains prepared aconite, ginger, and licorice. Ancient Chinese herbalists designed it for patterns of symptoms that primarily affect older adults, especially "frigid extremities"—that is, extremely cold hands and feet. The combination has also been used to treat abdominal pain, aversion to cold, a constant desire to sleep, a desire to sleep with the knees drawn up, diarrhea with undigested food particles, and a lack of thirst.

In this formula, aconite is used to jolt the body's energy processes when they are compromised by long illness. Aconite contains a potent analgesic agent, mesaconitine, which raises the threshold of pain and helps the body become attuned to both relaxation and stress. In laboratory studies, mesaconitine has been found to manipulate the brain's production of norepinephrine, one of the chemicals that excites the nervous system. During relaxation, mesaconitine decreases the brain's production of norepinephrine, while during stress, it increases the production of this brain chemical. Ginger and licorice moderate and soften the effects of aconite.

Modern traditional Chinese medicine (TCM) practitioners reserve this formula for chronic conditions in which the body's internal energy is severely compromised. It is a much more stimulating formula than Frigid Extremities Powder. (See FRIGID EXTREMITIES POWDER under The Formulas.) The conditions most commonly treated with this formula are persistent upset stomach, vomiting, diarrhea, some symptoms of hypothyroidism, cardiac insufficiency, and arthritis. TCM practitioners also use it to treat people who have had adrenal and pituitary insufficiency and hypothyroidism. Since the formula contains potentially toxic aconite, TCM practitioners and Chinese pharmacies normally sell the formula only after examining the patient. Other practitioners substitute another herb containing aconite, which is less toxic. Do not use this formula if you are anemic or have excessive thirst.

FRIGID EXTREMITIES POWDER

This traditional Chinese herbal formula contains whole bitter oranges, bupleurum, licorice, and peony. It was designed by ancient Chinese herbalists for symptoms including, as one might expect, coldness in the fingers and toes, possibly accompanied by a sensation of fullness in the chest.

In ancient times it was thought that "a clear energy firms up the four limbs." Energy was derived from food. Deficiencies in the energy of the hands and feet sometimes were thought to be caused by failures of digestion. Digestive processes could be restored by the herbs used in the formula. Therefore, this formula was, and is, used to treat cases of digestive diseases, such as gallstones, epigastric pain, diarrhea, and dysmenorrhea.

A chemical compound found in bitter orange, synephrine, stimulates the nerves that cause blood vessels to constrict—to "shut the gate"—in the femoral artery for blood flow to the legs, shunting blood flow to the heart, lungs, kidneys, and brain. This action may be adequate to increase circulation to the liver for the production of bile, needed for cleansing the gallbladder. Saikosides and other chemical constituents in bupleurum stimulate the pituitary gland to direct the adrenal glands to produce glucocorticoids, which reduce inflammation in cell studies. Licorice is useful for a number of digestive disorders. It soothes inflammation and protects the stomach and intestines from the effects of stomach acid. In fact, glycyrrhizinic acid was the first compound proven to promote the healing of ulcers. Unlike many ulcer drugs, glycyrrhizinic acid does not reduce acid production in the stomach, which would result in incomplete digestion. Instead, it increases the stomach's defense mechanisms by fortifying the stomach's protective mucous coating. Glycyrrhizinic acid also increases circulation to the cells lining the intestinal wall, boosting their supply of nutrients and oxygen. Finally, peony contains compounds that stimulate the reabsorption of collagen fibers that can block microscopic blood vessels. This helps repair damage to the blood vessels serving the gallbladder and bile duct caused by the passage of stones, as well increasing the general health of the liver.

The condition most commonly treated with this formula is gallbladder disease. Frigid Extremities Powder is also used to treat fibrocystic breasts, gastritis, hepatitis, mastitis, and peptic ulcer. Unlike Frigid Extremities Decoction, the formula is nontoxic and safe for use as an over-the-counter (OTC) formula. (See FRIGID EXTREMITIES DECOCTION under The Formulas.) Do not use this formula during pregnancy or if you have blood or kidney problems.

GASTRODIA AND UNCARIA DECOCTION

This traditional Chinese herbal formula contains the herbs eucommia, gardenia, gastrodia, hoelen, loranthus, polygonum vine, scutellaria, Sichuan ox knee root, and uncaria (a relative of cat's claw, also known as gambir), as well as finely pulverized abalone shell. Gastrodia, one of the two most important herbs in the formula, is one of the principal herbs in traditional Chinese medicine (TCM) for treating dizziness, headache, high blood pressure, joint pain, muddled speech, muscle spasms, seizures, and vertigo, especially as they relate to emotional tension.

Gastrodia encourages deep sleep and relaxes the central nervous system. It is especially effective in relieving muscle spasms in the face and nerve pain.

TCM practitioners use gastrodia together with uncaria in many formulas for the treatment of epilepsy. Research in Japan shows that these two herbs prevent seizures by increasing the brain's production of its own free-radical scavenger, superoxide dismutase (SOD). The two herbs together also prevent the activation of lipid peroxides, compounds that destroy cell walls. These actions have only been seen in cell lines, so it is not known if the herbal blend is effective for epilepsy, although it is used for this condition.

The most appropriate use of this formula is as a gentle treatment for headache or spasms that have been classified by a neurologist as borderline and not requiring prescription drug treatment. It is not a substitute for medically prescribed treatments for either condition. Check with your doctor first if you have regular headaches or frequent muscle spasms of the extremities.

Gastrodia is a relatively expensive herb. When using an over-the-counter (OTC) medicine that is labeled as including gastrodia, check the list of ingredients to make sure the manufacturer did not substitute the cheaper herb dendrobium.

GENTIANA LONGDANCAO DECOCTION TO DRAIN THE LIVER

This traditional Chinese herbal formula combines akebia, alisma, bupleurum, dong quai, gardenia, gentian, psyllium, rehmannia, and scutellaria.

The phrase *draining the liver* refers to reducing excess "heat" generated by emotional tension. In the theory of traditional Chinese medicine (TCM), anger, irritation, and stress lead to an unhealthy buildup of energy in a channel that passes over the external genitalia and the breasts to the eyes. The channel at the surface of the body is paired with a channel inside the body, starting at the eyes and crossing the head. When heat is constrained in these channels, it causes fever, inflammation, and swelling.

Ancient Chinese herbalists used this formula to treat a pattern of symptoms including bitter taste in the mouth, dizziness, headache, hearing loss, irritability, red and sore eyes, short temper, and swelling in the ears. They also used it to treat difficult or painful urination with a sensation of heat in the urethra, leukorrhea, and vaginal irritation. In women, the pattern of symptoms treated by this formula often includes a shortened menstrual period with unusually dark blood.

There has been only one scientific study of the effects of the formula as a whole. In cell and animal studies, Japanese scientists found that the formula alters the activity of digestive enzymes and slows the rate at which they break down proteins in food. The use of the formula in treating benign prostatic hypertrophy (BPH), ear infection, gallstones, herpes, hyperthyroidism, pelvic inflammatory disease (PID), tinnitus, urinary incontinence, swollen testes, and herpesvirus has to be understood either from the theory of TCM or from the properties of the herbs that go into the formula.

Akebia stops the process of inflammation in cells by deactivating hormones that would allow the capillaries to transport fluids to swell soft tissues. It may stimulate urination. It also sedates the central nervous system and reduces pain. Alisma contains complex polysaccharides that stimulate lymphatic cells to "eat" pathogenic bacteria and yeasts, especially in the urinary tract.

According to the *Japanese Pharmacopeia*, bupleurum stops allergies, aids fat metabolism, calms the central nervous system, induces interferon production for the body's response to cancer and viral infection, inhibits cyclic adenosine monophosphate (cyclic AMP or cAMP, a chemical that causes inflammatory reactions), prevents muscle spasms, prevents side effects of steroid medications, and relaxes smooth muscles. These actions have been demonstrated in cells but not in people yet. Bupleurum stops inflammation by blocking serotonin (also known as 5-hydroxytryptamine, or 5HT), a substance that "opens" the walls of capillaries to allow body fluids to swell into soft tissues. Gardenia teas stimulate the secretion of gastric juices and increase the activity of the muscles in the stomach that pass food down to the intestine. This herb also relieves fever caused by infection.

Gentian, also known as gentiana, helps ease not only gallbladder problems but also indigestion. The bitter taste of gentian triggers a reflex reaction that stimulates the production of saliva and gastric juices. Gentian also stimulates the production of bile. Although increasing the production of digestive juices stimulates both digestion and appetite, this formula is not typically used for these indications.

Of the all herbs in the formula, however, scutellaria has the greatest range of beneficial effects. The pituitary gland, located at the base of the brain, responds to the perception of stress by releasing adrenocorticotrophic hormone (ACTH), a chemical that starts the profound changes in body chemistry that make up the stress response. Laboratory studies have found that scutellaria stops the overproduction of ACTH. Scutellaria inhibits infections with *Staphylococcus aureus*, *Streptococcus pneumoniae*, *Pseudomonas aeruginosa*, *Corynebacterium diphtheriae* (the bacteria that cause diphtheria), and *Neisseria meningitidis* (the bacteria that cause gonorrhea). In one study, penicillin-resistant staph infections remained sensitive to scutellaria. Tinctures of this herb are effective against fungal infections of the skin and tongue.

You should not use this formula if you take medication for a seizure disorder, since it alters the fluid balance in the body and can change the concentration of seizure medications in the bloodstream. Long-term use is not advised. Do not use this formula if you have stomach or spleen ailments.

GINSENG DECOCTION TO NOURISH THE NUTRITIVE CHI

This traditional Chinese herbal formula contains astragalus, atractylodis, bitter orange peel, cinnamon, dong quai, ginseng, hoelen, licorice, peony, polygala root, rehmannia, and schisandra. The *nutritive chi* to which the formula's name refers is a flow of energy (chi) between the digestive organ, the "spleen," and the emotional organ, the "heart." The spleen, the organ believed in traditional Chinese philosophy to house intelligence, was thought to provide energy to the heart, the organ housing the emotions. If excessive deliberation taxed the spleen's energy, the heart also was deprived of energy, and emotional symptoms resulted.

Modern Japanese physicians use this formula to treat dry mouth and throat, dry skin, forgetfulness, hair loss, jaundice, shortness of breath, sores that will not heal, and tired limbs as symptoms accompanying a wide range of

The Mysterious Energy Known as Chi

In Eastern medicine, the natural energy known as chi (pronounced "chee") is the body's vital force, through which all the organs act in harmony to control the self and respond to the environment. Chi is considered to flow through a somewhat complicated system of five paired organs that control and supply one another in ways that reflect the movement of energy of both cosmic and microscopic levels. In the cosmos as a whole, the Five Elements—wood, fire, earth, metal, and water—both create and restrain one another through the action of heat. In the human body, each element is processed by one of the five organ systems: spleen/stomach, lung/large intestine, kidney/bladder, liver/gallbladder, and heart/small intestine. The energy associated with the organ system's activity then circulates up and down the body through precisely defined, but difficult to locate, energy channels, or meridians.

The importance of chi in modern traditional Chinese medicine (TCM) is not just as an explanation of how the body reacts to the Five Elements, but as a concept that unifies a pattern of symptoms. The liver channel, for instance, circulates energy over the breasts and the middle of the eyes to the crown of the head. An energy disturbance in this channel, therefore, can manifest itself in the liver, breasts, eyes, or crown of the head. Yellowing of the whites of the eyes, for example, is symptomatic of the liver disorder hepatitis. Breast pain may occur at the same time as headache in women with premenstrual syndrome (PMS). Especially in the early diagnosis of cancer, recognizing combinations of symptoms along the energy meridians makes TCM a useful complement to conventional medical treatment.

diseases. It is also used to increase the effectiveness of prednisolone (Pediapred, Prelone, and others), a steroid drug used to treat asthma, and cancer symptoms, but this was only shown to be true in cell studies. Human data for this use with prednisolone are lacking.

HOCHU-EKKI-TO

This Japanese herbal formula, also known as Tonify the Middle and Augment the Qi (or Chi) Decoction, combines astragalus, atractylodis, bitter orange peel, black cohosh, bupleurum, dong quai, ginseng, and licorice. Although the formula was originally used to treat prolonged infections causing fevers and chills, its most frequent application today is in the treatment of male infertility for which there is no readily discernible cause. It was also developed to relieve fatigue, boost immunity, and help relieve the symptoms of chemotherapy.

This product is studied more extensively than other Japanese herbal formulas in cell studies using human cells and in animals. However, clinical studies exist as well. In a clinical study in Japan, 20 percent of participating couples achieved conception within twelve weeks, and 51 percent of the men taking the formula had increased sperm counts. Laboratory studies indicate that the formula works by stimulating the production of proteins that enable sperm to reach functional maturity. The formula is particularly effective in alleviating male reproductive problems caused by chemotherapy with doxorubicin (Adriamycin, Rubex), but check with your doctor before using it. In a group of elderly patients complaining of general fatigue or weakness who took 7.5 grams of hochu-ekki-to experienced improvements in immunocological markers in the blood after four months.

Additionally, in human cell studies, hochu-ekki-to has been used to activate the immune system to attack certain kinds of cancer by increasing the number of NK (natural killer) cells, and to help the bone marrow recover after cancer treatment with either cyclophosphamide (Cytoxan, Neosar) or radiation therapy. If you have cancer, do not use the formula without checking with your physician first.

Hochu-ekki-to is available from practitioners of traditional Chinese medicine (TCM) for use as a tea. It does not interfere with hormonal treatments for infertile men.

HONEY-FRIED LICORICE DECOCTION

This traditional Chinese herbal formula contains cinnamon bark, gelatin, ginger, ginseng, jujube, licorice, marijuana seed (which is legal throughout the United States but nonetheless is usually labeled *linum*), ophiopogon, and rehmannia. Honey-fried licorice is licorice that has been caramelized to a reddish brown. Chinese herbalists still use this method of preparing the herb to treat digestive upsets. It also is used for nourishing the blood and maintaining optimal blood flow.

The formula can be understood in terms of its constituent herbs in cell studies. Cinnamon contains chemicals that inhibit a substance in the blood called thromboxane A_2. Thromboxane causes platelets in the blood to clump together. Counteracting this compound may lead to less clotting and a more normal blood flow.

Gelatin has several pharmacological actions. Its primary action, when the formula is taken for several weeks, is to stimulate hematopoiesis, the production of red blood cells and hemoglobin in the bone marrow. Gelatin not only stimulates the bone marrow to produce red blood cells, but also increases the rate at which the bones acrue calcium, potentially preventing osteoporosis. Gelatin helps muscle tissue to regenerate after injury. But these changes have been seen only in human cells and not in people.

Ginger has been found to inhibit the production of immune-system chemicals called cytokines in cell studies. This action reduces inflammation. This pharmacological effect makes ginger useful in treating a number of disorders marked by swelling and pain. Ginger also eases indigestion and nausea.

Ginseng reduces digestive upsets caused by emotional stress and may inhibit ulcer formation. Ginseng compounds even reduce *anticipated* stress. Studies have found that injected ginseng compounds increase the body's production of adrenocorticotropic hormone (ACTH) and certain steroid hormones, such as adrenaline. This stimulates the natural function of the body's stress-response system, which keeps the adrenal glands from burning out during prolonged periods of stress. This has not been demonstrated in humans.

Jujube contains some ascorbic acid. The immature fruit consists of 1 percent vitamin C, but this supplies less than 10 percent of the formula's recipe. The fruit also sweetens the formula and makes it less likely to cause stomach upset if overdosed.

Licorice is of special use in treating chronic fatigue syndrome (CFS). More than 95 percent of individuals with CFS, which is marked by overwhelming fatigue, have low blood pressure. Some physicians speculate that low blood pressure results in oxygen deprivation of brain cells, leading to depression and fatigue. One theory of this condition is that it stems from adrenal-hormone deficiencies that cause the body to lose both sodium and water, resulting in drops in both blood volume and blood pressure. Licorice is only 13.5 percent of the formula, so whether it works in people with CFS has not been demonstrated.

One of the chemical components of licorice can reverse the process of adrenal insufficiency. Glycyrrhizinic acid blocks the activity of an enzyme that otherwise would destroy the adrenal hormone cortisol. Proper cortisol levels in the bloodstream enable the kidneys to retain more sodium, and thus more water. This leads to higher blood pressure. Again, this was shown in cell studies but not in humans.

Ophiopogon has a number of effects on the cardiovascular system. It increases coronary blood flow, increases the vigor of heart muscle fibers, helps the heart deal with oxygen deprivation, and slowly elevates blood pressure. Rehmannia has a protective effect on the liver. The two herbs each provide 10 percent of the final product.

Both traditional and modern products based on this formula include marijuana seed. In Eastern medicine, marijuana seed is used only as a source of oils that prevent constipation. *Heat-treated* marijuana seed, imported from China, contains no psychoactive compounds, and is legal throughout the United States and Canada. It will not produce a "high," but will cause a false-positive urine test for marijuana, although sophisticated testing methods can distinguish use of marijuana seed from that of other plant parts.

Traditional Chinese medicine (TCM) practitioners use this formula, or modifications of it, for people whose symptoms include constipation, dry mouth and throat, insomnia, irritability, palpitations upon anxiety, shortness of breath, and/or weak pulse. The formula is used when the medical diagnosis is chronic fatigue with "dry" symptoms—dry skin, fever in the hands and feet, anxiety, insomnia, and irritability. It is also used to prevent weight loss in people with hyperthyroidism. Because the herbs used in the formula can stimulate estrogen production, Honey-Fried Licorice Decoction should not be used by women who have breast or endometrial cancer, endometriosis, uterine fibroids, or ovarian cysts.

HOXSEY FORMULA

The Hoxsey Formula was developed by Harry Hoxsey (1901–1974), an ex–coal miner who had dropped out of high school. Hoxsey often successfully treated cancer patients with a formula that he claimed had been passed down through his family. He engaged in a nationally publicized controversy with the president of the American Medical Association for over twenty years, and became the subject of both critical and complimentary books and films. Although there have been many variations of his formula, the Hoxsey combination most commonly used today contains barberry, burdock, casara sagrada, licorice, pokeweed, red clover, and stillingia.

Hoxsey Formula is under long-term study by the University of Texas School of Public Health. Unpublished results report that users of the formula include long-term survivors of advanced lung cancer, and a level-5 melanoma patient, a patient with recurrent bladder cancer, and a patient with labial (lip) cancer, all of whom went into remission. Given these types of cancer and the difficulty in treating them, the results are impressive. The University of Texas MD Anderson Cancer Center performed an extensive human study literature review of the Hoxsey treatment. Some benefit was seen in patients, but there were no controlled, matched patients with the same type of cancer, so it is difficult to interpret the results. A clinic in Tijuana, Mexico, run by Hoxsey's former nurse, claims

an 80 percent cure rate, but these claims have been neither confirmed nor refuted. Mildred Nelson, the former nurse, died in 1999.

Known characteristics of some of the herbs in the formula support its use in the treatment of cancer. Of the nine herbs in the blend, seven have been shown to have some anitcancer activity in cell studies. Barberry root is a source of berberine, which has known inhibitory effects on bladder cancer, colon cancer, glioblastoma (a type of brain cancer), leukemia, liver cancer, and myeloma cells. Berberine also increases the responsiveness of some kinds of cancer cells to the chemotherapy drug paclitaxel (Taxol) and improves the response of treatment-resistant liver cancer cells to chemotherapy. Burdock root increases the rate at which estrogen is excreted into the stool and lowers the amount of estrogen in circulation that might otherwise stimulate certain cancers of the breast, endometrium, or ovaries. One of the chemicals found in cascara sagrada, emodin, has been found in the laboratory to greatly enhance the effectiveness of conventional chemotherapies. It makes breast cancer cells more sensitive to paclitaxel (Taxol), and makes certain types of lung cancer cells more sensitive to cisplatin (Platinol) and doxorubicin (Adriamycin, Rubex). Do not use this formula with these drugs unless your physician agrees. Licorice may protect the body against a number of cancer-causing toxins. It prevents the formation of skin tumors in response to noxious chemicals in animals. Glycyrrhetic acid protects against tumor formation. It inhibits the cancer-causing effects of pollutants such as benzopyrenes and a chemical called aflatoxin that is found in improperly stored food grains. Pokeweed is being tested around the world as a potential treatment for leukemia. In laboratory tests, red clover blocks estrogen from stimulating breast cancer cells.

There are no known cases of toxic side effects from using Hoxsey Formula. Neither are there any chronic health conditions that are likely to be worsened by using the formula in the dosage recommended by its packagers and manufacturers. However, some ingredients of Hoxsey Formula can cause nausea, vomiting, and diarrhea if taken in larger quantities than advised. Barberry root can cause swelling of the kidneys and produces heart toxcitiy in rabbits. Toxic reactions have been reported, such as acne, erectile dysfunction (ED), and a mumps-like condition. Hoxsey Formula is not a substitute for medically supervised cancer treatment.

KIDNEY CHI PILL FROM THE GOLDEN CABINET

This traditional Chinese herbal formula contains alisma, cinnamon bark, cornelian cherry, dioscorea, hoelen, moutan peony, prepared aconite, and rehmannia. *Chi* refers to vital energy, and *The Golden Cabinet* was a fourth-century book explaining the highly esteemed herbal formulas of Zhang Zhongjing.

The ancient herbalist Zhang Zhongjing designed this

formula to treat diseases that cause symptoms such as back pain, a cold sensation in the lower half of the body, excessive urination or difficult urination occurring with edema throughout the body, tension in the lower abdomen, and weakness in the lower extremities.

In this formula, aconite provides pain relief. Aconite contains a potent analgesic agent, mesaconitine, which raises the threshold of pain and helps the body become attuned to both relaxation and stress. In laboratory studies, mesaconitine has been found to manipulate the brain's production of norepinephrine, one of the chemicals that excites the nervous system. During relaxation, mesaconitine decreases the brain's production of norepinephrine, while during stress, it increases the production of this brain chemical. Aconite also creates a sensation of warmth, useful in relief of symptoms of hypothyroidism. The other herbs in this formula stimulate urination to relieve accumulations of fluid.

The primary use of this formula is to correct conditions in which fluid has "poured into" the legs, making it difficult to walk. It is particularly appropriate for people who have leg pain or lower back pain. Other Western uses include diabetes, kidney disease, asthma, urinary retention, and hypothyroidism. It is not compatible, however, with many prescription medications.

While Kidney Chi Pill is used to treat *partial* seizure disorders for which other medication is not prescribed, anyone who is taking antiseizure medications should avoid it. The formula removes both fluid and minerals from circulation, which can cause bloodstream levels of prescription medications to become too concentrated. It is best to avoid food and drink around the time that the formula is consumed. Two of the ingredients in the formula can be toxic (rou gui [cinnamon] and fu zi [aconite]), so avoid taking too much Kidney Chi Pill. Despite having toxic herbs, the formula's herbs are combined to mitigate their toxicity when correctly prepared.

KUDZU DECOCTION

This traditional Chinese herbal formula contains cinnamon, ephedra, ginger, jujube, kudzu, licorice, and peony. It was originally formulated to treat a symptom pattern that included stiffness in the neck and upper back, and fever and chills without sweating. This formula contains ephedra. Ephedra is banned in the United States, though it is still allowed to be sold in dietary supplements sold by licensed practitioners in traditional Chinese medicine (TCM) formulations that are recommended for their TCM uses.

Kudzu may relieve tightness in the neck and back, and the other herbs in the formula may help increase circulation and relieve fever by inducing perspiration. In terms of TCM, the herbs of the formula act synchronously to "release" infection.

The description of an infection as being difficult to

release matches the symptoms of the early stages of herpes infection. The immune system vanquishes most viral infections, such as colds, within a few days to a few weeks. Some viruses, however—including herpesvirus, some hepatitis viruses, and HIV—can remain dormant in the body without causing symptoms for many years, only to be activated (or reactivated) when the body's overall resistance is weakened, when the infected area is exposed to ultraviolet light, or when the tissue containing the virus is mechanically damaged.

Researchers at Toyama University in Japan saw the connection between the two descriptions of symptoms and studied the use of Kudzu Decoction as a herpes treatment. Their research found that the formula neither kills the virus directly nor activates the body's immune system. Instead, Kudzu Decoction blocks the tissue-damaging effects of the reactivated virus in mice. In this way, the traditional Chinese herbal formula may treat one disease without creating a worse condition in its place, but there are no human studies to shown that this works in people.

Kudzu Decoction protects skin damaged by eczema or psoriasis. It is also used in everyday treatment in Japan for nasal allergy or colds accompanied by stiff neck or back, for diarrhea and food allergies in children, for ear infections, and for sinusitis. While this formula is extraordinarily nontoxic, it is important to drink at least eight glasses of water a day while taking bottled versions of the formula to avoid a small risk of dehydration.

LEDEBOURIELLA DECOCTION THAT SAGELY UNBLOCKS

This traditional Chinese herbal formula, also known by its name in Mandarin, *fang feng shong teng san*, combines atractylodis, dong quai, ephedra, epsom salts, forsythia, gardenia fruit, gypsum, ledebouriella, licorice, ligusticum, peony, peppermint, platycodon, schizonepeta, scutellaria, talc, and wine-treated rhubarb root. The most important of the seventeen herbs and minerals in the formula is ledebouriella. This formula contains ephedra. Ephedra is banned in the United States, though it is still allowed to be sold in dietary supplements sold by licensed practitioners in traditional Chinese medicine (TCM) formulations that are recommended for their TCM uses.

The Chinese name for ledebouriella, *fang feng*, literally means "guard against wind." In ancient Chinese medicine, *wind* was a symbolic as well as a literal term referring to any pernicious or pathogenic influence attempting to enter the body. Chinese physicians employed ledebouriella to expel "wind" from the exterior layers of the body to treat body aches, chills, fever, and headache. They also used the herb to expel "wind dampness," a condition believed to cause stiff joints, and "intestinal wind," a condition thought to result in recurrent, painful diarrhea with bright blood in the stool. In the literature of TCM, the herb's action is said to be *sage* in that it relieves the digestive tract of infection without purgation.

Ledebouriella has an inhibitory effect against some flu viruses as well as the bacteria that cause pseudomonas, shigella, and staph infections in laboratory studies. Taken in teas, it has been used to relieve fever. Ledebouriella teas also raise the threshold of pain—that is, they lower the sensitivity of the nervous system to pain. Chinese physicians have even found ledebouriella to be an effective antidote to arsenic poisoning.

The most common application of this formula today is for weight control. Obesity was essentially unknown in ancient China and Japan, but today it is more common in both of these countries. Japanese physicians have observed that the two "sage" effects of the formula act together to reduce weight, as shown in obese mice. The formula is especially helpful if symptoms include constipation, high blood pressure, chronic nasal congestion with thick discharge, sore eyes, or a tendency to flush in the face when excited or embarrassed.

Laboratory research has verified the formula's usefulness in the treatment of obesity. The formula activates energy-burning brown fat cells. Using the formula reduces both body fat percentage and total body weight.

Holistic physicians sometimes prescribe this formula to relieve diarrhea during withdrawal from morphine, a painkiller that also inhibits the transmission of nerve impulses to the smooth muscles lining the intestines. The use of this drug frequently leads to constipation. When people are weaned off morphine, they often experience the opposite symptom, diarrhea. Laboratory tests of Ledebouriella Decoction That Sagely Unblocks find that it may reduce the frequency and severity of diarrhea during morphine withdrawal.

For reasons that are not completely understood, ginger used in cooking or as a condiment or tea counteracts the medicinal effects of ledebouriella. You should not eat or otherwise consume ginger while taking this formula.

LICORICE, WHEAT, AND JUJUBE DECOCTION

This traditional Chinese herbal formula combines jujube, licorice, and wheat, common foodstuffs in northern China. Jujube and wheat are calming herbs whose effect on the central nervous system has been documented by science, and licorice settles stomach upset.

Practitioners of traditional Chinese medicine (TCM) have recommended this combination for centuries as a home remedy for emotional disorders causing disorientation, frequent attacks of sadness with crying spells, inability to control oneself, restless sleep, and frequent bouts of yawning. In the theory of TCM, this syndrome is attributed to anxiety, excessive worry, or pensiveness disrupting the flow of energy throughout the body. In early stages of the syndrome, the dominant symptoms are disorientation, impulsiveness, and fitful sleep. As the condition progresses, the "lost soul" produces attacks of unusual behavior related to a loss of self-control, such as crying or yawning.

Although the traditional interpretation of the effects of Licorice, Wheat, and Jujube Decoction is clearly poetic rather than scientific, there is some evidence for the ability of the formula to relieve depression. Wheat has pharmacological actions surprisingly similar to (although obviously far less strong than) those of opium. That is, alkaloids in wheat bind to the same receptor sites in the brain as opium, morphine, and heroin do. This may account for the calming effect of some so-called comfort foods, as well as for the psychological reactions sometimes experienced by people who are especially sensitive to wheat glutens.

This is an extraordinarily nontoxic formula, which is customarily given to children experiencing sobbing and loss of emotional control. It has been used to prevent bedwetting in children, but check with your child's pediatrician before using this formulation.

MAJOR BUPLEURUM DECOCTION

This traditional Chinese herbal formula contains bitter orange, bupleurum, ginger, jujube, peony, pinellia, rhubarb, and scutellaria. As its name suggests, its principal herb is bupleurum. In the terminology of traditional Chinese medicine (TCM), a *major* formula treats major symptoms that cause serious discomfort. Ancient Chinese herbalists designed this formula to treat bitter taste in the mouth, burning diarrhea or no bowel movements at all, continuous vomiting, despondency, fever and chills, and nausea. It was later used to treat women for what was referred to as a "lump-in-the-throat," which produced feelings especially related to sadness or depression.

There has been considerable scientific study of this formula as a whole. In rats, Major Bupleurum Decoction reduces the rate at which glucose enters the bloodstream from digested food after meals and increases the efficiency of insulin. It may be especially useful for the treatment of people who have diabetes with long-term gastrointestinal disorders such as gastroparesis. The formula also reduces the concentration of cholesterol in the bile, inhibiting the formation of gallstones.

Studies have found that Major Bupleurum Decoction is useful for people who have problems with both overweight and high cholesterol. A three-month course of treatment with this formula usually raises levels of high-density lipoprotein (HDLs, or "good") cholesterol and lowers low-density lipoprotein (LDLs, or "bad") cholesterol. It also was shown in cell lines to prevent free-radical reactions that can lead to atherosclerosis. Thus, Major Bupleurum Decoction's free-radical-scavenging action may reduce damage to nerve tissue after heart attack and stroke. It achieves this effect by scavenging oxygen-derived free radicals that are formed as blood circulation is restored.

TCM practitioners today use this formula to treat a wide range of conditions, including acute pancreatitis, occlusions of the bile ducts, gallstones, dysentery, food poisoning, gastroenteritis, hepatitis, malignant hypertension, migraine, peritonitis, pleurisy, fevers of malaria, and trigeminal neuralgia.

MAJOR CONSTRUCT THE MIDDLE DECOCTION

This traditional Chinese herbal formula consists of ginger, ginseng, maltose sugar, and prickly ash. The Chinese term *construct the middle* refers to the formula's use in stopping spasms and soreness in the middle of the body—that is, the abdomen and stomach. A *major* formula contains especially potent herbs for its purpose.

In animal studies, Japanese scientists have found that minutes after this formula is taken, the brain releases three proteins that control digestion and motion in the intestines: gastrin, motilin, and somatostatin. The secretion of gastrin ensures the normal production of stomach acids needed to digest food. Gastrin can react with the irritant chemical histamine, but the licorice in the formula blocks histamine. This may stop the production of quantities of stomach acid large enough to aggravate or cause ulcers. The somatostatin the brain releases in response to the formula also puts a brake on excessive acid production. Higher levels of motilin ensure that the digested food passes out of the stomach quickly, and that the stomach produces a minimal amount of acid. Regulating these proteins together offers significant relief of gastritis. However, there are no human studies available to confirm this.

In addition to helping stop production of excess acid in the stomach, this formula helps to ensure the smooth transit of digested food through the intestine. The herbs in this formula, especially ginger, help prevent intestinal blockages after surgery, but it has not been tested postoperatively in patients. Do not use this formula in this way unless your surgeon agrees.

Since this formula contains prickly ash, it should be avoided during pregnancy. Theoretically, the formula could stimulate immune processes that may be detrimental to the fetus.

MINOR BLUEGREEN DRAGON DECOCTION

This traditional Chinese herbal formula contains asiasarum, cinnamon bark, ephedra, ginger, licorice, peony, pinellia, and schisandra. In Chinese folk religion, the bluegreen dragon was the spirit of the east, a wood spirit responsible for generating clouds and for making waves on the sea. A major bluegreen dragon produced downpours of rain. A minor bluegreen dragon produced billowing waves on the sea. This formula was named after the minor bluegreen dragon for its ability to produce waves of movement in the chest, and possibly relieving congestion. This formula contains ephedra. Ephedra is banned in the United States, though it is still allowed to be sold in dietary supplements sold by licensed practitioners in traditional Chinese medicine (TCM) formulations that are recommended for their TCM uses.

Laboratory studies show that Minor Bluegreen Dragon Decoction is an effective preventive against influenza A, provided that it is administered four to seven days before exposure to the infection. Minor Bluegreen Dragon Decoction does not act directly on the virus, but rather stimulates the immune system to deal with the virus. Several tests, including a double-blind clinical study with 200 participants in Japan, found that Minor Bluegreen Dragon Decoction is effective against allergic rhinitis and allergic conjunctivitis. Although the formula is an antihistamine, it does not cause drowsiness or cardiac complications when used with other medications.

Because this formula contains several herbs that stimulate the production of estrogen, it should be avoided by women who have estrogen-stimulated cancers of the breast, endometrium, or ovaries, or who have melanoma, fibroids (uterine myomas), fibrocystic breasts, or premenstrual syndrome (PMS).

MINOR BUPLEURUM DECOCTION

This traditional Chinese herbal formula contains bupleurum, ginger, ginseng, jujube, licorice, pinellia, and scutellaria. It has become the most promising Eastern herbal formula for treating chronic viral infections and cancer.

A second-century Chinese herbalist named Zhang Zhongjing designed this formula for treating bitter or sour taste in the mouth, dizziness, dry throat, feeling of fullness in the chest, fever and chills, heartburn, irritability, nausea, reduced appetite, and vomiting. The symptoms were thought to occur as diseases progressed from acute to chronic. Over time, herbalists in China and Japan recognized that the formula was useful for treating infectious diseases that had weakened the body's defenses to reach the verge of progressing to chronic conditions. Modern Japanese researchers recognized that viral infections and cancer act in the same way.

Minor Bupleurum Decoction has become the treatment of choice for viral hepatitis B in Japan. Patients were followed for five years, and there was a one-third reduction in the incidence of liver cancer and a 40 percent reduction in death. The formula showed increases in the production of immune-system components that keep the virus from forming proteins and attack the virus directly. Today there is a vaccine for hepatitis B to prevent you from ever getting it.

The value of Minor Bupleurum Decoction in the treatment of liver disease is not limited to viral hepatitis.

Clinical trials have shown that the formula may be helpful in treating cirrhosis of the liver, and in cell studies the formula has been shown to slow or stop the development of liver cancer cells. In laboratory studies with animals, the formula stops the progression of hyperplastic alveolar nodules, or precancerous cells in the breasts, lungs, and ovaries. Minor Bupleurum Decoction is also effective against viruses other than those that cause hepatitis. In the laboratory, the formula produces a 50 percent reduction in the ability of HIV to replicate itself, a figure that jumps to 80 percent for leukemia viruses. The formula fights viruses by blocking an enzyme known as reverse transcriptase, an enzyme that viruses use to convert their genetic information into a form they can use to reproduce themselves. Studies at Columbia University show that Minor Bupleurum Decoction may be capable of lowering viral load in HIV-positive people who have not yet developed AIDS, although it is ineffective in stopping reproduction of the virus in people who already have AIDS. It is also under investigation to increase survival in patients with hepatitis C and liver cancer.

Traditional Chinese medicine (TCM) practitioners also use Minor Bupleurum Decoction in the treatment of asthma, although it was traditionally used for difficulty breathing, fullness of the chest, influenza, and bronchitis. This formula is also a part of a combination formula called *sairei-to.*

You should not use Minor Bupelurum Decoction if you have a fever or a skin infection. Taken long-term as a patent medicine rather than as a tea, this formula can cause headache, dizziness, and bleeding gums. These effects can be avoided if the formula is prepared from whole herbs as a tea. This formula also worsens side effects from the treatment of liver disorders with alpha-interferon.

Special caution is required in using this formula in the treatment of hepatitis C. Japanese physicians have reported sixty-six cases of interstitial pneumonia (pneumonia causing congestion lower in the lungs than in bronchitis) among people with hepatitis C who were being treated with this formula because of a unique complication of immune stimulation. This complication is not likely in people who do not have hepatitis C. Do not use this formula if you are pregnant or using interferon.

OPHIOPOGONIS DECOCTION

This Chinese herbal formula contains ginseng, jujube, licorice, the bulb of an Oriental lily known as ophiopogon, and pinellia. It was traditionally taken with rice porridge.

The second-century Chinese herbalist Zhang Zhongjing devised this formula to treat a condition then called "lung atrophy." The use of the formula was popularized and expanded in the fourth-century medical manual *Emergency Formulas to Keep Up One's Sleeve*, which recommended it for the treatment of digestive ailments. Practitioners of traditional Chinese medicine (TCM) today use the formula to treat ailments that cause coughing and spitting of saliva, a dry and uncomfortable sensation in the throat, dry mouth, red tongue, shortness of breath, and wheezing. The formula is used to treat a wide range of disorders of breathing or digestion, as well as the complications of drug treatment that interfere with breathing or digestion.

Modern science explains how Ophiopogonis Decoction could have an action on both the stomach and the lungs. Laboratory tests show that chemicals released by the formula increase the activity of beta-adrenergic nerves. These nerves relax the muscles lining the bronchial tubes, stimulate the burning of fat, and relax both the uterus and the lower gastrointestinal tract. Stimulating impulses along the beta-adrenergic nerves opens breathing passages in the lungs. Human studies have shown that this formula may be beneficial in treating nausea and vomiting (93 percent effective), morning sickness, dry mouth, gastritis (79 percent effective), peptic ulcer (95 percent effective), bronchitis, cough, and pneumonia.

At the same time the formula stimulates beta-adrenergic nerves, it inhibits the superior pharyngeal nerve. This is the nerve that causes the cough reflex. Unlike other drugs that suppress the cough reflex, such as codeine, Ophiopogonis Decoction seems to affect the superior pharyngeal nerve only during bronchitis or asthmatic attack. It probably does not activate the cough reflex in healthy people, but this has not been tested.

Ophiopogonis Decoction has been used in clinical tests for the management of Sjögren's syndrome, an autoimmune disease in which the body mistakes the salivary glands for invading infectious microorganisms. Ophiopogonis Decoction increases salivary secretion and prevents oral infection during Sjögren's syndrome.

Because the formula contains several herbs that stimulate the production of estrogen, it should be avoided by women who have estrogen-stimulated cancers of the breast, endometrium, or ovaries, melanoma, uterine fibroids, fibrocystic breast disease, or premenstrual syndrome.

OYSTER SHELL POWDER

This traditional Chinese herbal formula combines astragalus, ephedra, and wheat with finely pulverized oyster shell. Modern traditional Chinese medicine (TCM) uses it for symptoms including fatigue, irritability, lethargy, shortness of breath, and spontaneous sweating that worsen at night. Textbooks of TCM note that people who have these symptoms usually are also easily startled. This formula contains ephedra. Ephedra is banned in the United States, though it is still allowed to be sold in dietary supplements sold by licensed practitioners in TCM formulations that are recommended for their TCM uses.

The sages of Chinese herbal medicine understood this formula to work by "anchoring floating energies." *Floating energies* were displaced emotional energies that the body dissipated through nervous symptoms. The Chinese herbalists thought the formula acted primarily through its chief ingredient of the formula, oyster shell.

Today it is known that oyster shell is a mineral-balanced source of calcium, which is well known for its ability to relax tense muscles in cell studies. Wheat has pharmacological actions surprisingly similar to those of opium in laboratory studies. Opiumlike alkaloids in wheat bind to the same receptor sites in the brain as opium, morphine, and heroin in laboratory studies. This may account for the calming effect of some so-called comfort foods, for psychological reactions sometimes experienced by people who are especially sensitive to wheat glutens, and for the relaxing effects of this formula. The ingredients in the formula also act synergistically to reduce perspiration induced by emotional tension.

Two herbs make the formula useful for treating chronic fatigue syndrome (CFS) in cell studies. Astragalus stimulates components of the immune system that are depleted in people with CFS, especially the natural killer (NK) cells. It does this without stimulating the components of the immune system, especially the B cell. Ephedra raises blood pressure, which is often too low and poorly regulated in people with CFS. If you have CFS, speak to your doctor before using this product.

The medically defined condition most commonly treated with this formula is chronic fatigue. People who have celiac disease or allergies to shellfish or wheat should not use it.

PEONY AND LICORICE DECOCTION

This formula combines two herbs, peony and licorice. It is used to treat disturbances of the "liver channel," especially pain thought to be caused by rebellious emotions "stored" in the liver. When these emotions are released, they cause cramps and pain in all of the organs and parts of the body controlled by liver energies, including the abdomen, calves, and hands, and the breasts and external genitalia.

Modern research supports the traditional view of Peony and Licorice Decoction as a valuable aid to the reproductive system. Laboratory studies have revealed that the formula increases the body's production of dehydroepiandrosterone (DHEA), which is converted into estrogen. This action may make the formula useful in treating menopausal symptoms. It is thought to increase a woman's chances of becoming pregnant by influencing other hormone balances. It has also been used for normalizing the length of menstruation. In men, it decreases the production of testosterone, which can slow both benign prostatic hypertrophy (BPH) and the spread of prostate cancer.

Because Peony and Licorice Decoction stimulates estrogen production in women, it should not be used by women with estrogen-sensitive disorders, such as breast or uterine cancer, fibrocystic breast disease, uterine fibroids, or endometriosis. It also should be avoided by women who take birth control pills. It has been used for treating ovarian cysts, but it should not be used by those with polycystic ovarian syndrome.

PILL FOR DEAFNESS THAT IS KIND TO THE LEFT KIDNEY

This traditional Chinese herbal formula contains acorus, alisma, cornelian cherry, dioscorea, hoelen, magnetite (iron filings), moutan peony, rehmannia, and schisandra. The formula's quaint name derives from *The Yellow Emperor's Classic of Internal Medicine*, which said, "The kidney's chi [energy] goes through the ear. If the kidney is harmonized, the ear can hear the five tones." In Chinese medicine, the left kidney refers to the yin, or supportive, energies of the kidneys, while the right kidney refers to the yang, or circulating, energies of the kidney. When the left kidney chi is depleted, the function of hearing is inadequately supported.

Chinese herbalists designed this formula to treat continuous tinnitus that can be likened to the sound of swarming insects. It also treats blurry vision, hearing loss, insomnia, and irritability. It is not a treatment for tinnitus with abrupt onset or hearing loss related to an infection. This formula is a variation of Kidney Chi Pill without ingredients for pain relief. (*See* KIDNEY CHI PILL *under* The Formulas.)

PINELLIA AND MAGNOLIA BARK DECOCTION

This traditional Chinese herbal formula contains ginger, hoelen, magnolia bark, perilla leaf, and pinellia. A third-century classic of Chinese medical literature recommended this combination for "women who feel as if a plum pit were stuck in their throats." The condition, which of course can also be experienced by men, has come to be known in Eastern medicine as *plum-pit chi*. The corresponding term in English is "lump in the throat." The feeling that something is stuck in the throat is usually due to emotional upset.

The primary active ingredients of this formula are found in pinellia, which loosens the "lump in the throat" by preventing the transmission of impulses to the nerves that cause both the sensation of tightness over the larynx and the vomiting reflex. It also resolves phlegm accumulation in the lungs. The other nutrients in the formula restore bowel elimination, ease the liver, disperse stagnated water, and counteract nausea.

Today, this formula is most commonly used for symptomatic relief of anxiety and depression. Traditional Chinese medicine (TCM) practitioners also use it to treat chronic laryngitis, esophageal spasms, various gastrointestinal disorders related to chronic stress, hysteria, and sore throat. You should not use pinellia if you are experiencing any kind of bleeding. Use it with caution if you have a fever, and stop using it if any existing fever worsens.

Pinellia root contains compounds that are otherwise

nontoxic but that make the glaucoma medication pilo-carpine (in Betoptic Pilo, Ocusert, Pilopine, and Salagen) less effective. If you take pilocarpine, you should not take pinellia by itself. Formulas in which pinellia is combined with buffering herbs are safe for short-term use if you also take pilocarpine. It is best to avoid this formula during pregnancy, as some of the ingredients, such as magnolia bark, may be harmful, but most often only if they are taken in large doses.

PINELLIA DECOCTION TO DRAIN THE EPIGASTRIUM

This traditional Chinese herbal formula contains coptis, ginger, ginseng, licorice, chopped jujube dates, pinellia, and scutellaria. It was originally used to treat a pattern of symptoms including fullness and tightness of the area just above the navel with very slight or no pain, borborygmus (rumbling noises) with diarrhea, dry heaves or vomiting, and reduced appetite. In the experience of the ancient Chinese physicians who invented the formula, these symptoms most frequently resulted not from any infectious disease but rather from overdoses of stimulant laxative herbs.

Modern research has produced evidence confirming this formula's use in treating digestive upset in people with chronic bowel complaints, chronic hepatitis, early stage cirrhosis, and hypersecretion of acid from the stomach causing ulcers. Laboratory tests have shown in cells that the formula inhibits cyclic adenosine monophos-phate (cyclic AMP or cAMP), a chemical that instructs cells to make a series of hormones involved in inflammation.

Pinellia Decoction to Drain the Epigastrium also has a potential for a purely modern application. Researchers at Japan's Hoshi University have found that the formula is effective in preventing damage from radiation burns when it is taken orally after radiation exposure. However, this is in cells, and human data are lacking. This formula may help people undergoing treatment for cancer in that it slows diarrhea without affecting the motility, or propulsive power, of the intestines, so that constipation does not result if they accidentally take too much of the formula.

You should not use any formula containing pinellia if you have any kind of bleeding. Use pinellia with caution if you have a fever, and stop taking it if any existing fever worsens. Pinellia root contains compounds that are otherwise nontoxic but that make the glaucoma medication pilocarpine less effective. If you take pilocarpine (in Betoptic Pilo, Ocusert, Pilopine, and Salagen), you should not take pinellia by itself. Formulas in which pinellia is buffered by other herbs are safe for short-term use if you also take pilocarpine.

POLYPORUS DECOCTION

This formula contains alisma, gelatin, hoelen, a red clay known as kadinum, and the mushroom polyporus. It was developed in early Chinese medicine for a pattern of symptoms in which urinary difficulty is accompanied by fever and thirst. Secondary symptoms treated with the formula include cough, diarrhea, insomnia, irritability, and/or nausea.

According to the second-century sage of Chinese herbal medicine Zhang Zhongjing, the combination of symptoms for which Polyporus Decoction is appropriately given results from infection. Zhang's figurative description of the infectious process was that heat battles with water and disturbs the water pathways, resulting in urinary difficulty. Heat also gives rise to fever. When a person with a fever gives in to the desire to drink, fluids cannot be eliminated through the urine. Instead, they are eliminated through the stool, resulting in diarrhea. The principal herb in this formula, polyporus, imparts its energies to the water pathways and makes urination possible again.

The modern use of the formula has a more scientific basis. There is considerable clinical experience in Japan in the use of Polyporus Decoction to treat urinary tract infections (UTIs). Hospital tests record that over 90 percent of people with a combination of symptoms that modern Japanese doctors call "urethral syndrome"—painful urination and/or a sense of retained urine—found relief when taking this formula, without side effects.

The formula may stimulate the passage of kidney stones, but its use for this purpose is very dosage-specific. Modern Chinese formulas employ two to three times the amount of herb specified by Zhang Zhongjing. Clinical tests of Polyporus Decoction show that at low dosages, the formula relieves kidney stones without forcing the body to excrete vitamin C, unlike most medications for kidney stones. High doses of Polyporus Decoction, however, have no effect on kidney stones. Questions of dosage should be discussed with the traditional Chinese medicine (TCM) practitioner dispensing the formula, and if you are seeing a doctor for your kidneys, you should consult that professional as well.

TCM practitioners also use Polyporus Decoction to treat a range of other conditions in which nausea and vomiting are prominent symptoms. The formula is non-toxic and is compatible with prescription medications for diabetes, high blood pressure, and autoimmune diseases such as rheumatoid arthritis. However, do not use the formula in this way without consulting with your physician first. Polyporus Decoction should not be used while you are experiencing *acute* pain from kidney stones, but instead should be used as a long-term preventive measure.

ROBERT'S FORMULA

Robert's Formula is a combination of baptisia (wild indigo), cabbage powder, *Echinacea angustifolia*, geranium, goldenseal, marshmallow root, and slippery elm.

This formula has not been subjected to scientific testing,

but has long been a favorite of naturopathic physicians for the treatment of bowel disorders. Baptisia, or wild indigo, contains compounds that fight digestive infections and may increase the immune-stimulant effect of echinacea. Cabbage is a widely used treatment for peptic and duodenal ulcers. Clinical studies have found that it normalizes the secretion of stomach acid and digestive enzymes. *Echinacea angustifolia,* in addition to stimulating the immune system, is strongly anti-inflammatory. Geranium has an astringent action that causes proteins in the lining of the intestines to cross-link, promoting the healing of ulcers. Goldenseal contains berberine, which inhibits the growth of many disease-causing bacteria, and marshmallow root contains healing mucilages that coat the entire digestive tract. Additionally, marshmallow root has been shown to stimulate phagocytosis, the immune process in which cells called macrophages engulf and neutralize infectious microorganisms. Slippery elm has its own soothing mucilage.

Robert's Formula is available under many brand names in health food stores, such as Bastyr Formula. Additionally, it is possible to make the formula by combining equal portions of all the herbs except baptisia, of which one uses half as much. It is important to remember to take only 1 to 2 teaspoons of the mixture with ½ cup water daily, to avoid taking too much echinacea.

SAIREI-TO

Sairei-to is a combination of two traditional Chinese herbal formulas: Five-Ingredient Powder with Poria and Minor Bupleurum Decoction. (*See* FIVE-INGREDIENT POWDER WITH PORIA and MINOR BUPLEURUM DECOCTION.)

Japanese researchers have found that administering these two ancient formulas simultaneously produces benefits in the treatment of inflammation and stress that cannot be achieved with any other herbal treatment. Laboratory tests on guinea pigs have found that Sairei-to prevents recurrences of middle ear infection, especially when combined with antibiotic treatment. Extensive clinical tests at the University of Utah have found that the formula prevents chemical reactions that release inflammation-causing hormones in people with rheumatoid arthritis (RA). However, studies conducted in the United States did not yield favorable results in this population of RA patients—only five out of thirty benefited from Sairei-to. A Japanese clinical study has found that the combination allows much shorter periods of treatment when steroids such as prednisolone (Pediapred, Prelone, and others) must be given to children with kidney disease. The formula has been used to stop autoimmune reactions that cause repeated miscarriage and to induce ovulation in 70 percent of women with polycystic ovarian disease taking the formula in an attempt to become pregnant. Other laboratory cell studies have found that the formula protects the adrenal glands, hypothalamus, and pituitary gland

from burnout during steroid treatment and stress. Physicians at Holy Spirit Hospital in Tokyo have found that the formula prevents the buildup of scar tissue that can block the urinary canal after prostate surgery.

Any practitioner of traditional Chinese medicine (TCM) can provide this formula as a tea, although most prefer to make slight modifications to the traditional recipe for individual differences in symptoms. It also is possible simply to take standard dosages of over-the-counter (OTC) formulations of Five-Ingredient Powder with Poria and Minor Bupleurum Decoction, available from Chinese pharmacies in most larger cities, although the formulas have to be taken at the same time.

For people who also have hepatitis C, special caution is required in using Sairei-to in the treatment of any disorder. Japanese physicians have reported sixty-six cases of interstitial pneumonia (pneumonia causing congestion lower in the lungs rather than bronchitis) among hepatitis C patients being treated with one of the components of Sairei-to, Minor Bupleurum Decoction. This effect is due to a unique complication of immune stimulation by Minor Bupleurum Decoction. This complication is not likely to result from the use of Sairei-to by people who do not have hepatitis C.

SEVEN-TREASURE PILL FOR BEAUTIFUL WHISKERS

This traditional Chinese herbal formula contains amaranth, cuscuta, dong quai, hoelen, lycium, psoralea, and Solomon's seal. It is prepared with steamed and dry-heated sesame seeds. In ancient China, black whiskers were considered more attractive than gray, giving the seven-ingredient formula its colorful name. The ingredients focus on the kidneys and liver, which were thought to be related to graying hair and hair loss. Traditional Chinese medicine (TCM) practitioners today use this formula to treat premature graying of the hair in both men and women. The formula is considered especially effective for men who also suffer from loose teeth, lower back pain, and difficulties in achieving satisfaction in sexual intercourse.

The manner in which this formula works has not been scientifically explained, although it is likely to relate to the action of psoralens. These chemicals, found in psoralea, circulate through the bloodstream to the scalp, where they are activated by exposure to sunlight. The sun-activated psoralens change the immune system in the scalp in a way that may make immune cells known as T cells less active and less likely to destroy hair follicles. The formula also contains dong quai, which stimulates circulation to the scalp and may promote the health of existing hair follicles. Certain components of dong quai block the formation of prostaglandins, which may be involved in the destruction of hair follicles. These were done in cell lines, so the exact mechanism for humans is not known.

The properties of dong quai suggest that this formula, like all other treatments for hair loss, is likely to be more effective the sooner it is started after hair loss begins. In the United States, the formula is available from practitioners of TCM, who prescribe it for use as a tea.

SHIH QUA DA BU TANG

This is an important supplement for the treatment of symptoms related to cancer, and it contains ten herbs: astragalus, white atractylodis, cinnamon, dong quai, ginseng, hoelen, licorice, ligusticum, peony, and rehmannia. While it is usually identified by the phonetic spelling of its name in Mandarin, it is also known as All-Inclusive Great Tonifying Decoction, the free translation of its name in Chinese, and as Ten-Significant Tonic Decoction, the literal translation of its name in Japanese. The anonymous twelfth-century Chinese herbalist who designed this formula used it to treat symptoms that occur in any prolonged, serious illness, including continuous palpitations, easy fatigue in the extremities, lightheadedness, loss of appetite, excessive sweating, shortness of breath, and vertigo.

Even though this formula was invented nearly 900 years ago, clinical research has found that it is very useful as a supplemental treatment for a host of modern diseases that cause similar symptoms. The formula could be used as a general tonic for people with HIV/AIDS and chronic fatigue syndrome (CFS), but these are not its typical uses. More commonly, it is used for a weak heart, anemia, uterine bleeding, and chronic abscesses. It may benefit these conditions by stimulating the production of two important immune-system components: natural killer (NK) cells and a group of hormonelike chemicals known as the interleukins. However, the strongest actions of the formula are antitumor and anti-metastases.

This formula is most frequently used in the United States as a supplement during conventional medical treatment of cancer. The capacity of Shih Qua Da Bu Tang to support the immune system makes it perhaps the most versatile of all herbal formulas in cancer treatment. Tests at the University of Kansas have found that the formula prolongs survival time and minimizes side effects in a number of ways and for a number of different kinds of chemotherapy. Besides minimizing nausea, vomiting, and loss of appetite, the formula increases the effectiveness of the chemotherapy drugs cisplatin (Platinol), cyclophosphamide (Cytoxan, Neosar), fluorouracil (Adrucil), and mitomycin (Mutamycin) against many kinds of cancer cells. Administered after chemotherapy, the formula stimulates not only the immune system but also the production of red blood cells by bone marrow, and it may reduce drug-induced kidney damage. It helps minimize damage to the bone marrow, thymus, and spleen during radiation therapy. In one study, researchers in Japan gave Shih Qua Da Bu Tang to patients with advanced lung cancer for one year and patients lived longer. Improvement in anemia has also been reported in cancer patients.

Shih Qua Da Bu Tang is occasionally used to treat vitiligo when other measures fail, but no clinical studies are available. The usefulness of this formula in treating vitiligo is probably due to its content of dong quai. Coumarins supplied by dong quai stimulate circulation to the skin, while other compounds in the herb block the production of inflammation-generating prostaglandins that would normally be transported to the skin through the bloodstream. The net effect is that undesirable autoimmune agents are carried away from the skin while the production of new autoimmune agents is suppressed. Dong quai also inhibits the formation of skin-destructive antibodies at the very beginning of the inflammation process—that is, the herb may be more effective against vitiligo if it is used as soon as symptoms are noticed. Even if the formula is given after symptoms are established, the simultaneous pharmacological actions of the herbs in the formula may buy time for medical treatment to correct the imbalances that result in the disease. The formula is most often used for dry skin and night sweats rather than this condition, however.

This formula stimulates the production of B cells, immune-system cells that attack the body's own tissues in rheumatoid arthritis and related conditions. For this reason, people with rheumatoid arthritis, Sjögren's syndrome, lupus, and psoriatic arthritis, and especially people with myasthenia gravis, should not use it. Breast cancer patients should use this product with caution, as dong quai and ginseng may stimulate the growth of breast cancer cells.

SIX-INGREDIENT PILL WITH REHMANNIA

This traditional Chinese herbal formula contains alisma, cornelian cherry, dioscorea, hoelen, moutan peony, and rehmannia. Ancient Chinese herbalists designed it to treat a symptom pattern including dizziness, lightheadedness, night sweats, ringing in the ears or diminished hearing, and soreness and weakness in the lower back.

The condition most commonly treated with this formula is attention deficit disorder (ADD), although the traditional Chinese medicine (TCM) term is "slow mental development." It has been used for over 1,000 years in the treatment of children who experience any of the Five Delays:

- Delay in standing up.
- Delay in walking.
- Delay in the growth of hair on the head.
- Delay in the development of teeth.
- Delay in the development of speech.

Herbal practitioners in the United States offer anecdotal reports of success in using Six-Ingredient Pill with Rehmannia to treat the Five Delays in children with cerebral palsy or ADD, but no clinical studies exist for these conditions. The manner in which this formula affects intellectual development has not been scientifically determined, but is probably related to the action of compounds in hoelen. Some of the complex polysaccharides in hoelen likely induce changes in the production of cytokines, inflammatory chemicals associated with anxiety, memory loss, and seizures.

In addition, the herbs in the formula are all mildly diuretic but are also sources of potassium and trace minerals, exerting a beneficial influence on fluid balance in the inner ear for those with hearing impairment. In an extensive review on this formula, it has been shown to benefit patients with diabetes, infertility, prostatitis, stroke, and kidney problems. This formula stimulates the production of B cells, immune-system cells that attack the body's own tissues in people with rheumatoid arthritis (RA) and related conditions. For this reason, people with RA, Sjögren's syndrome, lupus, or psoriatic arthritis, and especially people with myasthenia gravis should not use Six-Ingredient Pill with Rehmannia.

TRIPHALA

Triphala, the most widely used ayurvedic herbal formula in the United States, consists of three fruits: amalaki, bibhitaki, and haritaki. These three herbs correspond to the three *doshas* (humors) of ayurvedic medicine. Amalaki is sour and is thought to balance the *pitta* (fire) humor. Bibhitaki is sweet and pungent, and balances the *kapha* (mucus) humor. Haritaki is bitter and balances the *vata* (breath) humor.

The formula is most frequently recommended for anemia, constipation, and obesity. Animal testing indicates that the formula taken as a whole slows down production of cholesterol in the liver, reducing and thereby lowering serum cholesterol.

No studies of the use of triphala in the treatment of constipation have been conducted, probably because the formula has been used for thousands of years as a strong laxative. The amalaki fruit in the formula may help prevent abdominal pain and spasms as the formula as a whole stimulates bowel movement. There are reports from India that a few weeks' use of the formula sometimes induces weight loss in obese people who also suffer from chronic constipation.

Triphala is frequently recommended by ayurvedic physicians as a *churna*, or powder, to be mixed with water, although it is much more palatable in pill or tablet form. Some adverse reations include intestinal gas, stomach upset, and diarrhea.

TRUE MAN'S DECOCTION TO NOURISH THE ORGANS

This traditional Chinese herbal formula contains atractylodis, chebula, cinnamon bark, dong quai, ginseng, licorice, nutmeg, opium poppy husk, peony, and saussurea. In traditional Chinese medicine (TCM), these herbs are considered tonics that dispel infection from the digestive tract and restore the body's fluid metabolism. This formula was named after one of the "eight immortals" in Chinese legend: Lü, the pure-yang true man. The *pure-yang* was an intense manifestation of energy that was capable of causing invaders (or infections) to flee. The *organs* are the five balanced energy systems to which TCM attributes the functions of organs as they are understood in Western medicine. *Nourishing* the organs provides them energy.

The formula is used today for syndromes in which the most prominent feature is chronic diarrhea, sometimes to the point of incontinence. Accompanying symptoms may include persistent abdominal pain that responds favorably to local pressure or warmth, fatigue, lack of strength in the legs, lower back pain, and a pale tongue. In terms of its pharmacological action, the formula can be considered a buffered form of paregoric, also based on opium. While the opiate blocks nerve impulses forcing urgent evacuation, ginseng stops neurochemical reactions that cause inflammation in cell line studies.

The conditions most commonly treated with this formula are chronic diarrhea in children and for adults, chronic colitis, chronic dysentery, and diarrhea. Check with your child's pediatrician before giving this formula to your child, as overdosing may result in potentially toxic and adverse side effects. It should not be used for more than two weeks at a time, since chronic use may mask symptoms of disease requiring medical attention. Do not consume alcohol, fish, or greasy foods when using this formula.

TRUE WARRIOR DECOCTION

This traditional Chinese herbal formula contains atractylodis, ginger, hoelen, peony, and prepared aconite. In Eastern tradition, the "true warrior" is the spirit of the north who manages fire and water. This formula, which was thought to increase yang ("masculine" or combative) energy and regulate urination, was named after that spirit.

Ancient Chinese herbalists designed this formula for a pattern of symptoms including abdominal pain, deep aching, heaviness in the extremities, and urinary difficulty. There may also be cough, dizziness, a heavy sensation in the head, palpitations, a swollen tongue with tooth marks, and vomiting.

Today, the formula has been used to treat anorexia and wasting, particularly when there is coldness in the hands and feet. Other uses include for kidney and liver failure and edema. The pharmacological properties of the herbs in this formula have been extensively researched. Aconite contains a potent analgesic agent, mesaconitine. This chemical raises the threshold of pain and helps the body attune itself to both relaxation and stress. In laboratory studies, mesaconitine manipulates the brain's production of norepinephrine, one of the chemicals that "excites" the nervous system. During relaxation, mesaconitine decreases the brain's production of norepinephrine, and during stress, mesaconitine increases norepinephrine. The changes in brain chemistry induced by aconite induce a sensation of warmth.

Ginger has been found to inhibit the production of immune-system compounds called cytokines in cell studies. These neurochemicals serve as a kind of molecular memory that conditions the nervous system to produce pain and tension again and again. Reducing the production of cytokines reduces inflammation and stimulates blood circulation. This property may make ginger useful for treating disorders marked by swelling and pain. Ginger also eases indigestion and nausea. Hoelen is calming, while peony contains compounds that repair damaged microscopic blood vessels in cells.

This formula is most often used for relief of symptoms of arthritis, for supportive care after radiation treatment, and in the treatment of Crohn's disease, Ménière's disease, high blood pressure, and hypothyroidism. If you take beta-blockers, a type of medication often prescribed for high blood pressure, you should not use this formula, as it counteracts the effects of these drugs.

VACHA RASAYANAS

Vacha Rasayanas are ayurvedic herbal mixtures containing various buffering and sweetening herbs with vacha, also known as sweet flag.

The principal herb of these combinations, vacha, is used to treat a broad range of brain conditions, especially related to aging. It works by protecting brain tissue from toxic free radicals, substances that are released from excess oxygen. When the flow of oxygen is restored to previously oxygen-deprived cells, these cells are temporarily unable to use all the oxygen available to them, and free-radical damage results. Tissue damage in the brain can lead to depression, as well as to memory loss or seizures, and can exacerbate situational depression due to the consequences of memory loss or seizures. Vacha helps to prevent these reactions. Although this is how the formula has been used traditionally, no clinical studies are available.

Vacha may reduce psychological disturbances during withdrawal from cocaine, heroin, and morphine. During the first one to ten days of withdrawal, an individual may experience intense drug cravings, nausea, and vomiting. Although vacha is legal in North America, many other countries ban the use of both vacha and calamus, vacha's American relative, in herbal medicine. Vacha Rasayanas should *never* be used without supervision of your physician.

WARM THE GALLBLADDER DECOCTION

This traditional Chinese herbal formula, also known as Bamboo and Hoelen Decoction, contains bamboo, both whole bitter orange and bitter orange peel, ginger, hoelen, licorice, and pinellia. In the terminology of traditional Chinese medicine (TCM), *warming* the gallbladder refers to

the treatment of a depletion of the chi (energy) generated by the gallbladder after a serious illness. The gallbladder drains the liver, which is thought to house emotional energy. Depletion of the gallbladder's chi keeps emotional energy locked in the liver, and results in insomnia with nervous stomach upset or peptic ulcer.

Bamboo is TCM's chief food and herb for the treatment of energy imbalances of the gallbladder as described above. Modern research in cell line studies has found that bamboo shoots are mildly antibacterial and antiviral, but that the healing chemicals derive not from the herb itself but from a fungus, *Shiraia bambusicola*, that naturally grows on it during storage.

Bitter orange not only settles the stomach but also regulates the central nervous system. It slows the heart rate and eases sleep. Unlike many drugs used for these purposes, it does not reduce circulation to the brain and kidneys. While one of the herb's chemical components, natsudaidain, is slowing the heart rate, it simultaneously makes the heart muscle beat more forcefully. At the same time, the chemical activates the alpha-receptors of the nerves that control tension in the femoral (leg) arteries so that circulation to the legs through the femoral arteries is reduced. This shunts blood to the top of the body where it is needed by vital organs. No human studies are available, but this formula is traditionally used for insomnia, breathing problems, and lung infections. Bitter orange peel contains other compounds that raise systolic blood pressure while not affecting diastolic blood pressure, increasing the heart's effective output, so use it with caution if you have high blood pressure.

Ginger has been found to inhibit the production of immune-system compounds called cytokines in cell studies. This action reduces inflammation and stimulates blood circulation, which is regulated in useful ways by chemicals from bitter orange. The synergistic action with bitter orange in this formula makes ginger useful in treating a number of disorders marked by swelling and pain. Ginger also eases indigestion and nausea.

Hoelen stimulates urination and helps protect the kidneys against stress from breakdown of proteins. It contains poriatin, which stops the production of cytokines, which in this case could be considered chemical messengers that immune cells use to coordinate attacks on kidney tissue. In addition, poriatin stops the activity of related chemical messengers that also cause destruction of kidney tissues, such as interleukins and tumor necrosis factor (TNF). But these observations were made in cells and not humans.

Licorice is useful for a number of digestive disorders. It soothes inflammation and protects the stomach and intestines from the effects of stomach acid. One of the compounds it contains, glycyrrhizinic acid, was the first substance proven to promote the healing of ulcers. Unlike many ulcer drugs, glycyrrhizinic acid does not reduce acid production in the stomach, which would result in incomplete digestion. Instead, it increases the stomach's defense mechanisms by stimulating the activity of mucus-producing cells to thicken the stomach's protective mucous coating. Glycyrrhizinic acid also increases circulation to the cells lining the intestinal wall, boosting their supply of nutrients and oxygen. However, licorice only compromises 7.5 percent of the formula, so all these benefits may not be realized.

Because the herbs used in this formula can stimulate estrogen production, you should not use Warm the Gallbladder Decoction if you have breast or endometrial cancer, endometriosis, uterine fibroids, or ovarian cysts. Do not use it if you are anemic.

WARM THE MENSES DECOCTION

This traditional Chinese herbal formula contains cinnamon bark, donkey-hide gelatin (which is, as its name suggests, a Chinese preparation of gelatin made from donkey hide), dong quai, evodia, ginseng, licorice, ligusticum, moutan peony, ophiopogon, peony, and pinellia. All of the herbs in this formula regulate and stimulate the flow of blood to the womb. In the terminology of traditional Chinese medicine (TCM), *warming* the menses refers to stimulating the flow of blood through its normal pathways. This action stimulates menstrual flow if a woman is not pregnant. During pregnancy, it removes obstructions in the "conception vessel" to supply nutrients to the developing fetus, but historically it has not been used during pregnancy.

Today, this formula is mainly used for irregular menstruation problems, chronic pelvic disease, and lower abdominal pain. It is also recommended for infertile women on the basis of its successful historic use. TCM also uses the formula to prevent infertility in men who have been infected with gonorrhea. Its application in the treatment of infertility may be partially explained by its action on the pituitary gland, which it causes to release pulses of the hormones that stimulate the production of eggs and sperm.

The recommendation of the formula for osteoporosis is based on preliminary scientific evidence. In laboratory studies, the formula prevents the erosion and pocketing of bone in animals deprived of estrogen. Japanese scientists believe that Warm the Menses Decoction is as effective as estrogen replacement in preventing osteoporosis.

Because some of the herbs in this formula stimulate estrogen production, women who have estrogen-sensitive breast cancers, endometriosis, or fibrocystic breast disease should use it with caution. It should not be used by women who take oral contraceptives.

WHITE TIGER DECOCTION

WHITE TIGER PLUS ATRACTYLODIS DECOCTION

WHITE TIGER PLUS GINSENG DECOCTION

White Tiger Decoction is a traditional Chinese herbal formula containing anemarrhena, gypsum, licorice, mirabilite, nonglutinous rice, and rhubarb. As their names

suggest, White Tiger Plus Atractylodis Decoction and White Tiger Plus Ginseng Decoction are modifications of the formula made by adding atractylodis and ginseng, respectively.

In Eastern mythology, the white tiger was the metal spirit of the west, whose appearance in the autumn heralded the end of summer's heat. The use of its name here is a metaphor for the action of the formula in reducing fever. The pathogenic influences against which the "white tiger" works are the four "greats": great (high) fever, great pulse, great sweating, and great thirst.

The pharmacological action of these formulas is surprisingly simple. All of their ingredients, except for the licorice and the rice, are either laxatives or diuretics, stimulating bowel movement or urination. The herbs eliminate heat by expelling stool, which, being in the core of the body, contains considerable body heat. The herbs slow the pulse and reduce sweating by reducing the amount of fluid in the body, while helping the body conserve potassium.

Anemarrhena accounts for the formulas' ability to relieve thirst. Laboratory experiments with test animals in Japan have found that this herb can lower blood sugar by increasing glycogen synthesis in the liver. Both hunger and thirst subside as blood sugar levels are lowered. The hypoglycemic characteristics of anemarrhena may make the formulas useful in the treatment of diabetes.

Atractylodis and ginseng are added to the formulas to treat additional symptoms that may occur in either uncontrolled diabetes or acute infection. Atractylodis relieves high fever and aversion to heat, marked irritability, profuse sweating, rapid pulse, red face, and severe thirst, plus a generalized sensation of heaviness and pain in the joints. Ginseng relieves fever, thirst, profuse sweating, and generalized weakness.

Some Japanese physicians use these formulas with steroid creams to treat skin allergies. You can take the formula as a tea and apply a steroid cream (for example, hydrocortisone) to the skin. These treatments act synergistically to stop oozing inflammation of the skin. The formulas are available for this purpose from practitioners of traditional Chinese medicine (TCM) and from Chinese pharmacies, and can be made into a skin-care cream by a compounding pharmacist. If one of the White Tiger Decoctions is compounded into a cream, it is applied between applications of the prescription steroid cream. If you need more than 6 to 7 doses, seek another evaluation by a natural practitioner or your own doctor. One ingredient, gypsum, has side effects—such as labored and difficulty breathing, rapid pulse, headache, and a generally cold feeling in the limbs—if too much is taken. You should stop using this formula at once if any of these symptoms occur.

YOGARAJ GUGGULU

Yogaraj Guggulu is an ayurvedic formula combining various flavoring herbs with the Indian herb guggul, also known as Indian bedellium. It is a special form of a churna (powder). To make a churna, an ayurvedic herbalist pulverizes selected herbs into a powder. To obtain a better fineness, the herbs are sifted through a piece of fine cloth, or *vastragalana*. The churna is bound together by the sticky guggul resin. Most formulations of yogaraj guggulu add a sugar syrup to the churna and guggul to make a dough.

Guggulu contains steroids known as guggulsterones, which, like other steroids, relieve inflammation. Yogaraj Guggulu is formulated for digestive problems accompanying depression, but also relieves inflammation of arthritis and muscle injury. This formula has traditionally been used for arthritis and muscle injury.

Several studies have found that guggul changes the way the body processes thyroid hormone, increasing the amount of thyroid hormone in circulation. For this reason, you should avoid Yogaraj Guggulu if you have hyperthyroidism. You should avoid this formula if you are taking beta-blockers, especially propranolol (Inderal, Inderide), or calcium channel blockers, especially diltiazem (Cardizem), for high blood pressure, since it can make these drugs less available to the body. Use it with caution if you have Crohn's disease or irritable bowel syndrome (IBS).

PART TWO

Herbal Prescriptions for Common Health Problems

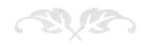

Introduction

The great strength of herbal treatment is that it can be used with conventional medicine in the treatment of almost every disease condition. However, you should always check with your physician before combining herbs with other medications, as there are known harmful interactions that can occur. Part One explained the principles of herbal healing and introduced its most commonly used herbs and herbal formulas. Part Two offers an A-to-Z listing of medical conditions that can be treated with these herbs and formulas. The listings in Part Two include not only age-old conditions that can be rationally treated with herbs, but also emerging conditions for which herbs are an important part of effective therapy.

The introduction of each entry is a basic overview of the disorder. Following are two groups of treatments, herbs and formulas. Only the best herbs and formulas for each condition have been listed, not all applicable therapies. When necessary, a list of precautions that ensure the safe use of the herbs is included, as is a list of herbs that people with the disease should avoid. This information is followed by recommendations of specific ways to counter a given disorder and considerations that discuss additional material of interest.

One word of caution: The herb ephedra is banned in the United States, except it is still allowed to be sold in dietary supplements sold by licensed practitioners in traditional Chinese medicine (TCM) formulations that are recommended for their traditional TCM uses. For this reason we have included formulas in this book that contain ephedra. If you are considering using one of the formulas in this book that contains ephedra, seek the advice of a TCM provider.

Every herb is recommended in its most appropriate form, whether capsule, compress, cream, granule, liposome, poultice, tablet, tea, or tincture, for the conditions for which it is indicated. The forms recommended in this book, however, are not usually the only forms that can be used beneficially. When a chemical constituent of an herb is specified, always use products labeled for the standardized ingredient, such as baicosides or ginkgolides or hypericin. Some herbs, such as milk thistle, are always best taken as a liposome. Other herbs, such as devil's claw and peppermint oil, must be taken in enteric-coated capsules. These restrictions are noted in the text. Otherwise, alternative forms of the herb, such as the substitution of a tincture for a capsule or a tea for a tablet, may be used beneficially. One cup of an herbal tea often substitutes for 250 milligrams of an herb extract. Of course, preparations meant to be applied to the skin, such as creams and poultices, cannot be substituted for herbs meant to be taken internally, such as capsules and tablets.

Product labels do not always explain dosages, so recommended dosages are listed throughout the text. It is important to remember, however, that the recommendation of a physician or professional herbalist, based on unique individual needs, always takes precedence over the recommendations in this book. It is helpful to remember that there is generally more leeway in dosing herbs than in dosing prescription medications. In most cases, taking a little more or a little less than the recommended amount will not interfere with the beneficial action of the herb.

In the long-term treatment of chronic conditions, it is especially important to choose a therapy in consultation with a doctor and a qualified herbalist. To ensure selection of the most beneficial therapy, many vendors who handle over-the-counter (OTC) versions of traditional formulas from ayurvedic and TCM, and all responsible providers of modern herbal formulas for serious conditions, will strongly recommend confirmation of the diagnosis by a health-care professional.

Herbs and formulas are not "tonics" to be indiscriminately substituted for prescription drugs. This being said, many herbal therapies and specific prescription medications interact positively for increased control of disease. Particularly in the treatment of allergy, asthma, arthritis, autoimmune diseases, cancer, and psoriasis, herbs may increase the effectiveness of medical treatments or reduce their side effects. Some prescription drugs have so many side effects that they cannot be used continuously. For these drugs, certain herbs and formulas may reduce the likelihood of relapse on the days or weeks the prescription drug is not taken.

In other cases, however, herbs can weaken the desired effect of prescription medications. While a number of possible interactions, along with possible side effects, are listed under the precautionary notes, these precautions cannot cover all possible unfavorable drug and herb interactions. If there is any reason to suspect that an unintended effect or drug interaction may occur, consult with a qualified herbalist or pharmacist.

Plan for improvement. To use these prescriptions for herbal healing successfully, it is essential to note one further rule: Avoid creating physiological imbalances by taking too much of an herb, or by taking an herb after it is no longer needed. After taking any herb or formula for three months, see a health-care professional for reassessment. As symptoms improve, it may be beneficial to continue with the same treatment or to start taking a different herb or formula. It also may be necessary to change or discontinue prescription medication. The doctor may determine that further treatment is not needed, depending on whether or not sufficient improvement has been made. If there are any questions regarding diagnosis or the propriety of any herb or formula, or any general questions about health, always consult a physician.

ACNE

Acne is a skin disorder characterized by the presence of blackheads, whiteheads, or pimples blocking the pores of the skin. It is the most common of all skin problems.

Acne does not result from dirty skin. Rather, it occurs when increased production of the male sex hormone testosterone stimulates the skin to produce vastly greater quantities of sebum, or oil. This hormone also stimulates the cells lining the hair shafts to produce keratin, a tough protective skin protein that can block the passage of sebum from the pores. The testosterone by-product dihydrotestosterone thickens the skin and toughens its underlying tissues. Other factors that contribute to the development of acne include heredity, stress, oily skin, and overgrowth of the yeast *Candida albicans*.

Acne lesions can progress to become nodules. These are tender accumulations of pus deep in the skin. Acne can also cause cysts (nodules that fail to drain) and pustules, which are deep-seated infections that break down the soft tissues below them. If cysts or pustules are left untreated or broken open, acne can lead to scarring and pitting.

The form of acne known as acne vulgaris (Latin for "common acne") is most common during puberty, the stage

Acne: Beneficial Herbs

Herb	Form and Dosage	Comments
Herbs to Be Applied Externally		
Calendula	Cream. Apply as directed on the label.	Promotes wound healing, prevents viral infection of broken skin. Especially useful during winter.
Lavender plus water or rosewater or witch hazel	Essential oil. Apply as a cold compress 2–3 times daily. (*See* COMPRESSES in Part Three.) Use 1 part essential oil to 10 parts diluting agent.	Relieves inflammation and pain.
Tea tree oil[1]	Lotion or ointment (2–5 percent oil). Apply as directed on the label.	Antiseptic.
Walnut leaf	Apply as a skin wash 2–3 times daily. (*See* SKIN WASHES in Part Three.)	An astringent that protects skin against allergens and infection.
Witch hazel	86 percent witch hazel extract in 14 percent alcohol. Use as directed on the label.	An antibacterial and astringent that stops oozing.
Herbs to Be Taken Internally		
Barberry[2] or coptis[2] or goldenseal[2] or Oregon grape root[2]	Tincture. Take 20 drops in ¼ cup water 3 times daily for up to 2 weeks.	Potent antimicrobial agent that stops oozing.
Echinacea[3]	*E. purpurea* tincture. Take 20 drops in ¼ cup water 3 times daily; or	Reduces inflammation, speeds healing.
E. angustifolia	tablets. Take 500 mg 4 times daily.	
Guggul	Guggulsterone tablets. Take 250–500 mg 3 times daily for 3 months.	Relieves infected cysts and nodules by stopping inflammation. Especially useful if skin is oily.
Milk thistle[4]	Silymarin gelcaps. Take 120 mg twice daily.	Helps remove excess hormones through the stool by increasing production of bile.
Saw palmetto	Extract capsules, preferably liposome. Take 320 mg daily.	Relieves acne in adult men who are not receiving testosterone therapy.
Vitex	Tablets. Take 175–225 mg daily.	Prevents premenstrual acne flare-ups by preventing production of dihydrotestosterone. May have to be used 3–6 months for best results.

Precautions for the use of herbs:

[1]People who are allergic to celery or thyme should not use tea tree oil products. Do not take this product internally.

[2]Do not use barberry, coptis, goldenseal, or Oregon grape root if you are pregnant or have gallbladder disease. Do not take these herbs with supplemental vitamin B_6 or with protein supplements containing the amino acid histidine. Do not use goldenseal if you have cardiovascular disease or glaucoma.

[3]Do not use echinacea if you have an autoimmune disease such as rheumatoid arthritis or lupus. Do not use it if you have a chronic infection such as HIV or tuberculosis.

[4]Milk thistle may cause mild diarrhea. If this occurs, decrease the dose or stop taking it.

of life in which the body creates the most testosterone. Testosterone production is heightened during puberty in both boys and girls. Despite the fact that the hormonal changes that cause acne occur in everyone who passes through puberty, not everyone develops acne, because each person's body chemistry is a little different. Also, there are significant differences between males and females in the amount of testosterone and dihydrotestosterone produced. Since males have significantly higher levels of both, acne is more common in boys than in girls.

As hormone levels stabilize after adolescence, acne also diminishes. Adults can still have flare-ups, however. For women, these flare-ups are often triggered by the premenstrual release of another hormone, progesterone. Since oral contraceptives contain progesterone, the use of birth control pills also can cause outbreaks, as can steroid treatment in men. Treatment with testosterone can cause or aggravate acne in people of any age and either sex.

Conventional medical treatments for acne include antibiotics and large doses of vitamin A. Each has drawbacks. Antibiotics are effective only if they are taken for long periods, and can lead to digestive disturbances, among other problems. Vitamin A supplements are generally safe when used as prescribed, but can cause liver damage in overdose and birth defects if there is an unexpected pregnancy. Isotretinoin (Accutane), a drug prescribed for severe acne, causes miscarriage and multiple birth defects if taken during pregnancy. It has other milder side effects as well, such as chapped lips and dry skin, which are counteracted by using moisturizing creams. Many herbal treatments do not carry these risks. Some herbs for acne are applied externally, while other herbs and formulas are taken internally. For best results, use both topical and internal treatment.

Herbs to Avoid

❑ If you have acne, you should avoid the following herbs: avena, chrysin, muira puama, pine pollen, Siberian ginseng, stinging nettle, and Tribestan, a trademarked extract of the herb *Tribulus terrestris*. All of these herbs either increase testosterone production or elevate testosterone levels in the bloodstream. (For more information regarding these herbs, *see* the individual entries *under* The Herbs in Part One.)

Recommendations

❑ Eat more fiber, either by eating fiber-rich foods such as whole-grain cereals and breads or by taking a fiber supplement. Burdock cereal, called goboshi in Japanese groceries, is a good source of fiber when eaten two to three times a week. Fiber absorbs waste testosterone in the intestines, which prevents the hormone from being reabsorbed through the intestinal wall. Always take fiber supplements separately from other supplements and medications.

❑ Eat more raw foods, such as almonds, beets, and spinach. These contain oxalic acid and may help the skin to clear and heal faster.

❑ Take 45 milligrams of zinc picolinate daily for six to twelve weeks. Zinc is involved in immune-system stimulation, protein formation, and wound healing. In clinical tests, it has been found to be as effective as the antibiotic tetracycline in relieving acne lesions. A 10 percent picolinic acid gel applied twice daily over the face is safe and effective in treating mild to moderate acne vulgaris.

❑ Drink eight glasses of water a day to ensure adequate hydration of the skin. The additional fluid in skin cells may help to open pores.

❑ If you eat sweets, eat them in small amounts over a period of several hours, rather than in large amounts all at once. Eating large quantities of sugar may aggravate acne by causing the body to produce excess insulin, which causes a burst of growth in the cells lining the pores and makes them close up.

❑ Do not squeeze pimples. This causes an increased risk of infection. Make sure your hands are clean before touching the affected areas.

Considerations

❑ Contrary to popular belief, there are no specific foods that cause acne (aside from the pore-closing effect of sugary foods eaten in large amounts). Even chocolate and nuts do

Acne: Formulas

Formula	Comments
Cinnamon Twig and Poria Pill	A traditional Chinese herbal formula used to treat acne if accompanying symptoms include a feeling of blood rushing to the head, facial redness, cough, and congestion. This formula is also used for acne that occurs with menstrual irregularities.
Peach Pit Decoction to Order the Chi	A kampo formula used by people with strong constitutions and ruddy complexions who tend to be constipated, and by women with menstrual problems.
Tang-Kuei and Peony Powder	A kampo formula that relieves acne caused by menstrual irregularities.
Triphala	An ayurvedic formula that promotes good digestion and stimulates hormone excretion.
Turmeric Rasayanas	An ayurvedic formula that contains turmeric, an antioxidant that stops inflammation. Other herbs in this formula are antibacterial and antiviral. This formula is traditionally taken with a teaspoon of honey.

not aggravate acne, although they can aggravate viral skin infections. (*See* HERPESVIRUS INFECTION.) An exception is the iodine found in seafood, which can bring on outbreaks in women who are sensitive to iodine. It is also possible for a specific food item (or many other substances, such as the balsams used in cosmetics) to trigger acne in cases of allergy. (*See* Food Allergies *under* ALLERGIES.)

❏ Long-term use of the antibiotic minocycline (Dynacin, Minocin) can result in blue pigmentation in the gums, known as the "blue smile." If your physician prescribes this drug for acne, discuss the possibility of alternating between antibiotic treatment and treatment with barberry, coptis, goldenseal, olive leaf extract, or Oregon grape root. In addition, taking 500 milligrams of vitamin C twice daily may reduce pigmentation. Do not interrupt antibiotic treatment without your physician's consent, however.

❏ Azelaic acid is a naturally occurring antibacterial compound proven in clinical tests to be as effective as the medications benzoyl peroxide, tretinoin (Retin-A), and tetracycline in controlling acne outbreaks. Use azelaic acid creams with the herbs listed above for maximum effect.

ACQUIRED IMMUNODEFICIENCY SYNDROME (AIDS)

See HIV/AIDS.

ALCOHOLISM

Alcoholism is a condition in which an individual depends on the daily consumption of alcohol to avoid the physical and psychological symptoms of withdrawal. Over time, an alcoholic individual tends to consume increasing quantities of alcohol, and to become more and more dependent on it.

In the United States, an estimated 17 million adults suffer from alcoholism or have alcohol problems, and the condition contributes to about 75,000 deaths a year. Men are twice as likely to be affected as women. Although most people are middle-aged by the time alcoholism becomes established, many younger people either are, or are becoming, alcohol-dependent. Alcohol-related automobile fatalities (alcoholism is said to be a factor in half of the annual fatal accidents in the United States), crime, diminished work productivity, and disrupted family lives make alcoholism a large-scale social problem as well as a health problem.

Alcoholism goes beyond simple intoxication. Intoxication is associated with discomfort, impaired judgment, poor coordination, and pain. Drinking to the point of intoxication is alcohol abuse, and while it is common among alcoholics, it does not necessarily signal alcohol dependency. Alcoholism always involves alcohol abuse, but does not necessarily cause discomfort, impairment, and pain every time the alcoholic drinks. Some alcoholics can drink heavily and still appear sober. One key symptom of

alcoholism is that the individual comes to need a drink for every mood—one to calm down, one to perk up, one to celebrate, one to deal with disappointment, and so on.

Long-term alcoholism is associated with a number of serious disorders. Its effects on the nervous system make an individual prone to psychological disorders such as depression. In addition, it greatly increases the risk of high blood pressure, erectile dysfunction (ED), stroke, and several types of cancer. Brain damage, liver disease, and kidney disease are other consequences of regular long-term alcohol consumption.

There are many indications that alcoholism is, at least in part, an inherited condition. The incidence of alcoholism is four times higher among biological children of alcoholic parents than among children of nonalcoholic parents. People in certain ethnic groups, especially Japanese and Korean people, seem to have lower rates of alcoholism than do people of other backgrounds. According to researchers, people of Japanese and Korean heritage do not have a gene that breaks down acetaldehyde, a chemical that is produced when the body processes alcohol and that causes headache, nausea, and redness in the face. As a result, they generally cannot tolerate more than one or two drinks at any given time, making them much less likely to develop alcohol dependence. The bodies of people of other ethnic backgrounds tend to be able to break down acetaldehyde very efficiently. They thus have a greater tendency toward alcoholism.

Alcoholism is usually treated through several different means. These usually include support and counseling. Sometimes the drug disulfiram (Antabuse) is prescribed. This drug induces extreme discomfort if alcohol is consumed. Herbal treatments offer a complement to conventional treatment, extending the usefulness of drugs to discourage the use of alcohol and protecting the liver from alcohol-induced disease.

Recommendations

❏ The most important step is to avoid all alcohol. This includes avoiding the alcohol found in some conventional medications and in herbal tinctures. It also means avoiding, to the extent possible, settings associated with drinking, such as bars and nightspots. There is no such thing as social drinking for someone with alcoholism.

❏ Eat several daily servings of dark green, yellow, or orange vegetables. The vitamin A in these vegetables may reduce cravings for alcohol, and could ease other complications of alcoholism, including sexual dysfunction. Eating a variety of meats, grains, and dairy will help maintain weight and provide essential nutrients that may have been lost from overconsumption of alcohol.

❏ To reduce depression, take omega-3 fatty acids daily. These essential fatty acids, found mainly in fish and krill oils, are essential for proper brain function.

Alcoholism: Beneficial Herbs

Herb	Form and Dosage	Comment
Kudzu	Tablets. Take 10 mg 3 times daily.	Helps deter alcohol consumption by producing nausea, swelling, and facial redness when taken before drinking.
Milk thistle[1]	Silymarin gelcaps. Take 600 mg (about 5 tablets) daily.	Prevents and treats cirrhosis and other liver disorders.
Reishi	Tablets. Take 3,000 gm 3 times daily.	Prevents alcohol-induced fatty liver and cirrhosis.
Soy lecithin[2]	Capsules. Take 1,500–3,000 mg daily.	Promotes liver cell regeneration and protects the liver from toxic damage.

Precautions for the use of herbs:

[1]Milk thistle may cause mild diarrhea. If this occurs, reduce the dosage or discontinue use.

[2]Soy lecithin may cause mild diarrhea when first used.

Alcoholism: Formulas

Formula	Comments
Kudzu Decoction	The principal herbal treatment in traditional Chinese medicine for alcoholism. If taken before drinking, it creates mild discomfort when alcohol is consumed.

❏ Take a multivitamin with extra thiamin and 30 milligrams of zinc daily. Many individuals with alcoholism have depleted stores of thiamin and zinc.

❏ Seek counseling to help resolve any psychological issues related to your alcoholism. In addition, support groups such as Alcoholics Anonymous can provide understanding and guidance from people who have battled the same problem.

Considerations

❏ People with a "sweet tooth" are at a greater risk for developing alcoholism. Studies done at the University of North Carolina found that 62 percent of alcoholic men liked the taste of a supersweet sugar solution, compared with 21 percent of those without a drinking problem. Animal studies show that a high sugar intake indicates a potential motivation to drink alcohol, but that actual alcoholism occurs only after many years of drinking.

❏ People in recovery from alcoholism are less likely to have seizures if their diets include adequate amounts of calories and protein. Dietary protein is essential for the normal functioning of a brain enzyme that recycles acetylcholine, which is essential for transmitting messages from nerve to nerve in the brain.

❏ Recovering alcoholics should avoid tranquilizers, because there is risk of substituting one addiction for another.

❏ *See also* CIRRHOSIS OF THE LIVER and HANGOVER.

ALLERGIC RHINITIS

See under ALLERGIES.

ALLERGIES

An allergy is an overreaction by the immune system to a normally harmless substance. Virtually any substance, natural or synthetic, can provoke an allergic reaction in susceptible individuals. This entry addresses food allergies and respiratory allergies, two of the most common types of allergies. It is also possible to be allergic to substances that come into contact with the skin. These are treated separately. (*See* ECZEMA.)

Food Allergies

Millions of people have allergic reactions to certain foods. Sometimes there is a delay between eating the offending food and experiencing the allergic reaction, which can make food allergies hard to pin down. Allergic reactions to food can cause a wide array of symptoms, including (but not limited to) gas, nausea, diarrhea, nasal congestion, swelling, fluid retention, itching, hives, and inflammation of the eyes. Food allergies also can contribute to chronic health problems, such as asthma. The foods responsible for allergies can be identified through allergy testing. (*See under* Recommendations, page 193.)

Food allergies occur when the immune system reacts to a normally benign component of food, most commonly a reactive protein or proteins. The proteins in corn, fish and shellfish, eggs, chocolate, citrus fruit, nuts, and berries are common triggers of food allergy. Some people have a severe allergic reaction to gluten, which is the major protein component of wheat and a number of other grains. This condition is called celiac disease. (*See* CELIAC DISEASE.) Other people have persistent yeast infections, which could leave them more prone to food allergies. (*See* YEAST INFECTION [YEAST VAGINITIS].)

Several factors predispose the immune system to react abnormally to food. One of these is known as leaky gut syndrome. This is a disorder in which the lining of the intestine becomes unusually porous, allowing substances to pass into the bloodstream, where they provoke allergic reactions. Some scientists believe that high levels of stress hormones reduce the body's ability to keep large food particles out of the bloodstream. However, the true leaky gut occurs when the intestine is deprived of food during illness such as in a hospital setting. Another possible factor in food allergy is an overabundance of the potentially tissue-destructive immune cells known as T-helper cells, without appropriate numbers of their counterparts, the T-suppressor cells. Circulating in the bloodstream and in the lymphatic channels serving the gut, the T-helper cells stimulate a strong allergic reaction that, if it goes unchecked by T-suppressor cells, provokes an allergic response. Other factors that may contribute to the development of food allergies are heredity and stress.

The terms *food allergy* and *food intolerance* are often used interchangeably, but they describe two separate conditions. Food intolerance occurs when the digestive tract lacks the enzymes necessary to properly break down food. An example of this is lactase deficiency, which causes the sufferer to experience abdominal tension, cramping, and diarrhea after consuming milk or dairy products. This condition is also referred to as lactose intolerance.

Food Allergies: Beneficial Herbs

Herb	Form and Dosage	Comments
Agrimony	Tea (loose), prepared by steeping 1½ tsp (1.5 gm) in 1 cup water. (*See* TEAS in Part Three.) Take 1 cup 3 times daily, between meals. Use for no more than 2 weeks at a time.	Helps to heal damaged mucous membranes and soothe bowel irritation.
Calendula	Tincture. Take 5 drops in ¼ cup water 3 times daily.	Prevents overgrowth of yeast in the bowel. Promotes digestion.
Chamomile	German chamomile (*Matricaria recutita*) tea bag, prepared with 1 cup water. Take 1 cup 3 times daily, between meals.	Soothes stomach irritation. Best when combined with agrimony.
Ginger	Tea (powdered), prepared by adding ⅓ tsp (1 gm) to 1 cup water. (*See* TEAS in Part Three.) Take 1 cup 3 times daily.	Settles the stomach. Deactivates inflammatory hormones.
Peppermint[1]	Enteric-coated oil capsules. Take 200–400 mg twice daily, between meals.	Relieves bowel inflammation, although it does not stop the allergic process itself.
Stinging nettle	Capsules. Take as directed on the label, before meals.	Studies show this herb may halt allergic reactions.

Precautions for the use of herbs:

[1]Do not use peppermint if you have a gallbladder disorder.

Food Allergies: Formulas

Formula	Comments
Kudzu Decoction	A traditional Chinese herbal formula used to treat diarrhea caused by food allergies. Helpful if allergies are accompanied by nervous tension.
Major Construct the Middle Decoction[1]	A traditional Chinese herbal formula used to treat spasmodic pain and diarrhea caused by food allergies.

Precautions for the use of formulas:

[1]Do not use Major Construct the Middle Decoction if you have a fever.

Unless otherwise specified, the herb dosages recommended here are for adults. Children under age six should be given one-quarter of the adult dosage. Children between the ages of six and twelve should be given one-half of the adult dosage. Formula dosages for children should be discussed with a knowledgeable health-care practitioner.

Recommendations

❏ Use of thymus extracts may improve the symptoms of food allergy and shorten their duration. These preparations act on the immune system, resulting in reduced production of the chemicals that cause allergic irritation. Take 750 milligrams once daily. Do not use thymus extracts if you are HIV-positive.

❏ Undergo allergy testing. These are blood tests to identify which foods cause allergies and how intense the allergic reaction is expected to be. A number of commercial laboratories have begun measuring IgG and IgA antibodies against foods. These are usually done by the ELISA method. However, there has been no confirmation of the validity of these testing procedures to identify food allergy. If you wish to read further about the rationale employed by laboratories performing these tests, you might visit one or two websites. An example of such a laboratory is US BioTek at www.USBioTek.com.

❏ Reduce your stress level as much as possible. (*See* RELAXATION TECHNIQUES in Part Three.)

❏ If lactose intolerance is a problem, read labels carefully. Various dairy-based additives, such as milk solids, are used in a wide variety of packaged foods. Casein, a milk protein, is also present in many processed foods, including prepackaged salmon, although it is in such small amounts it is unlikely to have an effect. It may help to try using supplements of lactase, the enzyme necessary for lactose digestion. These are available over the counter. If lactose continues to be a problem, you may wish to get a test verifying this condition. Be sure to take calcium and vitamin D supplements if you are avoiding dairy products altogether.

❏ Take three to five charcoal tablets or capsules as soon as allergic symptoms appear. They may absorb and arrest an attack in some cases.

❏ Often, foods a person craves or eats daily are the ones that cause a problem. Pay attention to your symptoms after consuming certain foods. Try omitting suspect foods from your diet for three to five days. If you see an improvement, stop consuming the offending food.

❏ If you are allergic to ragweed, do not eat cantaloupe. It contains some of the same proteins that ragweed does.

❏ Use only hypoallergenic dietary supplements.

❏ Always check food labels carefully for food additives, especially artificial colors, that may trigger reactions.

Considerations

❏ Two Japanese vegetables, pickled ginger and perilla, act to stop allergic reactions to seafood. These condiments traditionally are served with sushi, but they also can prevent reactions to other forms of seafood.

❏ If you are not allergic to seafood, consume it regularly. Women with the highest intake of omega-3 fatty acids from seafood had the lowest rate of allergic sensitization. If you do eat fish regularly, try not to eat just one type of fish—a variety is best. Also try to stay away from—or at least limit your intake of—fish that are known to be high in mercury, such as tuna and swordfish, to once a week.

❏ *See also* DIARRHEA and HIVES.

Respiratory Allergies

A respiratory allergy is a supersensitive reaction in the lungs, throat, and nasal passages to a normally harmless airborne substance. Both children and adults suffer from seasonal allergies to pollens from blooming plants and from allergies to animal dander, feathers, and a tremendous variety of environmental elements. Primary symptoms of respiratory allergies include sneezing, weeping and tearing of the eyes, coughing, runny nose, postnasal drip, and itching and irritation of the eyes, ears, nose, and throat. Secondary symptoms can include fatigue, headaches, nosebleed, and generalized itching. Respiratory allergies can also aggravate other health problems, including asthma, eczema, and acne.

The most common seasonal respiratory allergy, hay fever, is a creation of modern air pollution. In 1819, English physician and allergy sufferer John Bostock was able to find only twenty-eight other cases of hay fever among 5,000 people. Similarly, records indicate that hay fever was virtually unknown in America before 1850. Now, more than 30 million Americans sneeze, wheeze, and tear through the allergy season. The exact cause of respiratory allergies is unknown. Heredity seems to be a factor, however, and it is known that people who were breast-fed as babies are less likely than those who were bottle-fed to develop allergies. People seem to be most allergy-prone between the ages of fifteen and twenty-five, but new allergies can strike at any age.

An allergic reaction begins with the release of a burst of a chemical called histamine. Histamine is released into the bloodstream by a type of cell known as a mast cell when an allergen is detected. The bloodstream transports it to various kinds of effector cells, where it "docks" at the receptor sites on the membranes lining them. Activating effector cells in the central nervous system results in lowered blood pressure, which makes it difficult for the body to circulate fluids away from the lungs and sinuses. Activating effector cells in the smooth muscle cells lining the lungs results in increased air resistance within the breathing passageways. More important, activation of other effector cells stimulates secretions from the salivary glands and stomach lining, sedates the central nervous system, and causes fluid to flow into the sinuses and nasal passages. Drugs and environmental chemicals are more likely than environmental allergens such as pollen and dander to cause the release of the large amounts of histamine that cause severe allergic reactions—the reaction mechanism is the same, but reactions to chemicals tend to be more intense.

Most conventional allergy drugs act by blocking histamine from attaching to the receptor sites. The disadvantage of these drugs is that they can cross from the bloodstream to the brain, causing sleepiness and sedation. Using them can also actually perpetuate allergies. Some herbal therapies may shield the cells from the effects of histamine, and may not affect the brain. Many practitioners of traditional

Chinese medicine (TCM) report that a single course of treatment with the right herbs usually leads to remission of chronic allergies. While this result cannot be guaranteed, herbs can offer reliable relief from seasonal symptoms. Herbs and formulas recommended for seasonal allergies are not intended for constant, year-round use. Rather, you should start taking them one to two weeks before the beginning of the allergy season, and discontinue them one to two weeks after the expected end of the season.

Unless otherwise specified, the herb dosages recommended here are for adults. Children under age six should be given one-quarter of the adult dosage. Children between the ages of six and twelve should be given one-half of the adult dosage. Formula dosages for children should be discussed with a knowledgeable health-care practitioner.

Respiratory Allergies: Beneficial Herbs

Herb	Form and Dosage	Comments
Bupleurum[1]	Use in the form and dosage recommended by a TCM practitioner.	Prevents swollen nasal passages.
Chamomile	German chamomile (*Matricaria recutita*) tea bag, prepared with 1 cup water. Take 1 cup 2–3 times daily.	Reduces the intensity and duration of allergic reactions.
Chen-pi	Tincture. Take 10–15 drops in ¼ cup water 3 times daily.	Prevents allergic reactions.
Eucalyptus or thyme leaves	Whole dried herb. Soak 1 oz in 1 cup boiling water and inhale the steam. (*See* STEAM INHALATIONS in Part Three.)	Eases congestion.
Ginger	Capsules. Take 1,000 mg 3–4 times daily; Or Hexanol extract. Use as directed on the label.	Reduces allergic inflammation.
Horseradish	Prepared horseradish. Take ½–1 tsp daily until symptoms subside.	Relieves sinus congestion and helps to deter future allergy attacks.
Oligomeric proanthocyanidins (OPCs)	Grapeseed or pine-bark extract tablets. Take 150–300 mg daily.	Stops runny nose.
Quercetin[2]	Tablets. Take 125–250 mg 3 times daily, between meals, for 6–8 weeks before the allergy season begins.	Can help to prevent seasonal allergic reactions if started soon enough.
Rooibos	Tea bag, prepared with 1 cup water. Take 1 cup 1–3 times daily.	Acts as an antihistamine. Especially helpful if you also have food allergies.
Scutellaria[3]	Capsules. Take 1,000–2,000 mg 3 times daily.	Relieves headaches occurring with hay fever.
St. John's wort[4]	Capsules. Take as directed on the label.	An antihistamine that also reduces the risk of catching colds and flu.
Stinging nettle root	Capsules or tablets. Take 500–1,000 mg 3 times daily.	Can provide dramatic relief from hay fever. Stops runny nose.

Precautions for the use of herbs:

[1]Bupleurum occasionally causes mild stomach upset. If this happens, consult the TCM practitioner who dispensed it. Do not take bupleurum if you have a fever or are taking antibiotics.

[2]Do not take quercetin if you must take the immune-suppressing drug cyclosporine (Neoral, Sandimmune) or the calcium channel blocker nifedipine (Adalat, Procardia).

[3]Do not use scutellaria if you have diarrhea.

[4]Do not use St. John's wort if you are on prescription antidepressants or any medication that interacts with MAO inhibitors. Use it with caution during pregnancy. This herb may increase the chance of developing sun blisters if you are out in the sun for too long.

Respiratory Allergies: Formulas

Formula	Comments
Ephedra Decoction (Four Emperors Combination)[1]	A traditional Chinese herbal formula that stops wheezing. A variation—Ephedra, Apricot Kernel, Coix, and Licorice Decoction—is designed to lower fever in addition to treating other symptoms.
Ephedra, Asiasarum, and Prepared Aconite Decoction[2]	A traditional Chinese herbal formula that treats nasal congestion caused by allergy to cedar pollen when taken before start of cedar pollen season.
Kudzu Decoction	A traditional Chinese herbal formula that treats nasal allergy accompanied by stiff neck and upper back.

Precautions for the use of formulas:

[1]Do not use Ephedra Decoction if you are experiencing nausea or vomiting; if you have high blood pressure, anxiety, or heart disease; or if you take MAO inhibitors.

[2]Stop taking Ephedra, Asiasarum, and Prepared Aconite Decoction if fever occurs. This formula may cause a loss of sensation in the mouth and tongue.

Recommendations

❏ Use chamomile cream to relax muscles and make breathing easier. Apply the cream over the area of the diaphragm, the large muscle between the chest and the abdomen that controls breathing, all along the bottom of the rib cage.

❏ Use aromatherapy to open clogged nasal passages. Essential oils of eucalyptus, peppermint, and thyme are good for this purpose. (*See* AROMATHERAPY in Part Three.)

❏ Thymus extracts may improve the symptoms of nasal allergies and shorten their duration. These preparations act on the immune system, resulting in reduced production of the chemicals that cause allergic irritation. Take 750 milligrams once daily. Do not use thymus extracts if you are HIV-positive.

❏ Eliminate your exposure to allergens as much as possible. Keep carpets, rugs, and upholstered furniture clean, and have the furnace and air ducts in your home cleaned yearly. Encase your mattress, box spring, and pillows in allergen-proof covers. Install an air purifier with a HEPA filter, a special allergen-trapping filter, and use a vacuum cleaner equipped with a HEPA filter.

❏ Drink at least eight 8-ounce glasses of steam-distilled water a day. Do not drink tap water.

❏ If there is a cat in the house, eliminate the dander as much as possible. Cats produce an allergy-provoking protein in their dander that can stick to walls, curtains, and furniture. Give the cat a weekly bath—it may actually get used to the idea. There are also commercial products, such as Allerpet, that you apply to the cat in order to reduce the amount of dander. Ask your veterinarian for advice.

Considerations

❏ The usefulness of desensitization immunization, or "allergy shots," has long been debated. In this therapy, you receive injections containing increasing doses of the substances to which you are allergic. Over three to four years, about half of the people who take allergy shots overcome their allergies. When allergy shots fail to work, the problem usually is that the dosage is too low or the serum is improperly prepared.

❏ If your allergies are severe, wear long pants and long-sleeved shirts when spending time outside.

❏ Some people report that they have been cured of allergies after eating locally produced bee pollen or honey for several months. This should be done under a doctor's supervision, since you may have an intense reaction to pollen if you are strongly allergic. The pollen must be from local bees, and you should start consuming it well before the beginning of hay fever season. Start with ⅛ teaspoon daily, make sure you do not react to the pollen (or honey), then gradually work your way up to 1 teaspoon per day. Bee pollen and locally produced honey are usually available from beekeepers and health food stores.

❏ There is some evidence that allergies constitute a learned response. In one study, for instance, people who were allergic to real roses also had reactions to plastic roses, which presumably give off no allergy-inducing particles. Some scientists believe that conflict situations in which emotions cannot be expressed may cause the body to express its emotional state through allergic reactions, such as swelling, sneezing, and mucous secretion. The immune system "learns" this response and repeats it under similar circumstances. The personality type most associated with this kind of "learned" allergy is outwardly outgoing and positive, yet emotionally sensitive. For this type of allergy, hypnosis and psychological desensitization therapies may help.

❏ Clinical studies of the use of vitamin C in preventing hay fever have been inconclusive. However, taking doses of up to 1,000 milligrams of vitamin C may help, and it certainly will not hurt.

❏ Using a probiotic (*Bifidobacterium longum*) was shown to reduce symptoms of Japanese cedar pollinosis, which affects one in six people in Japan. In one study, participants experienced relief from symptoms such as watery eyes and were able to take less medication used to control allergies.

❏ In one study, spirulina, a blue-green alga, helped people who had allergic rhinitis by reducing nasal discharge, sneezing, nasal congestion, and itching.

❏ *See also* ASTHMA.

ALOPECIA

See HAIR LOSS.

ALZHEIMER'S DISEASE

Alzheimer's disease is a brain disorder that destroys memory and undermines personality. Some health-care professionals call it the disease of the twenty-first century in the United States, because doctors expect the number of people with this disease to grow as the population ages. There are currently about 5.1 million cases in the United States, and about 250,000 new cases are diagnosed annually.

Family history and advanced age are the two main risk factors for Alzheimer's disease, although it can strike at any age after the age of thirty. The illness begins slowly, usually manifesting itself initially as bouts of forgetfulness. These may be occasional at first, but eventually become more frequent. Ultimately, the disease progresses to a stage in which the individual must depend on others for all of his or her needs, both physical and mental. Before getting to this point, affected individuals experience a range of progressive symptoms that may include disorientation, dysphasia (the inability to find the right word), sudden and unpredictable mood swings, hallucinations or delusions, wandering without purpose, incontinence, and neglectfulness of personal hygiene. It is important to emphasize that occasional forgetfulness is by no means a sure indication of Alzheimer's disease. In the past there was no way to definitively test a living person for this disorder; diagnosis was based on symptoms and the elimination of other disorders that might cause them. However, today it is possible to determine if dementia is due to Alzheimer's disease 90 percent of the time.

Almost everything science knows about Alzheimer's disease comes from postmortem examinations. The first such examination was conducted in 1906 by Alois Alzheimer, for whom the disease is named. He noted unusual changes in brain tissue taken from a woman who had developed dementia at the age of fifty and died five years later. Alzheimer found that the tissue contained nerve cells with tangled fibers and clumps of degenerating nerve endings. Examination of people who have died of Alzheimer's disease has also revealed that their brain tissue contains higher than normal concentrations of the toxic metal mercury.

In Alzheimer's disease, brain cells disappear from both the cerebral cortex, a structure in the front of the brain that is the center of intellectual activity, and the hippocampus, a structure deep in the brain involved with memory and reasoning. As the cells malfunction and die, the connections between them are lost. This interferes with the intricate process of cell-to-cell communication.

Ginkgo: The Memory Herb and Alzheimer's Disease

Ginkgo biloba extract may help people with many diseases of senility, including Alzheimer's disease. This extract may increase the functional capacity of the brain through its effects on acetylcholine, a chemical that allows the nerve cells responsible for memory and reasoning to communicate with each other. In animal studies, ginkgo has been shown to make the hippocampus, the part of the brain most affected by Alzheimer's disease, more receptive to acetylcholine. It also may increase the ability of acetylcholine to transmit nerve messages, but this has not been shown in humans to date.

The benefits of ginkgo in treating the early stages of Alzheimer's disease have been demonstrated in several carefully controlled, double-blind studies. In one study, 216 people with either Alzheimer's disease or loss of mental function caused by multiple "mini-strokes" were given either 240 milligrams of ginkgo extract or a placebo daily for twenty-four weeks. The data from the 136 people who completed the study show that ginkgo was very useful in treating both kinds of dementia.

In another study, published in *The Journal of the American Medical Association* (*JAMA*), 202 people with Alzheimer's disease, at six research centers supervised by Harvard Medical School and the New York Institute for Medical Research, were given either 120 milligrams of ginkgo extract or a placebo daily for a year. Ginkgo treatment improved symptoms in 64 percent of those who received it, and there were no reports of side effects.

The authors of the study reported in *JAMA* did not find ginkgo to be a miracle cure, but they did find that its use was worthwhile. One of the scientists who conducted the study noted, "While the effect was modest, EGb 761 [ginkgo] reduced patients' cognitive decline and manifestations of dementia rated by the caregiver as compared with placebo, particularly for patients with a diagnosis of AD [Alzheimer's disease]. The mechanism of action is unclear but it is postulated to be related to the agent's [ginkgo's] antioxidant properties. Only a single dose was studied, drop-out rates were high, and longer-term follow-up will be important; but this agent is an intriguing addition to the drugs thought to be helpful for patients with AD."

A ginkgo extract may even be useful in preventing the development of Alzheimer's disease in the elderly. In one study, fewer women developed Alzheimer's dementia over seven years while taking the ginkgo extract, EGb 761. However, not all studies support a role for ginkgo for Alzheimer's patients. One study found no benefit in preventing cognitive decline—measured by memory, attention, visual-spatial construction, and language—in older adults compared to a placebo.

In addition to treating Alzheimer's disease, ginkgo could be useful if similar symptoms are caused by insufficient blood flow or depression misdiagnosed as Alzheimer's disease, but these conditions have not yet been studied. Discuss the use of ginkgo with your doctor before any type of surgical procedure. (For more information about ginkgo, *see* GINKGO BILOBA *under* The Herbs in Part One.)

Researchers have linked the cellular changes seen in Alzheimer's disease to a defect in a gene, called the apolipoprotein E (APOE) gene. This gene is responsible for the transport of cholesterol, an essential building material for all cell membranes, including those of nerve cells in the brain. Because cholesterol is soluble in fats but not in water, it needs a carrier molecule to circulate through the water-based bloodstream, so the liver attaches it to a water-soluble protein. When the resulting lipoprotein package arrives at a cell, the protein inserts itself into the cell membrane and unloads its cholesterol. The protein is then snapped off and recycled. In the brain tissue of people with Alzheimer's disease, the faulty APOE gene causes the carrier protein to be snapped off at the wrong place.

Immune cells circulating in the brain respond to the malformed protein as to a signal that something is wrong, and they attack the nerve cell. The problem is compounded when beta-amyloid, a type of protein that is potentially toxic, is created by the faulty protein break. As beta-amyloid disintegrates, it generates harmful free radicals, which in turn destroy cell membranes. The resulting mass of dead cells becomes entangled and forms a beta-amyloid plaque. Spiral filaments of protein form irregular circles around nerve cells and lead to the cells' death and destruction.

One of the most important uses of herbal treatment is as a complement to treatment with the pharmaceutical drug tacrine (Cognex). Herbal treatments may also be useful at earlier stages of the disease for retarding the progression of symptoms. Since people with Alzheimer's disease are usually prescribed drugs for other diseases as well, be sure to read all the information in Part One for any herb you are considering to avoid harmful herb-drug interactions.

Recommendations

❑ Use essential oil of rosemary in aromatherapy, or add 1 tablespoon (10 to 12 milliliters) of the oil to shampoo. The essential oil releases compounds that can be inhaled and that prevent the breakdown of acetylcholine. (*See* AROMATHERAPY in Part Three.)

❑ Take 1 gram of eicosapentaenoic acid (EPA) and docosahexaenoic acid (DHA) daily with a meal. In people with Alzheimer's disease, calcium enters brain cells and starts a series of chemical reactions that result in the formation of beta-amyloid, the toxic protein that forms plaques in the brain. DHA may limit calcium from entering cells and also stabilizes brain-cell membranes. In addition to taking EPA and DHA as a supplement, eat two to three servings of cold-water fish, such as salmon, sardines, or tuna, every week. Human studies show that people with higher levels of EPA and DHA have a lower risk of dementia.

❑ Take 2 grams of acetyl-L-carnitine (ALC) daily, between meals. ALC is a natural substance derived from the amino acid L-carnitine. It works with L-carnitine to help fatty acids cross into every cell in the body—including brain cells. Some studies have shown that ALC can slow

Alzheimer's Disease: Beneficial Herbs

Herb	Form and Dosage	Comments
Ashwagandha	Withanolide gelcaps. Take as directed on the label.	Reduces the brain's reliance on its own cells as a source of choline.
Brahmi concentrate	Bacoside tablets. Take 300 mg once daily.	Restores balance between brain proteins GABA and glutamate.
Butcher's broom	Ruscogenin tablets or capsules. Take as directed on the label.	Promotes healthy circulation.
Ginkgo[1]	Ginkgolide tablets. Take up to 500 mg once daily.	Has many beneficial effects on the brain and on circulation. (*See* "Ginkgo: The Memory Herb and Alzheimer's Disease" on page 196).
Gotu kola plus hawthorn	Tincture. Take 15 drops of each herb in ¼ cup water twice daily.	Reduces cholesterol plaques in blood vessels serving the brain. Normalizes the brain's use of oxygen.
Hawthorn	Tablets. Take 100–250 mg 3 times daily.	Reduces cholesterol plaques in blood vessels serving the brain.
Huperzine A	Tablets. Take as directed on the label.	Inhibits the breakdown of acetylcholine.
Rose hips	Fresh, natural vitamin C capsules (has a shelf life of 6 months). Take 1,000 mg daily.	A traditional Japanese remedy for memory loss caused by aging.
Soy isoflavone concentrate	Tablets. Take 100 mg once daily, before a meal.	Has effects similar to those of estrogen. May slow progression of the disease.
Soy lecithin[2]	Capsules. Take 15,000–25,000 mg (15–25 gm) daily.	Prevents brain tissue destruction under reduced-oxygen conditions. (*See under* Considerations, page 198.)

Precautions for the use of herbs:

[1] Avoid ginkgo if you are taking any type of blood-thinning medication. Discuss its use with your doctor before having any type of surgery.

[2] Soy lecithin may cause mild diarrhea when first used.

Alzheimer's Disease: Formulas

Formula	Comments
Biota Seed Pill to Nourish the Heart	Considered the most important traditional Chinese medicine herbal formula for age-related memory loss. It aids short-term memory.
Bupleurum Plus Dragon Bone and Oyster Shell Decoction[1]	A traditional Chinese herbal formula that reduces agitated behavior. A free-radical scavenger, it absorbs substances that would destroy nerve tissue.
Coptis Decoction to Relieve Toxicity	A traditional Chinese herbal formula that destroys harmful free radicals, preventing the damaging effects of both aluminum and D-aspartic acid from the artificial sweetener aspartame.
Eight-Ingredient Pill with Rehmannia	A traditional Chinese herbal formula that keeps blood sugar levels constant. Particularly useful for people who have both Alzheimer's disease and diabetes.
Gastrodia and Uncaria Decoction	A traditional Chinese herbal formula that increases both circulation to the brain and production of the brain's own free-radical scavenger, superoxide dismutase (SOD).
Settle the Emotions Pill	A traditional Chinese herbal formula that treats poor memory compounded by insomnia, dizziness, hot flashes, or dry mouth.

Precautions for the use of formulas:

[1]Do not use Bupleurum Plus Dragon Bone and Oyster Shell Decoction if you have a fever.

the progression of dementia, especially in people who have mild to moderate Alzheimer's disease.

❏ Take 1,000 milligrams of cytidine diphosphate choline (CDP) daily. In late-stage Alzheimer's disease, this nutrient enables the brain to produce more acetylcholine, the building block of healthy brain tissue. In early-stage Alzheimer's disease, it stops the immune system from producing interleukin-1B, a chemical that destroys brain tissue. If CDP is not available, take 4 grams of choline daily, with food.

❏ Take a good combination antioxidant supplement daily, as prescribed on the label. Although a direct link between increasing dietary antioxidants and controlling Alzheimer's disease has not been proved, it is likely that antioxidants may slow the progress of the condition. They also have many other benefits.

❏ Take a multivitamin with trace elements; such multivitamins have been shown to delay Alzheimer's disease.

❏ Eat a well-balanced diet with plenty of fiber to ensure an adequate supply of all nutrients and the healthy elimination of toxins.

Considerations

❏ Since soy lecithin provides nutrients that the prescription drug tacrine (Cognex) preserves, the two treatments are complementary. Lecithin may help mild to moderate cases. If there is no noticeable improvement within two weeks, this supplement should be stopped, since large doses of soy lecithin are expensive and may cause mild diarrhea. If diarrhea occurs, use food sources of lecithin, which include Brazil nuts, cowpeas (black-eyed peas), dandelion flowers, fava beans, lentils, mung beans, sesame seeds, and the Indian vegetable *alu methi* (fenugreek leaves).

❏ Practitioners of ayurvedic medicine recommend a diet rich in cumin, coriander, fennel, ginger, and turmeric for people with Alzheimer's disease. These spices contain natural antioxidants that may slow the progression of the disease.

❏ Avoid cigarette smoke, alcohol, and environmental toxins. According to a study published in the British medical journal *The Lancet,* smoking more than doubles the risk of developing dementia, including Alzheimer's disease.

❏ Vitamin B_{12} (cobalamin) deficiency may cause symptoms similar to those of Alzheimer's disease. Many elderly people have low B_{12} levels. Ask your doctor to measure your levels if you are concerned.

❏ *See also* MEMORY PROBLEMS.

AMEBIASIS

See under PARASITIC INFECTION.

ANEMIA

Anemia is a condition in which the blood is deficient in either red blood cells or hemoglobin, the iron-binding protein that transports oxygen through the blood. Red blood cells transport oxygen from the lungs to the tissues of the body, exchanging fresh oxygen for carbon dioxide, which is excreted by being exhaled. The symptoms of anemia result from a failure of the red blood cells to provide oxygen efficiently. These symptoms include pallor, breathlessness, weakness, a tendency to tire easily, loss of appetite, constipation, headaches, difficulty concentrating, and coldness of the hands and feet.

Iron-deficiency anemia occurs in 7 percent of children ages one to two years and 12 percent of females ages twelve to forty-nine years in the United States. Anemia can be diagnosed from laboratory tests that show a low level of total red blood cells or red blood cells of abnormal shape and size. Some people assume that anemia is always caused by "iron-poor" blood and that they need iron supplements. However, determining the cause of anemia is never a task for self-diagnosis. It is essential to conduct laboratory tests, especially tests that measure iron levels and iron-absorption ability, before trying to correct the problem.

The underlying cause of anemia may be excessive blood loss, excessive red blood cell destruction, or deficient red blood cell production. Factors that can contribute to the development of anemia include infections, medications, pregnancy, heavy and/or frequent menstrual periods, nutritional deficiencies, drug use, hormonal disorders, peptic ulcers, hemorrhoids, and liver damage. Most cases of anemia, however, result from deficient red blood cell production caused by nutrient deficiency, and are treated with nutritional supplementation. The three nutrients that are most frequently deficient are iron, vitamin B_{12} (cobalamin), and folic acid. Iron-deficiency anemia is a form of microcytic anemia, in which the red blood cells gradually shrink, until they become very small. Vitamin B_{12}, or pernicious, anemia is a form of macrocytic anemia, in which the red blood cells are very large.

Herbs to Avoid

❏ People who have anemia should avoid damiana, fennel, grapeseed extract, and rooibos. (For more information regarding these herbs, see DAMIANA, FENNEL SEED, and ROOIBOS under The Herbs in Part One.)

❏ Herbs containing high concentrations of tannins interfere with the absorption of iron supplements. Avoid taking iron supplements within two to three hours of using agrimony, chebula, gambir, green tea, uva ursi, white willow bark, or any form of St. John's wort other than hypericin-standardized capsules or tablets.

Recommendations

❏ Eat a diet rich in meats, poultry, and seafood. Each contains iron in its most absorbable form called heme iron. There are small amounts of iron, called non-heme iron, in plants and grains, but it is hard for the body to absorb this form of iron. Many people whose anemia is caused by iron-poor blood require iron supplements for a short time until iron stores return to normal. If the anemia isn't caused by iron deficiency, other treatments are available and vary by the cause.

❏ Avoid using bran as a source of fiber. Whole grains, especially wheat—unless they have been fermented in a sourdough process—contain large amounts of phytate, which interfere with iron absorption.

❏ Avoid coffee and tea. The tannins in coffee and the polyphenols in tea, including green tea and green-tea extracts, interfere with iron absorption.

❏ Limit or avoid foods containing oxalates, which inhibit iron absorption. Foods that contain significant amounts of oxalates include almonds, cashews, chocolate, cocoa, kale, rhubarb, soda, sorrel, spinach, Swiss chard, and most nuts and beans.

❏ Eat foods high in vitamin C to enhance iron absorption.

Anemia: Beneficial Herbs

Herb	Form and Dosage	Comments
Dandelion[1]	Tincture. Take 10–15 drops in ¼ cup water 3 times daily on an empty stomach.	Contains more iron, potassium, folic acid, and vitamin B_{12} than almost any other herb.
Stinging nettle	Capsule, juice, or tea. Take as directed on the label.	A rich source of iron, vitamin C, and chlorophyll that is effective for the treatment of iron-deficiency anemia.

Precautions for the use of herbs:

[1]Do not use dandelion if you have gallstones.

Anemia: Formulas

Formula	Comments
Four-Substance Decoction	A traditional Chinese herbal formula that treats all forms of anemia.

Considerations

❑ Over 75 percent of people undergoing chemotherapy experience some degree of debilitating fatigue, and over 60 percent list fatigue as their number-one problem. This fatigue may result from anemia. If you feel sluggish and are undergoing chemotherapy, ask your doctor whether you need iron supplementation. (*See* "Side Effects of Cancer Treatment" *under* CANCER.)

❑ To help prevent iron-deficiency anemia, prepare your food in cast-iron cookware. The small amount of iron that leaches out of iron pots during the cooking process is sufficient to avoid anemia, but is not so much as to cause iron overload. (*See* IRON OVERLOAD.) The amount of iron that enters the food from cookware is equal to the amount usually provided by iron supplements, and is adequate to treat all but the most severe cases of iron-deficiency anemia.

ANGINA

Angina is a syndrome of squeezing or heavy pressure-like pain in the chest caused by an insufficient supply of oxygen to the heart muscle. It can also be experienced as pain in the left shoulder blade, left arm, or jaw. The pain usually lasts from one to twenty minutes. It is typically brought on by physical exertion or stress and subsides with rest, because exertion and stress increase the heart's need for oxygen. Angina may be a precursor to heart attack, although many people have angina for years without experiencing damage to the heart itself.

Angina is almost always caused by atherosclerosis, the buildup of cholesterol-containing plaques in arteries. In people with angina, atherosclerosis narrows and eventually closes the coronary arteries, the blood vessels leading to the heart. Blockage of the coronary arteries in turn reduces the supply of blood (and therefore oxygen) to the heart. When the flow of oxygen to the heart is substantially reduced, or when there is an unusually high demand for oxygen in the heart, angina is the result. Angina may result from extreme hypoglycemia. That is because hypoglycemia can lead to increased production of hormones associated with stress, which can put a strain on the heart. There is another, rare form of the condition known as Prinzmetal's variant angina, which does not occur in a predictable pattern for chest pain. This unstable form of angina may be caused by exposure to cold, emotional stress, alcohol withdrawal, or medications that constrict blood vessels.

While severe angina can be relieved surgically, treatment for mild angina focuses on controlling high blood pressure and on lowering cholesterol through diet. Nutritional management of angina and coronary artery disease (CAD) consists of two strategies: removing the dietary factors that lead to angina and adding a healthy diet and dietary supplements that prevent it. The presence of cholesterol cannot be completely eliminated, since some cholesterol is absolutely necessary to the normal functioning of every cell in the body, but the activity of compounds that promote the formation of cholesterol plaques can be greatly reduced. The macrophages form a platform, called a foam cell, on which cholesterol can accumulate and later calcify in the artery wall. Being overweight and smoking cause an increase in plaque formation.

Dietary restriction alone may take two to five years to have an effect, but herbal medicine may help speed the process. Herbs may also help to prevent angina pain and reduce the frequency of attacks. People with angina must be especially careful, however, to take note of all precautions regarding the use of herbs (and other medications) that can produce dangerous interactions with nitroglycerin, which is used to treat acute attacks. It is best to discuss the use of any herbs, herbal formulas, or other substances with your physician before adding them to your treatment program.

Angina: Is Surgery Necessary?

Medical treatment of angina typically involves an angiogram, followed by angioplasty and stenting, or coronary artery bypass surgery, if lifestyle changes and medications don't work. An angiogram is an X-ray procedure in which dye is injected into the coronary arteries to locate blockages. These blockages are then most often opened with balloon angioplasty, a minor surgical procedure in which the diameter of the blocked artery is increased with the aid of a very small balloon attached to a flexible tube. The tube is threaded into the affected artery and the balloon is inflated to press atherosclerotic plaques back against the artery wall, compressing the blockage and increasing the amount of space available for blood to circulate. More difficult cases may involve coronary artery bypass surgery, a procedure in which a portion of a clean blood vessel from another part of the body—typically a segment of vein from the leg—is transplanted into the chest to construct an alternate route for circulating blood to reach the heart.

In the past, several clinical studies challenged the widespread use of angiograms, angioplasty, and coronary artery bypass surgery by cardiologists due to an increased risk of death and other complications. However, today, coronary angioplasty is a common procedure and serious complications are rare. Although today no deaths occur, 3 percent of people need coronary artery surgery because the stent didn't work, 4 percent have a heart attack, and less than 1 percent have a stroke. The risk of death within one year of having a coronary surgery procedure is increased over just taking heart medications, but 5 to 10 years later, the risk of death decreases. After having the procedure, 4 out of 100 people have angina again, and after five years 4 out of 100 need another operation. Today, treatments have improved. The method of treatment is up to your doctor and cardiologist. It is a good idea to discuss nonsurgical alternatives with your doctor before agreeing to any procedure, particularly if your condition is not critical. When diet and exercise and medications are not effective, many safe procedures are available.

Angina: Beneficial Herbs

Herb	Form and Dosage	Comments
Arjuna	Capsules. Take 500 mg 3 times daily.	Reduces the frequency of attacks. Lowers blood pressure and raises levels of high-density lipoprotein (HDL or "good") cholesterol.
Astragalus[1]	Capsules. Take 500–1,000 mg 3 times daily.	Provides strong pain relief.
Citrin	Tablets or capsules. Take as directed on the label.	A trademarked extract of the herb *Garcinia cambogia* that helps to prevent the buildup of fat in the body by inhibiting the synthesis of fatty acids in the liver.
Cordyceps	Tablet or tincture. Use as directed on the label.	Slows the heart rate, increases blood supply, and lowers blood pressure.
Dan shen[2]	Tea or tincture. Use only as directed by a health-care professional.	Relaxes muscle lining the coronary arteries. Reduces the heart's workload.
Hawthorn	Tablets. Take 100–250 mg 3 times daily. Use for at least 6–8 weeks to see results.	Stops chest pain that occurs after exertion.
Khella[3]	Khellin tablets. Take 20 mg daily.	Lowers blood pressure. Reduces hormonal reaction to stress.

Precautions for the use of herbs:

[1]Do not use astragalus if you have a fever or a skin infection.

[2]Avoid dan shen if you have an estrogen-sensitive disorder, such as breast cancer, endometriosis, or fibrocystic breasts.

[3]Khella makes the skin especially sensitive to ultraviolet light. While taking this herb, avoid tanning lamps and use sunblock when outdoors. Discontinue use if exposure to strong sunlight is unavoidable. Do not take this herb if you are taking the blood-thinner warfarin (Coumadin).

Angina: Formulas

Formula	Comments
Gastrodia and Uncaria Decoction[1]	A traditional Chinese herbal formula that increases blood flow to heart muscle and increases its resistance to oxygen deprivation. Also promotes deep sleep and relaxation, which leads to reduced stress hormone production.

Precautions for the use of formulas:

[1]Do not use Gastrodia and Uncaria Decoction if you are trying to become pregnant.

Herbs to Avoid

❑ Avoid ephedra, green tea (unless decaffeinated), maté, and all other herbs used as stimulants. Never use quebracho or yohimbe if you carry nitroglycerin tablets for relief of acute attacks. The combination of these herbs, or the drug yohimbine (Yocon, Yohimex), with nitroglycerin can be deadly. (For more information regarding these herbs, *see* EPHEDRA, GREEN TEA, MATÉ, and YOHIMBE *under* The Herbs in Part One.)

Recommendations

❑ If you have unstable angina—severe pain that occurs suddenly and recurs over days or even weeks—be sure to contact your doctor or go to a hospital for the first onset of pain. After you are out of immediate danger, you can consume at least 1,000 milligrams of vitamin C daily, most of it in the form of vitamin C–rich fruits and vegetables such as citrus fruits, cruciferous vegetables (broccoli, Brussels sprouts, cabbage, cauliflower, and kale), parsley, spinach, strawberries, and turnips. Vitamin C's antioxidant effect may reduce the production of inflammatory chemicals that set off spasms in the coronary arteries.

❑ Avoid consuming more than three or four servings of carbohydrates at any single meal. Instead spread out your carbohydrate consumption throughout the day. Eating a meal heavy in carbohydrates—such as grains, starchy vegetables, breads, or pasta—could exacerbate heart-related chest pains in people who have atherosclerosis. Such meals trigger the release of nitric oxide, a chemical that causes plaque-hardened arteries to contract.

❑ To avoid ingesting too much iron and copper, avoid multimineral supplements that contain these minerals.

❑ Limit your consumption of red meat, especially liver and other organ meats. Diets rich in vegetable proteins, seafood, and poultry have been shown to reduce the chances of recurrence of heart disease in patients with angina. In particular, supplementing with vitamins B and E has not been shown to prevent recurrence of disease in people with a history of heart problems. It is best to eat a diet rich in fruits, vegetables, and whole grains to get the needed essential micronutrients (vitamins and minerals).

❏ Perform moderate, gentle exercises, such as tai chi or yoga. Psychiatrist Jon Kabat-Zinn reports that the key to exercise for angina relief is "mindfulness." Slow, flowing, repetitive exercises that require mental focus distract the mind from pain and indirectly relieve overburdened coronary arteries. (*See* RELAXATION TECHNIQUES in Part Three.) Other exercise may be indicated, but check with your doctor before engaging in any activity.

Considerations

❏ Use treatments recommended for migraines to reduce the severity of Prinzmetal's variant angina. (*See* MIGRAINE.)

❏ Headaches that start during exercise and go away after rest may be a warning sign of angina. This is especially true for people who are over age fifty and for those with risk factors for heart disease: high blood pressure, diabetes, smoking, high cholesterol levels, or a family history of heart disease.

❏ Donating blood at least once every three years may offer some protection against both angina and heart attack—for nonsmokers, at least. (Benefits have not been demonstrated for smokers.) Donating blood depletes the body's supply of iron, which is needed to turn low-density lipoprotein (LDL, or "bad") cholesterol into arterial plaques.

❏ There is evidence that unstable angina may be the result of an allergic reaction to an unknown substance. Cardiologists find an increase in the levels of antibodies to allergens in the blood of people who have suffered attacks of unstable angina for more than twenty-four hours. (*See* ALLERGIES.)

❏ According to the U.S. Food and Drug Administration (FDA), taking one baby aspirin a day can reduce the risk of heart attack and stroke. Before starting any kind of aspirin regimen, talk to your doctor. Too much aspirin can cause stomach bleeding and/or ulcers.

❏ *See also* ATHEROSCLEROSIS; HEART ATTACK (MYOCARDIAL INFECTION); HIGH BLOOD PRESSURE (HYPERTENSION); and HIGH CHOLESTEROL.

ANKLES, SWOLLEN

Painless swelling of the ankles and feet is a common problem, particularly among older adults. Other possible causes include hormonal or salt imbalances, congestive heart failure, kidney disease, premenstrual syndrome, varicose veins, extensive burns or sunburn, generalized gonorrhea infection, injury, and insect bites or stings. A number of medications also can cause swollen ankles, including antidepressants, calcium channel blockers, chemotherapy agents, replacement estrogen or testosterone, oral contraceptives, and tamoxifen (Nolvadex).

Ankles swell when fluid moves from the capillaries into the surrounding tissue and stays there. If you squeeze a swollen ankle, the fluid will move out of the affected area, and a deep impression may be made that can last for a few moments. In addition to the ankles, the calves or even the thighs may be affected.

Herbal treatments for swollen ankles work over a period of three to six months. Other treatments, such as support stockings, can produce results in three to six weeks, which are then stabilized by the use of herbs. You should call a health-care provider immediately if swollen ankles are accompanied by shortness of breath, chest pain, difficulty speaking, inability to urinate, weight gain of more than six pounds (three kilograms) in three days or less, or an unusually slow or fast heartbeat.

Recommendations

❏ If you are overweight, lose weight. The extra stress of the weight worsens the swelling. Eating nutrient-rich foods like fruits, vegetables, whole grains, and dairy assures that you get all that you need with fewer calories.

Swollen Ankles: Beneficial Herbs

Herb	Form and Dosage	Comments
Butcher's broom	Ruscogenin tablets. Take 100 mg once daily.	Particularly effective for burning and itching.
Gotu kola[1]	Liposome tablets or capsules. Take 60–120 mg of asiatocides daily.	Stabilizes tissues supporting veins; increases oxygen transport.
Hawthorn	Solid capsules. Take 150–250 mg 3 times daily.	Strengthens fragile veins; increases tone of muscles supporting veins.
Horse chestnut[2]	Aescin tablets. Take up to 150 mg daily.	Makes blood vessels more elastic.
Oligomeric proanthocyanidins (OPCs)	Grapeseed or pine-bark extract tablets. Take 100 mg daily.	Improves blood-vessel strength and flexibility.

[1]Gotu kola should not be used if you are trying to become pregnant.

[2]Horse chestnut should not be taken internally if you are trying to become pregnant.

Be sure to eat protein at each meal from animal or protein-rich vegetable sources such as soy or legumes.

❑ Take a combination of vitamin C and 3,000 to 6,000 milligrams of citrus bioflavonoids daily. This combination is similar to a European nutritional supplement called Daflon, which has been found to be useful for treating swollen ankles.

❑ Avoid sitting or standing without moving for prolonged periods of time.

❑ Avoid putting anything directly under your knees when lying down. Do not wear constricting clothing or garters on your upper legs.

❑ Consult a health-care provider if swollen ankles are accompanied by swelling of the lower legs or feet; muscle or joint stiffness in arms and legs; trembling; problems in swallowing; pain or burning; bleeding, swollen, or tender gums; loss of balance; numbness or tingling of the hands or feet; vivid dreams; difficulty in urination; breast discharge; or hair loss.

Considerations

❑ A low-salt diet may help reduce fluid retention and decrease ankle swelling. This would mean mostly eating fresh foods rather than those in cans or packages. If you want packaged goods, look for those marked as "reduced sodium." Use salt for cooking and avoid using it at the table.

❑ Exercising the legs causes the fluid to work back into the veins and lymphatic channels so that the swelling goes down. The pressure applied by elastic bandages or support stockings can also help reduce ankle swelling.

ANXIETY DISORDER

Anxiety is a condition of inappropriate nervousness or fear. While fear is an appropriate and rational response to a real danger, anxiety usually lacks a clear or realistic cause. Symptoms of acute anxiety can include shortness of breath; heart palpitations; tingling sensations in the face, hands, and feet; tensing of the muscles; a claustrophobic sensation; hot flashes; and depression.

Some level of anxiety is normal and possibly even healthy because it helps the body stay alert to danger. But high levels of anxiety for long periods of time are not only unpleasant but can lead to significant health problems, such as chronic fatigue, diabetes, high blood pressure, and increased susceptibility to infection.

Anxiety Disorder: Beneficial Herbs

Herb	Form and Dosage	Comments
California poppy with corydalis[1]	Corydalis Formula. Take as directed on the label.	Treats anxiety without inducing drowsiness.
Chamomile	German chamomile (*Matricaria recutita*) tea bag, prepared with 1 cup water. Take 1 cup 3 times daily.	Relieves allergy and inflammation that aggravates anxiety.
Fennel	Tea. Take 1 cup before or after meals.	Relieves anxiety-related gastrointestinal upset and reduces flatulence.
Ginger plus	Tablets. Take 3,000 mg twice daily, with food.	Reduces anxiety by increasing flow of oxygen and nutrients to the brain.
ginkgo[2]	Ginkgolide tablets. Take 240 mg once daily.	
Ginseng	*Panax ginseng* tincture. Take as directed on the label.	Helps prevent anxiety during drug withdrawal.
Kava kava[3]	Kavapyrone tablets. Take 60–120 mg daily. Do not exceed 120 mg.	Relieves muscle tension and stops pain.
Passionflower	Tea bag, prepared with 1 cup water. Take 1 cup 3 times daily.	A calming agent that causes less drowsiness than prescription drugs.
Scutellaria[4]	Tablets. Take 250–500 mg 3 times daily.	Stops nighttime muscle cramps.
St. John's wort[5]	Tablets or capsules. Take as directed on the label.	Eases depression and helps to restore emotional stability.
Tilden flower	Tincture. Take 1–3 tsp (4–12 ml) with water three times daily.	Reduces the risk of migraine attacks during periods of anxiety.
Valerian	Valepotriate tablets. Take 50 mg 3 times daily.	Relieves panic attacks at night.

Precautions for the use of herbs:

[1]Do not use California poppy with corydalis if you are pregnant.

[2]Do not use ginkgo if you are taking blood-thinning medication. Discuss its use with your doctor before having any type of surgery.

[3]Kava kava increases the effects of alcohol and psychoactive drugs such as sedatives and tranquilizers. Avoid it if you are pregnant or nursing.

[4]Do not use scutellaria if you have diarrhea.

[5]Do not use St. John's wort if you are on prescription antidepressants or any medication that interacts with monoamine oxidase (MAO) inhibitors. Use it with caution during pregnancy. This herb may increase the chance of developing sun blisters if you are out in the sun for too long.

Anxiety disorders are classified as generalized anxiety disorder, in which symptoms last six months or more; phobias, in which anxiety is provoked by a specific situation, such as being at a height; or panic disorder, which is marked by panic attacks that occur for no obvious reason. In a panic attack, a person feels overwhelming dread and terror, often accompanied by feelings that he or she is going to die or go crazy. Anxiety also is associated with sleep disturbances, mood swings, forgetfulness, difficulty concentrating, and fatigue.

Psychological factors do play a role in anxiety, but this disorder has a nutritional basis as well. The key is a chemical called lactic acid, which is created when the body burns glucose, or blood sugar, without oxygen. This occurs, for example, when a person exercises so vigorously that he or she cannot catch breath. Lactic acid is changed into lactate and transported to the liver, where it is converted into harmless pyruvic acid. People who have panic disorders tend to suffer panic attacks when lactic acid is high in the blood. However, healthy individuals with no history of panic attacks are not affected by blood lactate levels. Stress and reactions to certain foods or drugs also can trigger anxiety. Other factors that can cause or contribute to anxiety include fatigue, malfunctions in brain chemistry, headaches, surges in adrenaline, and hypoglycemia (low blood sugar). Using recreational drugs, including marijuana, can cause panic attacks.

Conventional medicine uses both drug treatments and psychotherapy to treat anxiety. (*See under* Considerations, page 205.) If you are taking prescription medicine for anxiety, speak with your doctor before using an herbal treatment.

Herbs to Avoid

❏ Avoid ephedra, green tea (unless decaffeinated), and maté. (For more information regarding these herbs, *see* EPHEDRA, GREEN TEA, and MATÉ *under* The Herbs in Part One.)

Recommendations

❏ Try aromatherapy using essential oil of lavender. (*See* AROMATHERAPY in Part Three.) Lavender is a mild sedative that calms anxiety aggravated by caffeine consumption.

❏ To reduce lactate production, take 800 to 1,200 milligrams of any calcium and magnesium supplement daily. Also take a complete multivitamin with B-vitamin complex supplement daily.

❏ Avoid caffeine. Drinking coffee in the morning can lead to stress all day. As simple an act as avoiding coffee for one week can sometimes bring about significant relief of symptoms.

❏ Avoid alcohol and sugar. Reducing your intake of these substances, along with reducing caffeine consumption, can lower lactate production in the body.

❏ Get more exercise. Both moderate and vigorous exercise are effective at reducing anxiety, but the calming effect of vigorous exercise requires an after-workout rest period to take effect. Also, avoid working while you exercise. There is evidence that if you exercise and do mental work at the same time—such as reading school or job material while on an exercise bike—the exercise does not reduce anxiety levels. Remember, the idea of exercise is to relax.

❏ Use yoga to reduce anxiety, especially if you have a specialized form of anxiety known as obsessive-compulsive disorder (OCD). In some cases, people have been able to reduce or even eliminate medications after three to twelve months of weekly yoga. (*See* RELAXATION TECHNIQUES in Part Three.)

❏ If changes in diet and exercise do not help, consider meditation. Researchers have documented immediate benefits of this practice in terms of lowered blood pressure, decreased heart and respiratory rate, increased blood flow, and other measurable signs of the relaxation response. All

Anxiety Disorder: Formulas

Formula	Comments
Bupleurum Plus Dragon Bone and Oyster Shell Decoction[1]	A traditional Chinese herbal formula that treats insomnia, palpitations, and short temper caused by anxiety in people of robust constitution.
Coptis Decoction to Relieve Toxicity[2]	A traditional Chinese herbal formula that treats anxiety resulting in nervous excitement and rapid speech, with symptoms that include bleeding from the nose or gums, fever, headaches, and redness in the neck and face.
Pinellia and Magnolia Bark Decoction[3]	A traditional Chinese herbal formula that relieves "lump in the throat" and stomach upset accompanying anxiety.

Precautions for the use of formulas:

[1]Do not use Bupleurum Plus Dragon Bone and Oyster Shell Decoction if you have a fever.

[2]Do not use Coptis Decoction to Relieve Toxicity if you are trying to become pregnant.

[3]Do not use Pinellia and Magnolia Bark Decoction if you have a fever.

forms of meditation require regular, daily practice over a long period of time before they deliver rewards. (*See* RELAXATION TECHNIQUES in Part Three.)

❏ Consider talking to a therapist or other mental-health professional.

Considerations

❏ Most doctors treat anxiety and panic attacks with benzodiazepine tranquilizers or tricyclic antidepressants. These drugs can cause a number of side effects. In addition, the tranquilizers carry a high potential for addiction, and withdrawal can be emotionally and physically unpleasant. The antidepressants can sometimes cause the individual taking them to go from depression to manic excitement. This can make day-to-day functioning so difficult that anxiety actually becomes worse. However, many people have improved using antidepressant drugs. There are many drugs available in this class, so if you are having problems with one drug, ask your doctor if you can try another.

❏ Panic attacks may be accompanied by deficiency of omega-3 fatty acids. One, alpha-linolenic acid, an essential omega-3 fatty acid, is found in high concentrations in flaxseed oil. In one study, three out of four people with a history of agoraphobia (fear of going outdoors) improved after two to three months of taking 2 to 3 teaspoons of flaxseed oil daily. Physical signs of a deficiency of alpha-linolenic acid include dry skin, dandruff, brittle fingernails, and burning sensations in the skin. Another study found that using omega-3s from fish oil (3 grams a day) reduced anxiety levels in substance abusers.

❏ Postmenopausal women experienced temporary relief from anxiety but not long-term benefit from a proprietary extract blend of two herbs—*Magnolia officinalis* and *Phellodendron amurense.*

❏ Some authorities in natural medicine suggest taking supplemental gamma-aminobutyric acid (GABA) to prevent anxiety attacks. However, while GABA plays an important role in controlling anxiety by inhibiting nerves from excessive firing in the brain, there is little evidence that GABA reaches the central nervous system when taken orally.

❏ Studies conducted at Harvard Medical School suggest that wearing goggles or eye patches may reduce anxiety. Approximately 80 percent of subjects studied who had both anxiety and depression experienced heightened anxiety when one eye was covered and lessened anxiety when the other eye was covered. You can experiment with this at home by placing an eye patch over one eye (for no more than four hours at a time), judging any changes in your emotional state, and repeating the test by covering the other eye.

❏ *See also* STRESS.

ARRHYTHMIA, CARDIAC

See under CONGESTIVE HEART FAILURE.

ARTERIOSCLEROSIS

See ATHEROSCLEROSIS.

ARTHRITIS

See GOUT; OSTEOARTHRITIS; RHEUMATOID ARTHRITIS.

ASTHMA

The word *asthma* comes from the Greek term meaning "breathlessness." Asthma is a chronic respiratory disorder that causes acute attacks marked by shortness of breath; a feeling of being unable to get enough air no matter how hard one tries; coughing; expectoration of sticky, stringy sputum; and a feeling of tightness in the chest. These symptoms are followed by a prolonged phase marked by abnormal breathing sounds and wheezing.

Asthma constricts the muscles lining the small air passages, or bronchi, of the lungs, which keeps air from leaving the lungs. About 34 million Americans have asthma, and the incidence of this disorder is increasing. The underlying reason why some people develop asthma is unknown, although it seems likely that heredity, a history of allergies, and obesity may all play a role. The things that can trigger the acute attacks are easier to identify, though they vary from person to person. Common asthma triggers include exposure to cold air, emotional upset, exercise, infection, exposure to toxic chemicals, exposure to allergens, and stress of any kind.

Some physicians describe asthma as extrinsic or intrinsic. An extrinsic attack, now referred to as allergic asthma, is set off when a very small particle to which the body has been sensitized enters the lungs. This particle, or allergen, activates antibodies to produce massive amounts of a protein called immunoglobulin E (IgE). IgE binds to mast cells, specialized immune cells that are especially numerous in the lungs and nasal passages. When activated by IgE, mast cells release histamine, a chemical that causes the smooth muscles lining the bronchial passages to tighten, making breathing more difficult.

Histamine plays the same role in intrinsic asthma as in the extrinsic version. The onset of an attack triggers a surge in the production of leukotrienes, chemicals that are more potent than histamine in closing airways. There are no antibodies released, and this type of asthma is now just referred to as asthma. In sensitive individuals, leukotriene production is increased even more by the use of aspirin or nonsteroidal anti-inflammatory drugs (NSAIDs). Other triggers include cigarette smoke, cleaning agents, chest infections, stress, laughter, exercise, cold air, and food preservatives. In addition, some people with intrinsic asthma usually make less of the hormones that allow the bronchial muscles to relax.

The lungs are more susceptible to any type of asthma for several days after exposure to the air pollutant ozone and for several weeks after a viral infection.

Prescription drugs such as steroids, which are often prescribed for asthma, can have serious side effects, including changes in the skin and hair, reduced resistance to infection, swelling, and weight gain. However, they are needed by many individuals to avoid troubled breathing and trips to the emergency room. A number of herbal therapies may increase the effectiveness of steroid treatments so that they can be used in lower dosages, with fewer side effects.

It is important to remember that herbal medicine, including both single herbs and combination formulas, is most effectively used to prevent asthma attacks. The traditional Chinese herbal formulas listed here help minimize asthma with fewer side effects. These formulas must be

Asthma: Beneficial Herbs

Herb	Form and Dosage	Comments
Asmatica[1]	*Tylophora indica* capsules. Take 400 mg twice daily for 1 week, go off for 2 weeks, then take for another week, continuing this pattern as long as asthma symptoms persist.	An antihistamine and antispasmodic. Helps prevent acute attacks for up to 2 weeks after use.
Chamomile	German chamomile (*Matricaria recutita*) tea bags, prepared with 1 cup water. Take 1 cup 2–3 times daily.	A gentle antihistamine. Helps to prevent attacks.
Coleus	Forskolin dry extract from TR-Metro Natural Herbal Extracts. Take as directed on the label.	Helps to prevent asthma attacks. Recommended for people with high blood pressure.
Elderberry	Sambucol. Take as directed on the label.	Relieves nasal congestion and fever.
Ginger	Hexanol extract. Take as directed on the label.	Deactivates platelet-activating factor (PAF), which promotes allergic reactions.
Green tea	Tea bag, prepared with 1 cup water. Take 1 cup 2–3 times daily. To avoid dilution, do not use within 1 hour of taking other oral medications.	Contains theophylline, which opens bronchial passages.
Hawthorn	Capsules or tablets. Take 100–250 mg 3 times daily.	If you are using an inhaler for asthma, helps to prevent tissue damage in the heart, liver, and pancreas.
Hyssop	Tea bag, prepared with 1 cup water. Take 1 cup 2–3 times daily.	Relieves heavy, congested feeling in the chest.
Ipecacuanha	Tincture. Take as directed on the label.	Useful when there is marked overproduction of phlegm.
Khella[2]	Tincture. Take as directed on the label every 6 hours.	Prevents bronchial spasms.
Licorice[3]	Glycyrrhizin tablets. Take 200–800 mg daily, depending on the severity of symptoms. Use for 6 weeks, then take a 2-week break. Do not substitute deglycyrrhizinated licorice (DGL).	Stimulates mucus production to stop dry cough. Increases the effectiveness of steroid inhalers. Consume potassium-rich foods such as bananas or citrus juices, or take a potassium supplement, daily when taking this herb.
Lobelia[4]	Capsules or tablets. Take 500–1,000 mg 3 times daily. Take for no more than 2 weeks at a time. Product strength varies; take a lower dosage if recommended on the label.	Stops inflammatory reactions caused by dust, smoke, or chemicals.
Oligomeric proanthocyanidins (OPCs)	Grapeseed or pine-bark extract capsules or tablets. Take as directed on the label.	Helps prevent asthma attacks provoked by airborne allergens.
Quercetin[5]	Tablets. Take 125–250 mg twice daily, between meals.	Helps prevent attacks by relaxing bronchial passages.
Scutellaria[6]	Capsules. Take 1,000–2,000 mg 3 times daily, or forms and dosages as dispensed by TCM practitioner.	Prevents allergic reactions. Stops cell damage caused by dexamethasone.

Precautions for the use of herbs:

[1]Asmatica may cause reduced sensitivity to the taste of salt, slight nausea, and slight mouth soreness.

[2]Khella makes the skin especially sensitive to ultraviolet light. Avoid tanning lamps and use sunblock when outdoors, and discontinue use if exposure to strong sunlight is unavoidable. Do not take this herb if you are taking the blood-thinner warfarin (Coumadin).

[3]Do not use licorice if you have glaucoma, high blood pressure, or an estrogen-sensitive disorder such as breast cancer, endometriosis, or fibrocystic breast disease.

[4]Do not give lobelia to a child under age twelve.

[5]Do not use quercetin if you are taking cyclosporine (Neoral, Sandimmune) or nifedipine (Adalat, Procardia).

[6]Do not take scutellaria if you have diarrhea.

chosen with careful regard to the entire pattern of an individual's symptoms, preferably under the guidance of an herbal practitioner. Herbal treatments should not be used to treat acute asthma attacks. See a physician promptly if you experience an acute attack.

Unless otherwise specified, the herb dosages recommended here are for adults. Children under age six should be given one-quarter of the adult dosage. Children between the ages of six and twelve should be given one-half of the adult dosage. Formula dosages for children should be discussed with a knowledgeable health-care practitioner.

Recommendations

❏ Use essential oil of thyme in aromatherapy to ease congestion. (*See* AROMATHERAPY in Part Three.) Do not use this treatment during an acute asthma attack, however.

❏ Eat more fish. Cold-water fish is a rich source of omega-3 essential fatty acids, which are also found in oils from borage seed, evening primrose, flaxseed (linseed), and hemp. Consuming omega-3 oils can reduce the risk of asthma attacks by causing the body to produce a less inflammatory class of leukotrienes. Children taking a product of the omega-3 fatty acid eicosapentaenoic acid (EPA) and gamma-linolenic fatty acid experienced improved breathing and blood tests indicating that there was less asthma activity. Eating fish once a week has also been found to cut children's risk of getting asthma by one-third.

❏ Take antioxidant vitamins. Vitamin C (1,000 milligrams daily) may reduce the frequency of coughing by reducing the ability of dust and pollutants to irritate the bronchial passages. Vitamin E (400 IU daily) may ease the passage of phlegm. Beta-carotene is also a useful antioxidant for treating asthma. Preferably taken in the form of green leafy vegetables or yellow or orange vegetables and fruits, this nutrient may help to stop wheezing. One study found that asthmatic children benefited from a combination of vitamin C, zinc, and omega-3 fatty acids. Using all three was better than using any one singularly. Patients could breathe better and had reduced blood markers of inflammation.

❏ In addition to taking the antioxidant vitamins listed above, take 500 to 1,000 milligrams of magnesium daily if you have frequent acute attacks. However, this amount could induce diarrhea, so spread the amount throughout the day.

Asthma: Formulas

Formula	Comments
Arrest Wheezing Decoction[1]	A traditional Chinese herbal formula that treats asthma with wheezing, coughing, expectoration of large amounts of thick yellow sputum, simultaneous fever and chills, and labored breathing.
Ephedra Decoction[2]	A traditional Chinese herbal formula that is especially beneficial for children with asthma.
Ephedra, Apricot Kernel, Gypsum, and Licorice Decoction[3]	A traditional Chinese herbal formula that relieves asthma with nasal allergy or nasal flaring. Offers specific relief for sensitivity to cedar pollen.
Ephedra, Asiasarum, and Prepared Aconite Decoction[4]	A traditional Chinese herbal formula that relieves chronic coughing and wheezing. This formula is useful if there is a sensation of extreme cold and severe chills relieved by covering up, a mild fever with perspiration, and exhaustion.
Ginseng Decoction to Nourish the Nutritive Chi	A traditional Chinese herbal formula that may make it possible to reduce the dosage of prednisolone to manage asthma. Also likely to increase the effectiveness of hydrocortisone, methylprednisone, and prednisone.
Minor Bluegreen Dragon Decoction[5]	A traditional Chinese herbal formula that relieves asthma with copious production of white, stringy sputum.
Minor Bupleurum Decoction[6]	A traditional Chinese herbal formula that stops the reaction that leads to the release of inflammatory leukotrienes. This formula may make it possible to reduce prednisolone dosage. It is also likely to increase the effectiveness of hydrocortisone, methylprednisone, and prednisone.
Ophiopogonis Decoction[7]	A traditional Chinese herbal formula for asthma with coughing, spitting of saliva, dry and uncomfortable sensation in the throat, dry mouth, red tongue, shortness of breath, and wheezing.

Precautions for use of formulas:

[1]Do not use Arrest Wheezing Decoction if you have diarrhea or a fever.

[2]Do not use Ephedra Decoction if you are experiencing nausea or vomiting.

[3]Do not use Ephedra, Apricot Kernel, Gypsum, and Licorice Decoction if you are experiencing nausea or vomiting.

[4]Stop using Ephedra, Asiasarum, and Prepared Aconite Decoction if higher fever occurs. This formula may cause a loss of sensation in the mouth and tongue.

[5]Do not use Minor Bluegreen Dragon Decoction if you have a fever.

[6]Do not use Minor Bupleurum Decoction if you have a fever or a skin infection. Taken long term, it can cause headache, dizziness, and bleeding gums. Side effects can be avoided if the formula is taken as a tea.

[7]Do not use Ophiopogonis Decoction if you have a fever.

❏ Some people have reported benefit from using thymus extracts to improve symptoms and shorten the duration of asthma attacks. These preparations are thought to act on the immune system, resulting in lowered production of the chemicals that cause allergic irritation. Take 750 milligrams once daily. Do not use thymus extracts if you are HIV-positive, however.

❏ Be sure to drink eight 8-ounce glasses of water daily. Water helps to loosen phlegm and is particularly necessary after an asthma attack.

❏ Avoid eating before bedtime. Eating just before sleep may encourage the development of gastroesophageal reflux disease (GERD), which causes some people to wake up with a cough, sore throat, or hoarseness, even in the absence of other factors. GERD can cause acidic material to be sent into the back of the throat, from which it is inhaled into the lungs. Nineteen million Americans have GERD and as many as 70 percent of patients with asthma have GERD compared to 20 to 30 percent of the general population. GERD also greatly increases the risk of emphysema and pneumonia. GERD mainly occurs in adults who are overweight.

❏ Avoid sulfites. Sulfites are preservatives commonly used in making dried fruits and wine, and in restaurant salad bars. Sulfites may promote bronchial constriction that can induce acute attacks. The additive monosodium glutamate (MSG) may cause similar problems for some people with asthma.

❏ Avoid L-glutathione supplements. Doctors have found that glutathione inhalers cause bronchial constriction, and it is possible that glutathione tablets may have the same effect.

Considerations

❏ The bodies of children with asthma may not process the amino acid tryptophan properly. The body converts tryptophan into serotonin, a compound that, among many other things, may cause air passages to constrict. Children with this defect can benefit from a low-tryptophan diet, which eliminates tryptophan-rich foods such as turkey and milk. However, do not put your child on a low-tryptophan diet without talking to the child's pediatrician. All protein-rich foods contain tryptophan and it is an essential amino acid. Other options include: supplementation with vitamin B_6, since this vitamin helps the body break down tryptophan, and inhaled corticosteroids, which may exert their anti-inflammatory activity in the asthmatic airways in part by increasing enzymes to break down tryptophan.

❏ Deep breathing and other relaxation techniques, as well as yoga, can be useful for both adults and children who have asthma, even if it is possible to practice these techniques for only a few minutes a day. Relaxation and visualization techniques can be especially useful for controlling asthma attacks in children. In addition to building physical strength and flexibility, yoga teaches steady, controlled, deep breathing. (See RELAXATION TECHNIQUES in Part Three.)

❏ Children with asthma often experience improvement after massage therapy. In one study, thirty-two children with asthma were randomly assigned to receive either massage therapy or relaxation therapy for twenty minutes before bedtime each night for thirty days. The younger children (aged four to eight) who received massage therapy showed an immediate decrease in behavioral anxiety and stress hormone levels after massage. Also, their attitude toward asthma and their peak air flow and other lung functions improved over the course of the study. The older children (aged nine to fourteen) who received massage therapy reported lower anxiety after the massage, although their lung function did not improve as much. It appears that daily massage improves the size of the airway and control of asthma. (See MASSAGE in Part Three.)

❏ In children under age five, exposure to secondhand smoke does not in itself create severe asthma symptoms, but makes the development of mild asthma more likely. Once the child is no longer exposed to such smoke, prior damage can be partially compensated for by supplying adequate vitamin C and glutathione.

❏ Sensitivity to cat dander can be a problem even for people who do not have cats. Cat dander is spread from clothing of cat owners throughout almost all public places, especially airplanes and movie theaters.

❏ Some studies have found a link between asthma attacks, which may be immediate or delayed, and food allergies. However, the number of children with asthma that gets triggered by a food allergy is low. In one study, of 300 children who thought that they had food-induced asthma attacks, only 20 responded with the signs of a true food allergy. The authors recommend not putting children on an elimination diet because this could lead to unnecessary micronutrient deficiencies. In children with true food allergies, foods that are most likely to trigger immediate attacks are eggs, fish, shellfish, nuts, and peanuts. Foods most commonly associated with delayed attacks include milk, chocolate, wheat, citrus, and food colorings. (For more information, see Food Allergies under ALLERGIES.)

❏ Hypochlorhydria, or deficient production of gastric acid in the stomach, has been linked to asthma in both children and adults, as well as to a higher incidence of allergies. People with asthma who have this problem should take special care to identify and avoid allergenic foods.

❏ Yeast infection indirectly contributes to asthma. Yeast produces protease, which provokes allergic responses and increases the amount of IgE in circulation. Treating yeast infections can ease asthma in many cases. (*See* YEAST INFECTION [YEAST VAGINITIS].)

❏ The prescription blood pressure drug lisinopril (Prinivil, Zestril), as well as all of the blood pressure drugs known as beta-blockers, can aggravate asthma. If you have asthma and are taking any of these drugs, see your physician about an alternative medication, and explore herbal treatments for high blood pressure. (*See* HIGH BLOOD PRESSURE [HYPERTENSION].)

❏ Goose feathers can cause and aggravate lung ailments.

❏ *See also* Respiratory Allergies *under* ALLERGIES.

ATHEROSCLEROSIS

Atherosclerosis is a process in which cholesterol is deposited on the inside of blood vessels. This decreases their ability to supply tissues with blood, which can lead to a number of cardiovascular diseases. Atherosclerosis is the leading cause of death for both men and women in the United States. Symptoms of atherosclerosis can include high blood pressure, angina, and even heart attack and stroke. Underlying causes and risk factors for this condition include a family history of cardiovascular disease, high blood pressure, diabetes, obesity, abnormal cholesterol levels, and smoking.

When a blood vessel is injured by mechanical injury, high blood pressure, or infection, a chemical called platelet-activating factor (PAF) causes red blood cells to clump together to seal the leak in the vessel wall. PAF also stimulates the production of fibrous tissues over the injury site.

The presence of cellular debris attracts macrophages, immune cells capable of consuming dead tissue. The macrophages are sent to the injured vessel to clean up the debris. Hormones are released that increase the number of smooth muscle cells lining the injured part of the vessel wall. When the number of smooth cells increases, more cholesterol is pumped into the lining of the blood vessel. Cholesterol can accumulate on both muscle cells and macrophages, leading to the formation of a plaque. This process is accelerated by the presence of harmful free radicals, which are created by chemical reactions of oxygen with dietary copper and iron.

The plaque itself causes blood pressure to rise due to increased resistance of blood flow, causing further injury to the blood vessel and, in turn, further plaque formation. Over time, more and more macrophages may be attracted to the site of the injury, bringing more cholesterol to the smooth muscle tissues. If this state of injury and repair persists over a number of years, blood vessels can become completely blocked.

Recommendations

❏ Eat onions. Onions have many of the same cardioprotective effects as garlic when approximately 1 ounce (30 grams) per day is used in food preparation. You can eat your onions either raw or cooked, as you prefer. Because the key element here is the presence of sulfur, very mild onions, which are grown in sulfur-deficient soils, do not contain the compounds that counteract atherosclerosis and clot formation.

❏ If you do not take soy isoflavone concentrate as recommended under Beneficial Herbs on page 210, eat soy products on a regular basis. Scientists have found that the estrogen-like compounds found in soy, known as phytoestrogens, are effective in slowing the progression of atherosclerosis. Phytoestrogens reduce levels of low-density lipoprotein (LDL, or "bad") cholesterol and, unlike some estrogen replacement therapies used to treat menopause, can lower triglyceride (blood fat) levels that are often elevated in heart disease and diabetes. Soy is also a rich source of the amino acid arginine, which may keep blood cells from sticking to the inside of artery walls and forming clots. Soy may be especially helpful in controlling atherosclerosis for women who have diabetes. Soy protein has also been shown to increase the blood flow (a test called flow-mediated dilation) in postmenopausal women with elevated cholesterol levels.

❏ If you are not worried about consuming the extra calories, drink 12 to 14 ounces of purple grape juice or one glass of red wine daily. These beverages contain flavonoid compounds that stop the oxidation of LDLs as effectively as vitamin E. Moreover, flavonoids strengthen the muscle cells lining the arteries so that they can dilate the artery more easily, allowing freer circulation of blood. Supplements of vitamin C, zinc, and lycopene all have been shown to reduce oxidation of LDL cholesterol. In addition, a study found that green tea extract containing 583 milligrams of catechins lowered LDL and also induced weight loss and loss of body fat in obese people in Japan.

❏ Avoid organ meats, such as liver. Organ meats not only contain large amounts of cholesterol, but also are potent sources of iron. Excess iron, which may accelerate the process of atherosclerosis, can be removed through the use of chelation therapy.

❏ Walk or jog for exercise, but do not sprint. Sustained light or moderate exercise decreases the risk of LDL buildup on arterial walls. Short bursts of strenuous exercise, however, supply the blood with large amounts of oxygen, releasing harmful free radicals.

❏ Adopt as optimistic an attitude as possible. Feelings of hopelessness can accelerate the development of atherosclerosis in the carotid arteries, the large arteries in the neck that help carry blood to the brain. Finnish researchers have found that "negative expectation about oneself and the future" in men accelerates plaque development in the carotid arteries by about 20 percent, and is roughly as harmful to blood-vessel health as smoking a pack of

Atherosclerosis: Beneficial Herbs

Herb	Form and Dosage	Comments
Alfalfa[1]	Capsules. Take 500–1,000 mg daily.	Shrinks plaques. Lowers total cholesterol.
Andrographis	Standardized extract tablets. Take as directed on the label.	If you undergo bypass surgery, use this herb to help prevent the re-formation of cholesterol plaques.
Arjuna	Capsules. Take 500 mg 3 times daily.	Reduces frequency of attacks. Lowers blood pressure and raises levels of high-density lipoprotein (HDL, or "good") cholesterol.
Astragalus[2]	Capsules. Take 500–1,000 mg 3 times daily.	Prevents plaque formation after arterial damage caused by high blood pressure or infection.
Bilberry	Tablets. Take 240–360 mg daily.	Prevents plaque formation by strengthening arterial walls.
Bromelain[3]	Tablets. Take 250–500 mg 3 times daily, between meals.	Shrinks plaques. Stops clot formation and lowers blood pressure.
Chamomile	German chamomile (*Matricaria recutita*) tincture. Take ½–1 tsp (2–4 ml) in ¼ cup water 3 times daily.	An antioxidant that slows plaque formation.
Coptis[4]	Tincture. Take 15–30 drops in ¼ cup water 3 times daily for up to 2 weeks.	Stimulates the release of bile, which purges cholesterol from the body.
Dan shen[5]	Tincture. Use under professional supervision.	Reverses atherosclerotic damage. Lowers blood pressure.
Garlic[6] and fish oil	Enteric-coated tablets. Take 900 mg daily; or fresh garlic. Eat ½ clove or more in food daily. MaxEPA. Take as directed on the label.	Lowers cholesterol and triglyceride levels. Inhibits clot formation. Reduces both blood pressure and cholesterol levels.
Ginger	Tea (powdered), prepared by adding ⅓ tsp (1 gm) to 1 cup water. (*See* TEAS in Part Three.) Take 1 cup 3 times daily.	Reduces cholesterol levels. Stimulates uptake of oxygen by muscle tissue.
Green tea	Tea bag, prepared with 1 cup water. Take 1 cup 2–5 times daily. Do not use within 1 hour of taking other medications.	Keeps low-density lipoprotein (LDL, or "bad") cholesterol from being oxidized, a factor in plaque formation.
Hawthorn	Tablets. Take 100–250 mg 3 times a day.	Antioxidant. Increases the rate at which the liver converts LDL into HDL.
Khella[7]	Khellin tablets. Take 20 mg daily.	Increases the ratio of HDL to LDL.
Milk thistle[8]	Silymarin gelcaps. Take 120–300 mg daily.	An antioxidant. Stops plaque formation and lowers total cholesterol.
Polysaccharide kureha (PSK) and selenium	Tablets. Take 6,000 mg daily until cholesterol levels normalize. Take 200 mcg daily.	Protects immune cells in artery walls from free-radical damage. Enhances the effect of PSK.
Quercetin[9]	Tablets. Take 125–250 mg 3 times daily, between meals.	Antioxidant that prevents plaque formation.
Red yeast rice	Cholestin or Hong Qu. Take as directed on the label.	Naturally occurring chemicals that act in the same way as the prescription drug lovastatin (Mevacor), lowering LDL after 4–6 weeks' use.
Scutellaria[10]	Capsules. Take 1,000–2,000 mg daily.	Stimulates the release of bile.
Snow fungus	Tablets. Take 6–12 daily for at least 4 weeks.	Lowers total cholesterol.
Soy isoflavone concentrate	Tablets. Take about 3,000 mg once daily.	Prevents plaque formation; lowers LDL.
Turmeric	Curcumin tablets. Take 250–500 mg twice daily, between meals.	Helps prevent atherosclerosis in people with diabetes. A potent antioxidant.

Precautions for the use of herbs:

[1]Do not use alfalfa in any form if you have an autoimmune disease, such as lupus or rheumatoid arthritis.

[2]Do not use astragalus if you have a fever or a skin infection.

[3]People who are allergic to pineapple may develop a rash from bromelain. If itching develops, stop using it.

[4]Do not take coptis for longer than two weeks at a time. Do not use it if you are pregnant or have gallbladder disease. Do not take this herb with supplemental vitamin B_6 or with protein supplements containing the amino acid histidine.

[5]Do not use dan shen if you have an estrogen-sensitive disorder, such as breast cancer, endometriosis, or fibrocystic breast disease.

[6]Garlic counteracts the effects of *Bifidus* and *Lactobacillus* cultures taken as digestive aids. Consult a doctor before using garlic on a regular basis if you are on an anticoagulant drug such as warfarin (Coumadin). Discuss the use of garlic with your doctor before having any type of surgery.

[7]Khella makes the skin especially sensitive to ultraviolet light. Avoid tanning lamps and use sunblock when outdoors, and discontinue use if exposure to strong sunlight is unavoidable. Do not use khella if you take the blood-thinner warfarin (Coumadin).

[8]Milk thistle may cause mild diarrhea. If this occurs, decrease the dose or stop taking it.

[9]Do not use quercetin if you are taking cyclosporine (Neoral, Sandimmune) or nifedipine (Adalat, Procardia).

[10]Do not use scutellaria if you have diarrhea.

Atherosclerosis: Formulas

Formula	Comments
Dong Quai and Peony Powder	European studies of this traditional Chinese herbal formula indicate that it can stop excessive free-radical production in the cardiovascular system, stopping the process of atherosclerosis.

cigarettes a day. In women, atherosclerosis is more likely to be associated with suppressed anger and hostility. Relaxation techniques can be helpful. (*See* RELAXATION TECHNIQUES in Part Three.)

❏ Do not smoke, and stay away from secondhand smoke. As little as a half-hour in a smoke-filled room causes a serious drop in blood levels of such antioxidants as vitamin C. What's more, the smoke causes changes in cholesterol metabolism that encourage the deposit of LDLs on artery walls. If secondhand smoke is unavoidable, take 200 to 400 milligrams of vitamin C daily.

Considerations

❏ Doctors usually recommend that people with atherosclerosis eliminate major sources of dietary cholesterol as a way of stopping the disease process before it starts. Cholesterol-reducing drugs, which usually modify the way the liver processes cholesterol, may be prescribed as well.

❏ Some dietary fats are necessary. Include those from vegetable sources, and avoid trans fats. Limit your intake of saturated fats from animal sources by using low-fat dairy foods and trimming visible fat and skin from any animal meats. Include fish in your diet and take fish oil capsules, after checking with your doctor. One omega-3 fatty acid, eicosapentaenoic acid (EPA), has been shown to reduce the number of foam cells, thereby leading to a lower buildup of plaque in the blood vessels.

❏ Regular consumption of more than 50 grams of alcohol a day, roughly equivalent to two bottles of beer or two glasses of wine, is a "prominent risk factor for early atherogenesis [plaque development], surpassing even the effect of heavy smoking," according to an article in the journal *Stroke*. Moderate drinking has been shown to relax blood vessels and reduce heart disease risk, but check with your doctor to establish whether it is helpful for you.

❏ Infection with *Chlamydia*, a sexually transmitted microbe, could accelerate the process of atherosclerosis. When this germ invades the blood-vessel linings, the immune system sends cells to surround and digest the microorganisms. These immune cells attract cholesterol and eventually form the basis for plaque, which can lead to atherosclerosis. However, if chlamydia is treated, it is possible to virtually eliminate chlamydia infection as the cause of plaque formation.

(For information on controlling chlamydia, *see* GONORRHEA AND CHLAMYDIA.)

❏ Infection with *Helicobacter pylori*, the bacterium associated with peptic ulcers, may also trigger an immune response that may increase the risk of coronary artery disease. (*See* PEPTIC ULCER.)

❏ Sensitivity to pesticides may be linked to a higher than average risk of atherosclerosis. In the body, LDL cholesterol and phosphate-based pesticides are broken down by the same enzyme, paraoxonase. Exposure to pesticides may deplete this enzyme, leading to an increase of LDLs.

❏ Osteoporosis is a risk factor for atherosclerosis. Older women with the greatest loss of calcium from bone are also the women most likely to have calcium-containing cholesterol plaques in their carotid arteries. This effect can be offset, however, by vitamin D. Taking a vitamin D supplement is likely necessary, but get your blood vitamin D levels tested first to see if they are too low. Otherwise, expose your face and hands to direct sunlight for at least twenty minutes every day. (For more information, *see* OSTEOPOROSIS.)

❏ To make the blood less prone to clotting, anticoagulants such as aspirin are often prescribed by your doctor. For this treatment to be effective, supplemental vitamin K and foods rich in vitamin K must be avoided.

❏ *See also* HEART ATTACK (MYOCARDIAL INFARCTION); HIGH BLOOD PRESSURE (HYPERTENSION); HIGH CHOLESTEROL; and INTERMITTENT CLAUDICATION.

ATHLETE'S FOOT

Athlete's foot is an infection caused by the fungal organism tinea. It is commonly spread via the damp, moist floors of locker rooms and showers, and could spread quickly if the body's natural beneficial bacteria have been destroyed by the use of antibiotics or other drugs, or by radiation therapy. Medically known as *tinea pedis*, this condition begins as small, water-filled blisters that grow into inflamed patches accompanied by burning, itching, scaling, and cracking. Sometimes, patches of skin peel off over the area of inflammation. The particular fungus that causes athlete's foot flourishes on calluses and in any area of the foot that is difficult to dry, such as the skin between the toes.

Athlete's Foot: Beneficial Herbs

Herb	Form and Dosage	Comments
Black walnut	Tincture or tea. Use as a foot bath twice daily. (*See* FOOT BATHS in Part Three.)	Stops oozing from infected skin.
Calendula	Cream. Apply as directed on the label.	Heals cracked skin.
Goldenseal	Powder. Mix ½ tsp with ½ tsp arrowroot powder and apply to the feet before every sock change.	An antifungal that also fights secondary bacterial infections.
Tea tree oil[1]	Essential oil. Use as a foot bath twice daily. (*See* FOOT BATHS in Part Three.)	Relieves itching and burning.
Thyme	Essential oil. Apply 2–3 drops once daily.	An antifungal agent.

Precautions for the use of herbs:

[1]People who are allergic to celery or thyme should not use tea tree oil products. Do not take tea tree oil internally.

Not surprisingly, athlete's foot can be a serious infection among people whose immune systems are severely compromised. Even among people with normal immune systems, reinfection is common through the wearing of dirty socks that contain fungus spores. Wearing shoes and socks made of synthetic materials hinders air circulation and promotes dampness, increasing the severity of the infection.

A number of prescription and over-the-counter (OTC) drugs are available to fight athlete's foot, but some of these medications may cause problems. Side effects are minor and may include an allergy to the medication. These drugs should not be used during pregnancy or lactation. Herbal treatment may be effective for some cases of this disorder.

Recommendations

❑ Dry your feet thoroughly after showering or swimming. Use a new towel after each bath. The spaces between your toes can be dried with a hair dryer.

❑ Sprinkle baking soda on your feet to absorb moisture before putting on socks.

❑ Wash your bathtub or shower floor daily with a solution of 5 drops of coptis or goldenseal extract in 1 quart of water.

❑ Get rid of bath mats and wooden shower grids. They are breeding grounds for fungi and bacteria.

Considerations

❑ Keeping the feet dry is a more important consideration than keeping the feet cool in managing athlete's foot. Athlete's foot fungus can penetrate the skin in two to four days at temperatures ranging from 50 to 90°F (15 to 27°C) if the humidity of the air around the skin is 100 percent. If the humidity of the air around the skin is lowered just to 80 percent, the fungus does not penetrate the skin at all.

❑ The same fungus that causes athlete's foot also causes jock itch and ringworm. (*See* RINGWORM.) Men with athlete's foot who throw their gym clothes together in a bag and then wear them again risk contracting jock itch.

ATTENTION DEFICIT DISORDER/ATTENTION DEFICIT HYPERACTIVITY DISORDER (ADD/ADHD)

Attention deficit disorder (ADD) is a condition marked by learning disabilities, hyperactivity, and/or impaired judgment. Other symptoms include frequent forgetfulness, inability to focus on details or complete a task, excessive talking or interrupting, restless fidgeting, and problems with organizing activities. The best known form of ADD is attention deficit hyperactivity disorder (ADHD), which primarily affects children but also is present in adults. The hallmark of ADHD is constant motion and disruptive behavior. A less severe form, ADD without hyperactivity, also occurs in children. Because adults usually have developed some measure of coping skills, clinicians refer to both ADD and ADHD in adults as residual ADD.

ADHD is the most common neurological disorder among North American youngsters, affecting an estimated 9.5 percent of children four to seventeen years of age. Both ADD and ADHD tend to run in families, and boys with ADHD outnumber girls by at least three to one. It is estimated that 4.5 percent of adults have residual ADD.

Scientific study suggests that the common factor in all forms of ADD is a coordination failure within the brain. In order to focus on selected information from the outside world, certain brain regions must be activated while others are inhibited. The signals to these regions must be switched through a tiny brain area known as the locus ceruleus, which transmits information via a chemical messenger called norepinephrine. If anything goes wrong anywhere along the way, ADD or ADHD can result. Sugar consumption blunts the brain's responsiveness to norepinephrine and could contribute to the problem. In addition, it is possible that inflammation caused by allergies can lead to sensory overload, in which the brain receives more information than it can handle. Other factors believed to contribute to this disorder include neurological problems in the brain, family history, anxiety, oxygen deprivation at birth, lead poisoning, diet, and smoking by the mother during pregnancy.

Physicians most often prescribe psychostimulant or

antidepressant drugs. Oddly enough, long-term use of stimulant drugs may cause depression. This usually happens with long-acting stimulants. It is best to get screened for depression before starting any medication; however, if the depression is due to the ADD medication, switching to tricyclic antidepressants may be advised, but first speak to your doctor. Over time, psychostimulant drugs may become ineffective and cause a rebound effect, in which anger and frustration could reappear.

Unless otherwise specified, the herb dosages recommended here are for adults. Children under age six should be given one-quarter of the adult dosage. Children between the ages of six and twelve should be given one-half of the adult dosage. Formula dosages for children should be discussed with a knowledgeable health-care practitioner.

Recommendations

❑ Make sure a child with ADHD eats three balanced meals daily. Breakfast is particularly important and should

ADD/ADHD Beneficial Herbs

Herb	Form and Dosage	Comments
Avena	Tincture. Take 10 drops in ¼ cup water twice daily.	Reduces symptoms of withdrawal from methylphenidate (Ritalin). Relieves sadness and mild depression in adults.
Brahmi concentrate	Bacoside tablets. Take 300 mg once daily.	Improves attention and retention of new learning.
Chamomile[1]	German chamomile (*Matricaria recutita*) tea bag, prepared with 1 cup of water. Take 1 cup 1–2 times daily.	Relieves allergies, inflammation, and insomnia.
Ginkgo[2]	Ginkgolide tablets. Take 160–180 mg 3 times daily.	The best herb for adults with ADD.
Hawthorn	Capsules. Take 3–5 gm daily.	Relieves acting out, anxiety, and unrest in children. Stops inflammatory responses caused by allergies.
Lemon balm with valerian	Capsules. Take 240 mg 45 minutes before bedtime.	Hastens sleep and relaxes muscle tension without causing daytime drowsiness.
Lobelia[3]	Capsules. Take 500–1,000 mg 3 times daily. Take for no more than 2 weeks at a time. Product strength varies; take a lower dosage if recommended on the label.	For adults with ADD only. Especially useful if you also have asthma.
Oligomeric proanthocyanidins (OPCs)	Grapeseed or pine-bark extract tablets. Take 20 mg per 20 lbs body weight.	An antidepressant that does not cause emotional changes, hyperactivity, or drowsiness.
Passionflower	Tea bag, prepared with 1 cup water. Take 1–2 cups daily.	A calming agent that causes less drowsiness than prescription drugs.
Scutellaria[4]	Capsules. Take 1,000–2,000 mg 3 times daily.	Prevents allergic reactions.
Valerian root	Liquid extract, mixed in juice according to label directions. Take 2–3 times a day.	Used as a relaxant. Eases anxiety.
Wood betony	Low-alcohol tincture. Take as directed on the label.	For children with head or facial pain, or adults with high blood pressure.

Precautions for the use of herbs:

[1]Do not use chamomile on an ongoing basis. Avoid it if you are allergic to ragweed.

[2]Do not use ginkgo if you are taking blood-thinning medication. Discuss its use with your doctor before having any type of surgery.

[3]Do not give lobelia to a child under age twelve.

[4]Do not use scutellaria if you have diarrhea.

ADD/ADHD Formulas

Formula	Comments
Six-Ingredient Pill with Rehmannia (Rehmannia-Six Combination)[1]	A traditional Chinese herbal formula that treats developmental delays, as in speech and walking, and maintains brain-chemical function. Also effective for adults.

Precautions for the use of formulas:

[1]Do not use Six-Ingredient Pill with Rehmannia if you have an estrogen-sensitive disorder, such as breast cancer, endometriosis, or fibrocystic breasts.

include adequate protein. Children with ADHD may forget to eat, and school studies have linked hunger with absences, tardiness, and unruly behavior.

❑ Include in your diet cold-water fish such as tuna and salmon two times a week, as well as plenty of fruits, vegetables, beans, and natural whole grains. However, you should limit foods that contain natural salicylates, such as almonds, apples, apricots, berries, cherries, cucumbers, oranges, peppers, plums, and tomatoes.

❑ Take 250 milligrams of magnesium at night and 400 to 800 international units (IU) of vitamin E daily to ease sleep-disrupting muscle cramps if they occur in adults with ADD. Magnesium was also shown to improve attention, behavior, and emotional problems when combined with zinc and essential fatty acids of the omega-3 and omega-6 families.

❑ Use folic acid and iron supplements for children who have ADD/ADHD complicated by restless legs syndrome, in which the legs are "jumpy" at night. In one small study, children treated with prescription drugs for restless legs syndrome also showed reductions in ADHD symptoms. See the doctor about giving your child high-dose folic acid (35 to 60 milligrams daily). This is available only by prescription. Supplemental iron (200 milligrams ferrous sulfate, three times daily) used for no more than two to three months supports the action of folic acid. This is a very high dose of iron, so consult your child's physician first.

❑ A standardized extract of guarana was found to improve memory, increase alertness, and improve mood. Multiple doses were tested, but 75 milligrams seemed to provide the best results. In contrast, no benefit was seen in children with ADHD who took St. John's wort for eight weeks.

❑ Avoid sugar. Parents and clinical researchers alike note that aggressive and restless behavior could be tied to the amount of sugar a child with ADD/ADHD consumes. Sugar has no other nutrients except calories and is not needed by the body. However, a study published in the prestigious *New England Journal of Medicine* found no relationship between sucrose or aspartame on behavior and cognitive function in healthy children and those who were described by their parents as being sensitive to sugar.

❑ Avoid soft drinks, both sweetened and sugar-free. Soft drinks contain phosphates, which can displace calcium and magnesium in the body and weaken bones.

❑ Identify allergies and minimize or eliminate contact with allergens. Some children with ADD or ADHD are allergic to the blue, red, and yellow dyes used in food products. In one study, investigators in Australia found that food colorings caused changes in behavior—more irritability, restlessness, and sleep disturbances—when fed to hyperactive children in a controlled study. Other common allergens are citrus fruits, cow's milk, grapes, peanuts, and tomatoes. (*See* Food Allergies *under* ALLERGIES.) To avoid exposure to dyes, do not use highly processed foods, especially colored candies. Also, try avoiding the foods listed above for three to four days to see if a change in diet helps ease symptoms.

❑ If you are an adult with ADD, get more exercise to help manage the condition. Italian scientists have found that moderate exercise, such as jogging, for thirty minutes a day reduces brain excitability by 40 percent. The relaxing effects of exercise last for several hours to as long as a day. Children with ADD or ADHD also should get more exercise and avoid watching television and playing video games.

Considerations

❑ Seasonal affective disorder (SAD) is a condition misdiagnosed as often as ADD or ADHD. SAD is a form of depression induced by lack of sunlight and perhaps vitamin D. It occurs in winter months in northern latitudes, but can also occur in the summer months in hot areas of the southern United States, when children stay indoors to avoid the heat. If your child has ADD-like symptoms when forced to stay indoors, try letting him or her play outside when temperatures are moderate, or have the child sit under a full-spectrum lamp for at least forty-five minutes a day.

❑ Doctors have found that such nighttime breathing problems as sleep apnea and snoring aggravate ADHD. (*See* INSOMNIA.)

❑ Some adults with ADD find relief through pranayama, or ayurvedic breathing exercises. To perform pranayama, inhale deeply through the left nostril, with the right nostril closed, then exhale deeply through the right nostril, with the left nostril closed. Repeat this for a minimum of ten breaths and a maximum of ten minutes.

❑ Children who have difficulty controlling themselves in class may "glue" themselves to their computers or video games. Scientists have found a physiological reason for this behavior. People playing video games experience a surge of dopamine in the brain. This chemical enables the brain to exert fine control over movement. Dopamine levels remain elevated even after the game is over.

BAD BREATH

See HALITOSIS (BAD BREATH).

BALDNESS

See HAIR LOSS.

BASAL CELL CARCINOMA

See under SKIN CANCER.

BED-WETTING

Wetting the bed, also called enuresis, is an embarrassing problem that affects from 5 to 7 million children in the United States. Enuresis refers to the involuntary discharge of urine beyond the age when a child should be able to control urination, usually age six or older. Bed-wetting can be behavioral or physiological in nature. Sometimes an underlying condition is not identified. In these cases, bed-wetting seems to occur more often in children born to mothers younger than twenty, and to second- and third-born children. This condition almost always resolves itself as a child matures. However, if not properly handled, it can lead the child to suffer from emotional difficulties.

Current medical research offers several explanations of bed-wetting. Some studies indicate that this problem occurs if the kidneys have been damaged by infection and lose part of their reserve capacity. This is especially true if a child relapses into bed-wetting after having achieved bladder control. Other studies offer a hormonal explanation. Antidiuretic hormone is a body chemical that causes the kidneys to retain water. If this hormone is deficient, fluid flows from the kidneys into the bladder. Sodium flows into the bladder as well, and draws even more water with it. Since antidiuretic hormone is made in the brain, changes in brain chemistry associated with a stressful or scary situation decrease hormone production. Production of antidiuretic hormone can also be decreased by exposure to chemicals or nicotine from secondhand smoke. Other factors that can cause or contribute to bed-wetting include an unusually small bladder, very sound sleeping, consuming too much liquid before bedtime, emotional problems, stress, diabetes, and urinary tract infection.

There are drug treatments for bed-wetting, most notably desmopressin acetate (DDAVP) nasal spray, which is a synthetic form of antidiuretic hormone. There are situations, such as when a child is spending the night at a friend's house or going to camp, in which using desmopressin is preferable to using herbal medicine. On a long-term basis, however, herbal approaches may offer relief with fewer side effects and at a lower cost. Herbal treatments are best undertaken with a doctor's help, since a medical diagnosis is essential to determine the underlying cause of the problem. Seek the advice of the dispensing herbalist on a suitable child's dosage for formulas.

Recommendations

❑ If your child takes DDAVP, provide him or her with a low-salt diet that includes no salty foods such as pickles, processed meats, or salty snacks. If DDAVP is ineffective, the underlying problem could be an abnormality in the kidneys' ability to process sodium. The drug is very successful; 77 percent of children in one study showed improvements.

❑ Investigate the possibility of allergies, especially food allergies, which can cause bed-wetting. (*See* Food Allergies *under* ALLERGIES.) This is something that your child's doctor may not think of. However, one study demonstrated that there are provoking foods that trigger nighttime bed-wetting. Finding out which are the offending foods may help control the problem.

❑ Make sure there are ample opportunities for the child to urinate during the day. In a Swedish study, doctors followed twenty-two children with severe bed-wetting. Twelve went to the bathroom more often during the day, but received no other treatment, while ten children were

Bed-Wetting: Beneficial Herbs

Herb	Form and Dosage	Comments
Buchu or corn silk or oat straw or parsley	Take in the form and at the dosage recommended by a health-care professional.	These herbs are diuretics, so they promote emptying of the bladder before bedtime. Be sure to take them before 3:00 P.M.
Horsetail	Fluidextract. Take ¼–1 tsp (1–4 ml) 3 times daily.	An astringent that reduces urinary tract irritation.
Raspberry leaf	Tea bag, prepared with 1 cup water. Take 1 cup 1–2 times daily.	Traditional remedy that tones pelvic muscles.

Bed-Wetting: Formulas

Formula	Comments
Licorice, Wheat, and Jujube Decoction	A traditional Chinese herbal formula that treats bed-wetting aggravated by crying spells and depression.
Minor Construct the Middle Decoction	A traditional Chinese herbal formula that stops stomach spasms and increases bladder tone, allowing a child's bladder to hold more urine. Also relieves nervous stomach.

persuaded to make more trips to the bathroom and were either monitored with a moisture alarm or given DDAVP. The number of wet nights after one month decreased in all children, and the improvement continued for most of the children during the follow-up period.

❏ Make the bed in layers: plastic, sheet, plastic, sheet, plastic, sheet. This way the child can be taught to simply remove the top layer of plastic and sheet, toss them into the bathtub, and go back to sleep on "dry ground." This gives the child more independence and can reduce feelings of shame, since it is no longer necessary to wake a parent for help. And it works better than using pull-up diapers, which can make a child who wants to be a "big kid" feel like a baby. Using pull-ups also implies that, since the diaper will catch the urine, wetting the bed is not a problem that needs to be solved.

❏ Do not shame or ridicule the child for wetting the bed. That will only make matters worse.

Considerations

❏ Desmopressin acetate can work very quickly. The effect is canceled out, however, if the child consumes drinks that contain caffeine. Also, this drug is expensive. It is very safe but may cause transient headaches, nausea, or mild abdominal pain. In rare instances, desmopressin acetate may cause changes in blood pressure—either by raising it or lowering it for a short time—but this should resolve quickly by itself.

❏ Restricting fluids before bedtime doesn't work. Food becomes mostly liquid when it passes through the digestive system, and from there the fluid enters the bloodstream. Therefore, bed-wetting occurs during sleep even when liquids are restricted.

❏ Moisture alarms have long been a popular method of treatment. Unfortunately, the success of this method is limited to a few children, and it requires months of use. It works best for children who sleep very deeply. The alarm's effectiveness depends on the child's desire to get up at the first sense of wetness; in time the child learns to wake at the first feeling of urgency.

❏ Constipation often occurs in children who wet the bed and, in some cases, must be corrected before bed-wetting is overcome. (See CONSTIPATION.)

❏ Behavior modification by biofeedback may be helpful in some cases. For more information, contact the Association for Applied Psychophysiology and Biofeedback. (See Appendix B: Resources.)

❏ Some parents have success in teaching their children Kegel exercises, which strengthen the urinary sphincter. (See KEGEL EXERCISES in Part Three.)

❏ See also BLADDER INFECTION (CYSTITIS).

BELCHING

See under INDIGESTION.

BELL'S PALSY

Bell's palsy, also known as idiopathic palsy, is a temporary weakening of the facial nerve. Symptoms include facial paralysis or weakness, numbness, and, sometimes, dry eyes or mouth. The condition can also cause intense facial pain. Bell's palsy affects about 40,000 Americans a year, most commonly people between sixteen and fifty-nine years of age. The cause is not well understood, but the onset is often associated with a viral infection, particularly primary infection with herpes simplex type 1, auto-immune disease, or Lyme disease. It develops suddenly; sometimes it is preceded several hours beforehand by pain behind the ear on the affected side. The prognosis for individuals with Bell's palsy is generally very good. The extent of nerve damage determines the extent of recovery. Improvement is gradual and recovery times vary. With or without treatment, most people begin to get better within two weeks after the initial onset of symptoms and most recover completely, returning to normal function within three to six months. For some, however, the symptoms may last longer. In a few cases, the symptoms may never completely disappear. In rare cases, the disorder may recur, either on the same or the opposite side of the face.

One of the more disconcerting aspects of Bell's palsy is its effect on expression. Even in mild cases, the eyebrows may not lift symmetrically, and it may be impossible to smile and show your teeth. In other cases, the condition causes autonomic synkinesis, or "crocodile tears"—spontaneous crying with no emotional stimulus.

Many conditions besides Bell's palsy, some of them serious, can cause facial paralysis. For this reason, it is essential to avoid self-diagnosis of this condition. Because there is no specific test for this disorder, doctors generally diagnose it by eliminating other potential causes of symptoms, such as middle ear and parotid infections, stroke, cancer, mumps, and Lyme disease. Once Bell's palsy is diagnosed, various drug treatments may be used. Herbs may relieve specific symptoms.

Recommendations

❏ Do not delay treatment. The best time to start prescription drug treatment is during the first seventy-two hours after symptoms begin. The longer treatment is delayed, the more helpful herbs are as complements to prescribed medication.

❏ Practice proper eye care. Your doctor will probably prescribe eyedrops for use during the day, ointment for use at bedtime, and a gogglelike moisture chamber to be worn during the night. Do not scratch the cornea by patching or

Bell's Palsy: Beneficial Herbs

Herb	Form and Dosage	Comments
Cloves	Essential oil. Take 5–10 drops in ¼ cup water 3 times daily.	Increases the effectiveness of acyclovir (Zovirax).
Kudzu	Tablets. Take 10 mg 3 times daily.	Relieves muscle tension in the muscles of the face and neck not affected by palsy.
Licorice[1]	Glycyrrhizin tablets. Take 200–800 mg daily, depending on severity of symptoms. Use for 6 weeks; then take a 2-week break. Do not substitute deglycyrrhizinated licorice (DGL).	Prevents progression of palsy to paralysis; stops "crocodile tears." Consume potassium-rich foods such as bananas or citrus juices, or take a potassium supplement daily when taking this herb.

Precautions for the use of herbs:

[1]Do not use licorice if you have glaucoma, high blood pressure, or an estrogen-sensitive disorder such as breast cancer, endometriosis, or fibrocystic breasts.

Bell's Palsy: Formula

Formula	Comments
Ophiopogonis Decoction[1]	A traditional Chinese herbal formula that relieves dry eyes by increasing secretion to tears. Use this formula with the eye moisturizers described under Recommendations, page 216.

Precautions for the use of formulas:

[1]Do not use Ophiopogonis Decoction if you have a fever.

taping the eye itself. One easy way to keep an eye moist is to place a small piece of plastic wrap over the eye and apply it to the face with hairnet tape.

Considerations

❏ Some physicians prescribe a combination of an antiviral drug, acyclovir (Zovirax), with a steroid hormone, prednisone (Deltasone), for the treatment of Bell's palsy. Prednisone has potential side effects, among them high blood pressure, which can worsen the disease. If there is a question as to whether prednisone will be beneficial in your case, and your doctor has not prescribed it, try taking licorice for one month. Licorice contains glycyrrhizin, which may complement acyclovir in the same way prednisone does, but with fewer side effects. Monitor your blood pressure at least once a week when taking either licorice or prednisone, and inform your doctor if you have two or more consecutive readings over 140/90.

❏ Preexisting high blood pressure prolongs Bell's palsy and increases the risk it will recur. Check your blood pressure regularly. If you have readings exceeding 140/90 on two or more occasions, begin a program of blood pressure control. (*See* HIGH BLOOD PRESSURE [HYPERTENSION].)

❏ Electrical stimulation treatments, which may be offered to people with Bell's palsy as a possible therapy, unfortunately do not seem to correct this condition. There are even some indications that electrical stimulation can cause further nerve damage and delay healing.

❏ For reasons that are not entirely understood, Bell's palsy is extremely common in the Chinese city of Kunming, and acupuncturists in Kunming have developed extremely effective approaches to treating the disease. These approaches involve the technique of "pause and regress," in which needles are inserted, withdrawn, and replaced on acupuncture points over the parts of the face served by the facial nerve. Usually acupuncture is started on the side of the face that is not affected by palsy. It usually takes two weeks of daily treatment to see changes in symptoms. (*See* ACUPUNCTURE in Part Three.)

❏ Some people have derived benefit from vitamins including B_{12}, B_6, and zinc.

❏ Bell's palsy can be caused by Lyme disease. (See LYME DISEASE.)

❏ *See also* DRY MOUTH.

BENIGN PROSTATIC HYPERTROPHY (BPH)

The prostate is a walnut-sized gland that encircles the urethra, the tube through which urine passes. It produces seminal fluid, which forms the bulk of the ejaculate. BPH is a noncancerous condition in which the prostate becomes enlarged and presses on the urethra. BPH ordinarily does not arise until a man has reached middle age, usually at least age fifty.

In the beginning stages, there may be no symptoms. As the prostate grows, however, there may be difficulty in passing urine, frequent urination, and getting up at night to urinate. These symptoms can be aggravated by immobility, exposure to cold, or alcohol consumption. It can become difficult to achieve orgasm. As the prostate continues to swell, there can be pain or a burning sensation during urination, blood in the urine, and pain in the lower back or pelvis. Bladder infections and kidney disorders may develop. Since the symptoms of BPH are also seen in people with prostate cancer, they should always be brought to a doctor's attention.

BPH is linked to changes in hormonal levels that occur as a man ages. These changes cause the glandular tissue of the prostate to grow in the presence of testosterone, the primary male hormone. Conventional treatment consists of drugs and surgery. If you are using herbal formulas, you should consult with an experienced herbal practitioner.

Herbs to Avoid

❏ Men who have prostate enlargement should avoid the following herbs: American ginseng, cinnamon, cordyceps, epimedium, sarsaparilla, and Siberian ginseng. Ginseng should be used with caution. (For more information regarding these herbs, *see* AMERICAN GINSENG, CINNAMON, CORDYCEPS, EPIMEDIUM, GINSENG, SARSAPARILLA, and SIBERIAN GINSENG *under* The Herbs in Part One.)

Recommendations

❏ If erectile dysfunction (ED) occurs while using saw palmetto and pygeum, use micronized pollen instead. Take 3,000 to 4,000 milligrams in capsule form daily.

❏ Drink at least eight glasses of water daily. Dehydration stresses the prostate gland.

❏ Eat pumpkin seeds as a snack once or twice a week. Pumpkin seeds do not shrink an enlarged prostate, but they may help to restore normal flow of urine.

❏ Avoid bicycle riding and using exercise bikes, except for recumbent bicycles. Ordinary bicycle seats place pressure on the prostate.

❏ If you develop increased thirst, unintentional weight loss, or testicular pain, see a physician.

❏ Drink more unsweetened cranberry juice. This can protect against urinary tract infections, which have been linked to some forms of prostatitis.

BPH: Beneficial Herbs

Herb	Form and Dosage	Comments
Papain	Capsules. Take 500 mg 3 times daily for up to 2 weeks.	Relieves acute inflammation of the prostate.
Saw palmetto and	Capsules. Take 160 mg twice daily.	A combination that reduces inflammation and restores normal flow of urine.
pygeum and	Capsules. Take 50–100 mg twice daily.	
zinc picolinate	Tablets. Take 50–100 mg twice daily.	
Stinging nettle root	Capsules or tablets. Take 1,000–1,500 mg daily.	Blocks the action of growth hormone on the prostate. Restores normal urine flow.
Varuna	Tincture. Take as directed on the label.	Treats enlarged prostate in men who have consumed excess fat.

BPH: Formulas

Formula	Comments
Eight-Ingredient Pill with Rehmannia[1]	A traditional Chinese herbal formula that restores ease of urination.
Gentiana Longdancao Decoction to Drain the Liver	A traditional Chinese herbal formula that reduces incontinence caused by prostate enlargement or irritation. Treats symptoms that may accompany BPH, including headache, dizziness, hearing loss, bitter taste in the mouth, and emotional distress.
Sairei-to	A traditional Chinese herbal formula that is a combination of two commonly available formulas: Five-Ingredient Powder with Poria and Minor Bupleurum Decoction. This formula helps to reestablish normal urination after prostate surgery.

Precautions for the use of formulas:

[1]Eight-Ingredient Pill with Rehmannia should be used only if a definitive diagnosis of BPH has been made. It should *not* be used for prostate cancer.

❏ If your prostate is enlarged, be cautious about using over-the-counter (OTC) cold or allergy remedies. Many of these products contain ingredients that aggravate the condition and cause urine retention.

Considerations

❏ If there is severe obstruction of the urethra, surgery may be used to widen the opening. In addition, drugs are often prescribed to reduce prostate swelling. These drugs, however, can have a number of side effects, including a decrease in libido, and they may not always be effective.

❏ If the prostate is infected, treatment with antibiotics and analgesics may be necessary. (*See* PROSTATITIS.)

❏ Engaging in sexual intercourse while the prostate is infected and irritated may further irritate the prostate and delay recovery.

❏ Vasectomy for sterilization used to be linked to prostate cancer, but a recent National Cancer Institute panel conducted an extensive review and found no evidence of this relationship.

❏ All men aged forty or over should have a yearly rectal examination, during which the prostate gland is checked.

❏ *See also* ERECTILE DYSFUNCTION, PROSTATE CANCER, and PROSTATITIS.

BITE, INSECT

See INSECT BITES.

BLADDER CANCER

Bladder cancer is the sixth most common cancer in the United States. It usually strikes mature men who have been exposed to cigarette smoke and/or industrial carcinogens. Possible symptoms include blood in the urine, along with frequent, painful, and/or urgent urination.

Smoking causes about half of the deaths from bladder cancer among men (48 percent) and almost a third of bladder cancer deaths in women (28 percent). Other possible causes and risk factors for this disease include a history of working in the cigarette, rubber, or dye industries, which can lead to contact with the chemical 2-napthylamine; being white; being male over forty years of age; having a family member who has had bladder cancer; and having recurrent bouts of kidney stones or urinary tract infections. Bladder cancer may spread to nearby organs, such as the colon, and the pelvic bones.

The current understanding of bladder cancer is that it develops through at least a two-stage process at the cellular level. In the first stage, a cancer-causing agent destroys part of a gene known as gene p16. Damage to p16 causes no changes to the outside of the cell, so the immune system continues to treat it as if it were genetically healthy.

The damage to the DNA within the cell, however, induces the cell to make copies of itself, far in excess of the numbers needed to replace it. Using a test to measure p16 is a valuable biomarker to predict bladder cancer, prognosis, and clinical outcome.

The body has a second line of defense against genetic damage, gene p53. This gene serves as a "molecular patrolman" by making sure that defective cells do not multiply. However, gene p53 can also be damaged. Compromising p53, in the absence of other kinds of signals to the immune system, leaves the cancer cells free to multiply and spread. In addition, bladder cancers pick up hormonal signals to grow and multiply, especially from estrogen, the primary female sex hormone. (Men's bodies also produce estrogen, but in smaller amounts.) Fortunately, estrogen's effects occur slowly, so bladder cancer often produces visible symptoms that can be caught in time for effective medical treatment. Unlike p16, this gene is not as good a predictor of bladder cancer risk.

The mainstay of medical treatment for bladder cancer, besides surgery, is the chemotherapy drug cisplatin (Platinol) and its variations, along with other drugs. Some treatment regimens include immunotherapy, which gives concentrated amounts of synthetic versions of the chemicals the body uses to coordinate its immune defense. One major side effect of cisplatin is kidney failure, so new drugs are being explored.

Herbal treatments for bladder cancer are most effective when used in the context of conventional medical treatment. Since different herbs act on different phases of the disease process, you should consult with a knowledgeable herbalist who has experience in cancer care if you have questions about the use of herbs in your case.

Herbs to Avoid

❏ People who have bladder cancer should avoid raw shiitake mushrooms. Cooked shiitake do not pose a problem. People with bladder cancer should also avoid herbs that increase estrogen production: cordyceps, dan shen, fennel, licorice, and peony. (For more information on these herbs, *see* CORDYCEPS, DAN SHEN, FENNEL SEED, LICORICE, and PEONY *under* The Herbs in Part One.)

Recommendations

❏ To reduce the chance of bladder cancer recurring, eat one to two servings of cruciferous vegetables every day, such as broccoli, Brussels sprouts, cabbage, collard greens, radishes, turnips, and turnip greens. A recent study of 47,909 men found that eating broccoli and cabbage on a regular basis (five or more servings per week) significantly reduced the risk of bladder cancer. These foods are rich in carotenoids, which are particularly important for the prevention of bladder cancer.

❏ Reduce your consumption of charcoal-grilled meats and fish. These foods contain heterocyclic amines (HCA),

Bladder Cancer: Beneficial Herbs

Herb	Form and Dosage	Comments
Astragalus[1]	Capsules. Take 500–1,000 mg 3 times daily.	Activates p53, stimulates production of lymphokine-activated killer (LAK) immune cells.
Cat's claw[2]	Tincture. Take the dose recommended on the label in ½ cup water with 1 tsp lemon juice.	Raises white blood cell counts lowered by chemotherapy.
Garlic[3]	Enteric-coated tablets. Take at least 900 mg daily.	Reduces tumor size. A possible complement to immunotherapy.
Green tea	Capsules or tea. Use as directed on the label.	Has cancer-fighting properties and may cut off blood vessels that feed cancerous tumors.
Maitake	Maitake-D. Take 2,000 mg 3 times daily, before meals.	Reduces recurrence rate after surgery.
Quercetin[4]	Tablets. Take 125–250 mg 3 times daily, between meals.	Slows the growth of estrogen-activated cancers.
Red wine catechins	Resveratrol tablets. Take 125–250 mg 3 times daily between meals.	Retards cellular processes that cause tumor development and growth.
Siberian ginseng[5]	Pure *Eleutherococcus senticosus* extract. Take the dose recommended on the label in ¼ cup water.	Stimulates the immune system. Slows the growth rate of bladder cancer cells.

Precautions for the use of herbs:

[1]Do not use astragalus if you have a fever or a skin infection.

[2]Do not use cat's claw if you have type 1 diabetes. Do not use it if you are pregnant or nursing. Do not give it to a child under age six.

[3]Garlic counteracts the effects of *Bifidus* and *Lactobacillus* cultures taken as digestive aids. Consult a doctor before using garlic on a regular basis if you are on an anticoagulant drug such as warfarin (Coumadin). Discuss the use of garlic with your doctor before having any type of surgery.

[4]Do not use quercetin if you are taking cyclosporine (Neoral, Sandimmune) or nifedipine (Adalat, Procardia).

[5]Do not use Siberian ginseng if you have prostate cancer or an autoimmune disease such as lupus or rheumatoid arthritis.

Bladder Cancer: Formulas

Formula	Comments
CoD Tea	An Austrian formula that helps to stop tumor blood-vessel development, elevate mood, and relieve pain. This formula is best used with other therapies. Some people with late-stage bladder cancer have gone into remission after using this formula.
Coptis Decoction to Relieve Toxicity[1]	A traditional Chinese herbal formula that contains coptis, which stops cancer-cell multiplication, and scutellaria, which prevents immune-system damage caused by chemotherapy. Use this formula under a doctor's care after chemotherapy.
Essiac	There are isolated reports of remission from stage III bladder cancer after use of this American formula. This formula helps stop tumor blood-vessel development and spread and is best used with other therapies.

Precautions for the use of formulas:

[1]Do not use Coptis Decoction to Relieve Toxicity within 48 hours of taking cisplatin.

which are linked to bladder cancer. HCAs are formed from creatine, a protein that is destroyed by microwave cooking. Therefore, if you must eat charcoal-grilled meats or fish, microwave the meat for one minute before grilling. Or marinate the meat for at least three to four hours in sour cherry juice—researchers at Michigan State University have found that adding cherries to hamburger meat retards spoilage and largely eliminates the formation of HCA during grilling. Cherry burgers, which consist of ground beef mixed with a small amount of sour cherry pulp, are available in some stores (they do not taste like cherries).

❏ Drink more fluids, especially water. Drinking more fluids—at least eleven glasses versus five glasses or less—of any beverage has been shown to reduce the risk of bladder cancer in men by half, with water having the greatest effect. Cutting risk is an important consideration because bladder cancer has a higher rate of recurrence than other cancers.

❏ Adopt a healthy lifestyle of diet and regular exercise. Men with low-risk prostate cancer who changed their diet and began exercising had an increase in telomerase activity. Telomeres protect DNA, and when they shorten, this is a prognostic indicator of disease risk and life span. The enzyme telomerase blocks shortening.

❏ When possible, take showers instead of baths.

❏ Do not smoke or use smokeless tobacco.

❏ Cook with stainless-steel or glass cookware and wooden utensils. Other forms of cookware and utensils, such as plastic- and Teflon-coated pots and pans, have particles that can break off and get in the food.

❏ If you take vitamin C, do not use it in the form of sodium ascorbate. This form may cause a flare-up of symptoms. Natural vitamin C, such as acerola, does not have this effect.

Considerations

❏ Testing for bladder cancer has traditionally required cytoscopy, a procedure that requires sending a probe into the bladder through the urethra. This cumbersome and uncomfortable method does not catch early-stage tumors.

❏ The European drug Ukrain, a chemical combination of the herb greater celandine with the chemotherapy drug thiotepa, is a nontoxic treatment that may be effective against bladder cancer cells under laboratory conditions and has been remarkably effective in clinical use. The combination of the herb and the chemotherapy drug preserves the cancer-fighting effectiveness of the chemotherapy while stopping most side effects, especially depression of the immune system. It also preserves the DNA of healthy cells while disabling the DNA of cancerous cells. No human data are available to support its use.

❏ To learn about measures to reduce the side effects and increase the effectiveness of chemotherapy, *see* "Side Effects of Cancer Treatment" *under* CANCER. To learn about other herbal treatments that can prevent a cancer from developing its own blood supply, *see* CANCER.

BLADDER INFECTION (CYSTITIS)

Bladder infections, known medically as cystitis, are generally caused by bacteria. Bacteria can reach the bladder from the urethra or, much more rarely, through the bloodstream.

Symptoms of bladder infection include burning pain during urination and a frequent need to urinate; cloudy, dark, or foul-smelling urine; lower abdominal or back pain; and/or blood in the urine. There also may be fever and chills.

Bladder infections occur most often in women. Ten to 20 percent of all women have at least one bladder infection every year. Bladder infections occur when the natural balance of bacteria in the urethra has been disturbed. The body has defenses against infection, including urine with a normally favorable acid-base balance, and microbe-resistant properties of the bladder lining and, in men, the prostate fluid. Bladder infections typically only take hold when there is some injury to the urinary tract. This injury can occur during childbirth or intercourse, or it can be caused by structural abnormalities that block the free flow of urine. Other factors that can make a person more likely to develop a bladder infection include pregnancy, menopause, prostate infection, untreated diabetes, decreased immune function, and use of a diaphragm for birth control. Bladder infections are especially serious when a structural problem in the urinary canal causes urine to back up from the bladder to the kidneys. Urinary reflux is a relatively common complication of bladder infections in children, women, and older men. Recurring bladder infections increase the risk of kidney infection.

The conventional medical treatment for bladder infections is antibiotics. There is a growing concern, however, that antibiotic therapy actually increases the risk of recurrent bladder infection by giving rise to antibiotic-resistant strains of the bacteria *Escherichia coli* (*E. coli*). Antibiotic therapy may also eliminate the protective shield of normally occurring bacteria that line the external opening of the urethra. Speak to your doctor about antibiotics.

Use the herb or herbs indicated for the specific microorganism causing your infection, if you know what it is. The most common cause of bladder infections is *E. coli*. Otherwise, use the other herbs to ease specific symptoms. Barberry, coptis, goldenseal, Oregon grape root, and uva ursi are thought to be more effective if the urine is alkaline. To achieve this, limit your meat intake and take ¼ teaspoon (0.5 gram) of baking soda in ⅓ cup (70 milliliters) of water with every dose of herb. Eating fruits and vegetables also alkalizes the body.

Unless otherwise specified, the herb dosages recommended here are for adults. Children under age six should be given one-quarter of the adult dosage. Children between the ages of six and twelve should be given one-half of the adult dosage. Formula dosages for children should be discussed with a knowledgeable health-care practitioner.

Recommendations

❏ Drink plenty of liquids, including at least one 8-ounce glass of steam-distilled water every hour. The resulting increased urination may help to flush out bacterial infection.

❏ Avoid bladder irritants such as coffee, alcohol, caffeine, chocolate, sodas, citrus juices, and pepper (both red and black).

❏ Diet is very important in this condition. Foods to avoid include aged cheeses, alcohol, artificial sweeteners, coffee, nuts, cured meats, rye bread, onions, sour cream, soy, and yogurt.

❏ Avoid taking excessive amounts of zinc and iron supplements while you have a bladder infection. Taking too much can suppress the immune system, and stimulate bacteria growth.

Bladder Infection: Beneficial Herbs

Herb	Form and Dosage	Comments
Artemisia	Tincture. Take 20 drops in ¼ cup hot water 3 times daily for 21 days.	Treats *Klebsiella* infection, which is very difficult to treat with antibiotics.
Astragalus[1]	Capsules. Take 500–1,000 mg 3 times daily.	Treats *Proteus* infection, which can also cause kidney stones.
Barberry[2] or coptis[2] or goldenseal[2] or Oregon grape root[2]	Tincture. Take 20 drops in ¼ cup water 3 times daily for up to 2 weeks.	Activates the immune system. Useful if there is blood in the urine.
Birch leaf	Tea, made by soaking ½ oz (15 gm) of herb in 1 qt water. Use as a douche 1–2 times daily. (*See* DOUCHES in Part Three.)	Relieves bladder pain.
Buchu	Capsules. Take 500 mg twice daily.	Relieves burning sensation during urination.
Butcher's broom	Ruscogenin tablets. Take 10 mg daily.	Anti-inflammatory. Reduces urine retention.
Cranberry	Unsweetened juice. Drink 16 fl oz (500 ml) daily; or tablets. Take 250–500 mg 3 times daily.	Acts against bacteria by keeping them from "sticking" to the lining of the bladder.
Dandelion	Capsules. Take 500 mg 3 times daily.	Reduces urine retention.
Garlic[3]	Raw fresh cloves (preferred). Eat 2–3 in food daily; or tablets. Take at least 900 mg daily.	Increases production of "germ-eating" immune cells. Especially helpful for *Streptococcus* infections in children.
Java	Tea, made by soaking ½ oz (15 gm) of herb in 1 qt water. Use as a douche 1–2 times daily. (*See* DOUCHES in Part Three.)	Reduces urine retention. Stops spasms.
Marshmallow root	Tea. Drink 1 qt daily.	Inhibits bacterial growth by increasing the acidity of urine.
Uva ursi	Capsules. Take 500–1,000 mg 3 times daily.	Particularly effective against *E. coli* infections.

Precautions for the use of herbs:

[1]Do not use astragalus if you have a fever or a skin infection.

[2]Do not use barberry, coptis, goldenseal, or Oregon grape root if you are pregnant or have gallbladder disease. Do not take these herbs with supplemental vitamin B$_6$ or with protein supplements containing the amino acid histidine. Do not use goldenseal if you have cardio-vascular disease or glaucoma.

[3]Garlic counteracts the effects of *Bifidus* and *Lactobacillus* cultures taken as digestive aids. Consult a doctor before using garlic on a regular basis if you are on an anticoagulant drug such as warfarin (Coumadin). Discuss the use of garlic with your doctor before having any type of surgery. Raw garlic can cause heartburn and flatulence.

❏ To relieve the pain associated with bladder infection, take a twenty-minute sitz bath twice daily. Java tea can be helpful when added to the bathwater. Or you can add birch leaf along with 1 cup of vinegar. The vinegar acidifies the bath and kills bacteria, and also releases tannins in the birch leaf that coat the lining of the bladder. A woman should position her knees up and apart so that the water can enter the vagina. (*See* SITZ BATHS in Part Three.)

❏ Keep the genital and anal areas clean and dry. Women should wipe from front to back after emptying the bladder or bowels, empty the bladder before and after both exercise and sexual intercourse, and wash the vagina after intercourse. Condoms and spermicides increase the risk of urinary tract infections.

❏ Urinate every two to three waking hours.

❏ Do not use feminine hygiene sprays, packaged douches, bubble baths, tampons, sanitary pads, or similar products if they contain fragrances. These products contain balsam, which can activate allergies that increase irritation in the lining of the bladder and give bacteria new places to grow.

❏ If you are a woman who suffers from frequent urinary tract infections, use fragrance-free sanitary pads rather than tampons.

❏ Avoid holding in urine for long periods of time. This increases a woman's risk of bladder infection.

❏ If there is blood in the urine, consult a health-care provider.

Considerations

❏ Persistent bladder infections frequently result from a tenacious form of *Escherichia coli* (*E. coli*). This microbe contains a chemical that securely "glues" it to the bladder lining. Getting rid of *E. coli* sometimes requires antibiotics, but it is important not to let antibiotic treatment cause imbalances elsewhere in the body. While on antibiotics, take a daily dose of the "friendly" bacterium *Lactobacillus acidophilus*, either in yogurt (one serving daily) or in douche, suppository, or tablet form (follow label instructions). These friendly bacteria are also sold in capsules.

❏ Some people think that antibiotics may work more

quickly if the bladder lining is not irritated by allergens, which give the germs more places to infect. (*See* Food Allergies *under* ALLERGIES.)

❑ Bladder infection is not the only form of cystitis. Interstitial cystitis (IC) is a chronic, painful inflammatory condition in which tiny ulcers develop in the bladder lining. Individual symptoms vary from person to person, but the most notable symptom is pain, both pelvic pain and a frequent, urgent feeling described as "a hot poker on the bladder wall" or "razor blades in the bladder." For this reason, IC has also been called "painful bladder syndrome" or "irritable bladder syndrome." Women are ten times more likely than men to experience this. Birch leaf, buchu, and butcher's broom can all help relieve the underlying condition. In addition, marshmallow (althea) root can relieve irritation. Take 3 cups of the tea (prepared from tea bags) daily, or take 1 to 3 teaspoons of the tincture in ½ cup of water three times daily.

BLEEDING GUMS

See under PERIODONTAL DISEASE.

BLOATING

See under INDIGESTION; PREMENSTRUAL SYNDROME (PMS).

BLOOD PRESSURE PROBLEMS

See HIGH BLOOD PRESSURE (HYPERTENSION).

BLOODSHOT EYES

See under EYE PROBLEMS.

BLURRED VISION

See under EYE PROBLEMS.

BOIL

A boil, also known as a furuncle, is a deep-seated infection of an entire hair follicle and the adjacent tissue. A cluster of boils is called a carbuncle. A boil usually appears as a small rounded or conical nodule surrounded by redness, progressing to form a localized pus pocket with a white center. Tenderness, itching, mild pain, and swelling of nearby lymph glands may occur. The most common sites for boils are hairy parts of the body that are exposed to friction, such as the armpits, buttocks, groin, and neck, although they may appear in other places as well. Boils cause tenderness and pain, and can cause mild fever.

Almost all boils stem from infection with the bacterium *Staphylococcus aureus*, known commonly as "staph."

Staph may enter the skin through abrasions caused by friction, moisture, or pressure. Plugging the pores of the skin with cosmetics or petroleum jellies may trap the infection within, giving it an opportunity to multiply. Most boils heal within a week to ten days. Recurrent boils can be a sign of an underlying disease affecting immune response, such as anemia, diabetes, or HIV infection; chronic perspiration in the folds of the skin; or poor hygiene.

If boils do not begin to heal after two or three days of herbal treatment, consult a physician. Unchecked staph infections can spread to adjacent tissues, causing cellulitis, or enter the bloodstream, causing bacteremia. When boils do respond to treatment within two to three days, continue the treatment for seven to fourteen days, and at least two or three days after outward symptoms have disappeared.

Unless otherwise specified, the herb dosages recommended here are for adults. Children under age six should be given one-quarter of the adult dosage. Children between the ages of six and twelve should be given one-half of the adult dosage. Formula dosages for children should be discussed with a knowledgeable health-care practitioner.

Recommendations

❑ Be sure to eat leafy green vegetables or orange or yellow vegetables daily. These supply various forms of carotene, which supports the immune system.

❑ To improve the immune response, take 500 to 1,000 milligrams of vitamin C three times daily and 30 milligrams of zinc once daily.

❑ Eliminate any foods that may depress immune function, such as sugar and other simple carbohydrates, as well as all food allergens. (*See* Food Allergies *under* ALLERGIES.)

❑ To prevent the spread of infection, follow careful hygiene practices. Clean draining lesions frequently, and wash your hands thoroughly afterward. Change dressings often, and discard the dressings by placing them in a bag that can be sealed tightly. Do not reuse or share washcloths or towels. Wash clothing, washcloths, towels, sheets, or other items that contact infected areas in very hot (preferably boiling) water. Ask your doctor how to properly care for your boil.

❑ Keep the area as clean as possible. Avoid exercising until the boil heals so that sweat cannot cause additional irritation or cause the infection to worsen.

❑ To bring the boil to a head, apply hot Epsom salts packs. To make the pack, soak a washcloth in 2 tablespoons (10 grams) of Epsom salts per cup of hot water.

❑ Do not puncture or squeeze a boil prematurely.

❑ If a boil is recurrent, persistent, or extremely large, consult your physician.

Boil: Beneficial Herbs

Herb	Form and Dosage	Comments
Herbs to Be Applied Externally		
Coptis	Apply as a poultice twice daily. (*See* POULTICES in Part Three.)	Contains berberine, which is especially toxic to staph. Will not cause the boil to rupture.
Echinacea[1]	Liquid *Echinacea purpurea* extract or salve. Use as directed on the label.	An immune stimulant and anti-inflammatory.
Pau d'arco	Lotion or ointment. Apply as directed on the label.	Stimulates the production of bacteria-destroying immune cells called macrophages.
Slippery elm bark	Apply as a poultice twice daily. (*See* POULTICES in Part Three.)	Relieves inflammation.
Tea tree oil[2]	Lotion or ointment (2–5% oil). Apply as directed on the label.	Penetrates skin without irritation. Kills staph and 11 other boil-causing germs.
Herbs to Be Taken Internally		
Barberry[3] or coptis[3] or goldenseal[3] or Oregon grape root[3]	Tincture. Take 1–1½ tsp (4–6 ml) in ¼ cup water daily for up to 2 weeks.	Contains berberine, which is especially toxic to staph. May cause boils to rupture.
Burdock	Cereal (*goboshi* in Japanese groceries). Eat at least ⅓ cup daily.	Stimulates circulation to remove infectious toxins.
Dong quai	*Angelica sinensis* tincture. Take 15–20 drops in ¼ cup water 3 times daily.	Treats boils that occur at the site of traumatic injury.
Red clover	Tablets or capsules. Take as directed on the label.	Acts as a natural antibiotic and is good for bacterial infections. Cleanses the liver and the bloodstream.
Schizonepeta	Tea (loose), prepared by steeping 1 tsp (2 gm) in 1 cup water. (*See* TEAS in Part Three.) Take 1 cup 2–3 times daily.	Promotes drainage. Especially useful if chills or fever occurs.

Precautions for the use of herbs:

[1]Avoid echinacea if you have an autoimmune disease such as rheumatoid arthritis or lupus. Do not use it if you have a chronic infection such as HIV or tuberculosis.

[2]People who are allergic to celery or thyme should not use tea tree oil products. Do not take tea tree oil internally.

[3]Do not use barberry, coptis, goldenseal, or Oregon grape root if you are pregnant or have gallbladder disease. Do not take these herbs with supplemental vitamin B_6 or with protein supplements containing the amino acid histidine. Do not use goldenseal if you have cardiovascular disease or glaucoma.

Boil: Formula

Formula	Comments
Coptis Decoction to Relieve Toxicity[1]	Use this traditional Chinese herbal formula instead of coptis or related herbs when there is general fever or a sensation of heat in the boil.

Precautions for the use of formulas:

[1]Do not use Coptis Decoction to Relieve Toxicity if you are trying to become pregnant.

Considerations

❏ Barber's itch is a staph infection of the hair follicles in the bearded area of the face, usually the upper lip. Shaving aggravates the condition. Tinea barbae is similar to barber's itch, but the infection is caused by a fungus.

❏ Pseudofolliculitis barbae is a disorder that is an inflammation of one or more hair follicles and can occur anywhere on the skin. In this disorder, sometimes a beard hair grows into the adjacent hair follicle and forms a small curled mass. This mass then becomes chronically infected with any of a variety of bacteria. Shaving and scratchy clothing aggravate the condition. Use teas or tinctures instead of topical treatments to control both of these conditions. Keep the area clean.

BONE, BROKEN

See FRACTURE.

BONE CANCER

Bone cancer is not one disease but a collection of related diseases. The most common forms of primary bone cancer, or bone cancer that originates in the bone, are osteosarcoma, chondrosarcoma, and Ewing Sarcoma Family of Tumors. Secondary bone cancer is cancer that originates elsewhere in the body, such as a breast, lung, or prostate tissues. Bone cancer's most notable symptom is pain, but it is not always present. Only a doctor can diagnose bone cancer.

Osteosarcoma is the major form of primary bone cancer. Doctors are not sure what causes this disease. But since it most often affects adolescents, it may be related to the rapid bone growth that occurs between the ages of ten and nineteen years. It usually occurs in the knees and upper arm. Doctors usually treat osteosarcoma with surgery, radiation, and chemotherapy.

Probably the largest percentage of people who have bone cancer have secondary tumors. Cancers of the bladder, breast, kidney, lung, ovary, and prostate can all spread to bone. Even after these cancers establish themselves in bone, they could retain the characteristics they had in their organ of origin. Estrogen-stimulated breast cancer, for example, is still stimulated by estrogen when it spreads to bone tissue. The same is true of testosterone-stimulated prostate cancer.

Herbal medicines cannot replace medical treatment for bone cancer. However, herbal therapies can make conventional treatment of this disease more bearable. For maximum benefit, choose among the herbs in the appropriate categories after talking to a knowledgeable health-care provider. Especially in treating childhood bone cancer, always work with an herbal practitioner along with the physician; the dosages provided in this entry are meant for adults. In cases of secondary bone cancer, see the primary-cancer entry, such as breast or prostate cancer, for additional information and treatments.

Recommendations

❏ Get enough vitamin A and selenium, since these substances kill bone cancer cells in laboratory tests. Ensure an adequate supply of vitamin A by eating daily servings of dark green, yellow, or orange fruits and vegetables, and take 150 micrograms of selenium daily, or use a good multivitamin. Since selenium requires the help of vitamin E for its anticancer effect, also take from 200 to 400 international units of vitamin E daily.

Bone Cancer: Beneficial Herbs

Herb	Form and Dosage	Comments
Herbs That Increase the Body's Production of Interferon		
Bupleurum[1]	Tea prepared by traditional Chinese medicine practitioner; or Saikosaponin tablets. Take 300 mg 3 times daily.	Also prevents muscle spasms and steroid side effects.
Lentinan	Intramuscular injection, given by health-care provider.	Also activates natural killer (NK) and T cells against osteosarcoma.
Siberian ginseng[2]	Pure *Eleutherococcus senticosus* extract. Take the dose recommended on the label in ¼ cup water.	A natural complement to lentinan that also activates B cells.
Herbs That Stimulate the Immune System		
Astragalus[3]	Capsules. Take 500–1,000 mg 3 times daily.	Restores white blood cell count.
Maitake	Maitake-D. Take 2,000 mg 3 times daily, before meals.	Reduces tumor formation.
Scutellaria[4]	Capsules. Take 1,000–2,000 mg 3 times daily.	Kills bacteria and viruses in people with multiple myeloma.
Herbs That Prevent the Spread of Osteosarcoma to the Lungs		
Psoralea[5]	Psoralea seed, scurfy pea, or bu gu zhi capsules. Take 1,000 mg 3 times daily.	Contains compounds that prevent secondary lung cancer.

Precautions for the use of herbs:

[1]Bupleurum occasionally causes mild stomach upset. If this happens, speak with the dispensing herbalist about reducing the dose. Do not take bupleurum if you have a fever or if you are taking antibiotics.

[2]Do not use Siberian ginseng if you have prostate cancer or an autoimmune disease such as lupus or rheumatoid arthritis.

[3]Do not use astragalus if you have a fever or a skin infection.

[4]Do not use scutellaria if you have diarrhea.

[5]Psoralea increases sensitivity to sunlight. Use sunscreen and avoid exposure to the sun while using this herb.

Bone Cancer: Formulas

Formula	Comments
Ophiopogonis Decoction[1]	A traditional Chinese herbal formula that relieves dry mouth caused by chemotherapy or radiation treatment and also increases the effectiveness of various steroid drugs. This formula is particularly appropriate if there is coughing and wheezing.

Precautions for the use of formulas:

[1]Do not use Ophiopogonis Decoction if you have a fever.

Breast Cancer in Men

Breast cancer in men is rare and accounts for only 1 percent of all breast cancers. Thirty percent of the cases of breast cancer in men are in men with a family history for the disease in either his mother or father. According to the National Cancer Institute, in 2010, 1,970 new cases of breast cancer were identified in men. Because it is not often suspected as a cause of symptoms, it may be discovered at an advanced stage. Risk factors for breast cancer in men include high estrogen levels—often related to obesity, advancing age, family history, and radiation exposure. In general, the same treatments are used for men as for women, except that in men spread of the disease used to be treated by removal of the testes to eliminate the hormones that stimulate cancer growth. Now drugs know as luteinizing hormone-releasing hormone (LHRH) and analogs are used to lower male hormones produced by the testes such as testosterone.

Men who have breast cancer should consult with their physicians about the advisability of the herbs or formulas recommended for women to reduce estrogen production. Both men and women who have been exposed to the tropical disease *schistosomiasis* may benefit from the use of agrimony, as this disease can contribute to the development of both breast tumors and benign calcified cysts that appear as cancers on mammograms. Agrimony contains compounds that interrupt the life cycle of the parasite. It also stimulates B cells, immune-system cells that produce antibodies against cancer and various forms of infection. Take 1 cup of agrimony tea two to three times daily for up to three months. However, unless you have traveled to a region where you could contract this disease, it is very unlikely that this is a concern.

❑ Get twenty minutes of morning or evening sun daily. Sunlight helps the skin synthesize vitamin D, which regulates the reproduction of bone cells, slowing the rate at which bone cancer cells multiply. Adequate vitamin D is also found in most multivitamins.

❑ If you are taking psoralea, be sure to use sunscreen.

Considerations

❑ For measures to reduce the side effects and increase the effectiveness of chemotherapy, and for measures to reduce side effects of radiation therapy, *see* "Side Effects of Cancer Treatment" *under* CANCER.

BREAST CANCER

Next to non-melanoma skin cancer, breast cancer is the most common form of cancer among women, affecting one woman out of every eight at some point in life. Breast cancer also occurs among men, although at a much lower rate. (*See* "Breast Cancer in Men" below.) Symptoms include a lump or thickening in the breast; a clear, bloody, or yellow discharge from the nipple; and, only in rare instances, breast pain. Cancerous breast lumps are firm and do not shrink and expand with the menstrual cycle. While most lumps are not cancerous, any breast abnormality should be brought to the attention of a doctor.

Some of the major risk factors for breast cancer include age, family history, smoking, alcohol consumption, radiation exposure, and, in postmenopausal women, obesity. For women who do not smoke, however, the most important risk factor is exposure to the female hormone estrogen over the course of a woman's lifetime. Higher levels of estrogen in the bloodstream are associated with recurrence, resistance to treatment, and mortality. These cancers are called estrogen-dependent. Lifetime estrogen exposure is highest if menstruation starts at an early age, a woman bears children either late in life or not at all, menopause occurs late, and she uses estrogen replacement therapy (ERT).

Breast cancer is classified according to a multistage system that measures tumor size, the amount of lymph node involvement, and the absence or presence of metastases to other organs such as the bones, lungs, and liver. The main treatment is surgery. This ranges from lumpectomy, in which the lump itself is removed with a small amount of surrounding tissue, through more extensive operations to radical mastectomy, in which the breast, parts of the chest muscle, and armpit lymph nodes are removed. After surgery, radiation therapy or various forms of chemotherapy may be used.

One of the most useful treatments is hormonal therapy, including tamoxifen (Nolvadex). Estrogen interacts with an anticancer gene known as gene p53. This gene is a "molecular patrolman" that makes sure genetically defective cells do not multiply. Estrogen, however, promotes so much cellular growth within the breast that gene p53 cannot keep track of all the defective cells. Removing estrogen reduces the rate of cell growth so that this gene can do its job. Gene p53 is not alone in regulating cancer cells. Another gene, p21, stops the transformation of cells into a cancerous state even before they trigger the alarm for gene p53. Fortunately, isoflavones from both soy and kudzu activate p21 in cell studies. Ask your doctor about using either one of these, especially soy, as some oncologists don't want their patients to use these substances.

There are herbs and formulas that offset the side effects of chemotherapy and radiation therapy, as well as providing other benefits. Always use herbal medicine as part of a medically directed overall treatment plan for breast cancer.

Herbs to Avoid

❑ Women who have breast cancer should avoid the following herbs: cordyceps, dan shen, fennel, licorice, and peony. (For more information regarding these herbs, *see* CORDYCEPS, DAN SHEN, FENNEL SEED, LICORICE, and PEONY *under* The Herbs in Part One.)

Recommendations

❑ Avoid accumulating body fat; exercise and eat the right kind of dietary fat in appropriate quantities. This means you should limit your intake of red meat (and when you do eat it, trim visible fat), butter, and lard, especially

Breast Cancer: Beneficial Herbs

Herb	Form and Dosage	Comments
Astragalus[1]	Capsules. Take 500–1,000 mg 3 times daily.	Stops spread of cancers that respond to gene p53.
Cat's claw[2]	Tincture. Take as directed on the label in ½ cup water with 1 tsp lemon juice.	A potent immune stimulant.
Garlic[3]	Enteric-coated tablets. Take at least 900 mg daily.	Stops proliferation of estrogen-activated cancer cells, complementing tamoxifen.
Green tea	Catechin extract. Take 240 mg 3 times daily.	Blocks estrogen receptors, reinforcing action of tamoxifen.
Kudzu	Tablets. Take 10 mg 3 times daily.	Activates gene p21.
Lentinan	Intramuscular injection, given by health-care provider.	Activates lymphokine-activated killer (LAK) and natural killer (NK) immune-system cells to fight cancer.
Maitake	Maitake-D. Take 2,000 mg 3 times daily, before meals.	Stimulates the immune system. Slows tumor growth.
Milk thistle[4]	Silymarin gelcaps. Take 120–320 mg capsules daily.	Binds to estrogen receptor sites on cancer cells.
Mistletoe	Loranthus or mulberry mistletoe. Use only under professional supervision.	Complements chemotherapy by preventing immune suppression.
Quercetin[5]	Tablets. Take 125–250 mg 3 times daily, between meals.	Accelerates cancer cell death in treatment for multidrug-resistant cancer.
Red wine catechins	Resveratrol tablets. Take 125–250 mg 3 times daily.	Stops cellular processes that cause tumor development and growth.
Soy isoflavone concentrate	Tablets. Take 3,000 mg daily.	Blocks estrogen from cancer cells. Activates gene p21.
St. John's wort[6]	Capsules. Take 300 mg 3 times daily.	Prevents spread of cancer to tissues between chest wall and lungs.
Turmeric	Curcumin tablets. Take 250–500 mg twice daily between meals.	Activates p53; suppresses other genes that activate cancers.
Vitex	Capsule, tablet, or tincture. Use as directed on the label.	May inhibit the growth of breast cancer cells.

Precautions for the use of herbs:

[1]Do not use astragalus if you have a fever or a skin infection.

[2]Do not use cat's claw if you have to take insulin for diabetes. Do not use it if you are pregnant or nursing. Do not give it to a child under age six.

[3]Garlic counteracts the effects of *Bifidus* and *Lactobacillus* cultures taken as digestive aids. Consult a doctor before using garlic on a regular basis if you are on an anticoagulant drug such as warfarin (Coumadin). Discuss the use of garlic with your doctor before having any type of surgery.

[4]Milk thistle may cause mild diarrhea. If this occurs, decrease the dose or stop taking it.

[5]Do not use quercetin if you are taking cyclosporine (Neoral, Sandimmune) or nifedipine (Adalat, Procardia).

[6]Do not use St. John's wort if you are on prescription antidepressants or any medication that interacts with MAO inhibitors. Use it with caution during pregnancy. This herb may increase the chance of developing sun blisters if you are out in the sun for too long.

Breast Cancer: Formulas

Formula	Comments
Cinnamon Twig and Poria Pill	A traditional Chinese herbal formula that reduces the amount of estrogen in the bloodstream by acting on the ovaries.
Dong Quai and Peony Powder	A traditional Chinese herbal formula that is used for a wide range of conditions that benefit from reduced estrogen production. This formula is used by Japanese doctors to increase effectiveness of tamoxifen.
Essiac and Hoxsey formula	Long-used American formulas that reduce cancer cell activity. They also stimulate white blood cell production, which helps reverse white cell deficiency caused by chemotherapy.
Two-Cured Decoction[1]	A traditional Chinese herbal formula that reduces estrogen levels in women with breast cancer. Traditional use of this formula suggests it may stop spread to the lungs.

Precautions for the use of formulas:

[1]Do not use Two-Cured Decoction if you have a fever.

if you have not yet entered menopause, as these fats can promote cancer development. Instead, you should eat omega-3 fatty acids, the kinds of fats that protect against cancer. Omega-3s are found in fish oils—eating two to three servings of salmon, tuna, sardines, or other cold-water fish a week, or taking fish oil capsules, can supply the omega-3 you need. Other healthy fats include olive oil and similar monounsaturated fats. Overweight status increases risk of metabolic disorders such as diabetes and heart disease, but also for recurrence of breast cancer. In one study, women experienced a decrease in blood insulin and cholesterol levels by following a low-fat or low-carbohydrate diet. In another study, women with breast cancer who drank decaffeinated green tea (1 quart per day) had a slight reduction in body weight, significant increases in high-density lipoprotein (HDL, or "good") cholesterol, and better glucose control.

❏ Women who eat vegan diets, or diets that include no animal products at all, should consume plant oils on a daily basis. Laboratory research suggests that beta-sitosterol, a component of almost all vegetable fats, greatly reduces the growth of estrogen-stimulated breast cancer in cell studies. Also make sure you are getting adequate protein from legumes and beans.

❏ Eat fruits and vegetables that are rich in beta-carotene. On average, women with breast cancer tend to have lower levels of beta-carotene in their blood, although doctors cannot say whether this is a cause or a result of the disease. A small-scale study in Italy found that beta-carotene given with other, related carotene compounds increased the tumor-free period among women who had already had breast cancer. The safest and most effective way of maintaining healthy levels of beta-carotene is to consume three or more servings of dark-green, yellow, or orange vegetables and citrus fruits daily.

❏ Eat broccoli. Of all the cruciferous (cabbage family) vegetables, broccoli appears to have the greatest cancer-fighting potency. The act of chewing broccoli; releases

sulphoraphane, a compound that may help reduce cancer risk. It also has been shown to keep estrogen from binding to and stimulating the growth of breast cancer cells in cell studies. Sulphoraphane is produced in larger amounts when broccoli is eaten uncooked.

❏ Avoid fried foods and charcoal-grilled meats. Studies indicate that daily consumption of fried foods can raise the lifetime risk of getting breast cancer.

❏ Do not binge on sweets and starches. Eating a lot of sweet or starchy food at once causes the body to release a massive amount of the hormone insulin, which could accelerate the growth of breast cancer cells. There is some evidence that vitamin D can help transform breast cancer cells into healthy cells. However, there is no relationship between vitamin D levels in women with breast cancer and those who will have a recurrence of the disease. Nevertheless, it is important to maintain healthy vitamin D levels in the blood. Get your levels checked and take supplements as needed, per your doctor's advice.

❏ Make sure your diet includes fresh apples, cherries, grapes, plums, and all types of berries.

❏ Take extra fiber daily to maintain proper bowel function.

❏ Eat onions and garlic, or take garlic supplements.

❏ Relaxation techniques such as writing, meditation, yoga, or massage therapy can aid in battling breast cancer. (See MASSAGE and/or RELAXATION TECHNIQUES in Part Three.)

❏ For more information on estrogen and diet, including information on how fiber helps reduce estrogen levels, see ESTROGEN-REDUCING DIET in Part Three.

Considerations

❏ In one study, women with breast cancer experienced both increased and decreased immune function from ingestion of a liquid extract of maitake mushroom. Breast cancer patients should be aware that natural products are complex and can produce both beneficial outcomes and harmful ones.

❑ In one study, women who regularly used ginseng after breast cancer had slightly higher survival rates and a better quality of life compared to those who did not use ginseng.

❑ There are other herbal products that, while not available over the counter, may be worthy additions to a breast cancer treatment plan. However, none have published clinical studies and none can replace the regimen of your physician. Carnivora is a sundew extract that allows the immune system to "digest" cancer cells. It also prevents breast cancer from spreading to the lungs. The European formula Ukrain targets cancer cells for destruction while not affecting healthy cells. When used with vitamin C (1,000 milligrams daily), it has produced remission in early-stage breast cancer.

❑ Hormonal therapy uses drugs that act like estrogen within the body. They attach to cells at the same places estrogen does, but stimulate less cell growth. This gives genes p21 and p53 less work to do. Tamoxifen (Nolvadex) is a drug widely used after surgery for this purpose. However, while tamoxifen reduces the risk of breast cancer, it increases the risk of endometrial and, in rare cases, uterine sarcoma.

❑ The hormone melatonin may increase the effectiveness of tamoxifen. Used by itself or with astragalus, it may also increase the effectiveness and reduce the side effects of an immune-system component called interleukin-2 that is sometimes used in treatment. Do not use either without consulting with your physician.

❑ Laboratory tests have found that selenium and magnesium reduce the incidence of new breast cancers when taken with adequate dietary supplies of vitamins A, C, and E. Vitamin E is especially important for the anticancer action of selenium. While this vitamin has no direct effect on breast cancer, it may prevent the progress of mammary dysplasia, a precancerous condition of breast disease, to full-blown cancer. A dosage of 600 international units (IU) per day is adequate, along with daily doses of 150 micrograms (but no more) of selenium and approximately 1,000 milligrams of any magnesium supplement. In one study, women with BRCA1 mutation seem to benefit from selenium supplementation in particular to reduce damage to cellular DNA.

❑ Breast tissue is especially vulnerable to damage from the carcinogens in tobacco smoke at two points in a woman's life, during puberty and during pregnancy, when breast cells are actively dividing. Secondhand smoke exposure during these times increases the risk of cancer.

❑ Advances in genetic testing have allowed women to find out if they carry a defective gene, BRCA1, that predisposes them to breast cancer. Defects in this gene interfere with the ability of breast tissue cells to repair damage to their DNA, especially from radiation. On the basis of this information, many women have chosen to have prophylactic mastectomies, or operations to remove healthy breasts in order to prevent cancer. Traditional treatment may be effective for hereditary breast cancer and new procedures are being developed. The inability of the cells to repair their DNA stems from their oversensitivity to estrogen. For this reason, blocking the flow of estrogen to BRCA1-defective cells may reduce risk of hereditary breast cancer.

❑ Surveys have found that while nearly 25 percent of women perform breast self-examination seldom or never at all, as many as 18 percent examine their breasts daily or more often. Ironically, excessive self-examination also can interfere with effective treatment, since doctors making diagnostic decisions on the basis of these exams tend to falsely identify growths as cancer. If you are sufficiently concerned about breast health to make a daily exam, see a doctor for a complete workup. A breast cancer surgeon is the best person to give a breast examination.

❑ There appear to be differences in breast cancer risk based on race. In the United States, weight gain increases the risk of breast cancer among white women more than among African-American women. White women should make weight reduction their first priority, while eating a healthy diet and taking the proper supplements should be the first priority for African-American women.

❑ Do not take supplements containing iron. Iron may be used by tumors to promote growth.

❑ Folic acid has no effect on breast cancer in women who do not drink, but protects against breast cancer in women who drink more than 15 grams of alcohol (the equivalent of two to three drinks) per day. Doctors writing in *The Journal of the American Medical Association* (*JAMA*) recommend taking at least 300 micrograms of folic acid daily.

❑ Hormone replacement therapy may increase the risk of breast cancer in women who have never had breast cancer before. Speak to your doctor about the risks and benefits of this treatment for you. (For herbal treatments that can ease menopausal symptoms without increasing this risk, *see* MENOPAUSE-RELATED PROBLEMS.)

❑ If you experience itching, redness, and soreness of the nipples, especially if you are not currently breast-feeding a baby, seek evaluation by a physician.

❑ The stress of being diagnosed and treated for breast cancer in itself weakens the immune system. Psychological stress diminishes the capacity of natural killer (NK) and T cells to fight infection both during and after treatment for cancer. For this reason, stress management is extremely important to recovery. (*See* STRESS.)

❑ Lymphedema is a swelling of the tissues that may follow cancer surgery. (*See* LYMPHEDEMA.)

❑ For measures to reduce the side effects and increase the effectiveness when using chemotherapy, and for measures to help you cope with radiation therapy, see "Side Effects of Cancer Treatment" under CANCER. To learn about herbal treatments that can prevent a cancer from developing its own blood supply, see CANCER.

BREAST INFECTION

See MASTITIS.

BREAST PAIN

See under FIBROCYSTIC BREASTS; MASTITIS; PREMENSTRUAL SYNDROME (PMS).

BREAST-FEEDING-RELATED PROBLEMS

See MASTITIS.

BRONCHITIS AND PNEUMONIA

Bronchitis is an infection or irritation of the bronchi, the passageways from the windpipe to the lungs. Pneumonia is an infection or irritation of the lungs themselves. Both of these conditions are much more common in the winter.

Acute bronchitis usually follows a weakening of the immune system by a viral infection (such as a common cold), or exposure to noxious fumes or other irritants, or a combination of both factors. Fever usually occurs first, followed by a dry cough. The cough then becomes raspy, with much sputum production. Repeated airway inflammation may lead to chronic bronchitis, in which the airway walls enlarge. This narrows the passageway, making breathing more difficult. Symptoms range from persistent cough to difficulty in breathing, depending on the severity of the illness. Smoking, allergies, and asthma can all lead to chronic bronchitis.

Like bronchitis, pneumonia usually follows a viral infection or exposure to respiratory irritants. Pneumonia can also be caused by fluids or objects entering the lungs, as in cases of near-drowning or choking on a beverage or food, or by bacterial or fungal infections. Chills and fever are usually the first symptoms, followed by cough with sputum production, chest pain, and shortness of breath. Fatigue and muscle aches may be present.

The risk of bronchitis or pneumonia is higher after hospitalization, since a hospital stay often exposes the patient to a variety of germs and because hospital patients tend to spend long periods of time in a reclined position. Bronchitis and pneumonia are especially common among older adults, and pneumonia also tends to affect young children. People who have alcohol or drug abuse problems are at higher risk for these illnesses, as are people with AIDS, heart disease, or lung disorders.

Antibiotics may be prescribed for bronchitis and pneumonia. The person taking the drug may lose the beneficial intestinal bacteria that aid digestion, and probiotics may be helpful to restore the normal bacteria in the intestine. Antibiotic use can also allow drug-resistant strains of bacteria to develop.

The natural approach to treating bronchitis and pneumonia avoids creating new disease problems. Antibiotics are needed usually in the beginning of the diagnosis, but not for chronic bronchitis. It involves two goals: stimulating the normal processes that expel mucus, and stimulating the immune system to deal with viral infection. Expectorant herbs increase the fluidity and volume of phlegm, and stimulate cough. They are not cough suppressants, since cough suppression could trap phlegm in the bronchi and lungs. Use herbal treatments after receiving a definitive diagnosis, especially if there is a preexisting condition.

Unless otherwise specified, the herb dosages recommended here are for adults. Children under age six should be given one-quarter of the adult dosage. Children between the ages of six and twelve should be given one-half of the adult dosage. Formula dosages for children should be discussed with a knowledgeable health-care practitioner.

Recommendations

❑ Use essential oil of lavender in aromatherapy to ease breathing in chronic bronchitis. (See AROMATHERAPY in Part Three.) Or use steam inhalations of chamomile, elderberry flowers, and/or lemon balm to soothe irritation and relieve pain. (See STEAM INHALATIONS in Part Three.) If using chamomile, be sure to use German chamomile (*Matricaria recutita*), not Roman chamomile (*Chamaemelum nobile*).

❑ You can also use Tiger Balm, a camphor-and-menthol salve that relieves bronchial congestion by increasing blood circulation to the chest. Apply according to label directions.

❑ Eat a variety of vegetables. These are nutrient-rich and could support immune function. Avoid eating one to two hours before bedtime. Eating just before sleep may encourage the development of gastroesophageal reflux disease (GERD), which causes some people to wake up with a cough, sore throat, or hoarseness even in the absence of infection.

❑ Combine mustard seed plasters with postural draining. After removing the plaster, lie facedown on the edge of the bed, forearms on the floor for support. Maintain this position from five to fifteen minutes while expectorating into a basin or newspaper.

❑ To aid long-term recovery from viral bronchitis, avoid exposure to tobacco smoke, cold air, and air pollutants.

❑ Blow up a balloon a few times daily to aid in recovery. This helps to reduce the "breathless" feeling.

Bronchitis and Pneumonia: Beneficial Herbs

Herb	Form and Dosage	Comments
American ginseng[1]	*Panax quinquefolium* tincture. Take as directed on the label.	Clears bronchial passages and reduces inflammation.
and		
Siberian ginseng[2]	*Eleutherococcus senticosus* extract. Take as directed on the label.	
Bromelain[3]	Tablets. Take 250–500 mg 2–3 times daily, between meals.	Liquefies and decreases bronchial secretions. Prevents progression of sinusitis to bronchitis.
Coltsfoot[4]	Tea bag, prepared with 1 cup water. Take 1 cup 3 times daily. Discontinue after 1 week.	Relieves acute congestion and hoarseness.
Couch grass	Tea bag, prepared with 1 cup water. Take 1 cup up to 4 times daily.	Relieves inflammation.
Elderberry	Sambucol. Take as directed on the label.	Relieves nasal congestion and fever.
Elecampane	Tea bag, prepared with 1 cup water. Take 1 cup up to 4 times daily.	Gently stimulates coughing of mucus from the lungs; fights bacteria.
Fenugreek	Capsules or tea. Take as directed on the label.	Reduces the flow of mucus.
Lobelia[5]	Capsules. Take 500–1,000 mg 3 times daily. Take for no more than 2 weeks at a time. Product strength varies; take a lower dosage if recommended on the label.	Breaks up bronchial congestion; stops wheezing.
Osha	Tincture. Take 10–15 drops in ¼ cup water used as mouthwash.	Acts against viruses when used at first sign of bronchitis.
Plantain seed[6]	Tea bag, prepared with 1 cup water. Take 1 cup 3 times daily.	Coats sore throat and loosens phlegm.
Reishi	Syrup. Take ½ tsp (2 ml) 3 times daily.	Stimulates macrophages to fight bacterial infection; prevents secondary infection.
White mustard seed[7]	Apply as a plaster twice daily. (*See* PLASTERS in Part Three.)	Stimulates secretion of fluids into the lungs, making expectoration easier.

Precautions for the use of herbs:

[1]Do not use American ginseng if you have high blood pressure or a heart disorder.

[2]Do not use Siberian ginseng if you have prostate cancer or an autoimmune disease such as lupus or rheumatoid arthritis.

[3]People who are allergic to pineapple may develop a rash from bromelain. If itching develops, stop using it.

[4]In large doses, coltsfoot can cause bronchial passages to close, so do not take any more than is recommended. Do not give this herb to a child under age twelve.

[5]Do not give lobelia to a child under age twelve.

[6]Do not use plantain within one hour of taking other medications.

[7]Use white mustard seed plaster with care; when applied for too long, mustard plasters can cause skin ulcers. Do not place on varicose veins, and do not use if you have circulatory problems.

❑ Include garlic and onions in your diet. They contain quercetin and mustard oils, which have been shown to inhibit lipoxygenase, an enzyme that aids in releasing an inflammatory chemical in the body. These have not been shown to be effective in patients, although they are still healthy foods.

Considerations

❑ Some cases of bronchitis and pneumonia are not helped by antibiotics, since these drugs have no effect on viral infections.

❑ Especially in older persons, dental plaque can serve as a reservoir for the bacteria that may cause bronchitis. Regular dental cleanings can sharply reduce the incidence of bronchitis.

❑ Childhood trauma is statistically linked to chronic bronchitis in adulthood. Children who are exposed to physical, sexual, or emotional abuse; who witness domestic violence; or who are exposed to the mental illness, substance abuse, or criminal behavior of a household member are twice as likely to develop chronic bronchitis when they become adults. These findings indicate that reducing stress, particularly post-traumatic stress, will have a beneficial effect on chronic bronchitis. (*See* STRESS.)

❑ Natural eucalyptus throat drops from the Swiss company Ricola, found in health food stores and many drugstores, aid in opening air passages so that you can breathe better. You can also use eucalyptus essential oil to help break up mucus. Inhale a few drops several times a day.

❑ Do not swallow mucus. Dispose of it in a tissue.

Bronchitis and Pneumonia: Formulas

Formula	Comments
Ephedra Decoction[1]	A traditional Chinese herbal formula used if body aches and headache are troublesome. A variation—Ephedra, Apricot Kernel, Coix, and Licorice Decoction—is designed to lower fever, in addition to treating other symptoms.
Kudzu Decoction	A traditional Chinese herbal formula used if neck stiffness and muscle pain are prominent symptoms.
Minor Bluegreen Dragon Decoction[2]	A traditional Chinese herbal formula used for bronchitis marked by fever and chills, with chills predominating. This formula is more effective when taken hot as a tea than as a patent medicine.
Minor Bupleurum Decoction[3]	A traditional Chinese herbal formula that treats lingering cough. This formula is more useful when combined with Ephedra, Apricot Kernel, Coix, and Licorice Decoction or Minor Bluegreen Dragon Decoction.
Ophiopogonis Decoction[4]	A traditional Chinese herbal formula that treats spasmodic and mostly dry cough, dry and irritated throat, and laryngitis.

Precautions for the use of formulas:

[1]Do not use Ephedra Decoction if you are experiencing nausea or vomiting.

[2]Do not use Minor Bluegreen Dragon Decoction if you have a fever.

[3]Do not use Minor Bupleurum Decoction if you have a fever or a skin infection. Taken long term, it can cause headache, dizziness, and bleeding gums. Side effects can be avoided if the formula is taken as a tea.

[4]Do not use Ophiopogonis Decoction if you have a fever.

❑ Do not use cough suppressants if you have bronchitis. Coughing is necessary to eliminate mucous secretions.

❑ Avoid dairy products, processed foods, sugar, sweet fruits, and white flour, all of which can lead to the production of more mucus.

❑ Do not smoke, and avoid secondhand smoke. Exposure to cigarette smoke impedes the healing process.

❑ Wash your hands frequently to avoid spreading the virus.

❑ See also Respiratory Allergies under ALLERGIES; ASTHMA; COMMON COLD; EMPHYSEMA; HIV/AIDS; INFLUENZA; and SINUSITIS.

BRUISING

A bruise is an area of bleeding within the skin. The familiar symptoms include swelling, tenderness, and discoloration of the affected area—"black and blue marks." A hematoma is a large bruise that forms a lump. Most bruises form when a blow breaks the tiny capillaries within the skin, although bruises can form without a direct impact if the capillaries are weak.

Other than small bruises caused by identifiable injury, bruises are always medically significant and should be investigated. Bruises that are not caused by trauma may be symptoms of allergic reaction to a drug, autoimmune disease, a viral infection or illness affecting the blood's clotting ability, or excessive production of red blood cells. Bruises are not permanent and fade if the underlying cause is treated properly.

Unless otherwise specified, the herb dosages recommended here are for adults. Children under age six should be given one-quarter of the adult dosage. Children between the ages of six and twelve should be given one-half of the adult dosage. Formula dosages for children should be discussed with a knowledgeable health-care practitioner.

Recommendations

❑ Reduce black-and-blue bruises caused by trauma by applying ice packs to the injured area immediately after the injury and for the first day following. Use heat packs on subsequent days.

❑ Rub a sterile cotton ball soaked with distilled witch hazel on an injury to stop the swelling.

❑ Eat a lot of fresh, uncooked foods. People who do not eat enough of these foods can be prone to easy bruising.

❑ Call a health-care provider if there is sudden bleeding into the skin for no apparent reason, or if there is persistent, unexplained bruising.

Considerations

❑ Horse chestnut can be taken in the form of aescin tablets or cream to prevent bruising. Do not use this herb internally if you are trying to become pregnant.

❑ A rule of pediatrics for diagnosing bruises in infants is: "Kids who don't cruise seldom bruise." Bruising in infants who do not yet crawl calls for further investigation. Toddlers rarely bruise on the face, trunk, buttocks, or hands, although bruises on the shins and knees are common.

Bruising: Beneficial Herbs

Herb	Form and Dosage	Comments
Alfalfa	Tablets. Take as directed on the label.	Supplies beneficial minerals and vitamin K, which is needed for healing.
Arnica[1]	Cream. Apply as directed on the label 1–2 times daily.	Prevents the formation of blood clots and speeds healing.
Bromelain[2]	Tablets. Take 200–400 mg 3 times daily, between meals.	Accelerates healing of severe bruises. Especially useful for black eyes.
Horse chestnut	Aescin cream. Apply as directed on the label.	Stabilizes fragile capillaries damaged by trauma. Prevents both bruising and swelling.
Oregano	Oil. Apply topically to the bruise.	Helps with the healing process.
Yarrow[3]	Apply as a poultice twice daily. (*See* POULTICES in Part Three.)	Stops inflammation, restores circulation, and accelerates healing.

Precautions for the use of herbs:

[1]Do not apply arnica to broken skin or to an open wound, and do not take it internally. If a rash develops, stop using it. Do not use arnica if you are pregnant.

[2]People who are allergic to pineapple may develop a rash from bromelain. If itching develops, stop using it.

[3]If skin irritation occurs, stop using yarrow immediately.

❏ It generally takes from several days to about a week for a bruise to go through the healing process. If a bruise does not begin to heal within a week, you may want to have your doctor examine it.

BURNS

Burns are wounds to the skin caused by chemical or thermal (heat) injury. Every year, roughly 450,000 Americans suffer burns that are severe enough to require medical attention.

Burns are graded from first degree to third degree. In a first-degree burn, the skin is red but unbroken, and there is no danger of infection. In a second-degree burn, the skin is reddened and blistered. Often, there is a loss of fluid from the wound. In a third-degree burn, the entire thickness of skin is involved. The skin may be charred, but there may be little initial pain because of the loss of nerve endings. Severity is also judged by how extensive the burn is, based on the percentage of body surface involved. Both the degree and the extent of a burn must be considered in deciding the burn's severity.

Burned skin is initially free of contamination. However, bacteria, fungi, and viruses can enter the wound and cause infection. This invasion of microorganisms is accelerated by the fact that all the body's forms of immune resistance are lowered. The larger the burn, the more the immune system is disabled. The skin is a natural barrier to bacteria and the like, and in large body surface area burns, foreign contaminants can enter freely. If a burn is large and/or serious, see a physician at once or go to the emergency room of the nearest hospital. Once the wound is clean and you are stabilized, then you can use the herbs. If you are not sure, check with your doctor first.

Unless otherwise specified, the herb dosages recommended here are for adults. Children under age six should be given one-quarter of the adult dosage. Children between the ages of six and twelve should be given one-half of the adult dosage. Formula dosages for children should be discussed with a knowledgeable health-care practitioner.

Recommendations

❏ Do not attempt to treat a third-degree burn. Seek emergency treatment immediately. Do not remove clothing that is stuck to the burned area. A third-degree burn requires professional treatment.

❏ Cool a first- or second-degree burn (one in which the skin is intact) at once to reduce pain and swelling. Immerse the area in cool running water for as long as possible (until help arrives). Do not stop cooling prematurely. While cooling the burn, remove rings, wristwatches, belts, or anything else that could reduce circulation to the burn and cause swelling. Use herbal medicine for first- and second-degree burns where there are no open wounds. Larger burns require immediate medical attention.

❏ To remove hot tar, wax, or melted plastic from the skin, use ice water—but not ice—to harden the substance.

❏ Keep burns lightly covered to minimize the chance of infection.

❏ Watch for signs of infection, such as odor, pus, or extreme redness in the area of the burn. Protect the injury from sun exposure.

❏ Keep burn injuries elevated to minimize swelling and promote healing. This is especially important for burns on the hands, legs, or feet.

Burns: Beneficial Herbs

Herb	Form and Dosage	Comments
Herbs to Be Applied Externally		
Aloe	Gel. Apply as directed on the label.	Stops inflammation; accelerates healing.
Barberry[1] or coptis[1] or goldenseal[1] or Oregon grape root[1]	Ointment. Apply as directed on the label, for up to 2 weeks.	Fights staph and strep infections.
Blackberry or raspberry leaf	Apply as a cool compress made from bagged tea 2–3 times daily. (*See* COMPRESSES in Part Three.)	Contains tannins, which stop burns from oozing.
Calendula	Gel or ointment. Apply topically as directed on the label.	Effective as an anti-inflammatory agent and antiseptic.
Lavender	Essential oil. Apply to the burn as directed on the label.	The herb of choice for pain relief. Also an antiseptic.
St. John's wort	Cream. Apply as directed on the label.	Accelerates healing. Prevents staph infection.
Witch hazel	Eucerin. Use as directed on the label.	Reduces pain and swelling of sunburn.
Herbs to Be Taken Internally		
Astragalus[2]	Capsules. Take 500–1,000 mg 3 times daily.	Stimulates the immune system to fight infection without inflammation.

Precautions for the use of herbs:

[1]Do not use barberry, coptis, goldenseal, or Oregon grape root if you are pregnant or have gallbladder disease. Do not take these herbs with supplemental vitamin B_6 or with protein supplements containing the amino acid histidine. Do not use goldenseal if you have cardiovascular disease or glaucoma.

[2]Do not use astragalus if you have a fever or a skin infection.

❑ Don't diet while recovering from a burn. Extra protein is needed for tissue repair and healing. You also need to consume fruits and vegetables that are rich in vitamin C, since fresh produce also contains substances called bioflavonoids that make vitamin C more effective. A good multivitamin is also advised.

❑ Don't put butter on a burn. It does not accelerate healing (actually, it can trap heat and worsen a burn), and may contain bacteria.

❑ A white-oak compress stops oozing after the skin has healed enough to remove bandages. Make a compress with ½ ounce (15 grams) herb soaked in 1 cup of water. Apply two to three times daily. (For instructions for making compresses, *see* COMPRESSES in Part Three.)

Considerations

❑ Medical-grade dimethyl sulfoxide (DMSO) can reduce pain and accelerate healing, but should never be applied to an open skin area. Do not use commercial-grade DMSO, since it may contain impurities that are quickly transported through the skin to the bloodstream. The use of DMSO may produce a taste and odor similar to a combination of garlic and turpentine. This is temporary and is not a cause for concern.

❑ A modern Chinese herbal formula for severe burns, Moist Exposed Burn Ointment (MEBO), has been used successfully for third-degree burns to prevent scarring and disfigurement. Containing the active chemical compounds in coptis and scutellaria and formulated in a base of beeswax and propolis, MEBO is applied three times a day to burns without any debridement (removal of dead tissue) or exposure to air. However, it should be used only under a doctor's supervision.

BURSITIS

Bursitis is an inflammation of a bursa. The bursae are small fluid-filled sacs located between tendons and bones throughout the body. They help to promote muscular movement by cushioning against friction between the sharp edges of bones and other tissues. An inflamed bursa causes pain, tenderness to the touch, and limited range of motion. There also may be redness and swelling.

Most cases of bursitis result from flexing a joint with the same motion so many times that the bursae begin to break down. Occupational bursitis is not uncommon. The condition is sometimes identified by such familiar names as "housemaid's knee" (from too much kneeling), "policeman's heel" (from walking the beat), and "beat shoulder" (from too much shoveling) among coal miners. Bursitis most commonly develops in the shoulder, but it may also affect the knee, elbow, Achilles tendon, first joint of the big toe (bunion), or other areas. Chronic inflammation can occur with repeated attacks of bursitis.

Bursitis also can result from infections or sometimes from chronic inflammation caused by systemic diseases. Autoimmune diseases—such as rheumatoid arthritis,

Bursitis: Beneficial Herbs

Herb	Form and Dosage	Comments
Bromelain[1]	Tablets. Take 250–500 mg 3 times daily between meals.	Stimulates circulation and relieves swelling.
Ginger	Capsules. Take 3,000 mg twice daily with food. Use for at least 3 months; and	Stimulates circulation and reduces inflammation.
	Tea, prepared by adding ⅓ tsp (1 gm) powdered ginger to 1 cup water. Use as a compress 2–3 times daily. (*See* COMPRESSES.)	Helps to reduce inflammation.
Horsetail	Tea bag, prepared with 1 cup water. Take 1 cup 3 times daily.	Contains silica, necessary for tissue repair and healing.
Turmeric	Apply as a poultice twice daily. (*See* POULTICES in Part Three.) Do not substitute curcumin.	Offers pain relief like that of steroids, but without immune-system suppression.

Precautions for the use of herbs:

[1]People who are allergic to pineapple may develop a rash from bromelain. If itching develops, stop using it.

ankylosing spondylitis, and lupus—increase the risk of bursitis. Herbs treat symptoms of bursitis, but do not substitute for other forms of care. (*See under* Recommendations, below.)

Recommendations

❏ Rest until the pain goes away. The joint must be allowed to rest before healing can begin.

❏ Use gentle exercise to strengthen the affected area as pain and inflammation subside. If muscle atrophy has occurred from disuse or prolonged immobility, perform exercises designed to build strength and increase mobility. If bursitis has affected the knee, take care to avoid side-to-side motion while exercising. Modified exercise bikes are better than biking outdoors for bursitis of the knee. Seek the help of a physical therapist to avoid inflicting further damage.

❏ To recover from shoulder injuries, use the rest, ice, maintain mobility, and strengthen (RIMS) system. As soon as you feel shoulder pain, apply ice for thirty minutes, then let the shoulder rewarm for the next fifteen minutes. Continue this cycle for several hours, but be careful not to freeze the skin. Rest the shoulder for the next two days. After the rest period, gradually begin to strengthen the shoulder muscles. Light weightlifting, with an emphasis on a full range of motion, is recommended.

❏ See a doctor if fever accompanies pain in a joint. Fever can be a sign of an infection that needs direct treatment.

❏ Nonsteroidal anti-inflammatory drugs (NSAIDs) are often recommended until the pain and swelling subside.

Considerations

❏ Medical-grade dimethyl sulfoxide (DMSO) can reduce pain and accelerate healing. Do not use commercial-grade DMSO, since it may contain impurities that are quickly transported through the skin to the bloodstream. The use of DMSO may produce a taste and odor similar to a combination of garlic and turpentine. This is temporary and is not a cause for concern.

❏ Both acupuncture and shiatsu massage, in which acupuncture points are manipulated by finger pressure, are very effective for relief of pain. (*See* ACUPUNCTURE and MASSAGE, both in Part Three.)

❏ Bee venom therapy (BVT) or "bee-sting therapy" sometimes produces immediate remission from bursitis. Bee venom contains melittin, an anti-inflammatory compound that is approximately 100 times more potent than the steroid hydrocortisone, and adolapin, a compound known for its pain-relieving qualities. Allergic reactions to bee venom are rare; many people who think they have had them were actually stung by yellow jackets. To eliminate the risk of a serious allergic reaction, always take BVT from a qualified physician. For more information about this treatment, contact the American Apitherapy Society. (*See* Appendix B: Resources.) Clinical research on BVT is lacking, however.

❏ To avoid a bursitis flare-up in a susceptible joint, use creams made with the herb arnica before exertion to reduce the pain and stiffness experienced afterward.

❏ Inflammation at the back of the heel (Achilles bursitis) can be caused by landing hard or awkwardly on the heel, or by pressure from shoes that are too tight. Pain in the front of the heel (plantar fasciitis) is more likely to result from wearing shoes with poor arch support or stiff soles, repeated quick turns that put too much stress on the heel, or distance running.

❏ "Frozen shoulder" results from a combination of bursitis or tendinitis followed by development of a serious medical condition, such as heart attack or diabetes. In this condition, the bursae become surrounded with scar tissue and keep the joint from moving. Some cases of frozen shoulder resolve on their own in twelve to eighteen months. Herbal treatments may help to minimize pain.

❏ It can sometimes be difficult to differentiate between bursitis and tendinitis. Bursitis causes a dull, persistent ache that increases with movement, whereas tendinitis typically causes sharp pain on movement. Tendon inflammation may also result from calcium deposits that press against a tendon. Unlike tendinitis, bursitis is often accompanied by swelling and fluid accumulation. See a doctor to determine which condition you have so you are treated appropriately. (*See* TENDINITIS.)

CANCER

Cancer is a group of diseases in which genetically damaged cells multiply wildly, depriving healthy tissues of nutrients and oxygen. This section addresses cancer in general. Certain important types of cancer are treated individually elsewhere. (*See* BLADDER CANCER; BONE CANCER; BREAST CANCER; CERVICAL CANCER; COLORECTAL CANCER; ENDOMETRIAL CANCER; HODGKIN'S LYMPHOMA; KIDNEY CANCER [RENAL CELL CARCINOMA]; LEUKEMIA; LIVER CANCER; LUNG CANCER; OVARIAN CANCER; PROSTATE CANCER; SKIN CANCER; and STOMACH CANCER.)

Scientists now believe that there are as many types of cancer as there are people who have cancer, and that at any given time, many of us have some cancer cells somewhere in the body. However, most cancers are neutralized by the immune system, with the individual totally unaware of the potential disease. These would-be tumors are eliminated by each person's unique combination of defenses against cancer cells.

Cancer develops through a long series of steps that have to overcome these defenses. The first stage of carcinogenesis, or cancer formation, is initiation. This occurs if a cell's master code, its DNA, is injured by viruses, toxins, or radiation. The cell performs its normal functions and is not different from a normal cell in appearance, but it is vulnerable to change. The carcinogenic process can sometimes be halted at this stage through good diet. Foods rich in carotenoids, such as dark green leafy vegetables and yellow and orange fruits and vegetables; foods rich in sulphoraphanes, such as broccoli, cabbage, and Brussels sprouts; and foods and herbs rich in flavonoids, such as berries, green tea, and grapes, all could counteract cancer at the initiation stage. Tomato-based foods have been shown to reduce prostate-specific antigen (PSA) levels and the size of a tumor when ingested by men with prostate cancer. However, for most cancers, it is preferable to include these foods in your diet throughout a lifetime to reduce the chances of getting to this first stage of cancer development.

The next step of carcinogenesis is promotion. During this stage, the DNA-damaged cells are triggered by certain nutrients and their by-products to multiply. This stage can be triggered by arachidonic acid, found in meat and eggs and created from other fats rich in omega-6 fatty acids such as most vegetable oils, or by the hormone estrogen. During the promotion stage, minute precancerous masses have formed but are not yet malignant. An example of cancer in the stage of promotion is cervical dysplasia, or precancerous lesions of the skin such as actinic keratosis. Dietary emphasis on bromelain (or fresh pineapple) and quercetin (the flavonoid found in highest quantities in onion skin and blue-green algae) may be helpful at this stage.

The next stage of carcinogenesis is progression. During this stage, the formerly precancerous masses become cancerous and multiply wildly. This process consumes large quantities of arachidonic acid, the offending substance found in meat and eggs. Taking omega-3 fatty acids from marine sources causes a cascade of reactions that makes arachidonic acid less available to the newly cancerous cells. The lignans found in flaxseeds, legumes, soy, and nuts may also arrest this process, as can tangeritin, a chemical found in tangerines.

The fourth stage of carcinogenesis is invasion and

Warning Signs of Cancer

The list of possible causes and symptoms of cancer is so long that it would be impossible to mention them all here. However, the following risk factors and warning signs are among the most common:

Risk Factors:

- Age (growing older).
- Heredity (family history of cancer).
- Exposure to environmental pollutants.
- Certain infections (hepatitis, for example).
- Poor diet.
- Lack of physical activity.
- Overweight.
- Smoking.
- Alcohol consumption.
- Excessive sun exposure.

Warning Signs:

- Changes in bowel or bladder habits.
- A sore that does not heal.
- Unusual bleeding or discharge.
- Thickening or a lump in a breast or elsewhere.
- Indigestion or difficulty swallowing.
- Obvious changes in a wart or mole.
- A nagging cough or hoarseness.
- Persistent headaches.
- Unexplained weight loss or loss of appetite.
- Chronic bone pain.
- Persistent fatigue, vomiting, nausea.
- Persistent low-grade fever.
- Repeated infections.

Side Effects of Cancer Treatment

Sometimes, one of the most difficult aspects of dealing with cancer is coping with the side effects of treatment. There are two principal types of cancer treatment in conventional use today: chemotherapy and radiation therapy. Each poses unique challenges.

CHEMOTHERAPY

Chemotherapy is, as its name suggests, the chemical treatment of cancer and other conditions. The drugs used in chemotherapy are very powerful and can greatly help some people. However, the use of chemotherapy requires a careful consideration of whether its potential effects on the disease outweigh its potential disruption to health. Chemotherapy is best given at precisely the right time in the course of a disease to maximize benefits and minimize side effects.

Where and how chemotherapy is given varies, depending on which drugs are used and on the individual's condition. The treatment can be performed in a hospital, an outpatient clinic, a doctor's office, or even at home. The drugs may be given in a single dose each day, continuously over several days, once a week, or once a month. A course of treatment can last from several weeks to several years, and may be repeated if necessary.

If you need to undergo chemotherapy, herbal treatment may help reduce its side effects. This should not be surprising, since a large number of chemotherapy drugs are of herbal origin, including etoposide (Etopophos, Toposar, VePesid), paclitaxel (Taxol), vinblastine (Velban), vincristine (Oncovin, Vincasar), and vinorelbine (Navelbine).

This section lists, by drug, herb recommendations for several of the more commonly used chemotherapy treatments. These recommendations are additions to, rather than replacements for, standard chemotherapy drugs. No herbal treatment can replace chemotherapy that is medically required. Always use herbs in close cooperation with a physician. Unless otherwise noted, these herbs should be taken at the same time as chemotherapy treatments.

Considerations

☐ Nausea is a common chemotherapy side effect for which doctors often prescribe any of several antinausea agents, such as granisetron (Kytril) and ondansetron (Zofran). Some herbal agents that can help fight chemotherapy-induced nausea are astragalus, ginger, and the traditional Chinese herbal formula Shih Qua Da Bu Tang (also known as All-Inclusive Great Tonifying Decoction). Make astragalus tea using 1 ounce (30 grams) of loose tea in 3 cups of water and take 1 cup three times daily. (See TEAS in Part Three.) Take ginger in the form of hexanol extract, following the label directions. Use these remedies after consulting with your doctor and an herbal practitioner.

☐ A medication called Iscador, made from the herb mistletoe, is not approved for sale in the United States, but it is in Europe. The U.S. Food and Drug Administration (FDA) does not allow injectable mistletoe extracts to be imported or used in the United States except for clinical research. Iscador has been used in Europe since the 1960s and in Asia for even longer. Some experts believe that the side effects of Iscador are not nearly as bad as those of more traditional chemotherapy treatments.

Adriamycin. *See* **Doxorubicin.**

Cisplatin and Carboplatin

Cisplatin (Platinol) and carboplatin (Paraplatin) are used to treat cancers of the testes, bladder, cervix, stomach, prostate, breast, endometrium, and lung. Although these drugs can affect cancer cells and healthy cells alike, they are absorbed only by cells that are preparing

Cisplatin and Carboplatin: Beneficial Herbs

(Take under your doctor's supervision.)

Herb	Form and Dosage	Comments
Cat's claw[1]	Tincture. Take the dose recommended on the label in ½ cup water with 1 tsp lemon juice.	Normalizes white blood cell counts.
Quercetin[2]	Tablets. Take 125–250 mg 3 times daily, between meals.	Increases tumor-killing capacity of cisplatin while reducing its side effects.

Precautions for the use of herbs:

[1]Do not use cat's claw if you have to take insulin for diabetes. Do not use it if you are pregnant or nursing. Do not give it to a child under age six.

[2]Do not use quercetin if you are taking cyclosporine (Neoral, Sandimmune) or nifedipine (Adalat, Procardia).

Cisplatin and Carboplatin: Formulas

Formula	Comments
Shih Qua Da Bu Tang	A traditional Chinese herbal formula that stops anorexia, nausea, and vomiting; reduces kidney damage; and stimulates production of red blood cells. Stimulates the immune system, especially production of interleukins and natural killer (NK) cells. This formula is also known as All-Inclusive Great Tonifying Decoction.

(continued)

to make multiple copies of themselves. Since most healthy cells produce only a single replacement when they divide, these drugs do more damage to cancer cells than to healthy cells. Once the drug is absorbed, it "glues" strands of DNA together, so that cells cannot make the proteins they need to function and reproduce. Possible side effects include appetite loss, nausea and vomiting, peripheral neuropathy (tingling in the extremities), and low white and red blood cell counts. Kidney damage and hearing loss occur in fewer than 30 percent of the patients who take these drugs.

Cyclophosphamide

Cyclophosphamide (Cytoxan, Neosar) is used for chronic lymphocytic leukemia, Hodgkin's lymphoma, multiple myeloma, sarcoma, and cancers of the breast, cervix, lung, and ovary. It is also used to treat lupus. It keeps tumor cells from multiplying and works best when given with other chemotherapy drugs. Cyclophosphamide has no effect on cancer until it is activated by the liver, which means that it is necessary to have a healthy liver to benefit from the drug. The liver changes

Cyclophosphamide: Beneficial Herbs

(Take under your doctor's supervision.)

Herb	Form and Dosage	Comments
Alfalfa[1]	Capsules. Take 1,000–2,000 mg daily.	Reverses immune suppression in laboratory studies.
Aloe[2]	Juice. Take ¼ cup 2–3 times daily.	Enhances immune resistance. Increases the effectiveness of chemotherapy that combines 5-fluorouracil (5-FU) with cyclophosphamide.
Ashwagandha	Capsules. Take 1,000–2,000 mg twice daily.	Increases red and white blood cell counts.
Astragalus[3]	Fluid extract. Take 1–4 tsp (4–16 ml) 3 times daily.	Reverses immune suppression.
Cat's claw[4]	Tincture. Take the dose recommended on the label in ½ cup water with 1 tsp lemon juice.	Normalizes white blood cell counts.
Polysaccharide kureha (PSK)	Tablets. Take 6,000 mg daily. Start 1–2 weeks before treatment.	Reduces immune suppression.
Reishi	Tablets. Take 3 gm 3 times daily.	Increases counts of red and white blood cells.
Scutellaria[5]	Fluid extract. Take ¼–½ tsp (1–2 ml) 3 times daily. Start 1–2 weeks before treatment.	Reduces immune-system damage.
Turmeric	Curcumin tablets. Take 250–500 mg twice daily, between meals.	Helps prevent damage to lung tissue.

Precautions for the use of herbs:

[1]Do not use alfalfa in any form if cyclophosphamide is being used to treat a condition, such as lupus or rheumatoid arthritis, in which immune suppression is *desirable*.

[2]Do not take aloe vera juice internally if you have diarrhea.

[3]Do not use astragalus if you have a fever or a skin infection. Begin with the lowest dosage and, as long as no fever develops, move up to the highest dosage over a period of four days.

[4]Do not use cat's claw if you have to take insulin for diabetes. Do not use it if you are pregnant or nursing. Do not give it to a child under age six.

[5]Do not use scutellaria if you have diarrhea.

Cyclophosphamide: Formulas

Formula	Comments
Ginseng Decoction to Nourish the Nutritive Chi	A traditional Chinese herbal formula used to treat cancer patients who have anemia, forgetfulness, hair loss, jaundice, shortness of breath, and tired limbs.
Pinellia Decoction to Drain the Epigastrium[1]	A traditional Chinese herbal formula used to treat anorexia, feeling of obstruction below the heart, and vomiting. This formula also stops stomach "rumbling." It is most useful at the beginning of a course of chemotherapy.
Shih Qua Da Bu Tang	A traditional Chinese herbal formula that has been found to prolong survival time. This formula prevents kidney damage, stimulates blood-cell production, and reduces severity of anorexia, nausea, and weight loss; prevents the spread of colon cancer to the liver; and contains daidzein, which is active against leukemia and melanoma. This formula is also known as All-Inclusive Great Tonifying Decoction.

Precautions for the use of formulas:

[1]Do not use Pinellia Decoction to Drain the Epigastrium if you have a fever.

this drug into a chemical that is harmless to normal cells but destructive to tumor cells. Possible side effects include nausea and vomiting; suppression of red and white blood cell production; and in rare cases bladder irritation and bleeding may develop. There is a slight risk of infertility, and the development of secondary cancers such as leukemia or myelodysplasia, so speak to your doctor about these risks.

Recommendations

❑ Take 400 to 800 IU of vitamin E daily. Vitamin E may limit cyclophosphamide from encouraging the formation of tissue-damaging free radicals, especially in the lungs and the lining of the mouth.

❑ Take 150 micrograms of selenium daily before and during chemotherapy with cyclophosphamide. Selenium could reduce some of the toxicity of the drug without reducing its effectiveness.

❑ Take one or two tablets of *Lactobacillus*, the "friendly" bacteria that aid digestion, with food daily. Although this supplement has not been proved to have a positive effect on cancer by itself, it may help reduce diarrhea and indigestion associated with the drug.

Considerations

❑ If mouth ulcers are a major problem during cyclophosphamide treatment, consider eliminating barley, corn, wheat, and rye products from your diet. These grains contain proteins that can cause ulceration of the mouth in some people. Seek dietary counseling from your doctor to make sure you are not eliminating essential nutrients and calories.

Doxorubicin

Doxorubicin (Adriamycin, Doxil, Rubex) is used to treat acute leukemia, bladder cancer, Hodgkin's lymphoma, and cancers of bone, breast, cervix, endometrium, head and neck, liver, lung, ovary, and prostate. This drug tears apart strands of DNA in cells that are preparing to multiply. It affects both cancer cells and healthy cells that frequently reproduce, such as the bone cells that create blood cells. Possible side effects include nausea and vomiting, toxic effects on the heart, infertility, and low white blood cell counts.

Recommendations

❑ Take 400 to 800 IU of vitamin E daily starting the week before chemotherapy begins. Vitamin E deficiency is associated with increased heart damage from doxorubicin.

❑ Take 2,000 to 6,000 milligrams of vitamin B_3 (niacin) daily the week before treatment begins. Niacin may reduce doxorubicin's effects on the heart without reducing its effectiveness. Speak to your doctor first about taking this large dose.

❑ Take 150 micrograms of selenium daily before and during chemotherapy with doxorubicin. Selenium may reduce the drug's toxic effects on the heart.

❑ Take 500 milligrams of L-carnitine, which may protect the heart, three times a day during and after chemotherapy. In addition to L-carnitine, take 100 to 300 milligrams of coenzyme Q_{10} (Co-Q_{10}), which may allow heart cells to produce more energy during doxorubicin treatment.

Doxorubicin: Beneficial Herbs

(Take under your doctor's supervision.)

Herb	Form and Dosage	Comments
Jambul	Seeds. Use as desired in cooking daily.	Prevents heart and liver damage.
Milkthistle[1]	Silymarin gelcaps. Take 120 mg 3 times daily.	Prevents liver damage.
Schisandra[2]	Capsules. Take 100 mg 3 times daily.	Protects heart muscle.

Precautions for the use of herbs:

[1]Milk thistle can cause mild diarrhea.

[2]Do not use schisandra if you have gallstones or an obstruction of the bile duct. Do not use it if you are pregnant.

Doxorubicin: Formulas

Formula	Comments
Essiac and Hoxsey Formula	Modern herbal formulas that may help prevent liver damage.
Hochu-ekki-to	A traditional Chinese herbal formula that greatly reduces male infertility caused by doxorubicin treatment.
Six-Ingredient Pill with Rehmannia (Rehmannia-Six Combination)[1]	A traditional Chinese herbal formula that has been shown in animal studies to protect bone marrow, heart, kidney, and liver function during treatment.

Precautions for the use of formulas:

[1]Do not use Six-Ingredient Pill with Rehmannia if you have an estrogen-sensitive disorder, such as breast cancer, endometriosis, or fibrocystic breasts.

(continued)

5-Fluorouracil (5-FU)

This drug is used to treat cancers of the breast, colon, pancreas, and stomach; head and neck; and ovary. Topical uses include treating basal cell cancer of the skin and actinic keratosis. It keeps cancer cells from dividing by making it impossible for their DNA to unwind before cell reproduction. When used in topical cream form, its side effects can include dry, cracking, peeling skin and hyperpigmentation. When administered by injection, it can cause loss of appetite, nausea and rarely vomiting, diarrhea, and low white blood cell counts.

Recommendations

❏ Take 400 to 800 IU of vitamin E and 100 micrograms of vitamin K daily. Used together with 5-FU, these two vitamins may increase the anticancer effects of the drug without causing additional side effects. However, they can make the blood less able to clot. Be sure to inform your doctor if you are taking these vitamins, especially if surgery is required.

L-Asparaginase. *See under* LEUKEMIA.

Methotrexate

This drug is used to treat cancers of the breast, head and neck, lung, stomach, and esophagus. It also works for acute lymphoblastic leukemia, sarcomas, and non-Hodgkin's lymphoma. It acts by depriving rapidly dividing cells of the B vitamin folic acid. Although methotrexate affects all dividing cells, it does more damage to cancer cells than to healthy cells, which divide at a slower rate. Possible side effects include nausea, vomiting, mouth sores, poor appetite, and in fewer than 30 percent of patients, kidney toxicity, skin rash, hair loss, eye irritation, darkening of skin, and loss of fertility.

Recommendations

❏ Take 400 to 800 IU of vitamin E daily. This vitamin may help prevent drug-induced damage to the bone marrow and intestinal lining.

Mitomycin

Mitomycin (Mutamycin) is used to treat adenocarcinoma of the stomach and pancreas, and also anal, bladder, breast, cervical, colorectal, head and neck, and non–small cell lung cancers. It keeps cancer cells from making copies of themselves and makes them much more susceptible to radiation treatment. Mitomycin works best in tissues that are short on oxygen, such as tumors that have not yet developed their own blood supplies. Possible side effects include fever, hair loss, loss of appetite, nausea and vomiting, and suppression of white and red blood cell production. Lung and kidney damage are rare and found in less than 2 percent of patients.

5-Fluorouracil: Beneficial Herbs

(Take under your doctor's supervision.)

Herb	Form and Dosage	Comments
Coptis	Apply as a cold compress 2–3 times daily. (*See* COMPRESSES in Part Three.)	Increases the skin's permeability to topical 5-FU.
Lentinan	Intramuscular injection, given by health-care provider. Start 1–2 weeks before treatment.	Prevents immune-system damage.

5-Fluorouracil: Formulas

Formula	Comments
Shih Qua Da Bu Tang	A traditional Chinese herbal formula that has been found to prolong survival time. This formula prevents kidney damage, stimulates blood-cell production, and reduces severity of anorexia, nausea, and weight loss; prevents the spread of colon cancer to the liver; and contains daidzein, which is active against leukemia and melanoma. This formula is also known as All-Inclusive Great Tonifying Decoction.

Methotrexate: Beneficial Herbs

(Take under your doctor's supervision.)

Herb	Form and Dosage	Comments
Astragalus[1] and ginseng[1]	Tincture. Take 1–4 tsp (4–16 ml) in ¼–½ cup water 3 times daily. *Panax ginseng* tincture. Take 1–4 tsp (4–16 ml) in ¼–½ cup water 3 times daily.	A combination that has extended the lives of people with lung cancer treated with methotrexate.

Precautions for the use of herbs:

[1]With both astragalus and ginseng, begin with the lowest dosage. If no fever develops, increase to the highest dosage over a period of four days.

Mitomycin: Beneficial Herbs

(Take under your doctor's supervision.)

Herb	Form and Dosage	Comments
Cat's claw[1]	Tincture. Take the dose recommended on the label in ½ cup water with 1 tsp lemon juice.	Normalizes white blood cell counts.
Ginseng	*Panax ginseng* tincture. Take as directed on the label.	Makes cancer cells absorb mitomycin more rapidly.

Precautions for the use of herbs:

[1]Do not use cat's claw if you have to take insulin for diabetes. Do not use it if you are pregnant or nursing. Do not give it to a child under age six.

Mitomycin: Formulas

Formula	Comments
Shih Qua Da Bu Tang	A traditional Chinese herbal formula that has been found to prolong survival time. This formula prevents kidney damage, stimulates blood-cell production, and reduces severity of anorexia, nausea, and weight loss; prevents the spread of colon cancer to the liver; and contains daidzein, which is active against leukemia and melanoma. This formula is also known as All-Inclusive Great Tonifying Decoction.

Steroid Drugs: Beneficial Herbs

(Take under your doctor's supervision.)

Herb	Form and Dosage	Comments
Licorice[1]	Glycyrrhizin tablets. Take 200–800 mg daily, depending on the severity of symptoms. Use for 6 weeks, then take a 2-week break. Do not substitute deglycyrrhizinated licorice (DGL).	Contains compounds that increase the staying power of cortisol. Consume potassium-rich foods such as bananas or citrus juices, or take a potassium supplement daily when taking this herb.
Wild angelica[2]	*Angelica dahurica* tea (loose), prepared by steeping 1 tsp (2 gm) in 1 cup water. (*See* TEAS in Part Three.) Take 1 cup 2–3 times daily, between meals.	Reduces risk of fractures during steroid treatment.

Precautions for the use of herbs:

[1]Do not use licorice if you have glaucoma. high blood pressure, or an estrogen-sensitive disorder such as breast cancer, endometriosis, or fibrocystic breasts.

[2]Do not use wild angelica if you are pregnant.

Steroid Drugs

This family of drugs includes cortisone, dexamethasone, hydrocortisone, methylprednisone, prednisone, and prednisolone. These drugs may help the chemotherapy drugs that kill cancer cells work better, reduce inflammation, relieve sickness, and boost appetite. These drugs also reduce immune function, which is good for patients who have had an organ transplant. Possible side effects include indigestion, increased appetite and weight gain, changes in blood sugar levels, swollen hands and feet, high blood pressure, cataracts, glaucoma, irritability, insomnia, and increased vulnerability to infection.

Recommendations

❑ Limit salt and salty foods while using any of these drugs. Due to changes in the body's breakdown of cortisol, treatment with steroids may cause the body to retain both sodium and fluid. This can cause bloating, swelling, and high blood pressure.

Thiotepa

This drug is used to treat bladder and ovarian cancer, Hodgkin's and non-Hodgkin's lymphomas, and superficial tumors of the bladder. It

(continued)

Steroid Drugs: Formulas

Formula	Comment
Ginseng Decoction to Nourish the Nutritive Chi	A traditional Chinese herbal formula that increases the effectiveness of prednisolone.

Thiotepa: Beneficial Herbs

(Take under your doctor's supervision.)

Herb	Form and Dosage	Comments
Cat's claw[1]	Tablets. Take 500–1,000 mg daily.	Normalizes white blood cell counts.
Green tea	Tea bag, prepared with 1 cup water. Drink 2–3 cups daily. Do not use decaffeinated tea. To avoid dilution, do not use within 1 hour of taking other oral medications.	Contains caffeine, which increases the cancer-fighting effect of thiotepa.

Precautions for the use of herbs:

[1]Do not use cat's claw if you have to take insulin for diabetes. Do not use it if you are pregnant or nursing. Do not give it to a child under age six.

Vincristine: Beneficial Herbs

(Take under your doctor's supervision.)

Herb	Form and Dosage	Comments
Astragalus[1] and ginseng[1]	Tincture. Take 1–4 tsp (4–16 ml) in ¼–½ cup water 3 times daily.\n\n*Panax ginseng* tincture. Take 1–4 tsp (4–16 ml) in ¼–½ cup water 3 times daily.	Extends life in people with lung cancer treated with vincristine.

Precautions for the use of herbs:

[1]With both astragalus and ginseng, begin with the lowest dosage. If no fever develops, increase to the highest dosage over a period of four days.

acts by cross-linking strands of DNA in dividing cells, which prevents the cells from reproducing, and it affects more cancer cells than healthy cells. Thiotepa can cause inflammation of the mucous membranes (mouth sores) with high doses, low white blood cell counts and low red blood cell counts, nausea, vomiting, skin rashes, and bladder irritation.

Considerations

❑ Ukrain is a unique combination of thiotepa with a chemical derived from the herb greater celandine, which is a poppy plant. In animals, it promotes the death of cancer cells, but protects the DNA of healthy, dividing cells throughout the body, especially in the bone marrow where both white and red blood cells are formed. However, a review of seven randomized trials using Ukrain showed weak benefit, if any, and all of the studies were conducted at the institutions where Ukrain was developed. In addition, there is some evidence that celandine may cause hepatitis, so it should be avoided if your cancer is in or near the liver.

Vincristine

This drug is used to treat acute leukemia, Hodgkin's lymphoma and non-Hodgkin's lymphoma, neuroblastoma, Ewing's sarcoma, Wilms'

tumor, multiple myeloma, chronic leukemias, thyroid cancer, and brain tumors. It acts by stopping the unraveling of DNA that is necessary for the division of cells. Since cancer cells divide and multiply at a faster rate than healthy cells do, they are more affected by the drug. Possible side effects include loss of motor control due to nerve damage, constipation, abdominal cramps, weight loss, nausea and vomiting, diarrhea, taste changes, and anemia.

Recommendations

❑ Take 400 to 800 IU of vitamin E daily. This vitamin may reduce vincristine's toxic effect on the peripheral nervous system.

RADIATION THERAPY

Radiation therapy is part of conventional medicine's standard arsenal against cancer. It kills cells by promoting the formation of toxic free radicals, by-products of the use of oxygen in the body. The effects of radiation therapy are most pronounced in cells that are rapidly reproducing, such as cancer cells. The idea behind using this treatment is that more cancer cells than healthy cells are killed by the radiation.

Radiation can help eradicate cancers of the head and neck, skin and lips, breast, cervix and endometrium, and prostate; Hodgkin's lymphoma and local extranodal lymphoma; and retinoblastoma. It is

(continued)

Radiation Therapy: Beneficial Herbs

(Take under your doctor's supervision.)

Herb	Form and Dosage	Comments
Chaparral[1]	Extract. Take as directed on the label.	Helps to protect against harmful radiation.
Ginseng	*Panax ginseng* tincture. Take as directed on the label.	Protects the digestive tract from radiation injury.
Green tea	Catechin extract. Take 240 mg 3 times daily.	Protects the body from side effects of gamma radiation, including thyroid cancer.
Mistletoe	Loranthus or mulberry mistletoe. Use only under professional supervision.	Reduces risk of low white blood cell count. Prolongs survival time.
Pollen	Micronized in capsules. Take 3,000–4,000 mg daily.	Protects liver from antioxidant depletion.
Polysaccharide kureha (PSK)	Tablets. Take 6,000 mg daily.	Relieves pain, poor appetite, fatigue, weakness, and dry mouth and throat.
Slippery elm	Powder. Take 1–2 tsp in 1 cup cold water as often as desired.	Relieves dry mouth and sore throat. Safe to use during treatment.
Snow fungus	Snow fungus or yin mipian tablets. Take 6–12 daily before radiation for breast or uterine cancer.	Increases resistance to side effects.

Precautions for the use of herbs:

[1]Do not use chaparral on a regular basis, and do not take it daily for longer than one week. Long-term use may be harmful to the liver.

Radiation Therapy: Formulas

Formula	Comments
Pinellia Decoction to Drain the Epigastrium[1]	A traditional Chinese herbal formula that inhibits inflammation, and treats anorexia and vomiting.
Ten-Significant Tonic Decoction	A traditional Chinese herbal formula that prevents damage to the bone marrow, thymus, and spleen. This formula is also known as All-Inclusive Great Tonic Decoction.
Tonify the Middle and Augment the Chi Decoction	A traditional Chinese herbal formula that prevents deficiencies in white blood cells after treatment. This formula also activates immune-system cells called macrophages to fight bacterial infection.
True Warrior Decoction[2]	A traditional Chinese herbal formula that treats diarrhea without cramping.

Precautions for the use of formulas:

[1]Do not use Pinellia Decoction to Drain the Epigastrium if you have a fever.

[2]Stop using True Warrior Decoction if you develop a fever. This formula may cause a loss of sensation in the mouth and tongue.

not usually helpful in treating Wilms' tumor, colorectal cancer, soft tissue carcinoma, and embryonal carcinoma of the testes. It is also not typically useful for treating cancers that have metastasized.

Doctors try to aim radiation precisely at the cancer itself. Even so, it is impossible to not affect healthy cells. Radiation therapy inevitably causes a number of side effects, including fatigue, nausea and vomiting, headaches, loss of appetite, diarrhea, hair loss in treatment areas, dry mouth, swelling, trouble swallowing, and urinary and bladder changes. Different people experience different effects, depending on what part of the body is involved and how much radiation they receive. The side effects of radiation therapy may or may not be permanent, depending on the dose and the part of the body involved.

Unless directed by a physician to do otherwise, you should start herbal therapies after the last radiation treatment, so as to avoid counteracting the radiation's effects.

Recommendations

☐ Before taking radiation treatment for any kind of cancer, ask your physician for a frank assessment of the potential benefits and risks of radiation therapy for your type of cancer.

☐ Eat buckwheat, which is high in rutin, a bioflavonoid that may help protect healthy cells against radiation.

☐ Drink plenty of steam-distilled water.

(continued)

Considerations

❏ Lactose intolerance, which causes bloating, flatulence, and heartburn after consumption of dairy products, may occur during radiation therapy. If so, avoiding dairy products or taking a lactase enzyme supplement, such as Lactaid, can help. Make sure to consume a milk substitute such as soy milk if you don't take dairy.

❏ Dietary supplementation during radiation therapy requires careful consideration. Since radiation therapy depletes the body's stores of beta-carotene and vitamins C and E, it would seem natural to take supplements during radiation treatment. However, there is some evidence that the greater the body's stores of these free-radical

scavenging vitamins (and of the mineral selenium) during treatment, the larger the tumor will be after treatment. On the other hand, there is considerable laboratory evidence in animal studies that supplemental melatonin protects the whole body from side effects of radiation, and that vitamin A supplements may prevent lung damage. Do not take vitamin or mineral supplements during radiation treatment except on an oncologist's advice.

❏ Lymphedema is swelling of the tissues that may follow radiation therapy. (See LYMPHEDEMA.)

❏ For additional information on treating other possible symptoms caused by radiation therapy, see DRY MOUTH and MENOPAUSE-RELATED PROBLEMS.

metastasis. In this stage, the cancer cells break out of tissue boundaries and begin to intermix with cells in other organs. Tumor cells release corrosive enzymes that eat through the basement membrane separating the organ from the bloodstream until the cancer escapes. Resveratrol, tangeritin, and grapeseed extract have been studied and could prove to be helpful dietary interventions at this stage.

The fifth stage of carcinogenesis is migration, in which cancerous cells are transported through the blood vessels or lymph system to spread to distant areas. As in other stages of cancer development, omega-3 essential fatty acids may offset the ill effects of arachidonic acid.

Until recently, it was thought that the final stage of carcinogenesis was angiogenesis, the point at which a tumor forms its own blood vessels, just like those that supply healthy organs. For a tumor to grow beyond a width of about 2 centimeters, it must have its own blood supply. While this process must occur before the tumor grows any more than 2 centimeters it may begin when the tumor consists of as few as sixty to eighty cells. Some of the herbs listed in this section may counteract angiogenesis. This process is also retarded by the anthocyanins found in cherries, grapes, and plums, and the isoflavones found in soy. However, drugs are being developed to arrest this process, and these foods will likely be used mostly to complement them in the future.

In addition to the action of the immune system, attacking cancer cells in the same way that it attacks infectious microorganisms, there are genetic safeguards to catch the errors in DNA that propel this process. There are "watchdog" genes that "turn off" cancer cells unless the watchdog genes themselves are damaged. Certain herb compounds activate these genes in cell studies. In addition, most cells have an "address," specified by adhesion proteins that "glue" cells into their proper position. For a cancer cell to spread, it must have DNA instructions that allow it to break the bonds of that glue and to make new adhesion proteins before entering other tissues. Some herbal treatments, such as mistletoe (Iscador), and some foodstuffs, such as citrus pectin, provide lectins that compete with cancer's "glue" and prevent cancer cell adhesion. But, again, these actions were shown in cell studies and how it works in humans has not been studied.

The modern use of herbal medicine in cancer treatment relies on painstaking research. For example, scientists have identified compounds in herbs that protect the "watchdog" genes from damage. There are also herbal therapies that stimulate the immune system against cancer and keep cancer cells from establishing themselves in new tissues. Since treatment differs for each kind of cancer, this book discusses some of the most common cancers and recommendations for their treatment separately.

Herbal medicine is best used as part of a medically directed plan of treatment, which could involve some combination of surgery, chemotherapy, and radiation therapy. Despite the fact that most conventional cancer therapies damage at least as much healthy tissue as cancer tissue, these therapies can be very effective, even lifesaving. Many of the herbs and formulas within the individual cancer sections make taking harsh but necessary chemotherapy or radiation therapy easier. In addition, herbal treatments that can be used with conventional therapy for a number of different cancers are listed separately in their own sections. Always speak with your physician before using any herbal remedy if you are actively being treated for any type of cancer.

To overcome cancer, use every option that conventional and herbal medicine offer. The herbs listed may offer a measure of protection against recurrent cancers of most types; they could slow the process of angiogenesis in new tumors and ideally should be used before recurrent tumors reach a detectable size, if your doctor deems it appropriate. Other herbs that are appropriate to specific forms of cancer are listed in their entries. Do not hesitate to discuss any of the suggestions in this section or elsewhere in this book with an oncologist, and be sure to understand both the diagnosis and the forms of treatment to be used. Combining the doctor's expertise with natural medicine will provide the greatest opportunity for remission, recovery, and future health.

Considerations

❏ Regular exposure to secondhand smoke can increase a nonsmoker's chance of getting cancer by 20 to 30 percent.

❏ A review of forty-nine studies on mistletoe extract (Iscador) showed that when it was used as an adjuvant

Cancer: Beneficial Herbs

Herb	Form and Dosage	Comments
Herbs That Slow Angiogenesis		
Cat's claw[1]	Capsules. Take as directed on the label.	Enhances immune function and has antitumor properties.
Ginkgo[2]	Ginkgolide tablets. Take 40–60 mg 2–3 times daily.	Deactivates platelet-activating factor (PAF), needed for new blood-vessel growth of all kinds of solid tumors.
Ginseng[3]	*Panax ginseng* tincture. Use as directed on the label.	Has been shown to prevent angiogenesis in melanoma. May help prevent angiogenesis in other forms of cancer.
Green tea	Encapsulated extract or tea. Use as directed on the label.	Has powerful anticancer properties.
Kelp	As food. Eat 2 oz (50 gm) in a single serving several times a week.	Prevents angiogenesis by preventing fibrin formation.
Maitake or reishi or shiitake	Extract. Take as directed on the label.	These mushrooms have anticancer properties.
Milk thistle	*Silybum marianum* extract. Take as directed on the label.	Protects the liver and stimulates the production of new liver cells. Has shown anticancer effects against breast and prostate cancers.
Oligomeric proanthocyanidins (OPCs)	Grapeseed or pine-bark extract. Take as directed on the label.	Studies have shown the extract inhibits abnormal cell growth.
Olive leaf	Extract. Use as directed on the label.	Enhances immune system and has shown good results in fighting cancer.
Red clover	Extract or tea. Take as directed on the label.	Studies have shown that it helps to control cancer cells and keep them from spreading.
Turmeric	Curcumin. Take 250–500 mg twice daily, between meals.	Prevents angiogenesis by preventing fibrin formation.

Precautions for the use of herbs:

[1]Do not use cat's claw if you are pregnant.

[2]Do not use ginkgo if you are taking blood-thinning medication. Discuss its use with your doctor before having any type of surgery. Do not use it during chemotherapy or radiation therapy without your doctor's consent. The antioxidant properties of some of ginkgo's components may interfere with chemotherapy or radiation therapy.

[3]Do not use ginseng if you have a cancer of the endocrine glands.

Cancer: Formulas

Formula	Comments
Shih Qua Da Bu Tang	A traditional Chinese herbal formula found in clinical tests to slow or stop progress of a wide variety of cancers. This formula is also known as All-Inclusive Great Tonifying Decoction.

treatment for cancer patients, survival was increased in patients with tumors of the breast, stomach, lung, colon, ovaries, and skin.

❏ Essiac tea has a long history of use for many types of cancer, as does Ojibwa herbal tea, a Native American herbal tea that contains burdock root, slippery elm bark, and turkey rhubarb root.

❏ Kelp can help with the side effects of radiation therapy to some degree. Fresh kelp is best, but you can also used dried kelp from a health food store. Use it in cooking.

❏ Some patients with terminal cancer experienced reduced pain when using a blend of peony root, licorice root, and a Taiwanese tonic vegetable soup of lilii bulbus, nelumbo seed, and jujube fruit. If chronic pain is a concern, *see* PAIN, CHRONIC.

❏ For measures to reduce side effects and increase the effectiveness of chemotherapy, *see* "Side Effects of Cancer Treatment" in this entry.

❏ *See also* BLADDER CANCER, BONE CANCER, BREAST CANCER, CERVICAL CANCER, COLORECTAL CANCER, ENDOMETRIAL CANCER, HODGKIN'S LYMPHOMA, KIDNEY CANCER (RENAL CELL CARCINOMA), LEUKEMIA, LIVER CANCER, LUNG CANCER, OVARIAN CANCER, PROSTATE CANCER, SKIN CANCER, and STOMACH CANCER.

CANDIDIASIS

See YEAST INFECTION (YEAST VAGINITIS).

CANKER SORES (APHTHOUS ULCERS)

Canker sores are painful ulcers inside the mouth. They develop suddenly, usually in groups of two or three, but can appear singly. They burn and tingle, especially if you eat spicy or acidic foods. These sores can last from four to ten days.

Canker sores are frequently confused with cold sores, which are caused by viral infection (herpes). Canker sores have white middles with a red rim, while cold sores begin as red bumps and turn into blisters. Canker sores range in size from that of a pinhead to one inch (2.5 centimeters) or more. Recurrences are common with abnormally high stress levels or as a reaction to certain foods.

The exact cause of canker sores is not known, but it could be from a minor injury inside the mouth, food sensitivities to chocolate or coffee, or food allergy. Other causes include lack of vitamin B_{12}, zinc, or folic acid in the diet, *Helicobacter pylori* bacteria, hormonal shifts during menstruation, and use of toothpaste with sodium lauryl sulfate (SLS). Mast cells, the same cells that pour out inflammatory chemicals during allergic attacks, could also supply the chemicals that cause irritation in canker sores. Herbal remedies offer relief of pain.

Internal herb dosages recommended here are for adults. Children under age six can be given one-quarter of the adult dosage. Children between the ages of six and twelve should be given one-half of the adult dosage.

Herbs to Avoid

❏ If you suffer from canker sores, do not use feverfew. About one in ten people who take this herb experience irritation in the mouth that can be mistaken for canker sores. If you are taking this herb and develop mouth sores, stop taking it to see if the problem resolves. (For more information regarding this herb, *see* FEVERFEW *under* The Herbs in Part One.)

Recommendations

❏ Avoid chewing gum, lozenges, commercial mouthwashes, and tobacco. Also avoid coffee, citrus fruits, and foods that you know from experience trigger these sores.

❏ Take a high-potency multiple vitamin and mineral supplement daily. Canker sores have been linked to deficiencies of both the B vitamins (especially vitamin B_{12}) and iron. Check with your doctor to make sure you should take iron.

❏ Eat plenty of raw onions. Onions contain sulfur and have healing properties.

❏ Take one or two capsules of acidophilus daily during outbreaks. Break the capsules and apply the contents directly to the sores. Acidophilus may help to prevent and clear up canker sores. Emptying a capsule onto the sores at regular intervals is soothing. Avoid toothpastes that contain SLS. Research suggests that SLS may exacerbate canker sores. Instead, use a toothpaste such as Rembrandt Premium Whitening Mint Toothpaste, Macleans Toothpaste, or Biotene Dry Mouth Toothpaste. Avoiding SLS for at least three months may greatly reduce the risk of recurrent canker sores.

❏ If any kind of mouth sore does not heal, see your dentist.

Considerations

❏ Some suggest that an allergic reaction to gluten, a protein found in some grains, is involved in many cases of canker sores. However, one study found that people who had recurrent canker sores derived no benefit from a gluten-free diet. In gluten-sensitive people, eliminating gluten from the diet may result in some improvement. If the assay is negative, he or she may then recommend

Canker Sores: Beneficial Herbs

Herb	Form and Dosage	Comments
Goldenseal	Extract. Take ½ dropperful 3 times daily. Place it directly in the mouth and swish it around.	Heals mouth sores. Also can be used as a mouthwash added to water.
Licorice[1]	DGL tablets. Take 380 mg twice daily, before meals.	Provides same-day relief of pain. Promotes healing.
Myrrh	Tincture. Take 5 drops in ¼ cup warm water, used as a mouthwash 3 times daily.	Stops soreness and inflammation.
Quercetin[2]	Tablets. Take 125–250 mg 3 times daily, between meals.	Stops inflammation.
Rockrose	Extract. Use as a mouthwash.	Heals and eases the pain of mouth sores. Also known as sun rose.

Precautions for the use of herbs:

[1]Deglycyrrhizinated licorice (DGL), which is not useful for many conditions other than canker sores, does not require the precautions usually recommended for licorice. If you substitute whole licorice for DGL, follow the directions listed under Considerations for Use in LICORICE *under* The Herbs in Part One.

[2]Do not use quercetin if you are taking cyclosporine (Neoral, Sandimmune) or nifedipine (Procardia).

testing for food allergies. (*See* Food Allergies *under* ALLERGIES.) If food allergies are involved, canker sores may improve once offending foods are no longer eaten.

❑ Aside from allergies, stress is one of the most common causes of open mouth sores. (*See* STRESS.)

CARDIAC ARRHYTHMIA

See under CONGESTIVE HEART FAILURE.

CARDIOVASCULAR DISEASE

See ANGINA; ATHEROSCLEROSIS; CONGESTIVE HEART FAILURE; HEART ATTACK (MYOCARDIAL INFARCTION); HIGH BLOOD PRESSURE (HYPERTENSION); INTERMITTENT CLAUDICATION; STROKE.

CARPAL TUNNEL SYNDROME

Carpal tunnel syndrome (CTS) is a common, painful disorder that occurs because the median nerve in the wrist is compressed or damaged. The median nerve controls the thumb muscles. It is also responsible for sensation felt in the thumb, the palm, and the first three fingers of the hand. The carpal tunnel is a very small opening, about one-quarter inch below the surface of the wrist, through which the median nerve passes.

Carpal tunnel compression is not a nerve problem but the result of increased pressure on the median tendons in the carpal tunnel. Most likely the disorder is due to a congenital predisposition. Other factors include sprain or fracture, overactive pituitary gland, rheumatoid arthritis, low thyroid levels in the blood, and a cyst or tumor in the canal. Most people think that repetitive motions cause CTS. There is little clinical data to show that repetitive motion injury during work or leisure causes carpal tunnel. Repetitive movements cause bursitis or tendinitis, or writer's cramp, which is not CTS. That said, CTS is more common in industries such as manufacturing, sewing, finishing, cleaning, and meatpacking. In addition, it is more common in women and people with diabetes.

Symptoms of CTS can range from mild numbness

Carpal Tunnel Syndrome: Beneficial Herbs

Herb	Form and Dosage	Comments
Herbs to Be Applied Externally		
Arnica[1]	Cream. Apply as directed on the label.	Provides quick pain relief.
Cayenne[2]	Capsaicin cream. Apply as directed on the label.	Stops inflammation.
Chaparral[3] and/or osha[3]	Use as a hand bath no more than once a month. (*See* HAND BATHS in Part Three.)	Provides long-term inflammation relief.
Turmeric	Apply as a poultice twice daily. (*See* POULTICES in Part Three.)	Pain relief like that of steroids, but without immune-system suppression.
Wintergreen	Oil. Apply to painful areas.	Increases circulation; relieves muscle pain.
Herbs to Be Taken Internally		
Ashwagandha	Withanolide gelcaps. Take as directed on the label.	Relieves inflammation like aspirin does, but without stomach irritation.
Bromelain[4]	Tablets. Take 250–750 mg twice daily, between meals.	Stimulates circulation; relieves inflammation and swelling.
Butcher's broom	Ruscogenin tablets. Take 100 mg daily.	Stops swelling caused by repetitive motion stress.
Corn silk	Tea bag, prepared with 1 cup water. Take 1 cup 3 times daily.	Relieves CTS that worsens during premenstrual syndrome (PMS) or after eating salty foods. Also stops muscle cramps.
Devil's claw[5]	Enteric-coated capsules. Take 1,500–2,500 mg 3 times daily.	Relieves pain.
Skullcap	Extract. Take as directed on the label.	Relieves muscle spasms and pain.
St. John's wort[6]	Capsules. Take 300 mg 3 times daily.	Improves transmission over the median nerve.

Precautions for the use of herbs:

[1]Do not apply arnica to broken skin or to an open wound, and do not take it internally. If a rash develops, discontinue use. Do not use arnica if you are pregnant.

[2]Do not apply capsicum cream to broken skin. Avoid contact with the eyes or mouth.

[3]Chaparral and osha sensitize the skin to sunlight. Use a good sunscreen on all treated areas when outdoors. Do not take internally.

[4]People who are allergic to pineapple may develop a rash from bromelain. If itching develops, stop using it.

[5]Devil's claw can slow the heartbeat. Do not use if it you have congestive heart failure.

[6]Do not use St. John's wort if you are on prescription antidepressants or any medication that interacts with monoamine oxidase (MAO) inhibitors. Use it with caution if you are pregnant. This herb may increase the chance of developing sun blisters if you are out in the sun for too long.

and faint tingling to excruciating pain, accompanied by atrophy of the muscles in the thumb. Most commonly, CTS is experienced as burning, tingling, or numbness in the thumb and the first three fingers. The little finger is spared because it receives its nerve impulses from outside the carpal tunnel. The tingling is often referred to as feeling similar to the "pins and needles" associated with a limb "falling asleep," and it also involves a gradual weakening of the thumb. In the beginning, symptoms are often intermittent, but they become persistent as the condition worsens. CTS can affect both hands, but generally affects only one. Symptoms are often worse at night than in the morning, when circulation slows down. Pain may spread to the forearm and, in severe cases, to the shoulder.

While most of the herbal remedies for CTS relieve inflammation, one, St. John's wort, acts to reduce pain. Herbs applied topically and in baths and liniments offer fast relief; herbs taken internally improve symptoms of CTS over a period of several weeks.

Recommendations

❑ Take 25 milligrams of vitamin B₆ (pyridoxine) three to four times daily. Some believe that this vitamin may reduce the swelling associated with CTS. You can increase the effectiveness of vitamin B₆ by also taking a B-vitamin complex. Additional vitamin B₁ (thiamin) in the complex increases the uptake of B₆ and increases circulation. It may take up to three months to see results. A good multivitamin can be used in place of these single vitamins.

❑ Limit salt and foods that contain large amounts of salt. Salt promotes water retention and may aggravate CTS. Salt also counteracts prescription diuretics.

❑ Use bromelain to speed recovery from CTS surgery. Start taking bromelain three days prior to surgery and continue for at least three weeks afterward for maximum benefit. Talk to your surgeon before doing this.

❑ Try halting all repetitive finger movements for a couple of days to see if the CTS improves. If it does, try to spend less time performing tasks that aggravate CTS, such as by alternating tasks that require different motions. Many employers are now aware of the problems posed by repetitive motion injuries and are more likely to accommodate the needs of injured employees.

❑ To help prevent flare-ups of CTS, wear a splint. Splints, cloth-covered metal or plastic braces that support the wrist, are available at many pharmacies. Be sure to apply and wear the splint properly, since a poorly fitted splint can aggravate CTS. Wear the splint as often as possible (including while you sleep) for several days to see if your symptoms are reduced.

❑ Maintain proper keyboard posture. Sit up straight, with your weight slightly forward. Your feet should be flat on the floor or tilting comfortably on an adjustable footrest. An adjustable keyboard tray allows you to change hand position now and then, and helps keep your wrists straight, with your forearms horizontal and at a ninety-degree angle to your upper arms. Your elbows should be hanging by your sides in a relaxed position.

❑ Perform simple exercises while working at a keyboard. Every now and then, tilt your head slowly to each side, and then roll your shoulders twice forward and twice back. Squeeze your hands into tight fists and then stretch your fingers out as wide as they will go. Pull them back into fists and rotate your wrists a few times in each direction. If pain persists, consult a physical or occupational therapist.

❑ Try a different keyboard. Each brand has its own key touches and widths, some of which may feel better than others. If you can find a split keyboard, it may help keep your hands and arms at a more natural angle. There are also some new keyboards with unusual shapes, any of which may be more comfortable.

❑ Try to work in a warm, dry place. CTS is often aggravated by cool, damp conditions.

Considerations

❑ Physicians most often treat CTS with a combination of anti-inflammatory medications and splints. They also advise avoidance of any aggravating activity. (Steroid anti-inflammatory medications may have side effects that may be reduced with the appropriate use of herbs.) If medication and splints do not work, surgery may be recommended.

❑ Yoga can be useful in CTS. A study in *The Journal of the American Medical Association* (*JAMA*) found that a yoga-based exercise program—consisting of eleven yoga postures designed for strengthening, stretching, and balancing each joint in the upper body—done twice a week strengthened grip and reduced pain. The results of yoga were more beneficial than those of wearing a splint without doing the exercises. Also, acupuncture and chiropractic care have been shown to be beneficial.

❑ CTS usually involves only one hand. Pain and inflammation that involve both hands are more likely to be due to rheumatoid arthritis or some other disease caused by an overactive immune system. (*See* RHEUMATOID ARTHRITIS.)

❑ Always obtain a second opinion before opting for surgery. Many times it is performed unnecessarily.

CATARACTS

Cataracts are white, cloudy blemishes on the normally transparent lens of the eye. They progressively blur vision as the eyes become more and more unable to admit light properly. Besides blurred vision, symptoms of cataracts include difficulty focusing.

Cataracts are the leading cause of loss of sight in the United States. There are currently more than 22 million Americans with cataracts. Most of them have senile cataracts, or cataracts associated with aging. By age eighty, more than half of all Americans either have a cataract or have had cataract surgery. However, babies can be born with cataracts, termed congenital cataracts. Cataracts can be caused by a number of factors, including exposure to radiation and primarily sunlight, eye injury, and eye disease such as glaucoma. Aging and systemic disorders such as atherosclerosis and diabetes (with African-Americans being especially at risk) raise the risk of developing cataracts, as can the use of certain prescription drugs. These risk factors result in the formation of cataracts over a period of ten to twenty years through a process of free-radical damage to the proteins found in the lens. This process is analogous to the change that occurs in egg white when you boil an egg. These unstable molecules cause a cross-linking of proteins that eventually forms an opaque layer in the lens. Cataracts form only if the normal protective mechanisms of the lens cannot keep up with free-radical damage.

Herbal treatments usually have little effect on advanced cataracts. These must be treated with lens-replacement surgery. With developing cataracts, however, herbal treatments could extend the period before surgery becomes necessary. The development of cataracts also could be delayed or avoided by combining herbal treatment with diet, sun protection, and avoidance of certain common drugs, as noted below.

Herbs to Avoid

❏ People who have cataracts should avoid St. John's wort since it may sensitize the retina to sunlight and create further complications not directly related to the cataracts themselves. (For more information regarding this herb, *see* ST. JOHN'S WORT *under* The Herbs in Part One.)

Recommendations

❏ Take at least 1,000 milligrams of vitamin C, 200 to 600 international units (IU) of vitamin E, 250 milligrams of glutamine, and 150 micrograms (but not more) of the trace mineral selenium daily. These nutrients are all associated with a lower incidence of cataracts. Vitamin C has been shown to reduce the need for cataract surgery if used at a daily dose of 1,000 milligrams. Glutathione, which the body forms from glutamine when there is adequate vitamin C, plays a role in maintaining a healthy lens and preventing

Cataracts: Beneficial Herbs

Herb	Form and Dosage	Comments
Bilberry	Tablets or tea. Take as directed on the label.	Supplies bioflavonoids that aid in removing toxic chemicals from the retina of the eye. Use with vitamin C, up to 6,000 mg daily, in divided doses, to release pressure behind the eyes.
Corydalis	Use only under professional supervision.	Especially useful in diabetes.
Gentian[1]	Bitters capsules. Take as directed on the label.	Stops toxin creation. Especially useful for diabetic retinopathy.
Ginkgo[2]	Ginkgolide tablets. Take 40–60 mg 3 times daily.	Improves circulation within the eye, reducing free-radical damage.
Quercetin[3]	Tablets. Take 125–250 mg 3 times daily between meals.	Stops free-radical processes. Complements vitamin E and selenium.
Turmeric	Curcumin tablets. Take 250–500 mg twice daily between meals.	Stimulates production of an enzyme that prevents free-radical damage.

Precautions for the use of herbs:

[1]Do not use gentian if you have diarrhea.

[2]Do not use ginkgo if you are taking blood-thinning medication. Discuss its use with your doctor before having any type of surgery.

[3]Do not use quercetin if you are taking cyclosporine (Neoral, Sandimmune) or nifedipine (Procardia).

Cataracts: Formulas

Formula	Comments
Eight-Ingredient Pill with Rehmannia	A traditional Chinese herbal formula that balances mineral content of the lens, preventing cataract formation. This formula can delay cataract development by a decade or more, and is especially useful for cataracts caused by diabetes. Use for six months.

cataract formation. Vitamin E and selenium work together to prevent hydrogen peroxide, a major source of harmful free radicals, from forming in the fluid portion of the eye. Mixed tocopherols of vitamin E are better than just using alpha tocopherol.

❏ Eating a diet rich in fruits and vegetables has been shown to provide adequate important nutrients to protect against cataracts, especially vitamins E, C, and beta-carotene (and mixed carotenoids). In particular, diets rich in lutein and zeaxanthin are moderately associated with a reduced risk of cataracts in women, but this is likely true for men as well. Foods rich in these compounds include eggs, kale, spinach, turnip greens, broccoli, romaine lettuce, and Brussels sprouts.

❏ Avoid dairy products, saturated fats, and any fats or oils that have been subjected to heat, whether by cooking or processing.

❏ If you have cataracts, do not use antihistamines.

❏ Be sure to have eye examinations at least annually and any time you experience blurred vision.

❏ Use sunglasses to help protect your eyes from the sun's ultraviolet (UV) rays. It is important, though, to buy sunglasses specifically designed to block UV light.

Considerations

❏ Using steroids for asthma increases the lifetime risk of cataracts. The steroid beclomethasone (Beclovent, Vanceril, Vancenase, or Beconase) is associated with the formation of cataracts. Inhaler users have a higher risk of cataracts that develop on the back of the lens, where they are more difficult to treat. Researchers do not know the exact mechanism through which inhalers cause cataracts, but they believe that these drugs disturb the balance of calcium and potassium in the lens. Eating potassium-rich foods, such as fresh vegetables and fruit—especially bananas—can help restore potassium balance.

❏ The long-term use of aspirin may be linked to an increased risk of cataracts. Long thought to help protect against cataracts, using aspirin daily (as many people do to protect against heart attack) for more than ten years actually increases the risk. To avoid this complication, take an occasional "vacation" from aspirin, substituting herbs that also prevent blood clots. (*See* HEART ATTACK [MYOCARDIAL INFARCTION].)

❏ It appears that consuming too much vegetable oil, which is rich in linoleic increases the likelihood of developing cataracts. This relationship was seen in women but likely is true for men as well.

❏ Smoking, overconsumption of alcohol, and high triglycerides increase the risk of developing cataracts.

❏ *See also* ATHEROSCLEROSIS, DIABETES, and GLAUCOMA.

CELIAC DISEASE

Celiac disease is an ailment that occurs because of an inability to properly digest gluten, a protein complex found in wheat and other grains. The condition, which is also known as gluten-sensitive enteropathy, nontropical sprue, or celiac sprue, can occur at any age. Its symptoms, however, are most frequently noticed in infancy, when a child is first introduced to cereal foods. Exactly what makes some people unable to tolerate gluten is not understood, but heredity, emotional stress, and physical trauma may be involved in the genesis of this condition.

Gluten contains the protein alpha-gliadin. When a person who has celiac disease consumes this protein, the immune system is stimulated to produce large numbers of immune cells that attack the linings of the intestines. The resulting damage smoothes out the villi, or pockets through which nutrients enter the bloodstream. The villi are especially important for absorbing essential fatty acids, protein, minerals, and vitamins. If the villi are damaged or destroyed, the nutrients it contains stay in the stool. This leads to multiple mineral and vitamin deficiencies, as well as bulky, foul-smelling, frothy, greasy stools and diarrhea. The condition may also cause canker sores in the mouth and white flecks in the nails. Other symptoms of celiac disease include abdominal swelling, depression, fatigue, weight loss, nausea, irritability, and pain in the bones, joints, and/or muscles.

The more closely a grain is related to wheat, the more likely it is to cause symptoms in a person with celiac disease. Wheat, barley, oats, rye, and triticale all contain alpha-gliadin. Buckwheat (which is used in pancakes and Japanese soba noodles) and millet (found in some natural cereals) contain some alpha-gliadin, while rice and corn do not. Therefore, people who have this condition should avoid virtually all common grains except for rice and corn. In addition, extensive intestinal damage from celiac disease causes the intestine not to produce the milk-digesting enzyme lactase. As a result, people with celiac disease usually cannot tolerate milk products until the underlying celiac disease improves.

Since symptoms of celiac disease are triggered by certain foods, the essential part of the treatment is diet. It is necessary to avoid all sources of alpha-gliadin for life. Fortunately, symptoms usually improve within a few days of starting a gluten-free diet, although a small percentage of people who have celiac disease first see improvement only after twenty-four to thirty-six months on a restricted diet. Herbal remedies can ease symptoms, but no herb or other treatment substitutes for strict adherence to a diet free of grains that contain gluten.

The herb dosages recommended here are for adults. Children under age six can be given one-quarter of the adult dosage. Children between the ages of six and twelve should take one-half the adult dosage.

Celiac Disease: Beneficial Herbs

Herb	Form and Dosage	Comments
Alfalfa[1]	Tablets. Take 2,000–3,000 mg daily.	Supplies vitamin K, which is usually deficient in those with celiac disease.
Licorice	Deglycyrrhizinated licorice (DGL) tablets. Take 380 mg twice daily, before meals. Do not substitute whole licorice.	Provides pain relief.
Quercetin[2]	Tablets. Take 125–250 mg 3 times daily, between meals.	Stops secretion of inflammatory hormones.

Precautions for the use of herbs:

[1]Do not use alfalfa in any form if you have an autoimmune disease, such as lupus or rheumatoid arthritis.

[2]Do not use quercetin if you are taking cyclosporine (Neoral, Sandimmune) or nifedipine (Procardia).

Recommendations

❑ Most large supermarkets and specialty markets have an extensive line of gluten-free products. Other gluten-free foods and beverages include fresh meat, fish, poultry, fruits, most dairy products (unless you cannot tolerate them), potatoes, rice, vegetables, wine, distilled liquors, ciders, and spirits.

❑ Make rice and corn the main grains in your diet. Buckwheat and millet can usually also be tolerated in small quantities, but there is great variation among individuals. Other gluten-free substitutes include amaranth, arrowroot, quinoa, and tapioca.

❑ Avoid these: barley, bulgur, durum, farina, graham flour, rye, semolina, spelt, triticale, and wheat.

❑ Supplement your diet with omega-3 fatty acids, which are needed for the formation of hormones and pain-regulating chemicals. Fish oil and the fish itself are good sources.

❑ During the first sixty days of a gluten-free diet, take pancreatic enzymes—any capsule form including amylase, lipase, and protease—to bring about a more pronounced reduction in symptoms. After sixty days, however, there is no additional benefit in taking this supplement.

❑ You may have to avoid milk and other dairy products until the celiac symptoms improve. If symptoms resume after you return milk to your diet, the underlying problem may be a food allergy rather than celiac disease. (*See* Food Allergies *under* ALLERGIES.) Be sure to take calcium, magnesium, and vitamin D supplements to avoid deficiencies.

❑ Be sure to chew your foods thoroughly before swallowing. This will improve your intake of nutrients.

❑ Do not eat sugary products, processed foods, dairy products (if you can't tolerate them), bouillon cubes, chocolate, or bottled salad dressing, as these may contain hidden sources of wheat.

❑ Become a food sleuth, reading every food and drug label for both obvious and hidden sources of gluten. Obvious sources include any type of product made with wheat or another gluten-containing grain. Common sources of hidden gluten include caramel, gum, hydrolyzed plant protein (HPP), hydrolyzed vegetable protein (HVP), malt, maltodextrin, modified food starch, mono- and diglycerides, natural flavoring, soy sauce, texturized vegetable protein (TVP), and vinegar.

❑ If your child is a picky eater, try a grain-free diet for at least a week. If he or she becomes a better eater, the problem may be a mild form of celiac disease. Check with your pediatrician first.

❑ Iron deficiency anemia is common in children with celiac disease. Offer your child iron-rich foods such as red meat, poultry, and seafood and supplement with iron and folic acid, after speaking to your child's pediatrician.

Considerations

❑ If a child gets blisters and sores all over his or her mouth, he or she should be checked for celiac disease.

❑ Your doctor can order a test for gluten sensitivity that measures gluten antibodies in the saliva.

❑ Because celiac disease deprives the body of essential minerals, vitamins, proteins, and fatty acids, it is related to a broad range of other conditions, including malnutrition, which can cause stunted growth, loss of calcium in the bones leading to rickets and osteoporosis, cancer such as intestinal lymphoma and bowel cancer, and neurological complications such as seizure and peripheral neuropathy. People who have any of these diseases may profit by taking a blood test, the IgA antiendomysium test, for the presence of celiac disease. If the test is positive, going on a gluten-free diet can be beneficial.

❑ The proteins in wheat and milk are psychoactive—they act in much the same way as opiate drugs do, but to a much lesser extent. In people with healthy intestines, the psychoactive proteins are broken down into amino acids, but in people with celiac disease, they pass through the intestine in their psychoactive form. For this reason, celiac disease could be related to an attention deficit disorder with hyperactivity, bipolar mood disorder (manic-depressive disorder), depression, and schizophrenia. However, there are not enough studies available to be sure.

❏ *See also* CANKER SORES (APHTHOUS ULCERS); ECZEMA; and Food Allergies *under* ALLERGIES.

CELLULITE

Cellulite is a condition in which the skin appears dimpled. Fat cells beneath the skin become large, especially in areas of fat deposits. The result is ripples, bulges, and bumps on the surface of skin. The skin may feel like buckshot or sand when touched, causing pinching or pulling sensations. Cellulite can result in "mattress phenomenon," in which pinching the skin leaves a depression or indentation. This problem most often appears on the thighs, although it can appear on the hips, buttocks, abdomen, arms, or upper back. Women are much more likely to develop cellulite than men.

Cellulite may be caused by the body's inability to properly break down fat cells and make new ones. This disruption causes large fat cells to bulge near the skin's surface. Blood vessel changes may also be the cause, but mainly its etiology is unknown. Genes may play a part in whether or not you have cellulite. A poor diet, "fad" dieting, a slow metabolism, hormone changes, and even dehydration also may play a role.

The more extensive the area affected by cellulite, the longer treatment takes. Extensive cases usually take at least two months to respond to any kind of treatment, including herbal therapy.

Recommendations

❏ Beware of over-the-counter (OTC) treatments that promise quick results, especially those containing small amounts of many different kinds of fatty acids, which have no direct influence on cellulite. Some creams may even have side effects, such as skin reactions and rashes.

Considerations

❏ Losing weight can make cellulite deposits less noticeable. Exercising and being a healthy weight may also reduce the chances of developing this condition.

❏ A form of massage known as Endermologie (also called Lipomassage) may gradually reduce cellulite. The technique works by promoting circulation of fluids out of the spaces within the connective tissue. These treatments relax sore muscles and temporarily improve the appearance of cellulite. To maintain this improvement, it is necessary to continue the treatment. Cellulite treatment clinics may be found across the United States, Canada, and the United Kingdom. (*See* Appendix B: Resources.)

❏ Aminophylline, a component in asthma medications, is sometimes described as a "dream cream" for cellulite. It became popular after researchers at a medical meeting reported that some women who used the cream on their thighs for six weeks lost over an inch of fat. Although the cream does reduce cellulite, it can cause skin rashes, insomnia, and nervous irritability. The improvement in appearance that may be seen is probably due to smoother skin and perhaps less of a "cottage cheese" appearance. This effect may disappear when use of the cream is stopped.

❏ Newer techniques are being investigated, such as extracorporeal shock wave therapy combined with exercising the gluteal and thigh regions, dual-wave laser suction with massage, and radio waves with infrared light and tissue manipulation. These therapies have been shown to produce good results in less time than earlier methods.

CERVICAL CANCER

Cervical cancer is one of the most common cancers affecting women, although the rate has dropped over time as more women receive annual Pap smears. In this procedure, cells are taken from the surface of the cervix and examined for abnormalities. Pap smears are important because the early stages of cervical cancer usually produce no symptoms.

Cellulite: Beneficial Herbs

Herb	Form and Dosage	Comments
Gotu kola[1]	Liposome tablets. Take 60–120 mg daily.	Causes cellulite reduction.
Horse chestnut	Aescin cream. Apply as directed on the label.	Treats mattress phenomenon.
Kelp	As food. Eat 2 oz (50 gm) in a single serving. Limit use to once per week.	Stimulates the metabolism, which reduces the deposit of fat.

Precautions for the use of herbs:

[1]Do not use gotu kola if you are trying to become pregnant.

Cervical cancer has well-defined precancerous stages. It begins as cervical dysplasia, the appearance of abnormal cells on the surface of the cervix. Most cervical dysplasias form in response to infection with certain strains of human papillomavirus (HPV), a sexually transmitted virus that causes genital warts. A vaccine is available for females aged nine to twenty-six years to protect against two types of HPV infections that cause cervical cancer. While women who have had multiple sex partners have the highest rates of cervical cancer (as do those who begin sexual relations early in life), even women who are in lifelong monogamous relationships can develop the disease. Women who have sex with men who have had multiple partners are also at higher risk. For reasons that are not clear, there is a relatively high rate of cervical cancer among Native American women.

Another factor that increases the rate at which cervical dysplasia develops into cancer is use of birth control pills if they are used for more than five years. The risk decreases dramatically once the pills are no longer being taken. Oral contraceptives contain progesterone as well as varying amounts of estrogen. These hormones enable HPV to cause cancers and to poison gene p53, a gene that ordinarily ensures that genetically defective or cancerous cells do not multiply. While HPV-associated cancers may be started by estrogen, the hormone does not stimulate their growth once established. However, cervical cancer not caused by HPV infection (which is very rare) could be stimulated by estrogen. In these cases, reducing estrogen levels allows gene p53 to keep up with cell growth. Other factors that have been associated with cervical cancer include a weakened immune system, history of sexually transmitted disease, smoking, having taken DES (diethylstilbestrol) to induce pregnancy, first sexual intercourse before age eighteen, and having had more than five complete pregnancies.

Once cervical cancer grows and spreads enough to cause symptoms, it may cause abnormal vaginal bleeding, foul-smelling discharge, lower back or pelvic pain, and painful menstrual periods. Depending on its spread, cervical cancer is classified into stages 0 and I through IV. The extent of spread also determines which type of surgical procedures may be used. Such procedures range from removal of only a part of the cervix to removal of the entire uterus and its

Cervical Cancer: Beneficial Herbs

Herb	Form and Dosage	Comments
Aloe[1]	Juice. Take ½ cup (80 ml) 3 times daily.	Keeps the liver from processing certain toxins into carcinogenic forms.
Astragalus[2]	Capsules. Take 500–1,000 mg 3 times daily.	Increases production of immune-system chemical interleukin-2 (IL-2), which fights HPV. Activates gene p53.
Green tea	Catechin extract. Take 240 mg 3 times daily.	Deactivates plasmin, a substance that creates pathways for blood-vessel tumors.
Lentinan	Intramuscular injection, given by health-care provider.	Activates immune-system cells, lymphokine-activated killer (LAK) and natural killer (NK) cells, to fight cancer.
Polysaccharide kureha (PSK)	Tablets. Take 2,000 mg 3 times daily.	Stops tumor spread. Increases effectiveness of radiation therapy.
Snow fungus	Snow fungus or yin mi pain tablets. Take 6–12 tablets daily during radiation therapy.	Sensitizes cervical cancer cells to radiation therapy.
Turmeric	Curcumin tablets. Take 250–500 mg twice daily, between meals.	Activates gene p53.

Precautions for the use of herbs:

[1]Do not take aloe vera juice internally if you have diarrhea.

[2]Do not use astragalus if you have a fever or a skin infection.

Cervical Cancer: Formulas

Formula	Comments
Two-Cured Decoction[1]	This traditional Chinese herbal formula inhibits the development of cervical cancer and also reduces estrogen levels.

Precautions for the use of formulas:

[1]Do not use Two-Cured Decoction if you have a fever.

supporting structures. Lymph nodes in the groin also may be removed. In addition, chemotherapy or radiation may be used, although doctors usually try to avoid radiation in treating younger women, since it can damage the ovaries and induce menopause. Doctors sometimes try combining chemotherapy and radiation, an approach that usually does not alleviate symptoms or extend life. In these cases, immunotherapy is another option.

You should use herbal medicine as part of a medically directed overall treatment plan for cervical cancer. Herbal medicine can make chemotherapy or radiation treatment more bearable and effective, and increase the likelihood of achieving remission.

Recommendations

❑ Consume more dark green or yellow vegetables and fruits for their antioxidant content. A four-year study of 2,189 women with cervical cancer found that those who consumed these items frequently had a lower risk of developing invasive cancer. Compounds in these vegetables that are similar to vitamin A deactivate one of HPV's cancer-causing genes, although they are more effective in the disease's earliest stages. In one study, premenopausal women with cervical intraepithelial neoplasia who ate a diet high in fruits and vegetables were shown to form fewer free oxygen radicals that are known to damage the cervix and cause cancer. In another study, researchers looked at the diets of women and compared those who got cervical cancer and those who didn't. The women with cervical cancer had lower levels of antioxidants such as beta-carotene and vitamin E in the blood. Thus, it would seem that antioxidants play an important role in reducing the risk of cervical cancer.

❑ Fortify your diet with the antioxidant supplements vitamin E and glutamine. Taking 200 to 400 international units (IU) of vitamin E per day has been shown to provide a threefold decrease in the rate of invasive cancer. Lower levels of vitamin E have been found at every successive stage of cervical cancer—that is, the worse the cancer, the lower the tissue amounts of vitamin E. Similarly, scientists have found lower levels of the amino acid glutathione (and higher levels of the enzyme that destroys it) at every successive stage of the disease. Glutamine, taken at a dose of 250 milligrams a day, is an important antioxidant building block, especially if combined with 1,000 milligrams of vitamin C per day.

❑ Take thymic factor supplements to stimulate the immune system in cervical cancer. However, do not take thymic factors during chemotherapy with doxorubicin (Adriamycin) or cisplatin (Platinol), since the net effect of combining thymus supplements with these drugs is less than the effect of either thymus supplements or chemotherapy alone.

❑ If you smoke, quit, and avoid exposure to secondhand cigarette smoke. Cigarette smoke contains 4-(methylnitrosamino)-1-(3-pyridyl)-1-butanone, also known as NNK, which can interfere with the immune system, decreasing its ability to keep HPV in check and greatly increasing the risk of cervical cancer.

Considerations

❑ About 55 million Pap tests are performed each year in the United States. Of these, approximately 3.5 million (6 percent) are abnormal and require medical follow-up. An abnormal Pap smear does not mean a woman has cervical cancer. Only a small percentage of these women have cervical cancer, and most of those who do have it test positive for HPV. If a Pap test has shown abnormal cervical cells called atypical squamous cells (ASC), an HPV test can be done to help look for one or more high-risk types of HPV. If an HPV test shows that high-risk types of HPV are present, further testing, such as a colposcopy or cervical biopsy, may be recommended. Fortunately, there is now a more sensitive test for HPV infection. The Hybrid Capture II test detects 90 to 95 percent of cases of HPV infection compared to 75 to 80 percent for the Pap smear. This test is especially helpful if the results of a Pap smear are inconclusive.

❑ If cervical cancer in a younger woman must be treated surgically, a new operating procedure can preserve fertility. This procedure, known as a trachelectomy, removes the cervix while preserving the uterus. In the first twenty-six women who underwent the procedure, only one experienced a recurrence of the cancer. However, with the new vaccine, this procedure should not be necessary in the future. Advise your daughters and friends to get the vaccine to prevent this form of cancer.

❑ Women who take oral contraceptives who have cervical dysplasia are much less likely to develop more severe dysplasia or cancer if they take folic acid supplements. In one study of such women, 16 percent of those who did not take folic acid had more severe dysplasia after four months, while none of those taking folic acid (at a dosage of 10 milligrams per day) saw their conditions worsen.

❑ For measures to reduce the side effects and increase the effectiveness of chemotherapy and radiation therapy, see "Side Effects of Cancer Treatment" under CANCER. To learn about herbal treatments that can prevent a cancer from developing its own blood supply, see CANCER.

CHAGAS' DISEASE

See under PARASITIC INFECTION.

CHEMOTHERAPY SIDE EFFECTS

See "Side Effects of Cancer Treatment" under CANCER.

CHICKEN POX

See under HERPESVIRUS INFECTION.

CHLAMYDIA

See GONORRHEA AND CHLAMYDIA.

CHOLESTEROL PROBLEMS

See HIGH CHOLESTEROL.

CHRONIC FATIGUE SYNDROME

Chronic fatigue syndrome (CFS) is a state of overwhelming fatigue accompanied by a wide variety of physical and psychological complaints. More than 1 million Americans may have CFS; however, fewer than 20 percent of these cases have been diagnosed.

Symptoms of CFS vary greatly from person to person, but they can include the following: overwhelming tiredness that does not go away, even with rest; confusion; depression; difficulty thinking or concentrating; irritability; confusion and forgetfulness; fever; chills; pain in joints and lymph nodes; muscle weakness; sleep disturbances and feeling tired upon awakening after a night's sleep; and headaches. The fact that CFS symptoms mimic those of other conditions, such as depression, makes diagnosis difficult, as does the lack of a definitive test for CFS. Diagnosis is based on the elimination of other disorders and on the length and severity of the fatigue.

Virtually all cases of CFS arise suddenly in active people. It usually starts as a flulike illness the person vividly remembers as the onset of the disease. CFS has been connected to infection with human herpesvirus-6, as well as to cytomegalovirus and Epstein-Barr virus (EBV). It is likely that CFS results from a combination of factors, and may be related to age, prior illness, stress, environment, or genetics.

Chronic Fatigue Syndrome: Beneficial Herbs

Herb	Form and Dosage	Comments
Bitter melon[1]	Fruit, whole. Use ½–2 fruits in cooking daily. Use for 4 weeks; then discontinue for 4 weeks.	More effective than acyclovir (Zovirax) in killing herpesvirus.
Calumba	Tincture. Take ½–1 tsp (2–4 ml) in ¼ cup water 3 times daily, before meals.	Improves appetite without inducing constipation.
Clove	Oil. Take 10–15 drops in ¼ cup water 3 times daily.	Increases the effectiveness of acyclovir.
Dan shen[2]	Tincture. Take as directed on the label.	Increases available zinc. Sedates nerves that carry pain messages.
Echinacea[3] and/or	*Echinacea purpurea* tincture. Take as directed on the label.	Increases the activity of natural killer (NK) cells; fights secondary infection.
ginseng	*Panax ginseng* tea (loose), prepared by steeping 1 tsp (2 gm) in 1 cup water. (*See* TEAS in Part Three.) Take 1 cup daily.	Ginseng also controls emotional disturbances.
Lentinan	Powder. Take the dosage recommended by a health-care provider.	Reverses fever and fatigue. Activates T-helper cells.
Licorice[4]	Glycyrrhizin tablets. Take 200–800 mg daily, depending on the severity of symptoms. Use for 6 weeks; then take a 2-week break. Do not substitute deglycyrrhizinated licorice (DGL).	Helps the body conserve cortisol and maintain blood pressure. Fights depressions. Consume potassium-rich foods such as bananas or citrus juices, or take a potassium supplement daily when taking his herb.
Maitake	Maitake-D. Take 500 mg 3 times daily.	Stimulates general immune function; fights infection.
Oligomeric proanthocyanidins (OPCs)	Grapeseed or pine-bark extract tablets. Take 200 mg daily.	Antioxidant that lifts depression.
Scutellaria[5]	Capsules. Take 1,000–2,000 mg 3 times daily.	High zinc content. Antibacterial, antiviral.
Siberian ginseng[6]	Pure *Eleutherococcus senticosus* extract. Take the dosage recommended on the label in ¼ cup water.	Increases resistance to stress; increases activity on NK and T cells.
St. John's wort	Capsules. Take 900 mg of total hypericin daily.	Antidepressant. Also stops inflammatory reactions.

Precautions for the use of herbs:

[1]Do not use bitter melon if you have cirrhosis of the liver or a medical history of hepatitis or HIV infection compounded by liver infections.

[2]Do not use dan shen if you have an estrogen-sensitive disorder, such as breast cancer, endometriosis, or fibrocystic breasts.

[3]Do not use echinacea if you have an autoimmune disease such as rheumatoid arthritis or lupus. Do not use it if you have a chronic infection such as HIV or tuberculosis.

[4]Do not use licorice if you have glaucoma, high blood pressure, or an estrogen-sensitive disorder such as breast cancer, endometriosis, or fibrocystic breasts.

[5]Do not take scutellaria if you have diarrhea.

[6]Do not use Siberian ginseng if you have prostate cancer or an autoimmune disease, such as lupus or rheumatoid arthritis.

Chronic Fatigue Syndrome: Formulas

Formula	Comments
Calm the Stomach Powder	A traditional Chinese herbal formula that relieves fatigue with loss of taste, heavy sensation in the arms and legs, loose stools or diarrhea, nausea and vomiting, belching, and/or acid regurgitation.
Ginseng Decoction to Nourish the Nutritive Chi	A traditional Chinese herbal formula that treats chronic fatigue with weakness of the hands and feet.
Honey-Fried Licorice Decoction[1]	A traditional Chinese herbal formula that relieves chronic fatigue with symptoms that include dry skin and fever. This formula also relieves constipation and sluggish digestion.
Oyster Shell Powder	A traditional Chinese herbal formula that treats chronic fatigue with excessive sweating that is worse at night, and with possible palpitations.
Shih Qua Da Bu Tang	A traditional Chinese herbal formula that stimulates production of interleukins and NK cells. This formula is also known as All-Inclusive Great Tonifying Decoction.
White Tiger Decoction[2]	A traditional Chinese herbal formula that strengthens acyclovir's ability to stop herpesvirus from replicating itself.

Precautions for the use of formulas:

[1]Most manufacturers of Honey-Fried Licorice Decoction include the traditional marijuana seed. This does not produce a "high," but it will cause a positive urine test for marijuana, although sophisticated testing methods can distinguish medicinal from illicit use.

[2]Do not use White Tiger Decoction if you are experiencing nausea or vomiting.

The mechanisms of CFS are still being debated by doctors, and different explanations have emerged. Many doctors see CFS as a disorder in which the brain and the immune system are uncoordinated. Neurologist Jay Lombard and nutritionist Carl Germano describe it as a condition in which "the brain's master conductor misses a beat." According to this explanation, CFS seems to be caused, in large part, by a failure of the brain to stimulate production of cortisol, the hormone that allows the body to handle stress. Another common characteristic of people with CFS is an imbalance of an immune-system component, the T cells. In CFS, T cells are activated to fight a disease but are unable to "lock on" to their targets. Some researchers think this imbalance is related to a lack of available zinc compounds, as zinc is necessary for a healthy immune response.

Other factors that may contribute to or trigger CFS include viral infection, exposure to toxins, long-term stress, and anemia. There are also many other illnesses that can cause fatigue.

Several of the herbs recommended for CFS act by providing zinc. Other herbs counteract chronic viral infections underlying symptoms, act as general immune-stimulants, or relieve depression.

Recommendations

❏ Eat a healthy diet. Some reports have suggested that overgrowth of the yeast *Candida albicans* in the intestines is linked to chronic fatigue. This possibility spurred some to advocate special diets that recommend avoiding certain foods such as those containing gluten or sugar—even sugar from fruit. In a study of fifty-two individuals with chronic fatigue, half were assigned to a specially designed low-sugar, low-yeast diet and half followed a normal healthy diet plan. There was no apparent benefit to the special diet and it was hard for many people to follow, so they dropped out of the study early. It appears that a healthy diet is a better choice and offers a wider array of nutrients.

❏ Typical treatments for chronic fatigue include antidepressants such as low-dose tricyclics, cognitive-behavior therapy, meditation, and sleep management techniques.

❏ Eat more fish. Research indicates that supplementing the diet with omega-3 fatty acids and gamma-linoleic acid (GLA) significantly improves immune response in people with CFS. Get omega-3 fatty acids by eating two to three servings of cold-water fish (such as mackerel, salmon, or tuna) weekly, or by taking flaxseed oil and MaxEPA fish oil. Borage or evening primrose oil also is helpful.

❏ To maintain immune function, take zinc and vitamin C daily. For zinc, take 30 milligrams of either zinc glycinate or zinc histidinate daily, with food. Take 4 grams of vitamin C in two or more doses with food. Start with a lower dose and gradually add more. Use calcium ascorbate to help prevent stomach upset.

❏ To further support your immune system, use other antioxidant supplements. Harmful free radicals are generated by eating fatty foods (especially those cooked in old or rancid oils) and by exposure to cigarette smoke, environmental chemicals, and radiation. To deal with free radicals, the body creates the enzyme glutathione transferase, which deactivates toxic compounds that interfere with immune response. Take the following supplements to help maintain the body's supplies of glutathione: 200 milligrams of lipoic acid; 1 gram of N-acetylcysteine (NAC); and 150 to 200 micrograms of selenium (do not exceed 200 micrograms). Take these supplements with food.

❑ Take 200 milligrams of magnesium three times a day. One study revealed that people with CFS have lower amounts of magnesium in their red blood cells. CFS sufferers who take magnesium gain improved energy, better emotional states, and less pain. Green leafy vegetables, nuts, whole grains, and dried fruits are good sources of magnesium. Magnesium supplementation may cause diarrhea, so go slowly when adding it to your diet.

❑ Avoid chocolate, soft drinks, caffeine, and highly processed foods. These substances could deplete the body of magnesium, which leads to fatigue, and also are of low nutrient benefit.

❑ If you experience extreme fatigue after exercise, take 5 grams of creatine monohydrate on an empty stomach daily. Creatine is essential for proper muscle contraction. You should not take supplemental creatine, however, unless you have CFS and exercise regularly.

❑ Try to eliminate stress to the extent possible. (*See* STRESS.)

❑ Make sure that your bowels move daily. If necessary, add fiber to your diet.

Considerations

❑ Regular exercise can increase the infection-fighting effectiveness of natural killer (NK) cells. Light to moderate exercise is enough to stimulate immune function, although more vigorous exercise (such as training for a marathon) may be detrimental. One study found that immune function was significantly increased by the practice of tai chi, a martial arts technique that features movement from one posture to the next in a flowing motion resembling dance.

❑ A disorder that may be related to CFS is fibromyalgia, in which chronic muscle pain is the most prominent symptom. (*See* FIBROMYALGIA SYNDROME.)

❑ Taking regular cold or hot showers may help improve symptoms. Do not try this without talking to your physician first, however.

❑ Alternative therapies that are popular to help with the symptoms of CFS include biofeedback, deep breathing exercises, hypnosis, massage therapy, and yoga.

❑ Smoking or inhaling secondhand smoke can make symptoms worse.

❑ *See also* DEPRESSION, HERPESVIRUS INFECTION, and YEAST INFECTION (YEAST VAGINITIS).

CIRCULATORY PROBLEMS

See CONGESTIVE HEART FAILURE; HIGH BLOOD PRESSURE (HYPERTENSION); INTERMITTENT CLAUDICATION.

CIRRHOSIS OF THE LIVER

Cirrhosis of the liver is a condition in which the organ's outer layers develop nodules and fibrous scar tissue in response to repeated toxic damage. These nodules and fibers disrupt the blood supply to remaining healthy tissues in the liver. Eventually, cirrhosis leads to a loss of the liver's normal function.

Early cirrhosis may produce no symptoms. It may be discovered during a routine physical or through a blood test given for some other reason. The main symptoms of cirrhosis are weight loss, nausea, vomiting, jaundice, weakness, stomach pain, varicose veins, constipation or diarrhea, generalized itching, and reddening of the palms of the hands. Some people develop ascites, or abdominal swelling caused by fluid accumulation. If untreated, cirrhosis can lead to a decline in brain function caused by toxins that would normally be disposed of by the liver. It could also cause kidney failure or hepatic coma, and cirrhosis can lead to liver cancer.

While cirrhosis can be a result of hepatitis C infection, malnutrition, or chronic inflammation—and sometimes occurs for no identifiable reason—overwhelmingly, the most common cause of cirrhosis in North America is long-term overconsumption of alcohol. The amount and duration of alcohol abuse, rather than the type of alcoholic beverage consumed or the pattern of drinking (binge versus non-binge) determines the onset of cirrhosis. Women are more susceptible to this disease than men, probably because of differences in body weight and size.

Alcohol causes cirrhosis by overwhelming a key component of the liver's detoxification system known as the p450 enzymes. That leads to increased damage from harmful free radicals, which can attack liver cells. This enzyme prevents liver tissue from efficiently using oxygen and increases the production of collagen, a substance that becomes fibrous scar tissue. It also increases the rate at which the liver converts alcohol into acetaldehyde, a chemical that damages proteins.

Conventional treatment is more supportive than curative. The idea is to reduce the liver's workload as much as possible so that this resilient organ can repair itself, as long as too much tissue has not been destroyed. Standard treatment also addresses the symptoms and complications seen in cirrhosis. One approach to successful treatment, though, is helping the liver heal without activating the enzyme involved in cirrhosis development. Herbal medicines may support achieving this goal and can be used with conventional treatments. Be aware that some herbs may have a negative impact on the liver and/or interact negatively with conventional medicines. Always work

Cirrhosis of the Liver: Beneficial Herbs

Herb	Form and Dosage	Comments
Alfalfa[1]	Liquid or tablets. Take as directed on the label.	Helps build a healthy digestive tract and is a good source for vitamin K, which is deficient in most people who suffer from cirrhosis.
Green tea	Catechin extract. Take 240 mg 3 times daily; or tea bag, prepared with 1 cup water. Take 1 cup 3–5 times daily. To avoid dilution, do not use within 1 hour of taking other oral medications.	Treats infections that can cause or aggravate cirrhosis, including viral hepatitis.
Milk thistle[2]	Silymarin gelcaps. Take 600 mg daily.	May be able to reverse cirrhosis.
Schisandra	Capsules. Take 1,000–2,000 mg twice daily.	Protects against progression of cirrhosis to live cancer.
Soy lecithin[3]	Capsules. Take 1,500–3,000 mg daily.	Protects liver from damage by alcohol and other toxic chemicals.
Turmeric	Curcumin tablets. 250–500 mg twice daily, between meals.	Slows rate at which alcohol is converted into a toxic form within the liver.

Precautions for the use of herbs:

[1]Do not use alfalfa in any form if you have an autoimmune disease, such as lupus or rheumatoid arthritis.

[2]Milk thistle may cause mild diarrhea.

[3]Soy lecithin may cause mild diarrhea when you first use it.

with a qualified health-care practitioner. If you continue to drink, no herbal or conventional remedy will work.

Herbs to Avoid

❑ People who have cirrhosis should avoid bitter melon and wintergreen. (For more information regarding these herbs, *see* BITTER MELON and WINTERGREEN *under* The Herbs in Part One.)

Recommendations

❑ Eat a healthy diet including protein at each meal. Only with end-stage cirrhosis is too much protein possibly harmful. You need protein to heal the liver and support your other muscles, which could have an increased rate of wasting due to cirrhosis.

❑ Eat two to three daily servings of dark green, yellow, or orange vegetables for essential nutritional support.

❑ Eat the right kinds of fats in moderate amounts. Fat calories should total 30 percent of the diet. Fish oils (except for cod-liver oil), seeds, and nuts are the best sources of essential fatty acids, which are needed for cell protection. Saturated fats from meats such as beef, pork, and lamb, and the skin of poultry should be avoided.

❑ Drink grapefruit juice, which contains a substance that can decrease the enzymatic conversion of many potential toxins to toxic forms by the liver. Whether this actually works for cirrhosis is not known, but it is a healthy food that is good for the liver in general and can be included in the diet for that benefit alone. (Avoid grapefruit juice, however, if you are taking a calcium channel blocker for high blood pressure or—although this is unlikely in cirrhosis—if your doctor has given you any kind of anti-

coagulant drug.) Red chili peppers also contain a similar compound.

❑ Burdock root, dandelion, and red clover can aid in cleansing the blood, reducing the stress on the liver.

❑ Take 30 milligrams of zinc and 3,000 milligrams of vitamin C daily. Low zinc levels are associated with an increased risk of cirrhosis and with a reduced capacity for breaking down alcohol. Zinc, particularly if combined with vitamin C, greatly increases alcohol detoxification and survival in animal studies.

❑ Take calcium and vitamin D and eat a diet rich in these nutrients. Many patients with cirrhosis have bone loss. One study found no benefit from supplements alone, so inclusion of dairy and other foods with calcium and vitamin D at least once a day is a good idea.

❑ Use bovine (cow) colostrum supplements to slow the progress of cirrhosis. All mammals (including humans) produce colostrum. It is the first secretion from the mother's breasts after a baby's birth, and is a rich source of proteins and antibodies that provide temporary disease resistance until the infant's immune system begins to function. Bovine colostrum keeps the Kuppfer cells, immune cells distributed in layers throughout the liver, from becoming irritated by alcohol. Such irritation causes them to secrete collagen, which destroys circulation within the liver. However, there have not been any studies published on the use of these supplements for cirrhosis.

❑ Avoid alcohol in all forms. This includes the alcohol found in some conventional medications and in herbal tinctures.

❑ Visit the doctor for regular blood tests. These will show how the liver is healing.

Considerations

❑ People with cirrhosis who continue to drink are much worse off if they also consume a high-fat diet. The combination of excessive dietary fat and alcohol leads to the development of fibrous tissue in the liver. But the alcohol is the most poisonous thing you can consume, so stopping drinking is the first thing you should do.

❑ Be careful not to overeat. Overeating wears down the liver so that it may not be able to do its job as well as it should.

❑ Sometimes cirrhosis progresses to the point where cognition is impaired. In one study, the use of a probiotic, *Bifidobacterium*, and fructooligosaccharide (FOS) for thirty days reduced blood ammonia levels, thought to cause confusion, and tests of cognition in patients with hepatic encephalopathy improved. This alternative treatment worked as well or better than the standard therapy of lactulose (a synthetic sugar).

❑ Sometimes malnutrition arises in people who have cirrhosis resulting from liver cancer. Use of a snack that was enriched with branched-chain amino acids (i.e., leucine, isoleucine, and valine) improved the liver tissue so it didn't release toxic compounds such as ammonia—compared to a control group who did not get the snack and did not experience this improvement.

❑ For information on how to prevent cirrhosis from progressing to liver cancer, *see* LIVER CANCER.

❑ *See also* ALCOHOLISM and HEPATITIS.

COLD

See COMMON COLD.

COLD SORES

See under HERPESVIRUS INFECTION.

COLIC

Most babies go through periods when they seem to be abnormally fussy or they cry for no apparent reason, but true colic is a condition in which the baby cries for a long time no matter what the parent does. It can begin around three weeks after birth, but it usually stops when the child has reached the age of three to four months. It is rarely experienced by a baby older than six months.

The cause of colic is believed to be discomfort due to indigestion and gas. An infant doubles in weight during the first six months of life, and has to consume an enormous amount of food relative to his or her body weight to support such rapid growth. The sheer volume of food can cause indigestion. In addition, many infants swallow air during feeding, which can also cause stomach upset. Researchers have explored possible causes, including allergies, lactose intolerance, an immature digestive tract, maternal anxiety, and different ways a baby is fed or comforted.

When the child experiences gas pain, it is likely to be the worst pain of his or her life. The child shows distress in an arched back, a tense tummy with knees pulled up to the chest, clenched fists, and flailing arms and legs, all in addition to what seems like unstoppable crying. Suspect colic if the baby has crying bouts that last for several hours at a time and that always happen at the same time of day. The crying begins and ends abruptly, and the infant seems angry and struggles when held.

Most of the traditional home remedies for colic are herbal. While all of the herbal remedies recommended here are given to the baby, breast-feeding mothers should

Colic: Beneficial Herbs

Herb	Form and Dosage	Comments
Anise	Tea bag, prepared with 1 cup water. Take 1 cup (mother) plus 1 tsp (baby) 3 times daily.	A traditional colic remedy.
Chamomile[1]	German chamomile (*Matricaria recutita*) tea bag, prepared with 1 cup water. Take 1 cup (mother).	A traditional colic remedy. The effects of chamomile are cumulative. Effective treatment can take as long as 3 weeks.
Fennel seed[2]	Tea bag, prepared with 1 cup water. Take 1 cup (mother) plus 1 tsp (baby) 3 times daily.	Soothes colic. Also eases lactation, flavors breast milk.
Peppermint[3]	Tea bag, prepared with 1 cup water. Take 1 cup (mother) plus 1 tsp (baby) 3 times daily.	Stops cramping, diarrhea, and gas. Fights foodborne bacteria.

Precautions for the use of herbs:

[1]Chamomile should only be used by the nursing mother; it contains compounds that can cause allergic reactions in the baby.

[2]Do not take fennel seed if you have an estrogen-sensitive disorder, such as breast cancer, endometriosis, or fibrocystic breasts.

[3]Do not take peppermint if you have a gallbladder disorder.

take them as well. Be sure to note different dosages for mother and infant. Do not use any of these without consulting your infant's pediatrician or ob-gyn if you are breast-feeding.

Recommendations

❑ If you are a nursing mother, you can use tinctures, which are stronger, instead of teas. Take ½ to 1 teaspoon (2.5 to 5 milliliters) of tincture in ¼ cup of water three times a day. Because tinctures contain alcohol, they should not be given to infants.

❑ If a nursing child becomes colicky, simplify your diet so that you can keep track of his or her reactions when you eat certain foods. Even "perfect" babies can be sensitive to the foods their nursing mothers eat. The most common offenders are caffeine, chocolate, citrus fruit, cumin, curries, melon, pickles, salsas, and spicy foods. Also avoid gas-forming foods, such as beans, broccoli, Brussels sprouts, cauliflower, cucumbers, flaxseed, and green, red, or yellow peppers. In one study, breast-fed infants whose mothers excluded cow's milk, eggs, peanuts, tree nuts, wheat, soy, and fish from their diet cried less and were less fussy during the first six weeks of life.

❑ Promote growth of the "good" bacteria that help the body digest food. If breast-feeding, take ½ teaspoon (2 milliliters) of *Lactobacillus acidophilus* or *bifidus* powder twice a day. A bottle-fed infant should be given ⅛ teaspoon (250 milligrams) of powder dissolved in formula twice a day. Many formulas today include prebiotics that stimulate the growth of healthy bacteria.

❑ Try different ways to soothe the baby: cuddling and rocking, a warm bath, or playing either soft music or a recording of a heartbeat (a sound the baby heard in the womb).

Considerations

❑ Drug treatments for colic are usually harsh. A relatively mild treatment is simethicone (Mylicon Drops), which breaks the surface of gas bubbles and relieves pain. If large gas bubbles causing a bloated tummy are the primary problem, this may be a workable treatment, but do not give a child simethicone without consulting his or her pediatrician. One study found that breast-fed infants cried less with a natural probiotic, *Lactobacillus reuteri* (American Type Culture Collection Strain 55730). It performed as well as simethicone. Other drugs doctors give colicky babies include antiflatulents, antispasmodics, and sedatives. These drugs sometimes give quick relief, but are too strong for continuous use.

❑ In one study, using a combination of massage, a sucrose solution, herbal tea, and a hydrolyzed infant formula throughout the day resulted in fewer hours of crying. The best of these treatments was the hydrolyzed formula, but the researchers suggested all be used.

COLORECTAL CANCER

Cancer of the colon, or large intestine, and rectum is the most common digestive-tract cancer, striking more than 100,000 people a year in the United States. It generally affects those over sixty years of age, and there is a genetic link in some families. Other risk factors include being African-American, eating a diet high in red or processed meat, having colonic polyps, or having had breast cancer. Colorectal tumors can grow quite large without obstructing the bowel. Thus, they are often undetected until they have spread.

The symptoms of colorectal cancer include changes in bowel habits (diarrhea or constipation), vague abdominal pain, acid stomach, muscular tension and twitching in the abdomen, and, most notably, blood in the stool. Sometimes rectal bleeding cannot be seen, but can be detected by a home test kit available in drugstores. However, this test is often negative in colon cancer patients. (Blood in the stool can be caused by several intestinal conditions, so a doctor should always be consulted in cases of rectal bleeding.) Polyps—small, stalklike growths in the colon—also can cause bleeding. Polyps should be treated promptly, even if benign, because they can become cancerous as they enlarge. Colorectal cancers often start as polyps.

Colorectal cancer is associated with a high-fat, low-fiber diet. A lack of fiber allows stool to remain in the intestine for too long a period of time after each meal. In societies in which people normally eat a high-fiber, low-red-meat diet, colorectal cancer incidence is lower. The body does have certain defenses against colorectal cancer. One is gene p53, a "molecular patrolman" that stops defective cells from multiplying. Other genes and protective factors also slow or stop colorectal cancer. Some genes protect cells from the "bystander effect," or genetic damage that occurs when bacteria in the colon turn nitrates from food and nitrites added as food preservatives into harmful forms.

Several staging systems are used to classify colorectal cancer based on how far the cancer has spread, usually to the liver, lungs, or bones. Surgery is the main treatment. If cancer occurs in the rectum, doctors use surgical techniques designed to preserve normal bowel evacuation whenever possible. Chemotherapy and radiation therapy are also used, as is immunotherapy, in which concentrated amounts of the body's own immune-system chemicals, such as cetuximab (Erbitux) and bevacizumab (Avastin), are given.

Herbal treatments have been shown to work within the context of conventional therapy. Always use herbs as part of a medically directed overall treatment plan for colorectal cancer.

Herbs to Avoid

❑ People who have colorectal cancer should avoid aloe. (For more information regarding this herb, including the

Colorectal Cancer: Beneficial Herbs

Herb	Form and Dosage	Comments
Astragalus[1]	Fluidextract. Take ¼–½ tsp (1–2 ml) 3 times daily.	Stimulates two types of immune cells, T cells and lymphokine-activated killer (LAK) cells, to attack cancer.
Barberry[2] or coptis[2] or goldenseal[2] or Oregon grape root[2]	Tincture. Take 15–30 drops in ¼ cup water 3 times daily. Do not take any of these herbs daily for more than 2 weeks.	Contains berberine, which retards multiplication of cancer cells.
Garlic[3]	Enteric-coated tablets. Take at least 900 mg daily.	Inhibits bystander effect. Retards tumor spread.
Green tea	Catechin extract. Take 240 mg 3 times daily; or tea bag, prepared with 1 cup water. Take 3–5 cups daily. To avoid dilution, do not use within 1 hour of taking other oral medications.	Retards growth of nitrite-converting *Clostridium* bacteria in the colon.
Kelp	As food. Eat any quantity desired, but limit this to once per week.	Accelerates passage of food through intestines, which removes toxins via the stool.
Lentinan	Intramuscular injection, given by health-care provider.	Greatly increases effect of treatment with interferon or recombinant tumor necrosis factor (TNF).
Maitake	Maitake-D. Take 2,000 mg 3 times daily, before meals.	General immune stimulant. Slows growth of new tumors.
Polysaccharide kureha (PSK)	Tablets. Take 6,000 mg daily.	Reduces tumor spread to lymph nodes, peritoneum, lungs, and liver.
Quercetin[4] plus	Tablets. Take 125–250 mg 3 times daily between meals.	Deactivates enzymes that trigger tumor growth.
bromelain[5]	Tablets. Take 125 mg 3 times daily, between meals.	Increases absorption of quercetin.
Reishi	Tablets. Take 3 gm 3 times daily.	Stimulates production of immune-system chemical interleukin-2.
Soy isoflavone concentrate	Tablets. Take 3,000 mg once daily.	Contains daidzein, which inhibits colon cancer cells.
Turmeric	Curcumin tablets. Take 250–500 mg twice daily, between meals.	Activates gene p53.

Precautions for the use of herbs:

[1]Do not use astragalus if you have a fever or a skin infection.

[2]Do not use barberry, coptis, goldenseal, or Oregon grape root if you are pregnant or have gallbladder disease. Do not take these herbs with supplemental vitamin B_6 or with protein supplements containing the amino acid histidine. Do not use goldenseal if you have cardiovascular disease or glaucoma.

[3]Garlic counteracts the effects of *Bifidus* and *Lactobacillus* cultures taken as digestive aids. Consult a doctor before using garlic on a regular basis if you are on an anticoagulant drug such as warfarin (Coumadin). Discuss the use of garlic with your doctor before having any type of surgery.

[4]Do not use quercetin if you are taking cyclosporine (Neoral, Sandimmune) or nifedipine (Procardia).

[5]People who are allergic to pineapple may develop a rash from bromelain. If itching develops, stop using it.

Colorectal Cancer: Formulas

Formula	Comments
Alzium	A modern formula that has brought about remission when colorectal cancer has spread to the lung. In laboratory studies, it kills cancer cells that resist chemotherapy.
Minor Bupleurum Decoction[1]	A traditional Chinese herbal formula that complements steroid therapies for treatment of inflammation.

Precautions for the use of formulas:

[1]Do not use Minor Bupleurum Decoction if you have a fever or a skin infection. Taken long term, it can cause headache, dizziness, and bleeding gums. Side effects can be avoided if the formula is taken as a tea.

belief among some scientists that aloe-based laxatives might cause colorectal cancer, *see* ALOE *under* The Herbs in Part One.)

Recommendations

❏ To avoid recurrence of colon cancer, eat fiber-rich products at every meal as soon as possible after treatment. The minimum amount of daily fiber needed to protect against developing colorectal cancer is 30 grams, which can be obtained by eating a minimum of six to eight servings of whole grains, fruits, vegetables, or legumes (such as peas, lentils, or beans) each day. In one study, patients who ate the most fiber from fruits, vegetables, and whole grains had a 35 percent reduced chance of recurrence of colon cancer.

❏ Supplement your diet with omega-3 fatty acids by eating two to three servings of seafood weekly, or by taking fish oil capsules. Borage or evening primrose oil also may be helpful, but most of the research has focused on fish oil. Omega-3s activate gene p53, and increased omega-3 consumption can not only reduce the risk that cancer will develop and spread, it can also make colorectal cancer more responsive to chemotherapy with cisplatin (Platinol), doxorubicin (Adriamycin), or vincristine (Oncovin). Patients with anomalies in their rectal mucosa and cancer benefited from 2.5 grams of fish oil capsules and more (up to 7.7 grams) per day.

❏ Eat two to three daily servings of low-fat dairy products enriched with vitamin D. The kidneys turn vitamin D into a hormone that attaches to and deactivates colon cancer cells. Even modest amounts of vitamin D can hasten recovery from stage I colon tumors and produce a 50 percent reduction in the risk of developing new cancers. Even more effective is consuming a combination of calcium and vitamin D. Get your vitamin D levels measured to make sure that you have adequate amounts. There is a strong inverse association between blood vitamin D levels and the risk of developing colon cancer.

❏ Take 1,200 milligrams of calcium daily. Calcium supplements may reduce the risk of cancer development. Calcium combines with toxins to form insoluble soaps. These soaps are repelled from the lining of the digestive tract and are eliminated through the stool. Always take calcium supplements with magnesium to avoid creating an imbalance between the two minerals. Magnesium may cause diarrhea, so ingest small amounts at a time. Consuming adequate amounts of low-fat dairy products can obviate the need to use supplements, as they contain the right amounts of vitamin D, calcium, and magnesium.

❏ Take a complete mineral supplement containing copper but not iron. In cell studies, copper slows down the formation of "aberrant crypts," or cell abnormalities within the furrows normally found in the anal canal. Iron supplements may accelerate colon damage. Using multivitamins containing iron is fine, but speak to your doctor about your need for supplemental iron.

❏ Avoid red meat. A study published in *The New England Journal of Medicine* found that the relative risk of colon cancer in women who ate beef, pork, or lamb as a main dish every day is two and a half times that of women who ate such foods less than once a month. Processed meats and liver were also associated with increased risk, whereas eating chicken without skin and fish was related to decreased risk.

Considerations

❏ Aspirin slows the production of inflammatory prostaglandins. However, aspirin use can cause stomach bleeding, so a doctor should always be consulted before using aspirin therapy during treatment for cancer.

❏ Sulindac, a common prescription drug for arthritis pain, may act against precancerous conditions of the colon and rectum. Use of the drug has been associated with lowered risk of developing new polyps after colorectal surgery. If you have had colon surgery, or if you have desmoid (slow-growing) colorectal cancer, speak with your physician about treatment with sulindac.

❏ Recent studies have found that, at least for men, simply drinking more water greatly reduces the risk of developing colorectal cancer. A study in Taiwan found that men between the ages of thirty-three and eighty who drank more than eight glasses of water a day had a 92 percent lower risk of developing colon cancer than men who drank fewer than five glasses of water a day, even when all other factors were taken into account.

❏ Melanoma, a cancer that originates in the skin, may occur in the rectum. (*See* Melanoma *under* SKIN CANCER.)

❏ For measures to reduce the side effects and increase the effectiveness of chemotherapy and/or radiation therapy, *see* "Side Effects of Cancer Treatment" *under* CANCER. To learn about herbal treatments that can prevent a cancer from developing its own blood supply, *see* CANCER.

COMMON COLD

The common cold is a viral infection characterized by familiar symptoms: sore throat, headache, head and nasal congestion, coughing, watery eyes, and nasal discomfort with watery discharge and sneezing. As the cold progresses, the discharge becomes thicker. Throughout the course of a cold, the membranes lining the nasal passages are swollen. Headache, low-grade fever, and muscle aches may also be present.

Colds can be caused by a wide variety of rhinoviruses. Once a person has been infected with a particular strain of rhinovirus, he or she usually develops an immune defense to it. There are enough strains, however, that the average adult is exposed to one or two new ones every year. Young children, with their developing, uncoordinated immune systems, can have as many as seven colds a year. Exposure to new strains, combined with a general lack of immune resistance, sets the stage for a cold. Smoking, stress, and chronic lung disease all make a person more susceptible to colds.

The cure for the common cold continues to evade the best efforts of medical science. That is because the rhinovirus is well adapted to its human host. It plants itself on the adhesion molecules that attach immune-system cells to the lining of the respiratory tract. When the virus is attacked by the immune system, the body creates more cells that have to be held in place by more adhesion molecules. This gives the virus more places to grow. Eventually, the body defeats the virus by sloughing off the entire virus-cell mix into the nasal discharge associated with colds.

Unless otherwise specified, the herb dosages recommended here are for adults. Children under age six should be given one-quarter of the adult dosage. Children between the ages of six and twelve should be given one-half of the adult dosage.

Recommendations

❑ Use aromatherapy to help ease symptoms. (*See* AROMATHERAPY in Part Three.) Essential oil of yarrow helps reduce inflammation, while eucalyptus oil relieves congestion. Or use steam inhalations of chamomile, elderberry flowers, and/or lemon balm to soothe irritation and relieve pain. (*See* STEAM INHALATIONS in Part Three.) If you use chamomile, be sure to use German chamomile (*Matricaria recutita*), not Roman chamomile (*Chamaemelum nobile*).

❑ Take zinc lozenges at the first sign of a cold to "short-circuit" the infection process. Take 20 milligrams of zinc gluconate or acetate (other forms do not work) every two

Common Cold: Beneficial Herbs

Herb	Form and Dosage	Comments
Astragalus[1]	Capsules. Take 500–1,000 mg 3 times daily.	Keeps nasal-passage linings from letting in rhinoviruses.
Cat's claw[2]	Capsules. Take 2,000–3,000 mg daily.	Speeds rate at which the immune system gets rid of the virus.
Echinacea[3]	*Echinacea purpurea* extract tablets. Take at least 900 mg daily; or juice (Echinacin). Take 1 tsp (4 ml) 3 times daily.	Speeds recovery. Reduces risk of catching cold.
Elderberry	Sambucol. Take as directed on the label.	Promotes sweating and can help to break a fever. It also contains antioxidant flavonoids that protect cell walls against foreign substances.
Fenugreek and thyme	Fenu-Thyme from Nature's Way. Take as directed on the label.	Helps rid nasal passages of mucus.
Ginger	Tea, made by adding ⅓ tsp powdered ginger to 1 cup water. (*See* TEAS in Part Three). Drink 1 cup 2–3 times daily.	Stops head and chest congestion, malaise, and chills.
Horehound	Lozenges. Use as desired.	Breaks up nasal congestion.
Hyssop	Tea. Take 1 cup 2–3 times daily.	Acts as an expectorant and has antiviral properties.
Kudzu	Tablets. Take 10 mg 3 times daily.	For colds with sore neck or general muscle pain.
Osha	Tincture. Take 10–15 drops in ¼ cup water 3 times daily.	Useful if an ear infection is also present.
Shiitake	Tablets. Take 3 gm 3 times daily. Use mushroom in cooking as desired.	General immune stimulant. Good for colds that follow periods of stress.
Slippery elm bark	Powder. Take 1–2 tsp in 1 cup cold water as often as desired.	Relieves scratchy throat.
Tea tree oil[4]	Oil. Place 4–6 drops in ½ cup water and use as a mouthwash and gargle as often as desired.	Relieves sore throat.
Tilden flower	Liquid extract. Take ½–1 tsp (2–4 ml), 3 times daily.	Coats and soothes scratchy throat, and stops hacking cough without raising blood pressure.

Precautions for the use of herbs:

[1]Do not use astragalus if you have a fever or a skin infection.

[2]Do not use cat's claw if you have to take insulin for diabetes. Do not use it if you are pregnant or nursing. Do not give it to a child under age six.

[3]Do not use echinacea if you have an autoimmune disease such as rheumatoid arthritis or lupus. Do not use it if you have a chronic infection such as HIV or tuberculosis.

[4]People who are allergic to celery or thyme should not use tea tree oil products. Do not take tea tree oil internally.

to three hours for at least a day. Sweeteners such as mannitol and sorbitol may counteract the immune stimulant effect of zinc, so be sure to read the label if you use sweetened lozenges. These sweeteners also can cause intestinal discomfort.

❑ Take vitamin C to ease cold symptoms somewhat and decrease duration by about a day. Large doses (2,000 to 4,000 milligrams daily) are required. However, there is no consistent scientific evidence that taking vitamin C reduces the number of colds caught. Ask your child's pediatrician before using this amount in children.

❑ Unless fever is present, try to remain active. Activity helps to loosen fluids and mucus, making them easier to expel.

❑ To avoid infecting others and reinfecting yourself, wash your hands often and flush used tissues down the toilet.

❑ See a physician under any of the following conditions: if chest congestion develops; if a fever rises above 102°F (38.8°C) for more than three days; if white or yellow spots appear in the throat; if there are enlarged lymph nodes in the neck; or if there is wheezing or shortness of breath. Wheezing is a particularly serious symptom in childhood colds; it is a sign of an asthma attack. (Children who have not had asthma before usually have their first attack after a cold.)

❑ Do not give aspirin or any product containing aspirin to a child who shows symptoms of a viral infection. Aspirin use can result in Reye's syndrome, a potentially serious complication.

Considerations

❑ Echinacea is one of the most often used herbal remedies for the common cold. Some studies have found that echinacea prevents the symptoms of the common cold. However, in one study, even taking as much as 100 milligrams of echinacea three times a day at the onset of a cold did not reduce symptoms associated with a cold such as sneezing, nasal discharge, and hoarseness—or the duration of it. Another study found no benefit using 10 grams during the first twenty-four hours of a cold followed by 5 grams per day for the next four days. Illness severity and duration were not better for those who took the echinacea compared to those who took nothing. This study was funded by the National Institutes of Health's National Center for Complementary and Alternative Medicine.

❑ In one study, participants who took green tea (*Camellia sinensis*) capsules twice a day had fewer symptoms if they got a cold and got better faster compared to a placebo group.

❑ The oldest documented recommendation of chicken soup as a cold remedy is credited to Moses Maimonides, a theologian and physician who lived in the late twelfth century. Physicians at Mt. Sinai Medical Center in Miami tested the power of chicken soup for relief of a cold against plain hot and cold water, and chicken soup won hands down.

❑ Many people use over-the-counter (OTC) remedies to suppress cold symptoms so they can continue to go about their normal daily activities. Suppressing sneezes and mucus production could lengthen the amount of time the body needs to expel the virus.

❑ Colds and other viral respiratory infections are the most common diagnoses for which antibiotics are prescribed. But antibiotics cannot help fight a cold, since they are not effective against viruses. Moreover, unnecessary use of these drugs contributes to antibiotic resistance, a process in which bacteria become immune to the antibiotics needed to control them.

❑ The best way to fight a cold is to not catch one in the first place. Siberian ginseng has been shown to reduce the incidence of infection by over 95 percent. Take 1 cup of the tea (in bags) three times a day for eight to ten weeks before the colds season starts. And andrographis, when used throughout the cold season, reduces the risk of catching cold by more than 50 percent.

❑ Controlling colds is especially important for a child who also has an ear infection. A cold inflames and blocks the eustachian tube, which connects the throat and the ear. This changes the pressure in the inner ear so that bacteria are trapped and circulation of bacteria-removing lymph is cut off. The cold virus can then team up with the ear-infection bacteria to cause especially severe irritation of the middle ear. (*See* EAR INFECTION.)

❑ A cold can lead to sinusitis, an inflammation of the sinuses. The virus itself does not cause sinusitis, but irritates the linings of the sinuses so that bacterial infections can set in. (*See* SINUSITIS.)

❑ Especially severe symptoms may indicate presence of the flu. (*See* INFLUENZA.) Symptoms that are persistent or that occur at the same time each year may indicate an allergy. (*See* Respiratory Allergies *under* ALLERGIES.)

❑ If you have frequent bouts of cold and flu, you should have your thyroid function checked.

CONGESTIVE HEART FAILURE

Congestive heart failure is a condition in which the heart muscle is unable to pump blood fast enough to supply all the nutrients and oxygen needed by the body. About 550,000 new cases are diagnosed every year in the United States. Symptoms include fatigue and weakness, especially on exertion, and edema, or swelling associated with fluid retention. Fluid retention in the lungs can also cause shortness of breath.

The underlying causes of congestive heart failure may be acute or chronic. Acute failure is brought on by myocardial infarction, more commonly known as heart attack. Heart attacks that are "silent," in which no symptoms are present, can still produce heart failure. Acute heart failure can also occur after various infections of the heart muscle, which are collectively known as cardiomyopathy.

Chronic congestive heart failure is usually a long-term effect of high blood pressure, heart-valve problems, or previous heart attacks. Diabetes, hyperthyroidism, and extreme obesity can also cause chronic heart failure. Chronic lung disease, such as emphysema, and anemia are contributing factors.

Arrhythmia, a slow, fast, or irregular heartbeat, is another cause of chronic heart failure. Arrhythmia can be mild and nothing to worry about, or it can be a life-threatening health crisis. The most serious type of heartbeat irregularity is ventricular fibrillation, in which the heart cannot pass blood into the arteries because the beat is rapid, uncontrolled, and ineffective. A heartbeat that is too fast weakens the heart, and one that is too slow doesn't allow enough blood to get to the body, which can result in congestive heart failure.

Congestive heart failure is marked by heart enlargement and fluid retention. If the heart has to work too hard, it enlarges, just as other muscles enlarge during weight training. This helps the heart at first, but eventually the heart muscle weakens. The heart's pumping action decreases as a result. To aid a weakening heart, the body retains both sodium and fluid, which increases the amount of blood in circulation. Over time, the excess fluid seeps into the surrounding tissues, which causes edema.

Conventional therapy for congestive heart failure consists of treating any underlying disorders while also treating the heart failure itself. Treatment focuses on lifestyle changes, including smoking cessation and improved nutrition, and on the use of various drugs. For continuing care of congestive heart failure, use herbal medicine as part of a medically directed overall treatment plan. If acute symptoms occur, immediately seek professional help.

Herbs to Avoid

❑ People who have congestive heart failure should avoid turmeric and curcumin, a compound derived from turmeric. (For more information, see TURMERIC *under* The Herbs in Part One.)

Recommendations

❑ Use lemon balm (*Melissa officinalis*) to reduce the hormonal response triggered by stress. Take 1 cup of the tea (from bags) three times daily. (*See also* STRESS.)

❑ If sleeplessness is a problem, take 150 to 300 milligrams of valerian forty-five minutes before bedtime. (*See also* INSOMNIA.)

Congestive Heart Failure: Beneficial Herbs

Herb	Form and Dosage	Comments
Aconite[1]	Use only under professional supervision in carefully regulated doses.	Increases heart output. Relieves shortness of breath and edema.
Arjuna	Capsules. Take 500 mg every 8 hours.	Relieves pain. Helps heart muscle cells build up energy reserves.
Asparagus root	Tea (loose), prepared by steeping 1 tsp (1.5 gm) in 1 cup water. (*See* TEAS in Part Three.) Take 1 cup 3 times daily.	Increases urination, appropriate replacement therapy when prescribed diuretics are discontinued. Be sure to maintain adequate potassium levels when taking the commercial preparation Slo-K or by eating fruits and vegetables.
Astragalus[2]	Capsules. Take 500–1,000 mg 3 times daily.	Relieves pain on exertion.
Elecampane with guggul	Pushkarmoola rasayana. Usual dose is 1 tsp for each 50 lbs body weight daily.	Relieves shortness of breath on exertion. Gives better pain relief than nitroglycerin. Elecampane is also known as inula.
Hawthorn	Tablets. Take 100–250 mg 3 times a day.	Improves blood flow to the heart and cardiac enzymes, which measure damage to heart muscle.
Kudzu	Tablets. Take 10 mg 3 times daily.	Improves coronary circulation and reduces the heart's need for oxygen.
Motherwort	Liquid extract. Take ¼–1 tsp (1–4 ml) in ¼ cup water 3 times daily.	Strengthens but does not accelerate heartbeat. Useful if a nervous condition or an overactive thyroid exists.

Precautions for the use of herbs:

[1]Always use processed Asian aconite (*Aconitum carmichaeli*), not European aconite (*Aconitum napellus*). Large doses overstimulate the heart and can even cause ventricular fibrillation. Calcium can reverse this effect.

[2]Do not use astragalus if you have a fever or a skin infection.

❑ Use dandelion to relieve fluid retention after occasionally consuming salt to excess. Take 10 to 15 drops of the tincture in ¼ cup water three times daily between meals. Do not use if you have gallstones.

❑ If you are a woman past menopause who does not use estrogen replacement therapy (ERT), eat soy products such as tempeh and tofu liberally, or take kudzu. These products contain chemicals that, like estrogen, open and relax arteries. Talk to your doctor first about soy use before including it in the diet.

❑ Vitamin D seems to be of benefit for congestive heart disease patients. In one study, vitamin D_3 reduced inflammation in patients with this condition. Patients took 500 milligrams of calcium and 50 micrograms of vitamin D_3 for nine months. However, in another study a similar blend of calcium and vitamin D_3 did not improve bone health in patients with congestive heart failure compared to those taking 500 milligrams of calcium without vitamin D_3. Patients in both groups had fewer markers of osteoporosis. Given the contradictory results of these studies, speak to your doctor about how much you should take of these essential nutrients.

❑ Reduce sodium intake by eliminating salted foods, such as pickles, soy sauce, table salt, and most smoked fish and meats. This step alone causes many mild cases of heart failure to improve significantly. In more severe cases, there may be a need to eliminate commercially prepared breads, canned vegetables and soups, cheese, and canned beets.

❑ If you have mild congestive heart failure, take 500 milligrams of acetyl-L-carnitine three times daily. Carnitine increases the energy available to the heart muscle, resulting in a stronger heartbeat and a greater tolerance for physical exertion. The longer carnitine is used, the more dramatic the improvement. Laboratory tests find that carnitine may also be helpful in reversing heart damage caused by the chemotherapy agent doxorubicin (Adriamycin).

❑ If you are able to exercise, take 5 grams of creatine phosphate daily. Creatine has been shown to augment the endurance of both the heart and skeletal muscles by increasing muscle mass. One study found that taking 5 grams of creatine four times a day for six months along with typical congestive heart failure medication resulted in an increase in body weight and improvement in muscle strength.

❑ If swollen legs or ankles are a problem, take 4 grams of arginine daily. Arginine, an amino acid, may relieve edema that occurs after exercise or motion. It does not interfere with other medications.

❑ Avoid animal fats, such as butter or lard, as well as refined sugar, caffeine, tobacco, and alcohol. In one study, omega-3 fatty acids from fish oil (5 grams a day) enhanced heart contractions and increased blood flow and the size of the blood vessels in healthy subjects subjected to an exercise regimen. These results suggest that fish oil may help improve blood flow for patients with congestive heart failure.

❑ Should circumstances warrant it, consider asking a household member to learn cardiopulmonary resuscitation (CPR).

Considerations

❑ Hawthorn may be helpful to people with congestive heart failure who develop any kind of infectious disease. Less refined forms of the herb, such as hawthorn tea or juice, confer added benefits. Consult a physician immediately, however, if you experience swelling in the legs.

❑ A number of conventional drugs are used to treat heart failure. Diuretics remove water from the tissues, which increases urine flow. This action relieves edema. Vasodilators, such as the angiotensin-converting enzyme (ACE) inhibitors, relax the blood vessels, which allows more blood to reach the heart. Beta-blockers stabilize arrhythmias, and lower both blood pressure and the heart's need for oxygen. Other drugs control arrhythmias or increase the power of the heartbeat.

❑ Furosemide (Lasix), a diuretic widely prescribed for congestive heart failure, can produce dizziness and lightheadedness. In rare cases it may also cause muscle tenderness, nausea, or vomiting and ear ringing. These side effects may be corrected by taking vitamin B_1 (thiamin). A daily dosage of 200 milligrams also improves functioning of the left ventricle, the heart chamber that pumps blood throughout the body, in people with congestive heart disease.

❑ Magnesium is a potentially useful supplement, but not for everyone who has congestive heart failure. Magnesium supplements do not necessarily cause an increase of magnesium levels in the bloodstream. They are most useful for people who take ACE inhibitors and/or derivatives of the heart-rhythm stabilizer digitalis, such as digoxin (Lanoxicaps and Lanoxin). ACE inhibitors, while generally safe, can cause hormonal changes that keep heart cells from absorbing magnesium. Digoxin stabilizes heart rhythms but could destabilize magnesium balance. Magnesium supplements also seem to help people whose heart failure is caused by the heart-valve problem called mitral valve prolapse. A typical daily dosage is four tablets, each providing 100 milligrams of elemental magnesium. Magnesium is also of benefit to patients with heart failure because it lowers C-reactive protein, which is a biomarker of inflammation. In one study, patients lowered their C-reactive protein by taking 300 milligrams of magnesium citrate a day. Magnesium may cause diarrhea, so increase the dose slowly.

❑ The presence of heavy metals, especially lead, antimony, and mercury, may explain congestive heart failure that does not follow a heart attack or viral infection of the heart muscle. High concentrations of other metals, such as chromium, cobalt, and gold, could amplify the damage caused by antimony and mercury. These metals disable the mitochondria, which provide energy for cells. Co-Q_{10} may partially compensate for heavy metal exposure. This supplement, known by its chemical name ubiquinone, improves the heart's energy efficiency. One Italian study found that an average dosage of 100 milligrams per day for three months reduced fluid retention and stopped palpitations in more than 70 percent of the people who took Co-Q_{10}. But heavy metal was not necessarily the reason for the heart disease in this study. More harmful—and more common—toxins include alcohol, illegal drugs such as cocaine, and tobacco and chemicals from smoking.

❑ *See also* ANEMIA; ANGINA; ATHEROSCLEROSIS; DIABETES; HEART ATTACK (MYOCARDIAL INFARCTION); HIGH BLOOD PRESSURE (HYPERTENSION); HYPERTHYROIDISM; and OVERWEIGHT.

CONJUNCTIVITIS

See under EYE PROBLEMS.

CONSTIPATION

Constipation is the infrequent and difficult passage of stools. Although the frequency of elimination varies from person to person, constipation is medically defined as fewer than three bowel movements per week. Stomachache may also be present.

There are two main types of constipation. Acute constipation involves short-term bloating, discomfort, and inability to evacuate the bowels. Acute constipation in very rare cases may be caused by bowel obstruction, but is usually caused by failure to consume enough fiber or fluid, or to get adequate exercise.

Chronic constipation is the inability of the person to evacuate the bowels for three days or more over a period of months or years. In chronic constipation, the nerve endings in the rectum that trigger defecation can become desensitized either by the constipation itself or by long-term use of stimulant laxatives. People who cannot move about freely (generally older people who are infirm or people confined to bed) or people who ignore the urge to defecate may also experience chronic constipation. Chronic constipation may also be accompanied by anal fissures, or microscopic tears, caused by straining at stool. Other causes of chronic constipation include depression; stress; a low-fiber diet; pregnancy; spinal injuries; chronic illness, such as diabetes or kidney failure; disruption in usual routine, such as travel; the use of iron supplements and antacids; and the use of some prescription drugs, such as antidepressants or painkillers.

Constipation may cause other digestive problems, including indigestion, hemorrhoids, and flatulence. The pressure caused by straining at stool may cause diverticulitis, a condition in which pouches develop in the intestinal walls. Chronic constipation can cause or play a role in many other health problems, ranging from bad breath and body odor to insomnia and varicose veins. There may also be a link between long-term constipation and some forms of cancer.

There are several types of herbal laxatives. Bulking agents, as the name implies, add bulk to the stool, which makes it softer and easier to pass. They need to be taken with plenty of fluids. Stimulant laxatives cause the stool-retaining muscles in the intestines to relax and the stool-expelling muscles to contract. Still other laxatives increase bile flow into the intestines. Bile contains cholesterol, a fatty substance that lubricates the stool.

Recommendations

❑ If you are taking both a prescription medication and a laxative, you may need to take them at different times of the day. Many laxatives, herbal or otherwise, could affect the rate at which other oral medications are absorbed into the bloodstream, but always check with your doctor. One herbal tea, Smooth Move, was studied in eighty-six nursing home residents. During the first month there were significantly more bowel movements by the group that drank the tea than by the group that did not.

❑ Add more fiber to your diet, but do so gradually to avoid gas and bloating. Good sources include fresh fruits and vegetables (including those old standbys, prunes and figs) and whole grains. Apples, bananas, beets, cabbage, carrots, and citrus foods contain pectin fiber, which absorbs water in the intestines, making the stool softer and easier to pass. Flaxseed products, such as Uncle Sam's cereals, may be helpful.

❑ Drink at least eight to ten glasses of water a day. This is especially important if you are increasing your fiber intake. Warm water in tea, coffee, or soup is better than cold for promoting bowel movements.

❑ If increasing fiber is not enough to correct constipation, consider reducing your consumption of beef and dairy products, and increasing your intake of legumes to get enough protein. In one study, oat bran (5 grams a day) was shown to be of particular benefit to geriatric patients living in nursing homes.

❑ Eat small portions of food at a time. Do not eat large, heavy meals.

❑ Always move your bowels when you feel the urge. If chronic constipation is a problem, try to get into regular bowel habits by going to the toilet at the same time each day, even if there is no urge to defecate, and relaxing. (*See* BOWEL RETRAINING in Part Three.)

❑ If you have heart disease or risk factors for heart attack, use bulking agents instead of stimulant laxatives.

Constipation: Beneficial Herbs

Herb	Form and Dosage	Comments
Aloe (bitters)[1] or buckthorn[1] or cascara sagrada[1] or frangula[1] or senna[1]	Over-the-counter (OTC) tablets. Take as directed on the label.	Stimulant laxatives.
Dandelion[2]	Tincture. Take 20 drops in ¼ cup water 3 times daily on an empty stomach.	Increases bile flow into large intestine.
Ginger	Tea, prepared by adding ⅓ tsp (1 gm) powdered ginger to 1 cup water. (See TEAS in Part Three.) Take 1 cup 3 times daily.	Relieves muscle spasms accompanying constipation.
Hibiscus	Tea bag, prepared with 1 cup water. Take 1 cup 3 times daily.	Draws water into the intestine, softening stool.
Kelp	As food, eat 2 oz (50 gm) in a single serving. Limit this to once per week.	Bulking agent. Relieves stress on blood vessels lining rectum and anus.
Maté	Tea bag, prepared with 1 cup water. Take 1 cup 1–2 times daily.	Helps restore minerals lost after treatment with stimulant laxatives.
Milk thistle[3]	Silymarin gelcaps. Take 360 mg daily.	Increases bile flow into large intestine.
Psyllium seed[4]	Cereals and powders. Use as directed on the label.	Bulking agent. Soothes hemorrhoids. Does not cause cramping.

Precautions for the use of herbs:

[1]Long-term use (more than two weeks) of herbal stimulant laxatives is not recommended because the fluid drawn into the stool can result in depletion of electrolytes, especially potassium. Losses of potassium are even greater if aloe is taken internally with potassium-wasting diuretic drugs. Depletion of potassium due to the use of these herbs conceivably could lead to a toxic buildup of calcium in the bloodstream and kidney damage in women who take calcium carbonate (products such as Caltrate 600) for osteoporosis and use aloe laxatives on a regular basis. Even short-term use of herbal stimulant laxatives can result in dangerous potassium depletion and other serious mineral imbalances in people who take Cibalith-S, Eskalith, Lithobid, Lithonate, Lithotabs (all forms of lithium used in the treatment of bipolar disorder). You should not use herbal stimulant laxatives if you take potassium-depleting drugs, such as hydrochlorothiazide (HCTZ) or furosemide (Lasix).

[2]Do not use dandelion if you have gallstones.

[3]Milk thistle may cause mild diarrhea. If this occurs, decrease the dose or stop taking it.

[4]Do not use psyllium seed within one hour of taking other medications.

Constipation: Formulas

Formula	Comments
Cinnamon and Peony Decoction	A traditional Chinese herbal formula that treats constipation in which small quantities of loose stool are passed. Should be used by people who are in generally poor health and suffer stomach pain.
Major Order the Chi Decoction	A traditional Chinese herbal formula that treats constipation in which the person must strain to pass tough stools, especially if flatulence, abdominal pain, and a tense and firm abdomen are present.
Triphala	An ayurvedic formula that aids in the formation of odor-free, firm stools, especially if there is also gallbladder or liver disease.

Straining at stool can cause a heart attack in susceptible individuals. (See HEART ATTACK [MYOCARDIAL INFARCTION].) Some good choices include stool softeners (Peri-Colace) or laxatives (milk of magnesia).

❑ If you use laxatives, take *acidophilus* to replace the "friendly" bacteria. The continued use of laxatives cleans out the intestinal bacteria and leads to chronic constipation.

Considerations

❑ Be especially careful when taking antibiotics, which harm the friendly bacteria (*Lactobacillus acidophilus*) that normally inhabit the colon. Without the bacteria, stimulant herbal laxatives—such as aloe, buckthorn, cascara, frangula, and senna—will not work. To ensure the presence of helpful bacteria after antibiotic treatment, take 1 teaspoon of acidophilus daily at least six hours before taking a stimulant herbal laxative.

❑ New research is focusing on the use of other probiotics besides *Lactobacillus acidophilus*—whether or not antibiotics are being taken. In a large study, 300 people who had chronic constipation benefited from a blend of *Lactobacillus plantarum* and *Bifidobacterium breve* and a blend of *L. plantarum* and *B. animalis*. Within thirty days both combinations of probiotics helped participants have more frequent and softer bowel movements and the expulsion was easier.

❑ Recent research on exercise and constipation has provided mixed results. Some findings suggest that regular exercise can speed the passage of food through the digestive system, or "transit time," thereby easing constipation. But other findings suggest that exercise has no effect, or that it may even slow transit time, worsening constipation. In a study conducted at the University of California at Irvine, even "hard exertion" on an inclined treadmill for 3.2 miles (5 kilometers) daily did not relieve constipation in older people. The study suggests that regularity requires adequate fluid and fiber consumption.

❑ People who frequently feel constipated were more than four times as likely to develop colon cancer as those who did not complain of constipation, according to a report in the journal *Epidemiology*. Researchers speculate that constipation may increase the risk of colon cancer because the longer fecal material stays in the colon, the more toxins in the stool become concentrated.

❑ Cow's milk may cause constipation in children. However, the more likely cause is the lack of whole grains, fruits, vegetables, and adequate water. Make these changes in your child's diet—and also consult your child's pediatrician—before removing milk and dairy from the diet. For infants, breast-feeding or using cow's milk substitutes may relieve constipation, but for infants, the cause is usually dehydration.

❑ Constipation is common during toilet training. About one out of every five children experienced the problem for at least one month, according to a study in the journal *Pediatrics*. Many children are willing to use the toilet for urine, but not for a bowel movement. For successful toilet training, wait until the child expresses an interest and then gently guide him or her through the process, rewarding success, rather than scolding or punishing, and without referring to bowel movements as "dirty" or "stinky." A child should not be put into underpants until he or she understands that the toilet is for both urine and bowel movements.

❑ Foul-smelling stools and a burning feeling in the anus may be a sign of malabsorption and fat in the stool. Seek

medical attention if this problem persists for more than three days.

❑ If constipation recurs at irregular intervals, the problem may be irritable bowel syndrome. (*See* IRRITABLE BOWEL SYNDROME.)

❑ *See also* HEMORRHOIDS and INDIGESTION.

COUGH

A cough is the body's normal reaction to irritation in the throat, the bronchial tubes, or the lungs. Coughs are helpful because they expel mucus, bacteria, and other irritating substances from the respiratory tract. Coughing is a life-saving reflex when something gets stuck in the throat and blocks air passages.

Usually a cough signals a viral or bacterial infection, such as a cold or bronchitis. The immune system causes the bronchial tubes, lungs, and throat to attack the germs and get rid of them in a coating of mucus. Coughs that produce phlegm may be characteristic of respiratory infection. Coughs can also be caused by exposure to dust, cigarette smoke, polluted air, extremely dry air, or strong smells, such as that of ammonia. Coughs not caused by infection are more likely to be chronic and produce little phlegm. Other causes include asthma, allergic rhinitis, sinus problems, and esophageal reflux of stomach contents. In rare cases, it is caused by an aspiration of foreign objects into the lungs, and a chest X-ray is needed.

A brief bout of coughing in response to an infection or exposure to dust and pollution is a sign of health. Coughing is a problem if it fails to expel the offending substance or if it becomes continuous and interferes with eating, speech, or sleep. Chronic cough is also a symptom of a number of possible disorders, including allergies, chronic bronchitis or pneumonia, and tuberculosis. It can also be a side effect of certain medications, such as angiotensin-converting enzyme (ACE) inhibitors.

If you choose to use cough medicine, selecting the right one is important. For many coughs, however, just doing nothing is preferable so that mucus is removed from the

Croup

Croup is a form of viral laryngitis characterized by a "barking" cough, hoarseness, and high-pitched sounds when inhaling. Most frequently affecting children under age five, it is usually caused by a parainfluenza virus. The child may be restless, have a fever, and be working hard to keep breathing. Extra effort to breathe may be noticed as nasal flaring, the wider opening of the nasal openings during inhalation, increased use of the muscles of the neck and chest, and unwillingness to lie down, rest, eat, or drink. Children who have allergies or hay fever or who are on asthma medication are at the greatest risk for croup.

Home treatment for croup consists of providing either cool or warm humidified air. A hot shower can provide warm steam, and the child can be held in the bathroom for 20 minutes. (Do not place the child in the shower.) Taking the dry, warmly dressed child out into the cold air is also often helpful. Keep the child upright, offer fluids, encourage resting, and try over-the-counter (OTC) pain relievers such as children's acetaminophen.

Although viral croup usually goes away in three to seven days, severe difficulty breathing requires immediate medical treatment. Increasing difficulty breathing, bluish coloration of the skin, or dehydration requires immediate medical attention. See a doctor immediately if a child has a fever of 103.5⁰F or higher. Since the viruses that most frequently cause croup are the same that cause flu, herbal treatments for croup and flu are the same. (*See* INFLUENZA.)

lungs. This is especially true for those who have asthma or smoke. If you have high blood pressure, be careful, as many decongestants raise blood pressure. Some cough syrups suppress coughs and contain dextromethorphan. On March 2, 2011, the U.S. Food and Drug Administration (FDA) issued a safety alert about certain unapproved prescription cough, cold, and allergy products containing this drug in combination with other drugs. These products are not currently approved by the FDA for safety, effectiveness, and quality. The FDA took this action due to concerns about certain potential risks associated with use of these medications. These risks may include: the possibility of improper use in infants and young children; potentially risky combinations of ingredients; and patients receiving too much or too little of the medication because of problems with the way some "timed-release" products are made.

Expectorants are another kind of drug that thin mucus so it can be coughed up more easily. Drinking water also thins mucus. Expectorants should not be used to treat dry cough. Other treatments for cough work by "turning off" the part of the brain that causes the coughing response. Still others soothe the throat irritation caused by chronic cough. Some like camphor and menthol are used topically on the throat and chest. Although herbal treatments have fewer side effects than conventional remedies, they still must be chosen by the type of cough they are intended to treat.

Unless otherwise specified, the herb dosages recommended here are for adults, and some herbs are not suitable for children at all. (See the precautions at the end of the Beneficial Herbs table below.) Children under age six should be given one-quarter of the adult dosage. Children between the ages of six and twelve should be given one-half of the adult dosage. Formula dosages for children should be discussed with a knowledgeable health-care practitioner.

Recommendations

❑ Use essential oil of eucalyptus in aromatherapy to soothe throat irritation. (*See* AROMATHERAPY in Part Three.)

❑ Use eucalyptus, peppermint, rosemary, and sage together as a chest rub to relieve a child's cough and sore throat. Mix 5 drops of the essential oil of each herb into

Cough: Beneficial Herbs

Herb	Form and Dosage	Comments
Coltsfoot[1]	Tea bag, prepared with 1 cup water. Take ½ cup 2–3 times daily. Do not exceed the recommended dosage.	Relieves acute congestion and hoarseness lasting no more than 2–3 days.
Echinacea[2]	*Echinacea purpurea* tablets. Take 2,000 mg every 3 hours until symptoms improve.	Arrests both bacterial and viral infections that cause cough.
Fritillaria[3]	Ching chi hua tan tang syrup. Take as directed on the label.	Relieves sticky phlegm, snoring, and chronic sore throat.
Lobelia[4]	Capsules. Take 500–1,000 mg 3 times daily. Take it for no more than 2 weeks at a time.	Relieves dry, hacking cough.
Lungwort	Tincture. Take the dose recommended on the label 2–3 times daily for 3 days.	Good for children who have both cough and diarrhea.
Marshmallow root	Extract. Take 1 tsp (2 ml) in ¼ cup water 3 times daily. For children, use ¼ tsp (0.5 ml).	Relieves dry, hacking cough. Especially helpful for children. Also known as althea.
Mullein	Tea bag, prepared with 1 cup water. Take ½ cup 2–3 times daily.	For children at first sign of cough, before phlegm develops.
Peppermint[5]	Menthol lozenges. Use 1 per hour.	Suppresses cough reflex.
Reishi	Tablets. Take 3,000 mg 3 times daily.	Stops coughing if you have a cold and asthma at the same time.
Slippery elm bark	Tea (loose), prepared by steeping 1 tsp in 1 cup water. (*See* TEAS in Part Three.) Drink 1 cup as desired.	Coats and soothes sore throat.
Sundew[6]	Lozenges. Use 1 per hour, but not during acute cough.	Prevents coughing fits without causing sedation.
Wild cherry bark[7]	Over-the-counter syrup. Take the dose recommended on the label 2–3 times daily for 3 days.	Flavorful expectorant.

Precautions for the use of herbs:

[1]In large doses, coltsfoot can cause bronchial passages to close, so do not take any more than is recommended. Do not give this herb to a child under age twelve.

[2]Do not use echinacea if you have an autoimmune disease such as rheumatoid arthritis or lupus. Do not use it if you have a chronic infection such as HIV or tuberculosis.

[3]Do not use fritillaria if you have high blood pressure.

[4]Do not give lobelia to a child under age twelve.

[5]Do not take peppermint if you have any kind of gallbladder disorder.

[6]Do not give sundew to a child under age twelve.

[7]Do not use wild cherry bark if you are pregnant. Do not give it to a child under age four.

Cough: Formulas

Formula	Comments
Ephedra Decoction[1]	A traditional Chinese herbal formula that relieves colds in infants with acute congestion. This formula is also called Four Emperors Decoction. A variation of this formula, Ephedra, Apricot Kernel, Coix, and Licorice Decoction, is designed to lower fever, in addition to treating other symptoms.
Minor Bluegreen Dragon Decoction[2]	A traditional Chinese herbal formula that treats colds in infants and young children with cough, phlegm, and profuse, watery nasal discharge or phlegm.

Precautions for the use of formulas:

[1]Do not use Ephedra Decoction if you are experiencing nausea or vomiting.

[2]Do not use Minor Bluegreen Dragon Decoction if you have a fever.

3 tablespoons of olive oil and apply to the chest three times daily.

❑ Use antioxidant vitamins to soothe coughs. Taking 1,000 milligrams of vitamin C daily could reduce the frequency of a cough by reducing the irritability of the bronchial passages when faced with dust and pollutants. Taking 400 international units (IU) of vitamin E may ease the passage of phlegm. Beta-carotene, preferably obtained by eating plenty of green leafy vegetables or yellow or orange vegetables and fruits, stops wheezing.

❑ Avoid eating one to two hours before bedtime. Eating just before sleep may encourage the development of gastroesophageal reflux disease (GERD), which causes some people to wake up with a cough, sore throat, or hoarseness even in the absence of infection. Keep your head elevated if you have any type of reflux while sleeping. Antacids such as omeprazole (Prilosec) may help.

❑ To moisten the respiratory tract and thin mucus, use a cool-mist humidifier. Vaporizers and humidifiers are especially useful for children's coughs. Be sure to keep this equipment scrupulously clean (the instructions on the product should explain how) so that bacteria do not collect in it.

❑ Avoid exposure to cigarette smoke, either first- or secondhand.

❑ If a cough persists despite attempts to soothe it, see a doctor.

Considerations

❑ Siberian ginseng may be useful in preventing coughs caused by exposure to dust and drafts. Take 1 cup of the tea (from bags) per day, or use tinctures as directed on the label. Avoid this herb if prostate cancer or an autoimmune disease, such as lupus or rheumatoid arthritis, is present.

❑ Tobacco smoke is not the only cause of chronic cough in children. The presence of a furry pet or heating fuels such as bottled gas or paraffin also contribute to children's cough. Eliminate as many of these sources of irritation as possible.

❑ Some blood pressure drugs, such as fosinopril (Monopril) or lisinopril (Prinivil, Zestril), often cause chronic, dry, hacking coughs. If you experience hacking cough while taking blood pressure medication, see your physician about an alternative drug, and explore herbal treatments for high blood pressure. (*See* HIGH BLOOD PRESSURE [HYPERTENSION].) If you experience swelling of the lips, tongue, or throat after taking any blood pressure medication, with or without cough, seek immediate medical attention.

❑ *See also* BRONCHITIS AND PNEUMONIA; COMMON COLD; INFLUENZA; Respiratory Allergies *under* ALLERGIES; and STREP THROAT.

CROHN'S DISEASE

Crohn's disease is a condition in which severe inflammation causes ulceration of part or all of the digestive tract. The ulceration extends through the layers of the intestinal wall and may extend to the muscles, connective tissue, and lymph nodes below it. It is considered to be an inflammatory bowel disease. Crohn's disease, once rare, is becoming more common. It tends to run in families, and occurs more often among Jewish people than among members of other ethnic groups. It also is more common in Caucasians than in people of other races. The disorder generally appears before age thirty. Other risk factors include cigarette smoking, living in cities rather than the country, using the drug isotretinoin (Accutane) to treat acne, and using nonsteroidal anti-inflammatory drugs (NSAIDs). It is possible that Crohn's disease is caused by a virus or bacterium that the immune system cannot fight off.

Symptoms of Crohn's disease include diarrhea, abdominal pain and cramping, fever, headache, steatorrhea (passage of fatty stools that float), fatigue, loss of appetite, and unintended weight loss. There may also be rectal bleeding and ulceration of the intestinal wall. Nutrients are not properly absorbed, which can lead to malnutrition, and children with the disorder may not grow properly. Chronic bleeding may cause iron-deficiency anemia, and constantly open sores increase the risk of infection. Crohn's disease can result in bowel obstruction if scar tissue narrows the intestinal passageway. Fistulas (abnormal passageways) and abscesses (pockets of infection) also may develop. This disorder tends to follow a pattern of acute flare-ups followed by periods of remission that can last from months to years.

While surgery is an option in Crohn's disease, this disorder is often treated with drugs that relieve symptoms, including steroid drugs such as prednisolone. Other drugs used to treat Crohn's disease include anti-inflammatories such as sulfasalazine (Azulfidine), immune-system sup-

pressors such as infliximab (Remicade), and drugs to heal Crohn's-related fistulas such as cyclosporine (Gengraf). The herbs listed below can help relieve inflammation. They can also be used with prescription drugs; discuss the use of herbs with the prescribing doctor.

Herbs to Avoid
❑ People who have Crohn's disease should avoid burdock, echinacea, and pau d'arco. These herbs can trigger autoimmune reactions, which can cause relapses. (For

Crohn's Disease: Beneficial Herbs

Herb	Form and Dosage	Comments
Aloe[1]	Juice. Take 1 tbsp (10 ml) 3 times daily, just before meals.	Softens stools; speeds healing of intestinal ulcers.
Bromelain[2] or bromelain with papain[2]	Tablets. Take 250–500 mg 3 times daily, just before meals.	Aids digestion of proteins.
Fennel seed	Tea bag, prepared with 1 cup water. Take 1 cup 1–2 times daily.	Relieves constipation and gas.
Licorice[3]	Glycyrrhizin tablets. 200–800 mg daily, depending on the severity of symptoms. Use for 6 weeks; then take a 2-week break. Do not substitute deglycyrrhizinated licorice (DGL).	Protects digestive-tract lining from effects of excess acid. Consume potassium-rich foods such as bananas or citrus juices, or take a potassium supplement daily when taking this herb.
Marshmallow root	Powder. Take 3 tsp (10 gm) in 1 cup cold water 3 times daily.	Provides healing mucilages that form a protective layer within the digestive tract. Also known as althea.
Milk thistle	Silymarin gelcaps. Take 120 mg twice daily.	Stimulates release of bile, which dissolves fats and protects the intestinal lining.
Peppermint[4]	Enteric-coated oil capsules. Take 200–400 mg, between meals.	Stops muscle spasms. Stimulates release of bile.
Psyllium seed	Powder. Use as directed on the label. Do not use within 1 hour of taking other medications.	Absorbs excess water from stool.
Slippery elm bark	Powder. Take ½–1 tsp (1–2 gm) in ¼ cup hot water as often as desired.	Soothes inflammation and stops irritation of the mucous membranes.
St. John's wort	Fluidextract. Take 900–1,000 mg of total hypericin daily.	Regulates serotonin, a hormone that causes digestive irritation.

Precautions for the use of herbs:

[1] Do not take aloe vera juice internally if you have diarrhea.

[2] People who are allergic to pineapple may develop a rash from bromelain. If itching develops, stop using it.

[3] Do not use licorice if you have glaucoma, high blood pressure, or an estrogen-sensitive disorder such as breast cancer, endometriosis, or fibrocystic breasts.

[4] Do not use peppermint if you have any kind of gallbladder disorder.

Crohn's Disease: Formulas

Formula	Comments
Ginseng Decoction to Nourish the Nutritive Chi	A traditional Chinese herbal formula that relieves abdominal discomfort without causing sedation. Its use allows reduction in prednisolone dosage.
True Man's Decoction to Nourish the Organs[1]	A traditional Chinese herbal formula that treats diarrhea to the point of incontinence, with pus and blood in severe cases.
True Warrior Decoction[2]	A traditional Chinese herbal formula that treats unremitting diarrhea to the point of incontinence, which may be accompanied by pus and blood in the stool.

Precautions for the use of formulas:

[1] Avoid alcohol, wheat, cold or raw foods, fish, and greasy foods while using True Man's Decoction to Nourish the Organs. Do not use this formula if you have gallbladder problems, obstruction of the bile duct, or a tendency to retain urine. Do not use it if you are pregnant.

[2] Stop using True Warrior Decoction if you develop a fever. This formula may cause a loss of sensation in the mouth and tongue.

more information regarding these herbs, *see* BURDOCK, ECHINACEA, and PAU D'ARCO *under* The Herbs in Part One.)

Recommendations

❏ Eat a low-fat diet, except for sources of omega-3 fatty acids. These essential acids promote healing and ease inflammation. To get your omega-3s, use nonfat salad dressings mixed with flaxseed, walnut, wheat germ, or soybean oil. (Olive oil, a relatively healthy oil otherwise, does not have a beneficial effect on this disease.) Omega-3 oils are also found in cold-water fish; eat two or three servings of salmon or mackerel a week (although most seafood is good). In one study, moderate omega-3 intake from fish oil boosted the chances of remission from 26 to 59 percent. However, a newer study in more than 300 patients with Crohn's disease who were followed for more than four years showed no benefit from taking 4 grams of fish oil compared to a control group who did not get fish oil supplements. Limit margarine, butter, and fatty meats.

❏ Do not overdo carbohydrates in the diet. German studies have found that the best chances of continued remission are achieved by limiting simple carbohydrates (bread, pasta, potatoes, and rice) to about 400 calories daily and eliminating sugar altogether.

❏ During an acute attack, eat organic baby foods, steamed vegetables, and well-cooked brown rice, millet, and oatmeal. Seek medical attention if symptoms persist.

❏ Strictly avoid coffee (including decaffeinated coffee), all other sources of caffeine, and all stimulant drugs.

❏ If you are lactose intolerant, avoid milk and milk products, or use lactose-free products or soy-based ones.

❏ Avoid products sweetened with sorbitol, which draws fluid into the intestine and causes diarrhea. Sorbitol also interferes with protein absorption.

❏ If you have gluten sensitivity, avoid beer and baked goods. Some people with Crohn's disease are allergic to bakers' and brewers' yeasts. Avoiding these yeasts may make symptoms less severe.

❏ Use a heating pad to reduce abdominal pain.

❏ Do not use rectal suppositories that contain hydrogenated chemically prepared fats.

❏ To both keep the immune system in balance and reduce stress, get adequate aerobic exercise. Walking, jogging, and bicycling are all good.

Considerations

❏ Be aware that raw fruits and vegetables may be irritating while Crohn's disease is active.

❏ Some patients need supplemental iron, calcium, vitamin D, and B$_{12}$ intravenously. However, one group of investigators found that taking the usual amount of calcium and vitamin D found in three servings of dairy products or in supplements is adequate for patients with Crohn's disease, and that it does not help to take more. However, the patients in this study were in remission and it is possible that a person's needs may increase in the active state of disease. Ask your doctor if you would benefit from taking these nutrients.

❏ Probiotics have been studied in patients with Crohn's disease. One study looked at the effect of a probiotic, *Saccharomyces boulardii*, on strengthening the intestine wall to prevent toxins from permeating it. The bowel became less permeable in response to this probiotic after three months. Another study used a combination of probiotics (*Bifidobacterium and Lactobacillus*) and a prebiotic (psyllium) in Crohn's patients. The doses of each were very large—10 grams of psyllium and 45 billion cells of the probiotics, but the responses were impressive after about a year. The scoring system used to assess disease showed significant improvement, and many patients were able to use less steroid medication.

❏ Food allergies play a role in Crohn's disease. Undergo testing for food allergies and then adhere to an allergen-free diet. (*See* Food Allergies *under* ALLERGIES.) Many times people achieve remission only to have the disease return when they go back to their original diet. In one study, 84 percent of patients with Crohn's disease were found to have allergies to cheese and 84 percent to yeast. By changing their diet to remove these foods, the patients had 11 percent fewer stools and felt better.

❏ Yeast infections could indirectly aggravate Crohn's disease. Be sure to control any yeast infections as they emerge. (*See* YEAST INFECTION [YEAST VAGINITIS].)

❏ Try to reduce the effects of stress, which can aggravate Crohn's disease. (*See* STRESS.) Psychotherapy can help resolve emotional conflicts.

❏ It is important to remember that Crohn's disease tends to follow a pattern of flare-up and remission. As distressing as a flare-up can be, it is worth cultivating a positive mental state and working with practitioners who encourage you to experiment with different treatments in an effort to manage your own health. The potential for remission is always there.

❏ If Crohn's disease is active (with multiple flare-ups) for many years, bowel function gradually deteriorates. Surgery may be required to remove the diseased portion of the intestine. The surgery does not cure the disease, but it can relieve the symptoms. Five years later, at least 50 percent of those who undergo it are in good health and can work full-time without being restricted by diarrhea or pain.

❏ The symptoms of Crohn's disease are similar to those of irritable bowel syndrome. (*See* IRRITABLE BOWEL SYNDROME.)

CROUP

See under COUGH.

CUTS, SCRAPES, AND ABRASIONS

Cuts, scrapes, and abrasions are minor breaks in the skin caused by contact with sharp objects or by friction. Even simple cuts and scrapes can result in complications if there is infection or inadequate circulation. Symptoms of a local infection include a painful throbbing sensation, redness, and swelling of surrounding tissues, and heat in the wound.

If treatment is ineffective, or if the injury occurs on a part of the body affected by poor circulation, the result may be a skin abscess or skin ulcer. These conditions usually reflect problems elsewhere in the body and require medical attention. Herbal treatments may be used as primary treatment for uninfected closed cuts that heal within a few weeks. Any wound that is bleeding profusely, involves an extensive area, exposes internal organs, or is caused by an animal bite requires immediate professional treatment.

Dosages of herbs to be taken internally are for adults. A child under age six can be given one-quarter of the adult dose. A child between the ages of six and twelve can take one-half of the adult dose.

Recommendations

❑ To prevent infection, allow the injury to bleed a little so that germs are expelled. Then wash the area with soap and water or with hydrogen peroxide to clean out all visible dirt.

❑ Before treating a cut, wash your hands. Wash the wound thoroughly with mild soap and water; then apply antibiotic and herbal ointments and a clean bandage (unless no bandage is specified on the herb list).

❑ To stop moderate bleeding, apply direct pressure using a clean cloth. Do not apply a tourniquet. If the bleeding does not stop, seek professional help.

Cuts, Scrapes, and Abrasions: Beneficial Herbs

Herb	Form and Dosage	Comments
Herbs to Be Applied Externally		
Aloe	Gel. Apply to wounds that have begun to heal.	Good for frostbite, especially helpful if used with pentoxifylline (Trental).
Andiroba	Oil. Apply to wounds that have begun to heal.	Stops pain and inflammation; speeds healing process.
Bayberry or coptis or goldenseal or Oregon grape root	Apply as a cold compress once daily. (*See* COMPRESSES in Part Three.)	Stops bacterial infection of wounds.
Calendula	Cream. Apply as directed on the label, and cover with a fresh dressing daily.	Stops inflammation and stimulates production of collagen to cover broken skin. Helps to prevent infection. Good for wounds that are slow to heal.
Chamomile	German chamomile (*Matricaria recutita*) cream. Apply as directed on the label.	Prevents weeping from cuts and scrapes.
Comfrey[1]	Allantoin cream with aspirin. Apply with a fresh dressing daily.	Relieves pain and speeds healing of pus-filled wounds.
Sangre de drago[2]	Ointment. Apply without a dressing.	Forms an instant "second skin," protecting the wound and preventing infection.
St. John's wort	Oil. Apply with a fresh dressing daily.	Relieves pain and inflammation and helps prevent bacterial infection.
Herbs to Be Taken Internally		
Bromelain[3]	Tablets. Take 250–500 mg 3 times daily, before meals.	Relieves inflammation; speeds healing of skin abscesses and ulcers.
Gotu kola[4]	Liposome tablets. Take 60–120 mg daily.	Speeds healing of wounds and minimizes scar tissue.
Oligomeric proanthocyanidins (OPCs)	Grapeseed or pine-bark extract tablets. Take 100 mg daily.	Improves blood-vessel strength and flexibility. Helps slow-to-heal wounds.

Precautions for the use of herbs:

[1]Do not use comfrey if you are pregnant. Avoid contact with unaffected skin; allantoin may cause skin irritation. Wash your hands after application. Be especially careful not to rub your eyes with allantoin on your hands.

[2]Do not apply sangre de drago unless the wound has been cleaned.

[3]People who are allergic to pineapple may develop a rash from bromelain. If itching develops, stop using it.

[4]Do not use gotu kola if you are trying to become pregnant.

❏ If a cut, scrape, or abrasion is on the foot, avoid walking barefoot to avoid contact with tetanus bacteria.

❏ Do not probe a cut or remove embedded objects. Any wound that is deep and contains foreign objects requires professional attention. Do not attempt to clean a major wound after the bleeding has been brought under control.

❏ Do not breathe on an open wound.

❏ Keep local skin infections clean and dry, and apply antibiotic cream or ointment.

❏ To remove a splinter, use surgical-quality tweezers. The sort of tweezers used for plucking eyebrows is not adequate. Passing the tweezers through a flame is not adequate for sterilization; tweezers should be immersed in alcohol for at least twenty minutes prior to use. Surgical-quality tweezers are available from the Self-Care Catalog. (*See* Appendix B: Resources.) Pull the splinter out at the same angle it went in. If the splinter is just under the skin, use the tip of a sterilized needle to lift the splinter. Wash the area before applying ointments and a bandage.

Considerations

❏ A few drops of lemon juice applied to a cut or scrape will stop bleeding quickly.

❏ To prevent cuts and other injuries to children, keep knives, scissors, firearms, and breakables out of reach.

❏ Keep up-to-date vaccination records. A tetanus immunization (vaccine) is generally recommended every ten years.

❏ Consider taking a first-aid class, especially if there are young children in your household.

CYSTITIS

See BLADDER INFECTION (CYSTITIS).

DANDRUFF

Dandruff is a common scalp condition that occurs when dead skin is shed, producing irritating white flakes and, possibly, an itchy scalp. Ordinarily, dandruff results from excessive drying of the skin and overactivity of the oil glands, known as seborrhea, and may also be caused by an irritation from a yeastlike fungus called malassezia. Although dandruff is associated with the scalp, flakes may also appear on the face, nose, and eyebrows, as well as on the skin behind the ears, in the internal ear, and the skin of the trunk, particularly in creases.

Dandruff tends to run in families. Other causes and contributing factors include fatigue, stress, acne, obesity, hormonal imbalances, constant exposure to dry air, use of lotions that contain alcohol, and neurological conditions such as stroke, head injuries, and Parkinson's disease. Dandruff is not, however, the result of poor personal hygiene or the use of a dirty comb.

Sometimes switching to a less drying shampoo (so-called dandruff or medicated shampoos) is all that is needed to stop dandruff. If this does not work, then the best approach is to use herbal anti-dandruff shampoos and eat a balanced diet. If dandruff occurs with redness and severe skin irritation, it is a good idea to see a dermatologist to rule out a skin infection. Otherwise, a combination of nutritional and herbal treatments should bring improvement in six to eight weeks.

Recommendations

❏ To support healthy growth of skin, hair, and nails, take gamma-linolenic acid (GLA) daily. This essential fatty acid is found in black currant, borage, and evening primrose oils. It is usually taken in capsule form, 500 milligrams twice daily. Black currant oil is the most economical form for extended use. Flaxseeds, flaxseed oil, or fish oils from sardines or salmon also are excellent sources of the fatty acids that stop flaking.

❏ Wash your hair frequently, and use a non-oily shampoo. Use natural hair products that do not contain artificial chemicals. Avoid using irritating soaps and greasy ointments and creams.

❏ Do not use a shampoo containing selenium on a daily basis, even if it aids in controlling dandruff. Typically dandruff shampoos contain salicylic acid, coal tar, zinc, resorcin, ketoconazole, or selenium.

Dandruff: Beneficial Herbs

Herb	Form and Dosage	Comments
Burdock	Oil. Apply lightly (less than 1 tsp) to the scalp after shampooing and drying; and/or cereal (goboshi). Eat 1 serving (1 dry oz) daily.	Provides essential fatty acids for the skin.
Copaiba	Shampoo. Use daily as directed on the label; or oil. Add a few drops to commercial dandruff shampoo.	Stops inflammation and flaking.
Tea tree oil[1]	Oil. Add 2 tsp to 1 qt water and use as an after-shampoo rinse.	Eliminates fungal infection.

Precautions for the use of herbs:

[1]People who are allergic to celery or thyme should not use tea tree oil products. Do not take tea tree oil internally.

❏ Try rinsing your hair with vinegar and water instead of plain water after shampooing. Use ¼ cup vinegar to 1 quart of water.

❏ Do not pick at or scratch your scalp.

❏ Avoid eating fried foods, dairy products, chocolate, nuts, seafood, and foods containing refined sugar or flour.

Considerations

❏ Most commercial dandruff shampoos contain chemicals derived from coal tar. These shampoos can cause sensitivity to sunlight for twenty-four hours after use, and give the hair an orange-red tint. A few drops of copaiba oil added to the dandruff shampoo increase the effectiveness of the shampoo and reduce sensitivity to the sun.

❏ To make your own anti-dandruff shampoo, combine one part of propylene glycol (available from pharmacies) with four parts of baby shampoo, then add copaiba or tea tree oil. Propylene glycol, a form of glycerin, has antifungal properties and is the base of many skin creams and lotions.

❏ Dandruff in infants is known as cradle cap, and appears as thick, crusty, yellow scales on the child's scalp. Similar scales may be found on the eyelids, ears, and nose, and around the groin. To treat cradle cap, shampoo the baby's hair daily using a gentle shampoo, taking care to rinse off all the soap, and brush the hair after drying with a clean, soft brush. Massage the scalp gently with either your fingers or a soft brush to loosen scales and stimulate circulation. For difficult cases of cradle cap, apply a warm compress for up to an hour before shampooing (make sure it stays warm) or loosen the scales with mineral oil. (*See* COMPRESSES in Part Three.)

❏ Flaking associated with inflamed, weeping areas may be caused by eczema. (*See* ECZEMA.)

DEPRESSION

Almost everyone feels sad from time to time. A passing bad mood, however, is not clinical depression. Depression, one of the most common psychological disorders, can go unrecognized for years because it can produce so many different symptoms.

Symptoms of depression can include a consistently depressed mood, irritability, loss of interest or pleasure in all or nearly all activities, sleeplessness or a desire to sleep all the time, persistent feelings of guilt or worthlessness, fatigue, difficulty concentrating, a marked decrease or increase in appetite, suicidal thoughts, and physical complaints such as recurring headaches or backache.

One of the primary causes of depression is a shortage in the brain of a chemical called serotonin. Serotonin acts as a neurotransmitter, or a substance that carries impulses from one nerve cell to another. The brain and many other tissues in the body make serotonin from the amino acid tryptophan. The body's tryptophan supplies can run short for various reasons. These include stress-related hormonal changes, difficulty in getting tryptophan to cross from the bloodstream into the brain because of overabundance of other amino acids, and, in rare cases, dietary deficiency.

Depression is associated also with a deficiency in the brain's glial cells. These cells transport nutrients to the prefrontal cortex, the part of the brain that malfunctions during depression. Even with a greatly reduced number of glial cells, the brain is still able to get nutrients to the prefrontal cortex. If the allergy-provoking hormone histamine is present, however, the glial cells swell and are less effective. In addition, the glial cells carry fewer nutrients if reduced amounts of oxygen reach the brain, a reaction meant to protect the brain from disorders caused by free-radical damage.

Other factors associated with depression include tension, stress, traumatic life events, abuse, conflict, genetics, serious illness, and substance abuse. Nearly 30 percent of those with substance abuse are depressed. Other causes include hormonal problems especially related to the thyroid gland and early childhood trauma.

Psychotherapy is used to treat depression, as are a number of different drugs. While these drugs have helped many people, they do have various side effects, such as causing digestive problems, jitteriness, insomnia, and weight gain.

Most traditions of herbal healing share the view with modern psychiatry that depression is a physical condition that expresses itself in emotional symptoms. Single herbs are useful for long-term use in cases of mild to moderate depression, while formulas are best for depression accompanied by specific symptoms. No one should substitute herbal therapies for psychotherapy and/or prescribed antidepressants without first seeking guidance from both a doctor and an herbal medicine specialist. Immediately contact a suicide hot line or local emergency number if severe depression leads to thoughts of suicide.

Recommendations

❏ Maintain a cholesterol level as close to normal as possible. Especially in women between the ages of eighteen and twenty-seven, cholesterol levels below 160 milligrams per deciliter (mg/dL) are very strongly associated with anxiety and depression. Low cholesterol levels also aggravate major depression in people with panic disorder. While high cholesterol levels (200 to 220 mg/dL or more) do not prevent depression, severe diets to limit cholesterol can aggravate the condition.

❏ If you have both depression and any disease involving chronic inflammation, such as arthritis, supplement your diet with omega-3 essential fatty acids. Inflammatory illnesses could divert essential fatty acids from brain tissue. Eat two to three servings a week of cold-water fish (such

Depression: Beneficial Herbs

Herb	Form and Dosage	Comments
Ginkgo[1]	Ginkgolide tablets. Take 160–180 mg once daily.	Reverses depression, especially in older people on blood-pressure medication.
Kava kava[2]	Kavapyrone tablets. Take 60–120 mg daily. Do not exceed 120 mg.	Treats depression occurring with anxiety.
Lemon balm	Tablets or tea. Use as directed on the label.	Helps stomach and digestive organs during stressful situations.
Morinda	Capsules. Take 1,000–5,000 mg 3 times daily.	Relieves depression while enhancing male sexual function.
St. John's wort[3]	Capsules. Take 900 mg of total hypericin daily.	Useful if depression, tension, and exhaustion are combined.

Precautions for the use of herbs:

[1]Do not use ginkgo if you are taking blood-thinning medication. Discuss its use with your doctor before having any type of surgery.

[2]Kava kava increases the effects of alcohol and psychoactive drugs such as sedatives and tranquilizers. Do not use it if you are pregnant or nursing.

[3]Do not use St. John's wort if you are on prescription antidepressants or any medication that interacts with monoamine oxidase (MAO) inhibitors. Use it with caution if you are pregnant. This herb may increase the chance of developing sun blisters if you are out in the sun for too long.

Depression: Formulas

Formula	Comments
Biota Seed Pill to Nourish the Heart	A traditional Chinese herbal formula that treats age-related memory loss and accompanying symptoms of depression.
Bupleurum Plus Dragon Bone and Oyster Shell Decoction[1]	A traditional Chinese herbal formula that is particularly useful for treating depression accompanied by migraine headaches in men.
Coptis Decoction to Relieve Toxicity[2]	A traditional Chinese herbal formula that treats depression alternating with episodes of symptoms that include bleeding gums, fever, facial flushing, headaches, nervousness, or sinusitis.
Drive Out Stasis from the Mansion of Blood Decoction	A traditional Chinese herbal formula that is particularly useful for depression accompanied by migraine headaches in women, or for depression accompanied by extreme psychosomatic symptoms such as chest pain; chronic, piercing headache; and dry heaves.
Frigid Extremities Decoction[3]	A traditional Chinese herbal formula that treats depression accompanied by a queasy stomach.
Ginseng Decoction to Nourish the Nutritive Chi	A traditional Chinese herbal formula that contains small amounts of ginseng, which both softens the effects of stress and stimulates the immune system.
Licorice, Wheat, and Jujube Decoction	A traditional Chinese herbal formula that has calming actions similar to those of opium, but without causing addiction.
Pinellia and Magnolia Bark Decoction[4]	A traditional Chinese herbal formula that treats a condition in which internal stress or conflict causes a lump in the throat.
Restore the Spleen Decoction	A traditional Chinese herbal formula that treats depression that shows itself as anxiety, difficulty in maintaining concentration, fatigue of mind and body, and/or poor memory.
Vacha Rasayanas	An ayurvedic formula for depression that is associated with hyperactivity or drug dependence.
Yogaraj Guggulu	An ayurvedic formula used to treat depression occurring with loss of appetite and fluid retention, especially if there is also esophageal reflux, heartburn, or peptic ulcer.

Precautions for the use of formulas:

[1]Do not use Bupleurum Plus Dragon Bone and Oyster Shell Decoction if you have a fever.

[2]Do not use Coptis Decoction to Relieve Toxicity if you are trying to become pregnant.

[3]Stop taking Frigid Extremities Decoction if fever develops. This formula may cause a loss of sensation in the mouth and tongue.

[4]Do not use Pinellia and Magnolia Bark Decoction if you have a fever.

as salmon, tuna, or mackerel), or supplement your diet with flaxseed oil, MaxEPA fish oil, borage oil, or evening primrose oil (but fish oil and fish itself have been shown to be the most effective).

❑ In one study, patients who were depressed without other inflammatory conditions were less depressed and had better quality of life after eight weeks taking 2.5 grams of fish oil capsules.

❑ Take 200 micrograms of chromium twice daily, and 500 micrograms of vanadium—once daily, both with a meal. These minerals assist in regulating blood sugar levels and ensure a constant supply of glucose to the brain. Chromium also helps improve cognitive function and blood flow to the brain.

❑ Take 6 to 12 grams of inositol daily in two or three doses. This substance is a building block for chemicals that cause nerve transmissions to activate brain cells. If you are taking a comprehensive program of supplemental nutrition for depression, 6 grams may be enough to produce a positive effect. Otherwise, take 12 grams.

❑ Take 300 milligrams of phosphatidylserine daily. The brain depends on this compound more than any other cholesterol-based compound making up the lining of cells. It enables brain cells to use glucose efficiently and to capture and release neurotransmitters. It also protects cells from free radicals released when circulation to the brain is disturbed.

❑ If you suffer severe depression and cannot tolerate the side effects of conventional drug therapy, speak to your doctor about s-adenosylmethionine (SAMe). SAMe is a rapid, effective antidepressant with very few side effects. It acts by protecting brain cells against the effects of inflammation, and by increasing concentrations of the neurotransmitters serotonin and norepinephrine. Dosage must be set by a health-care professional. Do not give to a child under twelve.

❑ Get at least twenty minutes of sun exposure each day. Spending time in the sun slows the rate at which the brain breaks down serotonin. The brain equates spending time in dark places with sleep, for which less serotonin is needed.

❑ Exercise daily. Exercise, particularly outdoors in sunshine, increases serotonin levels in the brain. Regular vigorous physical activity causes the release of endorphins, the brain chemicals that are responsible for the so-called runner's high.

❑ Avoid tranquilizers, sleeping pills, recreational drugs, alcohol, and coffee. Especially avoid amphetamines, cocaine, barbiturates, and marijuana. All of these can make depression worse. Also avoid nasal decongestants containing the ingredient phenylpropanolamine, which has been known to induce psychiatric crises in people with depression or other mood disorders.

❑ Beware of prescription medications that may make you depressed. Physicians do not always mention that common antibiotics, blood-pressure drugs, corticosteroids, glaucoma drops, hormones, and medications to lower cholesterol can trigger depression.

❑ Do not hesitate to seek professional counseling, especially for depression marked by feelings of emotional disturbance or conflict.

❑ If you are nervous and wish to become more relaxed, consume more complex carbohydrates. For increased alertness, eat protein-based meals containing essential fatty acids. Salmon and all seafood are good choices. If you need your spirits lifted, you will benefit from eating foods like turkey and salmon, which are high in tryptophan and protein.

❑ Avoid processed foods.

❑ Avoid diet sodas and other products containing the artificial sweetener aspartame (NutraSweet, Equal). This additive may block the formation of serotonin and cause headaches, insomnia, and depression in individuals who are already serotonin-deprived.

Considerations

❑ There are several classes of antidepressant drugs. Fluoxetine (Prozac), paroxetine (Paxil), and sertraline (Zoloft) belong to the selective serotonin reuptake inhibitors (SSRIs). They keep nerve cells from absorbing serotonin, which keeps more serotonin in the gaps between nerve cells. SSRI use can cause wild dreams, hallucinations, and aggressive behavior, as well as sexual dysfunction, nausea, headaches, either insomnia or drowsiness, and diarrhea. Other classes of drugs act on serotonin and other brain chemicals. The tricyclic antidepressants—which include amitriptyline hydrochloride (Elavil), desipramine hydrochloride (Norpramin), and nortriptyline hydrochloride (Pamelor)—can cause constipation, dry mouth, and orthostatic hypotension, or a sudden drop in blood pressure when rising from a seated position. Use of the monoamine oxidase (MAO) inhibitors, such as phenelzine sulfate (Nardil) and tranylcypromine sulfate (Parnate), can lead to high blood pressure and changes in heart rate. MAO inhibitors also come with a fairly lengthy list of dietary restrictions (no pickles, certain cheeses, wine), and decongestants should be avoided.

❑ Antidepressant medications are often an effective way to treat depression and other mental disorders in children and adolescents. However, antidepressants do pose a risk of harmful side effects and complications. In fact, antidepressants are required to carry strong warnings about their possible link to suicidal behavior in children, adolescents, and young adults aged eighteen to twenty-four years. If your child is depressed, make sure you consult a health-care practitioner who is experienced in drug treatments for children.

❑ SSRIs exert effects for between four and six weeks after one stops taking them. During this period, they can produce dangerous drug interactions with either MAO inhibitors or certain herbal medications, such as St. John's wort.

❑ The discovery of the relationship between tryptophan and serotonin led to the beginning of an understanding of the relationship between food and mood. Tryptophan enters the brain more readily if blood sugar levels are high. When the extra tryptophan reaches the brain, it is turned into serotonin that stops depression. Bingeing on sugar during depression—which is not recommended—is in fact a form of self-treatment for the condition.

❑ Naturopathic medicine links depression to a shortage of a vitaminlike compound called tetrahydrobiopterin (BH4). This compound is needed for the creation of several neurotransmitters. Vitamin C, folic acid, and vitamin B$_{12}$ (cobalamin) may stimulate the body's production of BH4. B vitamins are also known to increase the effectiveness of tricyclic antidepressants.

❑ Some patients have benefited from acupuncture, which usually has no side effects. (See ACUPUNCTURE in Part Three.)

❑ Seasonal affective disorder (SAD) is a condition in which the body is not exposed to enough sunlight to maintain normal levels of serotonin. In North America, it occurs mostly in Canada and the states bordering Canada, and affects twice as many women as men. Fortunately, treatment of SAD is very simple. Spending thirty minutes a day under a full-spectrum lamp, or under very bright artificial light, or in a "light box," should begin to improve symptoms in three to four weeks. Avoid taking the sleep-regulating hormone melatonin while taking artificial light treatment; while taking melatonin at night could help, it can also make insomnia worse as days grow longer in late winter. For more information on SAD, contact the National Organization for Seasonal Affective Disorder (NOSAD). (See Appendix B: Resources.)

❑ Never use a light therapy box when taking khella, psoralea, or St. John's wort. These herbs may sensitize the retina to bright light and raise the risk of ocular damage from using the box. Do not use a light therapy box without your doctor's approval if you are taking any prescription medication that increases sensitivity to sunlight, such as fosinopril (Monopril) or lisinopril (Zestril, Prinivil), for high blood pressure, frequently prescribed for people who have both depression and high blood pressure.

❑ People with depression are more likely than other people to have various disturbances in calcium metabolism. Ask your doctor if you need calcium supplements.

❑ People who smoke are more likely than nonsmokers to be depressed.

❑ Steroid drugs and oral contraceptives may cause serotonin levels in the brain to drop.

❑ Music can have powerful effects on mood and may be useful in alleviating depression. Color also can have an effect. Many people feel better if they alter the predominant colors in their environment.

❑ See also ANXIETY, CHRONIC FATIGUE SYNDROME, INSOMNIA, and MEMORY DISORDER PROBLEMS.

DERMATITIS

See ECZEMA; HIVES.

DIABETES

Diabetes mellitus is a disorder in which the body is unable to regulate glucose, the fuel used by cells to produce energy, and insulin, a hormone that helps glucose enter cells. This causes glucose to accumulate in the bloodstream. The primary symptoms of diabetes are fatigue, hunger, thirst, increased frequency of urination, and unintended weight loss (in fact, you may lose weight even though you start to eat more than before). Acute blood sugar problems can lead to dizziness, sweating, and confusion.

There are two types of diabetes mellitus. In type 1 diabetes, formerly known as insulin-dependent or juvenile-onset diabetes, the body cannot produce enough insulin. Type 1 diabetes usually starts in childhood, although it can develop in adults. Treatment of type 1 diabetes always requires insulin by injections or a pump. Type 2 diabetes, also known as non-insulin-dependent or adult-onset diabetes, involves insulin resistance, a condition in which cells in the skeletal muscles and liver do not respond to insulin and cannot absorb needed sugars. This usually happens despite increased insulin production, so that the blood contains both too much insulin and too much glucose. In other words, the insulin is no longer working properly. Initial treatment of type 2 diabetes usually consists of weight

Risk Factors for Diabetes

Risk factors for type 1 diabetes include the following:

- Family history
- Genetics
- Geography (living farther away from the equator)
- Viral exposure, such as to Epstein-Barr virus
- Low vitamin D levels

Risk factors for type 2 diabetes include:

- Overweight
- Abdominal fat
- Inactivity
- Family history
- Race (including blacks, Hispanics, American Indians, and Asian-Americans)
- Age
- Prediabetes (where the blood sugar is higher than normal)
- Gestational diabetes (diabetes when you are pregnant)

loss, exercise, and oral drugs. Over time, if blood sugars are not carefully regulated, the bodies of people with type 2 diabetes also lose their capacity to make insulin, and insulin injections become necessary for them.

In type 2 diabetes, insulin made by the body can be rendered ineffective for a number of reasons. Obesity or high blood pressure can restrict the flow of insulin to muscle cells. Since fat cells may compete with other cells for insulin, having 300 times as many receptor sites for insulin as muscle cells, type 2 diabetes accelerates the accumulation of body fat, which in turn worsens the diabetes. Insulin is nature's storage hormone, so when it is in the blood, the body turns food including glucose into fat. Often the fat accumulates around the midriff. Insulin's effectiveness can be reduced by other factors, including hormonal reactions to stress and changes in female hormones. There are also relatively rare conditions in which liver and muscle cells can develop a deficiency of insulin receptor sites that makes them insensitive to insulin.

Diabetes has long-term complications unless blood-sugar levels are meticulously monitored and controlled. If sugars are allowed to soar, the brain, nerve tissues, and the lens of the eye—all of which absorb glucose without insulin's help—become saturated with glucose, which becomes toxic. This can result in diabetic neuropathy, a nerve disorder that can cause numbness, sensitivity, or pain; difficulty in swallowing or in controlling the bladder; atrophy of the nerves serving the digestive tract known as gastroparesis; and mild mania and mood swings. Visual problems can result from cataracts or diabetic retinopathy, in which blood vessels in the retina break.

Diabetes is a risk factor for atherosclerosis, the process in which cholesterol plaques develop in the blood vessels. The tendency of people with diabetes to develop poor circulation results in a dramatic increase in the risk of various cardiovascular problems. The risk of stroke more than doubles within the first five years of being treated for type 2 diabetes. About 75 percent of people with diabetes have some type of heart or blood-vessel disease. Diabetes may leave the skin vulnerable to infections and sores, including bacterial and fungal infections. The skin on the feet is prone to ulceration, cuts, and blistering. Diabetes can also cause erectile dysfunction (ED) through both poor circulation and damage to the nerves to the penis. In addition, years of stress caused by removing huge quantities of sugar out of the blood into the urine eventually causes the kidneys to "leak" protein and fail. The risk of dementia and Alzheimer's disease increases with prolonged periods of poor blood sugar control.

Almost every person who has diabetes sometimes finds his or her own blood sugars difficult to control. Almost every person who has diabetes at least occasionally "falls off the wagon" and consumes too much carbohydrates, resulting in blood sugars that are too high. There are also factors in diabetes management that are variable and difficult to manage. Foods do not release their sugars in the digestive tract in the same way every time; a very ripe apple, for example, will cause a faster surge in blood sugars than a slightly green apple. (A purely sugary food, such as a candy bar, on the other hand, produces the same detrimental effect every time.) Medications are usually absorbed to the same extent; absorption is influenced by the other contents of the stomach. There is up to 30 percent variability in the amount of insulin absorbed into the bloodstream even if the same dose is injected every time.

Managing diabetes requires thinking small. Small amounts of food—even the right food—keep sugars from surging. Small quantities of prescribed medication taken several times a day and small injections of insulin taken several times a day rather than in a single dose keep sugars at a more even level, but may result in more night-time low blood sugar episodes. Brief periods of exercise on a regular basis increase the chances of hypoglycemia appearing in the short term (a couple of hours afterward), but long-term, exercise is essential for good glucose control. If you are worried about this, monitor your blood sugars after exercise for up to three hours and consume food as necessary. Small mistakes in diabetes control have consequences for health.

Herbal treatment also has small but beneficial effects. Some herbal treatments can control blood sugar levels, while others may ease diabetic complications. A number of the herbs listed here have overlapping functions because, for reasons of availability or allergy or contraindications, one may need to change herbs from time to time. That is why it is always important to consult a doctor and herbal medicine specialist before using herbal remedies as part of an overall treatment program.

Herbs may be appropriate for type 1 or type 2 diabetes, or both. (For more complete discussions of the herbs recommended below, see the individual entries under The Herbs in Part One.) If your child has type 1 diabetes, consult the child's doctor before using herbs. Children are more susceptible to blood sugar swings than adults.

Unless otherwise specified, the herb dosages recommended here are for adults, and some herbs are not suitable for children at all. Children under age six can be given one-quarter of the adult dosage. Children between the ages of six and twelve can take one-half of the adult dosage. Formula dosages for children should be discussed with a knowledgeable health-care practitioner.

Recommendations

❑ To use astragalus and rehmannia together, thoroughly mix equal parts of the loose teas in a container. Place 1 teaspoon of the mixture in 1 cup of boiling water, steep for fifteen minutes, and strain before using.

❑ If you are experiencing weight gain while gaining control over blood sugar levels in type 2 diabetes, use pedra hume caa as a tea. Take 1 cup of tea made with 1 teaspoon (2 grams) of the herb three times daily. (See TEAS in Part Three.)

Diabetes: Beneficial Herbs

Herb	Form and Dosage	Comments
Treatments Appropriate for People with Type 2 Diabetes		
Agrimony	Tea (loose), prepared by steeping 1½ tsp (1.5 gm) in 1 cup water. (*See* TEAS in Part Three.) Take 1 cup 3 times daily.	Helps prevent progression of type 2 to type 1 diabetes.
Aloe[1]	Juice. Take 2–4 tbsp daily.	Stimulates insulin production without causing weight gain. Prevents high triglycerides.
Cajueiro	Tincture. Take as directed on the label.	Helps muscle and liver cells respond to insulin.
Garlic[2]	Fresh cloves, preferably raw. Eat 2–3 in food daily.	Stimulates insulin production; prevents insulin deactivation by the liver.
Nopal	Leaf. Use in cooking as desired.	Blocks the absorption of sugars. Also helps to prevent atherosclerosis.
Rehmannia and astragalus[3]	Tea. Drink 1 cup 3 times daily.	Treats blood-vessel complications.
Wild angelica[4]	*Angelica dahurica* capsules. Take 1,000–3,000 mg daily.	Reduces weight gain caused by oral diabetes medications.
Treatments Appropriate for People with Either Type 1 or Type 2 Diabetes		
Atractylodis[5]	Tea. Take as prescribed by dispensing herbalist.	Produces dramatic drops to normal if sugar levels are over 300 mg/dL. Also helps to protect against retinopathy.
Bitter melon[6]	Fruit, whole. Use 1–2 fruits in cooking daily. Use for 4 weeks; then discontinue for 4 weeks.	Increases the availability of glucose to muscles. Keeps sugars from being absorbed through intestine.
Bromelain[7]	Tablets. Take 250–500 mg 3 times daily, before meals.	Compensates for delayed movement of food from stomach due to nerve damage (gastroparesis).
Burdock	Cereal (*goboshi* in Japanese groceries), as desired.	Reduces after-meal sugar surges by providing fiber.
Chanca piedra	Tincture. Take as directed on the label.	Retards progression of neuropathy and retinopathy.
Chiretta	Tincture. Use as directed on the label.	Prevents after-meal sugar surges without increasing the risk of hypoglycemia.
Fenugreek	Seeds. Use 1 oz (25 gm) in cooking daily.	Slows absorption of sugars through intestine; sensitizes muscle to insulin. Also known as medhika.
Ginkgo[8]	Ginkgolide tablets. Take 40 mg 3 times daily or 60 mg twice daily.	Reduces blood-vessel damage and retinopathy risk.
Ginseng	*Panax ginseng* tincture. Take as directed on the label.	Prolongs effect of Lente and Ultralente insulin for types 1 and 2. Stimulates insulin production in type 2.
Green tea	Catechin extract. Take 240 mg 3 times daily; or tea bag, prepared with 1 cup water. Take 1 cup 2–5 times daily. To avoid dilution, do not use within 1 hour of taking other medications.	Slows sugar release from starchy foods. Also keeps blood from becoming "sticky"; protects against atherosclerosis and retinopathy.
Gurmar	Gymnemic acid or GS4. Take 400 mg daily.	Sometimes restores ability of pancreas to secrete insulin. Discourages cravings for sweets.
Jambul	Fruit pulp or seeds. Used in cooking as desired.	Reduces the risk of cataracts.
Juniper berries	Use as directed on the label.	Lowers blood glucose levels.
Licorice[9]	Glycyrrhizin tablets. Take 200 mg daily. Use for 6 weeks; then take a 2-week break. Do not substitute deglycyrrhizinated licorice (DGL).	Helps prevent cataracts. Consume potassium-rich foods such as bananas or citrus juices, or take a potassium supplement daily when taking this herb.
Pau d'arco	Tincture. Take as directed on the label.	Reduces spillover of glucose into the urine, lowering very high sugar levels. Also fights yeast infection.
Scutellaria[10]	Tablets. Take 250–500 mg 3 times daily.	High zinc content helps prevent atherosclerosis.

Precautions for the use of herbs:

[1] Do not take aloe vera juice internally if you have diarrhea.

[2] Garlic counteracts the effects of *Bifidus* and *Lactobacillus* cultures taken as digestive aids. Consult a doctor before using garlic on a regular basis if you are on an anticoagulant drug such as warfarin (Coumadin). Discuss the use of garlic with your doctor before having any type of surgery. Raw garlic can cause heartburn and flatulence.

[3] Do not use astragalus if you have a fever or a skin infection.

[4] Do not use wild angelica if you are pregnant.

[5] Do not use atractylodis if you have diarrhea or are sweating profusely.

[6] Do not use bitter melon if you have cirrhosis of the liver or a medical history of hepatitis or HIV infection compounded by liver infections.

[7] People who are allergic to pineapple may develop a rash from bromelain. If itching develops, stop using it.

[8] Do not use ginkgo if you are taking blood-thinning medication. Discuss its use with your doctor before having any type of surgery.

[9] Do not use licorice if you have glaucoma, high blood pressure, or an estrogen-sensitive disorder such as breast cancer, endometriosis, or fibrocystic breasts.

[10] Do not take scutellaria if you have diarrhea.

Diabetes: Formulas

Formula	Comments
Coptis Decoction to Relieve Toxicity[1]	A traditional Chinese herbal formula that treats yeast infections aggravated by diabetes, especially thrush and esophageal yeast infections causing heartburn.
Eight-Ingredient Pill with Rehmannia	A traditional Chinese herbal formula that lowers blood sugar, aids insulin regulation, and treats diabetic neuropathy in type 1 diabetes. It prevents eye and circulation problems.
Major Bupleurum Decoction[2]	A traditional Chinese herbal formula that reduces the rate at which glucose enters the bloodstream after meals and increases the efficiency of insulin. This formula is especially useful if diabetes occurs with long-term gastrointestinal disorders.
Minor Bupleurum Decoction[3]	A traditional Chinese herbal formula that reduces the rate at which glucose enters the bloodstream after meals. This formula is particularly useful if diabetes occurs either with HIV or as a complication of hepatitis infection.
Six-Ingredient Pill with Rehmannia[4]	A traditional Chinese herbal formula that treats symptoms that may accompany diabetes: lower-back soreness, lightheadedness, tinnitus, diminished hearing, night sweats, chronic dry or sore throat, toothache, or wasting.
White Tiger Plus Atractylodis Decoction[5]	A traditional Chinese herbal formula that lowers sugar levels by increasing the amount of sugar stored in the liver. It relieves cold feelings in the lower part of the body, a general feeling of heaviness, joint pain, and sweating.
White Tiger Plus Ginseng Decoction[5]	A traditional Chinese herbal formula that lowers sugar levels by increasing the amount of sugar stored in the liver. It relieves fever, thirst, profuse sweating, and generalized weakness.

Precautions for the use of formulas:

[1]Do not use Coptis Decoction to Relieve Toxicity if you are trying to become pregnant.

[2]Do not use Major Bupleurum Decoction if you have fever.

[3]Do not use Minor Bupleurum Decoction if you have a fever or a skin infection. Taken long term, it can cause headache, dizziness, and bleeding gums. Side effects can be avoided if the formula is taken as a tea.

[4]Do not use Six-Ingredient Pill with Rehmannia if you have an estrogen-sensitive disorder, such as breast cancer, endometriosis, or fibrocystic breasts.

[5]Do not use White Tiger Decoctions if you are experiencing nausea or vomiting.

❏ If food allergies or celiac disease is a problem with either type of diabetes, use wild yam (dioscorea) to lower blood sugars. Take 20 drops of tincture in ¼ cup of water three times daily after meals. Avoid overdosage, which can cause nausea.

❏ Milk thistle (silymarin) has been used to lower blood sugar levels in patients with type 2 diabetes. In one study, patients with type 2 diabetes who were taking other medications to lower blood sugar levels used 200 milligrams of silymarin three times a day. These patients had lower fasting blood sugar, total cholesterol, hemoglobin A1c (HgA1c), and triglycerides as well as healthy liver tests. Another group of patients with type 2 diabetes used 200 milligrams only once a day and had reduced fasting and postprandial glucose levels, and lower HgA1c and body mass indexes (BMIs). The patients in this study were already taking a drug to increase insulin secretions, glyburide (Micronase), and the silymarin enhanced the effect of the drug. Milk thistle may cause mild diarrhea when first used, especially if fatty foods are eaten.

❏ To reduce the pain associated with diabetic neuropathy, use cayenne in the form of capsaicin cream applied over the affected area (do not apply to broken skin). St. John's wort can also help; take 900 milligrams in capsule form for three to four weeks. St. John's wort has an action similar to the commonly prescribed amitriptyline (Elavil).

❏ Curcumin is thought to help control insulin and glucose levels in the blood.

❏ Ginseng is commonly used by people with diabetes to control blood sugar levels. However, one study found that the ginseng rootlets were more effective than other parts of the plant. One compound, Rg1, is found in higher amounts in the rootlets, and this is thought to be responsible for lowering blood sugar levels. Using 2 grams a day of the rootlets has been shown to be as effective as using 6 grams.

❏ Do not solely rely on herbs to control blood glucose levels. In an extensive review of the utility of using Chinese herbs to control blood sugar levels, although many were effective, most of the studies were poorly designed, making it difficult to confirm the proper doses and types of herbs that were most effective. Dietary control is more important in managing blood sugar levels than using herbs, but they can be used together.

❏ To avoid large fluctuations in sugar levels, try adopting a low glycemic-load diet. Foods included in this diet are any low-fat meats and dairy, which have virtually no impact on blood sugar levels. Vegetables and most fruits have very small effects. However, fruits have a bit more effect on blood sugar levels than vegetables and should be limited to two pieces a day. Whole grains raise blood sugar levels somewhat, and therefore they should be limited to one serving per meal. Also avoid refined flours and sugars, especially in between meals as snacks. One or two drinks containing alcohol with a meal slow the liver's ability to convert protein into glucose and could result in lower blood sugar, but this effect could be lost if simple carbohydrates (bread, pasta, and potatoes) or sweets are eaten. Dietary fat slows the absorption of sugars from food and also results in temporarily lower blood sugars; however, the temporary improvement in blood sugars is far more than offset by the long-term problems caused by overweight.

❏ Be sure to eat on a regular schedule—do not skip meals.

❏ Take 500 micrograms of vanadium and 50 to 100 milligrams of coenzyme Q_{10} (Co-Q_{10}) daily. Vanadium, a trace mineral, mimics insulin and prevents increases in blood sugar levels after carbohydrate consumption. Co-Q_{10} increases the formation of enzymes that help cells turn glucose into energy.

❏ Chromium (200 mcg) may also help lower blood glucose levels.

❏ Vitamin D may help patients with type 1 diabetes manage their blood sugar control, if they are vitamin D deficient. In one study, patients with type 1 diabetes who took 400 IU of vitamin D and 1,200 milligrams of calcium each day had lower HbA1c levels.

❏ Fish oil may improve blood flow, which is often impaired in diabetes. In one study, patients with type 2 diabetes who took 2 grams a day of fish oil for six weeks had improved blood flow relative to a placebo group. This suggests that long-term use of fish oil capsules and eating a seafood-rich diet would help protect the vascular system and keep blood flowing better.

❏ The way the body processes vitamin A and zinc is disrupted in type 1 diabetes. In one study, patients with this condition were given 10 milligrams of zinc and 6,250 international units (IU) of vitamin A. Improvements were seen in markers of heart disease risk such as increase in apoprotein A-1. These nutrients can easily be obtained from a daily multivitamin capsule.

❏ Do not use extra insulin to "cover" indulging in sweets. Extra insulin causes carbohydrates to be stored as glycogen in the liver, temporarily keeping blood sugars from going unusually high. In the long run, however, the liver has limited storage capacity and the stored sugar has to be burned off in exercise to keep sugars from surging after the next normal carbohydrate meal.

❏ If you are medically cleared for exercise, adopt the postal service motto of "Neither rain nor sleet nor snow, nor gloom of night . . ." with regard to daily workouts. Jogging, bicycling, and swimming are good aerobic exercise, helpful in "toning" the cardiovascular system. If finding time to exercise is a problem, perform (with your doctor's approval) anaerobic exercise instead. Strength-building exercises such as weightlifting, performed three to four times a week, create new muscle cells that use sugars and take excess insulin out of circulation. Both cardiovascular and muscle-building exercise programs reduce the need for insulin and prevent diabetic complications. Talk to your doctor about designing an exercise program that best suits your needs. Many people with diabetes who use insulin experience low blood sugar a couple of hours after exercise. Just be aware of this and watch for drops in blood sugar levels.

❏ Check sugar levels regularly at home, especially if making any medication (prescription or herbal) changes to your treatment program.

❏ Have annual eye exams and tests for kidney function. Get HbA1c tests every three months to monitor blood sugar control.

❏ Perform a daily foot inspection, and bring foot infections to the doctor's attention promptly.

❏ Always keep emergency glucose on hand if you are using insulin. If you feel unexpectedly faint, dizzy, or irritable, check your blood sugars. If your sugars are below 50 milligrams per deciliter (mg/dL), you are experiencing hypoglycemia and need glucose replacement. Take one tube of glucose gel, from three to five glucose tablets, or half a sugared (not sugar-free) soft drink, wait twenty minutes, and check your sugar levels again. Continue taking glucose as long as sugars remain below 70 mg/dL. If hypoglycemia occurs within three hours of taking an injection of "fast" insulin, you will need to monitor your sugar levels at least hourly until five hours after taking the injection.

❏ Supplement your diet with spirulina. Spirulina may help to stabilize blood sugar levels. Other foods that may help to normalize blood sugar include berries, dairy products, eggs, fish, garlic, sauerkraut, soybeans, and vegetables.

❏ If you have a child with diabetes, be sure his or her teacher knows how to respond to the warning signs of hypoglycemia and hyperglycemia.

Considerations

❏ Accu-Check Comfort Curve test strips can eliminate uncomfortable bruising caused by the finger pricking needed for blood tests. These strips use a smaller drop of blood and draw the sample into the test chamber by a wicking action, eliminating the need to squeeze out a drop. The curve of the strip fits the contours of the fingers, so it is possible to use more puncture sites and avoid calluses.

❏ Diabetes and depression often go together. Recovery from depression may improve diabetes symptoms without changes in body weight or diet. (*See* DEPRESSION.) If you feel sad for a long period of time, seek counseling. This is a very common problem and can be readily treated.

❏ Type 2 diabetes and constipation may go together. It is important to avoid stimulant laxatives for relief of constipation, since they cause fluctuations in fluid levels that also cause changes in blood sugar levels (mostly upward). Natural plants such as psyllium have been shown to lower blood sugar and address constipation.

❏ While type 2 diabetes mostly occurs in older adults, it can affect children as well. Any overweight child should receive a thorough physical examination, especially if there is unusual thirst as well as unusual hunger.

❏ If chronic pain is a concern, *see* PAIN, CHRONIC.

❏ Coronary artery disease is very common in people with diabetes. So is high blood pressure, which can lead to kidney disease.

❏ *See also* ATHEROSCLEROSIS, CATARACTS, DIABETIC RETINOPATHY, HIGH CHOLESTEROL, KIDNEY DISEASE, OVERWEIGHT, and YEAST INFECTION (YEAST VAGINITIS).

DIABETIC RETINOPATHY

Diabetic retinopathy is an eye disorder that affects the retina, the "projection screen" on which light that passes through the lens of the eye is thrown. In diabetic retinopathy, the capillaries that nourish the retina leak fluid or blood. This leakage results in inadequate circulation to the cells that respond to light and relay visual impulses to the optic nerve, which carries these impulses to the brain. Diabetic retinopathy is a common cause of blindness in people with severe diabetes. There usually are no symptoms until the individual begins to lose vision.

The risk factors for diabetic retinopathy include poorly controlled blood sugar levels, age, the length of time the

Diabetic Retinopathy: Beneficial Herbs

Herb	Form and Dosage	Comments
Bilberry	Tablets. Take 240–360 mg daily.	Helps prevent clotting in blood vessels serving the retina.
Chanca piedra	Tincture. Take 1 dropperful in ½ cup water twice daily.	Stops the formation of compounds that damage the retina.
Ginkgo[1]	Ginkgolide tablets. Take 160–180 mg once daily.	Prevents damage in retina cells responsible for distinguishing colors.
Hawthorn	Tablets. Take 100–250 mg 3 times daily.	Helps strengthen blood vessels supplying the eye's surface. Reduces blood-vessel response to emotional tension.
Jambul	Seeds. Use 2 tsp–1 tbsp (3–5 gm) in cooking daily.	Lowers blood sugars. Retards blood-vessel inflammation.
Oligomeric proanthocyanidins (OPCs)	Grapeseed or pine-bark extract tablets. Take 200 mg daily.	Antioxidant. Reduces blood-vessel inflammation.
Quercetin[2]	Tablets. Take 125–250 mg 3 times daily, between meals.	Slows formation of insulinlike growth factor I. Prevents blood clots.
Soy isoflavone concentrate	Tablets. Take about 3,000 mg once daily.	Slows formation of insulinlike growth factor I.

Precautions for the use of herbs:

[1]Do not use ginkgo if you are taking blood-thinning medication. Discuss its use with your doctor before having any type of surgery.

[2]Do not use quercetin if you are taking cyclosporine (Neoral, Sandimmune) or nifedipine (Procardia).

Diabetic Retinopathy Formulas

Formula	Comments
Eight-Ingredient Pill with Rehmannia	A traditional Chinese herbal formula that smoothes out blood sugar levels, providing tighter control. This prevents eye and circulation problems.

individual has had diabetes, and the presence of a "sticky" protein in the blood called glycosylated hemoglobin (HgA1c). Another risk factor for diabetic retinopathy is the presence of insulinlike growth factor I, a hormone produced in excess during diabetes. This hormone encourages the growth of fragile capillaries in the eye that easily break and leak fluid. Conventional treatment consists of laser surgery, which seals the leaking blood vessels.

Herbal treatments for diabetic retinopathy are primarily preventative. Herbs that provide large quantities of bioflavonoids strengthen the capillaries and may slow the progress of or prevent retinopathy. The best preventative for diabetic retinopathy, however, is careful control of blood sugars and regular eye exams to catch problems early.

Recommendations

❏ Follow the diet and exercise recommendations listed under DIABETES.

❏ Eat blackberries, blueberries, and cherries to the extent that they are allowed in your diet. These fruits contain proanthocyanidins similar to those in hawthorn, and may help strengthen the tiny blood vessels serving the retina.

❏ Take 1,000 milligrams of glutamine daily. Glutamine may slow or prevent damage to the retina, even after damage to the blood vessels serving it, by preventing free-radical damage. However, do not take glutamine supplements if you have cirrhosis of the liver or kidney problems, or if you have had Reye's syndrome.

❏ Don't skip insulin shots to try to lose weight. There are numerous reports in the medical literature, especially among teenagers and adult women, of people who developed diabetic retinopathy after reducing insulin dosage or skipping injections altogether as a form of weight control.

❏ Some people suggest that high doses of vitamin C may improve capillary strength and thus slow the progression of diabetic retinopathy. In one study, people with diabetes who used 1 gram a day of vitamin C had eye capillary strength returned to normal. If you take vitamin C, do not suddenly stop using it, as it could lead to a dramatic fall in blood levels and cause adverse effects to the retina.

❏ Make sure to have an annual eye exam to detect the onset of retinopathy. Laser surgery can help stem vision loss. Sometimes surgery is necessary, but prevention is a superior approach.

Considerations

❏ Tight control is a program of keeping as close to a normal (nondiabetic) blood glucose level as possible. Ideally this means levels between 70 and 130 mg/dL before meals and when you wake up, and less than 180 mg/dL two hours after starting a meal. You should set your goals with your doctor. Keeping a normal level all the time is not practical. And it's not needed to get results. Every bit

you lower your blood glucose level helps to prevent complications. Tight control can be confirmed by a blood test for HbA1c, or the percentage of "sticky" red blood cells. A reading below 7 percent confirms tight control. This program, now recommended for all people with diabetes, reduces the risk of retinopathy by about 60 percent.

❏ Tight control is one part of a larger overall program known as intensive therapy. This approach uses, in addition to tight control, a combination of diet, exercise, and medication to control high blood pressure. In a study of 166 people with diabetes, intensive therapy reduced the incidence of retinopathy by another 55 percent, in addition to producing even more dramatically lowered rates of nerve damage and kidney disease. The cost of tight control, however, is weight gain. Despite eating the same number of calories as people in a control group, and eating less fat, those on intensive therapy for two years gained an average of 9 pounds (4 kilograms) more than their counterparts in the control group. However, this effect can be offset by adherence to proper diet and exercise and possibly by using the herb wild angelica. (See DIABETES.)

❏ Although not a substitute for other treatments including surgery, acupuncture may help support normal circulation to the eye, which may favorably affect diabetic retinopathy. (See ACUPUNCTURE in Part Three.) Some have found that it may also lower eye pressures caused by glaucoma, which can accompany retinopathy. (See GLAUCOMA.)

DIAPER RASH

Researchers have conducted hundreds of studies to get to the bottom of diaper rash, also known as diaper dermatitis. Many of the studies simply confirm common sense: the wetter the diaper, the worse the diaper rash. A number of factors have been found to worsen diaper rash, including early introduction of cereals in the baby's diet and putting the baby to sleep on his or her back.

Diaper rash can be caused either by mechanical irritation or by infection. Contact diaper rash—that is, diaper rash caused by a reaction to stool, urine, soaps, disposable diapers, or plastic pants—produces redness and irritation. There may be swollen areas, and the skin may be dry and scaling, with discolored patches. Contact rash is often treated with zinc oxide, a standard drugstore remedy, and an ingredient in many products such as A + D Ointment, Balmex, and Desitin. Zinc oxide can also prevent diaper rash on non-irritated skin.

Infectious diaper rash can be caused by either yeast (*Candida albicans*) or bacteria (*Staphylococcus aureus*, commonly known as "staph"). Both infections make the skin bright red, shiny, and smooth, although staph may also cause small ulcerations to form. Candidal infections are generally treated with oral antifungal medications, while staph is treated with steroid creams instead of oral medications.

Diaper Rash: Beneficial Herbs

Herb	Form and Dosage	Comments
Calendula	Cream. Apply as directed on the label. Cover the entire rash.	Promotes wound healing; prevents viral infection. Mildly antibacterial.
Chamomile	German chamomile (*Matricaria recutita*) cream. Apply as directed on the label. Cover the entire rash.	Stops inflammation and allergic irritation.
Coptis	Finely ground powder. Apply ⅛ tsp in talcum powder over affected area.	Stops both staph and yeast infections. Can use goldenseal instead.
Licorice	Simicort cream. Apply as directed on the label. Cover the entire rash.	Fights inflammation.

It usually pays to have the rash diagnosed so the proper treatment can be used. For contact diaper rash, alternate any of the following herbs (except for coptis) with zinc oxide, using the zinc at one diaper changing and the herb at the next. To control infectious diaper rash, use coptis in addition to any prescription medication. All the herbs listed here are for external use only. Do not give any herbs to babies still in diapers until you speak with the child's pediatrician.

Recommendations

❏ To speed healing, wash the baby's bottom with an acidified liquid detergent, made by adding ½ to 1 teaspoon of lemon juice to the bathwater, but check with your pediatrician first.

❏ Make sure you use soft diapers. Scratchy diapers constantly irritate the skin.

❏ Because zinc oxide has a drying effect, do not apply it to cracked or dry skin.

❏ Your baby may be given an antifungal cream for candidal diaper rash (caused by yeast infection). Ask your doctor about the need for acidophilus supplements to reestablish a healthy bacterial balance in the baby's digestive system. Acidophilus (a supplemental form of the "friendly" microbe *Lactobacillus acidophilus*) helps keep harmful yeasts from taking root in the skin. Use ⅛ to ¼ teaspoon daily in formula.

Considerations

❏ It is vitally important that steroid drugs for diaper rash be given externally, and not orally or by injection.

❏ Children who wear disposable diapers may suffer from diaper rash more than children who wear cloth diapers. Diaper wipes also cause skin irritation, so use ones without scents.

DIARRHEA

Diarrhea is an increase in the fluidity, frequency, and volume of bowel movements. It may be accompanied by cramping, nausea, vomiting, thirst, or fever. Diarrhea is a common symptom that usually signifies a mild and temporary condition. However, chronic diarrhea requires medical attention. Diarrhea is also a concern if a person must maintain constant medication levels in the bloodstream, such as levels of lithium, antiseizure drugs, or diabetes medications.

Diarrhea can be caused by a number of disorders. One of the most common is food poisoning, in which various microorganisms attack the digestive system. Disorders that can cause diarrhea include AIDS; food intolerance; gallbladder or pancreatic disease; inflammatory bowel disease, such as Crohn's disease; and irritable bowel syndrome. Other factors that can cause or contribute to diarrhea include bowel surgery; chemotherapy or radiation treatment; consuming too much vitamin C, artificial sweeteners such as sorbitol, or caffeine; withdrawal from addictive drugs; some forms of cancer; and the use of laxatives that contain magnesium, phosphate, or sulfate.

In some cases, diarrhea may accompany fecal incontinence, in which the person cannot control bowel movements. This can result from surgery, spinal injuries, stroke, dementia, or damage to the nerves that serve the rectum.

Use any of the following herbs for diarrhea until symptoms subside. However, if diarrhea is chronic (lasting more than three days), consult a doctor. Unless otherwise specified, the herb dosages recommended here are for adults. Children under age six should be given one-quarter of the adult dosage. Children between the ages of six and twelve should be given one-half of the adult dosage. Formula dosages for children should be discussed with a knowledgeable health-care practitioner.

Recommendations

❏ Reduce your consumption of coffee and other sources of caffeine. Too much caffeine can cause diarrhea.

❏ Drink plenty of liquids, but nothing too hot or too cold. The prolonged loss of fluids as a result of diarrhea can lead to dehydration and loss of necessary minerals. Canned soup, which is high in sodium (salt), and orange juice, which is high in potassium, are good choices. Dilute the juice so that it is half water, half juice. Sip slowly.

Diarrhea: Beneficial Herbs

Herb	Form and Dosage	Comments
Agrimony	Tea (loose), prepared by steeping 1½ tsp (1.5 gm) in 1 cup water. (*See* TEAS in Part Three.) Take 1 cup 2–3 times daily.	"Tans" cells lining the intestine to prevent fluid from entering the intestines.
Bilberry	Tea bag, prepared with 1 cup water. Sip 1–2 cups throughout the day. Frequent, small doses are best.	"Tans" cells lining the intestine.
Chen-pi[1]	Tea (loose), prepared by steeping 1 tsp (2–3 gm) in 1 cup cold water. (*See* TEAS in Part Three.) Take 1 cup 3 times daily, before meals; or whole fruit, including peel. Dice finely and eat 1 bitter orange daily.	Relaxes smooth muscles lining the digestive tract. Also known as bitter orange.
Epimedium[2]	Use under the direction of a dispensing herbalist.	Relieves incontinence by encouraging tissue growth in sphincter muscles.
Fenugreek	Tea. Use as directed on the label.	Lubricates the intestines and reduces fever.
Marshmallow root	Tea. Use as directed on the label.	Helps calm the stomach and soothe intestinal problems.
Psyllium seed	Powder. Use as directed on the label. Do not use within 1 hour of taking other medications.	Absorbs water from stool. Soothes the intestinal lining.
Witch hazel	Tea (loose), prepared by steeping 1 tsp (0.5 gm) in 1 cup water. (*See* TEAS in Part Three.) Drink 1 cup 2–3 times daily.	"Tans" cells lining the intestine.

Precautions for the use of herbs:

[1]Do not use chen-pi if there is blood in the stool.

[2]Do not use epimedium if you have any kind of prostate disorder.

Diarrhea: Formulas

Formula	Comments
Five-Accumulation Powder[1]	A traditional Chinese herbal formula that treats diarrhea with abdominal pain, gurgling noises, and/or vomiting.
Five-Ingredient Powder with Poria	A traditional Chinese herbal formula that treats diarrhea with vomiting and difficulty in urination.
Kudzu Decoction	A traditional Chinese herbal formula that treats diarrhea in children caused by food allergies. Seek an herbalist's advice on a suitable child's dosage.
Major Ledebouriella Decoction[2]	A traditional Chinese herbal formula that reduces diarrhea during drug withdrawal. May cause a loss of sensation in the mouth and tongue.
True Man's Decoction to Nourish the Organs[3]	A traditional Chinese herbal formula that treats unremitting diarrhea to the point of incontinence. Not available as a patent medicine, but available from traditional Chinese medicine practitioners as variations on zhen ren yang rang tang.

Precautions for the use of formulas:

[1]Do not use Five-Accumulation Powder during menstrual periods.

[2]Stop taking Major Ledebouriella Decoction if fever occurs.

[3]Avoid alcohol, wheat, cold or raw foods, fish, and greasy foods while using True Man's Decoction to Nourish the Organs. Do not use this formula if you have gallbladder problems, obstruction of the bile duct, or a tendency to retain urine. Do not use it if you are pregnant.

❏ Avoid high-fiber foods, which may stress the digestive system. Instead, stick to foods that are easy to digest, such as cooked potatoes, rice, bananas, applesauce, or toast. Don't eat if you are not hungry. Some people have achieved relief using probiotic foods and supplements. In one study, green bananas containing a fiber called pectin helped control diarrhea in children by increasing the production of short-chain fatty acids in the intestine, which stimulates the growth of new colon cells and improves the absorption of fluids.

❏ Take steps to reduce your stress level. (*See* STRESS.) Constant stress can cause diarrhea.

❏ If you are taking very large daily doses (3,000 milligrams or more) of vitamin C, discontinue taking it altogether, and then gradually increase to 1,000 milligrams. In addition, take supplemental vitamin B_{12} (cobalamin) until the diarrhea clears, since the intestines are temporarily unable to absorb this nutrient.

❏ To prevent traveler's diarrhea, take bromelain tablets—250 milligrams three times a day beginning at least one day before traveling. Bromelain works by not allowing diarrhea-causing bacteria to "stick" to the intestinal wall. Bromelain is especially recommended for children who are traveling; the dosage for children is the same as that for adults, but check with the child's pediatrician first. People who are allergic to pineapple may develop a rash from taking bromelain. If itching occurs, stop using it.

❏ Use bismuth subsalicylate (Pepto-Bismol) for diarrhea prevention, if your doctor recommends it, but be aware that it can slow down bowel movements and potentially trap disease-causing microbes inside the intestines. Do not use any over-the-counter (OTC) drug to treat a child without speaking to a pediatrician.

Considerations

❏ If diarrhea is accompanied by painful cramps, the best treatment is opium, a time-proven remedy that is safe and effective if used in the proper dosage for a short period of time. The best preparation is deodorized tincture of opium (DTO), a concentrated extract available through a doctor's prescription. Alternatively, use camphorated tincture of opium (paregoric), taking 1 teaspoon of water with each teaspoon of the drug. Do not use this on a child without speaking to his or her doctor.

❏ If acute diarrhea occurs after consuming dairy products, lactose intolerance may be responsible. Lactose intolerance results from the lack of or a reduced production of the enzyme lactase, which breaks down milk sugars so they can pass through the intestinal wall. The sugars instead stay in the intestine and draw fluids into the stool, causing runny diarrhea. Lactose intolerance can be corrected with commercial products such as Lactaid.

❏ While milk may upset some people's digestion, it may actually be one of the best foods to give a child with diarrhea, provided the child does not have either lactose intolerance or a milk allergy. Milk contains opioids, compounds in the same chemical family as opium. These compounds stop cramping and slow the rate at which the stomach empties, thereby slowing diarrhea and easing cramps. Most children who have diarrhea can take at least some milk, especially if it's given with simple foods such as cream of rice or wheat.

❏ Bowel retraining can help people who have fecal incontinence. This differs from diarrhea, however. (See BOWEL RETRAINING in Part Three.)

❏ Breast-feeding has been shown to prevent diarrhea in infants, who can become easily dehydrated when they have this condition. An FDA-sponsored study of 500,000 households in the United States found that from 5 to 11 percent of all infants had diarrhea at some time between the ages of two months and seven months. However, among breast-fed children, this percentage dropped to between 1 and 2 percent. It is not necessary for the child to be exclusively breast-fed to be protected against diarrhea. Supplementing breast-feeding with formula, even daily, does not cancel out the protective effect of breast milk.

❏ Diarrhea that occurs in a child under age six is a cause for concern, and should be brought to a doctor's attention. In addition, a doctor should be consulted if diarrhea in an older child or adult is bloody, lasts more than three days or recurs, or is accompanied by cramping with weakness between attacks. In such cases, diarrhea is usually associated with an underlying condition. (See ALLERGIES; CROHN'S DISEASE; FOOD POISONING; and HIV/AIDS.)

❏ If diarrhea alternates with constipation, irritable bowel syndrome may be the problem. (See IRRITABLE BOWEL SYNDROME.)

❏ For measures to treat diarrhea that may accompany chemotherapy or radiation treatment, see "Side Effects of Cancer Treatment" under CANCER. In one study an herb, Agaricus sylvaticus fungus, from Brazil helped patients with colorectal cancer. Patients took 15 milligrams per pound of body weight, and not only did diarrhea abate but so did pain; they also slept better and experienced less postprandial fullness and abdominal distension. No such changes were observed in the placebo group.

❏ If diarrhea is chronic or recurrent, an underlying problem such as a food allergy, infection, or intestinal parasites may be the cause. Allergy testing can determine if you have any food allergies. A stool culture can be done to check for infection or the presence of parasites. More likely, the recurrence of diarrhea is related to poor sanitation or eating foods that have grown bacteria. Make sure you throw out cooked food after two days.

DRY MOUTH

Dry mouth, known medically as xerostomia, is a condition in which the salivary glands fail to work properly, which leads to a lack of saliva or reduced saliva production. It can be caused by various diseases and by a number of medical treatments, such as chemotherapy and radiation treatment. In addition, dry mouth is a side effect of more than 500 commonly used medications that are sold by prescription or over the counter. The most likely to cause dry mouth are drugs such as antidepressants and antianxiety drugs, antihistamines, decongestants, high blood pressure medications, antidiarrheals, and muscle relaxants. Dry mouth may make it hard to eat, swallow, taste, and speak. It can affect oral health by adding to tooth decay and infection.

Until recently, dry mouth was regarded as a normal part of aging, as was the resulting gum disease and loss of teeth. It is now known that healthy older adults produce as much saliva as younger adults. Dry mouth is not a normal condition at any age. However, because it is more common that older people will be using the medications that cause dry mouth, it is in fact seen more in older people. Whenever symptoms include burning of the tongue; difficulty in eating dry foods, wearing dentures, or speaking; frequent thirst; impaired taste; and/or dry cracked lips and dry skin at the corners of the mouth, the problem is likely to be dry mouth.

One of the most common medical reasons for dry mouth is Sjögren's syndrome, which results from an attack on the salivary glands by an overactive immune system. In addition to dry mouth and skin, this disease can result in dry, extremely painful eyes, with blurred vision; fatigue; recurrent canker sores; and, in women, a lack of vaginal lubrication. It can also affect the internal organs. Cavities and gum disease despite good oral hygiene are a warning signal of Sjögren's syndrome.

Herbal treatments for dry mouth either stimulate salivation or relieve inflammation. In using these treatments, the general rule is, within the limits recommended below, the more the better. The more the mouth is kept moist, the fewer the complications that will develop.

Recommendations

❏ To relieve dryness, sip water frequently. A little water taken frequently is better than a glassful of water drunk all at once.

❏ Avoid sugary snacks, caffeinated beverages, tobacco (smoked or chewed), and alcohol, all of which increase dryness in the mouth.

❏ Chew sugar-free gum. Chewing gum mildly stimulates the secretion of saliva.

❏ Use a saliva substitute. These commercially available products can be found in most pharmacies.

❏ Establish a good plaque-control program. Heavy plaque accumulations occur as the result of dry mouth. Use a fluoride rinse or brush-on fluoride before bed.

❏ Try breathing through the nose and not the mouth. Add moisture to the air at night by using a humidifier if you get congested.

❏ Both wheat germ and omega-3 fatty acids from fish oil have been shown to be effective at stimulating saliva production in patients with Sjögren's syndrome.

❏ For more information about Sjögren's syndrome, visit www.sjogrens.com.

Considerations

❏ Many doctors recommend pilocarpine for treatment of dry mouth caused by radiation treatment. The herbal extract

Dry Mouth: Beneficial Herbs

Herb	Form and Dosage	Comments
Prickly ash	Tincture. Take 10–20 drops in ¼ cup water 3–7 times daily.	Stimulates salivation in dry mouth caused by radiation treatment. Also prevents oral irritation.
Slippery elm	Tea (loose or bagged). Prepare as directed on the label and drink a cup as desired.	Reduces discomfort of mouth.
Solomon's seal	Probotannix capsules. Take 1,000–2,000 mg daily.	Relieves dry mouth caused by use of medications.

Dry Mouth: Formulas

Formula	Comments
Ophiopogonis Decoction[1]	A traditional Chinese herbal formula that increases salivary secretion and prevents oral infection.

Precautions for the use of formulas:

[1] Do not use Ophiopogonis Decoction if you have a fever.

jaborandi provides the same chemicals as pilocarpine (and was the original source of the drug). If you are having radiation therapy, check with your doctor first.

❏ Cancer therapies, especially radiation to the head and neck or chemotherapy, can cause dry mouth and other related problems, including tooth decay, painful mouth sores, and cracked and peeling lips. Before starting cancer treatment, it is important to see a dentist and take care of any necessary dental work. Your dentist can also show you how to care for your teeth and mouth before, during, and after cancer treatment to prevent or reduce the oral problems that may occur.

❏ Acupuncture treatments can increase salivary flow to relieve dry mouth after radiation treatment and in Sjögren's syndrome. (*See* ACUPUNCTURE in Part Three.) Typically, about twenty-four treatments are necessary to improve the condition. People who experience increased salivation after taking the herb-derived drug pilocarpine are the most likely to benefit from acupuncture.

❏ People who develop dry mouth as a side effect of medication or after treatment for cancer, or who have HIV, are especially at risk for thrush, an oral yeast infection. This condition appears as white blotches in the roof of the mouth. Thrush contained inside the mouth is painless, but may cause painful cracking of the skin at the corners of the mouth. (*See* YEAST INFECTION [YEAST VAGINITIS].)

DYSPEPSIA

See INDIGESTION.

EAR INFECTION

Next to the common cold, ear infections are the most commonly diagnosed childhood illness in the United States. More than three out of four kids have had at least one ear infection by the time they reach three years of age. The middle ear—which consists of three small bones behind the eardrum—transmits sound vibrations to the inner ear, which passes them on to nerve endings that carry them to the brain. Both viruses and bacteria can cause ear infections, which can also affect the outer and inner parts of the ear.

Otitis media, or middle-ear infection, is an inflammation of the middle ear, usually caused by bacteria, that occurs when fluid builds up behind the eardrum. Anyone can get an ear infection, but children get them more often than adults. Acute otitis media causes pain and throbbing in the ear, chills, fever, and redness and bulging of the eardrum. The eardrum may rupture, causing a bloody discharge. Chronic infections can cause hearing loss and complications that include fluid accumulations and acute mastoiditis, an infection of the bone behind the ear.

The viruses that cause upper respiratory infections such as colds also can cause middle-ear infections. Allergies can lead to ear infections as well. Allergies can inflame the eustachian tube, which connects the middle ear and the throat, or they can cause nasal passages to swell, trapping air and secretions in the middle ear. Sensitivity to allergens is increased by low humidity, and exposure to secondhand tobacco smoke and smoke from wood-burning stoves. Children who are bottle-fed, especially when lying down, tend to have more ear infections than do babies who are breast-fed.

Antibiotics are often used to treat ear infections, although that option is not always helpful. Infections that do not respond to antibiotics are treated with surgery, in which a plastic tube is placed in the ear to help drain fluid. Again, this treatment does not always help.

Allergy control and herbal medicine together may provide a safer, and effective, alternative for ear infections. However, if there is no improvement, see your doctor. The dosages given for internal remedies are for children; for the equivalent adult dosages, multiply by four. Formula dosages for children should be discussed with a knowledgeable health-care practitioner.

Recommendations

❏ Steam inhalations of chamomile, elderberry flowers, and/or lemon balm soothe irritation and relieve pain. (*See* STEAM INHALATIONS in Part Three.) If you use chamomile, be sure to use German chamomile (*Matricaria recutita*), not Roman chamomile (*Chamaemelum nobile*).

❏ Eat yogurt or take acidophilus supplements. Supplemental *Lactobacillus acidophilus* prevents antibiotic damage to the helpful bacteria residing in the digestive tract. It prevents stomach upset and hastens recovery from middle-ear infection.

❏ Use room humidifiers. Dry air, especially in winter, induces nasal swelling and reduces airflow to the eustachian tubes. This leads to increased secretions and an inability to clear fluid.

❏ Blow your nose very gently if you have an ear infection.

❏ Keep the ear canal dry. Retained soap and water in the canal can be dangerous. Put cotton in the ear canal when showering or bathing. Do not go swimming until healing is complete.

❏ Avoid unsanitary conditions. An ear infection may result from lowered resistance due to a recent illness. Nonprescription ear drops may relieve the pain. A nasal spray may help open up the eustachian tube and relieve the pressure.

❏ Do not give aspirin or any product containing aspirin to a child who shows symptoms of a viral infection.

Ear Infection: Beneficial Herbs

Herb	Form and Dosage	Comments
Echinacea[1] and goldenseal[1]	*Echinacea purpurea* and goldenseal formula. Take as directed on the label. Do not take on a daily basis for more than 2 weeks at a time.	Stops drainage; accelerates recovery.
Garlic	Oil.[2] Place several drops into the ear canal. (*See* GARLIC *under* The Herbs in Part One.)	An antibacterial.
Green tea[3]	Catechin extract. Take 240 mg once daily; or tea bag, prepared with 1 cup water. Take ½ cup once daily.	Helps children with viral infections and those with allergies or asthma.
Mullein	Oil.[2] Place several drops into the ear canal.	Soothes ear canal linings damaged by infection.
Olive leaf	Extract. Take as directed on the label.	Helps body to fight infection.
Pinellia	Ear drops. Use under professional supervision.	Relieves "oozing" infection in 1–2 days.
Scutellaria[4]	Fluidextract. Take ⅛ tsp (0.5 ml) once daily in ¼ cup water or juice.	Inhibits *Streptococcus* growth. Prevents viral infection of eustachian tubes.
St. John's wort	Oil.[2] Place several drops into the ear canal.	Relieves inflammation; kills viruses.

Precautions for the use of herbs:

[1]Do not use echinacea and goldenseal during pregnancy.

[2]When using oils as ear drops, always warm the oil to room temperature—do *not* use it cold. Plug the ear loosely with cotton after applying.

[3]Do not take green tea within one hour of taking other medications.

[4]Do not use scutellaria if you have diarrhea.

Ear Infection: Formulas

Formula	Comments
Gentiana Longdancao Decoction to Drain the Liver[1]	A traditional Chinese herbal formula suitable for adults, particularly if there is a bitter taste in the mouth, dizziness, headache, hearing loss, irritability, and/or sore eyes.
Kudzu Decoction	A traditional Chinese herbal formula suitable for children and adults. This formula activates the immune system against viral infection and stops inner-ear inflammation caused by food allergies.

Precautions for the use of formulas:

[1]Do not use Gentiana Longdancao Decoction to Drain the Liver if you are trying to become pregnant.

Aspirin use can result in Reye's syndrome, a potentially serious complication.

❑ Contact a health-care provider immediately if dizziness or hearing loss occurs, or if there is a bloody discharge or consistent ear pain stops suddenly. These symptoms are indications of a possible ruptured eardrum.

Considerations

❑ The problem in treating middle-ear infections with antibiotics is that the exact cause of the infection is often not identified. As a result, clinical studies have found that the most commonly prescribed antibiotic, amoxicillin (Amoxil and others), is no more effective than a placebo in actual use. Some strains of the germs that cause ear infections, such as *Haemophilus influenzae,* do not readily respond to medication. Other bacteria are becoming resistant to antibiotics, which are often misprescribed. Viral infections are not affected by antibiotics at all.

❑ Some have found *Echinacea purpurea* used by itself helps prevent infections from recurring. Use the liquid extract, ¼ teaspoon (1 milliliter) three times daily for up to two weeks. Avoid if you have gallstones, an autoimmune disease, or a chronic infection.

❑ Xylitol, an artificial sweetener, can inhibit the growth of *Streptococcus pneumoniae,* the germ that causes middle-ear infection in children. Xylitol is used in sugar-free gum. It is also found in plums, raspberries, and strawberries. Researchers at the Department of Pediatrics at the University of Oulu in Finland performed a randomized, double-blind, placebo-controlled study using chewing gum that contained either xylitol or regular sugar. The children in the study had to chew two fresh pieces of gum five times a day. At the end of a month, children who chewed the xylitol-sweetened chewing gum had 40 percent fewer ear infections. The scientists believe that xylitol retards the growth of the bacterium *S. pneumoniae* and thus prevents attacks of acute otitis media caused by this microorganism.

❑ Ear problems are more common in the homes of smokers.

❑ The lowest frequency of ear infection occurs in children who were breast-fed and who were not exposed to tobacco smoke as infants. Food allergies aggravate middle-ear infections. In one study, controlling food allergies eased symptoms in 86 percent of participants, while provoking food allergies worsened ear problems in 94 percent. (*See* Food Allergies *under* ALLERGIES.)

❑ Children who have had ear infections tend to be sensitive to high altitudes and cold. For these children, protective measures against colds, flu, and overexertion are advisable on ski trips.

❑ Young adults who had ear infections as children may be more likely to suffer hearing loss while using stereo headsets. Trauma caused by a too-loud stereo to the already injured ear can result in hearing loss and tinnitus. Whether you have had ear infections or not, sound that is too loud coming from a headset can cause deafness. (*See* TINNITUS [RINGING IN THE EAR].)

❑ Physician and complementary health-care expert Andrew Weil reports that cranial manipulation, practiced by some osteopathic physicians, is safe and "remarkably effective" for treating recurrent ear infections in children.

❑ "Swimmer's ear" is an infection of the outer ear caused by water becoming trapped in the ear canal. The best way to treat swimmer's ear is to avoid getting it in the first place, by wearing silicone or wax earplugs. If you do not use earplugs, you can try to head off the problem by using equal parts of white vinegar and rubbing alcohol. Gently rinse the ears with the mixture when you come out of the water, then gently dry the outer part of the ear with a cotton swab. Do not remove ear wax, because it helps protect the ear canal from moisture. Do not put anything in the ear—even a cotton swab.

❑ *See also* ASTHMA; and Respiratory Allergies *under* ALLERGIES.

ECZEMA

Eczema is a general term for a pattern of painful skin outbreaks. It causes some areas of skin to become dry, flaky, and red, and other areas to become inflamed, moist, oozing, and crusty. In chronic eczema, the cells of the skin may change color and become thick and scaly. Itching is often severe. Eczema leaves the skin open to infection from *Staphylococcus* (staph).

Eczema stems from an astonishingly broad range of causes, but it is usually the result of either atopic dermatitis or contact dermatitis. Atopic dermatitis is a persistent skin condition associated with allergy. Seventy percent of the people who have it also suffer from asthma, hay fever, or hives. It can occur anywhere on the body, but is most common on the face, neck, wrists, hands, and eyelids; behind the ears; and in the creases of the groin, knees, and elbows. Atopic dermatitis often starts in childhood, and children with this condition tend to have it over a wider area of skin than adults who develop the disease later in life. It can be caused by stress; rapid changes in temperature; certain foods such as eggs, milk, fish, soy, or wheat; low humidity; and long hot baths.

Another chronic form of eczema is contact dermatitis. This is a painful, weeping skin reaction caused by contact with an external agent. In North America, the most familiar agents are poison ivy and oak. Contact dermatitis results from exposure to other types of plants, as well as perfumes, industrial chemicals, dry-cleaning agents, certain metal alloys, wool, sweat, and latex. Allergies and hypochlorhydria, a condition in which the stomach fails to produce enough hydrochloric acid for proper digestion, may be contributing factors.

Both atopic and contact dermatitis cause changes in how the repair mechanism of the skin works. The repair process in the skin is permanently activated, but never completed. People with eczema regenerate skin faster than people without eczema, but the skin never acquires normal immune function. Standard drug therapy for eczema consists of steroids such as hydrocortisone.

Unless otherwise specified, the dosages for herbs used internally are for adults. Children under age six should be given one-quarter of the adult dosage. Children between the ages of six and twelve should be given one-half of the adult dosage. Herbs should not be used in children under age three. Formula dosages for children should be discussed with a Chinese medical—or other knowledgeable—health-care practitioner.

Recommendations

❑ To reduce inflammation, take MaxEPA or other fish oil supplements, which contain the important omega-3 fatty acids eicosapentaenoic acid (EPA) and docosahexaenoic acid (DHA). Borage seed oil, evening primrose oil, and flaxseed oil are other good sources of inflammation-reducing

Eczema: Beneficial Herbs

Herb	Form and Dosage	Comments
Herbs to Be Applied Externally		
Aloe	Gel. Use as directed on the label.	Relieves inflammation, by itself or with hydrocortisone creams.
Avena	Oat extract. Use in baths, as directed on the label.	Is soothing and anti-inflammatory.
Calendula or witch hazel	Cream, preferably in a choline base. Apply as directed on the label.	Reduces inflammation and redness.
Chamomile or chickweed or licorice	Cream, preferably in a choline base. Apply as directed on the label.	Prevents itching and stops hardening of the skin.
Copaiba	Oil. Apply to affected skin.	Provides quick relief of inflammation; antibacterial.
Marshmallow root	Cream. Apply as directed on the label.	Forms protective layer over skin; prevents infection. Also known as althea.
Rosemary	Tea. Use as a skin wash 2–3 times daily. (*See* SKIN WASHES in Part Three.)	Stimulates blood flow to skin. Prevents secondary infection.
Sangre de drago	Ointment. Apply as directed on the label.	Forms protective layer over skin; prevents infection. Shrinks damaged area.
Turmeric	Extract. Apply as a poultice twice daily. (*See* POULTICES in Part Three.)	Kills pain; promotes healing.
Walnut leaf	Extract. Apply as a skin wash 2–3 times daily. (*See* SKIN WASHES in Part Three.)	Protects against infection. Stops excessive sweating.
Witch hazel	Eucerin or any witch hazel cream in a phosphatidylcholine base. Use as directed on the label.	Relief of inflammation somewhat less than hydrocortisone, but without side effects.
Herbs to Be Taken Internally		
Burdock	Cereal (*goboshi* in Japanese groceries). Eat 1 dry oz daily; or tincture. Take as directed on the label.	Regulates the immune system. Reduces skin cell destruction.
Coleus	Forskolin tablets such as forskolin dry extract from TR-Metro Natural Herbal Extracts. Take 50 mg 3 times daily.	A potent herbal antihistamine. Stops inflammation process.
Oregon grape root[1]	Extract. Take as directed on the label.	Detoxifies the body and reduces inflammation.
Quercetin[2]	Tablets. Take 250 mg 3 times daily.	An antihistamine that stops inflammation.
Sarsaparilla	Capsules. Take 3,000 mg 3 times daily.	An anti-inflammatory.

Precautions for the use of herbs:

[1]Do not take Oregon grape root for longer than two weeks at a time. Do not use it if you are pregnant or have gallbladder disease. Do not take this herb with supplemental vitamin B_6 or with protein supplements containing the amino acid histidine.

[2]Do not use quercetin if you are taking cyclosporine (Neoral, Sandimmune) or nifedipine (Procardia).

Eczema: Formulas

Formula	Comments
Kudzu Decoction	A traditional Chinese herbal formula that protects eczema-damaged skin from the effects of herpes infection. This formula is especially useful for people who are HIV-positive.
Ledebouriella Decoction That Sagely Unblocks[1]	A traditional Chinese herbal formula that prevents allergic hypersensitivity. It soothes itching and makes sleeping easier, and is especially useful for children's eczema.

Precautions for the use of formulas:

[1]Do not use Ledebouriella Decoction That Sagely Unblocks if you are trying to become pregnant, or if you are experiencing nausea or vomiting.

gamma-linolenic acid (GLA), but are less effective and more expensive than fish oil. In one study, participants used 5.4 grams of DHA daily for twenty weeks and had an improvement in their eczema.

❏ Take 45 to 60 milligrams of zinc daily when eczema flares up; then reduce dosage to 30 milligrams a day when the condition clears. However, not all studies support a role for zinc in the treatment of eczema. In one study of more than fifty children with eczema (aged one to sixteen years), there was no benefit with 50 milligrams of zinc per day.

❏ Add brown rice and millet to your diet.

❏ You may try omitting certain foods from your diet, such as eggs, peanuts, soy foods, wheat, and dairy products one at a time and see if there is an effect. Make sure that you make up for any nutrients you lose if you are following an elimination diet. This is especially important for dairy products, which are the main dietary sources of calcium, magnesium, and vitamin D.

❏ Try keeping your house humidified and take fewer showers and baths. Showers and baths deplete the skin of natural oils.

❏ Manage stress. Stress hormones cause the immune system to secrete histamines and leukotrienes, chemicals that damage the skin. Stress-control methods such as biofeedback and progressive relaxation, practiced regularly over a period of several months, reduce both the severity and frequency of eczema outbreaks. (*See* STRESS.)

❏ Avoid moisturizing creams and lotions. Some of the moisturizers and emollients that work very well in normal skin inhibit the "barrier" function in eczema-affected skin, and encourage infection. Using "moisturizers" even causes cracking and peeling that can cause the skin to lose more moisture. To care for eczema-affected skin, use creams that preserve water content and stimulate normal cell growth of the skin.

❏ Avoid nickel if you are sensitive to it. Nickel jewelry, often used in body piercings, frequently causes skin allergy. One study looked at the effect of a low-nickel diet and disulfiram therapy (Antabuse) in people who were using steroids to control their nickel sensitivity. The drug was used because it is a known nickel chelator (gets the nickel out of the body). More than 90 percent of the subjects' eczema healed as a result. The combination of therapies may be a good alternative to steroids.

Considerations

❏ The short-term use of steroids often stops eczema outbreaks. However, long-term use can leave the skin fragile and thin, relieving the eczema but increasing the risk of skin breaks and infection.

❏ A number of herbal therapies provide antioxidant compounds that may slow the production of histamine and other inflammatory chemicals. Blackberries, blueberries, cherries, and raspberries; preparations of bilberry and hawthorn; and the herbal medicines pine bark and resveratrol all fall into this category. Using any of these foods or herbs can help people with eczema.

❏ Chemicals used in bubble-bath products may cause dermatitis and may even irritate the tissues of the lower urinary tract sufficiently to cause bloody urine. This is most likely to occur if you soak in treated bathwater for too long.

❏ Mothers who eat a diet rich in linoleic acid have babies with a higher risk of developing eczema. Linoleic acids are found in all vegetable oils, such as sunflower, safflower, canola, soy, and corn oils. Limit your intake of these if you are pregnant.

❏ Eczema is less frequent throughout childhood in children who have been breast-fed. A child who cannot be breast-fed should be fed as varied a diet as possible instead of being fed the same foods every day. Do not introduce food until the child's pediatrician says that it is all right. Some foods that may provoke eczema include cow's milk, eggs, and wheat, and these may be food allergens as well. However, a recent large-scale study on nearly 5,000 children indicated that delaying the introduction of solid foods beyond four months of age or removing allergenic foods from the diet had no effect on preventing eczema. Children under the age of three who have eczema usually have food allergies. (*See* Food Allergies *under* ALLERGIES.) Children over the age of three who have eczema usually have asthma, and are particularly likely to have allergies to dust mites and molds. (See Respiratory Allergies *under* ALLERGIES. Also *see* ASTHMA.)

❏ Adults with eczema could also be more prone to develop the disease-causing yeast *Candida albicans*. Treating yeast infections may reduce the allergic load on the body and reduce the immune system's hypersensitivity. (*See* YEAST INFECTION [YEAST VAGINITIS].)

❏ People with eczema who have underactive thyroid glands respond well to thyroid treatment, which balances immune function. (*See* HYPOTHYROIDISM.)

❏ If there are silvery, scaly bumps and raised patches of skin, psoriasis may be the problem. (*See* PSORIASIS.)

EDEMA

See ANKLES, SWOLLEN; LYMPHEDEMA. *See also under* PREMENSTRUAL SYNDROME (PMS).

EMPHYSEMA

Emphysema is a form of chronic obstructive pulmonary disease (COPD), in which the lungs become inelastic after years of exposure to cigarette smoke and air pollution. A person with emphysema cannot exhale without great effort. This is due to the fact that the alveoli, or air pouches, stay permanently open, and cannot squeeze out air for exhalation. As a result, stale air remains trapped in the lungs and no new oxygen can enter to meet the body's needs.

The most common symptom of emphysema is breathlessness, with coughing occurring after exertion, no matter how slight. Any physical exertion creates a sensation of a heavy weight on the chest. Symptoms may be subtle at first but worsen with time.

Most people who are diagnosed with emphysema are long-term cigarette smokers over age sixty. Long-term exposure to cigarette smoke depletes the lungs' ability to clear themselves of foreign particles such as dust, and these foreign particles compound the chronic inflammation caused by smoking. In a very few cases, young people and even children can develop emphysema due to a hereditary deficiency of a blood protein called antitrypsin, but the overwhelming majority of cases are due to smoking. (Only 2 to 3 percent of the population has antitrypsin deficiency.)

The primary use of herbal treatment in emphysema is in controlling immediate symptoms. Herbs are also very useful in preventing infection with colds and flu.

Recommendations

❑ First and foremost, avoid smoking and exposure to tobacco smoke. This action reduces the rate at which lung capacity is lost to the disease.

❑ To avoid putting any more stress on your lungs, try to avoid catching colds and the flu. *Echinacea purpurea*—at least 900 milligrams a day in capsule form, or 1 teaspoon (4 milliliters) of Echinacin juice three times daily—reduces the risk of catching cold, and speeds recovery from colds. Elderberry, in the form of Sambucol extract (take as directed), can help at the first signs of flu. Scutellaria, 1,000 to 2,000 milligrams three times daily, can prevent respiratory infections. Avoid echinacea if you have an autoimmune disease, and scutellaria if you have diarrhea.

❑ Get a flu shot once a year, in addition to a onetime pneumonia shot if your doctor agrees.

❑ If respiratory infections do develop, treat them as soon as possible, and see a doctor if the thickness or volume of sputum increases, or if there is fever or muscle pain.

❑ To help keep secretions fluid, drink at least eight glasses of water daily.

❑ Exercise moderately on a regular basis; walking is best. Arm exercises may place an extra exertion on the lungs. Ask your doctor if you are strong enough to do them.

❑ Eliminate aerosol sprays around the home. These include deodorants, hair sprays, and insecticides. Hair sprays can cause acute lung obstruction even in healthy people. It is also necessary to avoid perfumes and colognes.

❑ Eliminate as many other household chemicals as possible. Use an electric stove rather than a gas stove. Use ceramic tile, hardwood, or stone as flooring materials, since carpet can hold dust, mold, and cleaning chemicals. Do not use curtains and draperies, since they can also harbor dust. Use paint instead of wallpaper, since the glues used to hang the paper can contain chemicals that cause bronchial irritation.

❑ Avoid letting furry or feathered animals into your home or car. Their hair, dander, and feather dust can irritate the lungs.

❑ As much as possible, avoid polluted air. If your current working environment is dirty, dusty, or toxic to inhale, change jobs if at all possible.

Considerations

❑ Malnutrition is common in people with emphysema. Difficulty in breathing makes eating difficult and

Emphysema: Beneficial Herbs

Herb	Form and Dosage	Comments
Astragalus	Capsules or fluidextracts. Take as directed on the label.	Accelerates healing in the bronchial tubes and promotes better breathing.
Horsetail	Tincture. Take 10–20 drops in ¼ cup water, 3 times daily.	Loosens mucus.
Quercetin[1]	Tablets. Take 250 mg 3 times daily.	Increases the lungs' ability to deal with dust and particle pollution.

Precautions for the use of herbs:

[1]Do not use quercetin if you are taking cyclosporine (Neoral, Sandimmune) or nifedipine (Procardia).

unpleasant. For people whose weight is less than 85 percent of normal, there also may be protein deficiency. Using a protein drink called Immunocal can reverse protein deficiency and also measurably increase lung capacity. This drink is rich in cysteine, which helps protect and repair lung tissue. Any food you can get into your body if you are undernourished is encouraged. High-protein beverages such as milk shakes or smoothies with added whey protein are good choices.

❑ Emphysema and chronic bronchitis are separate disease processes, although many people suffer both conditions at the same time. Emphysema causes a more severe loss of breath than chronic bronchitis. The sputum in emphysema is scant and watery, but sputum in chronic bronchitis is copious and thick. (*See* BRONCHITIS AND PNEUMONIA.)

❑ Treating emphysema involves controlling other chronic respiratory diseases. (*See also* ASTHMA and Respiratory Allergies *under* ALLERGIES.)

❑ In some cases, a lung transplant may be considered. This is a highly invasive, complex procedure that carries substantial risk. It is a viable option for only a small percentage of people with emphysema.

❑ Supplemental oxygen can benefit anyone with impaired lung function. Long-term oxygen therapy combats erythrocytosis (an abnormal increase in red blood cells) and lowers the risk of heart failure.

ENDOMETRIAL CANCER

One of the most common forms of uterine cancer affects the lining of the uterus, the endometrium. Endometrial cancer usually strikes after menopause, and its primary warning sign is bleeding (before menopause, bleeding not related to the menstrual period). It can also cause pelvic pain and pain during intercourse.

The growth of endometrial cancer is thought to be stimulated by estrogen, but doctors don't know the true cause. Throughout a woman's reproductive life, the lining of the uterus grows and shrinks in response to rising and falling estrogen levels during the menstrual cycle. After menopause, most of the estrogen produced in a woman's body is produced by fat tissue. High-fat diets encourage the development of fat tissue and could increase the production of excess estrogen.

Endometrial cancer is diagnosed by examining a piece of endometrium, which is usually removed via a biopsy. The first line of conventional treatment is surgery, usually to remove the uterus, fallopian tubes, and ovaries. If the cancer has spread, chemotherapy or radiation therapy may be used. The doctor may also use hormonal therapy, in which a form of progesterone, another female hormone, is used to counteract the effects of estrogen.

Some herbal therapies for endometrial cancer may counteract estrogen and support the immune system. Others supplement conventional treatments. Always use herbal medicine as part of a medically directed overall treatment plan for endometrial cancer.

Endometrial Cancer: Beneficial Herbs

Herb	Form and Dosage	Comments
Alfalfa	Tablets. Take as directed on the label.	Good source of vitamin K and needed minerals, including iron.
Astragalus[1]	Tincture. Take 1–1½ tsp (4–6 ml) in ¼ cup water 3 times daily.	Slows spread of cancer; activates T and natural killer (NK) cells.
Cat's claw[2]	Tincture. Take the dose recommended on the label in ½ cup water with 1 tsp lemon juice.	Raises T cell counts.
Chamomile	German chamomile (*Matricaria recutita*) tea bag, prepared with 1 cup water. Take 1 cup 2–3 times daily.	Contains chemicals that prevent cancer cells from anchoring to new sites.
Garlic[3]	Enteric-coated tablets. Take at least 900 mg a day.	Retards angiogenesis and metastasis.
Green tea	Tea bag, prepared with 1 cup water. Take 1 cup 3 times daily. To avoid dilution, do not use within 1 hour of taking other medications.	Contains polyphenols, which block estrogen from tumors.
Polysaccharide kureha (PSK)	Tablets. Take 6,000 mg daily.	Shown to increase 3- and 5-year survival rates.
Soy isoflavone concentrate	Tablets. Take about 3,000 mg once daily.	Contains genistein, which inhibits growth of estrogen-dependent cancers.

Precautions for the use of herbs:

[1]Do not use astragalus if you have a fever or a skin infection.

[2]Do not use cat's claw if you have to take insulin for diabetes. Do not use it if you are pregnant or nursing.

[3]Garlic counteracts the effects of bifidus and *Lactobacillus* cultures taken as digestive aids. Consult a doctor before using garlic on a regular basis if you are on an anticoagulant drug such as warfarin (Coumadin). Discuss the use of garlic with your doctor before having any type of surgery.

Endometrial Cancer: Formulas

Formula	Comments
Augmented Rambling Powder	A traditional Chinese herbal formula that lowers estrogen levels. Appropriate for a range of conditions that cause increased menstrual flow and uterine bleeding.
Cinnamon Twig and Poria Pill[1]	A traditional Chinese herbal formula that lowers estrogen levels. Raises energy levels, restores appetite.
Dong Quai and Peony Powder[1]	A traditional Chinese herbal formula that lowers estrogen levels. Relieves fatigue.
Two-Cured Decoction[2]	A traditional Chinese herbal formula that lowers estrogen levels. Limits nausea and vomiting.

Precautions for the use of formulas:

[1]Since Cinnamon Twig and Poria Pill and Dong Quai and Peony Powder act on the ovaries, they will not help if you have had your ovaries removed.

[2]Do not use Two-Cured Decoction if you have a fever.

Herbs to Avoid

❑ Individuals who have endometrial cancer should avoid the following herbs: cordyceps, dan shen, fennel seed, licorice, and peony. (For more information regarding these herbs, see The Herbs in Part One.)

Recommendations

❑ Pay attention to diet. Proper nutritional requirements for cervical and endometrial cancer are very similar. (See CERVICAL CANCER.) To learn how to reduce estrogen levels through diet, see ESTROGEN-REDUCING DIET in Part Three.

❑ If you are receiving treatment for advanced endometrial cancer, take thymic-factor supplements before and during chemotherapy, but only after discussing this with your doctor. German research indicates that thymic factors "greatly reduce" the depletion of immune cells during chemotherapy for later-stage cancers of the uterus.

❑ Walk regularly. One study found that a moderate amount of brisk walking (a minimum of one mile a day, six days a week) reduces the risk of endometrial cancer. It is not necessary to go for long distances, since the beneficial effect of walking does not increase beyond a mile a day.

❑ Use a heating pad, a hot-water bottle, or a hot bath to help relieve pain.

❑ Avoid alcohol, caffeine, animal fats, butter, dairy products, fried foods, foods that contain additives, all hardened fats, red meats, poultry (except organically raised and skinless chicken or turkey), refined and processed foods, salt, shellfish, and sugar. The risk of endometrial cancer was found to be based on eating too many calories and cholesterol from meats. Limit calorie intake from all foods and rely on lean meats, skinless poultry, fish, and vegetables as your protein sources. Soy protein rich in isoflavones does not seem to affect the endometrial tissue and offers a good source of protein, but check with your doctor first to make sure soy is a good choice for you. Soy foods include miso and tofu. One study found that all animal proteins and fat increased the risk of endometrial cancer, while eating more fresh fruit, vegetables, and fiber decreased that risk.

Considerations

❑ Supporting the immune system is an important part of fighting endometrial cancer. Immune Support from Raintree Nutrition is a combination of South American herbs, including cat's claw, chuchuhuasi, macela, and mullaca, that is especially useful for treating immune deficiencies associated with this disorder. More information is available from their website at www.rain-tree.com.

❑ Lymphedema is a swelling of the tissues that may follow cancer surgery. (See LYMPHEDEMA.)

❑ For measures to reduce side effects and increase the effectiveness of chemotherapy and/or radiation therapy, see "Side Effects of Cancer Treatment" under CANCER. To learn about herbal treatments that can prevent a cancer from developing its own blood supply, see CANCER.

ENDOMETRIOSIS

Endometriosis is a chronic disease in which tissues that ordinarily develop in the inner layer of the uterine wall are deposited outside the uterus. These tissues form cysts, which may be found in the ovaries, uterine ligaments, fallopian tubes, colon, urethra, bladder, or vagina, and, in rare cases, the lungs and limbs. More than 5 million American women have endometriosis, which often runs in families.

The main symptom of endometriosis is pain: painful periods, pelvic and lower back pain, pain during ovulation, and pain during sexual intercourse. The pain may be barely noticeable, but more often is severe and debilitating. Endometriosis also causes inability to urinate, intestinal discomfort, and infertility. One-third to one-half of cases of infertility among menstruating women are caused by endometrial deformities. Because these symptoms are seen in a number of other disorders, an accurate diagnosis is very important.

Like the lining of the uterus, endometrial tissue outside the uterus responds to ovarian hormones by building up, breaking down, and bleeding. Endometrial tissues are more receptive to the hormone estrogen, but less receptive to the hormone progesterone. This makes them, in effect, permanently stuck in the first half of the menstrual cycle, constantly being stimulated to grow and divide by estrogen and never being instructed to stop by progesterone. Pregnancy, which stops the normal cycle, often brings relief from symptoms. For many women, though, this relief is only temporary.

There are a number of theories as to why endometriosis occurs. They range from the reflux menstruation theory, in which menstrual tissue flows back through the fallopian tubes and into the pelvic cavity, to the fetal defect theory, in which endometrial tissue attaches itself to the wrong body tissues before birth. It may also develop when one or more small areas of the abdominal lining turn into endometrial tissue. Both tissues—abdomen and endometrial—are descended from embryonic cells, with the potential to take on the structure and function of other tissues. The

result is that the abdomen cells behave like endometrial cells and cause endometriosis.

Conventional treatment of endometriosis consists of surgery and hormonal drugs. Herbal medicines may provide an adjunct or an alternative to standard medications, but have to be used for at least three months before improvements become noticeable.

Herbs to Avoid

Women who have endometriosis should avoid the following herbs: cordyceps, dan shen, fennel seed, licorice, and peony. (For more information regarding these herbs, *see* individual entries *under* The Herbs in Part One.)

Recommendations

❑ If you think you may have endometriosis, consult a gynecologist as soon as possible.

❑ Eat a diet that promotes lower body-fat levels, since fat produces estrogen. (For more information, *see* ESTROGEN-REDUCING DIET in Part Three.)

❑ If you do not take alfalfa in capsules, use alfalfa sprouts in salads and sandwiches to obtain close to the same benefits.

Endometriosis: Beneficial Herbs

Herb	Form and Dosage	Comments
Alfalfa[1]	Capsules. Take 1,000–2,000 mg daily.	Provides vitamin K for normal clotting of menstrual blood.
Green tea	Catechin extract. Take 240 mg 3 times daily; or tea bag, prepared with 1 cup of water. Take 1 cup 2–3 times daily. To avoid dilution, do not use within 1 hour of taking other medications.	Reduces formation of new endometrial cysts.
Jurubeba	Capsules. Take 1,000–2,000 mg daily.	Restores normal periods; relieves pain.
Turmeric	Curcumin tablets. Take 250–500 mg twice daily, between meals.	Supports liver function. Relieves pain and inflammation.
Vitex	Tincture. Take 1½ tsp in ¼ cup water 3 times daily.	Increases progesterone secretion. Especially useful if short periods occur.
Wild yam[2]	Tincture. Take 20 drops in ¼ cup water 3 times daily, after meals.	Especially useful for relieving pain that is worsened by lying down.

Precautions for the use of herbs:

[1]Do not use alfalfa in any form if you have an autoimmune disease, such as lupus or rheumatoid arthritis.

[2]Overdosage of wild yam can cause nausea. Be sure not to use an "herbal" product that contains synthetic progesterone while using this herb.

Endometriosis: Formulas

Formula	Comments
Dong Quai and Peony Powder	A traditional Chinese herbal formula that reduces production of both estrogen and inflammatory compounds in endometrial tissue without producing masculinizing side effects.
Four-Substance Decoction	A traditional Chinese herbal formula for relief of pain of endometriosis and fibroids.

❏ Women with endometriosis have increased free oxygen particles in the blood that stress and damage tissues. In one study, women with endometriosis had lower intakes of vitamins A, C, E, zinc, and copper compared to those without this condition. When the women with endometriosis were given an antioxidant-rich diet (rich in fruits and vegetables), the stress to tissues was reduced.

❏ Supplement the diet with omega-3 fatty acids by eating two to three servings of fish (such as salmon) weekly, or by taking MaxEPA fish oil. Borage or evening primrose oil could also be helpful. In laboratory studies, adequate supplies of omega-3 fatty acids stop the production of hormones that cause inflammation and stimulate growth of endometrial tissue.

❏ Limit consumption of coffee and other sources of caffeine. While it is not necessary to totally eliminate caffeine, a doubling in the risk of endometriosis occurs in women who consume 7 grams or more of caffeine a month (about four cups of coffee a day or more), compared to women who consume 3 grams (two cups of coffee a day or less).

❏ Use a heating pad, hot bath, or hot-water bottle to relax the muscles that cramp and cause pain.

❏ If you are taking medication for endometriosis, call your doctor immediately if there are any new or worsened symptoms, especially problems such as difficulty in breathing, or pain in the chest or legs. These symptoms may indicate that a blood clot is present. Frequent checkups are needed to watch for such possible side effects as osteoporosis. (See OSTEOPOROSIS.) Be aware that endometriosis symptoms often worsen temporarily when a woman starts taking medication.

Considerations

❏ Surgical options range from hysterectomy, in which the entire uterus is removed, to laparoscopy, in which the doctor removes abnormal tissue through a tube passed through a small incision (a procedure also used for diagnostic purposes). However, hysterectomy eliminates fertility, and either option may not provide a permanent solution because the underlying hormonal problems are still there. Surgery can also create painful abdominal adhesions. Hormonal therapies are used to stop ovulation and hormone production. However, such therapies can produce a wide array of side effects, from masculinizing changes (such as abnormal hair growth) to nausea, vomiting, vaginal dryness, and mood swings. Production of other hormones also can be affected.

❏ Regular exercise—forty minutes four times a week—prevents side effects from treatment with a drug called danazol (Danocrine). This drug "shuts off" normal hormonal cycles to control blood flow and pain and to keep abnormal tissue from spreading. Without exercise, the drug sometimes causes "masculinizing" side effects, such as a deepened voice, which are reversible when the drug is stopped. Regular exercise cuts the risk of these side effects in half. This drug is not usually the first line of treatment due to its side effects. Other drugs that are used more often include hormonal contraceptives, gonadotropin-releasing hormone (GnRH) agonist and antagonists, medroxyprogesterone (Depo-Provera), and aromatase inhibitors.

❏ Endometriosis is a benign (noncancerous) condition, but some research suggests that women who have endometriosis are at greater risk of developing breast cancer, melanoma, lymphoma, and ovarian cancer than women who do not have it.

❏ Adenomyosis is a condition similar to endometriosis in some respects, but it is confined to the uterus. This condition is common in women who have had several children. The uterine wall does not contract as it should, and blood flow continues after menstruation. Usual treatments include anti-inflammatory drugs, hormone medications, and hysterectomy.

ENLARGED PROSTATE

See BENIGN PROSTATIC HYPERTROPHY (BPH); PROSTATE CANCER; PROSTATITIS.

ENURESIS

See BED-WETTING.

EPILEPSY

See SEIZURE DISORDERS.

ERECTILE DYSFUNCTION

Erectile dysfunction (ED) is a condition in which a man does not have the ability to achieve or maintain an erection adequate for normal sexual intercourse. ED may be chronic or recurrent, or it may happen as a single isolated incident. This condition often results from both psychological and physical factors. Erections are made possible by a complex combination of blood vessel and nerve functions that are affected by hormones, especially the main male hormone, testosterone. An important part of the process is the production and release of nitric oxide, which allows the penis to fill with blood.

Anything that interferes with these interactions can interfere with erections. Diabetes, which leads to atherosclerosis and impaired circulation, is the most frequent cause of ED. ED can also be caused by high blood pressure and the medications given for it (and other drugs as well), insufficient testosterone production, hypothyroidism or hyperthyroidism, repeated infections of sexually transmitted diseases, excessive alcohol consumption, and smoking. Fatigue, overwork, and obesity can compound the problem. Conventional medicine treats ED with medication and erection-enabling devices.

Many of the factors associated with ED become more common with age. This explains why most men who suffer from at least occasional ED are older (although the condition also can affect younger men). While it often takes longer for older men to achieve erections, ED is not a normal consequence of aging. It is estimated that between 15 and 30 million men in the United States have some degree of ED.

No treatment for ED, whether herbal or conventional, should be undertaken until a complete physical examination is performed to see if there is an underlying disorder. Any of the herbal preparations listed here should be effective within three to four weeks of first use.

Herbs to Avoid

❑ Individuals who have ED should avoid vitex. (For more information regarding this herb, *see* VITEX *under* The Herbs in Part One.)

Recommendations

❑ To use muira puama most effectively, combine it with catuaba, iporuru, or yohimbe.

❑ Stop smoking, and avoid exposure to secondhand smoke. Smoking causes ED by several mechanisms, and the damage to the nitric oxide mechanism in the penis caused by smoking cannot be completely compensated for by Viagra or herbal remedies.

❑ If you have diabetes, pay close attention to regulating blood sugars. This means strictly limiting carbohydrates according to your doctor's orders and taking every prescribed insulin injection and oral agent. (*See* DIABETES.)

❑ Limit bicycle-riding sessions to one or two times per week, or consider using a recumbent bicycle, in which the rider lies down while pedaling. ED caused by pressure on the penis rubbing against the bicycle seat usually corrects itself after a six-week to three-month break from biking, but can be permanent.

❑ Seek counseling, if needed, to address psychological factors that can contribute to ED. Such factors include anxiety, depression, stress, guilt, and fear of intimacy.

Erectile Dysfunction: Beneficial Herbs

Herb	Form and Dosage	Comments
Ashwagandha	Encapsulated extract standardized for withanolides. Use as directed on the label.	Said to ensure potency and increase fertility.
Catuaba	Tincture. Take as directed on the label.	Strengthens erections. Increases erotic dreams and sexual interest.
Cistanche	Use as directed by a dispensing herbalist.	Enhances production of nitric oxide.
Damiana[1]	Tincture. Take ¼–½ tsp (1–2 ml) in ¼ cup water 3 times daily.	Increases stability of erection during intercourse. Aphrodisiac.
Epimedium[2]	Use as directed by a dispensing herbalist.	Increases blood flow to the penis. Stimulates the sensory nerves; increases sexual desire.
Ginkgo[3]	Ginkgolide tablets. Take 240 mg daily for at least 6 months.	Activates the release of nitric oxide from blood-vessel linings.
Ginseng[4]	*Panax ginseng* tincture. Take as directed on the label.	Promotes cell growth and healing in the sex organs.
Iporuru	Tincture. Take as directed on the label.	Produces stronger erections and greater numbers of viable sperm.
Morinda	Use as directed by a dispensing herbalist.	Antidepressant that increases erectile function. Also lowers blood pressure.
Muira puama	Tincture. Take as directed on the label.	Increases both libido and erectile strength (*see* Recommendations).
Yohimbe[5]	Tincture. Do not use tablets. (*See* Precautions, below.) Take as directed on the label.	Acts to increase blood flow into and reduce flow out of penis. It is more likely to be effective if you are fasting or if you eat a low-fat diet.

Precautions for the use of herbs:

[1]Do no use damiana if you are anemic or have chronic bleeding.

[2]Do not use epimedium if you have any kind of prostate disorder.

[3]Do not use ginkgo if you are taking blood-thinning medication. Discuss its use with your doctor before having any type of surgery.

[4]The aphrodisiac and potency-enhancing effects of ginseng are canceled out by the use of morphine and related drugs, including cocaine.

[5]Do not use "yohimbe" tablets. These often do not contain any actual yohimbe. *Never* take yohimbe and sildenafil (Viagra) within twelve hours of each other. Because yohimbe is a possible monoamine oxidase (MAO) inhibitor, avoid the following substances when using this herb: foods that contain tyramine (chocolate, most French cheeses, liver, organ meats, red wine), nasal decongestants, and weight-loss aids containing phenylpropanolamine. Do not use high doses of yohimbe, which can result in priapism, a condition characterized by a painful erection that requires surgery.

❏ Consult a urologist for testing to determine whether ED is caused by an underlying illness that requires treatment.

❏ Avoid stress. (*See* STRESS.)

Considerations

❏ The South American herb quebracho is another source of yohimbine, the anti–erectile dysfunction chemical found in yohimbe. Other herbs and supplements that have shown to be of benefit include Korean red ginseng; Kyo-Green, a green powdered drink; and an amino acid–like compound, L-citrulline.

❏ Sildenafil citrate (Viagra) works by relaxing blood vessels within the penis. Two other drugs have recently become available: tadalafil (Cialis) and vardenafil (Levitra). These three drugs can sometimes adversely affect the cardiovascular system, and can cause headache, digestive upsets, and vision problems, among other possible side effects. Some medications, such as nitroglycerin and anti-coagulants, interfere with drugs that treat ED, so speak to your doctor if you are using these or any other over-the-counter (OTC) medication, herb, or supplement before starting Viagra or any of the other ED drugs. Other treatments include drugs that are injected into the penis, penile implants, external vacuum-type devices, and testosterone replacement.

❏ In some cases, testosterone patches may be used to supply extra testosterone. These patches usually increase potency, but decrease fertility. Be sure to keep testosterone patches and creams away from children.

❏ Blood-pressure medications often cause erectile problems. Loss of potency caused by diuretics can be corrected in the short term by reducing total calorie intake. The resulting weight loss, over the long term, may make it possible to discontinue the blood-pressure medication under doctor's supervision. (*See* HIGH BLOOD PRESSURE [HYPERTENSION].)

❏ Urologists differ in the types of treatment they recommend for ED, but many opt first for nonsurgical treatment.

❏ *See also* ALCOHOLISM; ATHEROSCLEROSIS; HYPERTHYROIDISM; HYPOTHYROIDISM; and SEX DRIVE, DIMINISHED.

EYE PROBLEMS

Everyone experiences eye trouble at one time or another. Eyes that are bloodshot, blurry, dry, infected, irritated, itchy, sensitive to light, or ulcerated are among the most common health complaints. Chronic eye problems, such as farsightedness, nearsightedness, cataracts, and glaucoma, are usually caused by disorders in the eye itself. This section addresses some of the more common, relatively minor eye problems. A number of more serious disorders are discussed separately. (*See* CATARACTS; DIABETIC RETINOPATHY; GLAUCOMA; MACULAR DEGENERATION.)

The eyeball's tough outer layer is called the sclera, or the "white" of the eye. Beneath the sclera is the middle layer, the choroid, which contains the blood vessels that serve the eye. In the center of the sclera is the highly colored iris, and in the center of the iris is the pupil. Behind the iris is the lens. The front of the eye is covered by a transparent membrane called the cornea. At the back of the eye is the retina, a light-sensitive membrane that is connected to the brain by the optic nerve. Light passes through the cornea and is focused by the lens on the retina, which sends the image to the brain for processing.

The eye contains two important fluids. The aqueous humor, which fills the space between the cornea and the lens, contains all the components of blood except red blood cells. The vitreous humor is a jellylike substance that fills the back of the eyeball, in the space between the lens and the retina.

Herbal remedies for some of the most common (and least serious) eye complaints are covered in this section. In addition, a proper diet, especially one that includes natural antioxidants such as beta-carotene and vitamins C and E, can ease or slow the progression of many eye problems. Eat yellow, orange, or dark green vegetables daily to ensure an adequate supply of these nutrients.

Bags Beneath the Eyes

In the course of aging, the skin and the muscles underlying it can lose tone and sag. If fluids accumulate beneath the flaccid skin, bags beneath the eyes become noticeable. Possible causes of bags underneath the eyes include sleep deprivation, allergies, and aging.

Recommendations

❏ Avoid salt, both table salt and that found in prepared foods.

❏ Avoid drinking fluids before bedtime.

❏ Get adequate sleep.

❏ Refresh your eyes by placing a cloth dipped in very cold water over them for fifteen minutes once or twice daily. Wet tea bags or cold cucumber slices are also good.

❏ If you smoke, stop, and avoid secondhand smoke as much as possible.

Bloodshot Eyes

Bloodshot eyes occur when small blood vessels on the surface of the eye become inflamed. Inflammation of the capillaries on the surface of the eye can be caused by allergies or by exposure to airborne irritant chemicals. Other possible causes include eyestrain, fatigue, and disorders that impair circulation, including diabetes, high blood pressure, and high cholesterol.

Bags Beneath the Eyes: Beneficial Herbs

Herb	Form and Dosage	Comments
Siberian ginseng[1]	Pure *Eleutherococcus senticosus* extract. Take the dose recommended on the label in ¼ cup water.	Relieves puffiness associated with prolonged fatigue.

Precautions for the use of herbs:

[1]Do not use Siberian ginseng if you have prostate cancer or an autoimmune disease such as lupus or rheumatoid arthritis.

Bags Beneath the Eyes: Formulas

Formula	Comments
Unblock the Orifices and Invigorate the Blood Decoction	A traditional Chinese herbal formula that treats swelling or dark circles below the eyes accompanied by dark purple complexion, dizziness, headache, and ringing in the ears.

Bloodshot Eyes: Beneficial Herbs

Herb	Form and Dosage	Comments
Bilberry	Tablets. Take 250 mg 3 times daily.	Strengthens the linings of blood vessels.
Eyebright or mullein	Tea bag, prepared with 1 cup water, used as a compress. (*See* COMPRESSES in Part Three.) Apply lightly for 10–15 minutes 1–2 times daily.	Relieves inflammation.
Hawthorn	Tablets. Take 100–250 mg 3 times daily.	Counteracts allergic reactions. Strengthens linings of blood vessels; lowers blood pressure.
Raspberry leaf	Tea, used to make compresses. (*See* COMPRESSES in Part Three.) Apply to the eyes with the lids closed for 10 minutes or as needed.	Alleviates redness and irritation.

Bloodshot Eyes: Formulas

Formula	Comments
Augmented Rambling Powder[1]	A traditional Chinese herbal formula that relieves bloodshot eyes during premenstrual syndrome (PMS) by reducing estrogen production.
Cimicifuga and Kudzu Decoction	A traditional Chinese herbal formula that relieves bloodshot eyes caused by allergies.

Precautions for the use of formulas:

[1]Do not use Augmented Rambling Powder if you are trying to become pregnant.

Considerations

❏ While high blood pressure can lead to bleeding from the blood vessels serving the eyes, this usually occurs only after years of elevated pressure. (*See* HIGH BLOOD PRESSURE [HYPERTENSION].) If your pressure was normal the last time it was taken (providing that the last time was not years ago), the redness in your eyes is far more likely to be caused by irritation.

❏ *See also* DIABETES; HANGOVER; HIGH CHOLESTEROL; and Respiratory Allergies under ALLERGIES.

Blurred Vision

Vision can become blurred, causing objects to appear distorted or indistinct, for any number of reasons. Chronically blurred vision is usually caused by common vision defects such as farsightedness, nearsightedness, or astigmatism. Disturbances of the fluid balance in the eye also

Blurred Vision: Beneficial Herbs

Herb	Form and Dosage	Comments
Black cohosh	Tablets. Take 250-500 mg daily.	Relieves fluid imbalance during PMS.
Yarrow	Tea bag, prepared with 1 cup water. Take 1 cup 2–3 times daily	Strengthens muscles surrounding the eyes.

Blurred Vision: Formulas

Formula	Comments
Four-Substance Decoction	A traditional Chinese herbal formula that treats blurred vision that occurs during emotional tension or PMS. It may be necessary to take the formula for 2–3 months before results are noticeable.
Gastrodia and Uncaria Decoction[1]	A traditional Chinese herbal formula that treats blurred vision caused by high blood pressure.

Precautions for the use of formulas:

[1]Do not use Gastrodia and Uncaria Decoction if you are trying to become pregnant.

can cause blurred vision. These disturbances may be limited to the eye itself, as in eyestrain and excessive tearing, or they may reflect disturbances in fluid balance throughout the body, as in diabetes, high blood pressure, and premenstrual syndrome (PMS).

Recommendations

❏ Eat potassium-rich foods, such as apricots, avocados, bananas, blackstrap molasses, brewer's yeast, brown rice, dates, figs, dried fruit, garlic, nuts, potatoes, raisins, sea vegetables, winter squash, yeast, wheat bran, and yams. Potassium is essential for maintaining fluid balance within the eye.

❏ Take 10,000 to 50,000 international units (IU) of vitamin A daily for four weeks. Vitamin A is essential for regulating eye pressure and for forming pigments in the retina. Do not take more than 10,000 IU a day if you are or may become pregnant. The amount that is considered safe is 10,000 IU daily; if you are considering taking more than this, check with your health-care provider first.

❏ Take regular breaks if working at a computer or at any other eye-straining job.

❏ To relieve strain from close work or reading, frequently look away from reading matter or work to an object in the distance. Blinking the eyes also helps.

❏ Give your eyes intervals of restful darkness for at least fifteen minutes every day. Cover both eyes with cupped hands, making sure the palms do not rest on the eyeballs. Close the eyes, and make sure there is no tightness in the eyelids, brows, or fingers. Remain comfortable and relaxed by keeping the spine straight.

Considerations

❏ Laser surgery has a very high success rate, but it is important to determine whether you are a good candidate for this procedure. Review this thoroughly with your doctor.

❏ Blurring or loss of vision in one eye should never be ignored because it could be a sign of a stroke or transient ischemic attack, a short-term or "mini" stroke in which symptoms disappear within twenty-four hours. (*See* STROKE.)

❏ Blurred vision can also be a sign of uncontrolled or undiagnosed high blood sugar levels in people with diabetes. If blurred vision occurs with unusual thirst, hunger, large volume of urination, or unexplained weight loss, see a physician. (*See* DIABETES.)

❏ *See also* HIGH BLOOD PRESSURE (HYPERTENSION) and PREMENSTRUAL SYNDROME (PMS).

Conjunctivitis (Pinkeye)

Conjunctivitis, also known as pinkeye, is an inflammation of the membrane that lines the eyelid and wraps around to cover most of the white of the eye. Symptoms include an eye that appears swollen and bloodshot and feels itchy and irritated. Pus exuding from the inflammation site can cause "sticky eyes" after the eyes are closed for an extended period, such as during sleep.

Conjunctivitis is caused by viruses and bacterial infections. Bacterial conjunctivitis usually causes a heavier, stickier discharge. Allergies also can cause conjunctivitis, as can injury to the eye and exposure to eye irritants such as smoke and chemicals.

Conventional treatment for infectious conjunctivitis consists of warm compresses and, if bacterial infection is present, antibiotics. For allergic conjunctivitis, cold compresses and antihistamines are used.

The treatments listed below can be used by children, except for barberry, coptis, goldenseal, and Oregon grape root. Formula dosages for children should be discussed with a knowledgeable health-care practitioner. Remove contacts before using eyedrops or washes.

Recommendations

❑ If blurred vision or pain occurs, or if you wear contacts, seek immediate medical assistance.

❑ For bacterial conjunctivitis, apply plain hot compresses several times daily, since many of the germs that cause conjunctivitis cannot tolerate heat. (*See* COMPRESSES in Part Three.) To improve the effectiveness of this treatment, add tinctures of barberry, coptis, goldenseal, or Oregon grape root to the compress water. If the conjunctivitis persists, seek medical attention.

❑ If a *Staphylococcus* ("staph") infection is causing swollen eyelids, use a lotion made with madeira vine in addition to any prescribed antibiotics. Madeira, a folk remedy common in Mexico and the southern United States, is an antibacterial. If this remedy is not working, you may still need to go to a doctor for conventional treatments.

Conjunctivitis: Beneficial Herbs

Herb	Form and Dosage	Comments
Barberry[1] or coptis[1] or goldenseal[1] or Oregon grape root[1]	Tincture. Take 1–1½ tsp (4–6 ml) in ¼ cup water 3 times daily. Do not use these herbs for more than 2 weeks at a time.	Fights bacterial conjunctivitis.
Calendula	Eyedrops or washes. Used as directed on the label.	Antibacterial and antiviral. Helps reduce swollen eyelids.
Chamomile or	German chamomile (*Matricaria recutita*) tea bag, prepared with 1 cup water, used to make a compress. (*See* COMPRESSES in Part Three.) Apply for 10–15 minutes 2–3 times daily.	Reduce inflammation. Especially useful if you also have allergies.
Fennel seed[2]	Tea, used to make compresses. Apply 10–15 minutes 2–3 times daily.	
Eyebright	Eyedrops. Use as directed on the label.	A gentle antibacterial. Stops inflammation.

Precautions for the use of herbs:

[1]Do not use barberry, coptis, goldenseal, or Oregon grape root if you are pregnant or have gallbladder disease. Do not take these herbs with supplemental vitamin B$_6$ or with protein supplements containing the amino acid histidine. Do not use goldenseal if you have cardiovascular disease or glaucoma.

[2]Do not use fennel seed if you have an estrogen-sensitive disorder, such as breast cancer, endometriosis, or fibrocystic breasts.

Conjunctivitis: Formulas

Formula	Comments
Coptis Decoction to Relieve Toxicity[1]	A traditional Chinese herbal formula especially appropriate for treating infectious conjunctivitis. Use it for fever with sweating, and if the discharge from the eye is thin.
Dong Quai, Gentiana Longdancao, and Aloe Pill[1]	A traditional Chinese herbal formula that relieves systemic illness (as shown by dizziness, headache, and irritability) caused by eye infection.
Minor Bluegreen Dragon Decoction[2]	A traditional Chinese herbal formula used for fever without sweating, and if the discharge from the eye is thin.

Precautions for the use of formulas:

[1]Do not use Coptis Decoction to Relieve Toxicity or Dong Quai, Gentiana Longdancao, and Aloe Pill if you are trying to become pregnant.

[2]Do not use Minor Bluegreen Dragon Decoction if you have a fever.

Floaters: Beneficial Herbs

Herb	Form and Dosage	Comments
Dong quai	*Angelica sinensis* tablets. Take 250–500 mg daily.	Strengthens capillaries so they are not damaged by floaters.
Ginkgo[1]	Ginkgolide tablets. Take 40 mg 3 times daily or 60 mg twice daily.	Increases circulation within the eye, providing oxygen to the retina.

Precautions for the use of herbs:

[1]Do not use ginkgo if you are taking blood-thinning medication. Discuss its use with your doctor before having any type of surgery.

❏ If your eyelids are swollen, put a peeled, grated, fresh potato wrapped in gauze over your eye. It acts as an astringent and has a healing effect.

Considerations

❏ Conjunctivitis associated with hay fever may be treated with prescription drops containing steroids. (For herbal treatments that make steroid therapy more effective, *see* "Side Effects of Cancer Treatment" *under* CANCER.)

❏ *See also* Respiratory Allergies *under* ALLERGIES.

Floaters

Floaters are clear flecks and spots that move slowly through the visual field. They are caused by the accumulation of debris in the vitreous humor of the eye, the jellylike substance that fills the eyeball. The debris results when bits of the vitreous degenerate. Floaters tend to increase with age and to be more noticeable if you are nearsighted.

Recommendations

❏ It is normal to see several floaters from time to time, but if you suddenly see a lot of them, talk to an ophthalmologist. An increase in floaters may be a sign that the retina is separating from the back of the eyeball. If treatment is delayed, the retina may detach completely, a condition that requires immediate surgery.

FEVER BLISTERS

See under HERPESVIRUS INFECTION.

FIBROCYSTIC BREASTS

Fibrocystic breasts are characterized by the presence of round or oval lumps and/or cysts in the breast. The cysts are soft to firm in texture. Fibrous lumps are rubbery and move freely beneath the skin. (Cancerous lumps, in contrast, generally do not move freely under the skin.) These growths are frequently tender, usually in the week or so before menstruation begins.

More than half of all women have some degree of fibrocystic breasts, which often goes undetected. While the condition has been associated with breast cancer, there is no evidence that there is a connection. Any breast abnormality, however, requires medical examination. Conventional treatment consists of surgery and/or hormonal therapy.

A woman with fibrocystic breasts might start out in her late teens with a few lumps that become tender before her period begins. As she ages, the breasts become lumpier and more painful. Finally, as she reaches menopause, the discomfort becomes erratic.

Fibrocystic breasts occur because the body produces either too much estrogen or too little progesterone, the two main hormones that control the menstrual cycle. Estrogen stimulates tissue growth in the first half of the cycle. Progesterone regulates such growth in the second half. If a woman's body produces more estrogen than progesterone, stimulation exceeds regulation, and breast tissue grows. If a woman's breast cells are genetically coded to have more estrogen receptors, or docking points, than usual, fibrocystic disease develops.

Fibrocystic breast cells also respond to other hormones. A woman's body contains some testosterone, the main male hormone, and another hormone called aromatase converts testosterone into estrogen. One of the hormones induced by stress, PGE_2, makes aromatase more active in laboratory studies. Emotional tension and a diet that is high in simple sugar and undesirable fats—especially those in beef—could stimulate this hormonal overactivity, which also includes increased estrogen production. In addition, waste estrogen, which passes into the large intestine for elimination, can be reabsorbed into the bloodstream.

Most of the herbal remedies for fibrocystic disease slow estrogen production. A few, such as Dong Quai and Peony Powder, may help prevent "masculinizing" side effects of standard medical treatments by activating aromatase through certain biochemical pathways, as shown in cell studies. They can stimulate aromatase in such a way that it converts excess testosterone into estrogen, preventing growth of body hair and lowering of the voice, but not so that it creates excessive estrogen. All of the herbs recommended here must be used through several menstrual cycles, or for several months, to become fully effective.

Fibrocystic Breasts: Beneficial Herbs

Herb	Form and Dosage	Comments
Ginger	Tea, made by adding ⅓ teaspoon (1 gm) powdered ginger to 1 cup water. (*See* TEAS in Part Three.) Apply as a warm compress 3 times daily. (*See* COMPRESSES in Part Three).	Relieves pain. Stops production of hormones that cause swelling.
Green tea	Catechin extract. Take 240 mg 3 times daily; or decaffeinated tea bag, prepared with 1 cup water. Take 1 cup 2–3 times daily. To avoid dilution, do not use within 1 hour of taking other medications.	Reduces growth of existing cysts and formation of new cysts.
Kelp	As food. Eat 2 oz (50 gm) in a single serving. Limit this to once per week.	Increases bowel regularity, which reduces reabsorption of estrogen from the stool.
Kudzu	Tablets. Take 10 mg 3 times daily.	Keeps estrogen from activating cysts.
Soy isoflavone concentrate[1]	Tablets. Take about 3,000 mg daily.	Keeps estrogen from activating cysts.
Vitex	Tincture. Take 1½ tsp in ¼ cup water 3 times daily.	Balances estrogen and progesterone production; limits testosterone production.
Wild yam[2]	Tincture. Take 20 drops in ¼ cup water 3 times daily, after meals.	Useful for relief of pain and swelling. Also called dioscorea.

Precautions for the use of herbs:

[1]If concentrated soy isoflavones cause upset stomach, use kudzu instead.

[2]Overdosage of wild yam can cause nausea. Be sure not to use an "herbal" product that contains synthetic progesterone while using this herb.

Fibrocystic Breasts: Formulas

Formula	Comments
Augmented Rambling Powder[1]	A traditional Chinese herbal formula that lowers estrogen levels. Most useful if accompanying symptoms include dry mouth, blurry vision, sensation of pressure in the lower abdomen, difficult urination, and increased menstrual flow.
Dong Quai and Peony Powder	A traditional Chinese herbal formula that stops cyclical growth of breast tissue without having a masculinizing effect.
Two-Cured Decoction[2]	A traditional Chinese herbal formula that lowers estrogen levels.

Precautions for the use of formulas:

[1]Do not use Augmented Rambling Powder if you are trying to become pregnant.

[2]Do not use Two-Cured Decoction if you have a fever.

Herbs to Avoid

❑ Women who have fibrocystic breasts should avoid the following herbs: cordyceps, dan shen, fennel seed, licorice, and peony. (For more information regarding these herbs, *see* CORDYCEPS, DAN SHEN, FENNEL SEED, LICORICE, and PEONY *under* The Herbs in Part One.)

Recommendations

❑ Because estrogen is produced by body fat, eat a diet that does not promote excess body fat. (*See* ESTROGEN-REDUCING DIET in Part Three.) However, avoid diets that contain too little fat and cholesterol. Consuming at least 300 milligrams of cholesterol a day—that is, any diet other than a cholesterol-lowering diet—and more than 30 percent of total calories from fat—almost any American diet, including a vegan diet—protects against breast cysts.

❑ Soy protein seems to reduce the size of the fibroid and results in less tenderness. Ask your doctor about including soy in your diet if you do not already do so.

❑ To consume healthy sources of fat, eat two to three servings of cold-water fish (such as salmon) weekly, or take MaxEPA fish oil. Borage or evening primrose oil is also helpful. These foods and supplements contain omega-3 fatty acids, which complement the antiestrogenic activity of herbs by reducing the body's formation of hormones that cause pain and swelling.

❏ Consume 25 grams of fiber daily, preferably in the form of whole-grain cereals along with fresh fruits and vegetables. Fiber increases regularity, which reduces the amount of estrogen excreted into the stool that can be reabsorbed by the body.

❏ Take 50,000 international units (IU) of beta-carotene daily. The body turns beta-carotene into vitamin A, which causes breast cells to be less responsive to estrogen. Eat beta-carotene-rich foods as well—those that are orange or red such as winter squash, carrots, and tomatoes tend to be higher in beta-carotene.

❏ To protect breast tissue against harmful free radicals, take 100 international units (IU) of vitamin E daily.

❏ Avoid caffeinated medications (such as over-the-counter [OTC] medications for staying awake), chocolate, coffee, cola drinks, and tea. They all contain caffeine or related compounds that can aggravate fibrocystic breast disease, especially in the presence of emotional stress. However, data are conflicting. One study found that caffeine had no effect on the fibroids in the breast.

❏ If you take hormone therapy, be sure to exercise at least four hours a week. There is some clinical evidence that exercise counteracts "masculinizing" effects of hormone therapy.

❏ Do not take birth control pills that contain a high percentage of estrogen. Such pills can make symptoms worse.

Considerations

❏ Conventional treatment consists of surgery to either drain or remove cysts. This usually provides only temporary benefits since the underlying hormonal problems still exist. Hormonal therapy is designed to turn off the growth cycle initiated by estrogen. This often works, although some hormonal treatments may have masculinizing side effects, such as the growth of facial and body hair.

❏ Women who are iodine-deficient (a very rare occurrence) have breast tissue that is very sensitive to estrogen. A weekly serving of kelp, or the use of iodized salt, will usually correct iodine deficiency, but speak to your doctor first.

❏ Women who are sensitive to regular coffee are probably also sensitive to decaffeinated coffee, since decaf retains enough caffeine to affect sensitive people. There are many coffee substitutes available in supermarkets and health food stores, such as Cafix, Roma, and Teccino. Or use a caffeine-free herbal tea.

❏ Acupuncture is a useful complementary therapy for fibrocystic breasts. Unlike other treatments that focus on estrogen regulation, acupuncture modifies the tendency of the immune system to produce inflammatory chemicals that cause pain and swelling. Both traditional acupuncture and electroacupuncture are effective for this disease. (*See* ACUPUNCTURE in Part Three.)

❏ Some have reported good results using evening primrose oil to reduce the size of the cysts.

❏ *See also* PREMENSTRUAL SYNDROME (PMS).

FIBROIDS, UTERINE (UTERINE MYOMAS)

As many as three out of four women over age thirty-five have benign uterine growths known as fibroids or myomas. A fibroid is a well-defined, solid growth in the myometrium, or smooth muscle, supporting the uterus. Fibroids vary in size, from that of the period at the end of this sentence to that of a cantaloupe. Multiple fibroids may occur.

In many of the women who have them, fibroids produce no symptoms. The first symptom may be either pain at the beginning of the period or increased menstrual flow. Fibroids usually do not interrupt the menstrual cycle, but as they grow they can cause increased frequency of urination, bladder displacement, urine retention, and constipation. They can also cause infertility or miscarriage, pain during sexual intercourse, increased vaginal discharge, and, due to the bleeding, anemia. Sometimes a fibroid is forced partially through the cervix, loses its blood supply, and dies, resulting in a foul odor.

Fluctuations in levels of estrogen and progesterone, the two main female sex hormones, influence fibroids. Fibroid growth, like that of all uterine tissue, is stimulated by estrogen. Estrogen levels can increase for a number of reasons, including excess weight and the use of estrogen replacement therapy (ERT) during menopause. After menopause, when a woman's body produces as much as 80 percent less estrogen, fibroids shrink. And while all uterine tissue responds to estrogen, fibroid tissue is extrasensitive to progesterone.

Small fibroids may not need treatment, although they should be checked on a regular basis. Doctors are more likely to treat large and actively growing fibroids that are causing extensive bleeding; surgery and drugs (which may have such masculinizing effects as a deepened voice) are the most common options. Fortunately, fibroids are almost never malignant.

While herbal treatments used to control bleeding can work fairly quickly, those that control hormone levels usually bring noticeable results in approximately three months. Formulas relieve fibroids by balancing the body's production of estrogen and progesterone, and relieve combinations of symptoms in three to six months of use. Consult a health-care provider before using herbal medicine with prescription medications.

Uterine Fibroids: Beneficial Herbs

Herb	Form and Dosage	Comments
Black cohosh	Tablets. Take 250–500 mg daily.	Stops bleeding and relieves pain, especially leg pain.
Cinnamon	Oil, 5–10 drops every 15 minutes for up to 4 hours or until bleeding subsides.	A traditional American medicine for fibroid bleeding.
Dan shen[1]	Use only under professional supervision.	Treats congealed blood; dark, red clots during menses; and pelvic congestion.
Green tea	Tea. Take as directed on the label.	Powerful antioxidant with anticancer properties.
Reishi	Tincture. Take 1 tbsp (12 ml) in ¼ cup water 3 times daily.	Stops pelvic inflammation. Useful if there is also emotional tension.

Precautions for the use of herbs:

[1]Dan shen stops fibroid bleeding, but it increases bloodstream estrogen levels. Do not use it on an ongoing basis.

Uterine Fibroids: Formulas

Formula	Comments
Augmented Rambling Powder[1]	A traditional Chinese herbal formula that lowers estrogen levels. Most useful if accompanying symptoms include dry mouth, blurry vision, and difficult or painful urination.
Cinnamon Twig and Poria Pill	A traditional Chinese herbal formula that lowers estrogen levels without interfering with the menstrual cycle or encouraging weight gain.
Dong Quai and Peony Powder	A traditional Chinese herbal formula that reduces blood estrogen levels without having masculinizing effects. Also reduces the formation of inflammatory compounds in the uterus.
Four-Substance Decoction	A traditional Chinese herbal formula that treats both fibroids and endometriosis in women who are affected by poor diet or overwork.

Precautions for the use of formulas:

[1]Do not use Augmented Rambling Powder if you are trying to become pregnant.

Herbs to Avoid

❑ Women who have fibroids should avoid the following herbs: cordyceps, fennel seed, licorice, and peony. (For more information regarding these herbs, *see* CORDYCEPS, FENNEL SEED, LICORICE, and PEONY *under* The Herbs in Part One.)

Recommendations

❑ Because estrogen is produced by body fat, eat a diet that does not promote excess body fat. (*See* ESTROGEN-REDUCING DIET in Part Three.)

❑ Do not take oral contraceptives with a high estrogen content, unless your doctor recommends it. Consider barrier forms of contraception, such as a cervical cap, condoms and foam, or a diaphragm.

❑ Also avoid progesterone creams. Creams made with wild yam (dioscorea) are used by many women to treat menopausal symptoms. Such creams have no detrimental effects on uterine fibroids, and may actually stop bleeding and pain. However, some "dioscorea" creams contain progesterone that is not identified on the label, and which stimulates fibroid growth. Either use wild yam itself or use creams that are certified not to contain added progesterone. (*See* WILD YAM *under* The Herbs in Part One.)

Considerations

❑ Uterine bleeding can be a symptom of a number of different disorders, including cervical and uterine cancer. It should always be brought to a doctor's attention.

❑ In the past, it was a matter of general practice to remove fibroids surgically if the uterus was enlarged to the same extent it would be in the twelfth week of pregnancy. Increasingly, however, physicians are becoming reluctant to remove fibroids solely on the basis of the "twelve-week rule" unless they are causing medical problems. Since fibroids usually shrink with the onset of menopause, the condition may take care of itself over time, especially if herbal therapies are used to keep symptoms in check.

❑ High stress levels and excess weight work together to increase the risk of fibroids. Fortunately, improving any of these factors will decrease the risk of fibroids. (*See* STRESS.)

❑ A woman's chance of developing fibroids may be decreased if she avoids using oral contraceptives.

❑ Women with fibroids may have higher levels of human growth hormone in their bodies than other women do.

FIBROMYALGIA SYNDROME

Fibromyalgia is a complex syndrome marked by severe muscle pain that may be accompanied by other symptoms including abdominal pain, chest pain, depression, fatigue, low-grade fever, headaches, insomnia, irritable bowel syndrome, premenstrual and menstrual difficulties, and temporomandibular joint (TMJ) syndrome. In the United States alone, 10 million people suffer from fibromyalgia, the majority of them women between the ages of twenty and fifty. Symptoms generally appear gradually and become more intense as time passes.

The pain of fibromyalgia is often described as burning, shooting, stabbing, or throbbing. One of the hallmarks of this disorder is a set of nine "tender points"—points where the muscles are exceptionally sensitive to touch—in the back, buttocks, elbows, knees, neck, and thighs. Another important aspect of fibromyalgia is sleep disturbance. People with fibromyalgia get less rapid eye movement (REM) sleep, the sleep in which dreaming occurs. Deprivation of "dream time" leads to one awakening feeling tired, worn out, and in pain. Unfortunately, a cycle starts in which a day of fibromyalgia pain is followed by poor sleep, and poor sleep is followed by an even more painful day.

Despite hundreds of studies, there is no definite medical cause or cure for fibromyalgia. Some studies indicate that fibromyalgia is caused by a deficiency of the growth hormone somatomedin C. Other studies link the condition to an excess of the pain-transmitting nerve chemical substance P in the spinal cord. It may also be caused by low levels of serotonin and tryptophan, low blood flow to the hypothalamus in the brain, and abnormal cytokines, which are proteins related to stress and immunity. Still other studies associate fibromyalgia with problems in the processing of lactic acid, the chemical that produces a muscle "burn" after vigorous exercise. Fibromyalgia seems to run in families. For some the onset of fibromyalgia is slow; however, a large percentage of cases are triggered by an illness or injury that causes trauma to the body.

Herbal remedies for fibromyalgia are limited. St. John's wort can be used on a long-term basis to address the biochemical imbalances associated with the disease; other herbs are used for short-term relief of pain.

Recommendations

❑ Some have proposed that a vegetarian diet or a near-vegetarian one like the Mediterranean diet may help lessen some of the symptoms. In one study, a vegetarian diet was not effective for improving sleep or reducing fatigue, but it did seem to help with pain control in people with fibromyalgia. In another study, people with fibromyalgia who followed a vegetarian—mostly raw—diet showed improvements in the composite fibromyalgia score and quality of life, reduced shoulder pain, and increased flexibility. This diet consisted of raw fruits, salads, carrot juice, tubers, grain products, nuts, seeds, and a dehydrated barley grass juice product.

❑ Do not discontinue any prescription antidepressant medications you may be taking when starting to use St. John's wort, but speak to your doctor before taking the

Fibromyalgia: Beneficial Herbs

Herb	Form and Dosage	Comments
Boswellia	Take as directed on the label.	Good for morning stiffness and joint pain.
Cat's claw[1]	Capsules. Take up to 3,000 mg daily.	Numerous anecdotal reports of improvement in symptoms after approximately 3 months' use.
Kava kava[2]	Kavapyrone tablets. Take 60–120 mg daily.	Helps induce sleep. May be combined with passionflower or valerian.
St. John's wort	Hypericin capsules. Take at least 900 mg daily for 2–3 months.	Raises serotonin levels; restores sleep and eases pain.
Willow bark	Salicin tablets. Take as directed on the label.	Aspirin-like pain relief without risk of bleeding or stomach upset.

Precautions for the use of herbs:

[1]Do not use cat's claw if you have to take insulin for diabetes. Do not use it if you are pregnant or nursing.

[2]Kava kava increases the effects of alcohol and such psychoactive drugs as sedatives and tranquilizers. Do not use it if you are pregnant or nursing.

herb. The herb may complement and reinforce the effect of the drugs you are taking. Treatment, however, takes time. While a few people with fibromyalgia experience pain relief immediately, results usually take at least a month and frequently longer.

❑ Take 800 milligrams of the supplement S-adenosyl-methionine (SAMe) daily for at least six weeks to control symptoms. Five clinical studies show that SAMe relieves depression, fatigue, morning stiffness, muscular weakness, and pain in fibromyalgia. It is significantly more effective in treating the condition than transcutaneous electrical nerve stimulation (TENS), a popular treatment for the condition.

❑ Complement antidepressant therapy with 5-hydroxy-L-tryptophan (5-HTP) and magnesium. 5-HTP may increase the effect of St. John's wort and/or amitriptyline hydrochloride (Elavil). Take 50 to 100 milligrams three times a day, every other day for three months. Magnesium supplements may stimulate serotonin production and provide muscle cells with necessary energy, which helps to avoid a muscle burn. The best forms of magnesium for fibromyalgia are those bound to aspartate, citrate, fumarate, malate, or succinate, chemicals involved in the energy cycle of muscle cells. Take 200 to 250 milligrams three times daily. Magnesium may produce diarrhea, so start with less and gradually add more.

❑ Include pomegranates and pomegranate juice in your diet. They have anti-inflammatory and antioxidant properties.

❑ Drink plenty of liquids to help flush out toxins. The best choices are steam-distilled water and herbal teas. Fresh vegetable juices supply necessary vitamins and minerals, but eating whole fruits and vegetables is a better way to get these nutrients.

❑ Avoid alcohol, caffeine, and sugar.

❑ Even if it seems impossible, exercise daily. Pick exercises that do not use the most painful muscles. Increase your workout time from two or three minutes a day up to twenty or thirty minutes. While there may be some cardiovascular benefits to light exercise, the primary benefit is its effect on hormones and sleep.

❑ Be sure to get a thyroid function blood test. Hypothyroidism, or low thyroid activity, can cause symptoms that are very similar to those of fibromyalgia. (See HYPOTHYROIDISM.)

Considerations

❑ Since fibromyalgia is a complex process, simple pain relief with aspirin or such nonsteroidal anti-inflammatory drugs (NSAIDs) as acetaminophen is only partially effective. Treatment to restore normal concentrations of serotonin in the brain is necessary to stop the cycle of sleep deprivation and pain.

❑ Steroid drugs, such as hydrocortisone and prednisone, are often prescribed for fibromyalgia. Although useful for treating other kinds of pain, they are of little use in treating fibromyalgia and other drugs may be needed. There are several prescription drugs that are used for fibromyalgia, such as duloxetine (Cymbalta), pregabalin (Lyrica), and milnacipran (Savella).

❑ In one study, patients with fibromyalgia who used 10 grams of *Chlorella pyrenoidosa* for two to three months had improved quality of life and less pain and fatigue. The herb also lowered blood pressure and enhanced wound healing.

❑ Acupuncture relieves pain and produces measurable changes in concentrations of serotonin and substance P. No pain medication should be taken during an acupuncture session, but pain relief should be immediate afterward. (*See* ACUPUNCTURE in Part Three.) In addition, other therapies have been useful, such as aromatherapy, biofeedback, chiropractic manipulation, acupressure, and yoga.

❑ Studies are being conducted on the possible role of a genetic defect that interferes with the formation of adenosine triphosphate (ATP, the source of cellular energy) in this disorder.

❑ For more information on how to deal with chronic pain, *see* PAIN, CHRONIC.

❑ A disorder that may be related to fibromyalgia is chronic fatigue syndrome (CFS), in which fatigue is the most prominent symptom. (*See* CHRONIC FATIGUE SYNDROME.)

❑ Fibromyalgia can be associated with a number of disorders. (*See also* DEPRESSION, HEADACHE, INSOMNIA, IRRITABLE BOWEL SYNDROME, MENSTRUAL PROBLEMS, MIGRAINE, and PREMENSTRUAL SYNDROME [PMS].)

FLATULENCE

See under INDIGESTION.

FLOATERS

See under EYE PROBLEMS.

FLU

See INFLUENZA.

FOOD ALLERGIES

See Food Allergies *under* ALLERGIES.

FOOD POISONING

Food poisoning, also referred to as food-borne illness, is a result of eating contaminated food. Infectious organisms—including various bacteria, viruses, and parasites—or their toxins are the most common cause of food poisoning. Symptoms of food poisoning can include localized abdominal pain and cramping, severe diarrhea and/or vomiting, fatigue, fever, and nausea. One in six Americans suffer from food poisoning each year, according to the Centers for Disease Control and Prevention.

The symptoms of food poisoning can come on suddenly, generally within a few hours of eating contaminated food, and usually within forty-eight hours. Sometimes reactions will take longer, such as up to three days for *Salmonella* and *Rotavirus*, and eight days for *Escherichia coli* (*E. coli*). Symptoms may linger for several days, causing food poisoning to be mistaken for the flu. Unlike intestinal viruses, food poisoning produces localized abdominal pain, usually causes severe diarrhea and vomiting, and may cause fever (especially in children), blurred vision, and difficulty in breathing. Bloody diarrhea, diarrhea that lasts more than twenty-four hours, or fever above 102°F (39.8°C) requires immediate medical attention, especially in children or adults weakened by long-term illnesses.

Most cases of food poisoning result from food being improperly handled. It is an unpleasant fact that most cases of *E. coli* infection result from fecal contamination during slaughter or in the kitchen. Other common sources are unpasteurized milk and apple cider, alfalfa sprouts, and contaminated water. Kitchen utensils used on contaminated food can spread the microorganisms that cause food poisoning to uncontaminated food. Unwashed hands also can spread disease-causing microorganisms. For example, if a cook shapes hamburger patties from contaminated meat and then prepares salad vegetables without washing his or her hands, the microbes in the meat can contaminate the salad. Even if food is contaminated, thorough cooking kills germs before they can make illness-producing toxins,

provided the food is not left out of refrigeration for too long.

If diarrhea and vomiting are so profuse that they cause dehydration, taking drugs to stop fluid loss and to replenish lost fluids is medically necessary. Sometimes intravenous fluids and salts may be required. However, these measures treat only the symptoms, not the disease. Children and the elderly are more susceptible to dehydration, so seek medical attention immediately in these cases. Herbal treatments may act on the microbes themselves. However, not every herb treats every kind of food poisoning. For this reason, it is necessary to consider the differences among the kinds of microbial contamination. If symptoms indicate a form of food poisoning that can have serious consequences, such as severe dehydration, seek immediate medical attention.

Unless otherwise specified, the herb dosages recommended here are for adults. Children under age six should be given one-quarter of the adult dosage. Children between the ages of six and twelve should be given one-half of the adult dosage. Formula dosages for children should be discussed with a knowledgeable health-care practitioner.

Herbs to Avoid

❏ If you have food poisoning, you should avoid barberry, coptis, goldenseal, and Oregon grape root. These herbs contain berberine, which kills many of the kinds of microorganisms that cause food poisoning, especially shigella and staph. They also, however, slow the motion of the intestinal tract, locking the toxin-producing microorganisms inside, and therefore should be avoided in food poisoning. (For more information regarding these herbs, *see* BARBERRY, COPTIS, GOLDENSEAL, and OREGON GRAPE ROOT *under* The Herbs in Part One.)

Food Poisoning: Beneficial Herbs

Herb	Form and Dosage	Comments
Agrimony	Tea (loose), prepared by steeping ¾ tsp (0.75 gm) in ½ cup water. (*See* TEAS in Part Three.) Take 1 cup 1–3 times daily.	Relieves mild diarrhea in children; prevents fluid loss.
Clove	Oil. Take 10–15 drops in ¼ cup water once, at the first sign of symptoms.	Kills *Staphylococcus aureus*, found in contaminated eggs.
Fennel seed[1]	Tea bag, prepared with 1 cup water. Take 1 cup as desired.	Relieves intestinal inflammation.
Milk thistle	Silymarin gelcaps. Take as directed on the label.	Aids in liver and blood cleaning.
Peppermint[2]	Tea bag, prepared with 1 cup water. Take 1 cup as desired.	Stops growth of *Listeria* and *Salmonella*. Soothes intestinal irritation.
Slippery elm bark	Tea (loose), prepared by steeping 1 tsp in 1 cup water. (*See* TEAS in Part Three.) Take 1 cup, as desired, after diarrhea stops.	Coats and soothes the intestines.

Precautions for the use of herbs:

[1]Do not take fennel seed if you have an estrogen-sensitive disorder, such as breast cancer, endometriosis, or fibrocystic breasts.

[2]Do not use peppermint if you have any kind of gallbladder disorder.

Food Poisoning: Formula

Formula	Comments
White Tiger Decoction[1]	A traditional Chinese herbal formula that kills *Salmonella*. Best herbal formula for diarrhea that occurs after eating spoiled food.

Precautions for the use of formulas:

[1]Do not use White Tiger Decoction if you are experiencing nausea or vomiting.

Recommendations

❏ Use activated charcoal tablets before symptoms start if you suspect you have been exposed to food contamination. Activated charcoal may help to prevent toxins from being absorbed in the intestine.

❏ Use electrolyte-balanced drinks such as Gatorade for adults, or Lytren, Pedialyte, or Gastrolyte for children. But all fluids are of benefit and include others such as clear soda water, ginger ale, clear broths, and plain water. Drink 8 to 16 cups a day. For children, ask your child's pediatrician about how much fluid your child should consume.

❏ If you give a child anything by mouth during a bout of food poisoning, give very small quantities, a teaspoon (5 milliliters) or less. Adults tolerate larger amounts of fluid and more easily tolerate soft foods. Overfilling an inflamed stomach can result in spasms, which cause vomiting.

❏ Start back with solid food slowly by including easy-to-digest foods such as soda crackers, toast, gelatin, bananas, and rice. Until you feel better, avoid dairy, caffeine, alcohol, nicotine, and fatty and highly seasoned foods.

❏ Do not use over-the-counter (OTC) medicines to prevent diarrhea and vomiting, since diarrhea and vomiting can clear illness-causing germs from the system. However, excessive, prolonged, or violent vomiting or diarrhea can be controlled with a number of medications.

Considerations

❏ A number of over-the-counter (OTC) and prescription drugs are available to control diarrhea and vomiting. Loperamide (Imodium AD) controls frequent, watery diarrhea. This medication works by slowing the movement of the intestinal muscles. While it reduces the number of trips to the bathroom, it increases rather than decreases the concentration of toxins in the intestine. This drug also is not suitable for children. Dimenhydrinate (Dramamine) is useful for mild nausea and vomiting, but children under age two cannot take it. Stronger drugs to control vomiting include prochlorperazine (Compazine), promethazine (Phenergan), and trimethobenzamide (Tigan). These drugs are given as suppositories or by injection. Consult with your doctor before taking any of these drugs.

❏ Diarrhea medicines do not prevent traveler's diarrhea, although they may help ease any problems that develop. These medications trap the microorganisms that cause food poisoning in the intestine and therefore increase the concentration of microbial toxins, worsening rather than relieving symptoms.

❏ Some herbs are thought to prevent food poisoning. Cayenne pepper, eaten with food as desired, can kill the germs that cause botulism and waterborne diarrhea. One or more cups of green tea taken with meals can kill many different kinds of sickness-producing microbes. And perilla, a leaf served with shellfish in Japanese cuisine, lowers the risk of shellfish poisoning and prevents allergies to shellfish.

❏ Anyone who takes diuretics, which increase urination, needs to be cautious if vomiting and/or diarrhea occur. It may be necessary to stop taking the diuretic during an attack of food poisoning in order to avoid depleting body fluids.

❏ To avoid food poisoning from home-cooked meals, it is important to practice safe food-handling techniques. Always wash hands with soap and water before preparing food and before eating. Perishable food shouldn't be out of the refrigerator for more than two hours, and those two hours include all the time the food is left unrefrigerated, including time in the shopping cart or pickup counter and time spent going home. Raw foods should be kept separate from cooked foods, and meat, eggs, and seafood should always be cooked until thoroughly done.

❏ To avoid food poisoning from restaurant meals, it is a good idea to avoid all-day buffets, as the food often sits out for hours at a time. Lunch buffets also are high risk, since food often sits for longer periods at room temperature than it does at dinner buffets.

❏ Game meats are especially likely to harbor the bacteria that cause food poisoning, although the safety of game depends on the hunter's skill in both bringing down the animal and field-dressing the meat. Meat for jerky should be heated to at least 165°F (74°C) before drying.

❏ Honey is not good for babies. It can contain bacterial spores that may cause infant botulism, a rare but serious disease that affects the nervous system. Symptoms include weakness (your baby isn't able to suck or cry as usual), difficulty in swallowing, weak limbs or neck, and constipation lasting more than three days. See the pediatrician if your newborn shows these symptoms. Anyone with a compromised immune system, such as patients with HIV, also should not use honey.

❏ Black sludge in the food processor does not necessarily indicate spoiled food. Garlic and onions contain sulfur, which oxidizes to form a black, but harmless, sludge. To make sure the food processor is not contaminated, fill the bowl with boiling water and let the water stand for a few minutes. Simple rinsing may not kill all the bacteria. Many food processors can simply be put in the dishwasher, which may also help clean it.

❏ It is best to avoid fruits or vegetables that have been sprayed with the home and garden pesticide aldicarb (Temik), which can cause symptoms similar to those of food poisoning.

FRACTURE

A fracture is a break or crack in a bone. Fractures can occur in any bone in the body, but they are most common in the feet, ankles, hands, and wrists. Fractures often occur after a sports injury, a fall, or a traffic accident. Broken bones are called simple fractures if the skin is intact and compound fractures if the skin is broken. A compression fracture occurs when a vertebra collapses. A stress fracture is a small break in a bone resulting from prolonged or repeated force against the bone; it often occurs as the result of intensive athletic training. Any bone disease increases the risk of a fracture. One of the most common of these is osteoporosis, a disorder in which bones become thinner and more brittle than normal.

If there is a sharp cracking sound with an injury or a protruding, obviously broken bone, the nature of the damage is clear. In the absence of such clear signs, fracture should be suspected from the following symptoms: intense pain, pain that increases when weight or pressure is placed on injury, a body part that is deformed or immobile after injury, bruising or swelling (often severe), or a pocket of blood under the skin. Fractures that occur near joints are often mistaken for bad sprains. In some cases, only an X-ray can determine whether or not there has been a break.

Fractures are especially serious for older people. Broken bones can set off a cycle in which underlying health problems are compounded and new problems appear. Taking preventive measures is especially important as people age.

Emergency medical assistance is needed to set a broken bone and treat any associated injuries. After that, herbal and nutritional therapies can help ease pain and speed healing.

Recommendations

❏ Because an adequate calcium supply is important when recovering from a fracture, take from 1,000 to 2,000 milligrams of a calcium-magnesium supplement daily. Use calcium citrate malate, the form of calcium, from which the body absorbs the highest percentage of calcium. Other forms of calcium, such as calcium citrate and calcium carbonate, are also effective.

❏ Consume foods and nutrients that increase bone mineral density (the calcium in the bones), such as any dairy food, calcium supplements, animal proteins, and potassium from fruits and vegetables. In one study, the risk of stress fractures was reduced by 62 percent with each glass of skim milk consumed per day by young female

Fracture: Beneficial Herbs

Herb	Form and Dosage	Comments
Treatments That Strengthen Bone		
Hawthorn	Tablets. Take 100–250 mg 3 times daily.	Stabilizes collagen, the principal protein in bone.
Por huesos	Tea (loose), prepared by steeping 1 tsp (1 gm) in 1 cup water. (*See* TEAS in Part Three.) Take 1 cup 3 times daily, between meals.	Literally "for bones." Encourages formation of the matrix that supports bone growth.
Soy isoflavone concentrate	Tablets. Take about 3,000 mg daily.	Helps move calcium from the bloodstream into bone.
Treatments That Ease the Pain of Stress Fractures		
Andiroba	Oil. Apply to the skin over the fracture.	An anti-inflammatory. Increases circulation.
Arnica[1]	Cream. Apply to the skin over the fracture.	Prevents swelling.
Boswellia	Extract. Use as directed on the label.	Aids in recovery. Eases pain and acts as an anti-inflammatory.

Precautions for the use of herbs:

[1]Do not apply arnica to broken skin or to an open wound, and do not take it internally. If a rash develops, discontinue use. Do not use arnica during pregnancy.

cross-country runners. In another study, older participants (a group where protein malnutrition is common) took a protein supplement from whey and essential amino acids and in as little as seven days they gained weight.

❑ Based on a study in nearly 50,000 postmenopausal women, the best diet for preventing a fracture and maintaining an optimal mineral content in the bones is a low-fat diet (fat should be 20 percent of total calories consumed daily) and increasing intake of fruit and vegetables to more than five servings a day and grains to more than six servings a day.

❑ Eat leafy vegetables. Salad greens contain vitamin K, which helps bones use protein to construct the collagen "glue" that holds bones together. Vegetables that contain vitamin K include iceberg and romaine lettuce, broccoli, Brussels sprouts, cabbage, kale, and spinach.

❑ Include berries in your diet. Blueberries, cherries, and cherry juice contain anthocyanidins and proanthocyanidins, blue and red pigments that help stabilize collagen. This is especially important for vegetarians, either those who are recovering from a fracture or those who wish to prevent fractures, since eating animal—but not vegetable—protein has been shown to lower the risk of fracture in postmenopausal women.

❑ Eat raw oats. Raw oats contain silica, which may be helpful for forming bone matrix. Eat rolled oats soaked overnight to make muesli.

❑ To ensure adequate supplies of vitamin D, take 400 to at most 1,000 milligrams of vitamin D supplements daily. (Ask your doctor to measure your blood vitamin D levels to determine the correct amount that you need.) Vitamin D is needed for calcium to enter bones, and a deficiency of this vitamin is a major risk factor for both osteoporosis and bone fracture. The people most at risk for vitamin D deficiency are older adults who are unable to go outdoors and who do not consume dairy products enriched with this vitamin.

❑ Use clay poultices for bruises and swelling. (*See* POULTICES in Part Three.)

Considerations

❑ The entire process of healing a fracture can take several months. If a fracture still has not healed after three or four months, there are several devices used to speed the process along. One is the Sonic Accelerated Fracture Healing System (SAFHS), which uses ultrasound to stimulate bone growth. The other is a battery-powered electromagnet worn on the body. It also stimulates bone development. Both devices are available with a doctor's prescription.

❑ Women athletes in endurance training are at special risk of fractures, especially if they eat less than 2,000 to 2,800 calories per day. Regular workouts while dieting can interrupt the menstrual cycle and deplete a woman's body of estrogen, causing a risk of osteoporosis comparable to that of women after menopause. Women athletes who do not have regular periods should take a daily calcium supplement.

❑ Wild angelica (*Angelica dahurica*) may reduce fracture risk in women athletes with irregular menstrual cycles. It can also reduce the risk of fracture among people undergoing steroid treatment. One cup of tea should be taken two to three times a day; use 1 teaspoon (2 grams) of tea for every cup. (*See* TEAS in Part Three.) Wild angelica should not be taken during pregnancy. If you are without a period for more than two months, seek a doctor's help.

❑ Athletically active postmenopausal women may want to take the supplement monofluorophosphate (MFP) along with their daily calcium. Using the two nutrients together decreases the incidence of vertebral fractures whether or not estrogen replacement therapy (ERT) is used.

❑ There is evidence that vitamin A supplements can increase the risk of bone fracture. A Swedish study of 66,651 women found that every milligram (3,000 IU) of vitamin A taken over the minimum Recommended Daily Allowance (RDA) increases the risk of bone fracture by 68 percent. Taking excessive vitamin A reduces bone density, especially in the hip. Cod liver oil is an especially concentrated source of vitamin A, and should be avoided by athletes in training, people over age seventy, and people with osteoporosis. Beta-carotene did not have this effect.

❑ Drinking soda has no direct effect on bone, despite a common belief otherwise. Soda drinkers are only at higher risk for fractures if they fail to get adequate calcium in their diets.

❑ To prevent stress fractures during athletic training, it is important to build exercise intensity gradually. Stress fractures are more common among sedentary people who attempt a rigorous exercise program right off the bat. However, even among older people, regular weight-bearing exercise, such as light weightlifting, helps increase bone density and reduces the risk of fracture.

❑ *See also* OSTEOPOROSIS.

FUNGAL INFECTION

See ATHLETE'S FOOT; RINGWORM; YEAST INFECTION (YEAST VAGINITIS). *See also under* NAILS, INFECTED.

GALLSTONES

The gallbladder is a small, pear-shaped organ located beneath the liver on the right side of the abdomen. It stores bile, a yellow-brown fluid produced by the liver, and secretes bile into the small intestine to help digest fats.

The gallbladder is connected to the liver and the small intestine by a series of tubes known as the bile ducts. In roughly 20 million people these tubes are blocked by hard, crystalline structures called gallstones. People are more likely to develop gallstones as they age, and women are more prone to them than men.

Most gallstones are made primarily of cholesterol. They form when the bile contains too much cholesterol and not enough bile salts. Cholesterol stones also may form if the gallbladder fails to empty frequently enough, or if the liver fails to secrete certain proteins into the bile.

Other factors play a role in gallstone formation, but the exact cause is not clear. Obesity is a risk factor, probably because of excess cholesterol and because the pressure that fat tissue places on the gallbladder interferes with normal emptying. Very rapid, low-calorie diets also are frequently associated with gallstone formation. Additionally, increased levels of estrogen are related to an increased risk of stones. Pregnancy increases estrogen levels, as do hormone replacement therapy and hormonal contraceptives.

Gallstone attacks frequently come after a large, fatty meal that follows a period of fasting. The pain associated with gallstones, steady and severe, is located in the upper abdomen. The pain may last from one to four hours and then be followed by a residual mild ache or soreness that may persist for a day or so. Nausea, vomiting, and chills frequently accompany gallstone attacks, and blood tests show elevated amounts of the liver pigment bilirubin, which may be reflected in dark urine and jaundice. Most people, though, have "silent stones," or stones causing no symptoms. Gallstones that don't cause signs and symptoms, such as those detected during an ultrasound or computed tomography (CT) scan done for some other condition, typically don't require treatment. In some cases, people with silent stones may be given cholesterol-lowering medications.

Fever or chills with a gallstone attack indicates an underlying problem that requires medical attention. Approximately 700,000 Americans require the surgical removal of the gallbladder in any given year. Medications taken by mouth may help dissolve gallstones. But it may take months or years of treatment to dissolve gallstones in this way. An experimental treatment to inject gallstone medications directly into the gallbladder may dissolve gallstones more quickly. Tests are ongoing to determine whether this procedure is safe and effective. Medications for gallstones aren't commonly used and are reserved for people who can't undergo surgery.

Herbs used in gallstone treatment relieve the symptoms of cholecystitis, or gallbladder irritation, which include muscle spasms, pain, and general tension. There are two groups of herbs listed below, those that can be used during an acute attack and those that cannot. Check with your doctor before using the herbs in either group. Using the second group of herbs during an acute attack can result in a stone becoming stuck in the bile duct, a condition that requires immediate surgery.

Gallstones: Beneficial Herbs

Herb	Form and Dosage	Comments
Treatments That Can Be Used During an Acute Attack		
Peppermint[1]	Enteric-coated oil capsules. Take 200 mg 3 times daily.	Relieves mild spasms of the bile duct.
Prickly ash[2]	Apply as a plaster as needed. (*See* PLASTERS in Part Three.)	Temporarily relieves pain and spasms of the bile ducts.
Treatments That Cannot Be Used During an Acute Attack		
Alfalfa	Tablets or capsules. Take 1,000 mg with a glass of warm water twice a day.	Cleanses the liver and supplies necessary vitamins and minerals.
Boldo[3]	Tea (loose), prepared by steeping 1 tsp (1.5 gm) in 1 cup water. (*See* TEAS in Part Three.) Take 1 cup 3 times daily.	Stimulates bile production, flushing small gallstones out of the ducts.
Gentian[4]	Bitters capsules. Take as directed on the label.	Relieves inflammation; stimulates bile production.
Greater celandine[3]	Tincture. Take 15–30 drops in ¼ cup water 3 times daily.	Stimulates bile production; relieves bile-duct spasms.
Milk thistle[3]	Silymarin gelcaps. Take 600 mg daily.	Lowers cholesterol content of the bile.
Soy lecithin[3]	Capsules. Take 2,000 mg daily.	Reduces cholesterol production in the liver.
Turmeric	Curcumin tablets. Take 125 mg 3 times daily.	Inhibits formation of cholesterol crystals.

Precautions for the use of herbs:
[1]Peppermint should be used only during mild spasms. Do not use it when symptoms are absent, because it may slow the normal passage of bile.

[2]Do not take prickly ash internally.

[3]Boldo, greater celandine, milk thistle, and soy lecithin can cause mild diarrhea.

[4]Do not use gentian if you have diarrhea.

Gallstones: Formulas

Formula	Comments
Frigid Extremities Powder	A traditional Chinese herbal formula that treats gallbladder inflammation and gallstones. Especially useful if symptoms include coldness in the fingers and toes, abdominal pain, diarrhea, and a sensation of fullness in the chest.
Gentiana Longdancao Decoction to Drain the Liver[1]	A traditional Chinese herbal formula that treats gallbladder inflammation and gallstones. Especially useful if symptoms include bitter taste in the mouth, dizziness, hearing loss, irritability, pain in the area of the gallbladder, and sore eyes.
Major Bupleurum Decoction[2]	A traditional Chinese herbal formula that reduces concentration of cholesterol in the bile, which inhibits gallstone formation.

Precautions for the use of formulas:

[1]Do not use Gentiana Longdancao Decoction to Drain the Liver if you are trying to become pregnant.

[2]Do not use Major Bupleurum Decoction if you have a fever.

Herbs to Avoid

❑ Individuals who have gallstones should avoid gardenia and schisandra. (For more information regarding these herbs, *see* individual entries *under* The Herbs in Part One.)

Recommendations

❑ During an acute attack, apply hot compresses over the gallbladder, which is located on the upper right side of the abdomen right under the rib cage, until the pain subsides. (*See* COMPRESSES in Part Three.) Also apply compresses to the back and right shoulder blade.

❑ If you have an acute attack, drink 1 tablespoon of apple cider vinegar in a glass of apple juice. This should relieve the pain quickly. If the pain does not subside, go to a hospital emergency room to rule out other disorders, such as a heart problem.

❑ Lose weight if necessary, but do not go on a crash diet. Losing weight quickly—more than 1 to 2 pounds a week—can make gallstone problems worse, especially if a low-fat diet is used. Eat about one-third of the calories as fat. (If you eat 1,800 calories, then 600 calories are fat, or 67 grams of fat.) Following gastric bypass surgery for weight loss, patients have about a 70 percent chance of developing gallstones. If you have had the surgery and feel pain, discuss this with your doctor at once.

❑ Omega-3 fatty acids from fish oil may help to prevent gallstone formation, by reducing the cholesterol saturation of the bile in patients with gallstones.

❑ Peppermint oil capsules are used in Europe to cleanse the gallbladder.

Considerations

❑ Vegetarians run half the risk of gallstone formation as that of meat eaters. Vegetarians tend to weigh less than people who eat meat, which may reduce their risk. They also often eat fewer calories and less cholesterol.

❑ Constipation has been linked to the formation of gallstones. When constipation is successfully treated, the risk of gallstone formation may be reduced. (*See* CONSTIPATION.)

❑ Patients with high triglyceride levels often are prescribed a class of drugs called fibrates, which may increase the risk of gallstone formation.

❑ Gallbladder irritation, although not the stones themselves, can result from food allergies. One study found that every subject found complete relief from gallbladder pain when allergy-provoking foods were identified and eliminated from the diet. (*See* Food Allergies *under* ALLERGIES.)

❑ Rapid weight changes can cause gallbladder problems. A study published in the *Annals of Internal Medicine* revealed that so-called yo-yo dieting increases the risk of gallstones and the necessity for surgery by as much as 70 percent.

GAS

See under INDIGESTION.

GASTRITIS

Gastritis is a group of diseases that causes acid inflammation of the stomach lining. Symptoms include nausea, vomiting, and pain in the pit of the stomach or upper abdomen. Gastritis differs from peptic ulcer, which can cause the same symptoms. Gastritis does not usually result in a wound in the stomach wall, and seldom causes much bleeding.

For purposes of treatment, it is useful to think of gastritis as acute or chronic. Acute gastritis occurs immediately when an irritating chemical enters the stomach. Substances that can have this effect include aspirin, nonsteroidal anti-inflammatory drugs (NSAIDs), which are toxic to the stomach lining; histamine, which is produced in the body in response to allergens; and large quantities of stress hormones, which may be produced in response to trauma such as severe burns, major surgery, respiratory failure, or radiation therapy.

Fortunately, most cases of acute gastritis respond to antacids and antihistamines, usually given around the clock until symptoms subside. In as little as forty-eight hours the stomach lining begins to regenerate itself, and the crisis usually passes.

Chronic gastritis is more difficult to treat. In some cases gastritis is the body's response to an infection with *Helicobacter pylori*, which may break down the stomach's inner protective lining. Vulnerability to *H. pylori* may be hereditary, or it could be related to smoking or stress.

Some treatments include antibiotics such as clarithromycin (Biaxin) or metronidazole (Flagyl) to kill *H. pylori* if it is found in the digestive tract and is bothersome. Other people may need medications to block acid production and promote healing such as omeprazole (Prilosec). Antacids and medications to reduce acid production such as ranitidine (Zantac) may also be needed. Speak to your doctor about these medications.

Gastritis: Beneficial Herbs

Herb	Form and Dosage	Comments
Barberry[1] or coptis[1] or goldenseal[1] or Oregon grape root[1]	Tincture. Take 20 drops of any of these herbs in ¼ cup water 3 times daily.	Contains berberine, which kills *Helicobacter pylori*.
Calendula	Tea. Use as directed on the label.	Relieves stomach inflammation without reducing acid levels.
Carqueja	Tincture. Take as directed on the label.	An anti-inflammatory that reduces acid secretion.
Cat's claw	Capsules. Take 500–1,000 mg twice daily.	Stimulates immune defense against *H. pylori* infection. Relieves inflammation.
Espinheira santa	Tincture. Take as directed on the label.	Neutralizes stomach acid; stops spasms.
Licorice[2]	Glycyrrhizin tablets. Take 400 mg daily. Use for 6 weeks, then take a 2-week break. Do not substitute deglycyrrhizinated licorice (DGL).	Relieves inflammation. Consume potassium-rich foods such as bananas or citrus juices, or take a potassium supplement, daily when taking this herb.
Pau d'arco	Tincture. Take as directed on the label.	Antibacterial, anti-inflammatory. Stimulates blood flow to the stomach.

Precautions for the use of herbs:

[1]Do not use barberry, coptis, goldenseal, or Oregon grape root if you are pregnant or have gallbladder disease. Do not take these herbs with supplemental vitamin B_6 or with protein supplements containing the amino acid histidine. Do not use goldenseal if you have cardiovascular disease or glaucoma.

[2]Do not use licorice if you have glaucoma, high blood pressure, or an estrogen-dependent disorder such as breast cancer, endometriosis, or flbrocystic breasts.

Gastritis: Formulas

Formula	Comments
Augmented Rambling Powder[1]	A traditional Chinese herbal formula that treats gastritis associated with symptoms caused by emotional stress, such as migraine, eye pain, skin outbreaks on the cheeks, and pain or tenderness in the breasts.
Evodia Decoction	A traditional Chinese herbal formula that treats recurrent gastritis occurring with severe pain.
Five-Accumulation Powder	A traditional Chinese herbal formula that stops diarrhea accompanying gastritis attacks.
Major Construct the Middle Decoction	A traditional Chinese herbal formula that treats gastritis accompanied by anemia. Appropriate if there is belching of gastric acid, dull pain below the heart, and sloshing sounds in the stomach.
Minor Bupleurum Decoction[2]	A traditional Chinese herbal formula that treats gastritis with gallbladder disease or hepatitis. Protects the stomach lining and stops harmful gastric secretions.

Precautions for the use of formulas:

[1]Do not use Augmented Rambling Powder if you are trying to become pregnant.

[2]Do not use Minor Bupleurum Decoction if you have a fever or a skin infection. Taken long term, it can cause headache, dizziness, and bleeding gums. Side effects can be avoided if the formula is taken as a tea.

Recommendations

❏ Be sure to consume only properly handled, chilled, and cooked foods, and clean water. *H. pylori* contamination can persist in food, even if it is refrigerated, for several days. The infection can survive in fresh water for as long as a year.

❏ Fight bacteria with bacteria. One of the bacteria found in some yogurt cultures, *Lactobacillus gasseri*, reduces the amount of damage done to the lining of the stomach by *H. pylori*. Unfortunately, the more commonly known strains of *Lactobacillus* do not share this beneficial effect, so it is necessary to take yogurt or probiotic tablets that are labeled as containing *L. gasseri*. Others have found that *Bifidobacterium bifidum* YIT 4007 strain also improves symptoms associated with *H. pylori* gastritis.

❏ To fight chronic gastritis, be sure to take at least the minimum Recommended Daily Allowance (RDA) of B vitamins and calcium. If you are a woman who has not reached menopause, take the RDA of iron. Sometimes gastritis is self-limiting, especially in older people. If so much damage has been done to the lining of the stomach that it no longer secretes adequate acid, the stomach begins to heal. However, lack of acid makes it more difficult for the body to absorb B vitamins, calcium, iron, and vitamin K.

❏ Take small doses of vitamin C. Taking 500 milligrams of vitamin C a day may protect against the development of stomach cancer. Taking very large doses—that is, over 3,000 milligrams a day—may increase stomach irritation.

❏ Avoid spicy and salty foods, and eat moderate portions of other foods. Spicy and salty foods, and large portions of other foods, cause chronic inflammation of the stomach, which increases the risk of cancer.

❏ Eat smaller, more frequent meals if you experience frequent indigestion. Limit alcohol to one drink per day for women and two for men.

❏ Managing stress is key. Develop some coping strategies and consider meditation, yoga, or tai chi.

Considerations

❏ Prolonged, vigorous exercise can precipitate an attack of gastritis. This is due to inadequate circulation of blood to the stomach, rather than any direct action on *H. pylori* infection. However, moderate regular walking is good for other reasons, and controls weight, which may help ease pain.

❏ Eating broccoli or broccoli sprouts appears to help reduce *H. pylori*. In one study, people with *H. pylori* who ate 70 grams (about ½ cup) of broccoli sprouts had less *H. pylori* in the stomach. This reduction can lead to a reduced risk of stomach cancer. The other group ate alfalfa sprouts, which do not contain isothiocyanate sulforaphane, thought to be the active ingredient in the broccoli sprouts and broccoli spears; and had no change in the amount of *H. pylori* in the stomach.

❏ *See also* PEPTIC ULCER and "Side Effects of Cancer Treatment" *under* CANCER.

GASTROENTERITIS

See under FOOD POISONING.

GIARDIASIS

See under PARASITIC INFECTION.

GINGIVITIS

See under PERIODONTAL DISEASE.

GLAUCOMA

Glaucoma is a condition in which increased pressure within the eye causes tissue damage. While normal pressure is between 10 and 21 millimeters of mercury, glaucoma can raise this pressure to as high as 40 millimeters. Glaucoma usually affects people over sixty years of age and people at increased risk for this disorder include African-Americans; those with diabetes or high blood pressure; those with extreme nearsightedness or a family history of glaucoma; and those taking corticosteroid medications.

The eye produces a fluid called aqueous humor, which fills the eye's interior. In glaucoma, aqueous humor is produced faster than it can drain into the capillaries within the eye. The resulting increase in pressure damages both the capillaries and the nerve endings that carry vision impulses to the optic nerve, resulting in blindness. Glaucoma can occur because of tissue abnormalities or because the drainage mechanism is clogged with excess collagen, a protein that forms the eye's supportive structures.

There are two types of glaucoma. In chronic, or open-angle, glaucoma there is a persistent, moderate elevation of pressure. This form of glaucoma almost never causes symptoms until tissue destruction is advanced. The most pronounced symptoms are the loss of peripheral vision (the ability to see out of the corner of the eye) and difficulty adjusting to darkness. Other symptoms may include low-grade headaches and the need for frequent changes in prescriptions for corrective lenses.

Acute, or closed-angle, glaucoma is a medical emergency. This disorder produces severe, throbbing pain with markedly blurred vision. The pupil dilates and becomes fixed, and nausea and vomiting are common. People also may see halos and experience reddening of the eyes.

These symptoms call for immediate medical treatment, as irreversible blindness can result in less than forty-eight hours.

Conventional treatment of glaucoma uses surgery or various classes of drugs. Usually treatment starts with eyedrops, of which there are many different kinds, and your doctor will select the right one for you. The herbs and formulas listed here do not take the place of prescription medications, but, if used over a period of three to four months, help lower eye pressure and prevent progression of the disease. Using herbs and prescription drugs together, under the guidance of a health-care provider, is likely to provide the best control over glaucoma.

Herbs to Avoid

❏ People with glaucoma should avoid ephedra and licorice. (For more information regarding these herbs, *see* EPHEDRA and LICORICE *under* The Herbs in Part One.)

Recommendations

❏ Eat blackberries, blueberries, cherries, raspberries, or rose hips, or drink one glass of red wine a day. Like bilberry leaf, some berries and fruits and red wine contain flavonoid compounds that prevent further damage to the eye. To make flavonoids more effective, take 200 to 1,000 milligrams of vitamin C daily.

❏ People who eat lots of fruits and vegetables can have a nearly 30 percent reduced risk of glaucoma compared to those who eat fewer than one serving a day. In one study in women, eating carrots and peaches had the most pronounced effects on reducing glaucoma risks, but all fruits and vegetables were helpful.

❏ Take 200 to 600 milligrams of supplemental magnesium daily. Magnesium may lower eye pressure by relaxing the blood vessels supplying the eye. Four weeks' use should both lower pressure and slightly but measurably increase field of vision. Do not take this much all at once, as it tends to cause diarrhea.

❏ If you have type 2 diabetes, or if you are overweight, take vitamin B and chromium. Insulin stimulates collagen production, which could put people with type 2 diabetes at risk for glaucoma. This is also true of people who are overweight, since being overweight often leads to excess insulin production. Vitamin B_3 (niacin) may counteract insulin's effects on collagen. It is found in any complete B-vitamin tablet yielding at least the Recommended Daily Allowance (RDA) of the vitamin. Do not take too much, since vitamin B_3 aggravates glaucoma at daily dosages over 200 milligrams. Chromium is a more powerful fat burner and insulin-reducer than the B vitamins.

❏ Take 200 to 400 micrograms of chromium per day. This mineral complements the B vitamins by allowing the eye's focusing muscles to use glucose more efficiently.

Glaucoma: Beneficial Herbs

Herb	Form and Dosage	Comments
Bilberry	Tablets. Take 240–360 mg daily.	Helps prevent further blood-vessel damage in the eye. Helps maintain night vision.
Eyebright	Extract. Use as directed on the label.	Good for virtually all eye disorders.
Ginkgo[1]	Ginkgolide tablets. Take 240 mg in a single dose daily.	Helps prevent blood-vessel complications. Slows loss of peripheral vision.
Hawthorn	Tablets. Take 100–250 mg 3 times daily.	Contains substances that strengthen capillary walls.
Kudzu	Tablets. Take 10 mg 3 times daily.	Contains a natural beta-blocker, peurarin. Useful if pilocarpine fails.

Precautions for the use of herbs:

[1]Do not use ginkgo if you are taking blood-thinning medication. Discuss its use with your doctor before having any type of surgery.

Glaucoma: Formulas

Formulas	Comments
Five-Ingredient Powder with Poria	A traditional Chinese herbal formula that encourages urination, which drains fluid from the body and reduces pressure within the eye.

❏ Steroid drugs may bring about glaucoma by destroying collagen structures within the eye. If you must take prescribed steroid drugs, ask your physician to prescribe the smallest effective dosage for the shortest time possible.

❏ Avoid all sources of caffeine, including coffee, green and black tea, cola, and over-the-counter medications for staying awake. Both coffee and tea have been shown to raise eye pressure. Although one cup of either coffee or tea a day is not likely to have any significant effect on glaucoma, constant drinking of either beverage can make controlling eye pressure difficult.

❏ Avoid tobacco in all forms.

❏ If you do drink caffeinated beverages or smoke on a regular basis, do so on the day of your eye exam. This will produce a reading that is more normal for you.

❏ If the doctor approves, perform moderate exercise on a daily basis. In particular, body-inversion exercise, such as doing sit-ups on a slanted board, lowers eye pressure in some people with glaucoma.

❏ For more information and assistance, see the groups listed in Appendix B: Resources.

❏ Exercise regularly. Research has shown that people with open-angle glaucoma who exercise at least three times a week can reduce their intraocular pressure by 20 percent or more. If they stop exercising, the pressure begins to build up again. Exercise does not appear to have the same benefits for people with closed-angle glaucoma.

Considerations

❏ Physicians usually treat glaucoma with pilocarpine (Carpine) or a class of drugs known as beta-blockers, such as timolol (Timoptic). Pilocarpine and related drugs act by increasing the resistance of blood-vessel walls to fluids that might swell the eye. The beta-blockers lower blood pressure throughout the body, which relieves stress on the eye. If these drugs do not control glaucoma, physicians then add other drugs such as alpha-agonists, such as brinzolamide (Alphagan), to reduce production of aqueous humor (the watery fluid that fills the space between the cornea and the lens in the eye) and reduce pressure on the eye. These drugs tend to cause frequent urination. Also prescribed are eyedrops with prostaglandin-like compounds, such as latanoprost (Xalatan), and carbonic anhydrase inhibitors, such as dorzolamide (Trusopt).

❏ Beta-blockers can cause levels of low-density lipoprotein (LDL, or "bad") cholesterol, to rise, and levels of high-density lipoprotein (HDL, or "good") cholesterol, to drop. In addition, people who take beta-blockers for glaucoma are three times as likely to experience hip fractures. This is attributed to the dizziness and fainting experienced by some people who take these medications, especially during the first few weeks of treatment.

❏ If none of the drug treatments works, the next step is usually laser surgery. A procedure called laser trabeculoplasty burns new channels that allow the fluid to drain. This surgery does not work in all cases, though, and may have to be repeated.

❏ The chemotherapy drug mitomycin (Mutamycin) is sometimes used in conjunction with surgery for glaucoma. (For information on using herbs to avoid side effects of mitomycin, *see* "Side Effects of Cancer Treatment" *under* CANCER.)

❏ Eye pressures tend to be higher during the winter months than during the rest of the year. For this reason, it is especially important to avoid caffeinated beverages and to take appropriate nutritional supplements during the winter.

❏ Acupuncture sometimes can relieve elevated eye pressures and pain if other measures fail. The needles are not placed in or right next to the eye itself. Acupuncture is especially useful for people with diabetes who have glaucoma. (*See* ACUPUNCTURE in Part Three.)

❏ Allergic reactions to food can sometimes create an immediate increase in eye pressure of up to 20 millimeters (that is, to a pressure of 40 or higher), in addition to other allergic symptoms. (*See* Food Allergies *under* ALLERGIES.)

❏ Agents that act to dilate the pupils, such as ephedra and belladonna, should be avoided at all costs.

❏ If you are pregnant, do not drink alcohol. This can lead to your baby developing eye problems, including glaucoma.

❏ *See also* DIABETES, HIGH BLOOD PRESSURE (HYPERTENSION), and HYPOTHYROIDISM.

GLOMERULONEPHRITIS

See under KIDNEY DISEASE.

GONORRHEA AND CHLAMYDIA

Gonorrhea and a closely related disease, chlamydia, are the two most commonly reported infectious diseases in the United States. There are more than 300,000 new cases of gonorrhea reported each year. However, gonorrhea is substantially underdiagnosed and underreported, and the Centers for Disease Control and Prevention (CDC) estimates that there are approximately twice as many new gonorrhea infections each year as are reported.

Gonorrhea is caused by an infection with the bacterium *Neisseria gonorrhoeae*. In women, there may be no symptoms at all. If there are symptoms, they may include painful urination, vaginal discharge, and abnormal menstrual bleeding accompanied by discomfort around the anus.

In men, gonorrhea usually does cause symptoms, most notably painful urination and a thick discharge from the penis. Symptoms generally appear between two and fourteen days after sexual contact in men and from seven to twenty-one days after contact in women.

Once gonorrhea becomes established, it can spread, causing mild fever, achiness, and inflamed joints. In women, the spread of the disease from the cervix to the lining of the uterus is accelerated by the use of intrauterine devices (IUDs); menstruation also hastens the spread of the disease. Such spread can result in problems with fertility. Gonorrhea can spread within the male reproductive tract, causing infertility. In addition, men can experience a narrowing of the urethra.

The standard medical treatment for gonorrhea for adults is antibiotics, usually as an injection or as a single tablet taken by mouth. Typically the drugs are from a class called cephalosporins. Partners of people with gonorrhea should undergo testing, even if no signs are present. Babies born to mothers with it receive a medication in their eyes soon after birth to prevent infection. Chlamydia is usually caused by *Chlamydia trachomatis* or, in men, by *Ureaplasma urealyticum*. It produces symptoms similar to those produced by gonorrhea (the discharge in men tends to be thinner), can also cause infertility, and is treated in the same manner as gonorrhea.

These herbal remedies are to be used with antibiotics and are not substitutes for them.

Gonorrhea and Chlamydia: Beneficial Herbs

Herb	Form and Dosage	Comments
Andiroba and copaiba	Oil. Apply to irritated area as needed.	Relieves vaginal and rectal inflammation.
Arjuna	Capsules. Take 500 mg every 8 hours.	Contains luteolin, which kills gonorrhea bacteria.
Astragalus	Tincture. Use as directed on the label.	Helps protect the immune system.
Barberry[1] or coptis[1] or goldenseal[1] or Oregon grape root[1]	Tincture. Take 15–30 drops in ¼ cup water 3 times daily.	Contains berberine, which kills gonorrhea bacteria.
Epimedium[2]	Tablets. Take as directed on the label or by the dispensing herbalist. Use after suspected exposure.	Antibacterial. Stimulates urination to keep bacteria from attaching to the lining of the urethra.
Scutellaria[3]	Capsules. Take 1,000–2,000 mg 3 times daily.	May act against antibiotic-resistant strains of gonorrhea.

Precautions for the use of herbs:

[1]Do not use barberry, coptis, goldenseal, or Oregon grape root if you are pregnant or have gallbladder disease. Do not take these herbs with supplemental vitamin B_6 or with protein supplements containing the amino acid histidine. Do not use goldenseal if you have cardiovascular disease or glaucoma.

[2]Do not use epimedium if you have any kind of prostate disorder.

[3]Do not use scutellaria if you have diarrhea.

Gonorrhea and Chlamydia: Formulas

Formula	Comments
Dong Quai, Gentiana Longdancao, and Aloe Pill[1]	A traditional Chinese herbal formula that treats gonorrhea with accompanying herpes infection.
Eight-Ingredient Pill with Rehmannia (Rehmannia-Eight Combination)	A traditional Chinese herbal formula that increases urination, effectively flushing gonorrhea bacteria out of the genitourinary tract before they can cause damage. Use after suspected exposure.
Peony and Licorice Decoction[2]	A traditional Chinese herbal formula that treats gonorrhea complicated by cramping and abdominal pain or pain around the anus.

Precautions for the use of formulas:

[1]Do not use Dong Quai, Gentiana Longdancao, and Aloe Pill if you are trying to become pregnant.

[2]Do not use Peony and Licorice Decoction if you have an estrogen-sensitive disorder, such as breast cancer, endometriosis, or fibrocystic breasts.

Recommendations

❑ Take *Lactobacillus acidophilus*, the "friendly" bacteria that help the body digest food, every day. Eat one serving of yogurt daily, or take acidophilus capsules or tablets as directed on the label. Women can also use acidophilus as a vaginal suppository, after asking their doctor. These bacteria may reduce the chances of diarrhea associated with the use of antibiotics.

❑ Use a latex condom with nonoxynol-9 lubricant for sexual activity of any kind until the infection is gone completely, as gonorrhea is highly contagious. Be aware, though, that using a condom does not guarantee complete protection.

Considerations

❑ The gonorrhea bacterium, like many other bacteria, has developed an ability to resist treatment with ever-stronger classes of antibiotics, first to penicillin and then to tetracycline and, most recently, to spectinomycin. Therefore, it is important to complete any course of treatment (herbal or prescription) for gonorrhea. Ridding the body of the infection deprives the bacterium of opportunities to develop antibiotic resistance, and also ensures that it will not be spread to others.

❑ Several traditional Chinese herbal formulas can be used to treat the fertility problems that may result from gonorrhea infection. In women, Peony and Licorice Decoction increases estrogen production, which in turn increases the probability of conception, while Dong Quai and Peony Powder is used in Japan to prevent miscarriage. In men, Warm the Menses Decoction can reduce the risk of infertility. Gonorrhea must be treated with antibiotics as well.

❑ Many sexually transmitted diseases that once were in decline are now becoming more common. Many experts link this rise to the AIDS epidemic; because the immune system is compromised, AIDS increases susceptibility to disease of every kind.

❑ Infection with gonorrhea may predispose people infected with it to contracting HIV. Both are nearly preventable with proper condom use, however. (*See* HIV/AIDS.)

GOUT

Gout is a common form of arthritis caused by an excessive concentration of uric acid in body fluids. Uric acid is produced from the metabolism of purines, substances found in food. In people with gout, uric acid crystallizes in joints, tendons, kidneys, and other tissues, and causes inflammation, tissue damage, and pain. Gout mostly affects men between the ages of forty and fifty.

The first attack of gout is usually characterized by intense pain involving only a single joint. The first joint of the big toe is affected in nearly half of first attacks, and is involved at some time in most individuals with gout. As the attack progresses, the joint swells; the skin over the joint becomes red, tight, shiny, and sensitive to the touch, and fever and chills develop. First attacks usually occur at night and may be preceded by a specific event, such as eating too much red meat, drinking too much alcohol, or taking certain drugs and vitamins (including several forms of chemotherapy and overdoses of niacin). Obesity and crash dieting are also associated with gout.

The first attack is seldom the last. Most people who suffer a first attack will have another attack within a year. Affected joints can become immobile. Uric acid crystals form lumps in the kidneys, and some degree of kidney dysfunction occurs often in people with gout. There is also a greatly increased risk of kidney stones.

Conventional treatment uses various drugs to reduce both inflammation and uric acid production, by reducing acute attacks and preventing future attacks. These drugs include nonsteroidal anti-inflammatory drugs (NSAIDs), colchicine drugs if you can't take NSAIDs, and corticosteroids like prednisone, which reduce inflammation. To prevent complications associated with frequent attacks, you may be prescribed medications that block uric acid production, such as allopurinol (Zyloprim), and medications that improve uric acid removal, such as probenecid (Probalan). Along with these medications, gout can be treated with diet and lifestyle changes supported by herbal therapy.

Recommendations

❑ Eat a diet as low in purines as possible. While purines are found in all foods, it is especially important to limit protein intake. Completely avoid anchovies, baker's and brewer's yeast, herring, mackerel, sardines, and shellfish. Reduce consumption of other high-protein foods, such as meat, poultry, dried beans, and fish. Generally speaking, for a person weighing 150 pounds (70 kilograms), protein consumption should be limited to four to six ounces of protein foods daily. Also avoid asparagus and spinach.

❑ Eat a diet that emphasizes non-meat protein and whole, unprocessed foods, including nuts and seeds, vegetables, and whole grains. Also, tofu, eggs, and nut butters are good sources of protein.

❑ Eat cherries or take cherry extract. Eating half a pound (225 grams) of canned or fresh cherries a day has been shown to be a very effective means of preventing gout attacks. When fresh cherries are out of season, use cherry extracts or concentrates in tablet or tincture form, available from many health food stores. It is likely that cherries inhibit compounds that cause inflammation. This may reduce inflammation after uric acid builds up in a joint.

❑ To flush uric acid from the body, drink eight to sixteen glasses of water daily.

Gout: Beneficial Herbs

Herb	Form and Dosage	Comments
Bilberry	Extract. Take as directed on the label.	Provides powerful antioxidant compounds.
Bromelain[1]	Tablets. Take 250–500 mg 3 times daily, between meals.	Dissolves uric acid crystals. Brings relief to a joint also inflamed by injury.
Celery seed	Take as directed on the label.	Contains numerous anti-inflammatory compounds.
Devil's claw[2]	Enteric-coated capsules. Take 1,000–2,000 mg 3 times daily for up to 3 weeks.	Relieves short-term pain and inflammation.
Iporuru	Tincture. Take as directed on the label.	Stops acute inflammation.
Quercetin[3]	Tablets. Take 125–250 mg 3 times daily, between meals.	Keeps uric acid from forming.
Sarsaparilla	Capsules. Take 3,000 mg 3 times daily.	Reduces long-term frequency of gout attacks.

Precautions for the use of herbs:

[1] People who are allergic to pineapple may develop a rash from bromelain. If itching develops, stop using it.

[2] Devil's claw can slow the heartbeat. Do not use it if you have congestive heart failure.

[3] Do not use quercetin if you are taking cyclosporine (Neoral, Sandimmune) or nifedipine (Procardia).

❑ Avoid alcohol, since alcohol increases uric acid production.

❑ Coffee drinking, both regular and decaffeinated, produces lower uric acid levels in the blood. Don't start drinking coffee if you aren't already a coffee drinker, but continue drinking it if you are.

❑ Do not take more than 50 milligrams of vitamin B_3 (niacin) or 3,000 milligrams of vitamin C per day. In excess, these vitamins may compete with uric acid for excretion into the urine, and cause uric acid to accumulate in the body.

❑ Do not take aspirin or diuretics (water pills). These drugs may trigger a gout attack.

❑ Do not take supplements containing the amino acid glycine. Glycine can be converted into uric acid more rapidly in people who suffer from gout.

❑ Maintain a normal body weight. Obesity increases the risk of repeat gout attacks. (See OVERWEIGHT.) In one study, men with gout were shown to have a 30 percent higher risk of developing type 2 diabetes. Losing weight helps lower diabetes risk factors, such as high blood sugar levels.

❑ Try to de-stress using relaxation techniques such as deep-breathing exercises and meditation.

Considerations

❑ Allopurinol (Zyloprim) reduces uric acid formation. It is a highly effective drug but it can produce side effects, such as generalized rashes and breakdown of red blood cells. Another drug, colchicine, derived from the herb autumn saffron, eases acute gout attacks and prevents future attacks. While often quite effective, it too can have side effects. Colchicine is only used before starting a xanthine oxidase inhibitor regimen, which reduces new attacks.

❑ Steroids may be prescribed during acute attacks. (For more information about the side effects of this treatment, see "Side Effects of Cancer Treatment" under CANCER.)

❑ Gout can be a sign of lead poisoning, but mainly for people with poor kidney function. Make sure you are not using serving dishes or pitchers fired with a lead glaze for anything other than decorative purposes.

GRAVES' DISEASE

See under HYPERTHYROIDISM.

GUM DISEASE

See under PERIODONTAL DISEASE.

GUMS, BLEEDING

See under PERIODONTAL DISEASE.

HAIR LOSS

Everyone loses individual hairs—up to fifty scalp hairs a day—constantly. Hair loss only becomes noticeable if fewer hairs are produced after the old ones are shed, or if the new hair is weak and brittle. If hair falls out in patches, it is referred to as alopecia areata. Alopecia totalis means the loss of all the hair on the scalp, and alopecia universalis means the loss of all the hair on the body.

The most prevalent form of hair loss is androgenetic alopecia (AGA), more commonly called male pattern

Hair Loss: Beneficial Herbs

Herb	Form and Dosage	Comments
Biota	Tincture or scalp lotion, prepared by a compounding pharmacist or traditional Chinese medicine (TCM) practitioner.	Thickens existing hair and prevents further baldness.
Drynaria	Tincture or scalp lotion, prepared by compounding pharmacist or TCM practitioner.	Stimulates hair growth on portions of scalp affected by AGA.
Ginkgo	Ginkgolide tablets. Take 40–60 mg 2–3 times daily.	Improves circulation in the scalp.

Hair Loss: Formulas

Formula	Comments
Cinnamon Twig, Licorice, Dragon Bone, and Oyster Shell Decoction	A traditional Chinese herbal formula that treats hair loss in men and women. Especially appropriate if hair loss is accompanied by dizziness, insomnia, and/or palpitations. Also treats sexual difficulties in men. Available as a prescription from TCM practitioners.
Seven-Treasure Pill for Beautiful Whiskers[1]	A traditional Chinese herbal formula that treats hair loss and premature graying in both sexes. Available as a prescription from TCM practitioners.
Unblock the Orifices and Invigorate the Blood Decoction	A traditional Chinese herbal formula that treats hair loss in men and women who also have dark blue or purple patches on the skin, especially on the face and chest.

Precautions for the use of formulas:

[1]Do not use Seven-Treasure Pill for Beautiful Whiskers if you are suffering from constipation.

baldness. AGA occurs in response to the body's production of androgens, or male sex hormones, although the exact mechanism is not completely understood. It generally occurs in men who have a genetic tendency for baldness. Women also can have AGA, since their bodies also produce androgens, but are less likely to lose their hair completely.

Hair loss can occur for other reasons. Scalp infections such as ringworm can cause hair follicles to be damaged, leading to hair loss. Hormonal changes and imbalances due to pregnancy, childbirth, or discontinuation of birth control pills can cause temporary hair loss. Various drugs can accelerate hair loss, including chemotherapy agents, antidepressants, some blood-pressure and anti-inflammatory medications, and the gout medication allopurinol (Zyloprim). Severe illness, usually when accompanied by a high fever, can cause temporary hair loss. Alopecia areata, totalis, and universalis may be caused by overactivity of the immune system, including thyroid problems. T-helper cells signal other cells to dissolve dead hair follicles, while chemicals called cytokines regulate T cell activity. If cytokines are not produced properly and the action of the T cells is not checked, hair loss occurs.

Conventional medicine does offer drug treatments for hair loss. Herbal treatments for hair restoration should be undertaken in the context of comprehensive health-care under the supervision of an herbal practitioner. Complete restoration of hair using herbal therapy is rare, but is not unknown. The herbs listed here are meant for external use only. The formulas are to be taken internally.

Recommendations

❑ To combat hair loss resulting from nervous tension, renowned herbalist James Duke suggests using a shampoo made by mixing 2 tablespoons of dried carthamus with ⅔ cup olive oil. Apply and allow it to remain for fifteen to thirty minutes before rinsing.

❑ Avoid sweets and fatty foods. Poor diet may increase the production of insulin and insulinlike growth factors, which accelerate AGA at the crown of the scalp. However, a newer study found no relationship between blood insulin, cholesterol, glucose, or triglyceride levels (markers of insulin resistance) and androgenic alopecia. More study may be necessary to determine if there is any connection.

❏ If hair loss occurs with or shortly after an extended period of diarrhea, dizziness, leg cramps, and/or sexual problems, take thymopentin or thymic factors. This supplement seems to stop T cells from destroying the layer of skin cells immediately surrounding the hair follicle, and allows regrowth of hair. It is especially useful in women's hair loss during menopause.

❏ Include soy foods such as soybeans, tempeh, and tofu in your diet. Soy foods appear to inhibit the formation of dihydrotestosterone (DHT), a hormone implicated in the process of hair loss.

❏ Hair is fragile when wet. Gently pat your hair dry and squeeze out remaining moisture with a towel.

❏ If you are losing large amounts of hair, see a physician.

Considerations

❏ A combination of South American herbs—avena, catuaba, gervâo, muira puama, mutamba, sarsaparilla, and stinging nettle—from Raintree Nutrition frequently produces cosmetic improvements even in AGA of fifteen to thirty years' duration, and has the side effect of increasing erectile strength.

❏ A number of conventional drugs are used to fight hair loss, including minoxidil (Rogaine) and finasteride (Propecia, Proscar). The steroid drug prednisolone has shown some usefulness in reversing hair loss caused by immune-system factors.

❏ Telogen effluvium, or "patchy" hair loss, is usually triggered in women by a sudden hormonal change. This hormonal change may occur in response to a high fever, stress, nutritional deficiency, metabolic disturbances, discontinuation of oral contraceptives, abortion or miscarriage, childbirth, major illness, surgery, and trauma. The triggering event usually precedes hair loss and the resulting hair loss may persist for up to a month or two when new hair follicles become active again; full hair regrowth may take longer. Treating this kind of hair loss requires correcting the underlying hormonal imbalance, and medical testing to make sure the hair loss is not due to thyroid imbalance or chronic infection.

❏ Doctors sometimes prescribe steroids for patchy hair loss in both men and women. The treatments may produce immediate results, but baldness may recur if side effects require a reduction in steroid dosage. (For information on using steroids and herbs together, *see* "Side Effects of Cancer Treatment" *under* CANCER.)

❏ Hair loss can result from hypothyroidism. (*See* HYPOTHYROIDISM.)

HALITOSIS (BAD BREATH)

Halitosis, or disagreeable breath odor, happens to nearly everyone at one time or another. The most common cause is a specific food, especially cabbage, garlic, onions, and other vegetables, spices, and tobacco. Other causes include

Halitosis: Beneficial Herbs

Herb	Form and Dosage	Comments
Alfalfa	Tablets. Take 500–1,000 mg 3 times daily; or liquid. Take 1 tbsp in juice or water 3 times daily.	Supplies chlorophyll, which cleanses the bloodstream and colon, where bad breath often begins.
Barberry[1] or coptis[1] or goldenseal[1] or Oregon grape root[1]	Tincture. Place 3–4 drops in ¼ cup water and use as a mouthwash daily.	Kills *Escherichia coli*, the most common reason for denture odor.
Cat's claw[2]	Capsules. Take 500–1,000 mg twice daily.	Stimulates immune defense against *Helicobacter pylori* infection.
Chamomile	German chamomile (*Matricaria recutita*) tea bags, prepared with 1 cup water. Swish ½ cup around in the mouth and swallow 1–2 times daily.	Relieves inflammation and temporarily curbs bad breath due to gum disease.
Hawthorn	Tablets. Take 250 mg 3 times daily.	Helps keep gum tissue healthy.
Peppermint[3]	Tea bag, prepared with 1 cup water. Take 1 cup after a meal including garlic or onions.	Prevents lingering bad breath.
Tea tree oil[4]	Toothpaste. Use as directed on the label.	A powerful disinfectant with eucalyptus-like odor.
Turmeric	Tincture. Place drops in ¼ cup water and use as a mouthwash daily. Do not substitute curcumin for turmeric.	Prevents gum decay.

Precautions for the use of herbs:

[1]Do not use barberry, coptis, goldenseal, or Oregon grape root if you are pregnant or have gallbladder disease. Do not take these herbs with supplemental vitamin B$_6$ or with protein supplements containing the amino acid histidine. Do not take coptis for longer than two weeks at a time. Do not use goldenseal if you have cardiovascular disease or glaucoma. Do not take Oregon grape root for longer than two weeks at a time.

[2]Do not use cat's claw if you have to take insulin for diabetes. Do not use it if you are pregnant or nursing. Do not give it to a child under six.

[3]Do not use peppermint if you have any kind of gallbladder disorder.

[4]People who are allergic to celery or thyme should not use tea tree oil products. Do not take tea tree oil internally.

poor dental hygiene, cavities, throat or sinus infections, gum disease, dry mouth such as from Sjögren's syndrome, abscessed or impacted teeth, large doses of vitamin supplements, or (in children) a foreign body lodged in a nostril. Halitosis may result in disease—in about 10 percent of the cases—including cancer, metabolic disorders such as diabetes, kidney or liver failure, and GERD (gastroesophageal reflux disease). Medications used to treat high blood pressure, psychiatric problems, and urinary problems may also cause halitosis.

Bad breath that results from eating cabbage, garlic, or onions usually dissipates in a few hours. Lingering bad breath from eating these foods usually signals a digestive disturbance that allows odors from these foods to reach the breath.

Continuous bad breath usually signals a bacterial infection in the mouth, sinus, or digestive tract. While bad breath from oral infections can be masked, those that are produced by infection with *Helicobacter pylori* or tonsillitis does not go away unless the infection is controlled with medication. Herbal treatments can subdue this and other infections that cause bad breath.

Recommendations

❏ To reduce bad breath after eating garlic- or onion-laden foods, chew on a sprig of parsley or some fennel seeds. They freshen the breath and also aid in digestion.

❏ Drink plenty of fluids. A dry mouth intensifies bad breath. (*See* DRY MOUTH.)

❏ Make tongue cleaning a regular part of oral hygiene. To remove bacteria, use a tongue scraper, a metal instrument used to scrape the tongue once or twice a day, or brush the tongue with a germicidal toothpaste when brushing the teeth.

❏ Do not use commercial mouthwashes. The freshness they provide is temporary, and they can both irritate the inside of the mouth and pose a poisoning hazard to small children.

❏ Avoid foods that get stuck between the teeth easily or that cause tooth decay, such as meat, stringy vegetables, and sweets. Use dental floss twice a day to remove such foods.

Considerations

❏ Self-diagnosis does not always work for halitosis, especially if the individual suffers both halitosis and impaired sense of smell. In a physician's office, halitosis is diagnosed with a portable electronic monitor that measures the sulfides released by bacterial infections of the gums and intestines. This method gives a reliable way to measure progress in treatment.

❏ Certain diseases produce very distinctive breath and

body odors. Breath that smells like stale beer, even if a person does not drink beer, could be symptomatic of tuberculosis. A rotten egg smell may relate to liver failure. A fruity smell is the hallmark of extremely high blood sugars causing diabetic ketoacidosis. Bronchitis could smell like rotten fish. Other specific diseases may produce breath that smells like boiled cabbage, maple syrup, or chicken feathers. A sudden change in breath or body odor can be the very first sign of a health problem, so it is a good idea to see a doctor if the problem persists. Dental problems are more likely the cause than disease, however.

❏ Bad breath in children is frequently caused by postnasal drip. This also can cause bad breath in adults. (*See* Respiratory Allergies *under* ALLERGIES and COMMON COLD.)

❏ *See also* GASTRITIS, INDIGESTION, PERIODONTAL DISEASE, SINUSITIS, and STREP THROAT.

HANGOVER

Alcohol intoxication is the condition of discomfort, impaired judgment, poor coordination, and pain following acute overconsumption of the beverage alcohol. Intoxication should not be confused with alcoholism, in which the individual depends on regular alcohol consumption to prevent withdrawal symptoms. Intoxication is often, but not always, followed by hangover, which is marked by nausea, headache, and general malaise. These symptoms are produced by acetaldehyde, a chemical created when the body processes alcohol, that causes headache, nausea, and redness in the face. The body attempts to dilute acetaldehyde in the bloodstream by drawing fluids out of cells, dehydrating them and causing pain.

Hangover severity is related, at least in part, to genetics. Members of certain ethnic groups, especially people of Asian descent and Alaskan Natives, feel alcohol's effects to a greater degree and are more at risk for alcoholism because they do not have a gene that makes sufficient enzymes to break down acetaldehyde (a product of alcohol metabolism that is more toxic than alcohol itself). Members of other ethnic groups are genetically able to break down acetaldehyde very efficiently and thus feel alcohol's effects less. Most herbal treatments should be taken immediately after drinking to prevent or reduce hangover, instead of the next morning, and should be discontinued when the hangover subsides. The exception is Chinese senega root, which should be taken before alcohol is consumed. Because of alcohol's effects on driving ability, never drive after drinking, no matter what herbal therapies are used.

Recommendations

❏ Since hangover discomfort arises partially from dehydration, be sure to drink plenty of liquids. Having one

Hangover: Beneficial Herbs

Herb	Form and Dosage	Comments
Herbs That Can Help to Treat Hangover		
Ginseng	*Panax ginseng* tea (loose), prepared by steeping 1 tsp (2 gm) in 1 cup water. (*See* TEAS in Part Three.) Take 1 cup every 2 hours until symptoms subside.	Enhances breakdown of alcohol in the body.
Scutellaria[1]	Capsules. Take 100 mg 3 times daily.	In animal studies, prevents short-term memory loss due to alcohol intoxication.
Soy lecithin[2]	Capsules. Take 1,500–3,000 mg daily.	Relieves fatigue and corrects low blood sugar.
Herbs That Can Help to Prevent Hangover		
Aloe[3]	Juice. Drink ¼–½ cup before consuming alcohol.	Keeps alcohol from moving into the blood. Hastens recovery from intoxication.
Chinese senega root[4]	Tincture. Take 20 drops in ¼ cup water before consuming alcohol.	Contains compounds that can block alcohol absorption by about 90 percent. Does not necessarily reduce blood alcohol levels as registered by Breathalyzers, but does lower blood alcohol.

Precautions for the use of herbs:

[1]Do not use scutellaria if you have diarrhea.

[2]Soy lecithin may cause mild diarrhea when first used.

[3]Do not take aloe vera juice internally if you have diarrhea.

[4]Do not use Chinese senega root if you have gastritis or a peptic ulcer.

glass of water between each drink can lessen the hangover symptoms.

❏ Eat before drinking. It may help to have a glass of milk, which slows the absorption of alcohol by coating the stomach.

❏ Sip alcohol slowly when drinking. Choose beverages with fewer congeners (toxic chemicals that are formed during fermentation), such as vodka and gin, which are less likely to cause hangovers than those with more congeners, such as brandy and whiskey.

❏ Take a B-complex vitamin supplement plus extra thiamin (100 milligrams) to counter the B-vitamin depletion caused by alcohol.

Considerations

❏ The quality of the alcohol consumed is as important as the type consumed. Since alcohol is exempt from most labeling requirements, it may contain additives that may trigger asthma, migraines, and other reactions. Whenever possible, choose quality brands.

❏ Some people use nonsteroidal anti-inflammatory drugs (NSAIDs) such as Advil and Motrin to prevent hangovers. However, these types of medications can cause liver damage if they are taken with alcohol. If you are concerned, ask your doctor.

❏ *See also* ALCOHOLISM.

HAY FEVER

See Respiratory Allergies *under* ALLERGIES.

HEADACHE

Headaches are among the most common medical complaints. They can arise from numerous causes, including stress, depression, poor posture, jaw clenching, working in an awkward position or holding one position for a long time, eyestrain, hunger, fever, underlying infections, or illnesses.

The most common headaches are those caused by muscle tension in the head, neck, or shoulders, usually due to fatigue or stress. A tension headache is often accompanied by a feeling of tightness around the head, along with weakness or fatigue, and may worsen with sudden movement.

Intensely painful headaches can precede serious illness, particularly illness involving impaired circulation to the brain. Migraine headaches can bring excruciating pain, distortions in sensory perception, and episodes of complete debility lasting hours or days. (*See* MIGRAINE.) Other rarer causes of headache include infections of the ears, sinuses, or mouth; high blood pressure; glaucoma; allergies; brain tumors or abscesses; some drugs; and various foods, especially those containing the additive monosodium glutamate (MSG).

Use the herbs listed to relieve occasional headaches,

Headache: Beneficial Herbs

Herb	Form and Dosage	Comments
Cayenne	Powder. Mix with starchy food and eat. Use the smallest amount that causes a burning sensation.	Counter-irritant that relieves headache across the temples.
Chamomile	Tea. Use as directed on the label.	Relaxes muscles and soothes tension.
Codonopsis	Tincture. Take as directed by the dispensing herbalist.	Relieves headaches with high blood pressure, muscular tension, and indigestion.
Kudzu	Tablets. Take 10 mg 3 times daily.	Relieves headaches with muscle tension in the back of the neck.
Scutellaria[1]	Tincture. Take ½ tsp (2 ml) in ¼ cup water 3 times daily.	Relieves headaches associated with nervous tension.
Tilden flower	Fluidextract. Take ½–1 tsp (2–4 ml) in ¼ cup water 3 times daily.	Relieves headaches with high blood pressure.
Willow bark	Salicin tablets. Take 20–40 mg 3 times daily.	Provides lasting pain relief without stomach upset or changes in blood chemistry.

Precautions for the use of herbs:

[1]Do not use scutellaria if you have diarrhea.

Headache: Formulas

Formula	Comments
Cinnamon Twig Decoction	A traditional Chinese herbal formula that stops headache accompanied by nasal allergy or congestion, fever, or chills.
Cinnamon Twig Plus Kudzu Decoction	A traditional Chinese herbal formula that stops headache accompanied by nasal allergy or congestion, fever, or chills, along with the stiffness in the neck or back.
Gastrodia and Uncaria Decoction	A traditional Chinese herbal formula that relieves headaches with pain or twitches in the facial muscles, and headaches that come on very suddenly.
White Tiger Decoction[1]	A traditional Chinese herbal formula that relieves headache accompanied by bleeding gums or nose, fever, or irritability.

Precautions for the use of formulas:

[1]Do not use White Tiger Decoction if you are experiencing nausea or vomiting.

especially those that accompany specific disorders. Use the formulas to relieve recurrent headaches. Seek immediate medical attention for headaches that follow head injuries, or for severe headaches that appear very suddenly.

Recommendations

❏ For a quick reduction in headache pain, apply a light coating of lavender or peppermint oil to the forehead (and neck, if there is pain in the back of the head). Massaging in the oil is not necessary, although it might help.

❏ Use a cold washcloth or gel pack to help ease pain. Alternating with hot and cold washcloths may ease a tension headache.

❏ If you feel a headache coming on, drink a large glass of water every three hours until symptoms subside.

❏ To reduce the frequency of recurrent headaches associated with high blood pressure or atherosclerosis, take ginkgo tablets, 40 to 60 milligrams three times daily. Tell the doctor about use of this herb before any type of surgery, and do not use it if you take blood-thinning medications.

❏ For recurring nervous tension headaches (or migraines), try a four-week supplement program that includes 250 milligrams of magnesium, 25 milligrams of vitamin B$_6$ (pyridoxine), and 100 milligrams of 5-hydroxy L-tryptophan (5-HTP), each taken three times per day. Magnesium helps the blood vessels avoid painful constriction, and prevents overexcitement of brain cells. Magnesium can cause diarrhea, so start with a small dose and slowly increase it. Vitamin B$_6$ aids energy production within the blood vessels supplying the brain, supporting them and also helping them avoid painful constriction. 5-HTP is especially useful in treating chronic headaches in children, and headaches in adults if there is also sleep disturbance. Do not use 5-HTP in children without consulting a pediatrician. Take this supplement every other day for three months.

❏ For recurrent headaches, keep a diary of all foods eaten for several days to see if any specific food or foods are causing the problem.

❏ If you get a headache every time you exercise, see your health-care provider to rule out heart problems.

❏ To help prevent headaches, eat small meals and eat between meals to help stabilize wide swings in blood sugar. Include almonds, watercress, parsley, fennel, garlic, cherries, and pineapple in your diet.

❏ Consult a health-care provider if herbal and other therapies do not help, especially if any of the following symptoms occur: blurred vision, confusion, fever and neck stiffness, sensitivity to light, pressure in the sinuses or pressure behind the eyes that is relieved by vomiting, or pounding heartbeat.

❏ Maintain good posture habits.

❏ Be sure to get sufficient sleep.

❏ Some alternative therapies that have been beneficial include acupuncture, massage, deep breathing, biofeedback, and behavioral therapy.

Considerations

❏ In addition to headache relief, herbal medicine can be used for headache prevention. Ginger and quercetin both prevent headaches associated with allergy, and ginger also prevents headaches that occur as part of premenstrual syndrome (PMS). Take ginger in tea form, ⅓ teaspoon of powdered ginger in 1 cup of water three times daily. (*See* TEAS in Part Three.) Take quercetin tablets, 250 milligrams three times daily; do not take with cyclosporine (Neoral, Sandimmune) or nifedipine (Procardia). St. John's wort can prevent tension headaches. Use any product containing the dried herb as directed on the label.

❏ Stress is a common source of headaches. (*See* STRESS.) Manage your stress levels, as stress frequently triggers tension headaches in particular.

❏ If headaches persist, a variety of over-the-counter (OTC) and prescription drugs are available. Simple pain relievers such as ibuprofen (Advil) and naproxen sodium (Aleve) may be your first line of drugs. More severe cases, especially in those who experience migraine headaches and episodic headaches, may benefit from a class of drugs called triptans, and an injectable form of sumatriptan (Imitrex) may be used. Rarely are opiates or narcotics used because of the potential for dependency.

❏ *See also* MIGRAINE.

HEART ATTACK (MYOCARDIAL INFARCTION)

A heart attack, known as a myocardial infarction, occurs if the heart's blood supply is sharply reduced or cut off entirely. This deprives the heart of oxygen, which causes heart tissue to die if blood flow is not restored within minutes. In the United States, approximately 1.2 million people have heart attacks every year, and most of them die.

Symptoms of a heart attack include crushing, severe pain in the chest that can spread to the left arm, neck, or jaw, or the area between the shoulder blades. Other symptoms may include nausea, shortness of breath, sweating, and vomiting. The heart attack may be preceded by years of intermittent chest pain known as angina, in which a reduced amount of oxygen reaches the heart but no tissue damage occurs. In some cases, however, heart attacks do not produce pain. In such "silent" attacks, there may be a sensation like that caused by indigestion, or there may not be any symptoms at all.

Heart attacks can occur for several reasons, including arrhythmias, which are abnormal heart rhythms, and aneurysms, which are weak spots in blood vessels that may give way and disrupt blood flow. The vast majority of heart attacks, though, occur because an artery serving the heart becomes partially or completely blocked, generally by a blood clot. Usually the process of atherosclerosis has narrowed the affected artery. In atherosclerosis, excess cholesterol, immune-system cells called macrophages, and other materials gather into fatty plaques at the site of blood-vessel injuries. Other causes include age (over forty-five years for men and fifty-five years for women), family history of heart disease, lack of physical activity, obesity, and illegal drug use.

Maintaining healthy cholesterol and blood pressure levels can help prevent atherosclerosis. It is also important not to smoke, and to control diabetes. However, one can "do everything right" and have a heart attack, or "do everything wrong" and not have one. That is because atherosclerosis is only part of the process. The body can compensate for even severely narrowed arteries by creating new blood vessels to carry blood around the blockage.

The other part of the process is clot formation. Heart attacks occur if a blood clot develops rapidly at the site of a blood-vessel injury. Blood clots more readily under the influence of the stress hormones adrenocorticotropic hormone (ACTH) and epinephrine. However, these chemicals can cause only limited clotting unless another chemical, thromboxane, is produced. Thromboxane causes a protein "net" to be spun on which a clot can grow to an artery-clogging size.

This entry focuses on what you can do to help prevent

Heart Attack: Beneficial Herbs

Herb	Form and Dosage	Comments
Andrographis	Tablets. Take as directed on the label.	Helps prevent clogging of arteries and second heart attack after angioplasty.
Arjuna	Capsules. Take 500 mg 3 times daily.	Relieves pain. Helps heart muscle cells build up energy reserves.
Astragalus[1]	Capsules. Take 500–1,000 mg 3 times daily.	Improves circulation after heart attack; helps prevent second heart attack.
Bitter orange	Tea (loose), prepared by steeping 1 tsp (2–3 gm) in 1 cup water. (*See* TEAS in Part Three.) Take 1 cup 3 times daily, between meals.	Slows heartbeat without reducing circulation.
Cordyceps	Tablets or tincture. Use as directed on the label.	Lowers blood pressure and low-density lipoprotein (LDL, or "bad") cholesterol.
Garlic[2]	Enteric-coated tablets. Take 900 mg daily.	Reduces production of clotting factors.
Ginkgo[3]	Ginkgolide tablets. Take 120–160 mg daily.	Retards rapid heartbeat and resulting stress to the heart.
Ginseng	*Panax ginseng* tincture. Take as directed on the label.	Relaxes arteries; reduces hormonal stress reactions. Reduces heart's demand for oxygen after heart attack.
Hawthorn	Tablets. Take 100–250 mg 3 times daily.	Relaxes muscles surrounding arteries. Improves cardiac enzymes used to measure damage to heart muscle.
Kudzu	Tablets. Take 10 mg 3 times daily.	Improves coronary circulation; lowers the heart's need for oxygen.
Lemon balm	Tea bag, prepared with 1 cup water. Take 1 cup 3 times daily.	Lessens hormonal responses to environmental stress. Also called melissa.
Scutellaria[4]	Capsules. Take 1,000–2,000 mg 3 times daily.	Reduces overproduction of the stress hormone adrenocorticotropic hormone (ACTH).
Turmeric	Curcumin tablets. Take 250–500 mg twice daily, between meals.	Inhibits thromboxane formation.

Precautions for the use of herbs:

[1] Do not use astragalus if you have a fever or a skin infection.

[2] Garlic counteracts the effects of *Bifidus* and *Lactobacillus* cultures taken as digestive aids. Consult a doctor before using garlic on a regular basis if you are on an anticoagulant drug such as warfarin (Coumadin). Discuss the use of garlic with your doctor before having any type of surgery. (Raw garlic can cause heartburn and flatulence.)

[3] Do not use ginkgo if you are taking blood-thinning medication. Discuss its use with your doctor before having any type of surgery. Ginkgo is not useful for preventing heart attacks for people with diabetes.

[4] Do not use scutellaria if you have diarrhea.

Heart Attack: Formulas

Formula	Comments
Bupleurum Plus Dragon Bone and Oyster Shell Decoction[1]	Most useful Chinese herbal formula for controlling stress reactions that increase the risk of heart attack. Reduces the rate at which the body produces epinephrine in response to stress; treats general anxiety and muscular tension.

Precautions for the use of formulas:

[1] Do not use Bupleurum Plus Dragon Bone and Oyster Shell Decoction if you have a fever.

a heart attack. If you have already had a heart attack, the suggestions here may help you prevent a recurrence.

A program for preventing heart attack, therefore, consists of at least two parts. A key concern is stopping the process of atherosclerosis. A second and equally important concern is regulating the cardiovascular system's response to stress. Herbs are helpful in both parts of the cardiovascular risk prevention program, but if heart attack symptoms occur, seek immediate medical attention.

Recommendations

❏ Eat fiber-rich fruits, vegetables, and whole grains daily. Fiber reduces the amount of dietary cholesterol the body absorbs, and eating fiber lowers the risk of heart attack.

❏ Eat yellow or orange fruits or vegetables and green, leafy vegetables every day. These foods supply beta-carotene, which may reduce the risk of a first heart attack.

❑ Eat blackberries, blueberries, cherries, raspberries, or strawberries regularly. These berries and fruits contain substances that slow the process of atherosclerosis and give the cardiovascular system time to compensate for blockages in blood vessels.

❑ Consume omega-3 fatty acids, which change the form of thromboxane, making it less able to constrict blood vessels and produce a clot. Good sources include fish, at least three times a week, and fish oil capsules, about one a day. Limit servings of meat, fish, and poultry to eight ounces a day. A study of 4,800 people found that consuming diets rich in heme iron—the kind of iron found in meat and poultry—almost doubles the risk of heart attack, even after accounting for differences in cholesterol levels. Moreover, the first heart attack in people who consume lots of heme iron is more likely to be fatal.

❑ Avoid saturated fats, such as those found in meats and in butter, lard, and other solid fats. Men who eat 30 grams of saturated fat daily have twice the risk of heart attack as men who eat only 10 grams daily; in women, the risk increases by 50 percent.

❑ Do not smoke. Smoking constricts blood vessels and raises blood pressure. Even secondhand smoke increases the risk.

❑ Alcohol in moderation helps raise the high-density lipoprotein (HDL, or "good") cholesterol, and can lower the risk of heart attack. Men should have no more than two drinks a day and women no more than one. One drink equivalent is 12 ounces of beer, 4 ounces of wine, or 1.5 ounces of 80-proof liquor. Excessive drinking can raise your blood pressure and triglycerides, which are fats that clog arteries and increase your risk of a heart attack.

❑ Exercise regularly, but be careful to warm up and cool down before and after every exercise session. Any exercise is better than none at all. One study found that exercising as little as sixty minutes a week reduced the risk of cardiac arrest in men by 27 percent.

❑ To relieve stress and promote relaxation, add a few drops of lavender, sandalwood, or ylang-ylang essential oil to a bath. Or simply place a few drops on a tissue and inhale the aroma from time to time throughout the day.

❑ Take care of yourself by getting regular checkups to follow your blood cholesterol level and blood pressure, and to update medications.

❑ To help reduce stress, learn how to relax. (*See* RELAXATION TECHNIQUES in Part Three.)

Considerations

❑ Heart attacks most frequently occur in the morning. A quick hop out of bed can make even a healthy person feel woozy, as the cardiovascular system has to pump more blood to supply the brain. Moving from a prone to upright posture, straining to urinate or pass stool, drinking coffee, and beginning the day's activities all can increase stress hormone production and begin the process that causes a heart attack.

❑ Onions have many of the same heart-protective effects as garlic if taken in a dosage of approximately 1 ounce (30 grams) per day, either raw or in cooking. The key element in onions that relieves heart and artery disease, however, is sulfur. Onions grown in soils deficient in sulfur to provide an exceptionally mild taste do not contain the compounds that counteract atherosclerosis and clot formation.

❑ In one study, omega-3 fatty acids from fish oil supplements reduced the chance of dying from any cause and from developing heart-related events such as stroke in men who didn't have heart disease. The men in this study were at risk for a heart attack, and 2.7 grams of omega-3s each day seemed to improve their health. Eating fish and taking fish oil capsules is recommended to reduce the risk of a heart attack.

❑ Vitamin E does not reduce the risk of having a heart attack, but laboratory studies with animals suggest that it increases the likelihood of surviving a heart attack. Vitamin E also reduces the risk of heart attack in people with diabetes type 2. However, some studies show that taking more than 100 IU a day can increase your chance of dying from all causes. Consult your physician before taking vitamin E.

❑ One study in adult males showed that vitamins E and C did not reduce the chances of having a heart attack. This was a large study in more than 14,000 men who were followed over eight years. This study, and others, have shown that supplements of antioxidants usually are not effective in heart disease and it is better to get these nutrients from eating at least seven servings of fruits and vegetables a day.

❑ A deficiency of vitamin E and beta-carotene may predispose obese children to blocked arteries and heart disease later in life. At least two large clinical trials have shown that daily vitamin E supplements offer protection against heart disease in adults. It now appears that vitamin E supplements are appropriate for children. Ask your child's pediatrician before giving vitamin E to your child.

❑ Vitamin D levels do not seem to predict who will get a heart attack in people who already have heart disease. However, keeping your vitamin D levels in a normal range is important for reducing your risk of cancer.

❑ Elevated levels of the amino acid homocysteine are associated with increased risk of heart attack, but it is not yet clear whether elevated homocysteine causes heart disease or heart disease causes elevated homocysteine. However, supplementation with a combination of folic acid, vitamin B_6 (pyridoxine), and vitamin B_{12} (cobalamin) reduces homocysteine levels and may lower the risk of heart attack.

❏ Niacin is a proven, low-cost treatment for preventing second heart attacks. The drawback to using niacin is that it causes the face to flush twenty to thirty minutes after it is taken. Sustained-release forms of niacin allow this effect to be avoided, but can sometimes cause nausea, stomach upset, and liver damage, and should be avoided. A safer form of niacin, inositol hexaniacinate, is effective and may not be as damaging to the liver. For more information on using niacin, *see* Considerations *under* HIGH CHOLESTEROL.

❏ Arginine may be a good antioxidant to take if you have heart disease. In one study, people with existing heart disease took 3 grams of arginine for seven days and showed increased antioxidant capacity, which could reduce the risk of further heart disease. Another supplement, astaxanthin (Astaxin), taken in 2 to 4 milligram capsules, may also serve as an antioxidant and may be of help to people at risk for heart disease. Good sources of this compound include salmon, trout, shrimp, and lobster.

❏ Aspirin has a very mild blood-thinning effect in the body that reduces the chances of a heart attack. Many people take aspirin every day to reduce their risk. Ask your doctor whether you should take aspirin regularly. In rare cases, long-term use of aspirin has been linked to an increased risk of cataracts, especially cataracts on the back of the lens, which are difficult to treat. However, the benefit of aspirin for some patients far outweighs this rare risk.

❏ Treatment of infections is an important part of heart attack prevention. In rare cases, uncontrolled herpes infections increase the production of clotting factors in the blood and cause cells in the linings of blood vessels to multiply uncontrollably, closing the vessel. Treatment of gonorrhea and chlamydia reduces the risk of heart attack in infected individuals.

❏ It is highly recommended that at least one person in every household receive thorough training in cardiopulmonary resuscitation (CPR).

❏ There is ongoing debate about whether or not taking synthetic estrogen protects the heart after menopause. Some studies have suggested that it may, but there have also been studies showing it may actually increase the risk of a heart attack. Today, it is common practice not to use synthetic estrogen to lower a risk of heart disease, but only to manage symptoms associated with menopause.

❏ Studies have shown that people who take supplemental coenzyme Q_{10} (Co-Q_{10}) following a heart attack are less likely than those who did not to have a second attack within five years.

❏ Depression and heart attacks often go hand in hand. It is therefore wise to actively treat depression.

❏ Researchers have found that eating just an ounce of walnuts a day (about seven nuts) may reduce the risk of a heart attack by 8 to 10 percent.

❏ *See also* ANGINA and ATHEROSCLEROSIS.

HEART DISEASE

See ANGINA; CONGESTIVE HEART FAILURE; HEART ATTACK (MYOCARDIAL INFARCTION).

HEART FAILURE

See CONGESTIVE HEART FAILURE.

HEARTBURN

See under INDIGESTION.

HEAT STRESS

Heat stress occurs if physical activity during heat and humidity upsets the body's fluid balance. As air temperature and humidity increase, the body is less and less able to dissipate heat through perspiration. Higher temperatures also cause heat gain as the body absorbs heat from the sun.

Swelling is the mildest form of heat-related illness. It results from pooling of blood in the hands and feet when the blood vessels dilate in response to heat. Heat cramps are painful spasms of the skeletal muscles in the arms, legs, or abdomen. Fainting, or heat syncope, occurs with prolonged standing or upon sudden rising from a seated or lying position. Cramps occur if too much sodium has been removed from the body by sweat, and are a warning signal of heat exhaustion. Heat exhaustion occurs if a person experiences excessive sweating in a hot, humid environment, and fluids become depleted. Profuse sweating can continue even after the individual is moved to a cooler location, and there also may be several hours to several days of appetite loss, chills, dizziness, low blood pressure, racing pulse, muscular weakness, nausea, vomiting, and visual disturbances.

Heatstroke is a medical emergency in which the body's core temperature reaches 105°F (40.5°C) or more. At that point, internal production of heat exceeds the heat-relieving capacity of perspiration, and sweating stops. Disorientation, irregular heartbeat, and seizures may occur, and there is a sharply increased risk of heart attack and stroke. Heatstroke is more common in older individuals who stay indoors in buildings without air-conditioning during heat waves, but is more severe if it is caused by athletic activity in extreme heat. Call your doctor or go to the emergency room if your temperature reaches 104°F.

Herbal remedies can help treat milder cases of heat stress. If symptoms of heatstroke occur, seek immediate medical attention.

Heat Stress: Beneficial Herbs

Herb	Form and Dosage	Comments
Bitter orange	Tea (loose), prepared by steeping 1 tsp (2–3 gm) in 1 cup water. (*See* TEAS in Part Three.) Take 1 cup 1–2 times daily.	Helps maintain electrolyte balance.
Cayenne	Powder. Dissolve ½ tsp in 1 cup boiling water. Then take 1 tbsp of the mixture with 1 cup hot water, and drink slowly.	Relieves headache and fever, induces gustatory sweating.

Heat Stress: Formulas

Formula	Comments
Clear Summer Heat and Augment the Chi Decoction	A traditional Chinese herbal formula that treats heat stress accompanied by apathy, fever, profuse sweating, scanty and dark urine, shortness of breath, and thirst.

Recommendations

❏ Sip cool, slightly salty liquids. Do not try to force down large quantities of liquid.

❏ Lie down in a shaded place, preferably with your head lower than your feet.

Considerations

❏ Bitter orange tea may not only counteract heat stress, but may also help prevent this condition in people who have high blood pressure. It should be taken whenever heat stress is a possibility. However, if your blood pressure is high, you should take medications to reduce it, because the risk of stroke is greater.

❏ Eating hot peppers provokes a heat-related response, known as gustatory sweating, that prevents heat stress. Chili peppers increase perspiration if it is hot outside, but have no effect on perspiration if it is cold. As a result, a spicy meal eaten in Texas in July causes greater perspiration, but the same meal consumed in Alaska in January will have no effect on perspiration.

❏ It is important to drink water before work or exercise in heat, and to replace both water and electrolytes during activity. Before exercise, the necessary amount of sodium can be obtained through consumption of salty foods—using salt tablets is not necessary to avoid heat stress. When working or exercising, you can use sugar-sweetened electrolyte drinks, since many are designed to replace exactly what is lost in perspiration. One teaspoon of salt added to 1 quart of water may supply enough sodium to avoid cramps. However, you also are losing potassium, so the electrolyte drinks offer both and may be a better option.

❏ A number of drugs increase susceptibility to heat stress. This includes almost any psychoactive drug, such as alcohol, amphetamines, antidepressants, diuretics, lithium, seizure medications, and cocaine, heroin, and marijuana, as well as medications for allergies, Alzheimer's disease, asthma, high blood pressure, hypothyroidism, premenstrual syndrome (PMS), and Parkinson's disease. People with Alzheimer's disease, autism, or schizophrenia are at special risk for heat stress, since they may not be aware of or able to respond to symptoms.

❏ Being overweight puts a strain on your body to regulate its temperature and can cause the body to retain too much heat. Losing weight will help control this problem.

HEMOCHROMATOSIS

See IRON OVERLOAD.

HEMORRHOIDS

Hemorrhoids are swollen blood vessels in and around the anus. These blood vessels stretch under pressure in a manner similar to varicose veins in the legs. They are very common and can occur in anyone, but they appear more often in older people starting at age fifty. This happens because the veins to the rectum and anus are weakened and stretch with normal aging.

Symptoms of hemorrhoids include blood on the surface of the stool or on the toilet paper after a bowel movement, itching, leakage of feces, lump near the anus, itching and irritation in the anal region, swelling, and, sometimes, pain. Sometimes, however, there are no noticeable symptoms at all.

While hemorrhoids cause most cases of rectal bleeding, such bleeding can result from a number of conditions, and should always be brought to a doctor's attention.

Hemorrhoids: Beneficial Herbs

Herb	Form and Dosage	Comments
Herbs to Be Applied Externally		
Aloe	Gel. Apply directly to the irritated area.	Similar to aspirin, relieves pain and soothes the burning sensation.
Calendula	Cream. Apply to external hemorrhoids.	Relieves pain and inflammation.
St. John's wort	Oil. Use as an overnight retention enema (*see under* Recommendations, below).	Stops production of hormones that cause inflammation and swelling.
Witch hazel	Use as a poultice as needed. (*See* POULTICES in Part Three.) Or suppository. Use 1,000 mg 3 times daily.	Treats bleeding hemorrhoids. Also relieves pain and inflammation.
Herbs to Be Taken Internally		
Butcher's broom	Ruscogenin tablets. Take 100 mg once daily.	Particularly effective for burning and itching.
Dandelion[1]	Tincture. Take 10–15 drops in ¼ cup water 3 times daily.	Softens and lubricates stool.
Horse chestnut[2]	Aescin tablets. Take up to 150 mg daily.	Relieves swelling and inflammation. Makes blood vessels more elastic.
Horsetail	Tea bag, prepared with 1 cup water. Take 1 cup 3 times daily.	Helps relieve bleeding hemorrhoids. Mildly antibacterial.
Oligomeric proanthocyanidins (OPCs)	Grapeseed or pine-bark extract tablets. Take 100 mg daily.	Improves blood-vessel strength and flexibility.
Psyllium seed or plantain	Powder, as directed on the label. Avoid over-the-counter (OTC) laxatives that contain both cellulose and psyllium, since cellulose can cause itching. Do not use within 1 hour of taking other medications. Tea bag, prepared with 1 cup water; take 1 cup 3 times daily. Gentler alternative.	Soothes hemorrhoids; coats and protects bowel lining. Plantain is also called whole psyllium seed and is a gentler alternative.

Precautions for the use of herbs:

[1]Do not use dandelion if you have gallstones.

[2]Do not take horse chestnut internally if you are trying to become pregnant.

Conventional care of hemorrhoids includes the use of stool softeners, creams, and, in stubborn cases, surgery.

Internal hemorrhoids are located within the anal canal. External hemorrhoids are those that protrude outside the anus. Internal hemorrhoids that grow large enough to protrude from the anus are called prolapsed hemorrhoids, and can be extremely painful.

Both types of hemorrhoids result from increased pressure in the veins, such as that caused by pregnancy, obesity, chronic diarrhea, cirrhosis of the liver, or straining to pass hard stool. Sitting or standing for long periods of time and lifting heavy objects are other factors that can lead to the formation of hemorrhoids. Interestingly, hemorrhoids are essentially unknown in cultures in which people eat high-fiber diets and are physically active. Dietary fiber absorbs water, making the stools larger and easier to pass, and exercise stimulates defecation. The low-fiber, highly refined North American diet lacks fiber, which makes stools smaller and more difficult to pass. Some herbal treatments such as psyllium provide fiber, while other herbs are useful for soothing irritation or strengthening veins.

Recommendations

❑ To make an overnight retention enema, add 1 table-spoon oil to 1 pint distilled lukewarm water, and place in an enema bag. Just before going to bed, lie down on your right side, draw both knees toward the abdomen, and insert the nozzle. (It is a good idea to first lubricate the nozzle with vitamin E oil or a lubricant jelly.) Take a deep breath, which helps draw the greatest amount of fluid into the colon. Retain the fluid overnight, and expel it first thing in the morning. Do not give this to your child.

❑ If a food allergy is present, use a comfrey poultice to reduce inflammation. (*See* Food Allergies *under* ALLERGIES; *see also* POULTICES in Part Three.) Do not use comfrey during pregnancy.

❑ If using supplemental fiber, such as psyllium powder, be sure to increase your intake gradually. Taking too much right away causes painful bloating and gas, and may cause diarrhea. Psyllium has been shown to reduce the number of bleeding episodes and the number of hemorrhoid cushions that form in patients with internal bleeding hemorrhoids. It may take about two weeks before it works, so be patient.

❑ If you have bleeding hemorrhoids, see a doctor immediately to determine the cause of the bleeding. To treat them, eat foods such as alfalfa, blackstrap molasses, and dark green leafy vegetables, which are high in vitamin K.

❑ Use supplements designed to strengthen rectal blood vessels. Take 1,000 to 2,000 milligrams per day of a plant-based supplement called hydroxyethylrutoside (HER, or HER flavonoids) to heal hemorrhoids. If HER flavonoids are unavailable, take citrus bioflavonoids (rutin and hesperidin), 3,000 to 6,000 milligrams per day. An animal-based supplement called glycosaminoglycan (GAG, or aortic GAGs), taken in dosages of 100 milligrams per day, provides the protein building blocks for healthy veins and helps control pain.

❑ Cleanse the problem area often with warm water. To reduce swelling and relieve pain, take a hot bath for fifteen minutes each day without adding Epsom salts or bath beads, oils, or bubbles to the water. Or use a warm-water sitz bath to which you can add some white oak. (See SITZ BATHS in Part Three.) Do not use white oak or other sitz bath products if you have either weeping eczema or congestive heart failure.

❑ Wear cotton underwear, or make sure that the panty liner is cotton. Cotton has more "give" than other fabrics and is less likely to restrict circulation.

❑ Avoid harsh laxatives, most of which induce unnecessary straining at stool, often creating a diarrhea-like condition, all without providing the healthful benefits of natural products. Laxative products can also cause the bowels to become laxative-dependent, which interferes with normal functioning.

❑ Avoid prolonged straining at stool. Straining for more than five minutes is harmful to colorectal muscles and nerves. It can also increase stress on the veins of the rectum and worsens hemorrhoids. Straining can lead to diverticulosis—the formation of small blisterlike pockets in the colon walls that can become infected.

❑ Avoid reading in the bathroom. The veins and muscles serving the colon and rectum continue to be strained as long as the squatting position is maintained.

❑ Drink plenty of liquids, especially water (preferably steam-distilled). Water is the best, most natural stool softener in existence. It also helps prevent constipation.

❑ Learn not to strain when moving the bowels. Keep the bowels clean and avoid constipation. Don't sit on the commode for longer than ten minutes at a time, as this causes blood to pool in the hemorrhoidal veins.

❑ Sit on a soft cushion, not on hard surfaces. Use an ordinary cushion, not a doughnut-shaped one. The old-fashioned inflated doughnut cushion actually increases pressure on the hemorrhoidal blood vessels, aggravating the swelling and bleeding.

❑ Get regular moderate exercise.

Considerations

❑ In rare instances, zinc oxide from creams applied to hemorrhoids can cause a metallic taste in the mouth. If this happens, change creams. In very rare cases, overuse of zinc oxide creams can cause yellow eyes, yellow skin, and abdominal pain. In these cases, discontinue the cream and see a physician promptly.

❑ Treatments for hemorrhoids can reduce the risk of permanent fecal incontinence after childbirth, especially if you have an episiotomy or forceps are used during delivery. (See DIARRHEA.)

❑ Eating certain foods, especially beets, can cause the stool to become reddish and can be mistaken for blood.

❑ The most common cause of anal itching is tissue trauma resulting from the use of harsh toilet paper.

❑ See also CONSTIPATION.

HEPATITIS

Hepatitis is an inflammation of the liver. The liver can become inflamed as a result of chronic, excessive consumption of alcohol, exposure to toxic chemicals, or overdoses of some prescription drugs, but it is most commonly caused by viral infection. Most cases of viral hepatitis tend to be acute, that is, they generally last for a few weeks. Chronic hepatitis is an inflammation that lasts more than six months.

At least seven different hepatitis viruses cause liver infection, so blood tests are needed for an accurate diagnosis. While some forms can be spread through casual contact, the more serious forms are transmitted primarily through infusions of tainted blood, sexual contact, and, among intravenous drug users, sharing hypodermic needles. (See "The ABCs of Hepatitis," page 336.) Hepatitis symptoms vary widely. Initially they may include flulike complaints, such as malaise and loss of appetite. Later symptoms may include fever, nausea, sensitivity to light, vomiting, headache, swollen joints, dark urine, abdominal discomfort, and jaundice. Symptoms vary because the liver is an extremely robust organ, able to function even if large portions are destroyed.

In chronic hepatitis, the nutrients ordinarily distributed by the liver become unavailable. Low blood sugar levels and fatigue result. Chronic hepatitis also keeps the liver from breaking down the toxins it normally removes from

The ABCs of Hepatitis

Some viruses that can cause hepatitis, such as Epstein-Barr virus and cytomegalovirus, can cause other illnesses as well. In addition, there are at least seven viruses that exclusively infect the liver. They are identified as hepatitis A, B, C, D, E, F, and G.

The most common form of viral hepatitis, hepatitis A, is almost always a short-term, self-limiting illness. It is spread by person-to-person contact, or by contaminated food or water. Before symptoms arise, the infection can be halted with gamma-globulin injections.

Hepatitis B is a much more serious infection. Formerly known as serum hepatitis, it is spread by blood-to-blood contact or sexual contact with an infected person. Infected mothers can pass the virus to their babies during birth. In some parts of the developing world, hepatitis B is also spread by food and water contamination because of poor sanitation. While the virus sometimes persists for many years, most people recover within a year, compared with a usual recovery time of two months for hepatitis A. Hepatitis B can cause cirrhosis and an increased susceptibility to liver cancer. Fortunately, there is a highly successful vaccination for hepatitis B.

Hepatitis C (formerly called non-A, non-B hepatitis) is carried by nearly 4 million people in the United States alone. It is usually spread through transfusions or shared needles. Hepatitis C is a potentially deadly infection that is detected in the blood through a blood test that can verify that you have the virus, measure the quantity of the virus, and determine the genetic makeup of the virus. It has many of the same long-term consequences as hepatitis B, but now two vaccines have been approved to treat it—Incivek from Vertex Pharmaceuticals and Johnson and Johnson, and Victrelis from Merck.

Some cases of hepatitis are caused by four other viruses, hepatitis D, E, F, and G. Hepatitis D (formerly called delta hepatitis) and E (formerly called enteric hepatitis) are seldom encountered in North America, but are often epidemic in other parts of the world. The hepatitis D virus only multiplies in the presence of the B virus, and makes hepatitis B symptoms worse. Hepatitis E is sometimes epidemic in tropical areas after widespread flooding, especially in India and China. It produces symptoms similar to hepatitis B, such as jaundice and flulike aches, except that it is much more dangerous to pregnant women. Hepatitis F is an extremely rare strain of the virus that is found in the Far East. Hepatitis G is a mild form of the disease and does not seem to cause ongoing liver damage. However, if you have it, you should avoid alcohol and be sure to eat a balanced diet.

---

the body. The buildup of toxins in the bloodstream can result in depression, delirium, or loss of short-term memory. Toxic buildup of bile also can cause jaundice, a condition in which the skin and eyes turn any color from faint yellow to bright tangerine. Frequently, however, there is no change in skin color at all.

The destructive agent in viral hepatitis is not the virus, but rather the immune system itself. As long as the virus lies dormant in the liver cells, it is undetectable to the immune system. When the virus begins to multiply, however, immune-system cells engulf and destroy the cell. Thus, the immune response destroys liver tissue and causes the most serious symptoms of hepatitis. Asymptomatic viral hepatitis may wait for months or years for a trigger such as acute infection to manifest itself. This trigger stresses the liver and activates the infection. When that happens, symptoms appear. In a study in Hong Kong, a plant extract of *Fructus Schisandrae* (Wu wei zi) seemed to strengthen the immune system of people with hepatitis B.

Conventional treatment uses several different types of drugs. Be aware that some herbs may have a negative impact on the liver and/or interact negatively with conventional medicines. Always work with a qualified healthcare practitioner.

Recommendations

❑ If you are being treated for amebic hepatitis with a drug such as metronidazole (Flagyl), consult a traditional Chinese medicine (TCM) practitioner about taking a tea that combines dong quai, hoelen, and peony along with the prescription medication. This herbal combination may increase the effectiveness of the antiamebic drugs. A major study looked at all of the herb remedies for hepatitis C and found that a few were of benefit. Of benefit for suppressing the virus was silibinin. Some herbal blends such as Bing Gan Tang plus interferon had better clearance of the virus in the body. Another herbal mixture, Yi Zhu Decoction, showed viral clearance and normalization of liver function tests when combined with glycyrrhizin and ribavirin.

❑ Especially when symptoms are acute, take care to replace fluids by drinking vegetable broth, diluted vegetable juices, and herbal teas.

❑ Take 30 milligrams of zinc daily. The changes in virally infected liver cells that cause cirrhosis may involve an imbalance of zinc and copper, with copper in excess. Copper, an oxidant, can damage the walls of cells, and zinc displaces copper from the cells. However, hepatitis is not cirrhosis and you may not need to take this much.

❑ Take 500 to 1,000 milligrams of liver extracts daily. Over a period of three to six months, the use of liver extracts may lower liver enzyme levels.

❑ Avoid fatty foods entirely, and limit animal protein intake to between 3 and 6 ounces (about 100 to 200 grams) a day.

❑ Eat vegetable proteins such as soy and beans to maintain muscle mass.

❑ Avoid stale or moldy bakery products and grains. At least in laboratory studies, the fungus by-product aflatoxin amplifies the carcinogenic potential of hepatitis infection.

❑ Avoid alcohol in all forms, including that found in drugs and flavorings.

❑ If you are taking interferon for hepatitis B, make sure your doctor orders blood tests to monitor iron (ferritin) levels in your blood. Iron deficiency cuts the success rate

Hepatitis: Beneficial Herbs

Herb	Form and Dosage	Comments
Artichoke	Take as directed on the label.	Increases the effectiveness of liver function.
Hoelen and schisandra[1]	Tablets. Take 100 mg 3 times daily.	Stops inflammation caused by autoimmune reactions. Helps the liver to regenerate after viral infection. Protects the liver against toxins.
Licorice[2]	Glycyrrhizin tablets. Take 800 mg daily. Use for 6 weeks, then take a 2-week break. Do not substitute deglycyrrhizinated licorice (DGL).	"Locks" hepatitis B virus into cells and keeps it from spreading. Consume potassium-rich foods such as bananas or citrus juices, or take a potassium supplement, daily when taking this herb.
Ligustrum	Extract. Take as directed on the label.	An immune restorative and anti-inflammatory agent.
Milk thistle[3]	Silymarin gelcaps. Take 600 mg daily.	Promotes growth of healthy liver tissue; protects liver from free-radical damage. Relieves nausea.
Peppermint[4]	Enteric-coated oil capsules. Take 200 mg 3 times daily.	Relieves stomach upset and abdominal cramping.

Precautions for the use of herbs:

[1]Do not use schisandra if you have gallstones or an obstruction of the bile duct. Do not use it during pregnancy.

[2]Do not use licorice if you have glaucoma, high blood pressure, or an estrogen-dependent disorder such as breast cancer, endometriosis, or fibrocystic breasts.

[3]Do not use milk thistle if you are taking interferon for hepatitis B. This herb may cause mild diarrhea. If this occurs, decrease the dose or stop taking it.

[4]Do not use peppermint if you have any kind of gallbladder disorder.

Hepatitis: Formulas

Formula	Comments
Minor Bupleurum Decoction[1]	This traditional Chinese herbal formula interferes with viral reproduction and stimulates the immune system; relieves nausea. Prevents progression of hepatitis C. Especially useful in treating children; seek dispensing herbalist's advice on dosage.

Precautions for the use of formulas:

[1]Do not use Minor Bupleurum Decoction if you have a fever or a skin infection. Taken long term, it can cause headache, dizziness, and bleeding gums. Side effects can be avoided if the formula is taken as a tea.

of interferon treatment roughly in half. Your doctor will recommend treatments that can bring iron levels up to normal quickly if needed. Otherwise, do not take over-the-counter (OTC) iron supplements. Excess iron accelerates the progress of hepatitis infection to cirrhosis.

❏ Especially when traveling, be aware of the possibility of contaminated water or food grown in areas with polluted waters.

❏ Do not take any drugs that have not been prescribed by your doctor. Read package inserts carefully for information regarding liver toxicity.

Considerations

❏ Clinical studies find that milk thistle (silymarin) treatment can begin to reverse liver damage caused by chronic viral hepatitis in as little as seven days. In laboratory studies, silymarin stimulates the growth of healthy tissue and protects the cells of the liver from free radicals generated

by trace element imbalances caused by infection. When a group of patients with hepatitis C took 160 milligrams of *Silybum marianum* three times a day, they experienced a decrease in elevated liver function tests. However, the amount of virus in the blood did not decrease (called the viral load), indicating that milk thistle likely works as an antioxidant to protect the liver tissue but is not an antiviral agent.

❏ In one study, branched-chain amino acids such as leucine, isoleucine, and valine added to an evening snack as a supplement improved serum albumin levels and nitrogen balance, which are markers of improved nutritional status in patients with hepatitis C and cirrhosis.

❏ There are a number of conventional medicines used in hepatitis treatment. Steroids are sometimes used in more serious cases to suppress the immune system, and thus reduce tissue damage. Interferon, one of the body's own chemical defenders, is used for hepatitis B and hepatitis

C, and severe cases of hepatitis A. Interferons stop the growth of the virus over the long term in about 35 percent of people who use them. There are also a number of other drugs, known collectively as nucleoside and nucleotide analogues, designed to keep the virus from reproducing and/or causing active disease; they may be used with interferon in the form of antiviral "cocktails."

❏ Thymic factors may be helpful as a supplement for people with hepatitis C who are being treated with interferon.

❏ Monitoring the progress of treatment for hepatitis requires regular liver function tests, which can be done easily in any medical lab. A needle biopsy of the liver, a relatively safe and often painless day surgery, may be required. Carefully discuss the pros and cons of needle biopsy with the surgeon before consenting to the procedure.

❏ There is evidence that vitamin C, in a dosage of from 1,500 to 2,000 milligrams daily, can help prevent hepatitis in people exposed to the virus. Patients with hepatitis C benefit from not only vitamin C, but a cocktail of several antioxidants, such as lipoic acid, glycyrrhizin, schisandra, and L-gluthione. In one study, liver enzymes improved in 48 percent of the patients who received this mixture.

❏ In laboratory studies with mice, high cholesterol levels can render hepatitis-resistant mice vulnerable to hepatitis infection. As the liver cells absorb cholesterol, their outer walls become stiffer and expose more sites for the virus to take hold. Although there have been no studies of this phenomenon in humans, it may be that high cholesterol predisposes people to infection and reinfection with the hepatitis virus. (See HIGH CHOLESTEROL.)

❏ Today, the risk of getting hepatitis C from a transfusion is very small, because the blood supply is strictly tested. But those tests weren't available before 1992, so certain groups of people are more at risk for the disease. The U.S. Food and Drug Administration (FDA) recommends testing for anyone who ever injected drugs, even once; has had sex with an injecting drug user; hemophiliacs who used clotting factors before 1987; and recipients of pre-1992 organ transplants. An at-home hepatitis C test from Home Access is available. The kit is sold on the company's website, www.homeaccess.com.

❏ Hepatitis B vaccine has been successfully integrated into the childhood vaccination schedule, contributing to a 96 percent decline in the incidence of acute hepatitis B virus (HBV) in children and adolescents. It is recommended that children get their first vaccination at birth and complete the vaccine series by age six to eighteen months. Older children and adolescents who did not previously receive the hepatitis B vaccine should also be vaccinated. Currently, approximately 95 percent of new HBV infections occur among adults. Unvaccinated adults with behavioral risk factors or who are household contacts or sex partners of HBV-infected persons are at risk.

❏ There are vaccines against hepatitis A as well. Hepatitis A is a liver disease caused by the hepatitis A virus (HAV). Hepatitis A can affect anyone. Vaccines are available for long-term prevention of HAV infection in persons one year of age and older. Good personal hygiene and proper sanitation can also help prevent the spread of hepatitis A. However, adults traveling to certain parts of the world, such as Central or South America and Africa, should get vaccinated as well.

❏ If you require surgery and may need a blood transfusion, discuss this with your doctor or surgeon. You may be able to bank your own blood or the blood of a relative or friend before the procedure.

❏ If you have hepatitis C, it is best to take steps to reduce the level of iron in your body before starting any treatment. High iron levels inhibit therapy for the liver. One Japanese study compared removing blood on a biweekly basis to eating a low-iron diet in patients with chronic hepatitis C. Although it appears that patients did better with the removal of blood, a low-iron diet may still be of benefit. Today there are treatments for this condition, making iron overload less of a concern. Treatment options include a drug combination of boceprevir (Victrelis), ribavirin (Copegus, Rebetol), and peginterferon alpha-2b (PEG-Intron).

❏ For information on how to prevent cirrhosis from progressing to liver cancer, see LIVER CANCER; see also ALCOHOLISM and CIRRHOSIS OF THE LIVER.

HERPES ZOSTER

See under HERPESVIRUS INFECTION.

HERPESVIRUS INFECTION

There are a number of disease-causing herpesviruses. Herpes simplex virus 1 (HSV-1) causes mild skin outbreaks, generally in the form of cold sores (fever blisters) of the mouth and lips, though sometimes the genitals are affected. Herpes simplex virus 2 (HSV-2) causes more severe outbreaks, generally in the form of genital herpes, though sometimes the mouth is affected. Herpes varicella-zoster (herpes zoster) causes shingles and chicken pox. Herpes can also cause a painful eye disease called ocular keratitis. This is an infection of the white of the eye that can damage the cornea. Herpetic whitlow is an infection of the fingertip that can occur if the virus enters through a damaged cuticle, usually when a person touches an active herpes sore.

All three herpes infections can cause painful blisters. Herpes blisters are highly infectious until they are completely healed, which may take two to four weeks. Although herpes infections can be contagious even after healing, the rate of transmission drops dramatically at that point. In some cases, there are no symptoms.

HSV-1 initially produces burning or tingling around the lips and nose. In a few hours, this is followed by small red pimples and then by the blisters. There may be a mild fever and enlarged lymph nodes in the neck. Recurrences often happen after exposure to intense sunlight or sunburn. Outbreaks also can occur after other infections weaken the immune system.

The first symptoms of HSV-2 usually are noticed four to eight days after exposure. They include a burning or itching in the genital area, followed by the blisters that turn into red, painful sores that are easily infected. There may be pain upon urination, and fever, flulike symptoms,

and headache may also occur. Symptoms tend to be more severe in women. Outbreaks may be triggered by nerve damage, especially to the trigeminal nerve underlying the cheekbones, where HSV-2 frequently settles. (Dental procedures that disturb this nerve cause outbreaks in up to 40 percent of infected individuals.) HSV-2 can cause serious complications, including liver damage. An infected mother can pass the disease to her baby during birth, creating a risk of blindness or brain damage.

The first symptoms of shingles may include malaise, chills, fever, and intestinal or urinary difficulties. Three or four days later, the blisters develop, generally along the path of a nerve on one side of the trunk. Shingles often occur decades after a person had chicken pox, although

Herpesvirus: Beneficial Herbs

Herb	Form and Dosage	Comments
Herbs to Be Applied Externally		
Aloe or	Gel. Apply to the inflamed area.	Kills herpesvirus. Relieves inflammation.
St. John's wort	Cream. Apply to inflamed skin.	
Cayenne	Capsaicin cream. Apply to previously infected skin. Do not apply to active sores.	Relieves pain caused by nerve damage.
Copaiba	Oil. Apply to inflamed area.	Fast relief of inflammation. Prevents secondary infection.
Green tea	Tea bag, prepared with 1 cup water and used to make warm compresses. (*See* COMPRESSES in Part Three.) Apply 2–3 times daily.	Increases the effectiveness of topical interferon.
Lemon balm	Cream. Apply thickly to inflamed lips 2–4 times daily.	Reduces time needed to heal cold sores by roughly half. Reduces recurrences. Also known as melissa.
Papain	Cream. Apply to area of redness.	Relieves pain and inflammation.
Herbs to Be Taken Internally		
Acerola	Tablets, with vitamin C USP. Take as directed on the label.	Prevents blister formation; especially useful for mouth ulcers.
Astragalus	Take as directed on the label.	Enhances the immune system and acts as an antibiotic.
Bitter melon[1]	Tablets. Take as directed on the label. Use for 4 weeks, then discontinue for 4 weeks.	Kills acyclovir-resistant herpesviruses. Also known as momordica.
Cat's claw	Capsules or tincture. Use as directed on the label.	Has immune-enhancing properties and acts against viral infection.
Clove	Oil. Take 10 drops in ¼ cup water 3 times daily.	Increases the effectiveness of acyclovir without side effects.
Dendrobium	Tea (loose), prepared by steeping 1 tsp (2 gm) in 1 cup water. (*See* TEAS in Part Three.) Take 1 cup 3 times daily, between meals.	A remedy for mouth and lip sores activated by exposure to the sun.
Licorice[2]	Glycyrrhizin tablets. Take 400–800 mg daily, depending on the severity of symptoms. Use for 6 weeks, then take a 2-week break. Do not substitute deglycyrrhizinated licorice (DGL).	Kills herpes simplex and herpes zoster viruses. Consume potassium-rich foods such as bananas or citrus juices, or take a potassium supplement, daily when taking this herb.
Olive leaf	Extract. Take as directed on the label.	Helps curb the growth of viral diseases, including herpes.

Precautions for the use of herbs:

[1]Do not use bitter melon if you have cirrhosis of the liver or a medical history of hepatitis or HIV infection compounded by liver infections.

[2]Do not use licorice if you have glaucoma, high blood pressure, or an estrogen-dependent disorder such as breast cancer, endometriosis, or fibrocystic breasts.

Herpesvirus: Formulas

Formula	Comments
Gentiana Longdancao Decoction to Drain the Liver[1]	A traditional Chinese herbal formula that relieves symptoms of both herpes simplex and herpes zoster outbreaks, especially if there is eye irritation, fatigue, irritability, whitish vaginal discharge, painful urination, and inflammation in the ears.
Kudzu Decoction	Research shows that this traditional Chinese herbal formula prevents recurrences of HSV-1 and ocular keratitis.

Precautions for the use of formulas:

[1]Do not use Gentiana Longdancao Decoction to Drain the Liver if you are trying to become pregnant.

recurrences of the shingles themselves are rare. Possible complications include skin infections and lasting pain along the affected nerve.

The herpesvirus operates in two distinct modes. During acute infection, the virus reproduces and settles in adjoining tissues. After acute infection, it implants itself in the nerve tissue, where it does not attempt to reproduce. Only when the security of its "home" is threatened will the virus reactivate into a disease-causing form. Acyclovir (Zovirax) is the conventional drug most often used to treat herpes.

The key to managing herpes infections is making sure they do not implant themselves. A strong antibody response can keep the virus from entering cells. Some herbs may stimulate antibody production and may offer a first line of defense against the disease. After implantation, the aim of treatment is to destroy the virus without causing tissue damage.

Herbs to Avoid

❏ Individuals who have herpes infections should avoid dong quai and pinellia. (For more information regarding these herbs, *see* individual entries *under* The Herbs in Part One.)

Recommendations

❏ Eat a diet high in the amino acid lysine and low in the amino acid arginine. Arginine may stimulate the herpesvirus to multiply, while lysine interferes with the virus's ability to multiply. Foods high in lysine (to be included) include most vegetables, legumes, fish, turkey, and chicken. Foods high in arginine (to be avoided) include chocolate, almonds, peanuts, and most other nuts. You can also apply an L-lysine cream, available from health food stores, directly to inflamed skin. Or take an oral supplement of L-lysine.

❏ Take 50 milligrams of zinc daily. Zinc reduces the frequency, severity, and duration of herpes flare-ups.

❏ Use warm baking-soda baths to ease the pain and itching of genital herpes and to keep the area clean.

❏ Avoid sexual activity if genital sores are present.

❏ Inform your health-care provider if you are pregnant and know you have genital herpes. An attack that occurs late in the pregnancy may make it necessary for a cesarean section to be performed. On the other hand, a lack of lesions means that the risk to the baby is probably low.

❏ If an eye becomes infected, see a physician at once. This virus can cause a brain inflammation called encephalitis.

❏ Do not consume citrus fruits and juices while the virus is active.

❏ Drink steam-distilled water.

❏ Wear cotton underwear or underwear with cotton panty liners. Practice good personal hygiene—keep clean and dry.

Considerations

❏ Herbs may prevent outbreaks and reduce side effects. Licorice (*see* Beneficial Herbs, page 339) has been used as a "morning-after" treatment if herpes exposure is suspected. Cat's claw (1,000 milligrams twice daily) may prevent reinfection with herpes in people with AIDS. Scutellaria—from 1 to 1½ teaspoons of tincture in ¼ cup of water three times daily—may protect herpes-damaged skin against secondary infections.

❏ Eyewashes made with either coptis or prunella have been used to prevent herpes infections of the eye. Apply the wash by pouring ¼ cup of a coptis or prunella tea that has been cooled to room temperature over a partially open eye. (*See* TEAS in Part Three.)

❏ Standard medical therapy for chronic herpes infection is a group of drugs that includes acyclovir. Acyclovir destroys the virus, and is relatively safe. However, it cannot reach every herpesvirus in every cell, so reinfection is always possible unless, and sometimes even if, the medication is continued. A wide variety of herbs work with acyclovir to offer better protection against implantation than either herbs or acyclovir alone.

❏ In women, genital herpes infections increase the risk of cervical cancer. A woman with herpes should have Pap smears taken on a regular basis.

❑ Herpes infection increases the risk of atherosclerosis. Infection with the virus stimulates the smooth muscles lining arteries to grow cells around cholesterol plaques, narrowing the arteries. Be sure to maintain a good weight and heart-healthy diet, especially if you have herpes.

❑ Laboratory research suggests that capsaicin may be able to prevent outbreaks of genital lesions.

❑ Some physicians have used butylated hydroxytoluene (BHT) to treat herpes. This can have dangerous consequences, however, especially if taken on an empty stomach. Irritation and even perforation of the stomach can result.

❑ If chronic pain is a concern, *see* PAIN, CHRONIC.

HICCUPS

See under INDIGESTION.

HIGH BLOOD PRESSURE (HYPERTENSION)

Blood pressure—the force that circulating blood exerts against the walls of arteries—that is too high can cause arteries to narrow, which can lead to arteriosclerosis, heart attack, kidney disease, memory loss, and stroke. About one in three adults in the United States has high blood pressure, which often causes no noticeable symptoms. Only in severe cases are there outward signs, such as headache, sweating, rapid pulse, shortness of breath, dizziness, and visual disturbances. Most people with high blood pressure have primary (essential) hypertension, or elevated blood pressure that is not due to a single known cause. High blood pressure is more common among African-Americans than among members of other ethnic groups. It affects more men than women.

Doctors are not sure exactly what causes primary high blood pressure. There may be a genetic component, since it seems to run in families. But there may also be a lifestyle component, as high blood pressure has been linked to aging, diet, smoking, alcohol use, excessive caffeine and salt intake, and lack of exercise. Certain medications, such as birth control pills, can elevate blood pressure, as can pregnancy. Low vitamin D levels in the blood, stress, and chronic conditions such as diabetes also increase the chances that you will have high blood pressure.

Blood pressure is measured as a pair of numbers. The

High Blood Pressure: Beneficial Herbs

Herb	Form and Dosage	Comments
American ginseng	*Panax quinquefolium* tincture. Take as directed on the label.	Helps maintain healthy potassium levels.
Bilberry	Tablets. Take 240–360 mg daily.	Helps keep arteries flexible; prevents hypertensive damage to blood vessels in the eye.
Bitter orange	Tea (loose), prepared by steeping 1 tsp (2–3 gm) in 1 cup water. (*See* TEAS in Part Three.) Take 1 cup 1–2 times daily.	Lowers blood pressure while strengthening heartbeat.
Chanca piedra	Tincture. Take as directed on the label.	Lowers blood pressure and protects the kidneys, especially in salt-sensitive individuals.
Coleus	Forskolin extract. Take as directed on the label.	Lowers blood pressure while strengthening heartbeat and lowering pulse rate.
Corn silk	Tea bag, prepared with 1 cup water. Take 1 cup 1–2 times daily.	Stimulates urination without increasing potassium excretion.
Dong quai	*Angelica sinensis* capsules. Take 500–1,000 mg daily.	Prolongs resting period between heartbeats and lowers blood pressure.
Epimedium[1]	Use as directed by dispensing herbalist.	Lowers blood pressure and enhances male sexual capacity.
Ginseng	*Panax ginseng* tincture. Take as directed on the label.	Used as directed, lowers blood pressure; protects heart muscle; enhances sexual function in both men and women.
Hawthorn	Tablets. Take 100–250 mg 3 times daily.	Lowers both blood pressure and cholesterol levels.
Oligomeric proanthocyanidins (OPCs)	Grapeseed or pine-bark extract tablets. Take 200 mg daily.	Helps protect against complications of uncontrolled high blood pressure, especially in people with diabetes.
Reishi or shiitake	Fresh mushrooms or teas. Take as desired.	Lowers both blood pressure and cholesterol.
Scutellaria[2]	Capsules. Take 1,000–2,000 mg 3 times daily.	Dilates blood vessels and stimulates urination.

Precautions for the use of herbs:

[1]Do not use epimedium if you have any kind of prostate disorder.

[2]Do not use scutellaria if you have diarrhea.

High Blood Pressure: Formulas

Formula	Comments
Eight-Ingredient Pill with Rehmannia	A traditional Chinese herbal formula that reduces salt sensitivity and protects against kidney damage. Used if symptoms include dizziness, lightheadedness, night sweats, ringing in the ears or diminished hearing, and soreness and weakness in the lower back.

first number is the systolic pressure, exerted when the heart beats, and represents blood pressure at its highest. The second number is the diastolic pressure, exerted when the heart rests between beats, and represents pressure at its lowest. Pressure varies throughout the day in response to stress, activity level, and other factors. Normal readings for adults range from 110/70 mmHg to 140/90 mmHg, with 120/80 mmHg generally considered a good target, especially if you have another disease such as diabetes. Higher levels are tolerated in healthy individuals up to 140/90 mmHg. (The mmHg is millimeters of mercury—the units used to measure blood pressure.) Elevation of the diastolic pressure is of greater concern than that of the systolic pressure, with a diastolic blood pressure over 140 considered to be Stage 1 hypertension (140–159 mmHg) or Stage 2 hypertension (more than 160 mmHg).

Two factors contribute to many cases of primary high blood pressure. First, excessive blood levels of the hormone insulin stimulate the arterial walls to contract and cause the kidneys to retain sodium. Both actions increase pressure. Second, sodium is found in salt, and how strongly the kidneys react to sodium is determined by a person's salt sensitivity. In many people who have primary high blood pressure, an increase in blood-sodium levels leads to kidney production of angiotensin II, a substance that also stimulates the arteries to contract. Secondary high blood pressure is caused by kidney problems, adrenal gland tumors, use of illegal drugs like cocaine, and certain drugs such as birth control pills or decongestants.

Doctors urge people who have high blood pressure to lose weight, exercise, and cut salt consumption. If these measures don't work, doctors prescribe various drugs (*see* Considerations, page 343). Clinical researchers have found that herbal treatments lower blood pressure within a few days' use just as prescription drugs do, but the amount of the change is less. For this reason, herbal therapies are best for "borderline" cases. Herbal medicine may also be useful for people who know they are sensitive to salt or who suffer from depression.

Herbs to Avoid

❏ Individuals who have high blood pressure should avoid the following herbs: coltsfoot, dan shen, ephedra, licorice, and maté. (For more information regarding these herbs, *see* individual entries *under* The Herbs in Part One.)

Recommendations

❏ Use essential oil of lavender or lemon balm (melissa) in aromatherapy to relieve tension and lower blood pressure. (*See* AROMATHERAPY in Part Three.) There are also specific techniques that can help you relieve tension. (*See* RELAXATION TECHNIQUES in Part Three.)

❏ Reduce, but do not try to eliminate, salt from the diet. Start by excluding foods with visible salt, such as pretzels, potato chips, and salted nuts. Limit your consumption of very salty foods, such as olives, pickles, canned and smoked fish, and processed cheeses. By itself, eliminating added salt has a minimal impact on high blood pressure. Choose fresh foods such as fruits, vegetables, grains, and meat, all of which are very low in salt. Use salt to cook these foods and then make it a habit not to add salt at the table, and you'll be on your way to reducing salt in your diet.

❏ Increase potassium intake, since potassium counteracts sodium's pressure-raising effects. Potassium is found in all fruits and vegetables, including apricots, avocados, bananas, dates, dulse, figs, dried fruit, garlic, potatoes, raisins, sea vegetables, winter squash, and yams. More than five daily servings of fruits and vegetables are recommended. Potassium is also found in blackstrap molasses, brewer's yeast, brown rice, nuts, torula yeast, and wheat bran.

❏ Use moderate amounts of polyunsaturated fats (such as corn oil) in cooking to avoid weight gain. Supplementation with essential fatty acids in the form of omega-3s from fish oil, which can be taken in capsule form, 500 milligrams twice daily, may help lower blood pressure. Eating fish two to three times a week is also recommended.

❏ Discontinue use of all stimulants, including coffee and tobacco.

❏ Exercise regularly but moderately. Moderate exercise is more effective than vigorous activity, and injuries are more common while jogging than while walking, swimming, or cycling. After your pressure is under control, consult a physician about beginning a weight-lifting program. Weight lifting increases muscle mass, which helps the body use insulin and indirectly lowers blood pressure, and prevents long-term complications of high blood pressure. Taking long walks at a comfortable pace for thirty to sixty minutes each day reduces body fat, which lowers blood pressure.

❑ Monitor blood pressure at home daily. This gives immediate feedback on how well diet, exercise, herbs, and medication are working.

❑ Never discontinue a blood-pressure medication abruptly, especially if it is a beta-blocker. Gradually lowering the dose over a period of weeks prevents rebound hypertension, or blood pressure that goes higher when a medication is stopped than it was before treatment. Consult a physician before discontinuing any medication.

❑ Avoid foods such as aged cheeses, aged meats, anchovies, avocados, chocolate, fava beans, pickled herring, sherry, sour cream, wine, and yogurt.

❑ Keep your weight down. If you are overweight, take steps to lose the excess pounds.

❑ Be sure to get sufficient sleep.

Considerations

❑ Several classes of conventional drugs are used to fight high blood pressure. Diuretics remove water from the body's tissues and excrete it via the urine, which reduces the amount of fluid in the bloodstream. Beta-blockers cause the heart to slow down and lower its blood output, which reduces pressure (they also work well with diuretics). Other drugs inhibit angiotensin II production to relax blood vessels, and are called angiotensin-converting enzyme (ACE) inhibitors. These ACE inhibitors have been shown to work well with pycnogenol, a natural compound that has anti-edema effects. In one study, participants used 50 milligrams of pycnogenol three times a day with their drugs and their blood pressure went down. About 33 percent of patients with high blood pressure have some edema, and pycnogenol may help reduce it and lower blood pressure so that less of the ACE drugs are needed. The various drugs have different side effects, including fatigue, depression, fainting when rising from a seated position (orthostatic hypotension), and impaired male sexual function. Often drugs are combined, or a person must switch from one drug to another. Work with your physician to get the right mix of drugs for you. High blood pressure over time increases your risk of stroke.

❑ In the United States, African-Americans and Hispanics are more susceptible to developing high blood pressure than whites. One hypothesis is that darker skin absorbs less sunlight, which means it produces less vitamin D. Vitamin D deficiency causes the smooth muscles lining arteries to contract more readily and forcefully in response to such stress hormones as adrenaline. Since vitamin D deficiency is a known risk factor for high blood pressure, vitamin D supplements are probably especially useful to African-Americans and Hispanics with this condition. Eating vitamin D–enriched dairy products is also recommended. Read the label, because vitamin D is not added to all dairy products. There is also some scientific evidence that deficiencies in vitamin D contribute to salt sensitivity, and that adequate vitamin D supplies can reverse salt sensitivity. Although calcium and vitamin D are essential nutrients, long-term supplementation with 1,000 milligrams of calcium and 400 international units (IU) of vitamin D did not reduce blood pressure or the risk of developing high blood pressure in a study of more than 36,000 women.

❑ Sugar consumption by itself does not elevate blood pressure, but it may contribute to the development of sodium sensitivity. Animal studies suggest that consuming large amounts of table sugar can also reverse the beneficial effects of omega-3 fatty acids.

❑ Two herbs shown to reduce blood pressure in clinical trials are hawthorn and *Spirulina maxima*. In one study, people with high blood pressure took 1,200 milligrams of hawthorn and experienced small decreases, of 3 to 4 points, in blood pressure. Spirulina was used at 4.5 grams a day and people had reductions of 5 to 10 points in blood pressure.

❑ The Dietary Approach to Stop Hypertension (DASH) diet is rich in fruits, vegetables, and nuts, and low in processed foods. Eating processed foods and taking supplements of fiber, potassium, and magnesium (all of which are high in the DASH diet) does not work. There are other compounds in fresh foods that lower blood pressure.

❑ Kudzu may be an appropriate herbal treatment for nerve damage in people with a long history of high blood pressure. However, any herb or herbal formula taken for degenerative diseases affecting hearing or sight should not be used on a long-term basis. Instead, take one 10-milligram kudzu tablet three times daily for three to six months. Then replace it with another herb that has similar effects in consultation with an herbal practitioner. See a doctor for regular checkups.

❑ Ginkgo has not been shown to be effective in lowering blood pressure. In one study, taking 240 milligrams a day of ginkgo over six years did not lower blood pressure in people with high blood pressure compared to a control group who did not use ginkgo.

❑ In one study, use of a daily multivitamin and mineral supplement helped lower blood pressure in obese women who had an increased risk of a heart attack.

❑ Do not take antihistamines except under a physician's direction.

❑ Heavy snorers are more likely to have high blood pressure or angina than silent sleepers. Research suggests that some snorers may suffer from a malfunctioning of the part of the brain responsible for fluent breathing; this can put an unnatural strain on the heart and lungs due to oxygen shortage.

❑ Because the use of diuretic drugs causes increased urinary excretion of magnesium, it can cause hypomagnesemia in elderly people. Magnesium is needed in conjunction with calcium to prevent bone deterioration, as well as to maintain a normal heart rhythm and muscular contraction. Losses of potassium due to diuretics may be dangerous, causing heart malfunction. Herbal diuretics, such as celery seed, corn silk, horsetail, and juniper may be helpful, but most dietary potassium comes from eating many servings of fruits and vegetables. Consult your physician before using diuretics.

❑ Apple pectin may aid in reducing blood pressure.

❑ *See also* ATHEROSCLEROSIS; HEART ATTACK (MYOCARDIAL INFARCTION); HIGH CHOLESTEROL; and OVERWEIGHT.

HIGH CHOLESTEROL

Cholesterol is a fatty, waxy substance that occurs naturally in the body. Although cholesterol is often misunderstood as a toxic substance, the body needs it for everything from cell membrane creation to hormone production to nerve function. In fact, cholesterol is so important to health

High Cholesterol: Beneficial Herbs

Herb	Form and Dosage	Comments
Artichoke leaf	Cynarin tablets. Take 1,500 mg daily for at least 6 weeks.	Reduces cholesterol, triglycerides, and weight; increases HDL.
Asafoetida	Powder. Take 1 tsp (3 gm) daily.	Reduces total cholesterol levels elevated by excess dietary fat.
Cordyceps[1]	Tablets. Take 1,000 mg daily.	Lowers LDL and total cholesterol; raises HDL.
Garlic[3]	Enteric-coated tablets. Take 900 mg daily in at least 2 divided doses for 3–4 months.	Can lower total cholesterol by 9–12 percent.
Ginger	Pickled. Eat 2 tsp (5 gm) with food daily.	Reduces total cholesterol levels, especially levels elevated by butterfat.
Ginseng	*Panax ginseng* tincture. Take as directed on the label.	Lowers total cholesterol, LDL, and triglycerides.
Green tea	Tea bag, prepared with 1 cup water. Take 2–5 cups daily. To prevent dilution, do not use within 1 hour of taking other medications.	Lowers LDL while raising HDL.
Guggul[3]	Guggulsterone tablets. Take 25 mg 3 times daily for 3–4 months.	Lowers total cholesterol 9–18 percent; raises HDL.
Hawthorn	Tablets. Take 100–250 mg 3 times daily.	Helps the liver convert LDL into HDL.
Ho she wu[4]	Tablets. Take 1,500–2,500 mg daily.	Lowers total cholesterol levels. Also known as fo-ti.
Milk thistle[5]	Silymarin gelcaps. Take 300 mg daily.	Helps the liver convert LDL into HDL. Maintains general liver health.
Red yeast rice	Cholestin or Hong Qu. Use as directed on the label.	Contains a natural compound that acts in the same way as lovastatin (Mevacor), lowering LDL after 4–6 weeks' use.
Scutellaria[6]	Capsules. Take 1,000–2,000 mg daily.	Lowers total cholesterol.
Shiitake	Whole mushroom. Take ½–¼ oz (3–6 gm) in food daily.	Lowers LDL and raises HDL.
Snow fungus	Yin mi pian tablets. Take 6–12 daily for at least 4 weeks.	Lowers total cholesterol.
Soy lecithin[7]	Capsules. Take 1,500–3,000 mg daily.	Lowers LDL and raises HDL.
Spirulina	Take as directed on the label.	Lowers cholesterol.
Wild yam (dioscorea)[8]	Tincture. Take as directed on the label.	Raises HDL.

Precautions for the use of herbs:

[1]Do not use cordyceps if you have an estrogen-sensitive disorder, such as breast cancer, endometriosis, or fibrocystic breasts, or a testosterone-sensitive disorder, such as prostate cancer.

[2]Garlic counteracts the effects of *Bifidus* and *Lactobacillus* cultures taken as digestive aids. Consult a doctor before using garlic on a regular basis if you are on an anticoagulant drug such as warfarin (Coumadin). Discuss the use of garlic with your doctor before having any type of surgery.

[3]When using guggul, do not use crude guggulu, which can cause nausea, diarrhea, loss of appetite, and skin rashes.

[4]With ho she wu (fo-ti), do not use the unprocessed root, which can cause diarrhea and skin rashes. Very high doses can cause numbness in the arms and legs. Do not confuse this herb with Fo-Ti Tieng, a Chinese herbal medicine made from gotu kola.

[5]Milk thistle may cause mild diarrhea. If this occurs, decrease the dose or stop taking it.

[6]Do not use scutellaria if you have diarrhea, or if you have gallstones or bile duct disease.

[7]Soy lecithin may cause mild diarrhea when you first use it.

[8]Overdosage of wild yam (dioscorea) can cause nausea. Be sure not to use an "herbal" product that contains synthetic progesterone while using this herb.

High Cholesterol: Formulas

Formula	Comments
Bupleurum Plus Dragon Bone and Oyster Shell Decoction[1]	A traditional Chinese herbal formula that increases the ratio of HDL to LDL and reduces nervous tension that may contribute to high blood pressure.
Minor Bupleurum Decoction[2]	A traditional Chinese herbal formula that reduces atherosclerotic plaque formation by destroying toxic free radicals, which disables macrophages' ability to "dock" in artery linings. Increases the ratio of HDL to LDL.

Precautions for the use of formulas:

[1]Do not use Bupleurum Plus Dragon Bone and Oyster Shell Decoction if you have a fever.

[2]Do not use Minor Bupleurum Decoction if you have a fever or a skin infection. Taken long term, it can cause headache, dizziness, and bleeding gums. Side effects can be avoided if the formula is taken as a tea.

that up to 85 percent of the body's supply is made in the liver. Disturbances in the body's use of cholesterol can result in high cholesterol, or levels above those that doctors consider normal and safe. High cholesterol can lead to atherosclerosis, in which cholesterol gathers into artery-clogging plaques that can eventually plug arteries, impeding blood flow to the heart, brain, kidneys, genitals, and extremities. This process can lead to high blood pressure, mental impairment, and, often after many years, heart attack or stroke. High cholesterol levels can also lead to gallstones. Approximately one in every six adults—17 percent of the adult population in the United States—has high blood cholesterol. Anyone, including children, can develop high cholesterol. It greatly increases the risk for heart disease, the leading cause of death in the United States. Factors that can contribute to high cholesterol include heredity, diet, lack of exercise, smoking, and high blood-sugar levels.

Cholesterol, being fatty, cannot travel through the watery bloodstream by itself. Therefore, it is attached to a protein, forming a lipoprotein, for delivery to cells throughout the body. There are several different types of lipoproteins, but the two most important are low-density lipoprotein (LDL) and high-density lipoprotein (HDL). While LDL is thought of as "bad" cholesterol and HDL as "good" cholesterol, they are actually two stages in the body's use of the same substance, with LDL particles being much larger than HDL particles. The problem with cholesterol arises if LDL becomes "stuck" in the linings of arteries injured by high blood pressure or infection. This LDL attracts macrophages, immune cells that get their cholesterol supplies from LDL, which attach to the trapped LDL particles and become part of the growing plaque. The area of injury can grow larger and even harden with calcium deposits.

Doctors recognize that total cholesterol is not as important a measure of disease risk as the ratio of HDL to LDL. Doctors look for an LDL level under 130 milligrams per deciliter of blood (mg/dL), but lower levels are

more desirable (70 to 129 mg/dL) and an HDL level over 40 mg/dL, but 60 mg/dL and higher are most desirable. This represents an LDL/HDL ratio of 3.3 to 1 or lower, ideally less than 3.3 to 1.

Other factors increase the risk of disease if combined with high cholesterol levels. Triglycerides, a form of fat that often travels with lipoproteins, is a cause for concern if blood levels are higher than 200 mg/dL. In addition, disease risk is increased by untreated high blood pressure, and by factors that make the blood "sticky," including smoking and high blood sugar levels.

Herbal treatments can reduce total cholesterol, LDL cholesterol, and triglycerides, and a few, such as red yeast rice, may raise HDL. Most herbal treatments must be used for several months for their full benefit, although blood tests may show improved numbers in as little as three weeks.

Herbs to Avoid

❑ Gotu kola. For more information about this herb, see GOTU KOLA under The Herbs in Part One.

Recommendations

❑ Eat a diet that is low in both saturated fat and calories, and reinforce the effects of a healthy diet with exercise. Olive, canola, and peanut oils are good cooking choices. Trans fats have been removed from most foods, but look on the label just to be sure—they should be avoided.

❑ Use alfalfa sprouts in cooking, as they may help block the absorption of cholesterol from food.

❑ Consider taking a vitamin B_3 (niacin) supplement. Niacin is a proven, low-cost treatment for lowering LDL, raising HDL (sometimes), and reducing the production of blood clotting factors that cause heart attacks. The drawback to using niacin is that it causes flushing of the face twenty to thirty minutes after it is taken. Sustained-release forms do not cause this problem, but can cause nausea, stomach upset, and liver damage, and should be avoided.

A safer form of niacin, inositol hexaniacinate, does not cause liver damage, and is recommended. Start with a dosage of 500 milligrams three times per day with meals for two weeks, then increase to 1,000 milligrams three times per day. If taking niacin, inform your physician and ask to have your liver enzymes monitored. Also, do not use niacin with lovastatin (Mevacor) or with the natural supplement Cholestin. There have been several cases in which these combinations resulted in rhabdomyolysis, muscle destruction that progressed to kidney failure. To be safe, do not use niacin with the related drugs pravastatin (Pravachol) or simvastatin (Zocor) without informing your physician.

❏ Drink fresh juices, especially carrot, celery, and beet juices. Or eat the entire fruit or vegetable—not just the juice—to also get the fiber, which makes you feel fuller.

❏ Nuts are good, especially unsalted walnuts and almonds. Almonds are rich in the amino acid arginine. In one study, they were found to cut cholesterol levels by 16 points over a four-week period.

Considerations

❏ If cholesterol levels cannot be lowered through diet, doctors prescribe various types of cholesterol-controlling drugs. Some keep the liver from reabsorbing bile, which contains cholesterol, from the intestines. This forces the liver to remove cholesterol from the bloodstream in order to create more bile. Other drugs reduce cholesterol production within the liver itself. All these medications have possible side effects, ranging from digestive upsets to liver disturbances.

❏ People who have both high cholesterol and high triglycerides may benefit from supplementation with pantethine, the active form of vitamin B_5. In one clinical trial, a dosage of 900 milligrams per day lowered triglyceride levels by over 30 percent, total cholesterol levels by nearly 20 percent, and LDL levels by over 20 percent, all while raising HDL levels by nearly 25 percent. It is also especially useful for diabetics with high cholesterol and triglycerides, since it makes insulin more effective. For reasons that are not completely understood, the more common form of the vitamin, pantothenic acid, has little or no effect on blood fats, so be sure to use pantethine.

❏ Other supplements of value include artichoke, barley, and products containing beta-sitosterol, psyllium, garlic, oat bran, and sitostanol. Red yeast rice is popular and contains the same active compound as lovastatin, the bioactive ingredient in Mevacor. If you cannot tolerate this drug or other statins, red yeast rice, although natural, may cause side effects. The other problem is that the active amount of lovastatin varies widely among the products selling as red yeast rice. One in three of the twelve red yeast rice products looked at were found to contain toxins. Speak to your doctor before using red yeast rice.

❏ Some herbs that have been studied in clinical trials for lowering cholesterol include *Citrullus colocynthis* and a blend of *Salvia miltiorrhiza* and *Pueraria lobata* and other nutrients. Using 300 milligrams a day of *Citrullus colocynthis* reduced both total cholesterol and triglycerides in people who had high levels at the start of the study. In another study, the herbal blend called Danshen and Gegen in Chinese medicine was given to participants with high cholesterol for six months, and blood flow improved as a result of less cholesterol buildup in the blood vessels.

❏ Low cholesterol levels can also cause health problems. For instance, people with low cholesterol levels may be malnourished. If your level is too low, seek medical attention.

❏ Meat and full-fat dairy products are primary sources of dietary cholesterol. Whole grains, vegetables, and fruits are free of cholesterol. Consume low-fat dairy products, which are very healthy, and include fish or seafood such as salmon, mackerel, and herring at least three times a week.

❏ Sunlight—or rather, the lack of it—has been shown to have adverse effects on cholesterol levels and increases the risk of heart disease. However, it isn't really the sunlight, but the vitamin D that is needed. Take a supplement and eat foods rich in vitamin D, such as low-fat dairy products.

❏ Drink alcohol in moderation. This may increase your good cholesterol (HDL). This means no more than two drinks a day for men and one for women.

❏ *See also* ATHEROSCLEROSIS and HIGH BLOOD PRESSURE (HYPERTENSION).

HIV/AIDS

HIV is the human immunodeficiency virus, the virus that causes acquired immunodeficiency syndrome (AIDS). Millions of people worldwide now carry the virus. Many people who are HIV-positive look and feel healthy—only through blood testing can the presence of the virus be detected. Others have varying degrees of illness as a result, the most serious consequence of HIV infection being full-blown AIDS. This section treats HIV infection in the absence of AIDS and then discusses AIDS itself.

HIV Infection

HIV is the human immunodeficiency virus, the virus that causes AIDS. Millions of people worldwide now carry the virus, which is usually passed through sexual or blood-to-blood contact. Infected mothers can pass the virus to their children, either during birth or through breast-feeding. But today this is mostly prevented with drugs. It is not passed through coughing or sneezing, nor through everyday contact, such as shaking hands.

Most people who are infected with HIV are not aware at first that they have it. While the virus can sometimes cause a flulike illness two to four weeks after infection, it usually takes two to five years for symptoms—including oral thrush and other mouth lesions, intestinal parasites, prolonged and unexplained fatigue, swollen glands, unexplained fever lasting more than ten days, excessive night sweating, sore throat, and changes in bowel habits—to appear. Antigen tests can detect HIV infection before symptoms appear, but even frequent HIV testing usually cannot detect the virus in the first several months of infection. Once the virus does appear, doctors check an individual's viral load, or the amount of virus present in the bloodstream. In many cases, though, HIV is discovered only if the infected person develops one or more of the opportunistic infections or cancers associated with AIDS.

HIV affects immune-system cells called T cells. There are two types. T-helper cells, also known as CD4 cells, help the immune system respond against bacteria, viruses, and cancerous cells. T-suppressor cells stifle the immune system's response against these invaders, a process meant to keep the system from becoming overactive. The decrease in T-helper cells and the increase in T-suppressor cells results in an increased susceptibility to infections and cancer.

The key to understanding HIV infection is understanding that T-helper cells are destroyed not only by HIV, but also by the immune system itself. HIV changes the surface of T-helper cells so that they are recognized as foreign matter and eliminated by T-suppressor cells. As long as the immune system's response to the infected T-helper cells is not too strong, there is relatively little damage to the immune system as a whole. In this steady state, the symptoms of AIDS do not appear. Stimulating the immune system without regard to which components of the system will be activated, however, makes HIV worse, not better.

The precise relationship between HIV and the immune system was discovered when doctors gave tetanus booster, which acts as an immune-system stimulant, to volunteers

HIV Infection: Beneficial Herbs

Herb	Form and Dosage	Comments
Aloe[1]	Juice. Take ¼ cup (50–75 ml)1–2 times daily.	Soothes lining of digestive tract; increases nutrient absorption.
Astragalus[2]	Capsules. Take 500–1,000 mg 3 times daily.	Stimulates T-helper cells. Prevents strep infections.
Bromelain	Tablets. Take 250–500 mg twice daily, between meals.	A natural, nontoxic protease inhibitor.
Cat's claw[3]	Capsules. Take 1,000 mg twice daily.	Raises T cell counts that are below 400, but not those above 900.
Catuaba	Tincture. Take ½ tsp (2 ml) in ¼ cup water twice daily, or as directed on the label.	In laboratory experiments, causes HIV to become inactive. Prevents staph infections.
Garlic[4]	Enteric-coated tablets, 900 mg daily.	In laboratory studies prevents cell-to-cell transmission of HIV in the bloodstream.
Licorice[5]	Glycyrrhizin tablets. Take 50–75 mg daily. Use for 6 weeks, then take a 2-week break. Do not substitute deglycyrrhizinated licorice (DGL).	Increases T cell counts and preserves immune function. Consume potassium-rich foods such as bananas or citrus juices, or take a potassium supplement, daily when taking this herb.
Magnolia vine berries	Take as directed on the label.	Increase oxygen absorption and boost the immune system.
Maitake	Maitake-D. Take as directed on the label.	Toxic to HIV. Keeps the virus from entering cells.
Prunella[6]	Tea (loose), prepared by steeping 1 tsp–1 tbsp (3–9 gm) in 1 cup water. (See TEAS in Part Three.) Take 1 cup 3 times daily, between meals.	Keeps HIV from binding to and entering T cells.
Rooibos	Tea bag, prepared with 1 cup water. Take 1 cup 2–3 times daily.	Prevents HIV from binding to target T cells.
Shiitake	Shiitake mycelia or Lentinus edodes mycelia powder or capsules. Take as directed on the label.	Lowers viral load by preventing cell-to-cell transmission of virus.
Turmeric	Curcumin tablets. Take 250–500 mg twice daily between meals.	Most useful herbal HIV treatment (see Considerations).

Precautions for the use of herbs:

[1]Do not take aloe vera juice internally if you have diarrhea.

[2]Do not use astragalus if you have a fever or a skin infection.

[3]Do not use cat's claw if you have to take insulin for diabetes. Do not use it if you are pregnant or nursing. Do not give it to a child under age six.

[4]Garlic counteracts the effects of Bifidus and Lactobacillus cultures taken as digestive aids. Consult a doctor before using garlic on a regular basis if you are on an anticoagulant drug such as warfarin (Coumadin). Discuss the use of garlic with your doctor before having any type of surgery.

[5]Do not use licorice if you have glaucoma, high blood pressure, or an estrogen-dependent disorder such as breast cancer, endometriosis, or fibrocystic breasts.

[6]Do not use prunella if you are experiencing diarrhea, nausea, or vomiting.

with HIV. The doctors' expectation was that boosting the immune system would lower the amount of HIV in the volunteers' bloodstream. Instead, the amount of the virus present in the volunteers' blood increased 200 to 400 percent. Even worse, their remaining virus-free blood cells became more susceptible to HIV infection. On the other hand, medical attempts to depress the immune system in order to treat HIV have also failed.

One herbal approach to healing is to deal not with the immune system but with the virus itself (*see* Considerations). Before using any herbal therapy, be sure to discuss it with a physician, who can determine if a specific herb's effect is appropriate for any specific stage of the disease. Do not use herbs or any alternative supplement at the expense of your drug regimen. One study found that HIV-positive women were nearly twice as likely not to take their prescribed antiretroviral drugs if they were also using herbs and vitamins. Noncompliance with this medication regimen leads to increased resistance to drugs in the future.

Herbs to Avoid

❑ Individuals who have HIV infection should avoid St. John's wort because of the increased risk of sunburn. They also should use immune-stimulant herbs, other than cat's claw, with caution, and inform their physicians if using immune-stimulant herbs while on any kind of "cocktail" treatment. (For more information regarding individual herbs, *see* the relevant entries *under* The Herbs in Part One.)

Recommendations

❑ Take vitamin E. This vitamin may be able to slow the progression of HIV infection to AIDS. According to a report in the journal *AIDS*, those men with the highest blood levels of vitamin E experienced a 34 percent reduction in the risk of disease progression when compared with men who had the lowest blood levels of this vitamin. Studies in both humans and animals have shown that vitamin E supplements in doses of up to 800 international units (IU) per day can increase the immune response to foreign particles.

❑ Supplement the diet with a multivitamin and mixed natural carotenoids. Low blood carotene levels, which are common in HIV infection, predict early death. Taking these supplements may improve survival by correcting the deficiency of carotenoids in the blood.

❑ To boost the body's ability to fight harmful free radicals, take glutamine and vitamin C. Among people with very low T cell counts (under 200 cells per cubic millimeter of blood), glutamine supplements (200 milligrams daily) greatly increase survival time. This inexpensive and nontoxic treatment works by supplying an amino acid needed for the production of glutathione (GSH), the body's principal free-radical fighter. Vitamin C is a glutathione cofactor, or a substance that can make glutathione more effective. Take at least 200 milligrams daily, or eat fresh fruits and vegetables every day.

❑ Avoid factors that deplete the body's store of GSH. Ultraviolet radiation (usually from sunlight), or the consumption of alcoholic beverages or acetaminophen-containing drugs may lower GSH levels.

❑ Take 150 milligrams of lipoic acid three times a day. This free-radical fighter slows the destructive action of T-suppressor cells, and is toxic to HIV.

❑ Drink eight glasses of water daily. An adequate water supply can prevent kidney problems. This is especially important if you are taking indinavir sulfate (Crixivan).

❑ Get sufficient exercise. While immune suppression through the use of powerful drugs is harmful to people with HIV, immune suppression through strenuous exercise seems to help. People with HIV who exercise tend to have fewer complications and progress much more slowly to AIDS. Ask at a local health club about designing an appropriate exercise regimen.

❑ During the cold and flu season, use the herb scutellaria to prevent viral infections. Take one or two 1,000 milligram capsules three times a day.

❑ Avoid allergic situations. Allergies increase the speed at which HIV infection becomes AIDS. High levels of immunoglobulin E (IgE), the antigen the body makes in response to allergens, make progression to AIDS roughly four times more likely in any twelve-month period. In addition to

HIV Infection: Formulas

Formula	Comments
Minor Bupleurum Decoction[1]	A traditional Chinese herbal formula that can prevent the progression of HIV to AIDS. Does not interfere with T cell reproduction. Especially useful for people with AIDS who also have hepatitis.
Shih Qua Da Bu Tang	This traditional Chinese herbal formula is useful as a general tonic for people with HIV. Stimulates production of interleukins and natural killer (NK) cells. Also called All-Inclusive Great Tonifying Decoction.

Precautions for the use of formulas:

[1]Do not use Minor Bupleurum Decoction if you have a fever or a skin infection. Taken long term, it can cause headache, dizziness, and bleeding gums. Side effects can be avoided if the formula is taken as a tea.

working with the doctor to reduce the risk of allergic reactions to the drugs in your treatment schedule, avoid exposure to airborne and food allergens. (*See* ALLERGIES.)

❑ Avoid recreational drug use. Some drugs, notably cocaine and marijuana, may not affect HIV infection itself but can disable T cell response to other kinds of infections.

❑ Obtain as much fresh air and rest as possible, and moderate amounts of sunshine.

Considerations

❑ Of all the herbal products available for HIV infection, curcumin may be the most versatile for stopping the virus at every stage of infection. In laboratory studies, it deactivates the gene in HIV that takes the virus out of its dormant state. It contains chemicals that stop the action of integrase, an enzyme the virus needs to take over the DNA of an infected cell. And it prevents the production of tumor necrosis factor (TNF), a hormone that signals HIV if there are weakened or injured cells ready to be infected.

❑ In human trials, a combination of five Chinese herbs, namely *Glycyrrhiza glaba L.*, *Artemisia capillaris Thumb*, *Morus alba L.*, *Astragalus membranaceus (Fisch)*, and *Carthamus tinctorius*, taken three times a day (5 grams), was studied in people with HIV infection. The patients experienced reduced viral loads of between 14 and 35 percent. However, there was a surprising decrease in CD4 count, so this herbal combination is not being used routinely yet.

❑ Conventional drug treatments for HIV infection are aimed at keeping the HIV virus from reproducing and infecting cells. Many of these drugs act by inhibiting enzymes, such as protease and reverse transcriptase, that the virus needs to make copies of itself. Sometimes these drugs are combined into multidrug treatments called "AIDS cocktails."

❑ The ayurvedic herb guduchi may help prevent diabetes that may result from treatment with AIDS cocktails. Take ½ teaspoon of the powdered herb daily or use amrati rasayanas as directed on the label.

❑ Women who are infected with HIV are more likely to develop cell abnormalities that lead to cervical cancer. Women who have HIV infections should receive Pap smears on a regular basis. (*See* CERVICAL CANCER.)

❑ Yogurt with the probiotics *Lactobacillus rhamnosus* and *L. reuteri* helps resolve diarrhea and increase CD4 cell counts in patients with HIV/AIDS. In one study, all subjects who consumed yogurt with these probiotics had less diarrhea, flatulence, and nausea, and eleven out of twelve had CD4 counts that stayed the same or rose over one month.

❑ The only truly safe sex is sex between life partners who are HIV-free. Other than that, abstinence is the only way to avoid any chance of infection with a sexually transmitted disease (STD). While it doesn't offer 100 percent protection from HIV, a condom is the best option if you don't abstain. Changing partners particularly puts one at risk, and any exchange of body fluids is theoretically risky. Chronic, recurring vaginal yeast infections should be checked by a doctor. In rare cases, this can be a sign of HIV infection.

❑ *See also* HEPATITIS.

AIDS

AIDS (acquired immune deficiency syndrome) is a disease in which the immune system breaks down and fails to protect the body against infection. It develops as the result of infection with the human immunodeficiency virus (HIV). HIV usually is passed through sexual or blood-to-blood contact.

Doctors diagnose AIDS when a person's total count of T cells, the longest-living immune cells that orchestrate the immune response, drops to 200 or less (compared with from 1,000 to 1,500 in a healthy person). But doctors also take note of any decrease in the ratio of T-helper cells to T-suppressor cells. T-helper cells are those cells that mediate the immune system's chemical defenses against bacteria, viruses, and cancerous cells. T-suppressor cells, on the other hand, serve as a check on the T-helper cells' response to infection to prevent the destruction of healthy tissues. Doctors assay viral load, or the number of viruses present in the bloodstream.

The body's response to the initial HIV infection, and to the resulting loss of immune function, varies from person to person. In some people, the progression from HIV to AIDS follows a recognized pattern. Some infected people experience rashes or mild flulike symptoms three to six weeks after infection. These symptoms go away and there are no new signs of disease until there is a secondary infection with a different microorganism. At that point, HIV becomes symptomatic. This stage, once called AIDS-related complex (ARC), is now referred to as early symptomatic AIDS. However, in other people, the even more devastating symptoms seen in full-blown AIDS are the first symptoms of infection.

The decrease in T-helper cells and the increase in T-suppressor cells results in an increased susceptibility to infections and cancer. In up to 50 percent of all people with AIDS, the first symptom is *Pneumocystis carinii* pneumonia. This is a bacterial infection that takes hold in the body only in the absence of a normal immune defense. Many people develop Kaposi's sarcoma, a connective tissue cancer that causes purplish lesions and that is almost unknown except in people with AIDS. Other infections commonly experienced by people with AIDS include those caused by cytomegalovirus, Epstein-Barr virus (EBV), herpes, Salmonella, *Staphylococcus* (staph), *Streptococcus* (strep), tuberculosis, and yeasts. In addition to multiple infections, people with AIDS are subject to malnutrition. In time there

AIDS: Beneficial Herbs

Herb	Form and Dosage	Comments
Aloe[1]	Juice. Take ¼ cup (50–75 ml) 1–2 times daily.	Soothes lining of digestive tract; increases nutrient absorption.
Andrographis	Tablets. Take as directed on the label.	Decreases viral load; increases T-helper cell counts.
Astragalus[2]	Capsules. Take 500–1,000 mg 3 times daily.	Stimulates T-helper cells. Prevents strep infections.
Bromelain[3]	Tablets. Take 250–500 mg twice daily, between meals.	Natural, nontoxic protease inhibitor.
Cat's claw[4]	Capsules. Take 1,000 mg twice daily, or tincture, as directed on the label, taken in ½ cup water with 1 tsp lemon juice.	Raises T cell counts that are below 400, but not those above 900.
Catuaba	Tincture. Take ½ tsp (2 ml) in ¼ cup water twice daily, or as directed on the label.	Under laboratory conditions, causes HIV to become inactive. Prevents staph infections.
Epimedium[5]	Form and dosage recommended by traditional Chinese medicine practitioner.	Stimulates testosterone production and prevents muscle wasting.
Licorice[6]	Glycyrrhizin tablets, 50–75 mg daily. Use for 6 weeks, then take a 2-week break. Do not substitute deglycyrrhizinated licorice (DGL).	Increases T cell counts and preserves immune function. Consume potassium-rich foods such as bananas or citrus juices, or take a potassium supplement daily when taking this herb.
Maitake	Maitake-D, as directed on the label.	Toxic to HIV; keeps virus from entering cells.
Prunella[7]	Tea (loose), 1 tsp–1 tbsp (3–9 gm) in 1 cup water 3 times daily, between meals. (See TEAS in Part Three.)	Keeps HIV from binding to and entering T cells.
Rooibos	Tea bag, prepared with 1 cup water. Take 1 cup 2–3 times daily.	Prevents HIV from binding to T-helper cells.
Saw palmetto	Tablets. Take 320 mg twice daily, between meals.	Regulates testosterone; prevents muscle wasting.
Shiitake	Shiitake mycelia or *Lentinus edodes* mycelia powder or capsules. Take as directed on the label.	Lowers viral load by preventing cell-to-cell transmission of the virus.
St. John's wort[8]	Follow directions on the label.	Contains hypericin and pseudohypericin, which inhibits retroviral infections.
Turmeric	Curcumin tablets. Take 250–500 mg twice daily between meals.	Most useful herbal HIV treatment (*see* Considerations, page 351.)

Precautions for the use of herbs:

[1]Do not take aloe vera juice internally if you have diarrhea.

[2]Do not use astragalus if you have a fever or a skin infection.

[3]People who are allergic to pineapple may develop a rash from bromelain. If itching develops, discontinue use.

[4]Do not use cat's claw if you have insulin-dependent diabetes. Do not use it if you are pregnant or nursing. Do not give it to a child under age six.

[5]Avoid epimedium if you have any kind of prostate disorder.

[6]Do not use licorice if you have glaucoma, high blood pressure, or an estrogen-dependent disorder such as breast cancer, endometriosis, or fibrocystic breast disease.

[7]Do not use prunella if you have diarrhea, nausea, or vomiting.

[8]Do not use St. John's wort if you are on prescription antidepressants or any medication that interacts with monoamine oxidase (MAO) inhibitors. Use it with caution during pregnancy. This herb may increase the chance of developing sun blisters if you are out in the sun for too long.

usually is muscle wasting, persistent loss of body-weight mass, and chronic diarrhea, weakness, and fever.

There are a number of conventional drug treatments for AIDS that greatly extend the symptom-free period and life expectancy. It is now much like living with other chronic conditions like diabetes; each day you need to take medicines to remain healthy. Especially in the case of the AIDS cocktails, it is critical not to use herbs as alternatives to conventional treatment. The AIDS treatment regimen must be followed exactly even with herbal treatment; herbs may make its side effects more bearable and make relapses less frequent. Before using any herbal treatments for AIDS, be sure to discuss them with your physician, who can determine whether a specific supplement is appropriate within your overall treatment plan.

Herbs to Avoid

❑ Use immune-stimulant herbs, other than cat's claw, with caution, and inform your physician if using immune-stimulant herbs if you are on any kind of "cocktail" treatment. (For more information regarding individual herbs, *see* The Herbs in Part One.)

Recommendations

❑ To boost the body's ability to fight harmful free radicals, take glutamine, grapeseed extract, or Pycnogenol and vitamin C. Among people with very low T cell counts (under 200 cells per cubic meter of blood), glutamine supplements (200 milligrams daily) greatly increase survival time. This inexpensive and nontoxic treatment works by

AIDS: Formulas

Formula	Comments
Minor Bupleurum Decoction[1]	A traditional Chinese herbal formula that can prevent the progression of HIV infection to AIDS. Increases the ability of 3TC (lamivudine) or AZT (zidovudine) plus 3TC to stop HIV multiplication in T cells. Stops 90 percent of the activity of reverse transcriptase. Especially useful if there is also hepatitis infection (*See* HEPATITIS.)
Shih Qua Da Bu Tang	Useful as a general tonic for people with AIDS. Stimulates production of two immune factors, interleukins and NK cells, without affecting T cells directly.
True Man's Decoction to Nourish the Organs[2]	A traditional Chinese herbal formula used to treat unremitting diarrhea to the point of incontinence. Not available as a patent medicine, but widely available from traditional Chinese medicine practitioners as variations on zhen ren yang rang tang.
True Warrior Decoction[3]	A traditional Chinese herbal formula used to treat advanced stages of wasting and anorexia, with severe weakness and coldness in the hands and feet.

Precautions for the use of formulas:

[1]Do not use Minor Bupleurum Decoction if you have a fever or a skin infection. Taken long term, it can cause headache, dizziness, and bleeding gums. Side effects can be avoided if the formula is taken as a tea.

[2]Avoid alcohol, wheat, cold or raw foods, fish, and greasy foods while using True Man's Decoction to Nourish the Organs. Do not use this formula if you have gallbladder problems, obstruction of the bile duct, or a tendency to retain urine. Do not use it during pregnancy.

[3]Stop using True Warrior Decoction if fever occurs. This formula may cause a loss of sensation in the mouth and tongue.

supplying an amino acid needed for the production of glutathione (GSH), the body's principal free-radical fighter. Vitamin C is a GSH cofactor, or a substance that can make GSH more effective. Take at least 200 milligrams daily, or eat fresh fruits and vegetables every day.

❏ Avoid factors that deplete the body's store of GSH. Ultraviolet radiation (usually from sunlight), or the use of alcoholic beverages or acetaminophen, can lower GSH levels.

❏ Take 150 milligrams of lipoic acid three times a day. This free-radical fighter slows the destructive action of T-suppressor cells, and is toxic to HIV.

❏ Drink eight glasses of quality water daily. An adequate water supply can prevent kidney problems. This is especially important if you are taking indinavir (Crixivan).

❏ Make sure you meet all of your nutritional requirements. Increasing them will probably be necessary.

❏ During the cold and flu season, use the herb scutellaria to prevent viral infections. Take one or two 1,000-milligram capsules three times a day.

❏ Learn how to counteract stress. (*See* RELAXATION TECHNIQUES in Part Three.)

Considerations

❏ Of all the herbal products available for AIDS, curcumin may be the most versatile for stopping the virus at every stage of infection. It deactivates the gene in HIV that takes the virus out of its dormant state. It contains chemicals that stop the action of integrase, an enzyme the virus needs to take over the DNA of an infected cell, and it prevents the production of tumor necrosis factor (TNF), a

hormone that signals HIV if there are weakened or injured cells ready to be infected.

❏ The ayurvedic herb guduchi can help prevent diabetes that may result from treatment with AIDS cocktails. Take ½ teaspoon of the powdered herb daily, or use amrati rasayanas as directed on the label.

❏ For AIDS patients, a mixture of beta-hydroxy-beta-methylbutyrate (HMB), a metabolite of leucine, with L-glutamine and L-arginine was shown to markedly reduce muscle loss in patients who were wasting muscle. The patients, who took 3 grams of HMB and 14 grams each of glutamine and arginine for eight weeks, had increased CD4 counts as well as increased muscle mass. There were no changes in a placebo group in terms of muscle mass and CD4 count.

❏ People with AIDS who acquired the virus through sharing needles may be subject to vitamin A deficiencies. The best source of vitamin A for people with AIDS is a diet that includes daily servings of dark green, yellow, or orange vegetables and fruits.

❏ Do not smoke and stay away from people who do. Also avoid alcohol and anything else that can damage the liver.

HIVES

Hives, also known as urticaria, are raised, swollen, and itchy welts on the skin. They may expand and come together to form giant hives. Angioedema, a serious condition, is an eruption similar to hives but involves deeper structures of the skin. About 30 percent of adults with chronic urticaria also have angioedema.

Chronic hives are almost always associated with an identifiable allergy. Allergies result in the production of histamine, an inflammatory chemical that causes swelling. In adults, hives most often are caused by drug allergies. In children, hives most often are caused by food allergies, such as from shellfish, fish, peanuts, tree nuts, eggs, and milk.

Approximately 10 percent of the adult population is allergic to penicillin, an allergy that can cause angioedema or an even more serious allergic reaction known as anaphylaxis, which causes breathing difficulties and overall itching. Taking penicillin is not the only risk factor; allergy-provoking amounts of this drug have been found in frozen dinners, milk, and soft drinks.

Allergic sensitivity to aspirin is higher in people who have chronic hives than in people who do not. In addition to causing allergic reactions by itself, aspirin and other non-steroidal anti-inflammatory drugs (NSAIDs) increase the permeability of the lining of the intestine to other allergens from drugs and foods. Aspirinlike compounds (salicylates) also occur naturally in some herbs, such as willow bark.

Food additives are a major cause of chronic hives in children. In 1959, tartrazine (FD & C Yellow No. 5) was the first food additive reported to induce hives. (People who are allergic to tartrazine are usually also allergic to aspirin.) Prepared foods for children usually have higher tartrazine yellow content than prepared foods for adults.

Many people who have hives are allergic to benzoic acid and benzoates, preservatives added to fish and shrimp. Butylated hydroxyanisole (BHA) and butylated hydroxy-toluene (BHT) are antioxidants used in packaged foods, especially bread. They have been linked to chronic hives and other skin reactions on rare occasions. Sulfites are sprayed on fresh foods such as fruits and vegetables to keep them from discoloring, and are added to wine, beer, and some processed foods as preservatives. Sulfites induce hives, angioedema, and asthma in sensitive individuals.

Not all hives are caused by allergies. A form of hives known as dermographic urticaria occurs when moderate amounts of pressure are applied to the skin. These welts may appear as the result of contact with another person, bedding, furniture, jewelry, towels, or watchbands. They generally appear and subside quickly, but can last as long as forty-eight hours. Cold urticaria is a reaction caused by skin contact with cold air, water, or other objects. The lower the temperature, the faster the reaction, but the reaction is usually limited to the exposed area and symptoms subside in a few hours. Cholinergic urticaria, commonly known as prickly heat, results from overheating (such as a warm bath or sauna), consumption of spicy foods or alcohol, physical exercise, and/or emotional stress. It usually subsides in less than an hour. Contact with certain chemicals, such as latex, and animal dander can trigger hives.

Hives: Beneficial Herbs

Herb	Form and Dosage	Comments
Alfalfa	Tablets. Take as directed on the label.	Preventive blood tonic, cleans the blood and helps keep it free of toxins.
Aloe	Gel. Apply to inflamed area and cover with loose bandage or clean cloth.	Stops inflammation. Prevents infection. Especially effective for children with hives.
Black nightshade	Leaves. Wash and boil leaves in water, put on a cloth, and apply to the affected area.	Helps soothe the hives.
Chamomile	Dried whole German chamomile (*Matricaria recutita*), made into a bath, by soaking 2 oz (50 gm) in 2½ gal (10 L) warm water.	Relieves inflammation.
Stinging nettle leaf	Juice. Take 1 tbsp (12 ml) 3 times daily.	Accelerates healing of rash. Especially useful for reactions to shellfish.

Hives: Formulas

Formula	Comments
Four-Substance Decoction	A traditional Chinese herbal formula used to treat skin allergies and hives in women who also experience irregular menstruation. Especially appropriate if abdominal pain or general muscle tension is also present.
Ledebouriella Decoction That Sagely Unblocks[1]	A traditional Chinese herbal formula used for recurrent or persistent outbreaks of hives. Most used by people who have a tendency to constipation, high blood pressure, and/or overweight.

Precautions for the use of formulas:

[1]You should not use Ledebouriella Decoction That Sagely Unblocks if you are trying to become pregnant, or if you are experiencing nausea or vomiting.

Since hives can be a medical emergency, do not attempt to treat severe itching or swelling rashes over the entire body with herbal medications. Herbs should be used for mild cases that do not need strong medication (such as prickly heat) or for hard-to-treat cases that do not respond to antihistamine or steroid treatment, and for prevention.

Recommendations

❑ Try to identify the exact cause of your hives. If you do not choose to have testing for food allergies, it may help to keep a diary of all possible causes for a few days, including a diary of foods eaten. (*See* Food Allergies *under* ALLERGIES.) In one study, participants were given a modified food allergy diet that was low in food additives and histamine, and included some natural foods like fruits, vegetables, and spices. The diet only reduced chronic spontaneous urticaria in one-third of those who tried it over a three-week period.

❑ Avoid beans, eggs, fish, meat, milk, and nuts, which contain compounds that interact with the lining of the intestine and increase the absorption of allergens, if your doctor has confirmed that you have an allergy to one of these foods.

❑ Avoid prepared foods, which often contain additives.

❑ Avoid aspirin and other NSAIDs, especially if you are allergic to aspirin itself or to the food coloring tartrazine.

❑ If you are allergic to aspirin, avoid berries, dried fruit (especially prunes and raisins), and licorice and peppermint candies.

❑ If you are allergic to sulfites, buy organic produce, which usually is not sprayed with preservatives, and avoid wine and beer. In addition, take 200 micrograms of molybdenum per day. Molybdenum is a key component of the enzyme sulfite oxidase, which allows the body to convert sulfites into sulfates that can then be excreted through the urine.

❑ To reduce the risk of skin allergies, use stainless steel or 24 karat jewelry, especially in a freshly pierced opening. Nickel, used in 14 karat gold, can cause skin rash and hives. Also avoid nickel bra buckles, belt buckles, and watchbands. In one study, twenty-nine out of thirty participants with nickel sensitivity who followed a low-nickel diet combined with 0.1 milligram of nickel per day (a very low dose) had a reduction in hives, redness, and urticaria.

❑ Wear loose-fitting clothing.

❑ Take a cool shower if you see the first signs of hives appearing. Make sure that it is cool, not hot. This may slow the spreading of hives.

❑ If you have had hives for longer than six weeks, or if you are developing an acute case of hives, consult your health-care provider.

Considerations

❑ Catnip has been used in traditional medicine to prevent hives in children. Use ¼ teaspoon of the chopped herb in ¼ cup of water three times a day. (*See* TEAS in Part Three.)

❑ Quercetin may help with recurrent outbreaks of hives. Take 125 to 250 milligrams three times daily between meals for six to eight weeks. Do not take quercetin with cyclosporine (Neoral, Sandimmune) or nifedipine (Procardia).

❑ Ultraviolet (UV) light, from sunlight or tanning beds, helps some people with chronic hives. Dermographic and cold hives, and prickly heat, respond best to UV light.

❑ Anyone who experiences recurrent hives should wear a medical alert bracelet or carry a medical alert card to inform emergency care personnel of that fact. These devices can be obtained from Medic Alert. (*See* Appendix B: Resources.)

❑ Protein hydrolysates—compounds found in hair conditioners and shampoos—may be a source of allergic reactions. These compounds, including collagen, elastin, and keratin, are used in hair products that "restore body" to the hair. Allergic reactions to protein hydrolysates are likely to be especially severe in people who have eczema. (*See* ECZEMA.)

❑ Food additives cause harm in about 2 to 7 percent of children, based on a Danish study. Children were tested for various food additives that they were already thought to be allergic to. The offending agents were food colorings, food preservatives, and citric acid, all of which affected the skin.

HODGKIN'S LYMPHOMA

Hodgkin's lymphoma, formerly known as Hodgkin's disease, is a little-understood cancer of lymph tissue, the tissue that houses much of the body's immune function. This tissue is organized into lymph nodes found in various parts of the body. In North America, Hodgkin's lymphoma is more common in males.

Often the only symptoms of Hodgkin's lymphoma at first are night sweats with low-grade fever. In some people, there is a skin itch in the early stages. As the disease progresses, it causes increasing inflammation. The lymph nodes become swollen, and there may be coughing, chest pain, and bone pain. Because the initial symptoms resemble those of many other disorders, a positive diagnosis for Hodgkin's lymphoma can be made only by examining an enlarged lymph node.

Hodgkin's lymphoma could be caused by a virus, but no one knows for sure. Risk factors for getting the lymphoma include age (15 to 40 years and over 55) and family history. The body is more susceptible to Hodgkin's after infection with Epstein-Barr virus (EBV), mononucleosis, or HIV. It is also more common in those in higher socio-economic brackets and in people living in the United States, Canada, and northern Europe.

Although Hodgkin's lymphoma is a cancer of the immune system, it usually affects only one group of white blood cells. This cancer attacks B cells and causes them to develop abnormally. Normally the B cells work with T cells to fight infections. In Hodgkin's lymphoma, B cells become enlarged and instead of undergoing the normal cell cycle of life and death, these cells don't die, and they continue to produce abnormal B cells in a malignant process. These cells also attract other normal immune cells that cause the lymph nodes to enlarge. Hodgkin's lymphoma is classified into stages I through IV based on the number of lymph node regions involved. Medical treatment is set by stage.

Always use herbal medicine as part of a medically directed overall treatment plan for Hodgkin's lymphoma. Especially in treating childhood Hodgkin's lymphoma, always work with an herbal practitioner along with the physician; the dosages provided in this entry are meant for adults.

Recommendations

❏ Avoid vitamin C in the form of sodium ascorbate. This sodium salt of vitamin C can induce a flare-up of Hodgkin's symptoms. Natural vitamin C, such as acerola, does not have this effect.

❏ Avoid ham and liver. These meats have been associated with increased risk for developing Hodgkin's lymphoma, and may worsen symptoms.

Considerations

❏ Early stages of Hodgkin's lymphoma may be treated with radiation therapy. In later stages, when the lymph nodes and other organs are increasingly affected, chemotherapy is used. The preferred method of treatment is a chemotherapy regimen called ABVD, which includes the drugs doxorubicin (Adriamycin), bleomycin (Blenoxane), vinblastine (Velban), and dacarbazine (DTIC-Dome). Some people at high risk of disease are given BEACOPP, which is a regime of the drugs bleomycin, etoposide, doxorubicin, cyclophosphamide, vincristine, procarbazine, and prednisone. (For measures to reduce the side effects and increase the effectiveness of chemotherapy and radiation therapy, *see* "Side Effects of Cancer Treatment" *under* CANCER.)

❏ It is possible that nitrates and nitrites found in drinking water and cured meats such as hot dogs and ham increase the risk of non-Hodgkin's lymphoma. However, in a study conducted in Iowa on determining the risk of non-Hodgkin's lymphoma, there seemed to be no increased risk with drinking water with elevated nitrite levels or nitrite-containing foods such as red meat. But high intakes of cereals and breads that are rich in nitrites seemed to pose an increased risk.

❏ Eating fruits and vegetables may reduce the risk of developing Hodgkin's lymphoma even when there is a family history and a genetic predisposition. Green leafy vegetables, cruciferous vegetables such as broccoli and cauliflower, and zinc all seemed important to reduce risk.

❏ Beef spleen extracts may reduce the loss of immune defenses during chemotherapy and radiation treatment

Hodgkin's Lymphoma: Beneficial Herbs

Herb	Form and Dosage	Comments
Astragalus[1]	Capsules. Take 500–1,000 mg 3 times daily.	Stimulates T cells.
Siberian ginseng	Pure *Eleutherococcus senticosus* extract. Take as directed on the label in ¼ cup water.	Increases production and stimulates activity of T cells.

Precautions for the use of herbs:

[1]Do not use astragalus if you have a fever or a skin infection.

Hodgkin's Lymphoma: Formulas

Formula	Comments
Capital Chi Pill	A traditional Chinese herbal formula that relieves night sweats. Also effective for shortness of breath that may be accompanied by soreness and weakness in the lower back, lightheadedness, vertigo, tinnitus, or diminished hearing.
Six-Ingredient Pill with Rehmannia	A traditional Chinese herbal formula that relieves bone pain in the lower half of the body and spine.

for Hodgkin's lymphoma. The active protein is called thymopoeitein III, splenopentin, or Dac-SP5.

❏ Beef thymus extracts may reduce the risk of viral infection during treatment for Hodgkin's lymphoma.

HOT FLASHES

See under MENOPAUSE-RELATED PROBLEMS.

HUMAN IMMUNODEFICIENCY VIRUS

See HIV/AIDS.

HYPERACTIVITY

See ATTENTION DEFICIT DISORDER/ATTENTION DEFICIT HYPERACTIVITY DISORDER.

HYPERTENSION

See HIGH BLOOD PRESSURE (HYPERTENSION).

HYPERTHYROIDISM

About 1 percent of Americans suffer from hyperthyroidism, a condition in which the thyroid gland at the base of the neck becomes overactive. If this happens, the gland produces too much of the hormone thyroxine, which speeds up the body's functions. It occurs more often in women than men and runs in families. A blood test is used for diagnosis.

Graves' disease, also known as toxic diffuse goiter, is the most common cause of hyperthyroidism in the United States. This is an autoimmune disease in which the thyroid, mistakenly responding to immune-system signals, pumps more and more thyroxine into circulation.

In Graves' disease the appetite is disturbed, and there is weight loss, no matter how much food is consumed, because nutrients are poorly absorbed. Other symptoms include nervousness, irritability, insomnia, fatigue, and a constant feeling of being hot, with increased perspiration.

Graves' disease increases the frequency of bowel movements, decreases menstrual flow, and causes hair loss. It also induces rapid heartbeat, separation of the nails from the nail beds, hand tremors, changes in the thickness of the skin, and, sometimes, protruding eyeballs and disturbances of vision. The thyroid may swell as the disease progresses, forming a goiter.

Japanese researchers have linked Graves' disease to bouts of severe allergies, specifically to cedar pollen—although this is not the common thinking about how it is caused. Graves' disease has been linked in cell studies to a class of respiratory viruses known as the spumaretroviruses and a virus known as HTLV-1. Factors that may increase the risk for Graves' disease include being female and over twenty years of age, having been pregnant, and having been a smoker.

There are other forms of hyperthyroidism: Plummer's disease and a potentially dangerous form called toxic adenoma, which can cause mood swings, fever, extreme agitation, and weakness. Conventional treatment of hyperthyroidism consists of drugs and radiation therapy (*see* Considerations). If left untreated, all forms of this disease can lead to bone and heart disorders.

Herbs to Avoid

❏ Individuals who have Graves' disease should avoid the following herbs: aloe, American ginseng, astragalus, bamboo, burdock, chrysanthemum, echinacea, ginger, ginseng, lemon balm (melissa), Siberian ginseng, and wheat grass. (For more information regarding these herbs, *see* the individual entries *under* The Herbs in Part One.) There is no need to avoid these herbs if the hyperthyroidism is not caused by Graves' disease.

Recommendations

❏ Take 200 to 600 international units (IU) of vitamin E daily. Vitamin E may protect the linings of heart cells from free-radical damage. In studies of animals with hyperthyroidism, vitamin E normalizes heart rate and prevents arrhythmias. Ask your doctor before taking this high dose.

Hyperthyroidism: Beneficial Herbs

Herb	Form and Dosage	Comments
Bugleweed[1]	Tablets. Take as directed on the label.	Relieves nervousness, irritability, insomnia, fatigue, and increased perspiration.
Motherwort	Tea (loose), prepared by steeping 1 tsp (1.5 gm) in 1 cup water. (*See* TEAS in Part Three.) Take 1 cup 3 times daily.	Relieves heart palpitations.

Precautions for the use of herbs:

[1]Do not take bugleweed if you have been diagnosed with an underactive thyroid or Hashimoto's thyroiditis. Discontinuing this herb suddenly can result in a rebound reaction, in which symptoms become worse than they were before the herb was used. In very rare cases in which bugleweed has been used over a period of many years, goiter (thyroid enlargement) has been observed.

Hyperthyroidism: Formulas

Formula	Comments
Bupleurum Plus Dragon Bone and Oyster Shell Decoction[1]	A traditional Chinese herbal formula used if the primary symptoms are difficulties in concentration and speech, irritability, nervousness, and rapid pulse.
Eight-Ingredient Pill with Rehmannia	A traditional Chinese herbal formula that stops continuous sweating.
Gentiana Longdancao Decoction to Drain the Liver[2]	A traditional Chinese herbal formula used if the primary symptoms are irritability, headache, and short temper. Particularly useful for women who experience shortened periods.
Honey-Fried Licorice Decoction[3]	A traditional Chinese herbal formula that treats anxiety, irritability, and insomnia with weight loss.
Minor Bupleurum Decoction[4]	A traditional Chinese herbal formula that increases the effectiveness of the steroid drug prednisone. Relieves secondary symptoms, including chills alternating with hot flashes and nausea or acid stomach.
Ophiopogonis Decoction[5]	A traditional Chinese herbal formula that increases the effectiveness of the steroid drug methylprednisolone. Sometimes used to treat bulging eyes.

Precautions for the use of formulas:

[1]Do not use Bupleurum Plus Dragon Bone and Oyster Shell Decoction if you have a fever.

[2]Do not use Gentiana Longdancao Decoction to Drain the Liver if you are trying to become pregnant.

[3]Most manufacturers of Honey-Fried Licorice Decoction include the traditional marijuana seed. This does not produce a "high," but it will cause a positive urine test for marijuana, although sophisticated testing methods can distinguish medicinal from illicit use.

[4]Do not use Minor Bupleurum Decoction if you have a fever or a skin infection. Taken long term, it can cause headache, dizziness, and bleeding gums. Side effects can be avoided if the formula is taken as a tea.

[5]Do not use Ophiopogonis Decoction if you have a fever.

❏ Use scutellaria to prevent common viral infections without stimulating the immune system. Take one or two 1,000-milligram capsules three times daily. Do not use this herb if you have diarrhea.

❏ Eat plenty of the following foods: broccoli, Brussels sprouts, cabbage, cauliflower, kale, mustard greens, peaches, pears, rutabagas, soybeans, spinach, and turnips.

❏ Some people lose bone mass from hyperthyroidism. Make sure you get adequate calcium and vitamin D each day. You need 1,000 milligrams of calcium and at least 600 international units (IU) of vitamin D.

Considerations

❏ Conventional medicine treats hyperthyroidism with drugs that lower thyroxine output. Sometimes in cases of Graves' disease, radiation is used to destroy overactive thyroid tissue. This may result in underactive thyroid, and the lifelong need for thyroid supplements. (For measures to reduce the side effects and increase the effectiveness radiation therapy, see "Side Effects of Cancer Treatment" under CANCER.)

❏ Ironically, it is possible to have both Graves' disease and Hashimoto's thyroiditis, which causes underactivity of the thyroid, at the same time. (See HYPOTHYROIDISM.) Both conditions can occur with still other autoimmune diseases, including rheumatoid arthritis, lupus, chronic hepatitis, diabetes, pernicious anemia, and Sjögren's syndrome. People who have any of these diseases need periodic monitoring of thyroid function.

❏ Undiagnosed celiac disease often occurs with hyperthyroidism. (See CELIAC DISEASE.)

HYPOTHYROIDISM

Hypothyroidism is caused by reduced activity of the thyroid gland. This gland, which lies at the base of the neck, produces the hormone thyroxine, which regulates virtually all bodily functions. A lack of this hormone can cause these functions to slow down. Thyroxine deficiencies range from barely detectable (subclinical hypothyroidism) to severe (myexedema). About 5 percent of the U.S. population has hypothyroidism. Many cases of hypothyroidism are not detected, since the blood test used for diagnosis is not part of a standard physical examination.

Symptoms of hypothyroidism include depression, weight gain or difficulty losing weight, numbness and tingling in the feet and hands, constipation, fatigue, headache, menstrual problems, recurrent infections, swelling, sensitivity to cold, dry skin, dull or thinning hair, thinning of the eyebrows, and brittle nails. The tongue may thicken, and the quality of the voice may change. Women with hypothyroidism may be infertile.

Almost all cases of hypothyroidism occur as a sequel to an immune-system malfunction known as Hashimoto's thyroiditis. This is an autoimmune disease in which the thyroid, mistakenly responding to immune-system signals, becomes inactive. Fibrous tissue forms, and swelling and inflammation set in. This causes goiter, or an enlarged thyroid gland. The thyroid continues to function for a long time before the body suffers a thyroxine shortage. As a result, the disease can come on so gradually that the person is at first aware of only vague, low-grade symptoms.

Hypothyroidism can have other causes. Treatment of hyperthyroidism can destroy the thyroid gland. Problems in the pituitary gland can disrupt the supply of thyroid-stimulating hormone. In some parts of the world, iodine deficiency is a common cause of hypothyroidism.

Conventional treatment consists of replacing the missing thyroid hormone.

Herbs to Avoid

❑ Individuals who are in the early stages of hypothyroidism may be able to preserve remaining thyroid function by avoiding the following immune-stimulant herbs: aloe, American ginseng, astragalus, bamboo, burdock, chrysanthemum, echinacea, ginger, ginseng, kelp, lemon balm (melissa), motherwort, Siberian ginseng, and wheat grass. Individuals who have full-blown hypothyroidism should avoid fenugreek. (For more information regarding these herbs, *see* the individual entries *under* The Herbs in Part One.)

Recommendations

❑ Avoid consuming large amounts of soy foods, such as tofu or miso. These foods contain a chemical that interferes with the body's use of thyroid hormone.

❑ If taking the prescription drug thyroxine, you may ask your doctor about trying desiccated thyroid tablets, available over the counter in health food stores. These tablets provide all thyroid hormones except thyroxine, which is present only in trace amounts. Since these tablets do not contain thyroxine, they cannot be used in place of medically prescribed therapy.

❑ Limit processed and refined foods, including white flour and sugar.

❑ Do not take sulfa drugs or antihistamines unless specifically directed to do so by a physician.

Considerations

❑ Almost all cases of hypothyroidism require thyroid hormone replacement therapy. The replacement may be a mixture of several thyroid hormones, or just thyroxine, the main hormone. In most cases, therapy must be continued for life.

❑ You may experience symptoms of subclinical hypothyroidism, which produces no change in blood tests. Test for this condition by taking a body-temperature reading three mornings in a row. Before getting out of bed, hold a thermometer in either armpit for fifteen minutes, keeping as still as possible. Add the temperatures, and divide by three. If the average temperature is below 97.5°F, see the doctor. Women should avoid taking their temperatures while ovulating or during the first week of the menstrual period.

❑ Cessation of steroid treatment can produce temporary, reversible symptoms like those of hypothyroidism. Steroid drugs, such as cortisone, dexamethasone, hydrocortisone, and similar agents, are used for a wide variety of conditions. However, if you use a system where you

Hypothyroidism: Beneficial Herbs

Herb	Form and Dosage	Comments
Black cohosh	Tablets. Take as directed on the label.	Helps with symptoms.

Hypothyroidism: Formulas

Formula	Comments
Frigid Extremities Decoction[1]	A traditional Chinese herbal formula designed for a symptom pattern that includes extremely cold hands and feet, abdominal pain, aversion to cold, constant desire to sleep, diarrhea with undigested food particles, and a lack of thirst.
Kidney Chi Pill from the Golden Cabinet[1]	A traditional Chinese herbal formula that treats copious urination or urinary incontinence in hypothyroidism.
True Warrior Decoction[1]	This Chinese herbal formula is especially useful for treating abdominal pain and diarrhea.

Precautions for the use of formulas:

[1]With the formulas in this table, discontinue use if you develop a fever. These formulas may cause a loss of sensation in the mouth and tongue.

slowly taper off of these drugs, you should be able to prevent symptoms.

❏ Untreated hypothyroidism leads to higher low-density lipoprotein (LDL) levels and an increase in the rate at which cholesterol causes arterial plaques. (*See* ATHEROSCLEROSIS and HIGH CHOLESTEROL.)

❏ Lithium, a trace mineral used as a drug to treat bipolar mood disorder, can sometimes cause thyroid malfunction.

INDIGESTION

Indigestion, medically known as dyspepsia, is a term used to describe a variety of abdominal discomforts associated with eating. Some people experience indigestion as abdominal pain, pressure, or heartburn. Other people experience indigestion as belching, a feeling of excessive gas, or flatulence. Still others use the term to describe a vague feeling that digestion has not proceeded naturally or that they react badly to specific foods. Indigestion is one of the most common medical complaints in North America, with sales of over-the-counter (OTC) digestive aids running into the billions of dollars.

Indigestion can arise from a number of causes. Among the most common are obesity, poor diet, rushed meals, stress, and lack of exercise. A number of drugs, especially painkillers such as aspirin and ibuprofen, can irritate the lining of the stomach over time, and later lead to digestion problems. In addition, a number of illnesses can produce the same symptoms, including colitis, colorectal or stomach cancer, extremely high blood sugar levels, gallstones, gastritis, heart attack, hepatitis, intestinal obstruction, irritable bowel syndrome, and pancreatitis.

Chronic indigestion should always be brought to a doctor's attention. However, it is possible to distinguish simple indigestion from symptoms caused by other conditions. Indigestion occurs only after eating, and the pain it causes is dull rather than sharp. It spreads symmetrically to both the left and right of the abdomen and, if gas is not a problem, is felt above the navel. Pain below the navel is more likely to originate in the colon, while pain around the navel is usually associated with disorders of the small intestine. Pain caused by serious disease of the gallbladder, liver, or pancreas usually begins as an intense pain in a single spot that then spreads upward in the body.

Pain under the breastbone is especially significant. This pain may be caused by a malfunction of the esophagus, or by failures of circulation in and to the heart. Seek immediate medical attention if chest pain radiates to the jaw or arm; is viselike or squeezing in nature; or is accompanied by heartburn, dizziness, nausea, or cold sweats. In addition, consult a doctor if indigestion symptoms last longer than two weeks; if the pattern of symptoms changes noticeably; if abdominal pain persists longer than six hours; or if additional symptoms include unexplained weight loss, bleeding, or jaundice. Any loss of appetite, weight loss, vomiting, black or tarry stools, or jaundice (yellowing coloring around the eyes) requires immediate attention by a physician.

Some of the more common indigestion symptoms are covered in this section. For most types of indigestion, you should use the recommended herb after eating. In addition, a proper diet, especially if combined with a program of exercise and stress relief, can ease or prevent simple indigestion. Losing weight if you are overweight may also help. Do not overeat at any one meal; this worsens these conditions below.

Belching

A belch is a regurgitation of swallowed air. If excess air is swallowed, belching is the body's way of reestablishing normal pressure in the stomach. If the air cannot be expelled, it accumulates in the stomach and causes sharp pain. Predispositions to belching may include chronic anxiety, poorly fitting dentures, and postnasal drip, as well as drinking carbonated beverages or drinking through a

Belching: Beneficial Herbs

Herb	Form and Dosage	Comments
Chen-pi	Tea (loose), prepared by steeping 1 tsp (3 gm) in 1 cup water, (*See* TEAS in Part Three.)	Relieves belching, bloating, and gas. Also called bitter orange peel.
Fennel seed[1]	Tea bag, prepared with 1 cup water. Give an infant 1–3 tsp of tea.	For infants and babies. Relieves belching and gas in infants.
Ginger	Tea, prepared by adding ½ tsp (1 gm) powdered ginger to 1 cup water. (*See* TEAS in Part Three.) Take 1 cup as needed.	Relieves belching and stomach irritation.
Peppermint[2]	Oil. Take 10–15 drops in ¼ cup cold water.	The quickest herbal relief for belching for adults.

Precautions for the use of herbs:

[1]When using fennel seed, *never* give the essential oil to an infant. Always use tea.

[2]Do not use peppermint if you have any kind of gallbladder disorder or blockage of the bile ducts.

straw, eating rapidly, smoking cigarettes, or sucking on hard candy. Sometimes a person who belches a lot may have an upper GI (gastrointestinal) disorder such as peptic ulcer or GERD (gastroesophageal reflux disease).

Recommendations

❏ Avoid chewing gum, carbonated beverages, smoking, and consuming gas-producing foods and beverages.

❏ Lie on your side or on your back in a knees-to-chest position.

Considerations

❏ Chronic belching may be a sign of gallbladder disease, hiatal hernia, or peptic ulcer. Call a health-care provider if belching is persistent and unexplained or if it is accompanied by other symptoms.

Bloating and Flatulence

"Gas" causes a feeling of dull abdominal pain and bloating. The physiological process that produces feelings of bloating actually does not create more gas than is usually present in the lower digestive tract. Instead, it is a supersensitivity to gas that is only present in normal amounts.

Flatulence results from excess gas production. Breakdown of undigested foods causes gas. Such foods could include milk (the lactose in it), sorbitol, which is in many sugar-free gums and candies, starches such as potatoes and corn, and fiber from oats, peas, and most fruits. The gases involved include the odorless carbon dioxide and hydrogen, sometimes methane, and the odor-producing hydrogen sulfide.

Recommendations

❏ If you are prone to flatulence, avoid (in addition to beans) dates, figs, and prunes. Asparagus, onions, and whole wheat that is rich in fiber also may cause flatulence.

❏ For gas caused by swallowing air, eat slower, avoid gum chewing, and try to relax.

❏ Call a physician if flatulence is accompanied by pain or weight loss.

Considerations

❏ Intestinal gas may temporarily increase after starting a high-fiber diet.

❏ Many cooks use a four-step process for cooking beans and lentils to reduce their potential for causing flatulence:

1. Cover beans or lentils with water and boil three minutes.
2. Let beans or lentils soak in this water for four hours at room temperature.

Bloating and Flatulence: Beneficial Herbs

Herb	Form and Dosage	Comments
Angelica	*Angelica archangelica* oil. Take 10–15 drops in ¼ cup water.	Relieves feeling of fullness, flatulence, and mild spasms of the gastrointestinal (GI) tract.
Caraway	Oil. Take 10–15 drops in ¼ cup water.	Relieves feeling of fullness, flatulence, and mild spasms of the GI tract.
Chen-pi[1]	Tea (loose), prepared by steeping 1 tsp (3 gm) in 1 cup water. (See TEAS in Part Three.) Take 1 cup as needed.	Relieves belching, bloating, and gas. Also called bitter orange peel.
Cinnamon	Oil. Take 10–15 drops in ¼ cup water.	Relieves bloating, flatulence, and cramps.
Dandelion[2]	Tincture. Take ½ tsp in ¼ cup water.	Relieves feeling of fullness and gas.
Fennel seed[3]	Oil. For adults. Take 4–5 drops in ¼ cup water; or tea for infants. Give a baby 1–3 tsp.	Relieves feeling of fullness, gas, and belching.
Gentian[4]	Bitters capsules. Take as directed on the label.	Relieves bloating and gas after excessive consumption of fatty meats.
Hops[5]	Capsules. Take 500–1,000 mg 3 times daily.	Relieves stress-related digestive problems.
Horehound	Tea (loose), prepared by steeping 1 tbsp (4.5 gm) in 1 cup water. (See TEAS in Part Three.) Take 1 cup as needed.	Relieves feeling of fullness and gas.

Precautions for the use of herbs:

[1]Do not use chen-pi if there is blood in the stool.

[2]Do not use dandelion if you have gallstones.

[3]Do not take fennel seed if you have an estrogen-sensitive disorder, such as breast cancer, endometriosis, or fibrocystic breasts. Do not give essential oil to infants.

[4]Do not use gentian if you have diarrhea.

[5]Men should not take hops if erectile dysfunction (ED) is a problem. Women should not take it if they have an estrogen-sensitive disorder, such as breast cancer, endometriosis, or fibrocystic breasts.

3. Pour off soaking water.

4. Cook the beans or lentils in fresh water.

This method may leach out some of the complex carbohydrates that are fermented by bacteria in the large intestine and release gas.

❑ Another way to reduce flatulence caused by eating beans is taking Beano, a commercial preparation of the enzyme alpha-galactosidase. This enzyme breaks down the fermentable sugars in beans and many other fruits, grains, and vegetables.

❑ Flatulence after eating dairy products may be caused by lack of the digestive enzyme lactase. The commercial product Lactaid provides this enzyme and reduces flatulence, abdominal pain, and diarrhea caused by lactose intolerance.

❑ Milk products that are already fermented, such as yogurt, are less likely to cause gas even without the enzyme.

Heartburn

Heartburn is a sensation of warmth or burning beneath the breastbone or in the stomach above the navel. Heartburn pain can radiate to the neck and arms, mimicking heart pain caused by angina. Heartburn most often occurs after a person has eaten a large meal and then bends, stoops, or lies down. The change in position weakens the sphincter at the bottom of the esophagus, allowing acidic material from the stomach to back up into the esophagus. Aspirin, alcohol, spicy food, and citrus fruit juices may also induce heartburn, as can excess weight, overeating, stress, smoking, and pregnancy.

Recommendations

❑ Do not allow mealtime to become a rushed, stressful experience. Allow time for leisurely meals, and chew food carefully and thoroughly. Avoid conflicts during meals. Avoid excitement or exercise immediately after a meal.

❑ Eat smaller, more frequent meals, but make sure that this pattern doesn't cause weight gain. Excess pounds put pressure on the abdomen, pushing up the stomach and causing acid to back up into the esophagus.

❑ Avoid spicy food and fatty foods.

❑ Avoid eating cold food, especially ice cream, after a hot meal.

❑ Do not smoke, use alcohol, or chew gum.

❑ Use acetaminophen instead of aspirin.

❑ Sleep on the left, rather than right, side. The lower esophagus curves slightly to the left as it connects with the stomach. During sleep, the effects of gravity straighten out this curve, raising the potential for stomach acids to spill into the esophagus.

Considerations

❑ A calm environment and rest may help relieve stress-related heartburn. (*See* STRESS.)

❑ Some things you can do to de-stress include drinking peppermint tea and using relaxation techniques or cognitive therapy. Some have benefited from the herbal drug STW 5, which is a blend of peppermint and caraway. Yoga and meditation also may be of help. Two Chinese herbal medicines—Sho-hange-ka-bukuryo-to and Nichin-to—have been used to lower levels of cortisol, a hormone released when you feel stress.

❑ Review your medication use with your doctor and make sure you actually need everything you are taking. Many drugs have side effects in the GI tract and can cause heartburn. See if other options are available. If you are using selective serotonin reuptake inhibitors (SSRIs) for depression, know that these are likely to cause nausea and dyspepsia. In one study, an herbal blend called Gorei-san (TJ-17) helped patients taking SSRIs to feel better. The herbs in the blend include *Alismatis rhizoma, Atractylodis lanceae rhizoma, Polyporus, Hoelen,* and *Cinnamomi cortex.* Only five of the twenty patients did not get some improvement in their dyspepsia with the herbal blend.

❑ *See also* OVERWEIGHT.

Heartburn: Beneficial Herbs

Herb	Form and Dosage	Comments
Coptis[1] or goldenseal[1]	Tincture. Take 15–20 drops in ¼ cup water. Do not take for more than 2 weeks.	Stops heartburn associated with emotional tension.
Turmeric	Powder. Take 1 tsp in 1 cup cold water. Do not substitute curcumin.	Stops stomach irritation.

Precautions for the use of herbs:

[1]Do not use coptis or goldenseal if you are pregnant or have gallstones. Do not take these herbs with supplemental vitamin B$_6$ or with protein supplements containing the amino acid histidine. Do not take goldenseal if you have cardiovascular disease or glaucoma.

Hiccups: Beneficial Herbs

Herb	Form and Dosage	Comments
Galangal	Tea made by adding ¼–½ tsp (0.5–1.0 gm) powder in 1 cup water. (*See* TEAS in Part Three.) Take a cup as needed.	Stops inflammation that causes hiccups; relieves incomplete digestion.
Ginger	Tea, made by adding ½ tsp (1 gm) powdered ginger to 1 cup water. (*See* TEAS in Part Three.) Take a cup as needed.	Stops inflammation that causes hiccups; relieves incomplete digestion.

Hiccups

Hiccups are sudden, involuntary contractions of the diaphragm. They can occur in people of any age, but are more common in infants and small children than in adults. The most frequent causes of hiccups are indigestion and swallowing air while eating. If air is swallowed with food or drink, it has no place to go except back through the esophagus in the form of a hiccup.

Recommendations

❑ Before using any other hiccup remedy, try holding your breath while bearing down with the abdominal muscles. You can do this by pressing down on the abdominal muscles while breathing in and out of a paper bag held over the nose and the mouth. This raises the carbon dioxide level of the blood, calming the nerve and muscle irritability that causes hiccups. Do not use a plastic bag.

Considerations

❑ Hiccups can result from stress, excitement, temperature changes, use of barbiturates, and a variety of other triggers. If hiccups are chronic, consider factors other than stomach irritation.

INFERTILITY

As many as one out of every four American couples experiences infertility, defined as the failure to conceive after at least one year of unprotected intercourse. Sometimes this is due to problems with the male partner, sometimes with the female. In this section, the causes and treatments for infertility in men and women will be treated separately.

Infertility in Men

In men, infertility can be caused by a variety of injuries to and disorders of the sperm-producing organs, the testes. These include damage caused by mumps and certain other viruses; sexually transmitted diseases; radiation damage, whether through industrial accident or in the course of cancer treatment; exposure to environmental toxins; too much heat to the testicles, such as from staying in a sauna too long or wearing tight clothing that may increase the temperature of the scrotum area; prolonged cycling; the use of medications or recreational drugs, including alcohol, marijuana, heroin, or methadone; smoking; and the cancer treatments cyclophosphamide and doxorubicin hydrochloride (Adriamycin). In addition, systemic illnesses, including cancer of the male reproductive organs, cirrhosis of the liver, Hodgkin's lymphoma, sickle cell anemia, and acute fevers, can also lead to infertility. Deficiencies of vitamin C, selenium, zinc, and folate may contribute to infertility. Being overweight or older than thirty-five also increases the risk.

Infertility can also be caused by physical abnormalities. One is a vascular condition known as varicocele, in which blood accumulates in the testicles, a condition similar to varicose veins. It is fairly common, affecting 15 percent of men overall, and 40 percent of men with known infertility. However, it usually can be surgically corrected. Infertility can also result from blockage of the spermatic ducts, the tubes that carry sperm away from the testes. Sperm may also not be cooled adequately, which can lead to lower counts and potential infertility. This also can be corrected through surgery.

Infertility occurs if blood levels of testosterone, the main male sex hormone, are reduced, generally because illness or injury reduces blood flow to the testes. Lower levels of testosterone result in lowered sperm production. A man is most likely to be fertile if his ejaculate—the semen discharged in a single ejaculation—contains more than 39 million sperm. Even if a man produces enough sperm for conception, he may still be infertile if his sperm is not mobile or, in biological terms, motile. Sperm cells that are not motile cannot swim up into the woman's fallopian tubes, where conception generally occurs.

A complete medical exam should be done before any treatment for infertility is followed. However, despite the identification of various causes of infertility in men, almost half of all cases have no cause that can be pinpointed through examination. Some treatments that may be used include hormone injections and artificial insemination. Herbal therapies may be tried before attempting these procedures; the herbs recommended here may increase the number, motility, and viability of sperm.

Herbs to Avoid

❑ Men who have fertility problems should avoid jambul, neem, and vitex. Laboratory studies with extracts of

Infertility in Men: Beneficial Herbs

Herb	Form and Dosage	Comments
Astragalus[1]	Capsules. Take 1,000 mg 3 times daily.	Increases sperm motility.
Black cohosh	Capsules. Take 1,000 mg daily.	Increases motility and viability of sperm cells.
Dong quai[2]	Ferulic acid extract. Take as directed on the label; or tea. Take as directed by a traditional Chinese medicine practitioner.	Increases motility and viability of sperm cells.
Epimedium[3]	Use as directed by an herbalist.	Stimulates semen formation and nerve activity in the male sex organs.
Ginseng	*Panax ginseng* tincture. Take as directed on the label.	Increases the number and motility of sperm cells. Raises testosterone levels.
Yin yang-huo	Take as directed on the label.	May increase sperm count and semen density. Also known as horny goatweed.

Precautions for the use of herbs:

[1]Do not use astragalus if you have a fever or a skin infection.

[2]Use dong quai with caution if you are attempting to recover fertility after chemotherapy with bleomycin (Blenoxane). Some studies indicate that ferulic acid *increases* the risk of free-radial damage to sperm cells in men who are or who have been treated with this drug.

[3]Do not use epimedium for more than three months except as part of a TCM formula. There are no side effects, but the herb becomes less effective with continued use.

Infertility in Men: Formulas

Formula	Comments
Cinnamon Twig and Poria Pill	A traditional Chinese herbal formula that treats infertility due to varicocele; increases sperm count and sperm motility. Improves circulation in the lower abdominal region.
Hochu-ekki-to	Japanese herbal formula that helps sperm cells develop properly. Raises both testosterone levels and sperm counts. Also effective in alleviating infertility caused by the cancer treatment doxorubicin (Adriamycin).

echinacea, ginkgo, and St. John's wort indicate that these herbs contain chemicals that reduce the sperm's ability to penetrate the egg, but whether these herbs have the same effect in the human body is not known. (For more information regarding these herbs, *see* the individual entries *under* The Herbs in Part One.)

Recommendations

❑ Take 25 milligrams of zinc three times a day. For men with low testosterone levels, zinc supplements restore normal testosterone levels and increase both fertility and potency. For men with low semen zinc levels, zinc supplements may increase both sperm counts and fertility. Avoid taking too much zinc, since overdosage—several hundred milligrams daily—can depress the immune system. If taking zinc for more than a few weeks, take a mineral supplement that provides copper as well.

❑ Take 3,000 milligrams of L-carnitine daily. Taking this supplement for four months has been found to normalize sperm in men with low sperm quality, such as sperm that don't swim well.

❑ Do not smoke. Smoking has been implicated in low sperm counts, abnormal sperm shapes, and poor sperm motility.

❑ Do not use alcohol or marijuana, both of which have been implicated in infertility. Taking more than four drinks a day is directly toxic to sperm.

❑ Limit caffeine. There is some evidence linking lowered sperm counts to intake of more than two cups of coffee or four cans of cola a day.

❑ Avoid soaking in hot tubs. A hot soak even once or twice a week can significantly reduce sperm production.

❑ If you use a testosterone patch and are seeking to become a father, consult a physician. Testosterone therapy—as contrasted with treatments that increase the testes' ability to make testosterone—could reduce sperm counts. Anabolic steroids also reduce fertility.

❑ Some artificial lubricants can prevent the sperm from reaching the cervix. Saliva also may have a detrimental effect on sperm.

Considerations

❑ Injections of testosterone or other hormones do not increase male fertility and may even have feminizing side effects if the body converts the extra testosterone into female hormones. Other techniques that may be tried are in vitro fertilization or artificial insemination, in which either the man's or a donor's sperm is introduced directly into the woman's reproductive tract.

❑ The rain forest herb iporuru is a unique traditional treatment for infertile men in that it is taken by the female partner rather than the man. A plausible explanation for this effect is that the herb increases the receptivity of the cervix to sperm cells. The herb is also taken by men to increase their fertility. French scientists have proposed that men taking iporuru would have more viable sperm (and increased potency) through the action of yohimbine, a compound found in both iporuru and yohimbe.

❑ Vitamin B$_{12}$ (cobalamin) injections have been used to increase sperm counts. For treatment, consult a nutritionally oriented physician. Get a B$_{12}$ measurement of your blood first to see if you have low levels that could contribute to the problem.

❑ In one study, a combination of vitamin E and selenium improved sperm motility in infertile males.

❑ Acupuncture can be helpful in treating varicocele. (*See* ACUPUNCTURE in Part Three.) The treatments are not applied to the testicle itself.

❑ Because there are so many causes of infertility, in most cases, the opinion of a qualified health-care professional is needed.

❑ Marijuana and cocaine can lower sperm count.

❑ Sperm count reaches its highest level after two to three days of abstinence from any sexual activity, but sperm that remains in a man's body for longer than a month is less effective at fertilizing an egg.

Infertility in Women

Infertility in women can have many causes, including ovarian cysts and blockages of the fallopian tubes, endometriosis, hypothyroidism, and uterine fibroids. This section addresses infertility caused by ovulatory failure, or the failure of the ovary to release an egg.

In a woman of childbearing age, the ovaries normally release one egg per menstrual cycle. The pituitary gland, located beneath the brain, secretes follicle-stimulating hormone (FSH), which allows the egg to "mature" in the ovary. The pituitary also secretes luteinizing hormone (LH), which triggers ovulation. In addition, a form of estrogen called estradiol causes the uterine lining to thicken, which gives a fertilized egg a nutrient-rich attachment point in the womb. If an egg is not fertilized, the lining is broken down, both the egg and the lining are eliminated through menstruation, and a new cycle begins.

Anything that upsets this complex hormonal balance can interfere with ovulation. Stress, whether physical or psychological in origin, can disrupt the system. So can age, especially as a woman reaches her midthirties. Ovulatory failure also can occur for no detectable reason. Conventional medicine treats ovulatory failure with fertility drugs and in vitro fertilization.

The first step in dealing with infertility is to treat any reproductive-tract disorders that may be present. Single herbs may stimulate growth of the uterine lining, which increases the chances that a fertilized egg will attach to the uterus. Treatment to rebalance hormones, however, usually requires the use of multiple-herb formulas. Consult an herbal practitioner to determine the formula most likely to help, or consult a gynecologist regarding the type of hormonal balancing needed.

Herbs to Avoid

❑ Women who have a disorder of fertility should avoid the following herbs: amaranth (*achyranthis*), barley sprouts, blue cohosh, dong quai, gardenia, horse chestnut, neem, and snake gourd root. (For more information regarding these herbs, *see* the individual entries *under* The Herbs in Part One.)

Formulas to Avoid

❑ Women who are experiencing fertility problems should not take Augmented Rambling Powder. (For more information about this formula, *see* AUGMENTED RAMBLING POWDER *under* The Formulas in Part One.)

Infertility in Women: Beneficial Herbs

Herb	Form and Dosage	Comments
American ginseng	*Panax quinquefolium* tincture. Take as directed on the label.	Stimulates growth of the uterine lining.
Vitex	Tincture. Take 1 tsp in ¼ cup water daily.	Stimulates growth of the uterine lining.

Infertility in Women: Formulas

Formula	Comments
Cinnamon Twig and Poria Pill	A traditional Chinese herbal formula that stimulates ovulation. Increases blood levels of estradiol, FSH, and LH, and increases the weight of the uterus.
Peony and Licorice Decoction	A traditional Chinese herbal formula that increases chances of pregnancy, particularly for women with ovarian cysts. Acts by increasing the ratio of estradiol to testosterone and FSH to LH.
Warm the Menses Decoction[1]	A traditional Chinese herbal formula that treats infertility accompanied by bleeding between periods, extended menstrual flow, or irregular menstruation. Other symptoms include cold in the lower abdomen, dry lips and mouth, low-grade fever in the late afternoon, or warm palms and soles.

Precautions for the use of formulas:

[1]Do not use Warm the Menses Decoction if you have a fever.

Recommendations

❏ Do not try to have sex every day during ovulation. This could cause a drop in sperm count, which could be counterproductive to conception.

❏ Do not try to maintain an excessively low body weight, especially through vigorous exercise. Avoid regular exercise that is so vigorous that it interferes with the menstrual period and lessens fertility. Cutting back on exercise, or gaining 2 to 5 pounds (1 to 2 kilograms), may restore fertility, if you are underweight. Being overweight is also a risk factor for infertility.

❏ To the extent possible, avoid contact with chemical solvents and pesticides.

❏ Do not douche or use vaginal lubricants. These substances can slow down or kill sperm, making conception difficult or impossible. If lubrication is needed, baby oil and light vegetable oil are the best choices.

❏ Avoid all alcohol. Alcohol can prevent the implantation of a fertilized egg.

❏ Do not smoke, and avoid being around cigarette smoke.

Considerations

❏ Fertility drugs force the ovaries to release eggs. These drugs can not only have a number of different side effects, but could also increase a woman's risk of developing ovarian cancer if used over too long a period of time. If the drugs do not work, a woman can opt for in vitro fertilization. In this procedure, the ovaries are hormonally stimulated to release multiple eggs, which are then extracted, fertilized in a laboratory, and returned to the body. In vitro fertilization is expensive, but often covered by private insurance; however, it is not always successful.

❏ The diet of both the man and woman when trying to get pregnant is important. In one study, couples were asked to eat a Mediterranean diet and their chances of pregnancy increased by 40 percent. The diet that the couples ate was rich in fruits and vegetables, vegetable oils, fish, and legumes and was low in processed foods.

❏ Being overweight reduces the chances of conception. In a study of overweight women who had polycystic ovary syndrome and were having trouble getting pregnant, those who followed a structured exercise program and low-calorie diet had double the chance of ovulating compared to those who did not follow this regimen.

❏ Use of video display terminals is linked to infertility in women who have endometriosis. (*See* ENDOMETRIOSIS.)

❏ An underlying rare cause of infertility in women, especially those who have overactive thyroids, may be celiac disease. (*See* CELIAC DISEASE.)

❏ Infection with *Chlamydia,* the principal cause of pelvic inflammatory disease (PID), is another cause of infertility. (*See* PELVIC INFLAMMATORY DISEASE.)

❏ *See also* FIBROIDS, UTERINE (UTERINE MYOMAS); HYPO-THYROIDISM; and OVARIAN CYST.

INFLUENZA

Influenza, commonly called the flu, is a viral respiratory infection. The symptoms—fever, chills, muscle aches, headache, fatigue, weakness, nasal discharge, cough, and hot and cold sweats—are similar to those of a cold, except that flu symptoms tend to come on more suddenly and be more severe. The fatigue and weakness associated with the flu can last for several weeks after the initial infection.

The human body can build immunity to the influenza virus, which comes in two main strains, A and B. Flu epidemics generally occur during the winter.

Flu is transmitted through extremely small particles generated by coughs and sneezes. The virus begins to replicate within four to six hours of its arrival in the body, but the spread of infection sufficient to produce symptoms requires an incubation period of from two to three days.

The worse the case of the flu, the more likely it may be contagious. Medical treatment for flu consists mostly of pain relief, although some prescription medications are available.

Some people, such as older people, young children, and people with certain health conditions, are at high risk for serious flu complications. The best way to prevent the flu is by getting vaccinated each year. In 2009 to 2010, a new and very different flu virus (called 2009 H1N1) spread worldwide, causing the first flu pandemic in more than forty years. The seasonal flu vaccine protects against three influenza viruses that research indicates will be most common during the upcoming season. The Centers for Disease Control and Prevention (CDC) recommends that everyone six months of age and older get a seasonal flu vaccine. This includes all children aged six months up to their nineteenth birthday. Vaccination is especially important for children younger than five years of age and children of any age with a long-term health condition like asthma, diabetes, or heart disease. These children are at higher risk of serious flu complications if they get the flu.

Unless otherwise specified, the herb dosages recommended here are for adults. Children under age six should be given one-quarter of the adult dosage. Children between the ages of six and twelve should be given one-half of the adult dosage.

Recommendations

❑ Take hot chicken or turkey soup. This is grandmother's old remedy and it is still good today. Add a bit of cayenne pepper to help prevent and break up congestion.

❑ Use essential oil of yarrow in aromatherapy to soothe inflammation. (*See* AROMATHERAPY in Part Three.)

Influenza: Beneficial Herbs

Herb	Form and Dosage	Comments
Anise	Tea bag, prepared with 1 cup water. Take 1 cup 3 times daily.	Stimulates mucous secretion in the throat and lungs, and relieves unproductive cough.
Boneset	Take as directed on the label.	Works as an expectorant and eliminates mucus from the lungs.
Catnip	Tea bag, prepared with 1 cup water. Take 1 cup as desired.	Relieves digestive problems during flu attacks.
Cayenne	Powder. Add a pinch to soups and other foods.	Keeps mucus flowing, aiding in preventing congestion and headaches.
Echinacea[1] plus eupatorium[2]	*Echinacea purpurea* tablets. Take at least 900 mg per day. Tea (loose), prepared by steeping 1/3 oz (10 gm) in 1 cup hot water. (*See* TEAS in Part Three.) Take 1 cup 3 times daily.	Relieves flu symptoms. (*See under* Recommendations, above.) Increases the immune-stimulant effect of echinacea as much as 1,000 percent.
Elderberry	Sambucol. Take as directed on the label.	Speeds recovery from flu. Also prevents infection with flu.
Fritillaria[3]	Ching chi hua tan tang syrup. Take as directed on the label.	Relieves sticky phlegm, snoring, and chronic sore throat.
Garlic	Tablets. Take 900 mg daily; or fresh cloves. Use liberally in cooking.	Use this herb to prevent bacterial infections that may develop in addition to the flu.
Ginger	Tea (loose), prepared by adding 1/3 tsp (1 gm) powdered ginger to 1 cup water. (*See* TEAS in Part Three.) Take 1 cup 3 times daily.	Relieves chest and nasal congestion, scratchy throat.
Kudzu	Tablets. Take 10 mg 3 times daily.	Relieves muscle tension accompanying flu.
Licorice	Tea bag, prepared with 1 cup water. Take 1 cup 3 times daily for up to 2 weeks.	Accelerates healing. Also helps to prevent infection with influenza A.
Mullein	Tea bag, prepared with 1 cup water. Take 1 cup 3 times daily.	Soothes sore throat, encourages expectoration of phlegm.
Osha	Tincture. Take as directed on the label.	Contains Z-ligusticide, a compound that kills both A and B strains.
Tilden flower	Tea bag, prepared with 1 cup water. Take 1 cup 3 times daily.	Prevents headache, relieves scratchy throat.

Precautions for the use of herbs:

[1]Avoid echinacea if you have an autoimmune disease such as rheumatoid arthritis or lupus. Do not use it if you have a chronic infection such as HIV or tuberculosis.

[2]When using eupatorium, always use dried, not fresh, herb. The fresh herb contains tremetrol, which can cause nausea, stomachache, or vomiting.

[3]Do not use fritillaria if you are pregnant or nursing, or if you have high blood pressure.

❏ Do not take essential fatty acid supplements—such as fish oils, flaxseed oils, or gamma-linolenic acid (GLA)—during flu attacks. These oils are usually beneficial because they discourage the production of eicosanoids, which are involved in a wide variety of inflammatory reactions. During flu infection, however, inflammatory reactions are necessary to clear the virus from the body. In laboratory tests, using fish oils prolongs the time needed for animals to recover from the flu virus. After the flu, it is fine to begin using them again.

❏ Get adequate rest. Although keeping active during a cold is a good idea, it is important to remain relatively inactive during a bout of the flu.

❏ Do not give aspirin or any product containing aspirin to a child who shows symptoms of a viral infection. Aspirin use can result in Reye's syndrome, a potentially serious complication.

❏ If you are over sixty-five, see your health-care provider. Influenza can cause serious complications for people in this age group. In one study, residents of a nursing home who took L-cysteine and L-theanine (two amino acids) two weeks before they were inoculated for the flu virus responded better to the vaccination and had stronger immune systems to fight against the flu virus.

Considerations

❏ Green tea and scutellaria can prevent infections with either the A or B strain of influenza. Drink 2 to 5 cups of green tea daily when the flu is "going around," but do not use it within one hour of taking other medications. Take 1 to 1½ teaspoons (4 to 6 milliliters) of scutellaria tincture three times daily (do not use it if you have diarrhea).

❏ In one study, an herbal blend, Hochu-ekki-to, had no benefit in fighting off the flu compared to placebo.

❏ Vitamin C can be used to prevent the flu or to mitigate symptoms. Laboratory tests suggest that flu viruses are 10,000 times as infective if vitamin C levels are low. Take 2,000 to 4,000 milligrams daily. In one study, flu and cold symptoms were reduced by 85 percent in a group of over 400 students who took megadoses of vitamin C.

❏ In one study, vitamin D was effective in children who were not already taking vitamin D supplements and in those with asthma. The children received a high dose of 1,200 international units (IU) of vitamin D_3 from December to March. Do not do this without checking with your child's pediatrician.

❏ Probiotics have been shown to enhance the body's own immune response to fight off viruses like the flu.

❏ The A strain of flu can be treated with the prescription drug amantadine hydrochloride (Symmetrel), if taken within the first forty-eight hours of infection. This drug reduces the flu's duration by about 50 percent, although it can cause nervousness.

❏ Antibiotics are useless against viral illnesses like influenza. The best way to get rid of the flu or any other infectious illness is to attack it head-on by strengthening the immune system. The thymus and the adrenal glands are the power seat of the immune system. If the body is getting sick, or is already sick, it is under stress, and stress taxes the immune system. Some researchers have linked vulnerability to colds and flu to psychological stress.

❏ For most people, flu shots are recommended. Enhancement of immune function is also warranted. If you are allergic to eggs discuss with your doctor whether you should have a flu shot.

❏ See also COMMON COLD.

INJURIES

See BRUISING; BURNS; CUTS, SCRAPES, AND ABRASIONS; FRACTURE; MUSCLES, SORE; SHIN SPLINTS; SPRAINS AND STRAINS.

INSECT BITES

Bites and stings by insects, ticks, fleas, and spiders leave venom in the skin and cause a mild toxic reaction that produces itching or pain. Infected bites swell and become red the day after the bite, often after the bite seems to be healing. Insect bites are also a serious problem if the insect carries a disease, such as malaria, Lyme disease, or Rocky Mountain spotted fever.

Some people react to bites with allergic rashes. This can quickly progress to a dangerous condition known as anaphylactic shock, in which swelling blocks air passages. If a serious reaction to a bite occurs, seek professional help immediately. Use herbs preventively and over the long term to avoid reactions to insect bites.

Recommendations

❏ Use echinacea to help the immune system fight infected bites. Take ½ teaspoon (2 milliliters) of E. purpurea tincture in ¼ cup water four times daily for up to ten days. Do not use this herb for this purpose if you have an autoimmune disease, such as rheumatoid arthritis or lupus, or a chronic infection, such as HIV or tuberculosis.

❏ If stung by a honeybee, pull out the stinger immediately. If the stinger is removed before all the venom is pumped into the skin, the welt will be smaller and less painful. This will work with bumblebee stings also, although bumblebees seldom leave their stingers, while honeybees always do.

❏ Do not pull out a tick that is embedded in the skin. If ticks are removed in this way, the heads are often left behind. Instead, try to suffocate the tick by covering it

Insect Bites: Beneficial Herbs

Herb	Form and Dosage	Comments
Aloe	Gel. Apply as directed on the label.	An anti-inflammatory that helps to prevent infection.
Andiroba	Oil. Apply to the site of a tick bite while the tick is still attached.	Suffocates the tick, allowing it to fall from the skin cleanly. Eases inflammation.
Calendula	Ointment. Apply as directed on the label.	Acts as an insect repellent and counter-irritant.
Comfrey[1]	Allantoin cream. Apply to spider bites after cleaning and disinfection.	Accelerates tissue healing.
Copaiba	Oil. Apply to rash from fire ant stings.	Relieves pain and irritation, speeds healing, and prevents infection.
Sangre de drago	Ointment. Apply to spider bites after cleaning and disinfection.	Forms an instant "second skin," protecting the wound and preventing infection.
Tea tree oil[2]	Oil. Apply full strength to infected bite.	A topical antiseptic to fight and/or prevent infection.

Precautions for the use of herbs:

[1]Do not take comfrey internally. Do not use it in any form during pregnancy. Avoid contact with unaffected skin to prevent irritation, and wash your hands after applying the cream. Especially avoid touching your eyes if there is any cream residue on your hands.

[2]People who are allergic to celery or thyme should not use tea tree oil products. Do not take tea tree oil internally.

with petroleum jelly or mineral oil. If the tick does not release at once, wait twenty minutes and pull it out with surgical tweezers, being careful that all parts of the tick are removed. Surgical-quality tweezers are available from the Self Care Catalog. (*See* Appendix B: Resources.)

❑ Wash any insect bite with soap and water, and then disinfect the area with either rubbing alcohol or hydrogen peroxide.

❑ To avoid mosquitoes, wear light-colored clothing; mosquitoes are attracted by dark colors. Loose-fitting clothing creates barriers of air between fabric and skin that mosquitoes cannot bite through.

❑ For flea control, dust upholstery, drapes, and carpets with neem powder, available at home and garden centers. Try keeping pets outside the house, if possible, and wash pet bedding in hot water and detergent once a week. Once a flea infestation is under control, vacuuming every other day may help remove the eggs that fleas lay in the carpet. Get rid of the vacuum bag each time, because the fleas hatch inside. When washing the floor, pay special attention to baseboards and under the furniture. Shampoo the carpets or bring in a professional steam cleaner at least twice a year.

❑ Rub a cut onion on an insect bite to provide a powerful antioxidant treatment.

❑ Avoid using perfume, hair spray, and other cosmetics. These attract insects.

Considerations

❑ Some herbs can help repel insects before they have a chance to bite. Citronella oil, rubbed on exposed skin before going outdoors, is a natural insect repellent that is safe for children and pregnant women. Pennyroyal, made into a skin wash, is another good insect repellent. (*See* SKIN WASHES in Part Three.) Keep citronella away from the eyes, and never use pennyroyal internally. Garlic, consumed in food, can produce a body odor that repels insects (although it might repel people as well).

❑ Some herbalists believe that certain herbs may reduce the risk of anaphylactic shock in people allergic to insect bites and stings. If taken on an ongoing basis, ginseng may reduce susceptibility to anaphylactic shock by counteracting inflammation. Make ginseng tea by using 1 teaspoon (5 grams) of sliced *Panax ginseng* root in 1 cup of water once a day. (*See* TEAS in Part Three.) Children under age six should be given ¼ cup, and children from ages six to twelve should be given ½ cup. Another herb, licorice, helps prevent fluid from accumulating in the lungs. It also reduces the rate at which the body breaks down epinephrine, a medicine used to combat anaphylactic shock that may be self-administered by means of an epinephrine pen (Epi-Pen). Take 800 milligrams of glycyrrhizin tablets once a day (children aged six to twelve, 400 milligrams) for four weeks after an attack. Do not give licorice to children under age six. Do not use in lieu of your medication and do not take substances known to induce allergies.

❑ Electric insect-repelling devices ("bug zappers") are not recommended. They kill biting bugs, but not black flies and mosquitoes, which cause many if not the majority of the most uncomfortable bites. Moreover, many of the insects they do kill are an important part of the daily diet of birds. If you feel you must use one of these devices, do not place it near children's play areas, barbecue grills, or picnic tables. When insects like houseflies get zapped, the parts can spray as far as seven feet, spreading bacteria and viruses.

❑ *See also* LYME DISEASE.

INSOMNIA

Insomnia is a state of inadequate sleep. It may take the form of an inability to fall asleep, or of a tendency to wake up in the night and be unable to go back to sleep. Although older people tend to sleep less than younger people, insomnia is a problem for people of all ages. And both age groups need the same amount of sleep for optimal health. Conventional medicine uses tranquilizers and other sleep aids to ease insomnia.

Insomnia may be transient, lasting from one to several nights. This is usually caused by short-term stress, changes in schedule or surroundings, or jet lag. Insomnia may be short-term, persisting for between a few days and three weeks. This is caused by protracted stress, such as surgery or short-term illness.

After three weeks, insomnia is considered to be chronic. Chronic insomnia, which can persist for months or years, is caused by a fundamental imbalance in the body or the emotions. Anxiety, depression, and chronic pain can contribute to chronic insomnia, as can some medications. Breathing difficulties also can lead to insomnia. Such difficulties include sleep apnea, in which the sleeper stops breathing momentarily throughout the night. Another possible cause of insomnia is restless legs syndrome, which causes uncomfortable, "jumpy" sensations in the legs.

Unless otherwise specified, the herb dosages recommended here are for adults. Children under age six should be given one-quarter of the adult dosage. Children between the ages of six and twelve should be given one-half of the adult dosage. Formula dosages for children should be discussed with a knowledgeable health-care practitioner.

Recommendations

❑ If repeated nightmares are a problem, use ho she wu (fo-ti). Take 500 milligrams two to three times daily. Do not use unprocessed root, which can cause diarrhea and skin rashes. Very high doses can cause numbness in the arms and legs.

❑ To help relieve anxiety, especially the stress of new surroundings, use lemon balm (melissa). Take 1 cup of the tea (using two bags instead of one) two to three hours before bedtime.

❑ To induce relaxation, especially if sinus pain is causing sleeplessness, use lavender oil in aromatherapy, or take 1 to 4 drops of the oil on a sugar cube. (*See* AROMATHERAPY in Part Three.) Just be sure the lavender oil you use has calming effects; for example, Spanish lavender is a stimulant, and should be avoided.

Insomnia: Beneficial Herbs

Herb	Form and Dosage	Comments
Chamomile	German chamomile (*Matricaria recutita*) tea bag. Prepare with 1 cup water. Take 1 cup 2–3 hours before bedtime.	Helps calm people under stress. Especially good for children.
Hops[1]	Capsules. Take 500–1,000 mg 3 times daily.	Especially useful for insomnia accompanied by indigestion.
Kava kava[2]	Kavapyrone tablets. Take 60–120 mg daily.	Relaxes the skeletal muscles; sedates the central nervous system.
Passionflower[3]	Tea bag, prepared with 1 cup water. Take 1 cup 2–3 hours before bedtime.	Induces muscle relaxation and sleepiness without causing next-morning drowsiness.
Rooibos	Tea. Prepare and take as directed on the label.	Induces sleep. Also stops generalized inflammation and pain.
Schisandra[4]	Tincture. Take 1 tsp (4 ml) in ¼ cup water 3 times daily.	Increases the effectiveness of the benzodiazepines chlordiazepoxide (Librium) and diazepam (Valium), allowing for lower drug dosages.
St. John's wort	Capsules. Take 900 mg of total hypericin daily.	Increases the amount of time spent in deep sleep (but not total sleep).
Valerian	Valepotriate tablets. Take 50–100 mg on an empty stomach, 1 hour before bedtime.	Reduces time required to fall asleep without next-morning "hangover."
Wild lettuce	Tincture. Take ¼–1 tsp in ¼ cup water. Use a low dosage for children under age three.	Encourages sleep after colds, flu, or overexcitement. Stops irritable cough.

Precautions for the use of herbs:

[1]Men should not take hops if erectile dysfunction (ED) is a problem. Women should not take it if they have an estrogen-sensitive disorder, such as breast cancer, endometriosis, or fibrocystic breasts.

[2]Kava kava increases the effects of alcohol and such psychoactive drugs as sedatives and tranquilizers. Do not use it if you are pregnant or nursing.

[3]Passionflower increases the effects of alcohol and such psychoactive drugs as sedatives and tranquilizers.

[4]Do not use schisandra if you have gallstones or an obstruction of the bile duct. Do not use it during pregnancy.

Insomnia: Formulas

Formula	Comments
Bupleurum Decoction to Clear the Liver[1]	A traditional Chinese herbal formula that treats insomnia generated by constant emotional stress, particularly if accompanied by bad breath, flushed cheeks, severe headaches, hearing loss, or ringing in the ears.
Cinnamon Twig Decoction Plus Dragon Bone and Oyster Shell	A traditional Chinese herbal formula for men who have insomnia accompanied by depression, dream-filled sleep, feelings of frustration, and palpitations.
Coptis Decoction to Relieve Toxicity[2]	A traditional Chinese herbal formula that treats insomnia accompanied by redness in the face, a feeling of blood rushing to the head, high blood pressure, and possibly chronic constipation.
Gastrodia and Uncaria Decoction	A traditional Chinese herbal formula that encourages deep sleep and relaxes the central nervous system. Also increases blood flow to the heart muscle.
Licorice, Wheat, and Jujube Decoction	A traditional Chinese herbal formula that treats insomnia in children who are awake all night crying.
Pill for Deafness That Is Kind to the Left Kidney	A traditional Chinese herbal formula that relieves insomnia caused by tinnitus.
Polyporus Decoction	A traditional Chinese herbal formula that treats insomnia accompanied by nausea or vomiting.
Warm the Gallbladder Decoction[3]	A traditional Chinese herbal formula that relieves insomnia in people who have not completely recovered from a cold or lung infection and are troubled by coughing and sputum production. Also known as Bamboo and Hoelen Decoction.

Precautions for the use of formulas:

[1]Do not use Bupleurum Decoction to Clear the Liver during pregnancy.

[2]Do not use Coptis Decoction to Relieve Toxicity if you are trying to become pregnant.

[3]Do not use Warm the Gallbladder Decoction if you have a fever.

❏ To relax tense muscles, take 1,000 milligrams of a calcium and magnesium supplement at bedtime. The citrate and gluconate forms of calcium are the best absorbed. This combination may also help prevent nighttime leg cramps.

❏ Eliminate stimulants, including caffeine, cold medications, and tobacco.

❏ Avoid alcohol. Although using alcohol can reduce the amount of time needed to fall asleep, the resulting dehydration can interrupt sleep. This is true also for infants who nurse after their mothers have consumed alcohol.

❏ Take a warm bath before bedtime to relax tense muscles.

❏ If possible, keep a regular routine of going to bed at the same time every night.

❏ Keep the bedroom dark. Light activates kidney function and increases the urge to urinate. Turning on the light in the middle of the night disrupts the biological clock. Too-frequent interruptions of the sleeping pattern can lead to chronic insomnia.

❏ Do not try to sleep with cold feet. Placing a hot water bottle at the feet, or wearing socks, helps induce sleep more quickly.

❏ Avoid over-the-counter (OTC) sleep aids, unless suggested by your doctor. However, lack of sleep is often debilitating and effective treatments should be sought out.

❏ In the evening, eat bananas, dates, figs, milk, nut butter, tuna, turkey, whole-grain crackers, or yogurt. These foods are high in tryptophan, which promotes sleep. Eating a grapefruit half at bedtime also helps.

❏ Go to bed only when you are sleepy.

Considerations

❏ If there is no obvious underlying physical cause of insomnia, doctors treat this condition with a variety of mild tranquilizers and antidepressants. In addition to other side effects, some of these drugs can be habit-forming, and some can cause daytime sleepiness.

❏ Drugs for asthma, high blood pressure, and Parkinson's disease frequently cause insomnia and/or nightmares. If you experience insomnia while taking prescription drugs for these conditions, consult a physician.

❏ Chemotherapy and interferon therapy interact with the immune system and alter the sleep-wake cycle. If you are taking either chemotherapy or interferon treatment for cancer, be sure to speak with a physician about timing treatments so that they do not interfere with sleep.

❏ In one study, some adults with insomnia experienced improvements with a tart cherry juice blend from Cherry-Pharm Inc. The people who took the beverage had fewer minutes awake after going to bed.

❏ Interruption in a regular exercise routine frequently results in "withdrawal symptoms," including insomnia. Fortunately, all that is needed to reverse withdrawal insomnia is to resume exercise.

❏ A form of sleep apnea called obstructive apnea, in which the throat or upper airway becomes blocked, is linked to excess body weight. (*See* OVERWEIGHT.) Being overweight without apnea also increases the chances of insomnia.

❏ A lack of sleep may cause premature aging. Experts recommend getting at least eight hours of sleep a night at any age.

❏ *See also* ANXIETY DISORDER; DEPRESSION; PAIN, CHRONIC; and RESTLESS LEGS SYNDROME.

INTERMITTENT CLAUDICATION

Circulation problems are generally caused by arteries that are too narrow to carry adequate amounts of blood. Arteries become narrow if cholesterol gathers in the artery linings to form plaques, which can then calcify into blood-vessel blockages. This process, known as arteriosclerosis, can lead to intermittent claudication, a painful circulation problem in the legs. The most common symptom of this condition is a pain, ache, cramp, numbness, or sense of fatigue in the muscle of the leg. It occurs after exercise and goes away after rest. This recurring sensation occurs down the leg from the site of the plaques that are blocking circulation. Sometimes, pain occurs as high as the thighs and buttocks, but more often it is felt below the knees. In advanced cases, the toes and feet may be constantly cold. The pain may occur at night if the legs are stretched out flat, and only be relieved when they are lowered—which may be difficult to do because of the pain.

Drug treatments of circulatory problems in the leg may not be successful, but there are other options, such as surgery and use of a hyperbaric chamber, to help leg ulcers heal. Some herbal supplements can bring substantial relief. Herbal medicine for intermittent claudication should always be used under a doctor's supervision, since some herbs magnify the effect of blood-thinning drugs. Treatment is also needed for the underlying cause or causes of the arterial blockages.

Recommendations

❏ Take 300 to 600 international units (IU) of vitamin E for at least three months to improve walking distance and stimulate blood flow. However, be sure to inform your doctor you are taking vitamin E before any planned surgery or if you are taking any medication to thin the blood.

❏ Take omega-3 fatty acids to reduce the risk of worsening heart disease. However, omega 3s did not show any benefit specifically related to intermittent claudication in a review of six studies in more than 300 people. Nevertheless, it is prudent to include two or three servings of cold-water fish (such as mackerel, salmon, or tuna) in your diet weekly. Your doctor may also suggest that you take a fish oil capsule to improve blood flow.

❏ After consulting with the doctor, exercise thirty to forty-five minutes daily, stopping when pain begins and resting until it goes away. Bicycle riding (including stationary bicycles) and swimming are less likely to cause pain than walking.

❏ Since circulatory problems anywhere in the leg affect the feet, be sure to practice proper foot care. Keep the feet dry and clean. Wear well-fitting, protective shoes, and avoid elastic support hose, as they reduce blood flow to the skin.

❏ If pain occurs at rest, try using a canopy, available through many medical supply houses, over the feet to relieve the weight of bed covers.

❏ If you smoke, stop. Nicotine causes tension in the linings of the arteries, which reduces circulation.

Considerations

❏ When circulatory problems in the legs occur in someone who is overweight, weight loss sometimes can dramatically improve symptoms. Losing weight takes pressure off the dural sheath that surrounds the arteries, allowing them to expand to supply more blood for walking and exercise. Low-calorie diets are necessary for weight loss until circulation is restored. (*See* OVERWEIGHT.)

❏ Some people with intermittent claudication have seen improvement in blood flow with folic acid supplements.

Intermittent Claudication: Beneficial Herbs

Herb	Form and Dosage	Comments
Ginkgo[1]	Ginkgolide tablets. Take 40–60 mg 2–3 times daily for at least 6 weeks.	Increases pain-free walking distance. Prevents further plaque buildup.
Prickly ash	Tea (loose), prepared by steeping 1 tsp (3 gm) in 1 cup water. (*See* TEAS in Part Three.) Take 1 cup 3 times daily.	Increases pain-free walking distance. Relieves coldness in feet and toes.

Precautions for the use of herbs:
[1]Do not use ginkgo if you are taking blood-thinning medication. Discuss its use with your doctor before having any type of surgery.

Iron Overload: Beneficial Herbs

Herb	Form and Dosage	Comments
Milk thistle[1]	Silymarin gelcaps. Take 120 mg 3 times daily.	Prevents liver damage; stops iron from promoting atherosclerosis. (*See under* Considerations, below.)

Precautions for the use of herbs:

[1]Milk thistle may cause mild diarrhea. If this occurs, decrease the dose or stop taking it.

❑ Varicose veins in men are a signal of future circulation problems and coronary heart disease. Men over the age of forty who have varicose veins should take all necessary steps to manage cholesterol. (*See* VARICOSE VEINS.)

❑ Poor circulation can be due to any number of reasons, so it is important to see a doctor if it becomes persistent.

❑ *See also* ATHEROSCLEROSIS, DIABETES, HIGH BLOOD PRESSURE (HYPERTENSION), and HIGH CHOLESTEROL.

IRON OVERLOAD

Iron overload, or hemochromatosis, is a hereditary disease in which the body stores so much iron that it begins to "rust," with the iron degrading cell membranes in the liver, pancreas, and heart. Over 1 million people in the United States alone have full-blown iron overload disease, and another 30 million carry a gene that causes a milder form of the condition.

The risk of iron overload disease is highest for people who have close family members (parent or sibling) who have been diagnosed with the disorder. The disease is caused by inheriting a gene called HFE. If both parents pass the mutated HFE gene to you, you may develop hemochromatosis—but not always. There may be spotting or darkening of the skin. Iron overload is a lifelong condition, but symptoms usually do not begin to appear until about age forty. Men are much more susceptible to this disease than women.

A medical diagnosis of full-blown iron overload disease can be made after a needle biopsy of the liver. A blood test for ferritin, however, may show high iron levels that are associated with increased risk for complications even if the liver biopsy itself does not show excessive amounts of iron. Genetic testing can confirm if you are a carrier of the HFE gene.

Conventional treatment of iron overload consists of phlebotomy, or the taking of blood at regular intervals. Left untreated, this condition can lead to cirrhosis, diabetes, and heart disease. However, if it is detected and corrected early, serious symptoms do not appear. Effective treatment, though, requires phlebotomy. For this reason, herbal medicine and other treatments cannot substitute for phlebotomy, although they may accelerate recovery from iron overload when used as supplemental therapies.

Recommendations

❑ To reduce iron intake, limit servings of meat, fish, and poultry to one per day, and do not eat organ meats at all. Heme iron, the kind of iron found in meat, not only contributes to iron overload disease, but also increases the risk of heart attack. Raw shellfish can cause infections, so it should be avoided. Do not take vitamin C supplements, especially with food. This nutrient increases iron absorption. If you want to eat or drink foods with vitamin C, such as oranges or orange juice, do so in between meals. However, eating two or more non-citrus fruits, such as bananas and pears, can help lower the ferritin levels in people with iron overload.

❑ Consult an alternative health-care practitioner about using chelation therapy to supplement phlebotomy. Note that chelation therapy removes iron from circulation much more slowly than phlebotomy does.

Considerations

❑ The principal medical treatment for iron overload is a modern update on the traditional use of leeches—phlebotomy. The standard medical treatment for hemochromatosis is to remove 1 pint (500 milliliters) of blood once or twice a week until iron levels return to normal. People with hemochromatosis typically have 25 grams (25,000 milligrams) of excess iron in their systems. Each phlebotomy session removes approximately 250 milligrams of iron. It takes about ten to thirty minutes to remove 1 pint of blood. Once your iron levels return to normal, you may need blood drawn only four to six times a year.

❑ Milk thistle (silymarin) may be used as an adjunct to phlebotomy and a low-iron diet. Silymarin may relieve some symptoms within the first two or three days of use.

❑ *See also* HEART ATTACK (MYOCARDIAL INFARCTION).

IRRITABLE BOWEL SYNDROME

Irritable bowel syndrome (IBS) is a condition in which the rhythmic muscular contractions of the digestive tract become irregular and uncoordinated, and the normal movement of food and waste material is impaired. For reasons unknown, IBS is more common in women between the ages of twenty and thirty, and it occurs five to six times more often among people of Jewish ancestry than among people of other ethnic backgrounds. It also runs in families.

Symptoms of IBS include diarrhea alternating with constipation, lasting for six months or more; intermittent abdominal tenderness; bloating and abdominal distention; gas; nausea and vomiting; and loss of appetite. Eating may result in intense pain that is relieved by moving the bowels. There may be mucus in the stool.

Although the physical cause of IBS is not known, predisposing factors may include a low-fiber diet, emotional stress, and hormonal changes in women. Some foods, such as chocolate milk and alcohol, may trigger IBS. Carbonated beverages and some fruits and vegetables may lead to bloating. People with IBS often are "bowel conscious"—they are more sensitive than other people to motion and sensations within the digestive tract.

Physical digestive disorders must be ruled out before the doctor can make a firm diagnosis of IBS, which does not involve an observable physical illness. In conventional medicine, this disorder is treated with drugs that relieve symptoms. Herbs also relieve symptoms, generally with fewer side effects.

Herbs to Avoid

❑ Individuals who have IBS should avoid ephedra and maté. (For more information regarding these herbs, *see* The Herbs in Part One.) All stimulant herbal formulas should also be avoided.

Recommendations

❑ Avoid insoluble fiber from roughly processed foods, such as bran. Although some doctors recommend a low-fiber diet for IBS, modest amounts of soluble fiber from fruits and vegetables may correct both constipation and diarrhea. Speak to your doctor first before changing your diet.

❑ Avoid coffee (both regular and decaf), tea, and tobacco. They contain chemicals that change pressure within the intestines, and cause bloating and flatulence.

Irritable Bowel Syndrome: Beneficial Herbs

Herb	Form and Dosage	Comments
Alfalfa	Liquid or tablets. Use as directed on the label.	Contains vitamin K needed to build intestinal flora for proper digestion, and chlorophyll for healing and cleansing the bloodstream.
Asafoetida	Tincture. Take ½–1 tsp (2–4 ml) in ¼ cup warm water 3 times daily.	Relieves gas buildup and intestinal inflammation.
Calendula and dandelion and fennel and lemon balm and St. John's wort	Tinctures. Mix equal parts of all and take 1 tsp (4 ml) in ¼ cup water 3 times daily for 15 days. Store in a tightly sealed glass container.	Relieves either constipation or diarrhea. Especially useful for chronic IBS.
Chamomile	German chamomile (*Matricaria recutita*) tincture. Take ½–1 tsp (2–4 ml) in ¼ cup warm water 3 times daily.	Stops gastrointestinal spasms. Relieves nausea.
and ginger	Tincture. Take as directed on the label.	
Lemon balm	Tea, made by steeping 2 tea bags in 1 cup water. Take 1 cup 3 times daily.	Relieves gastrointestinal spasms.
Milk thistle	Silymarin gelcaps. Take 120 mg once daily.	Stimulates bile production, which relieves constipation.
Peppermint[1]	Enteric-coated oil capsules. Take 200–400 mg as needed.	Relieves spasms, especially after medical exams.
Psyllium seed	Ground seeds. Take 1 tbsp (15 gm) soaked in 1 cup cold water overnight. Do not use within 1 hour of taking other medications.	Provides bulking fibers to control diarrhea.
Rosemary	Tea, made by steeping 1 tsp (2 gm) dried herb, crushed just before use, in 1 cup water. (*See* TEAS in Part Three.) Take 1 cup as needed.	Relieves cramps and spasms.
Slippery elm bark	Tea, made by steeping 1 tsp (2 gm) in 1 cup cold water. (*See* TEAS in Part Three.) Take 1 cup as desired.	Causes the stomach to produce protective mucus.
St. John's wort	Tincture. Take ¼ tsp (1 ml) in ¼ cup water daily.	Relieves gastrointestinal inflammation.
Valerian	Tincture. Take ¼–¾ tsp (1–3 ml) in ¼ cup water, 3–4 times daily.	Stops gastrointestinal spasms; eases sleep.

Precautions for the use of herbs:

[1]Do not use peppermint if you have any kind of gallbladder disorder.

Irritable Bowel Syndrome: Formulas

Formula	Comments
Calm the Stomach Powder	A traditional Chinese herbal formula that relieves spastic abdominal pain.
Four-Gentlemen Decoction	A traditional Chinese herbal formula that treats loose stools (but not digestive-tract pain) in people with low and soft voices, pallid complexions, and weakness in the limbs.
Minor Construct the Middle Decoction	A traditional Chinese herbal formula that treats symptoms including intermittent, spasmodic abdominal pain and reduced appetite. There may also be cold hands and feet, dry mouth and throat, irritability, low-grade fever, or palpitations.
Pinellia Decoction to Drain the Epigastrium[1]	A traditional Chinese herbal formula that treats symptoms including diarrhea with rumbling in the lower digestive tract, fullness and tightness over the stomach with little pain, and reduced appetite.
Robert's Formula	Traditional naturopathic remedy for inflammatory bowel disease. Stimulates the immune system to fight intestinal infections and has a direct antibacterial effect. Soothes irritation, reduces gas.

Precautions for the use of formulas:

[1]Do not use Pinellia Decoction to Drain the Epigastrium if you have a fever.

❏ Some people need to avoid cottage cheese, chocolate milk, and ice cream that has been stabilized with carrageenan (check the label). The digestive process breaks down this seaweed extract into compounds that may irritate the colon.

❏ Avoid products sweetened with sorbitol. This sugar alternative is poorly absorbed through the intestinal lining and so remains in the gut to be digested by bacteria, a process that forms gas. Eating foods sweetened with sorbitol can cause bloating, flatulence, and abdominal pain.

❏ Try eliminating wheat, including wheat bran, from the diet. Reactions to wheat are common both in IBS and in a condition with very similar symptoms, celiac disease. (*See* CELIAC DISEASE for a list of foods that may contain gluten, the substance in wheat that causes digestive problems in susceptible people.) Do not make this change in your child's diet without consulting with a pediatrician.

❏ Take 30 to 45 milligrams of zinc picolinate daily, as well as the recommended dosage of any multivitamin supplement containing folic acid and vitamin B$_{12}$ (cobalamin), daily. Deficiencies of these nutrients are common in IBS. Zinc picolinate is better absorbed than other forms of zinc by people with IBS.

❏ Take 350 to 700 milligrams of Pancreatin or a similar pancreatic enzymes three times per day between meals. Pancreatic extracts help promote digestion and reduce inflammation.

❏ Take a milk-free acidophilus supplement between meals. *Acidophilus*, the "friendly" bacteria that aid in digestion, compete against bacteria that may cause or aggravate IBS. It also helps the intestine handle "gassy" foods that supply needed fiber.

❏ Chew your food well. Do not overeat or eat in a hurry.

❏ Wear loose-fitting clothing. Do not wear anything that is tight around the waist.

❏ Do not eat right before going to bed. Wait one to two hours after eating before lying down.

Considerations

❏ Gastroesophageal reflux disease (GERD), which commonly occurs with IBS, is a condition in which stomach contents back up into the esophagus, causing heartburn. Reflux disease is aggravated by foods and beverages that directly irritate the esophagus, including alcohol, chocolate, citrus juices, coffee, peppermint (although not enteric-coated tablets, which dissolve in the intestines), and tomatoes. Avoid these items if burping and belching with heartburn is a problem.

❏ Emotional trauma appears to play an important role in the development of IBS after an intestinal infection. People who develop IBS more frequently experience traumatic life events, such as bereavement or the breakup of a relationship. Stress management begun as soon as IBS symptoms are noticed may slow or reverse the development of the disease. (*See* STRESS.)

❏ People who have IBS may also have asthma or gastritis. (*See* ASTHMA and GASTRITIS.)

❏ An imbalance of intestinal flora is common in people with IBS. Usually, the pathogenic flora outnumber the friendly bacteria.

❏ People with IBS should receive regular physical examinations. This disorder has been linked to a higher than normal incidence of colon cancer and diverticulitis.

❏ Many people with IBS have experienced improvements in symptoms with traditional Chinese medicine (TCM). However, some Chinese herbal remedies have been tested and have not been shown to be effective in improving symptoms associated with IBS. The herbs that were not effective were *Curcuma xanthorrhiza* and *Fumaria officinalis*. Peppermint appears to be effective short-term as an antispasmodic (causing less rumbling in the intestine).

❏ Relaxing with yoga or hypnosis has been shown to be of benefit.

❏ Probiotics such as *Bacillus coagulans* have been shown to reduce the daily number of bowel movements in patients with IBS. A combination of probiotics and prebiotics (fiber) helps reduce symptoms such as nausea, indigestion, and watery diarrhea in people with IBS.

❏ The symptoms of IBS are similar to those of Crohn's disease. (*See* CROHN'S DISEASE.)

KIDNEY CANCER

(RENAL CELL CARCINOMA)

There are several types of cancer that affect the kidney, but the most common type is called renal cell carcinoma. It appears twice as often in men as in women and generally strikes people in their late fifties. The causes of kidney cancer are not exactly known, but an increased risk is associated with smoking and high-fat diets.

Blood in the urine, flank pain, and an abdominal mass that the doctor can feel are the three main symptoms of kidney cancer, although all three symptoms seldom occur together. While blood in the urine is the most common symptom, it is by no means a sure sign of kidney cancer.

Kidney stones; infections of the kidney, bladder, and urethra; and urinary tract injuries also can cause bleeding. A cancer diagnosis must be confirmed by a biopsy.

Kidney cancer is classified according to systems that measure tumor size and extent of spread. This form of cancer tends to spread early in its development, especially to the bones, brain, liver, and lungs. It also disables the immune system, which makes treatment more difficult. In early stages, the kidney and adjacent lymph nodes may be removed. In later stages, surgery can remove the affected kidney or remove the tumor from the kidney. Chemotherapy is sometimes used, although kidney cancer is resistant to most drugs. Newer treatments for kidney cancer include immunotherapy, such as the immune component interleukin-2 (IL-2), to boost immune function.

Herbal therapy should always be used as part of a medically directed overall treatment program for kidney cancer, especially since making immunotherapy bearable is an important use of herbs in this disease.

Herbs to Avoid

❏ If you have kidney cancer, you should avoid maté. This herb also increases the risk of developing kidney cancer, especially among people who eat beef daily. (For more information regarding this herb, *see* MATÉ *under* The Herbs in Part One.)

Recommendations

❏ Drink grape juice. There is some evidence from cell line studies that grape juice may serve as an antidote for food toxins causing kidney and liver cancer.

❏ Use of supplemental L-carnitine may reduce (but not eliminate) the swelling associated with IL-2 therapy. Take 500 milligrams three times daily.

Kidney Cancer: Beneficial Herbs

Herb	Form and Dosage	Comments
Astragalus[1]	Capsules. Take 500–1,000 mg 3 times daily.	Stops the spread of kidney cancer. Stimulates the immune system to produce T and natural killer (NK) cells.
Cat's claw[2]	Tincture. Take the dosage recommended on the label in ½ cup water with 1 tsp lemon juice.	Stimulates NK cell production.
Lentinan	Intramuscular injection, given by health-care provider.	Activates lymphokine-activated killer (LAK) and NK cells to attack kidney cancer cells.
Licorice	Glycyrrhizin tablets. Take 600 mg daily. Use under professional supervision.	Reduces inflammation. Has eliminated tumors in laboratory animals.
Reishi	Tablets. Take 3 gm 3 times daily.	Stimulates production of interleukin-2 (IL-2). Helps reduce swelling.
Siberian ginseng	Pure *Eleutherococcus senticosus* extract. Take as directed on the label in ¼ cup water.	Can be useful for cancers that respond to immunotherapy.

Precautions for the use of herbs:

[1]Do not use astragalus if you have a fever or a skin infection.

[2]Do not use cat's claw if you have to take insulin for diabetes. Do not use it if you are pregnant or nursing. Do not give it to a child under six.

Kidney Cancer: Formula

Formula	Comments
Shih Qua Da Bu Tang	A traditional Chinese herbal formula that stimulates production of interleukins and NK cells. Prolongs survival time and minimizes side effects of cancer treatment, including treatment with fluorouracil.

Considerations

❏ Immunotherapy is the use of agents that stimulate the immune system. Interferon-alpha slows the growth of cancer cells, and alters their surfaces so that immune-system cells called macrophages can recognize and destroy them. Interleukin-2 (IL-2) activates two kinds of immune-system cells—tumor-infiltrating lymphocytes (TIL) and lymphokine-activated killer (LAK) cells—that attack cancer cells, and other parts of the immune system that fight infection. Sometimes the hormone melatonin is used with IL-2 for increased effectiveness. While these therapies do help some people, they have side effects that may be severe enough to stop treatment. These effects include swelling caused by IL-2, and loss of appetite, fatigue, fever and chills, and nausea caused by interferon-alpha. Using the two therapies together has shown positive results, but also combines the side effects. Numerous clinical studies are ongoing, so speak to your doctor if you wish to learn more or participate in a study.

❏ Eating a healthy diet is an important way to help prevent kidney cancer. Eating five servings of fruits and vegetables daily may reduce the risk of developing kidney cancer by about 80 percent, and that risk can be further reduced by avoiding the fat found in whole milk and butter. The best vegetables appear to be those that are orange or dark green in color. It is also a good idea to avoid eating too much protein. Although an independent connection between protein consumption and kidney cancer has not been clearly established, high protein consumption may cause other kidney problems. Eating protein from legumes seems to reduce the risk of developing kidney cancer, and peas and lentils provide an excellent source of protein.

❏ Some people believe that kidney cancer is caused by eating too many refined cereals and starchy foods. However, one study found no relationship between the intake of these foods and the risk of kidney cancer.

❏ Use over-the-counter (OTC) analgesics sparingly. Aspirin, acetaminophen, and caffeine in OTC drugs should be used with caution. Heavy coffee consumption (seven or more cups a day) may raise the risk of kidney cancer.

❏ In one study, the effect of Haishengsu, an extract of *Tegillarca L. granosa*, was shown to increase remission rates in people undergoing immunotherapy for advanced renal cell cancer. The patients who were given this herb ate more, gained more weight, and had a better quality of life compared to a group who did not get this herb.

❏ Alternative activities such as art therapy, dance movement, exercise, meditation, music therapy, and relaxation exercises have all been used successfully by patients with this condition.

❏ For measures to reduce side effects and increase the effectiveness of chemotherapy and/or radiation therapy, *see* "Side Effects of Cancer Treatment" *under* CANCER. To learn about herbal treatments that can prevent a cancer from developing its own blood supply, *see* CANCER.

KIDNEY DISEASE

The main function of the kidneys is to eliminate wastes and to regulate fluid balance in the body. A number of disorders can cause the kidneys to malfunction.

The basic functional unit of the kidney is the nephron. It contains structures that filter out wastes from the blood, retain essential nutrients, and concentrate the remaining fluid into urine, which passes into the ureters and then the bladder.

The most easily recognized symptom of nephritis, or kidney inflammation, is blood in the urine. Bloody urine should always be brought to a doctor's attention, as it appears in a number of urinary tract disorders. Kidney damage is sometimes signaled by swelling, as the kidneys cannot move fluids out of the body. If advanced nephritis cripples the kidneys' ability to retain protein, the urine can actually take on a gel-like appearance. Other symptoms of kidney disease can include abdominal pain, loss of appetite, back pain, chills, fever, fluid retention, and nausea.

Kidney disorders can be roughly divided into two categories, acute and chronic. The acute disorders are caused by infection, last for relatively short periods of time, and cause relatively few side effects. Chronic disorders, though, have more long-lasting consequences. Idiopathic rapidly progressive glomerulonephritis (IRPG) is a collection of diseases that cause the kidneys to leak massive quantities of protein into the urine. It may be caused by an autoimmune disease such as lupus or scleroderma, in which the immune system attacks the body's own tissues. It is also caused by type 1 and type 2 diabetes, high blood pressure, kidney stones, and kidney infections. Nephrotic syndrome also causes the kidneys to lose protein. In addition, it can cause mineral deficiencies and swelling. It can arise from many of the same conditions that cause IRPG.

Conventional medicine uses drugs and other treatments for kidney disease. Herbal therapy for kidney disease should always be used as part of a medically directed overall treatment plan that includes conventional treatment. The formula listed below is especially helpful for kidney disease in children; seek the advice of the dispensing herbalist on a suitable child's dosage.

Recommendations

❏ Avoid adding salt to your diet, especially if there is high blood pressure. (*See* HIGH BLOOD PRESSURE [HYPERTENSION].) Many convenience foods such as frozen dinners, canned soups and vegetables, and processed meats and cheese are loaded with sodium.

❏ Eat a low-protein diet by restricting consumption of meat, fish, dairy products, and dried beans. Restricting dietary protein limits the amount of urea, a protein by-product, the kidneys have to cleanse from the bloodstream, and allows them to heal if blood pressure is also controlled. It is important to understand, however, that a low-protein diet is not always synonymous with a high-carbohydrate diet (that is, more than 600 calories per day from carbohydrates). Total calories as well as total protein may have to be adjusted to prevent the progression of kidney disease. You should get the advice of a dietitian on what to eat for your condition and current weight.

❏ Take 200 to 400 international units (IU) of vitamin E and any supplemental source of omega-3 fatty acids daily. Vitamin E helps slow the progression of the disease in a cell model, and omega-3 fatty acids may offer additional protection.

❏ Take chitosan as directed on the label. In lab studies, this fiber supplement shifts the burden of excreting nitrogen found in dietary protein from the kidneys to the intestines, and slows the course of proliferative glomerulonephritis.

❏ Include in your diet legumes, seeds, and soybeans. These foods contain the amino acid arginine, which is beneficial for the kidneys.

❏ Choose foods that are lower in potassium; a dietitian can help you, but some examples are apples, cabbage,

Kidney Disease: Beneficial Herbs

Herb	Form and Dosage	Comments
Abuta	Capsules. Take 1,000–2,000 mg daily. Use for up to 2 weeks at a time.	Antibacterial and anti-inflammatory. Prevents bleeding in mild kidney disease.
Bupleurum[1]	Use forms and dosage recommended by a traditional Chinese medicine practitioner.	Prevents protein loss and resulting tissue damage.
Dandelion root	Extract. Take as directed on the label.	Aids in excretion of the kidneys' waste products and is very beneficial for nephritis.
Hoelen[2]	Dried or fresh herb. Eat ⅛–¼ oz (3–6 gm) in food daily.	Immune suppressant that prevents lesions in kidney tissue.
Marshmallow root	Tea. Drink 1 qt daily.	Helps cleanse the kidneys.
Uva ursi	Arbutin tablet. Take 400–700 mg daily. Use for up to 2 weeks at a time.	Antibacterial and anti-inflammatory. Prevents bleeding in mild kidney disease.

Precautions for the use of herbs:

[1]Bupleurum occasionally causes mild stomach upset. It this happens, speak with the dispensing herbalist about reducing the dose. Do not take bupleurum if you have a fever or are taking antibiotics.

[2]Do not use hoelen if you have a long-term illness that causes excessive urination. In such cases, use Five-Ingredient Powder with Poria. (*See under* Formulas, below.)

Kidney Disease: Formulas

Formula	Comments
Sairei-to	A combination of two traditional Chinese herbal formulas. Five-Ingredient Powder with Poria helps promote fluid flow in the kidney, and increases the effectiveness of prednisone. Minor Bupleurum Decoction prevents tissue damage, enhances the effectiveness of immunotherapy, and reduces cholesterol in kidney tissue.

carrots, green beans, and strawberries. Foods with high potassium that you should avoid are bananas, oranges, potatoes, spinach, and tomatoes.

Considerations

❑ Standard medical treatment for chronic kidney disease includes drugs to control blood pressure, lower cholesterol, relieve anemia, reduce swelling (diuretics), and prevent bone loss (calcium and vitamin D). Steroid drugs, such as prednisone, which dampens the immune system, and/or cyclophosphamide, which may inhibit capillary formation and thus reduces bleeding, are also used. Treatment with these drugs increases the risk of infection. Other treatments include dialysis, in which a machine takes over the blood-cleansing function, and kidney transplantation.

❑ Some patients with poor kidney function experience anemia; one common drug is erythropoietin, which causes the body to produce more red blood cells to assure that adequate oxygen gets to every tissue in the body. In one study, people who were not responding to erythropoietin were given the Japanese herbal remedy Juzen-taiho-to and they had better blood counts (less anemia) as a result.

❑ People who have diabetes should have annual blood tests for creatine. High levels of this substance indicate kidney damage, which is a common complication of diabetes. People with diabetes who do not have kidney disease do not need to follow a low-protein diet, although all people who have diabetes must monitor carbohydrates carefully. (*See* DIABETES.)

❑ Infectious diseases, such as measles, scarlet fever, and tonsillitis, may damage the kidneys if they are not treated properly and completely.

❑ Recurrent urinary tract infections indicate the possibility of a serious underlying problem. See your health-care provider.

❑ For measures to reduce side effects and increase effectiveness when using steroid drugs, *see* "Side Effects of Cancer Treatment" *under* CANCER.

KIDNEY STONES

Kidney stones are crystals that form in the kidneys or the bladder. These crystals are composed of calcium salts, uric acid, or struvite, a kind of crystal that contains magnesium. A passed stone's appearance is a clue to its composition. Calcium stones—the most common kind—may be mulberry-shaped. Uric acid stones are shaped like footballs and are reddish-brown or tan. Struvite stones are the color of maple syrup and are faceted.

Kidney stones usually cause no symptoms until they are dislodged. A dislodged kidney stone can cause excruciating, radiating pain originating in the flank or kidney area, along with chills, fever, nausea, vomiting, profuse sweating, frequent urination, pus and blood in the urine, and odorous or cloudy urine. Struvite and uric acid stones may form "staghorns" that embed the stone into the kidney. Embedded stones also can cause extreme pain. These form in response to an infection and grow quickly.

Possible causes of kidney stones include Cushing's syndrome, or overactive adrenal glands; and sarcoidosis, an autoimmune disease. Cystinuria, or elevated levels of the amino acid cystine in the urine, is very rare and hereditary, and may cause kidney stones. Diet is another important factor in the formation of kidney stones. Stones can form in response to hepatitis and bacterial urinary tract infections, which can infect the stones themselves.

Kidney Stones: Beneficial Herbs

Herb	Form and Dosage	Comments
Aloe[1]	Juice. Take ¼ cup daily. Do not use for more than 2 weeks at a time.	Contains aloemannan, which slows rate of crystal formation.
Birch leaf	Tea bags, prepared with 1 cup water. Take 1 cup 3 times daily.	Stimulates urination and stops spasms.
Chanca piedra	Tincture. Take as directed on the label.	Dissolves calcium stones.
Khella[2]	Khellin in any standardized form. Take 20 mg daily.	Helps the urinary tract heal after passage of a stone.
Marshmallow root	Tea. Drink 1 qt daily.	Helps cleanse the kidneys and to expel kidney stones.
Varuna	Tea (loose), prepared by steeping 1 tbsp (5 gm) in 1 cup water. (*See* TEAS in Part Three.) Take 1 cup 3 times daily.	Inhibits an enzyme essential for the formation of calcium oxalate stones.

Precautions for the use of herbs:

[1]Aloe has laxative effects if taken in dosages larger than those recommended. Do not use if you are menstruating, have rectal bleeding, or are taking any kind of diuretic.

[2]Khella makes the skin especially sensitive to ultraviolet light. Avoid tanning lamps and use sunblock when outdoors, and discontinue use if exposure to strong sunlight is unavoidable. Do not take this herb if you are taking the blood-thinner warfarin (Coumadin).

Kidney Stones: Formulas

Formula	Comments
Polyporus Decoction	A kampo formula that relieves nausea and vomiting accompanying acute attacks. Prevents urinary tract infection. Provides relief from painful urination and a sensation of retained urine.

The diagnosis of kidney stones is made by locating the stone or by ultrasound, in which sound waves are used to produce a "picture" of the urinary tract. Small stones may be simply monitored to see that they do not grow. Large stones may be treated with lithotripsy, in which high-frequency sound waves are used to crush the stone. If lithotripsy does not work, surgery may be necessary. Herbal therapies should be used preventively, rather than during acute attacks.

Recommendations

❑ Use the Japanese beverage lisymachia or kinsenso tea, available from Japanese grocery stores, to increase urination and help the kidneys flush out small stones. Take 1 to 2 cups daily for three to four months.

❑ Drink black or green tea each day; it could reduce the risk of kidney stones. However, tea contains a lot of oxalic acid, so ask your doctor if this is a specific concern for you.

❑ Lemon juice and orange juice could reduce the risk of kidney stones. Citric acid reduces calcium levels, leading to formation of fewer stones.

❑ Eat adequate amounts of fiber. Low fiber consumption is associated with a high risk of stone development.

❑ Use any magnesium supplement that does not include calcium. Magnesium may reduce the rate at which the digestive tract absorbs calcium and lower the concentration of calcium in the urine.

❑ To avoid the formation of new stones, do not consume large amounts of alcohol or fat.

❑ Avoid high-protein and "crash" diets. They may increase the acidity of the urine, which can promote the development of some types of stones.

❑ Limit vitamin C supplementation to 2,000 milligrams or less daily for periods up to two weeks at a time, taking care to drink at least eight glasses of water daily. Higher dosages, continuous use of vitamin C, or use of vitamin C during periods of dehydration may contribute to stone formation. In people who are prone to developing stones and even in those who aren't, taking 2,000 milligrams a day increased urinary oxalate and Tiselius Risk Index (a marker of who will get kidney stones).

❑ To prevent new calcium stones from forming, limit dairy products, meats, beet greens, black tea, cocoa, chocolate, tea, okra, sweet potatoes, cranberries, nuts, parsley, pepper, spinach, Swiss chard, and especially rhubarb. These foods have oxalic acid, which may increase stone formation.

❑ To prevent new uric acid stones from forming, avoid purine-rich foods, such as anchovies, herring, mackerel, sardines, shellfish, and yeast.

❑ To prevent new struvite stones from forming, limit foods that contain the amino acid methionine, such as dairy products (except whole milk), fish, garbanzo beans (chickpeas), lima beans, mushrooms, and all nuts except hazelnuts and sunflower seeds.

❑ Drink water before, during, and after exercise, especially in hot weather. Calcium stones form more easily after exercise because physical activity causes a short-term acidity of the bloodstream. Drinking extra water partially offsets this effect. Drink a lot of water—2½ quarts a day. Use only distilled water for drinking and cooking. Add trace mineral drops to your drinking water.

❑ If you have a family history of kidney stones, take calcium supplements with meals. When you consume calcium-rich foods with oxalates, they bind together and are expelled in the stool, lessening your risk of kidney stones. Calcium supplements should be avoided only by those with a personal history of kidney stones.

Considerations

❑ Women who have both kidney stones and bone loss from osteoporosis can use calcium supplements, but have to be careful about what supplements they use and what they eat. A low-oxalate diet—no beet greens, parsley, rhubarb stems, spinach, and Swiss chard—combined with no more than 1,000 milligrams of calcium citrate daily helps osteoporosis without increasing the formation of new kidney stones. Dietary calcium from foods does not affect stone formation as much as taking calcium as supplements. Continue with calcium-rich foods to protect your bones unless your doctor advises against it. Supplements of calcium should be taken with meals. If you use calcium supplements, be sure to increase your intake of water, potassium, and phosphorus to reduce the risk of stone formation.

❑ Children with kidney stones especially benefit from an increase in dietary potassium intake. Citrus fruits or juices, bananas, and green leafy vegetables should be part of the child's daily diet.

❑ In some cases, drinking coffee, tea, and wine may lower the risk of kidney stones, while drinking grapefruit juice may increase it.

❑ The measures used to treat kidney stones and to prevent recurrences depend on the nature of the stone, so it is important to take any stone you pass to your health-care provider for analysis. There is some evidence that vitamin C is sometimes converted to calcium oxalate, which can become concentrated in the urine. This is a condition known as ascorbate-induced hyperoxaluria. For some people, this may result in the formation of kidney stones. This is rare, however. Such a response to vitamin C may be genetically determined, so if you have a family history of kidney stones, screening for ascorbate-induced hyperoxaluria is recommended. Alternatively, taking vitamin B_6 and magnesium may reduce oxalate stone formation.

❑ *See also* BLADDER INFECTION (CYSTITIS), HEPATITIS, and YEAST INFECTION (YEAST VAGINITIS).

LARYNGITIS

Laryngitis is a loss of voice caused by irritation, infection, or overuse of the vocal cords. The voice may sound weak, breathy, scratchy, or husky.

A wide range of disorders, ranging from cancer to smoking, can cause changes in voice quality. However, most cases of laryngitis are associated with allergies, asthma, colds, and flu, since any acute infection of the upper respiratory tract makes the mucosa lining the vocal cords vulnerable to injury. Coughing and clearing the throat, especially with exposure to tobacco smoke, irritate the vocal cords and may worsen or provoke hoarseness. Emotional distress can interfere with fine motor control of the voice box muscles. Stresses on the musculoskeletal system may cause problems with the voice. Many cases of laryngitis are associated with the upward movement of stomach acid after eating. The different causes of laryngitis produce variations in symptoms. Intermittent, unpredictable laryngitis is usually caused by allergies. Other respiratory disorders can cause hoarseness, excessive phlegm, and throat clearing that can last for a period of several days. Severe breathiness, or loss of air while speaking, may be asthma. Laryngitis that is more of a problem in the morning or that goes away after talking for a while is often associated with reflux of gastric acid. Hormonal conditions may produce volume disturbance, that is, an inability to speak loudly or softly. A tickle in the throat is a sign of irritation of the edges of the vocal cords. Pain while using the voice may be caused by excessive muscular activity in the neck.

Unless otherwise specified, the herb dosages recommended here are for adults, and some herbs are not suitable for children at all. Children under age six should be given one-quarter of the adult dosage. Children between the ages of six and twelve should be given one-half of the adult dosage. Formula dosages for children should be discussed with a knowledgeable health-care practitioner.

Laryngitis: Beneficial Herbs

Herb	Form and Dosage	Comments
Bibitaki	Tea (loose), prepared by steeping 1 tsp in 1 cup water. (*See* TEAS in Part Three.) Take 1 cup 3 times daily.	Relieves laryngitis associated with sore throat.
Coltsfoot[1]	Tea bag, prepared with 1 cup water. Take ½ cup 2–3 times daily.	Relieves hoarseness and acute congestion lasting no more than 2–3 days.
Couch grass	Tea (loose), prepared by steeping 1–3 tsp (2–6 gm) in 1 cup water. (*See* TEAS in Part Three.) Take 1 cup 3 times daily.	Loosens phlegm and makes speaking easier.
Fritillaria[2]	Ching chi hua tan tang syrup. Take as directed on the label.	Relieves laryngitis with sticky phlegm, snoring, and sore throat.
Lobelia[3]	Capsules. Take 500–1,000 mg 3 times daily. Use for no more than 2 weeks at a time.	Relieves laryngitis with dry, hacking cough.
Marshmallow root	Extract. Take 1 tsp (2 ml) in ¼ cup water 3 times daily. For children, use ¼ tsp (0.5 ml).	Relieves laryngitis with dry, hacking cough. Also called althea.
St. John's wort	Capsules. Take at least 900 mg daily for 2–3 months.	Relieves laryngitis and vocal pain associated with fibromyalgia.

Precautions for the use of herbs:

[1]In large doses, coltsfoot can cause bronchial passages to close, so do not take any more than is recommended. Do not give this herb to a child under age twelve.

[2]Do not use fritillaria if you are pregnant or nursing, or if you have high blood pressure.

[3]Do not give lobelia to a child under age twelve.

Laryngitis: Formulas

Formula	Comments
Pinellia and Magnolia Bark Decoction	A traditional Chinese herbal formula that treats "lump in the throat" caused by internal stress or conflict.

Recommendations

❑ The first, and best, treatment for laryngitis is to rest the voice. Avoid speaking and singing while the vocal cords hurt. Inhaling steam in a steam room or using a vaporizer also can help.

❑ Avoid eating immediately before speaking or singing. A full stomach can interfere with abdominal support, and the contraction of the abdominal muscles can result in reflux of gastric acids.

❑ Avoid chocolate and ice cream, especially before vocal performances. Although the exact reason why these foods frequently cause laryngitis is not known, allergy is likely.

❑ To treat laryngitis caused by reflux of stomach acid, avoid eating for three to four hours before going to bed, and elevate the head of the bed—propping up the head with pillows is not sufficient. It is important to treat the underlying condition. (See GASTRITIS.)

❑ Breathe through the nose. This allows air to be filtered, warmed, and humidified.

❑ Avoid tobacco smoke. Also keep in mind that marijuana smoke is even more irritating to the vocal cords than tobacco smoke, since marijuana smoke is unfiltered.

❑ Especially if you speak or sing often, keep the abdominal muscles toned with regular exercises such as sit-ups.

❑ Be sure to drink eight or more glasses of water daily when traveling by plane. Not only is the air in planes extremely dry, but cabin noise may force passengers to speak loudly. Avoid alcohol.

❑ Use antihistamines with caution for sore throat and postnasal drip. These agents can cause drying, which leads to decreased lubrication of the vocal folds, increased throat clearing, and frequent coughing.

Considerations

❑ It is important to avoid overtreating laryngitis. Antibiotics are of limited or no value in treating most cases, since laryngitis is rarely the result of bacterial infection. Vocal nodules, scars on the vocal cords, usually go away through voice therapy alone and rarely require surgery.

❑ Speaking or singing when you have a head cold will not harm your voice. However, taking high doses of vitamin C (5 to 6 grams or more daily) to prevent colds can lead to mild dehydration and cracking of the voice. If you are taking high doses of vitamin C, be sure to drink eight or more glasses of water daily.

❑ Coffee and other caffeine-containing beverages aggravate gastric reflux and seem to alter mucosal secretions, leading to frequent clearing of the throat in some people. On the other hand, lemon juice and herbal teas are both felt to be beneficial to the voice. Lemon acts as a demulcent, thinning mucosal secretions.

❑ Alcohol abuse damages the voice. Lack of coordination and decreased awareness of vocal stress lead to cumulative damage. In addition, cocaine is extremely irritating to the mucosal linings of the vocal cords and also causes loss of vocal control.

❑ Removal of the tonsils can alter the voice by changing the configuration of the vocal tract. In addition, scarring may alter muscle function in the voice box. It generally takes from three to six months for the voice to stabilize or return to normal following tonsillectomy.

❑ Laryngitis in women is not uncommon in the immediate premenstrual period, and is believed to be associated with hormonal changes. (See PREMENSTRUAL SYNDROME [PMS].) Contraceptive pills relieve some of these symptoms, but oral contraceptives also harm voice range and character in women taking them. The voice should be monitored carefully if oral contraceptives are used.

❑ Female singers and other women who are voice professionals with endometriosis may not be treated with testosterone, even at low dosages. Testosterone therapy can cause irreversible vocal unsteadiness, rapid changes in timbre, and lowering of the fundamental voice frequency. (See ENDOMETRIOSIS.)

❑ Laryngitis can be an indicator of systemic disorders. Even mild hypothyroidism can cause hoarseness, vocal fatigue, muffling, a loss of vocal range, a feeling of having a lump in the throat, or a feeling of having a veil over the voice. Being overweight and frequently feeling cold, along with laryngitis, is a strong indicator of underactive thyroid. Debilitating conditions such as chronic anemia or chronic viral infection may be noticed first as vocal fatigue. Myasthenia gravis may present itself as the voice breaking into high or low registers. (For more information, see ANEMIA, HYPOTHYROIDISM, and MYASTHENIA GRAVIS.)

❑ *See also* ALLERGIES; ASTHMA; COMMON COLD; COUGH; INFLUENZA; and STREP THROAT.

LEUKEMIA

Leukemia is an overall name for a group of cancers that originate in the blood-producing cells of the bone marrow. Most leukemias are classified by two major criteria: the cell of origin (lymphoid or myeloid) and the course of the disease (acute or chronic). Acute leukemias tend to develop more rapidly than chronic forms.

The two main acute leukemias are acute lymphocytic leukemia (ALL) and acute myelogenous leukemia (AML). ALL is the most common leukemia in children but it is also the rarest overall. Acute myelogenous leukemia is more common and occurs at all ages but is most common in adults aged sixty-five years and older. Symptoms include fatigue; weight loss; shortness of breath; blood in the stool, urine, or sputum; easy bruising; repeated infections; slow wound healing; and nosebleeds. Acute leukemia tends to spread to the liver, lymph nodes, and spleen.

The two main chronic leukemias are chronic myelogenous (or granulocytic) leukemia (CML) and chronic lymphocytic leukemia (CLL), both of which occur mainly in

Leukemia: Beneficial Herbs

Herb	Form and Dosage	Comments
Boswellia	Boswellin. Take as directed on the label.	Stops uncontrolled growth cycle of leukemia cells in lab tests.
Dong quai	*Angelica sinensis* fluidextract. Take ½ tsp (2 ml) in ¼ cup water 3 times daily.	Protects healthy white blood cells during chemotherapy.
Garlic	Enteric-coated tablets. Take at least 900 mg daily.	Induces apoptosis (cellular suicide) of leukemia cells in laboratory tests.
Green tea	Catechin extract. Take 250 mg 3 times daily; or tea bag, prepared with 1 cup water. Take 1 cup 2–5 times daily. To prevent dilution, do not use within 1 hour of taking other medications.	Supplies free-radical scavengers. Stops proliferation of cancer cells.
Hawthorn	Capsules. Take 3–5 gm daily.	Contains rutin, which accelerates death of leukemia cells.
Kelp	Take at least ¼ cup one day per week.	Stimulates the immune system to fight leukemia.
Kudzu	Tablets. Take 10 mg 3 times daily.	Contains daidzein, which stops growth of certain strains of leukemia cells.
Polysaccharide kureha (PSK)	Tablets. Take 6,000 mg daily.	Stops invasion of normal tissues by leukemia cells.
Red wine catechins	Resveratrol tablets. Take as directed on the label.	Reverses genetic damage that causes healthy cells to turn cancerous.
Turmeric	Curcumin tablets. Take 250–500 mg twice daily, between meals.	Causes death of leukemia cells. (*See under* Recommendations, page 382.)
Zedoary root	Tea (loose), prepared by steeping 1 tsp (1gm) in 1 cup water. (*See* TEAS in Part Three.) Take 1 cup 3 times daily.	Contains elemene, which stops division of leukemia cells in laboratory tests.

Leukemia: Formulas

Formula	Comments
Essiac	A modern herbal formula that contains aloe-emodin, which kills some strains of leukemia cells in laboratory tests.
Hoxsey Formula	A modern herbal formula that contains berberine and emodin, which kill certain strains of leukemia cells under laboratory conditions.
Minor Bupleurum Decoction[1]	A traditional Chinese herbal formula that is especially appropriate for people who also have either HIV or hepatitis. Reduces the rate at which some leukemia-causing viruses can reproduce, without interfering with T cell reproduction.
Polyporus Decoction	A traditional Chinese herbal formula that stops reproduction of some kinds of leukemia cells. Useful if other symptoms include urinary difficulty accompanied by fever and thirst, sometimes with diarrhea, nausea, cough, or insomnia.

Precautions for the use of formulas:

[1]Do not use Minor Bupleurum Decoction if you have a fever or a skin infection. Taken long term, it can cause headache, dizziness, and bleeding gums. Side effects can be avoided if the formula is taken as a tea.

adults. The symptoms tend to be more subtle than those of acute leukemia, and include abdominal fullness, a "rundown" feeling, sweating, and easy bruising. The spleen, where chronic leukemia concentrates its effects, may be enlarged, causing a feeling of fullness in the left side of the abdomen. Diagnosis of the precise form of leukemia in each case is made by taking a bone marrow biopsy. Chemotherapy is the main conventional treatment for leukemia.

Different types of leukemia have different risk factors. In adults, smoking is associated with all forms. Some types are associated with environmental hazards, such as exposure to industrial solvents or radiation (including radiation treatment for other forms of cancer). Others are linked to genetic disorders such as Down's syndrome. Still others are linked to a family history of leukemia.

All forms of leukemia increase the number of white blood cells and decrease the number of red blood cells. White blood cells are essential for fighting infection. While the total number of white cells rises dramatically in leukemia, the bone marrow fails to produce all the different kinds of white cells the body needs to fight infection. At the same time, the body's resources for producing red blood cells are consumed by the production of the cancerous white blood cells. In particular, the bone cannot produce platelets, which stop bleeding.

Herbal medicine should be part of a medically directed overall leukemia treatment program. Especially in treating childhood leukemia, always work with an herbal practitioner along with the physician; the dosages provided in this entry are meant for adults.

Recommendations

❏ Take a multivitamin with vitamin D. In laboratory conditions, vitamin D helped return leukemia cells to a normal growth cycle and gave them a growth advantage over cancerous cells. The effects of vitamin D also enhance the leukemia-fighting effects of curcumin and green tea polyphenols, according to laboratory studies. It also increases the leukemia-fighting effects of lycopene, the red pigment found in tomatoes. Bone damage often occurs in children with leukemia, so it is important to make sure they consume 2 to 3 servings of milk a day, take calcium and vitamin D supplements, or both. Speak to your child's oncologist regarding what is best for your child.

❏ Supplement your diet with omega-3 fatty acids, which are needed for the formation of hormones and pain-regulating chemicals. Flaxseed oil and fish oil are good sources. Omega-3 fatty acids make leukemia cells more susceptible to vitamin D. The beneficial effects of omega-3 fatty acids are most pronounced in AML.

❏ Take 250 to 500 milligrams of coenzyme Q_{10} (Co-Q_{10}) daily. This supplement helps the heart recover from the effects of chemotherapy, and helps prevent virally induced leukemia.

❏ Avoid slimming diets after treatment for leukemia. Restricted food intake can deprive the body of essential micronutrients it needs to stay in remission.

Considerations

❏ In leukemia treatment, different types of drugs and administration methods are used for different specific diseases. Chemotherapy-resistant leukemias may be treated with interferon, a naturally occurring immune component. In addition, there are targeted therapies that use drugs such as imatinib (Gleevec). Imatinib is in a class of medications called protein-tyrosine kinase inhibitors. It works by blocking the action of the abnormal protein that signals cancer cells to multiply. This helps stop the spread of cancer cells. Doctors sometimes treat cases that do not respond to these methods with a stem cell transplant.

❏ Asparaginase (Elspar) is a drug used to treat ALL that kills leukemia cells by breaking down the amino acid asparagin (the amide of aspartic acid), which healthy tissues can create on their own but which leukemia cells need to obtain from the bloodstream. Without asparagine, cells cannot multiply. After completing the asparaginase phase of chemotherapy, use whole-soy products, such as tofu or cooked soybeans, in your daily meal plans. (Be sure to use cooked soybeans, as raw beans can cause the breakdown of red blood cells.) Soy is a rich source of natural L-asparagine, which may replace asparagine depleted by the drug. However, do not give soy foods to children under age six, since soy contains a chemical that interferes with the mechanisms that inhibit leukemia-cell growth.

❏ Bone marrow transplants for acute leukemia can—in rare cases—transfer celiac disease from the donor to the recipient. (See CELIAC DISEASE.)

❏ Japanese clinical tests in cell lines have found that the traditional Chinese herbal formula Shih Qua Da Bu Tang (All-Inclusive Great Tonifying Decoction) prevents leukemia caused by chemotherapy for other forms of cancer. (See SHIH QUA DA BU TANG under The Formulas in Part One.)

❏ In one study, patients with myelogenous leukemia who were undergoing chemotherapy took a probiotic called Enterococcus faecium M-74. The strain was well tolerated but was not effective at reducing low blood counts and fever due to chemotherapy. It is possible that other healthy probiotics may work better than this one.

❏ For measures to reduce side effects and increase effectiveness when using chemotherapy, see "Side Effects of Cancer Treatment" under CANCER.

LEUKODERMA

See VITILIGO.

LIVER CANCER

Liver cancer is usually an end result of another liver disorder, such as hepatitis C or cirrhosis, or the spread of cancer from another part of the body, such as the colon or breast. Factors that can contribute to the development of liver cancer include alcohol, exposure to carcinogens such as aflatoxin, and a history of hepatitis. Possible symptoms include abdominal pain, a severe form of abdominal swelling known as ascites, jaundice, weakness, and loss of both appetite and weight. However, these symptoms usually appear only when the disease is advanced. The liver may be enlarged, and hard masses may be present. A diagnosis of liver cancer is confirmed by biopsy.

Surgery may be used for localized growths, although liver cancer often occurs as multiple tumors. A number of different chemotherapy drugs may be used. In addition, doctors may employ a targeted drug therapy, such as sorafenib (Nexavar), which is designed to interfere with a tumor's ability to generate new blood vessels.

For information about appropriate treatment of secondary liver cancer, see the appropriate entry for the type of primary cancer involved, such as breast cancer or lung cancer. Be aware that some herbs may have a negative impact

Liver Cancer: Beneficial Herbs

Herb	Form and Dosage	Comments
Astragalus[1]	Capsules. Take 500–1,000 mg 3 times daily.	Stimulates lymphokine-activated killer (LAK) cells to attack tumors.
Barberry[2] or coptis[2] or goldenseal[2] or Oregon grape root[2]	Capsules. Take 500 mg of any of these herbs daily.	Herbs that contain berberine, which stops multiplication of liver cancer cells.
Cinnamon	Freshly grated. Eat at least 1 tsp daily, in food.	Deactivates plasmin, a substance that allows cancer cells to invade healthy tissues.
Lentinan	Injection, given by health-care practitioner.	Slows the growth of liver tumors.
Reishi	Tablets. Take 3 gm daily.	Helps to stop the progression of liver cancer.
Scutellaria[3]	Capsules. Take 1–2 gm 3 times daily.	Induces death of liver-cancer cells. Stops chemotherapy-caused immune-system damage.
Soy lecithin[4]	Capsules. Take 3,000 mg daily.	Stops free-radical reactions in cancer development.

Precautions for the use of herbs:

[1]Do not use astragalus if you have a fever or a skin infection.

[2]Do not use barberry, coptis, goldenseal, or Oregon grape root if you are pregnant or have gallbladder disease. Do not take these herbs with supplemental vitamin B_6 or with protein supplements containing the amino acid histidine. Do not use goldenseal if you have cardiovascular disease or glaucoma.

[3]Do not use scutellaria if you have diarrhea.

[4]Soy lecithin may cause mild diarrhea when you first use it.

Liver Cancer: Formulas

Formula	Comments
Essiac	A North American formula that helps to stop cancers from developing their own blood supplies and using glucose efficiently. Also stimulates production of white blood cells, making it useful during chemotherapy.
Major Bupleurum Decoction[1]	A traditional Chinese herbal formula that controls symptoms of liver cancer, including alternating fever and chills, bitter taste in the mouth, nausea, continuous vomiting, burning diarrhea or no bowel movements, fullness in the chest with or without pain, and irritability.
Minor Bupleurum Decoction[2]	A traditional Chinese herbal formula that controls progression of liver cancer. Keeps cancer cells from multiplying without reducing production of blood cells. Also prevents the progression of chronic hepatitis to liver cancer. Also known, for this application, as Xiao Chai Hu Tang.

Precautions for the use of formulas:

[1]Do not use Major Bupleurum Decoction if you have a fever.

[2]Do not use Minor Bupleurum Decoction if you have a fever or a skin infection. Taken long term, it can cause headache, dizziness, and bleeding gums. Side effects can be avoided if the formula is taken as a tea.

on the liver and/or interact negatively with conventional medicines. When dealing with cancer, you should always work with a qualified health-care practitioner.

Recommendations

❑ Use safflower and perilla oils in salad dressings and for cooking. These oils are rich in the polyunsaturated omega-6 fatty acids that suppress the development of liver cancer in laboratory tests. On the other hand, avoid supplemental omega-3 fatty acids, such as MaxEPA and fish oil, since these fatty acids can promote the spread of cancers to the liver.

❑ Eat foods rich in the amino acid arginine, such as chocolate, coconut, hazelnuts, and sunflower seeds; all protein sources are rich in this amino acid as well. Animal studies show that supplementation with arginine prevents the growth of liver tumors without depriving the rest of the body of essential protein.

❑ Eat Jerusalem artichokes. They contain inulin, which in laboratory tests slows the growth of liver tumors.

❑ Avoid the supplement s-adenosyl methionine (SAMe). In animal tests, methionine stimulates the growth of liver cancers. Use the following methionine-rich foods in limited quantities (no more than one serving per week): dairy products except whole milk, fish, garbanzo beans, lima beans, meat, mushrooms, and all nuts except coconut, hazelnut, and sunflower seeds.

❑ If you have any chronic liver disease and develop itching all over, see a physician who will order an alpha-fetoprotein test. This itching, caused by bile salts accumulating near the surface of the skin, can be a symptom of the early stages of liver cancer.

Considerations

❑ People who have fevers or are receiving interferon cannot take Minor Bupleurum Decoction, but they can take the herb milk thistle. Silybinin, a chemical in milk thistle, protects the liver's Kuppfer cells from inflammation. These specialized immune cells engulf foreign matter in the liver, and also play a role in destroying cancer cells that have entered the bloodstream. Silybinin acts without interfering with tumor necrosis factor (TNF), an immune-system chemical that accelerates the destruction of cancer cells. This herb is available in a standardized form that delivers 120 milligrams of silymarin in a 500-milligram capsule. It is also possible to use 500-milligram capsules of milk thistle seeds themselves. Take either form three times daily. Or make milk thistle tea by placing ⅓ to ½ ounce (12 to 15 grams) of seed in 2 cups (500 milliliters) of boiling water, and allowing it to steep for forty-five minutes. Strain and drink one-third of the tea in three doses per day. Since milk thistle tinctures are made with alcohol, people with liver cancer must avoid them. There are no human data on using silymarin to treat liver cancer. However,

those with end-stage liver disease had reduced tumor activity from getting an under-the-skin (subcutaneous) injection of an extract of mistletoe herb.

❑ In one study, a traditional Chinese medicine herb, *Bletilla striata*, worked to shrink the liver tumor, decrease the blood levels of alpha fetoprotein, and improved survival in patients compared to a control group.

❑ Several herbs have been shown to lower the risk of developing liver cancer in laboratory studies. Bitter orange contains monoterpenes, which stop liver tumors before they can get started. Take 1 cup of the tea daily; use 1 teaspoon (2 to 3 grams) per cup. (*See* TEAS in Part Three.) Green tea prevents liver cancer development—as long as viral hepatitis is not present—if soy lecithin is also taken. Drink 2 to 5 cups of green tea a day, or take 250 milligrams of green-tea catechins three times daily. Licorice and scutellaria have been used together in tea form to help prevent hepatitis C from progressing to liver cancer, but there are no current human studies to support this. Take 1 cup of each (from bags) daily. Avoid licorice in cases of glaucoma, high blood pressure, or disorders affected by estrogen, such as diseases of the female reproductive system. Use for six weeks, then take a two-week break. Consume a potassium-rich food, such as bananas or citrus juices, or take a potassium supplement, daily when taking this herb. Avoid scutellaria during diarrhea.

❑ To lower the risk of developing liver cancer, take 150 micrograms of selenium (any form except seleno-methionine) daily on an ongoing basis. A clinical trial in China involving over 100,000 people found that taking supplemental selenium reduced the rate of liver cancer by 35 percent over an eight-year period. When the selenium supplement was discontinued, liver cancer rates began to rise again. However, this study was conducted in a region of China where selenium intake is inadequate. If this study had been conducted in the United States where there is no selenium deficiency, the study would not have shown a decrease in liver cancer. Selenium may be helpful for people infected with hepatitis B, however.

❑ Smoking, drinking, and inadequate vitamin A intake increase the risk of liver cancer in people infected with hepatitis B. The effect is especially severe for men who smoke more than ten cigarettes per day. Eating one to three servings of leafy green, yellow, or orange vegetables per week provides sufficient A vitamins to reduce the risk of liver cancer as much as 80 percent among men who have hepatitis B.

❑ The grain contaminant aflatoxin greatly increases the risk of developing liver cancer. It causes mutations in the p53 gene, which "patrols" for and deactivates developing cancer cells. Always consume only fresh cereals and flour products. Also, eat green leafy vegetables on a daily basis. Animal studies indicate that chlorophyll reduces the cancer-causing capacity of aflatoxin.

❑ Patients with liver cancer have derived benefit in controlling pain through acupressure, acupuncture, deep breathing exercises, music, and massage.

❑ For measures to reduce the side effects and increase the effectiveness of chemotherapy and/or radiation therapy, see "Side Effects of Cancer Treatment" under CANCER. To learn about herbal treatments that can prevent a cancer from developing its own blood supply, see CANCER.

❑ See also CIRRHOSIS OF THE LIVER, ALCOHOLISM and HEPATITIS.

LIVER DISEASE

See CIRRHOSIS OF THE LIVER; HEPATITIS; LIVER CANCER.

LUNG CANCER

Lung cancer is one the most common forms of cancer; every year it is diagnosed in approximately 100,000 men and 90,000 women in the United States. The most significant risk factor is smoking—smokers are ten to twenty times more likely to get lung cancer. Passive exposure to secondhand smoke increases one's risk approximately 20 to 30 percent. Exposure to asbestos, pollution, or industrial metals also increases risk of developing this disease, as does radon gas exposure. Family history of lung cancer, and other lung diseases, such as chronic obstructive pulmonary disease (COPD), are also risk factors. More people in the United States die from lung cancer than any other type of cancer. This is true for both men and women.

Symptoms of lung cancer include cough, bloody or rusty sputum, hoarseness, and wheezing. There may be chest pain that radiates from the shoulder to the arm, as well as shortness of breath, loss of appetite, fever, and/or weight loss. The symptoms often appear late in the course of the disease. Most lung cancers take one of two main forms: small cell lung cancer usually found in heavy smokers and non–small cell lung cancer, which is an umbrella for several types, including squamous cell carcinoma, adenocarcinoma, and large cell carcinoma. In addition, cancers that originate elsewhere in the body may spread to the lung.

Many lung cancers can be detected by chest X-ray. In some cases, a CAT (computerized axial tomography) scan, which is more sensitive, is needed to find small tumors. The diagnosis must then be confirmed via a biopsy. At that

Lung Cancer: Beneficial Herbs

Herb	Form and Dosage	Comments
Aloe[1]	Juice. Take ¼ cup (60 ml) daily.	Stops processes that convert chemicals in tobacco smoke into carcinogens.
Astragalus[2]	Capsules. Take 1,000 mg 3 times daily.	Stimulates T cells and lymphokine-activated killer (LAK) cells to attack lung cancer.
Astragalus[2] and ginseng	Tincture. Take ½ tsp (2 ml) in ¼ cup water 3 times daily. *Panax ginseng* tincture. Take ½ tsp (2 ml) in ¼ cup water 3 times daily.	Stimulates the immune system. Can greatly increase longevity if chemotherapy is given.
Cat's claw[3]	Tincture. Take the dose recommended on the label in ½ cup water with 1 tsp lemon juice.	Immune stimulant. Reportedly has brought about some remissions from lung cancer.
Cayenne	Powder. Use at least 1 tbsp in cooking daily.	Stops conversion of a chemical in tobacco smoke to its carcinogenic form.
Espinheira santa	Tincture. Take as directed on the label.	Toxic to several kinds of lung cancer cells.
Lentinan	Intramuscular injection, given by health-care provider.	Increases survival time in secondary lung cancer.
Polysaccharide kureha (PSK)	Tablets. Take 6,000 mg daily.	Extends longevity if radiation therapy is given.
Psoralea[4]	Psoralea seed, scruffy pea, or bu gu zhi capsules. Take 1,000 mg 3 times daily. Use under professional supervision.	Contains compounds that inhibit lung cancer.
Scutellaria[5]	Capsules. Take 1,000–2,000 mg 3 times daily.	Stops inflammatory processes. Relieves cough.
Soy isoflavone concentrate	Tablets. Take 3,000 mg daily.	Induces death of lung cancer cells.
Turmeric	Curcumin tablets. Take 250 mg 3 times daily.	Activates cancer-disabling gene p53 to fight small cell lung cancer.

Precautions for the use of herbs:

[1]Do not take aloe vera juice internally if you have diarrhea.

[2]Do not use astragalus if you have a fever or a skin infection.

[3]Do not use cat's claw if you have to take insulin for diabetes. Do not use it if you are pregnant or nursing. Do not give it to a child under age six.

[4]Psoralea increases sensitivity to sunlight. Use sunscreen and avoid exposure to the sun while using this herb.

[5]Do not use scutellaria if you have diarrhea.

Lung Cancer: Formulas

Formula	Comments
Six-Ingredient Pill with Rehmannia[1]	A traditional Chinese herbal formula that significantly increases life expectancy in Chinese clinical tests involving people with lung cancer who also underwent chemotherapy or radiation therapy.

Precautions for the use of formulas:

[1]Do not use Six-Ingredient Pill with Rehmannia if you have an estrogen-sensitive disorder, such as breast cancer, endometriosis, or fibrocystic breast disease. Do not use it if lung cancer is secondary to cancer of the breast, cervix, or uterus.

point the cancer is classified according to tumor size and how extensively it has spread.

Conventional treatment includes surgery for small, localized tumors. However, since lung cancers usually spread before they are detected, the main treatments are chemotherapy, using a wide variety of drugs, and radiation therapy. Radiation therapy directed to the lung cancer part of the lung and newer drugs that target the tumor also are used.

Always use herbal medicine as part of a medically directed overall treatment plan for lung cancer. In cases of secondary lung cancer, see the primary-cancer entry, such as BREAST CANCER, for additional information and treatments.

Recommendations

❏ The most obvious step is, if you smoke, stop, and avoid all secondhand tobacco smoke. Continued exposure to tobacco smoke makes it that much harder to overcome the cancer, and may promote the development of other lung disorders that can further reduce lung capacity.

❏ Eat parsley daily. It contains myristicin, which, in preliminary cell studies tests, activates the detoxifying enzyme glutathione S-transferase (GST) and reduces the formation of lung tumors.

❏ Take the recommended daily dosage of any folic acid supplement, unless you are receiving chemotherapy with MTA, UFT, tegafur, or fluorouracil (which act by depriving cancer cells of folic acid). A study at the New England Medical Center found that lung-cancer survivors who took folic acid supplements had an average cancer-free period of forty-one months, compared with eleven months for those who did not. For additional benefits, also take 500 milligrams of vitamin B_{12} (cobalamin). These vitamins, used together, may help prevent lung damage in smokers.

❏ Take natural sources of gamma-linolenic acid (GLA), such as borage seed oil or evening primrose oil, except during chemotherapy with cisplatin. GLA encourages the growth of healthy cells and stops the growth of lung cancer cells in a laboratory setting, but interferes with the ability of cisplatin to kill cancer cells. Fish oil supplements also seem to be of benefit to patients with lung cancer. It

seems that the fish oil works as an immune-modulator by making the immune system stronger. In one study, taking 2 grams of fish oil three times a day with celecoxib (Celebrex), a drug that also favorably affects immune function, made the patients feel less tired and increased their appetites.

❏ Avoid taking vitamin E during chemotherapy for drug-resistant cancer. Vitamin E protects cancer cells from agents that make them more sensitive to doxorubicin hydrochloride (Adriamycin) and vinblastine sulfate (Velban).

❏ A diet high in fruits and vegetables is associated with a reduced risk of lung cancer.

Considerations

❏ To help prevent lung cancer, include apples, black tea, carrots, and tomatoes in your diet. One Swedish study found that eating carrots was the most important factor in avoiding lung cancer among people who had never smoked. Among women, consumption of lycopene, which is found in tomatoes, is associated with lowered risk of lung cancer. Drinking two or more cups of black tea daily reduces the risk of developing lung cancer, especially in light smokers, and eating apples, in one study, reduced the risk of developing lung cancer by over 50 percent.

❏ Women, in particular, should avoid eating well-done, fried red meat. A study by the National Cancer Institute found that every ⅓-ounce increase in average daily consumption of well-done, fried red meat increased lifetime risk of contracting lung cancer by 4 to 9 percent, with the increase in risk becoming greater as more fried meat was consumed.

❏ Take 150 to 200 micrograms of selenium daily, especially if you smoke. In one study, those taking 200 micrograms of selenium a day had a 25 percent lower risk of getting lung and other cancers such as colon and prostate. However, taking more than 200 micrograms had no additional effect on reducing lung cancer risk. Low selenium levels, especially in combination with low vitamin E levels and heavy smoking, are strongly associated with increased risk of lung cancer. But do not take beta-carotene supplements if you smoke. Studies have found that such supplements have no preventive value against lung cancer and may even increase the risk of lung cancer in men who smoke. That is because beta-carotene converts some of the toxic chemicals found in tobacco smoke into a carcinogenic form. This effect is likely only to occur if consumption of beta-carotene is not balanced by consumption of the other carotenes naturally occurring in fruits and vegetables. Instead of taking supplements to get your beta-carotene, eat more fruits and vegetables.

❑ For measures to reduce side effects and increase the effectiveness of chemotherapy and/or radiation therapy, *see* "Side Effects of Cancer Treatment" *under* CANCER. To learn about herbal treatments that can prevent a cancer from developing its own blood supply, *see* CANCER. Other things that the American College of Chest Physicians has found helpful for patients with lung cancer include acupuncture, hypnosis, massage, meditation, and yoga.

LUPUS

Lupus (systemic lupus erythematosus, or SLE) is a chronic inflammatory condition that affects connective tissue. For some people, the first sign of the disease is a butterfly-shaped rash over the nose and cheeks that looks a bit like the facial markings of a wolf. This is the reason the disease is termed lupus, which in Latin means "wolf." Another form of lupus, discoid lupus erythematosus (DLE), primarily affects the hair follicles and skin on the scalp, and two other forms, subacute cutaneous lupus erythematosus (SCLE) and acute cutaneous lupus erythematosus (ACLE), affect only the skin.

About 90 percent of all people who have lupus are women. Most are young adults. Genetic factors play a strong role in lupus. But there are other risk factors associated with this disorder, including stress, infections, severe drug reactions, and viral infection.

Because lupus affects many parts of the body, it produces many different symptoms. These include scaling skin lesions, nausea, headaches, diarrhea and/or constipation, malaise, fatigue, weight loss, a red rash, mouth sores, and a heightened sensitivity to the sun. Mental symptoms include confusion, irritability, and depression. Attacks of lupus can induce arthritis, with both swollen joints and fever, and can destroy tissues in the lungs, spleen, heart, and brain, and especially the kidneys. Not everyone experiences all of these symptoms, however, and the range and variability of symptoms can make lupus a difficult disease to diagnose.

Lupus: Beneficial Herbs

Herb	Form and Dosage	Comments
Chamomile	German chamomile (*Matricaria recutita*) tea bag, prepared with 1 cup water. Drink 1 cup as desired.	Stops formation of the tissue-destructive hormone IL-8.
Codonopsis	Tablets. Take 1 gm 3 times daily.	Decreases the formation of antibodies that target DNA in healthy cells.
Feverfew[1]	Capsules. Take 1,000 mg daily for as long as symptoms persist.	Relieves inflammation and pain in joints.
Hawthorn	Tablets. Take 100–250 mg 3 times daily.	Relieves fatigue caused by exercise or exertion.
Hoelen[2]	Tea, brewed with 1 cup water and a tea bag containing 1.5 gm hoelen for 20 minutes. Take 1 cup 3 times daily.	Regulates the immune system to stop inflammation. Particularly protects kidney tissue.
Licorice[3]	Glycyrrhizin tablets. Take 200–800 mg daily, depending on the severity of symptoms. Use for 6 weeks, then take a 2-week break. Do not substitute deglycyrrhizinated licorice (DGL).	Relieves pain and inflammation. Increases effectiveness of steroids, especially prednisolone. Consume potassium-rich foods such as bananas or citrus juices, or take a potassium supplement, daily when taking this herb.
Milk thistle	Silymarin gelcaps. Take as directed on the label.	Cleanses and protects the liver.
Stinging nettle root[4]	Capsules or tablets. Take 600–900 mg daily.	Stops arthritic inflammation and pain; may prevent tissue damage.
Tripterygium[5]	Tincture. Take as directed on the label.	"Retires" tissue-destructive T cells. Contains chemicals more potent than steroids and cyclophosphamide.

Precautions for the use of herbs:

[1]Discontinue use of feverfew if any signs of allergic reactions occur.

[2]Do not use hoelen if you have a long-term illness that causes excessive urination.

[3]Do not use licorice if you have glaucoma, high blood pressure, or an estrogen-dependent disorder, such as breast cancer, endometriosis, or fibrocystic breasts.

[4]Be sure to use the root, not the leaf, of stinging nettle. The leaf stimulates urination, which can increase discomfort in men with enlarged prostates.

[5]Men seeking to become fathers should not use tripterygium. Tinctures of this herb temporarily reduce sperm counts. Counts usually return to normal 2–4 weeks after the herb is discontinued.

Lupus: Formulas

Formula	Comments
Ginseng Decoction to Nourish the Nutritive Chi	A traditional Chinese herbal formula that increases the effectiveness of prednisolone. Many patent medicines offer a variation that substitutes codonopsis for the traditional ginseng (*Panax ginseng*). This substitution of a cheaper herb actually makes the formula more effective for lupus.
Sairei-to	A combination of two traditional Chinese herbal formulas: Five-Ingredient Powder with Poria and Minor Bupleurum Decoction. Reduces the number of antibodies that destroy skin DNA and relieves pain and swelling.

Lupus is caused by a misdirected attack by the body's white blood cells on its own organs. This happens when the immune system produces antibodies, which normally attack infectious microorganisms that "lock on to" and attack DNA in the skin cells. In some people with lupus, another immune-system component called the T cell becomes involved. If this happens, the immune response is even stronger than normal, and greatly increases the severity of symptoms.

Because DNA is normally contained within the cells, the antibodies are activated only if skin cells are damaged by some other event, such as sunburn or the natural aging process. For this reason, lupus is characterized by periodic attacks followed by remissions. Without treatment, however, each subsequent attack produces worse symptoms than the episode preceding it.

Conventional medicine uses drugs to control lupus. Herbal medicine's ability to make steroid drugs more effective is one of its most helpful modern applications in treating lupus. This minimizes the side effects of the drugs and extends lupus control over days when steroids are not taken.

Herbs to Avoid

❏ People with lupus should use any immune-stimulating herb with caution. Herbs that stimulate the immune system's response to infection also stimulate the production of interleukins, which cause inflammation and tissue death. People with lupus should also avoid alfalfa, ephedra, and ginkgo. (For more information regarding these herbs, *see* ALFALFA, EPHEDRA, and GINKGO *under* The Herbs in Part One.)

Recommendations

❏ To fight infections without stimulating the components of the immune system that aggravate lupus, use astragalus or scutellaria. In laboratory studies, astragalus increases activity of natural killer (NK) cells, which fight infection. For people who are responding well to steroid drugs, taking astragalus may reduce the risk of infection, especially when infections are "going around." Take 500 to 1,000 milligrams of the freeze-dried herb in capsules three times daily. However, be sure to let the doctor know

if you are taking astragalus, since it increases the body's response to steroids. Do not take astragalus for more than two out of every four weeks, and avoid it altogether if not taking steroids. Scutellaria inhibits several types of bacterial infections in cell line studies, including staph and strep. Take 250 to 500 milligrams of the powdered solid extract three times daily. Do not use this treatment if you have diarrhea.

❏ For colds and coughs, use fritillaria. Take the syrup (Ching chi hua tan tang) as directed on the label. Do not use fritillaria if you have high blood pressure, or if pregnant or nursing.

❏ Avoid alfalfa sprouts as well as herbal products made from alfalfa. Instead, try sunflower sprouts or broccoli sprouts. Other tasty sprouts are buckwheat sprouts, sometimes used in Japanese cuisine, and radish sprouts, which many people find refreshingly spicy.

❏ Take 500 milligrams of black currant oil twice daily. This oil is a particularly useful source of an essential fatty acid, gamma-linolenic acid (GLA), which helps reduce inflammatory reactions. In one study, patients with lupus and kidney damage were given 30 grams of ground flaxseed daily for one year. Unfortunately, a lot of people dropped out, so the results were hard to interpret, but those who stayed in the study showed improvement in creatinine levels in the blood, an indicator of better kidney function. In another study, taking 3 grams of fish oil a day produced significant improvements in several markers of disease burden, which indicate how sick a patient is.

❏ Take 200 to 600 international units (IU) of vitamin E several times a week. One study showed that the combination of vitamin E (800 IU) and vitamin C (500 milligrams) daily reduced markers of lipid peroxidation, which means there is less damage to tissues in the body by free oxygen radicals. However, there was no improvement in blood flow or reducing the risk of heart disease, which is common in these patients. At least once or twice a week, get vitamin E from vitamin-rich foods such as nuts and seeds rather than from a supplement.

❏ Take 500 milligrams of L-carnitine daily if you experience fatigue after physical exertion. L-carnitine may help the heart muscle use fats to produce energy. The supplement may also protect the heart from damage during treatment with the drug cyclophosphamide.

❏ Avoid sunburn by avoiding sun exposure between 10 A.M. and 3 P.M. If you must be outside during these hours, wear pants (not shorts), a long-sleeved shirt, and a hat, and use sunscreen on all exposed skin.

❏ Include in your diet brown rice, fish, green leafy vegetables, nonacidic fresh fruits, oatmeal, and whole grains.

❏ Get your iron from food sources, not from supplements, unless you have been diagnosed with anemia by a health-care professional. Get plenty of rest and regular moderate exercise that promotes muscle tone and fitness.

❏ If you take birth control pills, speak to your doctor about switching to another form of contraception. Birth control pills may cause lupus to flare up.

Considerations

❏ Mild cases of lupus are treated with painkillers such as aspirin or ibuprofen. Other methods involve treating specific signs and symptoms, such as joint pain with nonsteroidal anti-inflammatory drugs (NSAIDs) and skin rashes with corticosteroids. Treatments for aggressive lupus include high-dose steroids and immunosuppressive drugs such as cyclophosphamide (Cytoxan) and azathioprine (Imuran). Although these drugs are useful in preventing lupus attacks, they have many side effects.

❏ Lupus and its treatments make weight control very difficult. The disease tends to destroy organ and muscle cells but not fat cells, so it is not only possible but likely that a person with lupus will lose weight and gain fat at the same time, even if exercising dietary restraint. (For additional information on weight control, see OVERWEIGHT.)

❏ If chronic pain is a concern, see PAIN, CHRONIC.

❏ See also KIDNEY DISEASE.

LYME DISEASE

Lyme disease is a chronic inflammatory disease caused by the bacterium *Borrelia burgdorferi,* which is transmitted by the bite of a deer tick or black-legged tick. Lyme disease was first described in the United States in the town of Old Lyme, Connecticut, in 1975, but it has now been reported in most parts of the country. Most cases occur in the Northeast, upper Midwest, and Pacific Coast. Mice and deer are the most commonly infected animals that serve as host to the tick.

Lyme Disease: Beneficial Herbs

Herb	Form and Dosage	Comments
Cat's claw[1]	Capsules. Take 2,000 mg daily.	General immune stimulant.
Echinacea[2] plus ginseng	*Echinacea purpurea* tincture. Take as directed on the label. *Panax ginseng* tea (loose), prepared by steeping 1 tsp (2 gm) in 1 cup water. (See TEAS in Part Three.) Take 1 cup daily.	A combination that increases activity of immune cells called natural killer (NK) cells. Fights secondary infections. Ginseng also controls emotional disturbances.
Kudzu	Tablets. Take 10 mg 3 times daily.	Relieves tension in the muscles of the face and neck.
Lentinan	Powder. Use the dosage determined by your health-care provider.	Reverses fever and fatigue. Activates T-helper cells.
Licorice[3]	Glycyrrhizin tablets. Take 200–800 mg daily, depending on severity of symptoms. Use for 6 weeks, then take a 2-week break. Do not substitute deglycyrrhizinated licorice (DGL).	Helps to prevent progression of neurological symptoms. Counteracts chronic fatigue. Consume potassium-rich foods such as bananas or citrus juices, or take a potassium supplement, daily when taking this herb.
Maitake	Maitake-D. Take 500 mg 3 times daily.	Stimulates general immune function; fights infection.
Red clover	Extract. Take as directed on the label.	Cleanses the bloodstream.
Scutellaria[4]	Capsules. Take 1,000–2,000 mg 3 times daily.	An antibacterial and antiviral.
Siberian ginseng[5]	Pure *Eleutherococcus senticosus* extract. Take as directed on the label.	Increases resistance to stress. Increases activity of NK and T cells.
St. John's wort	Capsules. Take 900 mg of total hypericin daily.	An antidepressant. Also stops inflammatory reactions.

Precautions for the use of herbs:

[1]Do not use cat's claw if you have to take insulin for diabetes. Do not use it if you are pregnant or nursing.

[2]Avoid echinacea if you have an autoimmune disease such as rheumatoid arthritis or lupus. Do not use it if you have a chronic infection such as HIV or tuberculosis.

[3]Do not use licorice if you have glaucoma, high blood pressure, or an estrogen-dependent disorder, such as breast cancer, endometriosis, or fibrocystic breasts.

[4]Do not use scutellaria if you have diarrhea.

[5]Do not use Siberian ginseng if you have prostate cancer or an autoimmune disease such as lupus or rheumatoid arthritis.

Lyme disease is difficult to diagnose because its symptoms mimic those of many other diseases. Usually a "bull's-eye" rash—a round, red mark with a white center—occurs at the site of the bite. (The bite may go unnoticed, especially if no rash develops, because the deer tick is so small.) As the infection spreads through the bloodstream and lymphatic system, secondary symptoms develop. These include fatigue, headache, heart palpitations, muscle pain, nausea and vomiting, neck stiffness, and blurred vision, as well as a general feeling of malaise. In rare instances, Lyme disease can also produce symptoms similar to those of chronic fatigue syndrome (CFS), such as severe fatigue, and neurological symptoms, including impaired speech, facial paralysis, drooping eyelids, hallucinations, and abnormal sensitivity to light.

Lyme disease is usually treated with a fourteen- to twenty-one-day course of antibiotic therapy. The herbs mentioned here support the antibiotics. If the disease is untreated, about two-thirds of those infected develop recurring arthritis years later.

Recommendations

❑ Ensure adequate levels of vitamin A by consuming one to three servings of dark green, yellow, or orange fruits or vegetables daily. Laboratory studies with animals show that vitamin A deficiencies aggravate arthritis in Lyme disease.

❑ Take the Recommended Daily Allowance (RDA) of vitamin D (included with a multivitamin), which has been shown to prevent the development of arthritis in Lyme disease in laboratory studies.

❑ When walking or hiking in tick-infested areas, tuck long pants into socks to protect the legs, and wear shoes (not sandals) and long-sleeved shirts. Ticks show up on white or light colors better than on dark colors, making them easier to remove from clothing. Remove ticks immediately by using tweezers, pulling carefully and steadily. (*See also* INSECT BITES.)

❑ Try to reduce the number of ticks on your property. Chemical insecticides are not recommended; pyrethrum is relatively safe.

❑ Include plenty of garlic in your diet or take garlic supplements. It is a natural antibiotic and immune-booster.

❑ Take hot baths or whirlpool treatments. Heat relieves joint pain.

❑ If you are being treated for Lyme disease and are not getting better, consider having yourself tested again. False-positive results are possible, and you may actually have a different problem.

Considerations

❑ Motherwort, if taken within the first ten days after a tick bite, prevents secondary viral infections in laboratory

studies. Take ¼ to 1 teaspoon (1 to 5 milliliters of fluidextract) in ¼ cup water three times a day.

❑ In 2002, the Lyme disease vaccine was discontinued due to lack of demand. Today the disease is easily and effectively treated using antibiotics, so there is no need for a vaccine.

❑ Russian investigators have had success in using water extracts of blueberries in stimulating the immune systems of laboratory animals to deal with tick-borne infections. Regular consumption of blueberries during tick season may contribute to disease resistance.

❑ Antibodies are not always present at detectable levels in people with active Lyme disease, and antibodies may be bound with bacteria so that they are not detectable through most blood tests. Information about state-of-the-art blood testing for Lyme disease is available from the Lyme Disease Information Resource. (*See* Appendix B: Resources.)

LYMPHEDEMA

Lymphedema is swelling caused by the inability of lymph, the clear fluid that bathes all of the body's cells, to circulate properly. Normally, lymph collects in lymph vessels, which return this fluid back to the bloodstream. These vessels contain valves that allow for one-directional flow. If the lymphatic vessels are blocked, the fluid remains in the tissues, causing swelling. Infections, which stimulate the immune system to produce lymph, aggravate this condition, and lymphedema in turn creates the conditions under which infections are more likely to occur.

Most cases of lymphedema occur when parts of the lymphatic system—the lymph vessels and nodes, small structures in which lymph is filtered—are removed as part of cancer surgery. If a tumor and the adjacent lymph nodes are removed, the natural drainage of lymphatic fluid through that area is blocked. Fluid accumulates and becomes stagnant in the tissues of the limb closest to the obstruction. The limb may then swell to several times its normal size. Lymphedema is made even worse by recurrence of cancer, as tumors attract sodium and cause fluid retention.

Herbs and nutritional supplements may be helpful in managing edema but should not be used by themselves. Massage, compression garments, exercise, and prescription drugs together with herbs and supplements offer maximum relief for this disease.

Recommendations

❑ Reduce swelling through the following measures (discuss them in detail with your physician first):

❑ Massage, particularly a specialized form of light-pressure massage called manual lymph drainage.

❑ Compression garments (replaced every three to six months) that cover and apply pressure to affected limbs.

Lymphedema: Beneficial Herbs

Herb	Form and Dosage	Comments
Bromelain[1]	Tablets. Take 250–500 mg 3 times daily, between meals.	Reduces swelling, breaks up immune complexes that cause inflammation.
Butcher's broom	Ruscogenin tablets. Take 100 mg once a day for at least 3 months.	Strengthens walls of lymph vessels; relieves swelling and inflammation.
Ginger	Tea, made by adding ⅓ tsp (1 gm) powdered ginger to 1 cup water. (*See* TEAS in Part Three.) Take 1 cup 3 times daily.	Increases circulation; reduces inflammation.
Horse chestnut[2]	Aescin cream. Apply as directed on the label; and aescin tablets. Take 150 mg daily.	Reduces swelling and strengthens lymphatic vessel walls.
Oligomeric proanthocyanidins (OPCs)	Grapeseed or pine bark extract tablets. Take 200 mg daily.	Reduces blood-vessel inflammation.

Precautions for the use of herbs:

[1]People who are allergic to pineapple may develop a rash from bromelain. If itching develops, stop using it.

[2]Do not take horse chestnut if you are trying to become pregnant.

❏ Compression pumps, which move excess fluid toward still-functioning lymph vessels.

❏ Flexibility, aerobic, and weight-training exercises.

❏ The supplement Varicosin, which combines butcher's broom, gotu kola, and horse chestnut extract, may be substituted for any of its individual herbs.

❏ Take 500 milligrams of rutin twice daily, which may strengthen lymph-vessel walls.

❏ Take the enzyme preparation Wobenzym as directed on the label. In an Austrian clinical test involving women who had breast cancer surgery, a combination of Wobenzym with manual lymph drainage reduced arm size, lessened pain, and improved skin condition in less than two months' use.

❏ Do not try to reduce swelling by drinking less water. Drink 1 ounce (20 milliliters) of water daily for every 2 pounds (1 kg) of body weight. For instance, a person weighing 128 pounds should drink 64 ounces, or 8 cups, of water daily.

❏ Keep the affected limb clean. Make certain all fabric in contact with the skin is regularly laundered, including bandages and compression garments.

❏ If you get a cut, scrape, or other break in the skin on an affected limb, apply a topical antibiotic and notify your physician at once.

Considerations

❏ Losing weight helps reduce symptoms associated with lymphedema. In one study, women with this condition who followed a twelve-week weight reduction diet for healthier eating lost weight and had reduced arm size. In another study, women with lymphedema ate either a low-calorie diet or a low-fat diet. Both regimens resulted in significant weight loss, lower body mass index (BMI), and reduced skinfold thickness measurements at four sites, which indicated fat stores were reduced. In both groups, the more weight the women lost, the more they also lost volume in the arms and the less pain they had.

❏ A study reported in *The New England Journal of Medicine* stated that only 25 percent of those women taking oral coumarin drugs experienced significant relief of symptoms. However, using herbs or drugs containing coumarin both internally and externally at the same time increases their effectiveness in reducing swelling 150 to 300 percent over either form of application used by itself. One approach is to take a prescribed coumarin medication orally while at the same time using a horse chestnut or sweet clover cream topically. This is not a typical approach to care, however, so speak to your doctor first.

❏ Compression stockings are very helpful in managing leg edema. A Japanese study found that nineteen out of twenty people who used compression stockings kept their leg edema from getting worse, while only one in four who did not use compression stockings did so.

❏ When hospitalized, people who have undergone lymph node removal should not have medications administered by IV or injection into the affected arm. The arm also should not be used for blood pressure measurements, allergy testing, or drawing blood.

❏ Barometric pressure is reduced at high altitudes, which can make lymphedema worse. Wearing a compression garment is extremely important if you travel by air or hike at high altitudes.

MACULAR DEGENERATION

The retina is the "screen" at the back of the eye on which light that enters the eye is thrown. Macular degeneration is the progressive destruction of the macula, the part of the retina responsible for fine vision. It is the leading cause of vision loss among people over age fifty-five in North America.

There are two forms of macular degeneration: dry (atrophic) or wet (exudative). In the dry form, which is more common, cells in the macula accumulate sacs of debris called drusens. These drusens swell and block off circulation to the microscopic blood vessels that serve the macula. In the wet form, blood vessels themselves swell, and unnecessary vessels form beneath the retina. These vessels leak fluid and may bleed, which causes scarring. Laser surgery may be used to destroy the leaking blood vessels, although this surgery is not suitable for everyone.

Aging, atherosclerosis, a diet low in fruits and vegetables, high blood pressure and cholesterol levels, and smoking all contribute to blood-vessel damage in the eye. As blood vessels are damaged, less oxygen reaches the retina, and the blood vessels constrict to preserve the available oxygen. If normal blood flow is restored from time to time, the vessels don't relax right away, and oxygen-rich blood gathers in the retina. As a result, toxic free radicals, which are oxygen-based, accumulate and cause damage. Heredity also seems to play a role in this disorder.

Herbal treatments may help to stop the breakage of blood vessels and to preserve night vision and the ability to see in bright light. Ongoing use of herbs is necessary, and safe, for macular degeneration.

Recommendations

❏ Eat spinach and corn regularly. These vegetables are sources of the compounds lutein and zeaxanthin, which are similar to vitamin A, and spinach contains beta-carotene as well. Eating 2 ounces (60 grams) of spinach daily and substituting corn flour for wheat flour (150 grams, or 5 ounces daily) for three to four months may increase the thickness and health of the macula. Orange peppers, kiwi fruit, grapes, summer squash, orange juice, and egg yolks are also useful sources of lutein and zeaxanthin. Any foods with a variety of colors help contribute to eye health.

❏ Taking a high-dose formulation of antioxidant vitamins and zinc may reduce the progression of dry macular degeneration to vision loss, according to research by the National Eye Institute (NEI). In its research, the NEI used a formulation that included 500 milligrams vitamin C, 400 international units (IU) vitamin E, 15 milligrams beta-carotene, 80 milligrams zinc, and 2 milligrams copper.

❏ A healthy diet helps slow the progression of vision loss, including using whole grains over refined grains, avoiding saturated fats, and including seafood such as salmon, sardines, and tuna regularly in the diet. In one study, patients with age-related macular degeneration who took 720 milligrams of eicosapentaenoic acid (EPA) and 480 milligrams of docosahexaenoic acid (DHA) daily for six months experienced a buildup of these omega-3 fatty acids in the red blood cells. This study should prompt new research on how these fats can slow the progression of the disease.

❏ To get the best results from surgery, try to maintain good circulatory health. This means keeping high blood pressure, if present, under control, and keeping cholesterol and triglyceride levels down. (*See* HIGH BLOOD PRESSURE [HYPERTENSION] and HIGH CHOLESTEROL.)

❏ Avoid alcohol, cigarette smoke, all sugars, saturated fats, and foods containing fats and oils that have been subjected to heat and/or exposed to the air, such as fried foods, hamburgers, luncheon meats, and roasted nuts.

Considerations

❏ Japanese researchers are exploring the use of interferon, a substance produced by the immune system, to reverse the overgrowth of blood vessels. Shiitake mushroom increases the body's own production of interferon in laboratory studies. Take 3 grams of shiitake in tablet form three times daily.

❏ Although sun exposure is a key part of macular degeneration development, there are factors that predispose an individual to sun injury. People who have blue eyes are

Macular Degeneration: Beneficial Herbs

Herb	Form and Dosage	Comments
Bilberry	Tablets. Take 120 mg 3 times daily.	Stimulates production of rhodopsin, a pigment essential to night vision.
Ginkgo[1]	Ginkgolide tablets. Take 120–160 mg in 2–3 doses daily.	Stops breakage of blood vessels. Increases oxygen supply to the eye.
Oligomeric proanthocyanidins (OPCs)	Grapeseed or pine-bark extract tablets. Take 200 mg daily.	Reduces sensitivity to glare and bright lights. Helps macular tissue adjust to oxygen fluctuations.
Quercetin[2]	Tablets. Take 125–250 mg 3 times daily, between meals.	Protects the macula from effects of low oxygen levels and neurological poisons.

Precautions for the use of herbs:

[1]Do not use ginkgo if you are taking blood-thinning medication. Discuss its use with your doctor before having any type of surgery.

[2]Do not use quercetin if you are taking cyclosporine (Neoral, Sandimmune) or nifedipine (Procardia).

more susceptible to macular damage. In addition, sensitivity to glare, or a tendency to burn instead of tan, is a factor in macular degeneration development. Total number of hours of exposure to the sun does not predict the risk of macular degeneration; in fact, people with macular degeneration spend less time in the sun than people who do not have the disease.

❏ If you burn rather than tan, wearing UV-blocking sunglasses is an important way of protecting against macular degeneration. Be sure to get sunglasses made to block ultraviolet (UV) light. Regular sunglasses can cause more harm than good; the dark lenses cause the pupil to dilate, admitting more light, but do not filter out the macula-damaging UV rays.

MALARIA

See under PARASITIC INFECTION.

MASTITIS

Nursing mothers can develop mastitis, an infection of the milk ducts. Diabetes increases the risk of developing all types of infections, including mastitis. As a result, women who have diabetes are more likely to be affected by mastitis than women who do not.

Mastitis can be caused by either *Staphylococcus* (staph) or by an infectious yeast called *Candida albicans*. The first symptom of mastitis caused by staph infection is fatigue. This is followed about twenty-four hours later by breast swelling and inflammation, and by fever. Other possible symptoms of mastitis include redness in the breast; yellow, puslike secretions from the nipple; and flulike symptoms.

The infection usually occurs when the naturally occurring bacteria on the mother's skin and the baby's skin pass through cracks in the mother's nipples. Conventional medicine uses antibiotics to treat mastitis. Doctors usually recommend that mothers with either type of mastitis continue nursing. The exception is if an abscess, or a localized collection of pus, forms. If this happens, the concentration of infection may harm the baby, causing pneumonia and even lung abscesses. In the case of breast abscess, herbal treatments are inappropriate. Swift antibiotic action is needed for the health of both mother and baby. For staph mastitis without abscess, herbal treatments may reduce breast inflammation and pain, but your doctor still may recommend antibiotics.

Recommendations

❏ To make a marshmallow root bath, place 2 tablespoons (10 grams) of powdered marshmallow root in 1 quart (1 liter) of boiling water. Allow the mixture to cool, and steep overnight. Add the infusion to a sink full of warm water. Immerse and massage the breasts. Wash carefully before nursing your baby.

Mastitis: Beneficial Herbs

Herb	Form and Dosage	Comments
Treatments for Use by Nursing Mothers		
Aloe	Gel. Apply to inflamed breasts.	An antibacterial. Relieves pain.
Calendula	Cream. Apply to sore nipples after every feeding.	A gentle antibacterial. Relieves pain and inflammation.
Coix	Cereal (available in Japanese groceries as *hatomugi*). Eat 1 oz (30 gm) daily.	Reduces pain and swelling. Increases lactation.
Fenugreek	Tea bag, prepared with 1 cup water. Take 1 cup 3 times daily.	Increases milk volume.
Marshmallow root	Tincture, used in a bath. (*See under* Recommendations, above.)	Relieves excess milk accumulation and stops pain. Also known as althea.
Schizonepeta	Cream. Apply to cracked skin.	Relieves pain and inflammation.
St. John's wort	Oil. Apply to dry, cracked nipples.	An antiviral. Relieves pain and inflammation.
Viola	Tea (loose), prepared by steeping 1 tbsp (3 gm) in 1 cup water. (*See* TEAS in Part Three.) Take 1 cup 3 times daily.	Treats enlarged, painful breasts, especially if accompanied by constipation and headache.
Treatments for Use by Mothers Who Are Not Nursing		
Barberry[1] or coptis[1] or goldenseal[1] or Oregon grape root[1]	Tincture. Take 20 drops of any of these herbs in ¼ cup water 3 times daily.	Kills candida, staph, and a wide variety of other bacteria.
Tea tree oil[2]	Oil. Apply to dry, cracked skin.	Kills *E. coli* and staph infections.

Precautions for the use of herbs:

[1]Do not use barberry, coptis, goldenseal, or Oregon grape root if you are pregnant or have gallbladder disease. Do not take these herbs with supplemental vitamin B_6 or with protein supplements containing the amino acid histidine. Do not use goldenseal if you have cardiovascular disease or glaucoma.

[2]People who are allergic to celery or thyme should not use tea tree oil products. Do not take tea tree oil internally.

❏ Wash hands thoroughly before and after handling the breasts.

❏ Make sure the breast is completely emptied, as any buildup of milk worsens the problem. Use a breast pump if the child does not drink all the milk. Nurse or pump at least once a day.

❏ Drink plenty of fluids.

❏ A mother who has a high fever, along with other symptoms of mastitis, should see a doctor.

Considerations

❏ Mastitis is frequently treated with cephalexin (Keflex) and dicloxacillin (Dycill). In many cases, these antibiotics are very effective, although their overuse in veterinary medicine, especially in animals used for food, has created some strains of staph that do not respond to antibiotics. If women are allergic to these, erythromycin can be used.

❏ Men who have diabetes also can develop mastitis, since in diabetes extra sugar is present in all the body's tissues. Men respond better to antibiotic treatment for mastitis than women.

❏ Most minor infections heal by themselves in a few days. More severe ones can heal in about a week if treated with antibiotics.

MEASLES

Measles (rubeola) is a highly contagious viral infection that produces a characteristic red, splotchy rash. The rash appears about four days after the initial symptoms, which include fatigue, fever, irritability, cough, runny nose, sneezing, and red, irritated eyes. The rash erupts on the forehead and spreads downward over the face, neck, trunk, limbs, and feet. Fevers can run as high as 105°F (40.6°C). The disease runs its course in about ten days. People with measles can infect others five days after they have been exposed to the disease (more than a week before symptoms appear) until five days after the rash breaks out. German measles (rubella) is a similar illness that is less contagious and produces milder symptoms.

Measles, long thought of as a childhood illness, is prevalent among children in developing countries. However, since vaccination has been available beginning in 2000 in the United States, a much larger percentage of people in North America who get measles have been adults who were never exposed to, or vaccinated for, the disease, or who have low vitamin A levels. Also, those who travel abroad are more likely to get it. Measles causes more severe symptoms in adults than in children, and the vaccine can sometimes cause mild symptoms associated with the disease that clear up within a few days.

Recovering from measles provides lifetime immunity from future infection. The disease also causes immune-system changes that may have some beneficial effects, in that it may reduce the risk of developing asthma and hay fever. In rare cases, however, recovery from measles can be complicated if the immune system overreacts and fails to "turn off" after it has contained the virus. This can cause damage to the lungs, eyes, heart, liver, kidneys, or brain.

Measles: Beneficial Herbs

Herb	Form and Dosage	Comments
Licorice[1]	Glycyrrhizin tablets. For post-vaccination symptoms. Take 200–800 mg daily, depending on the severity of symptoms, for up to 1 week. Use as needed until the rash disappears.	Eases joint pain and fever after vaccination. Consume potassium-rich foods such as bananas or citrus juices, or take a potassium supplement, daily when taking this herb. Relieves external inflammation without affecting internal immune processes.
Lobelia[2]	Extract. Take ½ tsp every 4–5 hours.	Helps relieve pain.

Precautions for the use of herbs:

[1]Do not use licorice if you have glaucoma, high blood pressure, or an estrogen-dependent disorder such as breast cancer, endometriosis, or fibrocystic breasts.

[2]Do not give lobelia to a child under age twelve, except under the direction of a doctor.

Measles: Formulas

Formula	Comments
Kudzu Decoction	To be used after possible exposure, but before symptoms appear. A traditional Chinese herbal formula that can moderate symptoms by supplementing the antiviral activity of the immune system.

Conventional treatment for measles consists of using non-aspirin painkillers to ease pain and reduce fever.

Internal herb dosages recommended here are for adults. Children under age six should be given one-quarter of the adult dosage. Children between the ages of six and twelve should be given one-half of the adult dosage. Formula dosages for children should be discussed with a knowledgeable health-care practitioner.

Recommendations

❏ Take vitamin A supplements, 400,000 international units (IU) per day for two days, to reduce the risk of complications. Vitamin A deficiency is associated with dry eyes and eye damage caused by measles. Only use this vitamin if symptoms appear after known exposure to measles, since it can interfere with the immune response if taken too early. (Pregnant women should not take vitamin A, since high dosages of this vitamin can harm the baby.) Vitamin A is only effective in the presence of zinc, so take 30 to 60 milligrams of zinc at the same time. This is for adults only; children should only get vitamin A as part of a multivitamin.

❏ Do not give aspirin or any aspirin-containing product to a child who shows symptoms of a viral infection. Aspirin use can result in Reye's syndrome, a potentially serious complication.

❏ Drink plenty of fluids such as water, juices, herbal teas, and vegetable broths.

❏ Avoid processed foods.

❏ Rest until the rash and fever have disappeared.

❏ Do not send a child who has had measles to school until seven to nine days after the fever and rash have disappeared.

Considerations

❏ Allergic reactions to mumps-measles-rubella (MMR) vaccine in children that are severe enough to require emergency room treatment are rare, affecting approximately one in a million people given the vaccine. Milder reactions—such as pain, redness, swelling, and fever of up to 103°F (39.5°C)—are much more common but are usually temporary. The risk of allergic reaction to MMR shots may be reduced by giving the child fermented foods that contain live *Lactobacillus* bacteria, such as yogurt or sauerkraut, for two to three days before injection, but ask the pediatrician before doing this.

❏ A "combination" vaccine called MMRV, which contains both MMR and varicella (chickenpox) vaccines, may be given instead of the two individual vaccines to children twelve years of age and younger. The first dose of MMRV vaccine has been associated with rash and higher rates of fever than MMR and varicella vaccines given separately. Rash has been reported in about one person in twenty and fever in about one person in five. Seizures caused by a fever are also reported more often after MMRV. These usually occur five to twelve days after the first dose.

❏ Measles vaccinations are more likely to have serious side effects in adults. Women who are pregnant or could become pregnant within three months should not be vaccinated. The same is true for men and women who have uncontrolled tuberculosis or are receiving chemotherapy. Otherwise, people who were born after 1957 and have never had measles should consult a physician about vaccination. This is particularly true for those people who travel to areas of the world where measles is still common.

❏ Antibiotics are useless against viruses, so they are not called for unless complications occur.

MELANOMA

See under SKIN CANCER.

MEMORY PROBLEMS

Occasional lapses of memory are an almost universal condition among people of all ages. Chronic memory problems, however, most often occur among older people, and can cause considerable anxiety and concern.

While memory loss is most commonly associated with Alzheimer's disease and stroke, this problem can be caused by other disorders as well. Brain tissue can be damaged by toxic free radicals, which are produced by normal body processes. Impaired circulation can reduce the flow of oxygen and nutrients to the brain. (*See* ATHEROSCLEROSIS.) Thyroid disease and low blood sugar levels also may affect memory.

The ability to remember can be affected by a variety of other factors. Some of these are short-term and reversible situations, such as infections, metabolic problems such as of the thyroid, nutritional deficiencies such as too little vitamin B_{12}, drug reactions, poisoning, brain tumors, lack of oxygen to the brain (anoxia), and heart and lung problems. Anxiety and depression (and the drugs used to treat them) may cause memory problems, as can drug and alcohol use. Certain prescription drugs can affect memory, including blood pressure medications, painkillers, antihistamines, and muscle relaxants. Toxic metals, such as aluminum, lead, and arsenic, could impair memory if they accumulate to a toxic degree in the body. Stress can affect memory, both through its physical effects and because it makes a person less likely to concentrate on the matter at hand. Poor nutrition can also play a role. The first step in dealing with memory loss involves a full examination, so that obvious physical causes can be ruled out.

Neither herbs nor any other treatments for memory problems work immediately. Several weeks to several months of use is almost always necessary for noticeable improvement.

Memory Problems: Beneficial Herbs

Herb	Form and Dosage	Comments
Ashwagandha	Withanolide gelcaps. Take as directed on the label.	Principal ayurvedic herb for chronic memory loss.
Brahmi Concentrate	Bacoside tablets. Take 300 mg once daily.	Restores balance between brain proteins gamma-aminobutyric acid (GABA) and glutamate.
Garlic	Enteric-coated tablets. Take as directed on the label.	Possesses memory-enhancing properties.
Ginkgo[1]	Ginkgolide tablets. Take up to 500 mg once daily.	Improves learning ability and memory, especially under conditions of anxiety.
Gotu kola[2]	Liposome tablets. Take 60–120 mg daily.	Protects the blood vessels supplying the brain. Useful during stress.
Hawthorn	Tablets. Take 100–250 mg 3 times daily.	Improves circulation in blood vessels serving the brain.
Soy lecithin[3]	Capsules. Take 15,000–25,000 mg (15–25 gm) daily.	Reduces memory loss in smokers and in people with high blood pressure.

Precautions for the use of herbs:

[1]Do not use ginkgo if you are taking blood-thinning medication. Discuss its use with your doctor before having any type of surgery.

[2]Do not take gotu kola if you are trying to become pregnant.

[3]Soy lecithin may cause mild diarrhea when you first use it.

Memory Problems: Formulas

Formula	Comments
Biota Seed Pill to Nourish the Heart	Considered the most important traditional Chinese herbal formula for age-related memory loss; aids short-term memory.
Bupleurum Plus Dragon Bone and Oyster Shell Decoction[1]	A traditional Chinese herbal formula that reduces agitated behavior. A free-radical scavenger, it absorbs substances that would destroy nerve tissue.
Coptis Decoction to Relieve Toxicity[2]	A traditional Chinese herbal formula that destroys free radicals, preventing the damaging effects of D-aspartic acid from the artificial sweetener aspartame and aluminum.
Eight-Ingredient Pill with Rehmannia	A traditional Chinese herbal formula that keeps blood sugar levels constant. Particularly useful for people who have hypoglycemia or diabetes.
Gastrodia and Uncaria Decoction[3]	A traditional Chinese herbal formula that increases both circulation to the brain and production of the brain's own free-radical scavenger, superoxide dismutase.
Settle the Emotions Pill	A traditional Chinese herbal formula that treats poor memory compounded by insomnia, dizziness, hot flashes, or dry mouth.

Precautions for the use of formulas:

[1]Do not use Bupleurum Plus Dragon Bone and Oyster Shell Decoction if you have a fever.

[2]Do not use Coptis Decoction to Relieve Toxicity if you are trying to become pregnant.

[3]Do not use Gastrodia and Uncaria Decoction if you are trying to become pregnant.

Recommendations

❏ Use unsaturated (liquid) fats in cooking. Monounsaturated fatty acids in olive oil and polyunsaturated fatty acids from vegetable oils seem to help memory deficits because they are better for the heart than saturated fats from animal sources.

❏ If over age sixty-five, take 200 to 400 international units (IU) of vitamin E and 1,000 milligrams of vitamin C daily, and obtain beta-carotene from your diet by eating five to seven servings of dark green, yellow, or orange fruits and vegetables weekly. Adequate levels of these three antioxidant vitamins are associated with free recall, recognition, and vocabulary in adults over age sixty-five. Of these vitamins, vitamin E is the most important.

❏ Take 2,000 milligrams of the amino acid tyrosine daily. This protein component may lower systolic blood pressure and improve short-term memory and attention. It is especially helpful for correcting memory problems during conditions of short-term emotional stress.

❏ Forget about losing your memory. Anxiety about memory sometimes can be a greater problem than actual memory loss, especially in younger people. Recall of facts or events is easiest if the emotional mood at the time of attempted recall is the same as the emotional mood at the time the fact or event occurred. Anxiety weakens memory of all but distressing memories.

❑ Include blueberries and spinach in your diet. Some researchers believe that flavonoids found in these foods may aid in memory retention.

❑ Keep yourself physically active. This increases blood flow to the brain.

Considerations

❑ Recall is slower after eating very large quantities of carbohydrate, that is, more than 150 grams (ten to twelve servings of carbohydrate in a single meal. The sugars released into the bloodstream change mood, which affects recall of facts. Protein consumption and exercise, or their lack, do not similarly affect memory.

❑ Memory and attention problems in school-aged children are sometimes associated with caffeine withdrawal. This effect is observed in children who consume as little as 120 to 145 milligrams of caffeine a day, the amount in one cup of coffee or two and a half 12-ounce cans of a soft drink.

❑ The nutrient tryptophan may help correct alcohol-induced memory impairment, especially visual memory.

❑ The vitamin thiamin, taken in a dosage of 500 milligrams per day, may help restore memory in people recovering from cocaine addiction.

❑ The trace element boron seems to be important to memory, attention, and motor skills. This trace element is abundant in legumes and nuts, which also provide vitamin E. Many calcium supplements contain boron, as it also strengthens the bones.

❑ In one study, a vitamin and mineral drink that included guarana (a natural form of caffeine) helped improve memory testing of accuracy and speed in healthy volunteers. This result suggests it may be prudent if your memory is failing to take a multivitamin/mineral mixture with caffeine or guarana, if you can tolerate these two substances.

❑ Ginkgo is one of the most commonly used herbs for memory. In one study, 80 milligrams of a ginkgo extract taken three times a day seemed to slow the progression of memory loss, but only if the full dose was taken every day for forty-two months.

❑ Frequent consumption of curry containing turmeric may slow memory loss associated with aging. In an elderly Asian population from Singapore, those who used more of the spice turmeric, which contains curcumin, had better memory than a group that rarely used this spice in cooking.

❑ Parents of children addicted to video games, take heart. Scientists have found playing in a virtual environment may improve memory and cognitive skills. Video games may help rehabilitate adults who have developed memory problems.

❑ Human growth hormone (HGH) has been shown to improve brain function. Fountain of Youth Technologies has a safe gel and cream designed for external use that is absorbed directly into the bloodstream. (*See* Appendix B: Resources.)

❑ The keys to having a good memory are in attitude and approach. As we age, our attitudes change. Our ability to remember isn't affected as much as we think. It is the change in our motivation to remember things that is probably the larger factor.

❑ *See also* ALZHEIMER'S DISEASE and STROKE.

MÉNIÈRE'S DISEASE

Ménière's disease is an inner-ear disorder that causes attacks of vertigo, or dizziness, and loss of balance. The vertigo may be accompanied by nausea and vomiting, and there may be a sense of fullness in the ear. Milder forms of the disease cause only slight difficulty in concentration, discomfort in the head, and momentary dizzy spells. Severe forms of the disease cause profound dizziness, ringing in the ears, and, eventually, deafness. Once deafness occurs, attacks of dizziness cease. In most people, Ménière's disease affects only one ear, although it is possible to have it in both ears. Conventional medicine uses drugs and diet to control this disorder; in advanced cases, surgery may be necessary.

In Ménière's disease there is an accumulation of lymph in the inner ear, an organ important to both hearing and balance. The swelling damages the delicate hairs with which the ear detects sound. They also change the flow of fluid in the ear so that it cannot adjust to rapid changes in body position, such as getting out of bed or rising from a chair. Changes in spinal-fluid pressure aggravate the condition.

Because no single cause has been identified, it is likely that the disease is caused by a combination of factors, including blocked drainage in the ear caused at birth or otherwise, abnormal immune system, allergies, viral infections, genetic predisposition, and head trauma. The inner ear is a cluster of passages and cavities called a labyrinth. Outside the inner ear is made of bone and inside is a soft structure, which is smaller but shaped like the bony part. In the soft part is a fluid that is lined with hairlike sensors that respond to fluid. These sensors work only when the fluid volume is correct, with the right pressure and chemical composition. If any of these are disrupted, Ménière's disease can occur.

As with conventional medicine, early herbal treatment of Ménière's disease is essential. Once deafness occurs,

Ménière's Disease: Beneficial Herbs

Herb	Form and Dosage	Comments
Butcher's broom	Ruscogenin capsules or tablets. Take as directed on the label.	Combats fluid retention and improves circulation.
Goldenseal[1] and scutellaria[2]	Tincture. Take 1–1½ tsp (4–6 ml) of both herbs in ¼ cup water 3 times daily.	Controls infection and circulates lymph away from the inner ear.
Licorice[3]	Glycyrrhizin tablets. Take 200–800 mg daily. Use for 6 weeks, then take a 2-week break. Do not substitute deglycyrrhizinated licorice (DGL).	Increases effectiveness of steroid treatments. Consume potassium-rich foods such as bananas or citrus juices, or take a potassium supplement, daily when taking this herb.
Siberian ginseng	Pure *Eleutherococcus senticosus* extract. Take the dosage recommended on the label in ¼ cup water.	Deactivates mast cells, which cause inflammation.

Precautions for the use of herbs:

[1]Do not take goldenseal for longer than two weeks at a time. Do not use it if you are pregnant or have cardiovascular disease, gallbladder disease, or glaucoma. Do not take goldenseal with supplemental vitamin B_6 or with protein supplements containing the amino acid histidine.

[2]Do not use scutellaria if you have diarrhea.

[3]Do not use licorice if you have glaucoma, high blood pressure, or an estrogen-dependent disorder, such as breast cancer, endometriosis, or fibrocystic breasts.

Ménière's Disease: Formulas

Formula	Comments
Bupleurum Plus Dragon Bone and Oyster Shell Decoction[1]	A traditional Chinese herbal formula that treats Ménière's disease if secondary symptoms include constipation, agitation, inability to turn the torso, rapid pulse, and/or a sensation of heaviness throughout the entire body.
Five-Ingredient Powder with Poria	A traditional Chinese herbal formula that treats Ménière's disease caused by trauma or accompanying fever; other symptoms include headache, irritability, strong thirst but with vomiting after drinking, and/or urinary difficulty.
True Warrior Decoction[2]	A traditional Chinese herbal formula that treats Ménière's disease accompanied by cold sensations in the body, swelling, and urinary difficulty, but no pain.

Precautions for the use of formulas:

[1]Do not use Bupleurum Plus Dragon Bone and Oyster Shell Decoction if you have a fever.

[2]Stop using True Warrior Decoction if fever occurs. This formula may cause a loss of sensation in the mouth and tongue.

attacks of dizziness cease, but the damage cannot be corrected.

Recommendations

❏ When symptoms first appear, take 3 milligrams of melatonin daily for up to a month. This hormone seems to activate the white blood cells in the inner ear to recognize and dispose of collagen.

❏ Avoid sugar and highly processed carbohydrates. Some people with Ménière's disease have abnormalities in insulin production, along with either slightly high or slightly low blood sugar levels. Reducing consumption of sugar could help symptoms. Sugar-free diets may be good for sufferers of Ménière's disease who do not respond to other forms of treatment. Some people also respond to supplemental calcium (1,000 milligrams or more daily)

and vitamin D (no more than 800 international units [IU] daily), which should be tried for three months.

❏ Maintain a low-fat diet and avoid fried foods, monosodium glutamate (MSG), alcohol, or anything containing caffeine.

❏ Limit sodium intake to 1,500 milligrams a day (about 1 teaspoon). Avoid caffeine. Stop smoking and avoid allergens.

❏ As much as possible, reduce the anxiety in your life. Stress is a major trigger in Ménière's disease.

Considerations

❏ Conventional medical treatment of Ménière's disease has used drugs combined with a low-salt diet to reduce both inflammation and the amount of fluid circulating in the body. Unfortunately, these measures do nothing to help people who have already lost their hearing. More recently, doctors have used antibiotic therapy to alter the mineral balance of the fluid within the inner ear, which alleviates swelling. Overdoses may cause hearing loss. If drug treatment fails, surgery may be used to ease vertigo and, if possible, preserve hearing.

❑ Some doctors recommend a high-protein, low-refined-carbohydrate diet because they have found that people with this disorder have high blood insulin levels. High insulin levels impair circulation. Researchers in Sweden have tested a specially processed cereal that can increase the body's ability to make antisecretory factor, a protein known to affect transport of nutrients in the intestine. The flow of these nutrients is impaired in Ménière's disease and this special cereal reduced vertigo, which is common in this disease, in 14 out of 27 patients compared to only 2 out of 27 in the placebo group.

MENOPAUSE-RELATED PROBLEMS

Menopause starts twelve months after menstruation ends. It occurs after a period of several years in which production of the main female hormone, estrogen, diminishes, a period known as the climacteric. Unless brought about

by injury, surgery, or chemotherapy, the climacteric (also called perimenopause) usually begins in the midforties. Menopause usually is complete by age fifty to fifty-five.

During the climacteric, the ovaries greatly reduce their estrogen production (although small amounts are produced by other bodily tissues), while the production of other hormones greatly increases. As a result the menstrual cycle starts to shorten. Eventually, the period becomes irregular—sometimes longer, sometimes much shorter. The vagina and fallopian tubes shrink, vaginal lubrication decreases, and the ligaments supporting the uterus and vagina lose their strength.

It is important to remember that menopause is not a disorder, but a natural part of life. Nevertheless, it can produce symptoms that range from mildly uncomfortable to extremely distracting, and that affect each woman differently. Many women experience hot flashes, which generally occur in the first two years. Other symptoms include spontaneous sweating, heart palpitations, urinary urgency, head and body aches, fatigue, mood swings, nervousness, depressed feelings, deficiencies in concentration and memory, and insomnia. Backache and a tendency to develop back sprain are common. The skin becomes drier. Sex drive may either increase or decrease.

The decline in estrogen production has other important

Menopause-Related Problems: Beneficial Herbs

Herb	Form and Dosage	Comments
Aloe	Gel. Apply to the vagina at night.	Relieves vaginal dryness.
Black cohosh	Tablets. Take 500–1,000 mg daily.	Increases vaginal lubrication; relieves headaches and muscle pain; stops irregular bleeding.
Blue cohosh[1]	Tablets or capsules. Take 250 mg 3 times daily.	Relieves hot flashes.
Calendula	Cream. Apply as directed on the label.	Relieves vaginal itching.
Damiana[2]	Tincture. Take ½ tsp (2 ml) in ¼ cup water 2–3 times daily.	Restores sexual desire. Reduces hot flashes.
Dong quai[3]	*Angelica sinensis* extract tablets. Take 250–500 mg daily.	Increases circulation and protects the heart. Increases effectiveness of other herbal treatments.
Ginseng plus	*Panax ginseng* tincture.	Stops hot flashes, increases ovarian estrogen production in early menopause.
vitamin E	Take as directed on the label. Take 800 IU daily.	Increases the effects of ginseng.
Red clover	Capsules. Take 500 mg 1–2 times daily.	Relieves abdominal pain. A mild estrogen stimulant.
Sarsaparilla	Fluidextract. Take 1 tsp (4 ml) 3 times daily.	Restores libido in women with low testosterone levels.
Saw palmetto	Capsules. Take 160 mg 1–2 times daily, between meals.	Counteracts effects of excessive testosterone without reducing sex drive.
Stinging nettle leaf	Capsules. Take 500 mg 1–2 times daily.	Relieves blurred vision. Stimulates urination.
Valerian	Valepotriate tablets. Take 50–100 mg on an empty stomach, 1 hour before bedtime.	Relieves nervous tension and insomnia.
Vitex[4]	Tablets. Take 250–500 mg daily.	Stops hot flashes, sensation of movement in the skin, dizziness, and depression.

Precautions for the use of herbs:

[1]Do not take blue cohosh if you are pregnant or if you are experiencing excessive menstrual bleeding.

[2]Do not use damiana if you are anemic or have chronic bleeding.

[3]Different forms of dong quai have different effects on the uterus. Be sure to use the form specified.

[4]Vitex has been known to stimulate the release of multiple eggs from the ovary, potentially resulting in multiple births. If you are still ovulating and do not wish to become pregnant, use reliable birth control.

Menopause-Related Problems: Formulas

Formula	Comments
Augmented Rambling Powder	A traditional Chinese herbal formula that relieves menopausal problems compounded by emotional distress.
Bupleurum and Cinnamon Twig Decoction[1]	A traditional Chinese herbal formula that treats eye problems (myopia spuria), headache, hot flashes, and spontaneous sweating. Not appropriate for women who exercise more than 1 hour per day or those who do not exercise at all.
Cinnamon Twig and Poria Pill	A traditional Chinese herbal formula that treats hot flashes accompanied by abnormal genital bleeding or pelvic congestion.
Dong Quai and Peony Powder	A traditional Chinese herbal formula that treats hot flashes accompanied by muscle tremor and/or fluid retention.
Eight-Ingredient Pill with Rehmannia (Rehmannia-Eight Combination)	A traditional Chinese herbal formula used if there is sensitivity to cold in the hands and feet, dry and itchy skin, impaired vision and hearing, and/or abnormalities in urination.
Hochu-ekki-to	A Japanese herbal formula that is especially appropriate if the predominant symptom is fatigue and/or loss of muscle tone. Useful for incontinence and prolapse of the uterus. In formulas for menopause, it is sometimes identified as Center-Supplementing Chi-Boosting Decoction.

Precautions for the use of formulas:

[1]Do not use Bupleurum and Cinnamon Twig Decoction if you have a fever.

effects. The bones no longer retain as much calcium and phosphorus. A condition called osteoporosis can result, in which the bones become soft, and even minor stresses can result in fractures. Decreased estrogen production is also associated with an increased risk of heart disease. The ovaries form estrogen from low-density lipoprotein (LDL), the "bad," artery-clogging kind. This action decreases the ratio of LDL to "good," artery-clearing high-density lipoprotein (HDL).

One treatment for menopausal symptoms is estrogen replacement therapy (ERT), which has recently gone out of favor, as it does not seem to have the heart-protective effects it was thought to have and may increase the risk of breast cancer. However, hormone estrogen replacement is still the most effective treatment, so consult your physician to assess your specific risk factors. Some women with menopausal symptoms find relief using herbal medicine alone. However, herbal therapies can be used to supplement ERT, or ERT can be used to supplement the herbs discussed in this entry. Phytoestrogens (plant estrogens) elevate hormonal levels. Estrogen-like substances from plant sources bind to estrogen receptor sites and may help to reduce the effect of low estrogen, including hot flashes and bone loss. An added benefit is protection against clogged arteries that aids in protecting the heart. Foods rich in phytoestrogens include soy, rye, chickpeas, clover, and flaxseeds. Either kind of treatment usually takes several months to work.

Recommendations

❑ If vaginal irritation is a problem, take 3,000 milligrams of evening primrose oil daily. (For information about bladder or yeast infections, *see* BLADDER INFECTION [CYSTITIS] and YEAST INFECTION [YEAST VAGINITIS].)

❑ To stop hot flashes, try breathing exercises. Deep, slow breathing can reduce hot flashes by calming the central nervous system. (*See* RELAXATION TECHNIQUES in Part Three.)

❑ For vaginal dryness, try Replens vaginal lotion, and use lubricant jellies (such as K-Y Brand Jelly) before sexual intercourse. Occasionally, a topical estrogen cream (prescribed by a physician) can restore normal lubrication to vaginal tissue, although some of the estrogen will be absorbed into the bloodstream.

❑ Get regular moderate exercise. Learn to strengthen your pelvic floor to correct urinary incontinence. Don't smoke.

❑ Avoid stress as much as possible. Try yoga.

❑ Drink 2 quarts of quality water each day to help prevent drying of the skin and mucous membranes.

Considerations

❑ Phytoestrogens in certain foods, such as soybeans, chickpeas, flaxseed, whole grains, and some fruits and vegetables, may relieve hot flashes and other menopausal symptoms. But these foods have a weak estrogen effect and may increase the risk of breast cancer. Speak to your doctor before using these foods or taking supplements with phytoestrogens in them.

❑ Black cohosh is widely used in Europe and is also popular in the United States. However, one study found no benefit in terms of changes in blood hormone levels, abnormal bleeding, and vaginal dryness when it was used alone, with soy, or with other herbs. The women assigned to the hormone replacement therapy group did experience beneficial changes.

❑ Other supplements such as wild yam, chasteberry, licorice, and dong quai, which are also used by some for menopausal symptoms, have less scientific support for their use. However, general symptoms of anxiety and depression were improved in patients in late perimenopause who used a blend of St. John's wort and chasteberry for sixteen weeks.

❑ In one study, two Chinese herbal blends (Kunbao Pill and Modified Xiaoyao Pill) worked better relieving symptoms of menopause such as anxiety and bad temper as well as lowering total cholesterol and increasing the HDL, or "good," cholesterol levels when used in combination. These women also received psychological counseling. In another study, an herbal Chinese blend called Geng Nian Le helped women near menopause to have fewer symptoms of depression according to a standardized test called the Hamilton Depression Scale.

❑ In hormone replacement therapy, estrogen and another female hormone, progesterone, are taken in a carefully balanced monthly cycle. Oral estrogen replacement therapies (ERT) may not be well tolerated. Estrogen replacement given via vaginal suppositories may cause breast discomfort and bloating. Worst of all, ERT is associated with an increased risk of breast cancer and possibly increased heart disease risk. Speak to your doctor about the risks and benefits of hormone replacement. Raloxifene (Evista) is a drug that mimics estrogen's beneficial effects on bone density in postmenopausal women, and does not have the associated risk of estrogen. Unlike estrogen, however, it has been shown to lower the risk of breast cancer, and it may lower the risk of uterine cancer.

❑ The hormonal changes of menopause frequently cause prolapse of the bladder, bowel, uterus, and/or vagina. Prolapse is a loosening and falling down of tissues or organs due to the force of gravity and stretching. Severe prolapse may require surgery, but milder cases of vaginal prolapse can be corrected with Kegel exercises. (*See* KEGEL EXERCISES in Part Three.)

❑ Oryzanol, a rice-bran extract found in many over-the-counter (OTC) formulas for menopause-related symptoms, may help tone the muscles that hold the uterus and bladder in place. It has the added benefit of lowering total cholesterol and triglycerides while raising levels of HDL cholesterol.

❑ Smoking is associated with early menopause.

❑ Frequent sexual intercourse can help relieve vaginal dryness.

❑ Some women think that it is more important to replace progesterone than estrogen. Natural progesterone cream is a good way to do this.

❑ Saliva testing may be used instead of blood testing for determining hormone levels because it measures only levels of active hormone. You can ask your doctor to order this type of test, but many doctors use blood tests.

❑ *See also* HIGH CHOLESTEROL and OSTEOPOROSIS.

MENSTRUAL CRAMPS

See under MENSTRUAL PROBLEMS; PREMENSTRUAL SYNDROME (PMS).

MENSTRUAL PROBLEMS

Every month, as part of the menstrual cycle, a woman's body sheds the tissues that line the uterus. This occurs because the body must prepare every month for a possible pregnancy, and does so by growing a thicker, spongier uterine lining meant to nourish a growing fetus. If no pregnancy occurs, this lining is not needed and breaks down.

Three problems associated with menstruation are absence of periods (amenorrhea), pain before or during the beginning of the period (dysmenorrhea), and unusually heavy bleeding (menorrhagia). Periods can stop because of hormonal imbalances or strenuous exercise. Menstrual pain, which is quite common, can be accompanied by nausea, vomiting, diarrhea, headache, dizziness, and blurred vision. In primary dysmenorrhea, no physical cause of the pain can be identified. In secondary dysmenorrhea, the pain is associated with an observable physical condition, such as endometriosis, uterine fibroids, adenomyosis (a condition in which tissue in the lining of the uterus grows into the muscle walls of the uterus), pelvic inflammatory disease, or cervical stenosis. A heavy period involves bleeding more heavily—which may mean passing large clots, needing to change protection during the night, or soaking through a sanitary pad or tampon every hour for two to three hours in a row—during menstrual cycles of normal length unless caused by another disorder, such as endometriosis or uterine fibroids. Conventional treatment of these conditions varies with each specific disorder.

Primary menstrual pain and heavy bleeding are usually related to the production of inflammatory substances called series-2 prostaglandins. These hormonelike compounds produce pain by causing uterine contractions to increase, and heavy bleeding by promoting inflammation and clotting in the uterine lining. Both herbs and formulas may have to be used for three to four months before results are apparent. Use of the menstrual-pain herbs is tied to a regular monthly cycle; if periods are irregular, see a doctor. These treatments should be used only after secondary causes, such as endometriosis, are ruled out.

Recommendations

❑ Eat the right kinds of fats. The prostaglandin imbalances that cause both menstrual pain and heavy periods result from an imbalance in the types of fats in the diet. In the modern Western diet, there is a deficiency of omega-3

Menstrual Problems: Beneficial Herbs

Herb	Form and Dosage	Comments
Treatments That Stop Excessive Bleeding		
Agrimony[1]	Tea (loose), prepared by steeping 1 tsp (1 gm) in 1 cup water 3 times daily. (*See* TEAS in Part Three.)	A traditional Chinese remedy for heavy menstruation.
Cinnamon	Oil. Take 15–30 drops in ¼ cup water up to 3 times daily.	Stimulates blood flow out of uterus. Stops heavy periods and abnormal bleeding.
Shepherd's purse	Tincture. Take 1½–2 tsp (6–8 ml) in ¼ cup water 3 times daily for 3 months.	Stops excessive bleeding.
Treatments That Reduce Menstrual Pain		
Amaranth[2]	Tea (loose), prepared by steeping 1 tbsp (4–5 gm) in 1 cup water. (*See* TEAS in Part Three.) Take 1 cup 3 times daily.	Relieves menstrual pain. Also called niu xi or tu niu xi.
Dong quai[3]	*Angelica sinensis* extract tablets. Take 250–500 mg daily. Use during first 14 days of cycle for 3–4 months.	Regulates menstrual function.
Treatments That Restore Normal Length of Menstrual Period		
Blue cohosh[4]	Tablets. Take 250 mg 3 times daily.	Shortens long periods. Increases menstrual flow.
Dan shen	Tea (loose), prepared by steeping 2 tbsp (5–6 gm) in 1 cup water. (*See* TEAS in Part Three.) Take 1 cup 3 times daily for up to 3 months.	Restores periods after amenorrhea.
Morinda	Tea (loose), prepared by steeping 1 tsp (2 gm) in 1 cup of water. (*See* TEAS in Part Three.) Take 1 cup 3 times daily.	Restores normal periods. Corrects urinary incontinence.
Vitex[5]	Tablets. Take 250–500 mg daily. Use during last 14 days of cycle for 3–4 months.	Lengthens short periods. Decreases menstrual flow.

Precautions for the use of herbs:

[1]Do not use agrimony for more than two weeks in any month.

[2]Do not use amaranth if you are trying to become pregnant.

[3]Different forms of dong quai have different effects on the uterus. Be sure to use the form specified.

[4]Do not take blue cohosh if you have excessive menstrual bleeding.

[5]Vitex has been known to stimulate the release of multiple eggs from the ovary, potentially resulting in multiple births. If you do not wish to become pregnant, use reliable birth control while taking this herb.

Menstrual Problems: Formulas

Formula	Comments
Formulas That Reduce Menstrual Pain	
Augmented Rambling Powder[1]	A traditional Chinese herbal formula that treats menstrual pain with tenderness in the breasts and lower abdomen, irritability, edema, headache, and digestive disturbances at the beginning of the period.
Cinnamon Twig and Poria Pill	A traditional Chinese herbal formula that stops sharp, severe pain with discharge of clotted blood.
Formula That Regulates Menstrual Flow	
Four-Substance Decoction	A traditional Chinese herbal formula that regulates blood flow to relieve either heavy periods or lack of periods. Most useful if symptoms include general fatigue.

Precautions for the use of formulas:

[1]Do not use Augmented Rambling Powder if you are trying to become pregnant.

essential fatty acids, substances that promote healing and calm inflammation. These fatty acids are found in flaxseed and flaxseed oil, but they are not in the bioactive form, meaning that they cannot readily make prostaglandins. Eating seafood and taking fish oil capsules corrects the problem faster and with fewer calories (you need to consume ten times the amount of safflower oil per every calorie of fish oil). At the same time, eating less polyunsaturated fat from grain oils like corn and safflower will also help. One study found that adolescents with menstrual problems who took 2 grams of fish oil containing vitamin E showed a marked improvement in their symptoms according to the Cox Menstrual Symptom Scale. The benefits were apparent after two months of taking the fish oil capsules.

❑ Dairy products may reduce symptoms. In a survey conducted on women with menstrual problems, those who consumed three or four servings a day of dairy products compared to those who ate none had fewer symptoms, such as bloating and pain.

❑ Take from 500 to 1,000 milligrams of vitamin C three times a day. This vitamin may help stabilize fragile capillaries that may break and bleed, and could contribute to heavy menstrual bleeding.

❑ Use a heating pad or a hot water bottle to help ease menstrual cramps.

Considerations

❑ Conventional treatment of amenorrhea consists of treating any underlying hormonal disturbances. Treatment of primary dysmenorrhea consists of painkillers and, if needed, bed rest. If a narrow cervix is discovered, it may be dilated. Treatment of primary menorrhagia consists of using female hormones, such as those used in birth control pills, to correct the hormonal imbalance linked to prostaglandin production.

❑ Heavy athletic training, particularly if dietary protein is inadequate, may cause amenorrhea. Introducing one rest day a week and using sports protein supplements usually restores regular periods in young women athletes within three to four months.

❑ *See also* ENDOMETRIOSIS; FIBROIDS, UTERINE (UTERINE MYOMAS); PELVIC INFLAMMATORY DISEASE; and PREMENSTRUAL SYNDROME (PMS).

MIGRAINE

Migraine is commonly thought of as the ultimate headache. Attacks are excruciatingly painful and recurrent, but can occur without pain. Symptoms include temporary slurring or loss of speech; distortion of sight, with "shooting stars" and kaleidoscopic color patterns; temporary paralysis; short-term memory loss; nausea; and tenderness in neck and scalp.

Migraine may be heralded by an aura or prodrome, which may be experienced as a "curtain falling" over the field of vision or as a wave of inexplicable depression and emotional pain. Migraines may last for a few hours or a few days, and may occur a few times a year or every day. If untreated, the duration of a migraine is usually seventy-two hours. The first attack usually occurs between the ages of ten and thirty, but many people "outlast" migraines by the age of fifty. Since the blood-vessel changes that occur in the brain during migraine are influenced by estrogen, more women are affected than men.

Noise and other forms of environmental disturbance aggravate migraine. Other factors that can trigger a migraine include hormonal changes in women, such as fluctuations in estrogen levels; certain foods, such as beer, wine, and aged cheeses; changes in sleeping patterns; and changes in the weather. Until recently, migraines were thought to be caused by spasms of the blood vessels supplying the brain. However, they are likely caused by changes in the trigeminal nerve, a major pain pathway. Imbalances in brain chemicals such as serotonin may also be involved. Serotonin levels drop with migraines, so this may trigger the release of substances called neuropeptides, which travel to the brain's outer covering, resulting in a headache.

Migraine treatment has improved and many options are available. Conventional treatment of migraine uses painkillers (if the headache is mild enough) and drugs meant to redirect blood flow. Some migraine sufferers are treated successfully with antiseizure medication, although these drugs must be used very carefully, as in high doses they can cause nausea, diarrhea, and cramps.

Herbs are able to complement standard treatments and to complement each other. Except for cayenne, which is taken at the beginning of an attack, use any of the herbs listed below on an ongoing basis to prevent migraines. When using formulas, matching the formula to the overall symptom pattern is essential; see an herbal practitioner.

Recommendations

❑ To relieve migraine pain, use a formula that combines feverfew with willow bark, such as Migracin, according to the label directions. Feverfew by itself may be useful if you are also taking a selective serotonin reuptake inhibitor (SSRI) for depression. (*See* Considerations, page 405.) However, in a review on the use of this herb, no benefit was seen over placebo in over 300 patients from five studies. When feverfew was prepared as an extract using CO_2 (MIG-99), however, migraine sufferers who used 6.25 grams a day prophylactically for twenty-eight days had three times fewer attacks than those in a placebo group.

❑ Avoid foods containing the amino acid tyramine. These include anchovies, beer, hard cheeses, chocolate, corned beef, dried meats, fava beans, fermented beans such as miso and soy sauce, lima beans, pickled herring,

Migraine: Beneficial Herbs

Herb	Form and Dosage	Comments
Cayenne	Powder. Mix with starchy food. Use the smallest amount that causes a burning sensation on the tongue.	Produces changes in nerve fibers that prevent them from transmitting migraine pain.
Dong quai	*Angelica sinensis* capsules. Take 500–1,000 mg daily.	Prevents migraine attacks, especially those related to premenstrual syndrome (PMS).
Feverfew[1]	Freeze-dried leaf in capsules. Take 25 mg daily and increase to 100 mg daily after 2 weeks.	Prevents migraine attacks by stopping release of serotonin. (*See under* Recommendations, page 403).
Ginkgo	Extract. Take as directed on the label.	Enhances cerebral circulation.
Quercetin[2]	Tablets. Take 125–250 mg 3 times daily, between meals.	Prevents migraine attacks, especially those triggered by food allergies.
Tilden flower	Fluidextract. Take 1 tsp (4 ml) 3 times daily.	Prevents and treats migraines associated with high blood pressure.

Precautions for the use of herbs:

[1]Do not take feverfew if you are pregnant. Stop using it if you have an allergic reaction.

[2]Do not use quercetin if you are taking cyclosporine (Neoral, Sandimmune) or nifedipine (Procardia).

Migraine: Formulas

Formula	Comments
Bupleurum Plus Dragon Bone and Oyster Shell Decoction[1]	A traditional Chinese herbal formula used especially in modern Japan to treat migraines caused by environmental stresses, such as weather changes, noise, allergens, and drafts.
Four-Substance Decoction	A traditional Chinese herbal formula that relieves migraine with dizziness, blurred vision, lusterless complexion and nails, general muscle tension, lower abdominal pain, and irregular or absent menstruation.
Gastrodia and Uncaria Decoction[2]	A traditional Chinese herbal formula that is especially useful for preventing migraines with severe visual disturbances.
Major Bupleurum Decoction[3]	A traditional Chinese herbal formula that relieves migraine with alternating fevers and chills, bitter taste in the mouth, nausea, and either burning diarrhea or severe constipation.

Precautions for the use of formulas:

[1]Do not take Bupleurum Plus Dragon Bone and Oyster Shell Decoction if you have a fever.

[2]Do not take Gastrodia and Uncaria Decoction if you are trying to become pregnant.

[3]Do not take Major Bupleurum Decoction if you have a fever.

red wine (white wine can be used in moderation), sardines, sauerkraut, and yeast. Although a single serving of a tyramine-containing food such as chocolate may not provoke a migraine, excessive consumption of these foods can increase the frequency of attacks. Other foods may trigger migraines, so learn what foods you are sensitive to and avoid them.

❏ Avoid bingeing on sweets or starches. The temporary "sugar buzz" is followed by hypoglycemia (low blood sugar), which may trigger migraine attacks.

❏ Eliminate coffee and other sources of caffeine from the diet. Once you are off caffeine, you may be able to use coffee as a treatment for migraine. Drink one or two cups of strong coffee at the first sign of an attack; then lie down in a dark, quiet room.

❏ Take fish oil containing docosahexaenoic acid (DHA) and eicosapentaenoic acid (EPA). A useful dosage is 1,000 milligrams of fish oil for every 10 pounds (5 kilograms) of body weight. Fish oil modifies the production of prostaglandins, hormonelike substances generated in the linings of blood vessels in the brain that may exacerbate migraine symptoms. Interestingly, when adolescents with recurring migraines took either fish oil capsules or olive oil capsules, they had fewer attacks, and those they did have were shorter and less severe. It may be that a combination of fish oil and olive oil would work best to reduce migraine attacks. Using olive oil in salads and consuming seafood is also prudent.

❏ Take 800 to 1,000 milligrams of any calcium-magnesium supplement daily. Many naturopathic doctors report that migraines become less frequent if people take supplemental calcium. The effect of calcium is amplified by vitamin D, so make sure that the supplement has both nutrients. Drinking milk (cow's or soy) will also provide the needed calcium and vitamin D. Research shows that women who have premenstrual syndrome (PMS) suffer fewer migraines if they take supplemental magnesium.

❏ Speak with your doctor about taking vitamin B$_2$ (riboflavin) to prevent migraines. In a European clinical trial, a high dosage of riboflavin, 400 milligrams per day, used for three months, reduced the frequency of migraines by 50 percent in those people who respond to it (about two-thirds of those who took it). Riboflavin is inexpensive and readily available, and produces side effects—mild diarrhea and increased urination—in only about 4 percent of the people who take it. A dosage this large, however, requires a doctor's prescription and must be taken for about a month before it has an effect.

❏ Coenzyme Q$_{10}$ (Co-Q$_{10}$) levels have been found to be low in people who experience migraines. In a study of over 1,500 children and adolescents with migraines, nearly 40 percent had Co-Q$_{10}$ levels in the blood that were too low. When those who had low levels took about 50 to 150 milligrams a day of Co-Q$_{10}$, the frequency of headaches was reduced, there were fewer debilitating days, and the levels of Co-Q$_{10}$ in the blood increased.

❏ Ask your doctor about taking a children's aspirin every other day. In low doses, aspirin may reduce the frequency of migraine attacks.

❏ Do not take the prescription painkiller Fiorinal on a regular basis, unless your doctor recommends it. It contains an addictive barbiturate (butalbital) and caffeine, in addition to aspirin. There are many other options available and this drug is not often used.

❏ Include almonds, almond milk, watercress, parsley, fennel, garlic, cherries, and fresh pineapple in your diet.

❏ Get regular moderate exercise.

❏ Avoid loud noises, strong odors, and high altitudes.

❏ Do not smoke and avoid secondhand smoke.

Considerations

❏ The Headache ICE-PILLO is a horseshoe-shaped collar containing a frozen gel pack. Applying the pack to the back of the head at the first sign of a migraine attack may reduce its duration and severity.

❏ People who experience migraine may also experience chronic depression. The antidepressants known as SSRIs—including Celexa, Paxil, Prozac, and Zoloft—are sometimes used to treat migraines, but not much anymore because in rare instances they can provoke severe migraines with symptoms similar to those of stroke. This effect can be even worse for people taking both an SSRI and the prescription medication sumatriptan (Imitrex). If a first migraine occurs during treatment with an SSRI, be sure to inform your physician immediately. People with migraines who take SSRIs should also take feverfew,

which prevents surges in serotonin levels. It is more common to be prescribed tricyclic antidepressants such as amitriptyline (Elavil), nortriptyline (Pamelor), and protriptyline (Vivactil). These are considered the first line of treatment to reduce migraines by affecting serotonin and other brain chemicals. (For information about herbal antidepressants that do not cause migraine pain, *see* DEPRESSION.) It is wise to prevent migraines by taking the prescribed medicine from your health-care provider.

❏ Some women who suffer from migraines should not use high-estrogen birth control pills. However, others have derived benefits.

❏ Coital headache—that is, migraine pain occurring during sexual climax—affects both sexes. Coital headache accompanied by nausea, vomiting, visual disturbances, loss of motor control, or loss of consciousness should always be brought to a doctor's attention.

❏ Scientific studies of chiropractic manipulation of the neck as a treatment for migraine have found that chiropractic reduces the severity, although not the frequency, of migraine attacks. Other treatments that have been shown to help include muscle relaxation exercises, acupuncture, biofeedback, and massage. Getting enough sleep may also help.

❏ Children with migraines frequently benefit from training in progressive relaxation, usually given by a psychologist or licensed therapist. (*See* RELAXATION TECHNIQUES in Part Three.)

❏ The effectiveness of acupuncture as a treatment for migraine is closely linked to the psychological state of the person receiving it. Researchers have found that extroverted people are much more likely to benefit from acupuncture for headaches than introverted people, and that response to acupuncture is better if the person has been having attacks for only a few months. (For more information, *see* ACUPUNCTURE in Part Three.)

❏ A recent study of reflexology—the application of pressure to spots on the soles of the feet that correspond to various parts of the body—as a therapy for migraine found that 80 percent of people experienced reduced symptoms, and 20 percent were able to discontinue all (including herbal) medications after three months of weekly treatment. Researchers believe that reflexology helps migraine sufferers interpret body signals and avoid migraine triggers.

❏ Migraine headaches in women may result from hormonal changes during the menstrual cycle. After menopause, the headaches may decrease.

❏ Music has a calming effect and can help to relieve migraines.

❏ Caffeine has been found to be a very safe and effective method for increasing pain relief. Adding caffeine to over-the-counter (OTC) pain relievers has been shown to make pain relievers 40 percent more effective in treating headaches.

❏ Migraines can be triggered by food allergies, and may be relieved by identifying and avoiding problem foods. (*See* Food Allergies *under* ALLERGIES.)

MONONUCLEOSIS

Mononucleosis, nicknamed mono, is an acute viral infection typically caused by the Epstein-Barr virus (EBV). Since the infection is transmitted by saliva, it is frequently referred to as "kissing fever." It can be transmitted through the sharing of food or eating utensils and sexual contact. The virus can also be airborne. While peak incidence occurs in fifteen- to seventeen-year-olds, the infection may occur at any age. It is most often diagnosed in people between the ages of ten and thirty-five.

The infection usually begins slowly with fatigue, malaise, headache, and sore throat. A moderate to high fever develops. The sore throat becomes progressively worse, often with enlarged tonsils covered with a whitish-yellow fibrous discharge. The lymph nodes in the neck are frequently enlarged and painful, and the spleen often becomes enlarged.

A pink measleslike rash may occur in some cases of mono and is more likely if you take the medicines ampicillin or amoxicillin for a throat infection. (Antibiotics should *not* be given without a positive strep test.) Fever usually abates in ten days, and swollen lymph glands and spleen heal in four weeks. Fatigue may linger for two to three months. Mononucleosis generally goes away on its own, but it may leave the body vulnerable to other chronic conditions.

There are no prescription antiviral treatments for EBV, but herbs may help with symptoms. Seek emergency medical assistance if there is a sharp, sudden pain in the left upper abdomen. This could indicate a ruptured spleen, which requires emergency surgery.

Recommendations

❏ Be sure to get plenty of rest, especially if your liver and spleen are enlarged.

❏ Treat swollen lymph glands with ice packs.

❏ Do not give aspirin or any aspirin-containing product to a child who shows symptoms of a viral infection. Aspirin use can result in Reye's syndrome, a potentially serious complication.

❏ Do not strain when having a bowel movement, as this may injure an enlarged spleen.

❏ Eat protein-rich foods. Protein is needed to stimulate the formation of antibodies that protect against complications such as hepatitis and jaundice.

❏ Drink plenty of fluids, such as water and fruit juices, to help relieve fever and sore throat. Gargling with salt water several times a day may also relieve a sore throat. Use ½ teaspoon of salt for every 8 ounces of water.

❏ Ease back into your normal routine, which could take a few weeks, particularly getting back to an exercise regimen. It may take two to three months until you are completely back to normal. Resuming a normal life too soon can result in a relapse.

Considerations

❏ Chronic EBV infection may produce symptoms similar to those of Sjögren's syndrome, but without raising antibody counts in blood tests that confirm a Sjögren's diagnosis. There is a different antibody test to show the presence of EBV. In addition to other treatments, a three- to six-month course of treatment with scutellaria may help relieve Sjögren's-like symptoms, which include dry eyes, mouth, and skin.

❏ EBV infection leaves a long legacy of unbalanced production of B and T cells in the immune system. If the immune system is weakened by organ transplant, chronic infection, or HIV, you may become sicker.

Mononucleosis: Beneficial Herbs

Herb	Form and Dosage	Comments
Astragalus	Tablets. Take as directed on the label.	Boosts the immune system.
Gleditsia	Tablets. Take as directed on the label.	Contains saponins that kill EBV. Also called zao jiao ci.
Olive leaf	Extract. Take as directed on the label.	Helps inhibit the growth of viruses that cause diseases such as mononucleosis.
Scutellaria[1]	Tincture. Take 1–1½ tsp (4–6 ml) 3 times daily.	Contains baicalin, which kills EBV.

Precautions for the use of herbs:

[1]Do not use scutellaria if you have diarrhea.

Morning Sickness: Beneficial Herbs

Herb	Form and Dosage	Comments
Chamomile	German chamomile (*Matricaria recutita*) tea bag, prepared with 1 cup water. Take 1 cup as desired.	Stops gastrointestinal (GI) spasms.
Ginger	Tea, prepared by adding ⅓ tsp (1 gm) powdered ginger to 1 cup water. (*See* TEAS in Part Three.) Take 1 cup as desired.	Stops nausea. (*See under* Considerations, below.)
Raspberry leaf	Tea bag, prepared with 1 cup water. Take 1 cup as desired.	Stops diarrhea.

❑ Adequate rest, exercise, and nutrition are essential for the maintenance of general health and the prevention of mononucleosis.

MORNING SICKNESS

For a pregnant woman with morning sickness, the taste, sight, or smell of food can cause nausea, vomiting, and excessive salivation. Although called "morning" sickness, this condition can occur at any time of the day. It typically begins at four to eight weeks into the pregnancy and continues for up to sixteen weeks. Overall, the condition is most common in women who become pregnant before age thirty, but about 50 to 70 percent of all pregnant women experience nausea and vomiting at some point.

Why some women experience morning sickness and others do not is not clear, but the condition may be beneficial to the developing embryo. Through a mechanism that is not fully understood, nausea and vomiting may stimulate the production of estrogen. Estrogen thickens the lining of the uterus and stimulates the growth of blood vessels serving the placenta, which nourishes the infant.

While the herbal treatments recommended above are both safe and effective, it is important to remember that they are intended to treat, rather than prevent, symptoms. Do not take any of these herbs on a continuous basis—that is, two or three times daily—during early pregnancy. Always check with your obstetrician before using any of these treatments.

Recommendations

❑ Neutralize excess stomach acid by eating a few whole-grain crackers or whole-wheat toast in the morning. Drinking lemon juice in water also will help neutralize stomach acid, as will eating pickled or raw ginger.

❑ Eat small, frequent meals.

❑ If nausea and vomiting continue beyond sixteen weeks, see a doctor. About 1 to 2 percent of pregnant women develop an especially severe form of morning sickness known as hyperemis gravidarum, in which nausea and vomiting continue beyond sixteen weeks, and result in weight loss and electrolyte disturbances. Sometimes it is necessary to provide intravenous fluids and nutrition if

the problem persists. In one study, more than 60 percent of women who required intravenous nutrition due to hyperemis gravidarum had blood levels of key vitamins and minerals—such as vitamins B$_6$ and C and calcium—that were below normal. Intravenous feeding alleviated the nausea and vomiting and corrected the vitamin levels in the blood.

❑ Do not go without food or drink because of the nausea.

❑ Do not sit up or get out of bed too quickly.

Considerations

❑ The use of ginger during pregnancy, once a source of controversy among herbalists, has been extensively studied. Drinking as many as ten cups of ginger tea a day is considered relatively safe and should have no effect on either the development of the child or the possibility of miscarriage. However, speak to your doctor first before consuming large quantities of ginger tea.

❑ While morning sickness may be a mechanism that protects the baby, women who do not experience nausea and vomiting during pregnancy have no special reason to fear a problem pregnancy. Persistent stories claiming that not having morning sickness means the child will be born with a birth defect are not true.

❑ The additional estrogen production during morning sickness in pregnancy may aggravate estrogen-related diseases after pregnancy. This effect may be canceled out by breast-feeding, which reduces the production of estrogen, especially with the first child.

MOTION SICKNESS

Motion sickness is the queasiness some people experience in a moving vehicle or while watching a simulation of movement. Queasiness can become headache, dizziness, nausea, vomiting, cold sweats, excessive salivation, fatigue, loss of appetite, and even a total loss of coordination. Motion sickness can occur while riding in all common forms of transportation, while on amusement-park rides, and while playing video games. The more the "ride" is curvy and bumpy, the worse the symptoms.

Motion Sickness: Beneficial Herbs

Herb	Form and Dosage	Comments
Black horehound	Take as directed on the label.	Reduces nausea.
Fennel seed[1]	Tea bag, prepared with 1 cup water. Take 1 cup as desired.	Relieves lingering nausea.
Ginger	Tea (powdered), prepared with ⅓ tsp (1 gm) powdered ginger and 1 cup water. (*See* TEAS in Part Three.) Take 1 cup as desired; or tincture. Take as directed on the label.	Relieves symptoms more effectively than Dramamine.
Peppermint[2]	Tea bag, prepared with 1 cup water. Take 1 cup as desired; or tincture. Take as directed on the label.	Relieves nausea, upset stomach, and gas.

Precautions for the use of herbs:

[1] Do not take fennel seed if you have an estrogen-sensitive condition, such as breast cancer, endometriosis, or fibrocystic breasts.

[2] Do not take peppermint if you have a gallbladder disorder.

The underlying cause of motion sickness is a disturbance in the labyrinth of the inner ear, which is responsible for equilibrium and balance. Uneven motion causes an interruption of blood supply to the ear, which results in a jumble of signals to the brain. The eyes and sensory nerves send additional information to the brain, which can aggravate the symptoms produced by the signals from the inner ear. Even with the eyes closed, moving the head from side to side can make symptoms worse. Offensive odors, sights, and sounds contribute to motion sickness.

Although motion sickness is not a psychosomatic illness, it has a strong psychological component. Past episodes of motion sickness train the brain to "expect" upset stomach and vertigo. Therefore, treating motion sickness attacks prevents future attacks. If severe symptoms appear within a few seconds, or if there is chest pain or loss of muscle control on one side of the body, the problem is not motion sickness. Seek medical help immediately.

Unless otherwise specified, the herb dosages recommended here are for adults. Children under age six should be given one-quarter of the adult dosage. Children between the ages of six and twelve should be given one-half of the adult dosage. Formula dosages for children should be discussed with a knowledgeable health-care practitioner.

Recommendations

❑ Look straight ahead. Glancing from side to side in particular worsens symptoms, while keeping the gaze fixed ahead relieves them. On a ship, stay on deck and look at the horizon; on a plane, sit near the wing.

❑ If symptoms are not too severe, place some kind of weight in your lap. This may prevent the draining of blood away from the head, which helps provide the inner ear with needed circulation. Or you could lie down.

❑ Drink adequate fluids before and during the trip, but avoid loading the stomach with greasy foods, salty foods, or alcohol. Instead, eat a bulky source of slowly released carbohydrate, such as whole-grain cereals or breads before traveling, and nibble on crackers or whole-grain breads during the trip.

❑ Try sipping green or ginger tea during long trips. Sucking on a fresh lemon also may calm the stomach.

❑ Do not read while traveling.

Considerations

❑ To prevent chronic motion sickness, take 240 milligrams of ginkgo extract once a day. Discuss the use of ginkgo with your doctor before having any type of surgery, and avoid it entirely if you are taking a blood-thinning medication.

❑ Chronic motion sickness may be helped with prism eyeglasses, more commonly used for the treatment of learning disabilities.

❑ Use forms of transportation that have a fairly smooth motion, such as buses and trains.

❑ Motion sickness from playing video games and training in simulators worsens with repeated exposure.

❑ Motion sickness attacks usually become less severe with age. People who have problems with motion sickness as children usually "outgrow" attacks by their mid-twenties.

❑ Sailing can cause motion sickness that may trigger migraine in people who otherwise do not get migraine headaches. These headaches occur regardless of the hormonal factors that usually trigger migraine.

❑ Chewable papaya tablets can be helpful.

MOUTH AND GUM PROBLEMS

See CANKER SORES (APHTHOUS ULCERS); DRY MOUTH; HALITOSIS (BAD BREATH); PERIODONTAL DISEASE. *See also* information on cold sores *under* HERPESVIRUS INFECTION.

MULTIPLE MYELOMA

See under BONE CANCER.

MULTIPLE SCLEROSIS

Multiple sclerosis (MS) is a disease of the central nervous system, where the body's own immune system attacks itself. Nerve cells are sheathed in a substance called myelin. In MS, there is chronic inflammation and destruction of these sheaths. This leaves the underlying nerves vulnerable to damage, which can result in scarred areas called plaques. No one knows exactly how many people have MS. It is believed that, currently, there are approximately 250,000 to 350,000 people in the United States with MS diagnosed by a physician. This estimate suggests that approximately 200 new cases are diagnosed each week.

The symptoms of MS may be dramatic or mild, and depend on which nerve fibers in the brain or spinal cord are damaged. Common problems include weakness of the limbs; loss of dexterity; muscular stiffness, tremors, and the recurrent stubbing of the big toe due to "foot drop," or a weakness in which the toes drag on the ground in walking. There may also be blurred vision or partial blindness, facial pain, dizziness, tingling, numbness, and spasms. Urinary or bowel dysfunction may occur. Mental symptoms, such as mood swings, may occur. Almost all cases of

MS are marked by fatigue and heat sensitivity, that is, the appearance or worsening of symptoms after exposure to heat (such as a hot shower).

MS may occur as relapsing MS, in which acute attacks lasting from days to weeks are followed by some degree of recovery; chronic progressive MS, in which symptoms become gradually worse without periods of stability; or inactive MS, with fixed areas of damage that do not worsen with time. The varied nature of this illness means that there is no one test that can detect it. Diagnosis depends on observation of the disease and testing to rule out other causes.

MS is much more common in temperate climates than in tropical ones, and marked differences in the prevalence of MS exist between different ethnic groups. It occurs more frequently in Scandinavia and northern Europe, while it is virtually unknown in sub-Saharan Africa and almost completely unknown in Japan. In addition, being female, between the ages of twenty and forty, and having a family history increase your risk.

While the exact cause of MS is unknown, scientists currently believe that MS requires a combination of genetic predisposition and a triggering factor, usually a viral infection in late childhood. In MS, the infection causes the body to create misdirected immune-system cells called T cells, which secrete tumor necrosis factor (TNF). TNF, in turn,

Multiple Sclerosis: Beneficial Herbs

Herb	Form and Dosage	Comments
Alfalfa	Liquid or tablets. Take as directed on the label.	Provides good source of vitamin K.
Ginkgo[1]	Ginkgolide tablets. Take 160–180 mg once daily.	Improves blood flow to the brain. Helps prevent relapses.
Soy lecithin[2]	Leci-PS tablets. Take 300 mg daily.	Reduces TNF production.

Precautions for the use of herbs:

[1]Do not take ginkgo if you are taking blood-thinning medications. Discuss the use of this herb with your doctor before having any type of surgery.

[2]Soy lecithin may cause mild diarrhea when first used.

Multiple Sclerosis: Formulas

Formula	Comments
Four-Substance Decoction	A traditional Chinese herbal formula that provides symptomatic relief of blurred vision and dizziness.
Ginseng Decoction to Nourish the Nutritive Chi	A traditional Chinese herbal formula that increases the effectiveness of prednisolone.
Ophiopogonis Decoction[1]	A traditional Chinese herbal formula that relieves respiratory distress (coughing, wheezing) accompanying MS. Increases the effectiveness of steroid drugs.
Sairei-to[2]	This is a combination of two commonly available traditional Chinese herbal formulas: Five-Ingredient Powder with Poria and Minor Bupleurum Decoction. It increases the effectiveness of prednisone.

Precautions for the use of formulas:

[1]Do not use Ophiopogonis Decoction if you have a fever.

[2]Do not use Sairei-to if you are taking alpha-interferon.

signals other immune-system cells called macrophages to attack the nerve cells. This leads to an abnormal blood-brain barrier that is "opened" by extremely small blood clots, which allows toxic chemicals to enter the brain. However, thus far this has only been seen in a laboratory model.

There is no one conventional treatment for MS (*see under* Considerations, this page). Herbal therapies are being used experimentally in treatment. Always speak to a doctor before taking these therapies, and use them under the guidance of an herbal practitioner.

Herbs to Avoid

❑ People who have MS should avoid cistanche, ginseng, and maitake. Cistanche and ginseng, like sildenafil (Viagra), relax the penile artery, but also stimulate the production of proteins that activate the immune system to attack nerves. (For more information regarding these herbs, *see* the individual entries *under* The Herbs in Part One.)

Recommendations

❑ Follow a low-fat diet, but be sure to get enough essential fatty acids. A study of 150 people with MS found that consuming fewer than 200 calories (or 10 percent of total calories) a day in fat greatly reduced the rate of disability from the disease. On the other hand, scientists believe that one reason MS is rare in Japan is that the traditional Japanese diet is rich in essential omega-3 fatty acids, which are vital for nerve health. In one study, patients with MS who went on a low-fat diet (15 percent of total calories) and took fish oil capsules had fewer relapses as well as improvements in many symptoms according to two scales that are used by doctors to assess how someone with MS is doing over one year. Another group ate 30 percent of calories from fat and used olive oil in cooking. This group also had less fatigue and a decrease in the number of relapses but did not get other benefits on the scales for MS symptoms.

❑ Fight carbohydrate cravings with 5-HTP. The urge to consume sugar-rich foods is a sign that the brain may be experiencing a shortage of the amino acid tryptophan, which enters the brain more readily if blood sugar levels are relatively high. Without tryptophan, the brain cannot make serotonin, which helps control mood. Supplementing with 5-HTP may allow the brain to make serotonin, without binge eating, to raise both sugar and tryptophan levels.

❑ Be careful in the sun. The mechanisms the body uses to cope with heat are compromised in MS, and some sunbathers who have MS have even died of heat exhaustion. However, sun exposure allows the body to make vitamin D, which is important for MS patients, especially in children who are still growing. In one study, a group of young patients with MS had half as many relapse incidents when they took daily supplements of magnesium, calcium, and vitamin D. Adults should probably take these supplements

as well because it is likely that these nutrients are important for the development and structure of myelin.

❑ Eat plenty of raw sprouts and alfalfa, plus foods that contain lactic acid, such as sauerkraut and dill pickles. Also good are "green drinks" that contain plenty of chlorophyll.

❑ Drink at least eight 8-ounce glasses of quality water each day to keep yourself hydrated.

Considerations

❑ Steroid drugs, such as prednisone (Deltasone), are used to reduce symptoms during MS relapses, but also can cause a number of side effects. (*See* "Side Effects of Cancer Treatment" *under* CANCER.) Other drugs and treatments such as plasma exchange are used to reduce the frequency of relapses or to protect myelin from destruction. Plasma exchange mechanically separates your blood cells from your plasma, which has been shown to help patients with MS who do not respond to steroids.

❑ Researchers in Scandinavia have long used essential fatty acid supplementation to treat MS and to reduce the frequency of exacerbations.

❑ According to the New Jersey College of Medicine, X-ray irradiation of the lymph glands and the spleen may halt the progress of MS in rare cases. However, radiation exposure depresses the immune system.

❑ If chronic pain is a concern, *see* PAIN, CHRONIC.

MUMPS

Mumps is a viral disease causing acute and painful inflammation of the salivary glands and sometimes other glands in the body. The virus is passed through infected saliva. First symptoms can include headache, chills, loss of appetite, malaise, and, if the body's immune resistance is especially low, fever. For many people, however, the first symptom is the swelling of the salivary glands, the mumps, which generally starts about a day after any initial symptoms.

Once in the body, the virus incubates for twelve to twenty-five days before the swelling appears. A person can infect others for about five days before the mumps appear until about nine days afterward. This disease appears most often in children, but can occur in adults as well. Adults with mumps tend to experience greater discomfort and suffer more complications. Complications of mumps are potentially serious, but rare—and your odds of contracting mumps aren't very high. Mumps was common until the mumps vaccine was licensed in the 1960s. Since then, the number of cases has dropped dramatically. Because outbreaks of mumps still occur in the United States and mumps is still common in many parts of the world, getting a vaccination to prevent mumps is important.

About 25 percent of males past puberty who get mumps experience swelling of the testicles (orchitis). Shaking chills and high fevers are frequent, and may be accompanied by headache, nausea, and vomiting. Usually testicular swelling eases after seven to nine days. Even if the testicles atrophy after the infection runs its course, complete infertility is rare whether or not both testicles are inflamed. Other, rarer, complications include inflammation of the brain, pancreas, or ovaries, hearing loss, and miscarriage. The current scientific understanding of mumps is that the immune system both defends against the virus by producing interferon, and causes the pain and swelling characteristic of the disease by needlessly activating other immune-system components called T cells.

Conventional treatment consists of using aspirin or other painkillers to ease pain and reduce fever. Young children should not take aspirin if they have a fever because aspirin use can result in Reye's syndrome, a potentially serious complication. Herbal therapies should be used only until the swelling subsides. Children under age six should be given one-quarter of the adult herb dosage. Children between the ages of six and twelve should be given one-half of the adult dosage. Formula dosages for children should be discussed with a knowledgeable health-care practitioner.

Herbs to Avoid

❑ People who have mumps should avoid echinacea, which activates T cells. (For more information about this herb, see ECHINACEA under The Herbs in Part One.)

Recommendations

❑ Eat mostly juiced or soft foods while your glands are swollen.

❑ To relieve the pain of swollen glands, use either warm or cool compresses, depending on what feels best.

❑ Do not give any product containing aspirin to a child who shows symptoms of a viral infection. Aspirin use can result in Reye's syndrome, a potentially serious complication.

❑ Do not consume coffee, dairy products, tobacco, or white flour or sugar. Avoid acidic foods, such as pickles and citrus fruits or juices, as they are likely to cause discomfort.

❑ Stay warm and dry and get plenty of rest.

❑ Drink plenty of pure water and fresh juices to keep the body well hydrated and to flush the system clean.

Considerations

❑ Bed rest cannot prevent testicular swelling, contrary to popular belief, but can ease testicular pain.

❑ Allergic reactions to mumps-measles-rubella (MMR) vaccine in children that are severe enough to require emergency room treatment are rare, affecting approximately one in a million people given the vaccine. Milder reactions—including pain, redness, swelling, and fever of up to 103°F (39.5°C)—are much more common. The risk of allergic reaction to MMR shots may be reduced by giving

Mumps: Beneficial Herbs

Herb	Form and Dosage	Comments
Elder flower	Tea bags. Take as directed on the label.	Helps reduce fever.
Siberian ginseng[1]	Pure eleuthero extract. Take as directed on the label in ¼ cup water.	Increases interferon production. Use as soon as possible after exposure.
Yarrow	Tea. Take as directed on the label.	Reduces fever and inflammation and is a good lymphatic cleanser.

Precautions for the use of herbs:

[1]Do not use Siberian ginseng if you have prostate cancer or an autoimmune disease, such as lupus or rheumatoid arthritis.

Mumps: Formulas

Formula	Comments
Kudzu Decoction	A traditional Chinese herbal formula that can moderate symptoms by supplementing the antiviral activity of the immune system.
Minor Bupleurum Decoction[1]	A traditional Chinese herbal formula that relieves pain and swelling, and prevents progression of viral diseases.

Precautions for the use of formulas:

[1]Do not use Minor Bupleurum Decoction if you have a fever or a skin infection.

Sore Muscles: Beneficial Herbs

Herb	Form and Dosage	Comments
Amor seco	Tea bags. Take 1 cup 3 times daily. Prepare as directed on the label.	Especially useful for sore back muscles.
Arnica[1]	Cream. Apply 1–2 times daily.	Relives pain and stiffness.
Cayenne[2]	Capsaicin cream. Apply as directed on the label.	Relieves pain.
Tolu balsam	Resin. Apply 1–3 times daily.	Relieves pain and stiffness.

Precautions for the use of herbs:

[1]Do not apply arnica to broken skin or to an open wound. Do not take arnica internally. If a rash develops, stop using it. Do not use arnica if you are pregnant.

[2]Do not apply cayenne to broken skin. Avoid contact with eyes and mouth.

the child fermented foods that contain live *Lactobacillus* bacteria, such as yogurt or sauerkraut, for two or three days before the injection.

❏ Because complications are more common if this disease is contracted in adulthood, immunization should be considered for any adult who has not had mumps or who has not already been vaccinated against it.

❏ In most U.S. states, immunization against mumps is required before a child can be admitted into public kindergarten.

MUSCLE INJURY

See MUSCLES, SORE; SPRAINS AND STRAINS.

MUSCLES, SORE

Sore muscles are muscles that are compressed out of their usual shape during the course of exercise, reducing circulation to them. Muscle pain goes away as circulation is restored to the muscle, and inflammatory hormones are carried away by the bloodstream. Like "burning" muscles caused by anaerobic exercise, sore muscles usually heal by themselves, but the process may be accelerated.

Recommendations

❏ For muscles that are sore immediately after a workout, apply moist heat. After a day's rest, do gentle stretching exercises to restore blood circulation.

Considerations

❏ Massage is a standard and effective method of easing muscle pain. (*See* MASSAGE in Part Three.)

❏ Some experts recommend a cold-water soak for sore muscles. This will not reduce pain, but it will reduce stiffness and preserve range of motion.

❏ *See also* FRACTURE.

MYASTHENIA GRAVIS

Myasthenia gravis (MG) is a condition in which there is fluctuating weakness of commonly used muscles. Weakness occurs if the nerve impulse does not adequately reach muscle cells. This is caused by a blockage of neurotransmitters, the chemicals that transmit signals from nerve cells to muscle cells. The blockage may occur if the immune system produces high levels of antibodies, which could destroy muscles receptor sites for a neurotransmitter called acetylcholine. With fewer receptor sites, the muscles receive fewer signals, resulting in muscle weakness.

The precise cause of autoimmune disorders such as MG is unknown. Especially in older men, MG is associated—in about 15 percent of cases—with tumors of the thymus, an immune-system organ in the upper chest. It also occurs with, but is not necessarily caused by, hyperthyroidism and pernicious anemia.

MG primarily affects vision and breathing. There is usually double vision, difficulty maintaining a steady gaze, and drooping of the eyelids. Attempts to swallow frequently result in choking or gagging. Muscle weakness or paralysis that worsens with exertion later in the day may be a problem, although this can usually be relieved with rest. Difficulty in chewing, climbing stairs, lifting objects, and talking may also develop. While remissions can occur, the disease is progressive unless medically treated.

A number of conventional treatments are used for MG; herbal therapies should be included as part of an overall treatment plan. Seek emergency medical assistance if difficulties in breathing occur.

Herbs to Avoid

❏ People who have MG should avoid aloe, burdock, maitake, schisandra, Siberian ginseng, and snow fungus, and especially cat's claw and echinacea. These herbs stimulate the production of antibodies to nerve tissue. (For more information regarding these herbs, *see* ALOE, BURDOCK, MAITAKE, SCHISANDRA, SIBERIAN GINSENG, and SNOW FUNGUS, *under* The Herbs in Part One.)

Myasthenia Gravis: Beneficial Herbs

Herb	Form and Dosage	Comments
Astragalus[1]	Capsules. Take 500–1,000 mg 3 times daily.	Reduces concentrations of antibodies that cause myasthenia gravis (MG). (*See under* Considerations, below.)
Soy lecithin[2]	Capsules. Take 1,500–3,000 mg daily.	Provides materials needed for repairing nerve tissue.

Precautions for the use of herbs:

[1]Do not use astragalus if you have a fever or a skin infection.

[2]Soy lecithin may cause mild diarrhea when first used.

Myasthenia Gravis: Formulas

Formula	Comments
Hochu-ekki-to	A Japanese herbal formula that reduces concentrations of MG-causing antibodies while stimulating other immune cells. Helps prevent bacterial infection and certain kinds of cancer.

Recommendations

❏ Avoid L-carnitine. This supplement can aggravate double vision in MG.

❏ If eating is difficult, chew slowly and rest between bites. Eat small portions of juiced and soft foods, and avoid such sticky foods as peanut butter. Be sure to sit up straight while eating.

❏ Get adequate rest throughout the day. Close your eyes for a few minutes each hour or lie down several times a day.

❏ Avoid factors that can worsen MG-related weakness, including infections, extremes of heat or cold, and stress. (*See* STRESS.)

Considerations

❏ In MG the severity and extent of muscle weakness vary greatly from person to person. As a result, there is no one best way to treat this disorder. Conventional treatment includes drug therapy, the replacement of antibody-laden blood plasma with clean artificial plasma, surgery to remove the thymus gland (in about 15 percent of patients), and the immune suppressant azathioprine (Imuran). Imuran treatment can be highly effective if begun early, although it is difficult to determine its proper dosage. In other cases, steroids are used to suppress the immune system; however, they can cause an increased risk of infection, liver damage, and cancer. (To learn how to ease the side effects of steroid treatment, *see* "Side Effects of Cancer Treatment" *under* CANCER.) Drugs such a pyridostigmine (Mestinon) enhance communication between nerves and muscles. They don't cure the underlying disease but improve how people feel. Side effects include gastrointestinal (GI) upsets, excessive salivation, and frequent urination.

❏ Although astragalus is an immune stimulant in many conditions, it is an immune suppressant in MG. In one study that compared a control group of people treated with either cobalt-60 or dexamethasone with people treated with astragalus, the herb significantly reduced nicotinic acetylcholine receptor antibodies, a measure of the disease's severity. Unlike many other immune-stimulant herbs, astragalus does not stimulate the production of macrophages, which are necessary to provoke a series of immune reactions that create antibodies that destroy nerve tissue. Astragalus is a principal component of the traditional Chinese herbal formula Tonify the Middle and Augment the Chi Decoction, which has similar effects on MG but even greater effects against infection.

❏ Anesthesia and treatments for severe pain in people with MG are difficult because the same dosage must stop pain in both damaged and healthy nerve fibers. Acupuncture can be used to reduce pain if pain-relief drugs cannot be used. (*See* ACUPUNCTURE in Part Three.)

❏ *See also* HYPERTHYROIDISM, LUPUS, and RHEUMATOID ARTHRITIS.

MYOCARDIAL INFARCTION

See HEART ATTACK (MYOCARDIAL INFARCTION).

NAILS, INFECTED

Bacterial, fungal, and viral infections of the nails cause discoloration, distortion, deterioration, and pain. Fungus is the most common reason for infection of the nails, however. Nail infections become increasingly common with age. People treated with steroid drugs are at special risk for nail infections, as are people who take antibiotics.

Bacteria may cause painful pockets of infection in surrounding skin; severe infection may result in the loss of the nail plate. Bacteria can also create a reservoir of infection that can spread to other parts of the body. Fungi, molds, and yeasts, which also produce changes in the color, texture, and shape of the nails, usually enter the nail when it is cut, crushed, or exposed to irritating chemicals. Yeast infections are more common in fingernails than in toenails and in women than in men. Viral warts may cause a change in a nail's shape or cause skin to grow under the nail. Nail infections are more than just a cosmetic problem, since thickened and painful nails may limit mobility, interfere with circulation, and aggravate diabetic ulcers.

Nail infections are notoriously difficult to treat (*see under* Considerations, page 415). This is because people who get chronic nail infections tend to have a quirk of the immune system that creates many of the antibodies that generate irritation, but few of the macrophages that surround and dispose of infectious microbes. Herbal treatment helps compensate for this immune imbalance, and also is directly antibacterial and antifungal.

Recommendations

❑ Take *Lactobacillus* daily, especially if you have been taking antibiotics. *Lactobacillus* may help restore beneficial bacteria in the intestine.

❑ For weak, brittle nails, take 500 milligrams of black currant oil twice a day; results require about two months of use. Taking gelatin as a supplement does not strengthen nails.

❑ Avoid tight-fitting shoes or gloves. The immune system requires good circulation to the fingers and toes to fight nail infections. Wear loose-fitting rubber gloves to protect hands from overexposure to water. Wear cotton or wool socks to allow moisture to escape from your feet.

❑ Exercise care in using communal lavatories and showers. Most of the microorganisms that cause nail infections thrive in moist, warm conditions.

❑ Avoid the use of sodium hypochlorite solutions (such as Clorox) to treat infected nails. Sodium hypochlorite can be extremely irritating to the skin, even if diluted. Some people are especially sensitive.

❑ Tincture of iodine is a traditional remedy for fungal infections of the nails. Apply tincture of iodine per label directions daily until improvement is noted. In addition, a vinegar soak may help cure nail fungus. Soak feet or hands for fifteen to twenty minutes in 1 part vinegar and 2 parts warm water. Others have had success using Vicks VapoRub directly on the affected nail.

❑ Keep hangnails clipped. Wash your hands carefully after clipping infected nails.

❑ Do not bite, pick at, or tear your nails. Nail biting can be a sign of anxiety, chronic stress, or uncontrollable

Infected Nails: Beneficial Herbs

Herb	Form and Dosage	Comments
Barberry[1] or coptis[1] or goldenseal[1] or Oregon grape root[1]	Tincture. Take ¼–½ tsp (1–2 ml) in ¼ cup water 3 times daily.	Contain berberine, which kills bacteria and fungal nail infections.
Bloodroot	Salve. Use as directed on the label.	Stops bacterial infections at nail borders.
Coix	Cereal (available in Japanese groceries as hatomugi). Eat 1 oz (30 gm) daily.	Stimulates the immune system to fight viruses that cause warts under nails.
Echinacea	*Echinacea angustifolia* tincture. Take as directed on the label.	Controls *Pseudomonas*, which causes greening of the nails.
Pau d'arco	Capsules. Take as directed on the label; or tea. Use as a hand bath. (*See* HAND BATHS in Part Three.)	Stimulates immune system to destroy yeast cells.
Scutellaria[2]	Tincture. Take ½ tsp (2 ml) in ¼ cup water 3 times daily.	Kills many bacteria and fungi that infect nails.
Tea tree[3]	Oil. Apply full strength to affected nails once daily in the evening.	Controls yeast infections under the nails in 3–6 months.
Walnut leaf	Homemade salves. Apply to nails daily (commercially available in Canada).	Astringent. Prevents new yeast cells from "rooting" in the nail as old yeast cells die.

Precautions for the use of herbs:

[1]Do not use barberry, coptis, goldenseal, or Oregon grape root if you are pregnant or have gallbladder disease. Do not use these herbs daily for more than two weeks. Do not take these herbs with supplemental vitamin B_6 or with protein supplements containing the amino acid histidine. Do not use goldenseal if you have cardiovascular disease or glaucoma.

[2]Do not take scutellaria if you have diarrhea.

[3]People who are allergic to celery or thyme should not use tea tree oil products. Do not take tea tree oil internally.

compulsion. In extreme cases, psychological help may be necessary. (*See also* ANXIETY DISORDER and STRESS.)

❏ Some professional manicure businesses have been cited for not meeting health codes. If you have professional manicures, always insist on sterile instruments or bring your own to ensure that they are free from bacteria and disease. Use isopropyl alcohol to sterilize your instruments.

❏ If you have diabetes, see your health-care practitioner if your cuticles become inflamed, because the infection can spread.

Considerations

❏ Nail infections are often treated with prescription antifungal drugs such as terbinafine (Lamisil) or itraconazole (Sporanox). Clinical tests have found that tea tree oil, in addition to having no side effects, is at least as effective as the most often prescribed medications for yeast infections of the nails. Herbal treatments also have the advantage of not interacting with medications for asthma, high cholesterol, and aftercare of heart attack, unlike the prescription drugs used for this disorder.

❏ Many times deteriorating nails reflect an underlying health problem. Valve problems in the heart, cancer or chronic infection in the lungs, and other conditions that reduce the amount of oxygen in the blood may produce "clubbing" of the nails, in which the contour of the nail looks like the back of a teaspoon. Thyroid diseases, including both hypothyroidism and hyperthyroidism, may produce brittle nails, or nails that separate from the nail plate. Severe illness or surgery may produce Beau's lines, which are horizontal depressions in the nails. Vitamin deficiency or malnutrition of any sort can cause loss of luster or brittle nails, as can chronic hepatitis.

❏ Chronic exposure to nail polish or moisture may produce brittle nails with peeling of the edge of the nail.

❏ Nail problems that develop while dieting may indicate insufficient protein intake. Replace one carbohydrate serving with one protein serving daily if nail problems develop.

❏ Yellow nails that grow slowly could be a symptom of lymphedema rather than infection. Taking 800 international units (IU) of vitamin E daily, or applying a vitamin E cream to the affected nail, will help slowly reverse the condition. (For more information, *see* LYMPHEDEMA.)

❏ Yeast can infect the skin and other tissues. (*See* YEAST INFECTION [YEAST VAGINITIS].)

NAUSEA

Nausea is the unpleasant sensation of feeling as though one needs to vomit, which may or may not be followed by actual vomiting. In varying degrees, nausea is associated with increased perspiration, increased salivation, pallor, trembling, urgent defecation, and loss of appetite.

Although nausea is associated with the digestive tract, it is experienced in the brain. Nausea occurs when a chemical messenger known as 5HT3 binds to receptors in the area of the brain responsible for the sensation of nausea, an area known as the "trigger zone." Therefore, while nausea can be provoked by such digestive-tract disturbances as insufficient secretion of stomach acids, food poisoning, gallbladder problems, and appendicitis, it can also be caused by a variety of conditions not associated with the digestive tract. Stress, hormonal changes induced by chemotherapy or radiation treatment, uncontrolled diabetes, congestive heart failure, Ménière's disease, migraine, and motion sickness are just a few of the conditions that commonly cause nausea. Morphine and synthetic painkillers frequently cause nausea as well.

Sudden, severe, unexpected nausea requires medical attention. Herbs can be used on an ongoing basis to relieve other cases of chronic, mild nausea. Unless otherwise specified, the herb dosages recommended here are

Nausea: Beneficial Herbs

Herb	Form and Dosage	Comments
Chen-pi (also called bitter orange peel)[1]	Tea (loose), prepared with 1 tsp (3 gm) tea and 1 cup water. (*See* TEAS in Part Three.) Take 1 cup 3 times daily between meals.	Relieves nausea, bloating, belching, and flatulence.
Chiretta	Tincture. Take 10 drops in ¼ cup water, before meals.	Stops nausea by increasing production of bile, gastric juices, and saliva.
Ginger	Tea, prepared by adding ⅓ tsp (1 gm) powdered ginger to 1 cup water. (*See* TEAS in Part Three.) Take 1 cup 3 times daily.	Stops production of chemicals that activate the trigger zone.
St. John's wort	Tincture. Take as directed on the label.	Binds to $5HT_3$ receptors in the brain.

Precautions fort the use of herbs:

[1] Do not use chen-pi if you have bloody stool.

415

for adults. Children under age six should be given one-quarter of the adult dosage. Children between the ages of six and twelve should be given one-half of the adult dosage. Formula dosages for children should be discussed with a knowledgeable health-care practitioner.

Herbs to Avoid

❏ People who have nausea should avoid using the following herbs internally: butcher's broom, ephedra, horse chestnut, prunella, and uva ursi. (For more information regarding these herbs, *see* individual entries *under* The Herbs in Part One.)

Recommendations

❏ Do not use bicarbonate of soda to control nausea (although it may help other forms of indigestion). Not only does it not relieve nausea, but it blocks the action of St. John's wort and the prescription anti-nausea agent ondansetron (Zofran).

❏ Avoid overdoses of mineral supplements, especially those containing copper. As little as 10 milligrams of copper a day can cause nausea. But overdoses of any nutrient may contribute to nausea. Always take supplements with meals.

❏ Eat crackers or whole-wheat toast.

❏ Make sure you get enough liquids.

Considerations

❏ For ways to relieve nausea related to specific conditions, *see* CELIAC DISEASE; CONGESTIVE HEART FAILURE; GALLSTONES; HEPATITIS; MÉNIÈRE'S DISEASE; MIGRAINE; MORNING SICKNESS; MOTION SICKNESS; PARASITIC INFECTION; and VOMITING. *See also* "Side Effects of Cancer Treatment" *under* CANCER and Food Allergies *under* ALLERGIES.

NEPHRITIS

See under KIDNEY DISEASE.

NERVOUSNESS

See ANXIETY DISORDER; STRESS.

NOSEBLEED

Nosebleeds occur when the delicate capillaries in the nasal linings rupture. This can arise from a number of causes, most commonly through breathing dry air or nose picking. Other nosebleeds are caused by irritation of the mucous membranes lining the nasal passages and sinuses. Nosebleeds can also occur as a result of sudden change in atmospheric pressure, blowing the nose too forcefully, or an underlying illness.

Often, injury-related nosebleeds produce what looks like a lot of blood, although the amount of blood usually lost is slight. Irritation nosebleeds involve chronic, light bleeding. Nosebleeds that are severe and last longer than twenty minutes require emergency attention, as it may interfere with breathing.

The preparations listed here are appropriate for chronic, light nosebleeds that have no known cause and thus are assumed to be associated with irritation, or with emotional or hormonal factors (*see* Recommendations, page 417). Use any of these therapies until nosebleeds no longer recur. Unless otherwise specified, the herb dosages recommended here are for adults. Children under age six should be given one-quarter of the adult dosage. Children between the ages of six and twelve should be given one-half of the adult dosage. Formula dosages for children should be discussed with a knowledgeable health-care practitioner.

Nosebleed: Beneficial Herbs

Herb	Form and Dosage	Comments
Agrimony	Tea (loose), prepared with 1½ tsp (1.5 gm) and 1 cup water. (*See* TEAS in Part Three.) Take 1 cup 3 times daily.	Encourages clot formation. Especially useful for children's nosebleed.
Alfalfa[1]	Capsules. Take 1,000–2,000 mg daily; or fresh sprouts. Eat a handful or so daily.	Provides vitamin K for normal blood clotting.
Calendula (also called marigold)	Cream. Rub into the nostril.	Prevents infections. Promotes healing.
Oligomeric proanthocyanidins (OPCs)	Grapeseed or pine-bark extract tablets. Take 200 mg daily.	Antioxidant. Reduces blood-vessel inflammation.
Shepherd's purse	Tincture. Take 1½–2 tsp (6–8 ml) 3 times daily.	Stimulates constriction of the smooth muscles that surround blood vessels.

Precautions for the use of herbs:

[1]Do not use alfalfa if you are taking warfarin (Coumadin) or any other prescription or herbal blood-thinner. Do not take this herb if you have lupus or if you are pregnant.

Nosebleed: Formulas

Formula	Comments
Augmented Ophiopogonis Decoction[1]	A traditional Chinese herbal formula traditionally used to treat nosebleeds occurring during the menstrual period. Also useful in treating nosebleeds that occur at other times when estrogen levels are high, and those associated with use of birth control pills.
White Tiger Decoction[2]	A traditional Chinese herbal formula that stops a nosebleed caused by high blood pressure or that occurs with emotional stress.

Precautions for the use of formulas:

[1]Do not take Augmented Ophiopogonis Decoction if you have a fever.

[2]Do not take White Tiger Decoction if you are nauseous or if you are vomiting.

Recommendations

❑ Assess whether the nosebleed requires medical attention. Anterior nosebleeds are those in which bright red blood flows from one or both of the nostrils if the person stands or sits, although it may flow into the throat if the person lies down. This type of nosebleed can be frightening, but usually is not serious and can be self-treated. Posterior nosebleeds, on the other hand, require urgent medical attention. In this kind of nosebleed, blood, usually dark red, comes from the rear of the nose and runs down the back of the mouth into the throat, no matter what position the person is in. Posterior nosebleeds are more common in older people and among people with high blood pressure.

❑ Use horsetail tincture to treat a minor nosebleed. Wet a piece of gauze with a mixture of 10 drops of horsetail tincture added to ¼ cup of cold water. Place the gauze in the bleeding nostril and pinch the nostril closed. After ten minutes, slowly remove the gauze from the nostril.

❑ Do not lie flat on your back if you have a nosebleed. Blood that runs into the throat can cause choking or vomiting.

❑ Place cold compresses around your neck and calves. This reduces circulation to the head and slows bleeding.

❑ If nosebleeds are frequent, avoid aspirin and fruits and vegetables that contain aspirin-like chemicals, including apples, apricots, bell peppers, all berries, cloves, cherries, cucumbers, grapes, mint, pickles, plums, raisins, and tomatoes.

❑ Avoid taking more than 800 international units (IU) of vitamin E daily. Taking more than this amount can increase bleeding.

❑ When you sneeze, cover your mouth, but keep it open.

❑ To counteract dryness in the nasal passages, use nasal irrigation. Spray plain warm water into your nostrils two to three times daily.

❑ In winter months, maintain indoor humidity with a humidifier or by using steam heat. This prevents drying, cracking, and bleeding of the sinuses.

❑ Do not blow your nose for at least twelve hours after a nosebleed stops. Doing so may dislodge the blood clots that stanch bleeding.

❑ If you have frequent nosebleeds, see your doctor. Frequent nosebleeds may be a sign of high blood pressure. (*See* HIGH BLOOD PRESSURE [HYPERTENSION].)

❑ Use hawthorn to help prevent nosebleeds caused by high blood pressure. Take 100 to 250 milligrams of the tablets three times daily.

Considerations

❑ Nosebleeds are more common in children than in adults, in part due to children's tendency to place fingers and other objects in their nostrils. The mucous membranes lining the nose are thinner in children than in adults and thus more prone to damage.

❑ High estrogen levels increase the flow of blood from the mucous membranes in the nose. This is why nosebleeds are more common during pregnancy. Oral contraceptives also can contribute to nosebleeds.

❑ The risk of serious nosebleeds increases with hemophilia, Hodgkin's lymphoma, rheumatic fever, vitamin C deficiency, or the prolonged use of nose drops or nasal sprays.

❑ *See also* Respiratory Allergies *under* ALLERGIES.

OBESITY

See OVERWEIGHT.

OSTEOARTHRITIS

Osteoarthritis (OA) is the most common disorder in the world—nearly everyone has some degree of it by age sixty.

It results from wear and tear on joints, and is more common in those who weigh more. Injury and an inherited defect in the protein that forms cartilage also play roles in its development. Obesity, bone deformities, or having other disease such as gout, rheumatoid arthritis, or Paget's disease are also contributing factors. The hands and the weight-bearing joints—the knees, hips, and spine—are the areas most often affected.

Arthritic joints are painful and stiff, and lose their flexibility. The pain of OA can range from mild to excruciating. The bones can become deformed, often quite badly, even if the person experiences no pain. If the deformity is bad enough, the affected joint's range of motion can be severely limited.

OA primarily affects the synovial pads that line the bones within the joint. Over time, stress breaks down collagen, a protein found in the pads. With age, the ability to produce new collagen decreases. As the pads wear away, the bones rub together, causing pain and inflammation.

OA can also occur if there is traumatic stress on a joint, such as fracture or surgery.

Conventional treatment for OA depends on a variety of painkillers, both prescription and over-the-counter (OTC) (see under Recommendations, below). Formulas are used to treat symptom patterns, while individual herbs can control individual symptoms.

Recommendations

❑ Use every available alternative to aspirin, nonsteroidal anti-inflammatory drugs (NSAIDs), and steroids for pain control. Some evidence based on animal and cell studies suggests that these painkillers may have a destructive effect on cartilage. Aspirin and NSAIDs suppress the joint's ability to manufacture cartilage-building proteins, and they deactivate enzymes that are essential for making chondroitin, an important cartilage component. The more the joint has been damaged by OA, the more it absorbs NSAIDs that damage it even further, starting a spiral of

Osteoarthritis: Beneficial Herbs

Herbs	Form and Dosage	Comments
Alfalfa	Capsules. Take as directed on the label; or fresh sprouts. Eat a handful or so daily.	Contains all the minerals essential for bone formation.
Ashwagandha	Withanolide gelcaps. Take as directed on the label.	Anti-inflammatory effect similar to aspirin, without stomach irritation.
Boswellia[1]	Boswellin capsules or tablets. Take as directed on the label.	Relieves swelling and inflammation.
Cat's claw[2]	Capsules. Take 1,000–2,000 mg 3 times daily.	Relieves swelling and inflammation.
Cayenne[3]	Capsaicin cream. Apply as directed on the label.	Causes temporary skin pain that counteracts joint pain.
Chaparral and/or osha[4]	Tea. Use in a hand bath no more than once a month. (See HAND BATHS in Part Three.)	Stops inflammation.
Copaiba	Tincture. Take as directed on the label.	Relieves arthritic inflammation.
Devil's claw[5]	Enteric-coated capsules. Take 1,500–2,500 mg 3 times daily.	Relieves pain.
Feverfew[6]	Freeze-dried leaf in capsules. Take 25 mg daily and increase to 100 mg daily after 2 weeks.	Anti-inflammatory. Also reduces headache symptoms.
Ginger	Tea, prepared by adding ⅓ tsp (1 gm) powdered ginger to 1 cup water. (See TEAS in Part Three.) Take 1 cup 1–2 times daily.	Stops production of inflammatory chemicals.
Hawthorn	Tablets. Take 100–250 mg 3 times daily.	Helps stabilize collagen, protecting joints from wear.
Turmeric	Powder. Apply in a poultice twice daily. (See POULTICES in Part Three.)	Relieves pain as effectively as steroid drugs without weakening the immune system.
Willow bark	Salicin tablets. Take 20–40 mg 3 times daily.	Pain relief similar to aspirin, but longer-lasting and without stomach irritation.
Yucca	Saponin extract. Take 3–6 drops in ¼ cup water twice daily.	Prevents inflammation. Stops circulation of toxins to the joint.

Precautions for the use of herbs:

[1]Do not take boswellia if you are pregnant.

[2]Do not take cat's claw if you take insulin for diabetes. Do not use this herb if you are pregnant or nursing.

[3]Do not apply cayenne to broken skin. Avoid contact with eyes and mouth.

[4]Chaparral and osha sensitize skin to sunlight; use sunscreen on the treated area when you are outdoors. Do not take these herbs internally.

[5]Devil's claw can slow heartbeat. Avoid this herb if you have congestive heart failure.

[6]Discontinue taking feverfew if you have an allergic reaction.

Osteoarthritis: Formula

Formula	Comments
True Warrior Decoction[1]	A traditional Chinese herbal formula designed to treat people who have aching bones and joints, aversion to cold, and cold extremities. Used if the primary symptom is swelling.

Precautions for the use of formulas:

[1]Discontinue using True Warrior Decoction if you develop a fever. This formula may cause a loss of sensation in the mouth and tongue.

pain and tissue destruction. Steroid inflammatory drugs are even more destructive, causing chondroitin-making cells to die at five times the normal rate. However, if using these drugs is the only way you can continue to exercise and live a normal life, it may be worth the risks.

❏ Avoid aspartame. While there is scientific evidence that aspartame can relieve arthritis pain (from a clinical study conducted by a scientist who noticed that his arthritis pains went away whenever he had a Diet Coke), aspartame has been shown in cell studies to have many of the tissue-destructive effects of aspirin and NSAIDs. However, using other artificial sweeteners such as Splenda helps people lose weight, which may ease symptoms of OA.

❏ Take at least 200 milligrams of s-adenosylmethionine (SAMe) daily. SAMe reduces swelling and crepitation (the creaking sound made by arthritic joints), and improves mobility and range of motion. SAMe helps control pain like NSAIDs without damaging cartilage or irritating the stomach, although in some cases it can cause nausea.

❏ Since SAMe is not effective for OA if there is vitamin B_{12} (cobalamin) or folate deficiency, take supplements of these vitamins. One milligram per day of each vitamin is sufficient.

❏ Take 1,200 milligrams of chondroitin sulfate and 1,500 milligrams of glucosamine sulfate daily. These substances may help joint repair. Taking glucosamine supplements may reduce pain as effectively as taking ibuprofen without tissue damage, although not as quickly. Chondroitin, although poorly absorbed through the digestive tract, is useful in increasing the effect of glucosamine. However, the results of a two-year study on slowing the progression of joint erosion in the knees showed that most participants did not see benefit in the combination of the two ingredients. Still, many people do get relief from a combination of glucosamine and chondroitin, so it's reasonable to try it and see if it works for you.

❏ Chondroitin and glucosamine may be made more effective by supplementation with 200 to 300 milligrams of magnesium ascorbate daily. This triple combination is especially helpful in treating OA of the knee and lower back.

❏ Another natural compound that has been shown to be effective for reducing pain from osteoarthritis of the knee is methylsulfonylmethane (MSM). In one study, patients who used 3 grams twice a day (6 grams total) had less pain and better physical function at the end of twelve weeks and there were no side effects.

❏ Vitamin D may be of benefit. Take 400 to a maximum of 1,000 international units (IU) of vitamin D daily. This can be as part of a calcium supplement or a multivitamin. Taking more than 400 milligrams may not be of benefit. Get your vitamin D levels tested to figure out your true needs.

❏ Eat foods rich in vitamin K, such as alfalfa, blackstrap molasses, and dark green leafy vegetables. Together, vitamins D and K may be helpful in preventing severe OA of the hip joints and knees.

❏ Soak in hot water and hot whirlpool baths as often as possible to prevent pain. Relieve acute pain and swelling with ice packs over "hot" joints.

❏ Exercise to keep joints as mobile as possible, but avoid putting stress on the joints. For aerobic exercise, swim or do exercises in warm water; see if a community pool in your area has an aquacise program designed for people with joint problems.

❏ Avoid wearing high-heeled shoes. High heels place stress on the knee joint and accelerate degeneration of the joint.

❏ Eat fresh pineapple frequently. In cell studies, bromelain, an enzyme found in pineapple, has been shown to reduce inflammation. To be effective, the pineapple must be fresh, as freezing and canning destroy enzymes.

❏ Reduce the amount of fat in your diet. Limit consumption of dairy fat and red meat. Use low-fat dairy products and increase your intake of poultry and seafood. Also avoid caffeine, citrus fruits, paprika, salt, tobacco, and everything containing sugar.

Considerations

❏ Overweight people with OA generally find that symptoms improve as they lose weight. (See OVERWEIGHT.)

419

Even if weight loss is not possible, however, OA symptoms improve with exercise and lowered body fat; that is, increasing muscle mass while maintaining weight.

❑ Maintaining muscle strength through regular exercise may slow the progress of OA. Professionally supervised stretching exercises and weight training reduce pain and increase flexibility for OA in the hip and knee, although the benefits are modest.

❑ If blood is too acidic, the cartilage in the joints may begin to dissolve. The joints lose their normal smooth sliding motion, bones rub together, and the joints become inflamed, causing pain. Acidic blood is best corrected by eating a diet rich in fruits and vegetables.

❑ In one study, taking extra vitamin E (500 IU) each day for two years had no effect on knee cartilage loss in patients with osteoarthritis of the knee. Vitamin E is an essential nutrient and is best obtained from the diet or taking it as part of a multivitamin pill.

❑ In one study, a natural product called Phytalgic, containing fish oil, vitamin E, Urtica dioica (stinging nettle), and zinc, was tested in patients with OA of the hip or knee for three months. People who got the natural product had less stiffness and more mobility, and were able to use fewer NSAIDs. These benefits were not seen in the placebo group.

❑ Lyme disease can mimic arthritis, causing many of the same symptoms.

❑ To learn how to deal with chronic pain, *see* PAIN, CHRONIC.

❑ *See also* RHEUMATOID ARTHRITIS.

OSTEOPOROSIS

Osteoporosis is a condition in which the bones become porous and easily broken. Osteoporosis can affect men, but the overwhelming majority of people who have osteoporosis are women who are past menopause. Usually there are no symptoms until a severe backache, which indicates a fractured vertebra, or hip fracture occurs. This happens because osteoporosis causes the loss of minerals from the pelvis and spine, which can be seen on an X-ray. Fractured vertebrae can cause a decrease in height. Curvature of the spine and a change in posture can be indicative of osteoporosis.

People often think of bone as a dry, inert substance, but

Osteoporosis: Beneficial Herbs

Herb	Form and Dosage	Comments
Alfalfa[1]	Capsules. Take 1,000–2,000 mg daily; or fresh sprouts. Eat a handful or so daily.	Provides vitamin K_2, which stimulates regrowth of bone.
Feverfew[2]	Encapsulated freeze-dried herb. Take as directed on the label.	Good for pain relief and acts as an inflammatory.
Hawthorn	Tablets. Take 100–250 mg 3 times daily.	Stabilizes collagen.
Por huesos	Tea (loose), prepared with 1 tsp (1 gm) tea and 1 cup water. (*See* TEAS in Part Three.) Take 1 cup 3 times daily, between meals.	"For bones" is the literal translation of the name of this herb. Encourages formation of the matrix that supports bone growth.
Soy isoflavone concentrate	Tablets. Take approximately 3,000 mg daily.	Helps move calcium from the bloodstream into bones.

Precautions for the use of herbs:

[1]Do not use alfalfa if you are taking warfarin (Coumadin) or any other prescription or herbal blood-thinner. Avoid this herb if you have lupus or if you are pregnant.

[2]Do not take feverfew if you are pregnant.

Osteoporosis: Formulas

Formula	Comments
Eight-Ingredient Pill with Rehmannia or Shih Qua Da Bu Tang or Warm the Menses Decoction[1]	In laboratory studies, these traditional Chinese herbal formulas prevent the erosion and pocketing of bone in animals deprived of estrogen. Japanese scientists believe any of these three formulas is as effective as estrogen replacement in preventing osteoporosis. (*See under* Considerations, page 421.)

Precautions for the use of formulas:

[1]Do not take Warm the Menses Decoction if you have a fever.

in fact it is a living tissue richly supplied with blood vessels and nerves. The same process the body uses to repair broken bones is also used to replace bone tissue over time, completely regenerating the entire skeleton every several years. Bone is broken down and built up at about the same rate in middle adulthood, but as a person ages, bone loss starts to exceed bone replacement.

In the bone regeneration process, two types of cells—cells that dissolve bone, called osteoclasts, and cells that build bone, called osteoblasts—work together to break down old bone and build up new bone. Osteoblasts secrete collagen, a tough, flexible protein that acts as a framework on which the calcium crystals that give bones their strength are deposited.

Osteoporosis often occurs after menopause because hormones regulate the regeneration of bone. Since every cell in the body requires calcium, a fall in bloodstream calcium levels triggers the production of hormones that direct osteoclasts to break down bone and release calcium into the bloodstream. Estrogen deficiency, such as that which occurs at menopause, makes osteoclasts more sensitive to the hormone that causes bone breakdown. Small, fine-boned people are more prone to developing osteoporosis than are larger-boned people. Also, poor dietary and lifestyle habits, as well as a lifetime of insufficient calcium intake, also play roles in the development of this disorder.

Herbs to Avoid

❏ People who have osteoporosis should avoid coleus (forskolin). (For more information regarding this herb, *see* COLEUS *under* The Herbs in Part One.)

Recommendations

❏ One of the most useful form of calcium for supplementation is calcium citrate malate, the form of calcium that is most absorbed by the body. Take any calcium-magnesium supplement providing at least 1,000 milligrams of calcium citrate daily. This form is expensive, however, and other forms work just as well as long as you use them daily.

❏ Eat a diet rich in calcium and vitamin D. In one study, eating fortified dairy products and following a healthy diet was shown over thirty months to increase body mineral density of the spine, arm bones, and the body overall compared to a group that did not follow a healthy diet high in calcium and vitamin D.

❏ A salad each day helps keep fractures away. This is because salad greens contain vitamin K, which helps bones use protein to construct the collagen "glue" that holds them together. Vegetables that contain vitamin K include iceberg lettuce, broccoli, Brussels sprouts, cabbage, kale, romaine lettuce, and spinach. As little as one serving a day of any of these vegetables can reduce the risk of fractures.

❏ Other foods may also help prevent fractures. Blueberries, cherries, and cherry juice contain anthocyanidins and proanthocyanidins, pigments that give them their blue and red colors. Like similar pigments in the herb hawthorn, these natural coloring agents stabilize collagen. Raw oats contain silica, (a naturally occurring form of silicon), which is essential for forming the bone matrix into which calcium crystals are deposited. Eat rolled oats as porridge or soaked overnight to make muesli.

❏ Silicon (Si) is the most abundant trace element in the diet after iron and zinc. The dietary consumption of silicon and other trace minerals may help increase bone mass, while deficiencies in this mineral may reduce bone density. Some water from artesian aquifers is rich in silicon. In one study, postmenopausal women who drank 1 quart a day for twelve weeks experienced an increase in silicon in the urine compared to a group that got low-silicon, purified water. Although no markers of bone health changed, these data were promising and this water may serve as a prevention or treatment to drug therapy for osteoporosis. Ask your doctor if you should use silicon supplements and for the correct dose for you.

❏ Avoid vitamin A supplements. A Swedish study of a pool of 66,651 women found that every milligram (3,000 IU) of vitamin A taken over the minimum Recommended Daily Allowance (RDA) increases the risk of bone fracture by 68 percent. Taking excessive vitamin A reduces bone density, especially in the hip. Cod liver oil is an especially concentrated source of vitamin A, and should be avoided by athletes in training and older people (especially women), as well as by people with osteoporosis. Beta-carotene is safe to take, as are foods that naturally contain vitamin A. Look for a multivitamin that uses beta-carotene rather than vitamin A.

❏ Exercise regularly after your doctor gives you an okay. In older people, progressive strength training and light weight lifting have been demonstrated to be safe and effective forms of exercise that reduce the risk of falling and increase bone mineral density, strengthening bones. In those people who cannot do weight exercises, tai chi—a form of gently rhythmic exercise—improves balance and confidence, and reduces the risk of falls.

❏ Include garlic and onions in your diet, as well as eggs (if your cholesterol level is not too high). These foods contain sulfur, which is needed for healthy bones.

Considerations

❏ Over 600 articles in the medical literature support the observation that plant-derived estrogens, or phytoestrogens, serve the same physiological functions as estrogen in the human body. In the body, estrogen and receptor sites on cells act like a car ignition—estrogen turns the osteoclast's "key," killing the ignition and stopping the breakdown of bone. Most phytoestrogens have a molecular structure that is very similar to the forms of estrogen naturally circulating in the bloodstream, which allows phytoestrogens to also serve as keys. In one study, post-menopausal women who consumed between 80 and 120 milligrams of soy isoflavones per day showed improvements in several areas, including new bone growth and increased bone mineral density in the femur and cortical bone.

❏ Though most cases of osteoporosis result from estrogen deficiency, both poor diet and drug treatment can cause the disease in both women and men. Osteoporosis is aggravated by acidosis—a condition in which body fluids become overly acidic—caused by not consuming enough fruits and vegetables. People who are bulimic or have anorexia nervosa tend to develop osteoporosis more frequently than the general population. Osteoporosis can also be caused by the use of corticosteroid drugs.

❏ Many people used to think that a high-protein diet caused osteoporosis. However, in one study, eating a high-protein diet compared to a low-protein diet (about 118 grams a day of protein as opposed to 48 grams of protein) caused an increase in calcium absorption and calcium lost in the urine in postmenopausal women. The net effect was no impact on bone formation. A high-protein diet is safe for the bones and a good way to lose weight. Protein increases the acid in the blood, which may be why it was thought to increase risk. Fruits and vegetables can counterbalance the acid buildup from animal protein. It is good to mix animal and vegetable sources of protein in your diet.

❏ It is important for bone health to engage in an exercise regime when you are dieting. In one study, postmenopausal women who participated in an aerobic exercise program while losing weight increased bone mineral density.

❏ Vitamin D deficiency is a major risk factor for both osteoporosis and bone fracture. The body manufactures its own vitamin D, but this process requires exposure to at least twenty minutes of sun daily on a regular basis and may increase the risk of skin cancer. The people most at risk for vitamin D deficiency are older people who are unable to go outdoors and who do not consume vitamin D–enriched dairy products. It is easy to get adequate vitamin D from supplements; try to take vitamin D with calcium.

❏ Vegetarians should be sure to consume proanthocyanidin-rich foods (see under Recommendations, page 421).

❏ In Europe, physicians are finding that using phytoestrogens and estrogen replacement therapy (ERT) together reduces the amount of estrogen replacement medication needed to prevent the loss of calcium. (See MENOPAUSE-RELATED PROBLEMS.)

❏ Both men and women slowly lose bone as they age. A woman may lose approximately 50 percent of her trabecular bone (spongy bone) and 30 percent of her cortical bone thickness over a lifetime—about half is lost during the first ten years after menses have ceased. Men lose far less.

❏ Carbonated soft drinks contain high amounts of phosphates. These cause the body to eliminate calcium as the phosphates themselves are excreted, even if calcium must be taken from the bones to do this.

❏ See also FRACTURE.

OSTEOSARCOMA

See under BONE CANCER.

OVARIAN CANCER

Approximately 14 out of 1,000 women in the United States will contract ovarian cancer at some point in life. The risk of developing this form of cancer increases with estrogen replacement therapy (ERT) use, family history of ovarian cancer, history of another cancer of the rectum or uterus, and never having been pregnant.

The symptoms of ovarian cancer are abdominal swelling, masses in the abdomen, bleeding, lower back pain, and urinary difficulties. Benign ovarian cysts can also cause these symptoms. (Sudden, sharp, and severe pain is usually caused by an ovarian cyst.) Because the symptoms of ovarian cancer overlap with several other conditions, this cancer is difficult to detect early and is frequently diagnosed only at an advanced stage.

A firm diagnosis is made by biopsy, although a number of other tests may be performed. Ovarian cancer is classified into stages I through IV by the extent of spread and by the type of cell from which it originated. It most often spreads to nearby organs within the abdomen, and then to the liver, lungs, or bones.

A number of conventional treatments are used for ovarian cancer (see under Considerations, page 423). Some ovarian cancers involve a defect in the "cancer-patrol" gene p53, a gene that is also important in controlling most kinds of cancer occurring in the breast, cervix, colon, lungs, and prostate, and in all strains of small cell lung cancer. Herbal treatment is most likely to be helpful in these cases. Always use herbal medicine as part of a medically directed overall treatment plan.

Herbs to Avoid

❏ Women who have ovarian cancer should avoid the following herbs: cordyceps, dan shen, fennel, licorice, and peony. (For more information regarding these herbs, see individual entries under The Herbs in Part One.)

Recommendations

❏ Use both quercetin and soy isoflavones. Laboratory studies at the Indiana University School of Medicine have found that quercetin and genistein, a key soy isoflavone, enhance each other's effects.

Ovarian Cancer: Beneficial Herbs

Herb	Form and Dosage	Comments
Astragalus	Capsules. Take 500–1,000 mg 3 times daily.	Increases production of immune-system chemical interleukin-2 (IL-2), which fights human papillomavirus (HPV). Activates gene p53.
Espinheira santa	Tincture. Take as directed on the label.	Slows growth of ovarian tumors.
Green tea	Catechin extract. Take 250–500 mg daily.	Deactivates plasmin, which helps tumors spread.
Mistletoe	Loranthus or mulberry mistletoe. Use only under professional supervision.	Greatly increases survival time in advanced ovarian cancer.
Polysaccharide kureha (PSK)	Tablets. Take 6,000 mg daily.	Simulates production of immune agent IL-2.
Quercetin[1]	Tablets. Take 125–250 mg 3 times daily, between meals.	Stops chemical signals that give ovarian cancer cells a growth advantage over healthy cells.
Soy isoflavone concentrate	Tablets. Take 3,000 mg daily.	Interrupts multiplication of ovarian cancer cells. (*See under* Recommendations, page 422).
Turmeric	Curcumin tablets. Take 250–500 mg twice daily, between meals.	Activates gene p53. Prevents inflammation.

Precautions for the use of herbs:

[1]Do not take quercetin with cyclosporine (Neoral, Sandimmune) or nifedipine (Procardia).

Ovarian Cancer: Formulas

Formula	Comments
Coptis Decoction to Relieve Toxicity	A traditional Chinese herbal formula that helps stop the multiplication of many types of ovarian cancer cells and prevents damage to the immune system from chemotherapy. This formula can be used during chemotherapy to reduce side effects.

❏ Take 200 micrograms of selenium daily. Selenium supplements are especially useful for women with ovarian cancer who are undergoing multidrug chemotherapy.

❏ Avoid weight-loss diets and fasts. Although certain kinds of fat restriction reduce the risk of developing ovarian cancer, calorie restriction after the disease has developed may accelerate the disorder's progress.

Considerations

❏ Surgery is the first line of treatment for ovarian cancer. In addition to the ovary, the uterus and fallopian tubes also may be removed, as may the membrane that lines the abdomen. After surgery, physicians give combinations of chemotherapy, immunotherapy, and radiation therapy. In recent years, the trend has been to use multiple chemotherapy drugs, including cisplatin (Platinol), cyclophosphamide (Cytoxan), doxorubicin hydrochloride (Adriamycin), and 5-fluorouracil (Adrucil) in various combinations over a longer period of time. The use of extended chemotherapy often harms the immune system and the bone marrow.

❏ The dietary factors that contribute to the risk of ovarian cancer are more specific than those for other cancers.

Vegetable fiber decreases risk by approximately 60 percent for each 10-gram increase in the average daily amount of vegetable fiber consumed (about that found in five to seven servings of vegetables). Each increase in daily saturated fat consumption of 10 grams (about 100 calories) increases risk of developing ovarian cancer approximately 20 percent; consumption of unsaturated fats neither increases nor decreases risk. Cholesterol from eggs, but not from other sources, increases risk of developing ovarian cancer approximately 40 percent for each 100-milligram increase in average daily consumption (about half of an egg). (Increased risk is also associated with total cholesterol levels over 200 mg/dL.) In addition, habitual consumption of more than two alcoholic drinks per day is associated with increased risk.

❏ Some fruits and vegetables are rich in isoflavones (soy) and flavonoids (blueberries, red onions, apples), and increasing their consumption can reduce the risk of developing ovarian cancer by 50 percent.

❏ Adequate levels of selenium not only support treatment for ovarian cancer but also reduce the risk of developing this disease. Low levels of selenium have been associated with a greater risk of ovarian cancer. A daily dosage of between 150 and 200 micrograms is enough.

❏ In one study, women who used B-complex vitamins, vitamin E, and beta-carotene for more than ten years had a one-third to one-half reduced risk of ovarian cancer compared to those who did not use these supplements.

❏ For measures to reduce side effects and increase effectiveness when using chemotherapy or radiation therapy, *see* "Side Effects of Cancer Treatment" *under* CANCER. To learn about herbal treatments that can prevent a cancer from developing its own blood supply, *see* CANCER.

OVARIAN CYST

The ovaries are made up of follicles, each of which contains an egg. Once a month, a follicle ruptures and releases an egg. Ovarian cysts are enlarged follicles that have failed to rupture. Often, ovarian cysts cause few symptoms. Some women, however, experience generalized aching, heaviness, disruption of the menstrual cycle, back pain, abdominal pain, and pain during sexual intercourse.

If discomfort is slight, and the size of the cyst is less than two centimeters, physicians typically wait two or three periods before deciding how to treat the cyst. Functional cysts are small and usually disappear within several menstrual cycles. Pathological cysts, which are caused by disease, require medical intervention. This includes cysts that result from a disorder called polycystic ovarian disease, in which the ovaries contain many cysts and high levels of male hormones are present. Twisting of an ovary by a cyst can cause sudden, extreme pain and necessitate surgery.

In most cases of ovarian cysts, the woman's body produces enough or even too much estrogen, but produces it at the wrong time in her menstrual cycle. Therefore, the first step in treatment is to reduce estrogen overproduction. If needed, drugs such as birth control pills are used to regulate hormone balances.

Herbal therapies have to be used on a long-term basis, at least three months, before changes in symptoms can be expected. They can be used with short-term birth control pills and hormone-regulating drugs as well; discuss such usage with a doctor.

Herbs to Avoid

❏ Forskolin, a preparation made from coleus, counteracts the effect of oral contraceptives used to treat ovarian cysts. People who have ovarian cysts should avoid the following herbs entirely: cordyceps, dan shen, fennel seed, licorice, moutan, and peony. (For more information regarding these herbs, *see* individual entries *under* The Herbs in Part One.)

Recommendations

❏ If necessary, lose weight, since fatty tissues make estrogen. (*See* OVERWEIGHT. *Also see* ESTROGEN-REDUCING DIET in Part Three.) Be sure to not lose muscle mass, which is counterproductive, so include about 30 grams of protein at each meal.

❏ Get regular exercise, both aerobic exercise, such as walking or bicycling, and resistance exercise, such as weight lifting. Muscle toning increases the sensitivity of muscle tissue to insulin, reducing the amount of insulin available to stimulate the growth of ovarian cysts. Exercise programs must be maintained for at least six months before cysts begin to shrink.

❏ Avoid melatonin and selenium supplements. Preliminary studies in dairy cattle indicate that an excess of melatonin or selenium may be involved in the formation of ovarian cysts.

Considerations

❏ Wild yam (dioscorea) may be useful for relieving pain that is worsened by doubling over or lying down but eases with motion or when stretching out or bending backward.

Ovarian Cist: Beneficial Herbs

Herb	Form and Dosage	Comments
Dong quai[1]	*Angelica sinensis* freeze-dried root in capsules. Take 500–1,000 mg daily. Take during 2 weeks after period; then discontinue for 2 weeks.	Relieves pain caused by ovarian cysts.
Milk thistle[2]	Silymarin gelcaps. Take 120–240 mg daily.	Counteracts liver damage from pioglitazone (Actos), rosiglitazone (Avandia), and troglitazone (Rezulin).
Wild yam (dioscorea)[3]	Tincture. Take as directed on the label.	Treats cramping caused by ovarian cysts. (*See under* Considerations, above.)

Precautions for the use of herbs:

[1]Different forms of dong quai have different effects on the uterus; be sure to use the form specified.

[2]Milk thistle can cause mild diarrhea.

[3]Taking too much wild yam (dioscorea) can cause nausea. Do not use wild yam (dioscorea) products that are mixed with synthetic progesterone.

Ovarian Cist: Formulas

Formula	Comments
Augmented Rambling Powder[1]	A traditional Chinese herbal formula that lowers estrogen levels. Use this formula if symptoms include dry mouth, blurry vision, lower abdominal pressure, difficult urination, and increased menstrual flow.
Cinnamon Twig and Poria Pill	A traditional Chinese herbal formula that reduces bloodstream estrogen levels. Use this formula if symptoms include weakness, lack of appetite, and fatigue.
Dong Quai and Peony Powder	A traditional Chinese herbal formula that reduces both the amount of estrogen in circulation and the formation of inflammatory compounds in the tissue lining the uterus. Unlike some treatments, this formula does not have a "masculinizing" effect.
Peony and Licorice Decoction[2]	A traditional Chinese herbal formula that corrects abnormal hair growth (hirsutism) in women with long-term polycystic ovarian disease.
Two-Cured Decoction[3]	A traditional Chinese herbal formula that reduces estrogen levels. Use this formula if symptoms include coughing that produces large amounts of easily expectorated phlegm, and/or vomiting and nausea.

Precautions for the use of formulas:

[1]Do not use Augmented Rambling Powder if you are trying to become pregnant.

[2]Use Peony and Licorice Decoction with caution, since it acts by converting testosterone, which causes hirsutism, into estrogen, which may aggravate ovarian cysts. Use under the supervision of an herbal practitioner, and only until symptoms are reversed or up to six months. Do not use this formula for ovarian cysts not associated with polycystic ovarian disease.

[3]Do not use Two-Cured Decoction if you have a fever.

❑ To counteract ovarian cysts, women are usually told to take estrogen-based contraceptive pills. The use of these pills reduces your risk of ovarian cancer. In addition, drugs are used that help regulate the balance between two other sex hormones, luteinizing hormone (LH) and follicle-stimulating hormone (FSH), which together control the release of eggs from the ovaries.

❑ Women who take seizure medications, particularly sodium valproate (Depakote), may develop problems with ovarian cysts. Women who take such drugs should avoid weight gain—although this task is made more difficult by the drugs themselves—and get regular exercise.

❑ Ovarian cysts are a frequent cause of infertility. (*See* Infertility in Women *under* INFERTILITY.)

OVERWEIGHT

For adults, overweight and obesity ranges are determined by using weight and height to calculate a number called the body mass index (BMI). BMI is used because, for most people, it correlates with their amount of body fat. An adult who has a BMI between 25 and 29.9 is considered overweight. An adult who has a BMI of 30 or higher is considered obese. It is important to remember that although BMI correlates with the amount of body fat, BMI does not directly measure body fat. As a result, some people, such as professional athletes, may have a BMI that identifies them as overweight even though they do not have excess body fat.

Excessive weight is usually as body fat, and this is a health problem because it can lead to a number of serious disorders, including heart disease, diabetes, stroke, high blood pressure, and certain kinds of cancer. Overeating, lack of exercise, heredity, diabetes, hyperinsulinemia, emotional tension, and boredom all can contribute to excess weight. Weight loss is the most easily understood principle of health. All that is necessary to lose weight is to make sure that the calories consumed in food are fewer than the calories spent on exercise and daily activities. That is because excess calories, no matter what their source, are turned into fat before being stored. Therefore, simply eating less can allow one to lose weight and keep it off for a few weeks or months. Maintaining weight loss for a lifetime is, unfortunately, much more complicated. Losing and regaining the same twenty pounds is a common theme in many weight-loss histories.

Regaining lost weight does not simply reflect a lack of willpower. The body makes the hormones insulin and leptin in proportion to the amount of stored body fat. After a few weeks of dieting, the body starts making less insulin and leptin. If the brain receives less of these hormones, it activates appetite centers.

Compounding the difficulty are changes in the body's energy requirements after weight loss. Many diet experts have speculated that the body learns to use food more efficiently during diets. The idea is that dieting slows down resting metabolism so that, for example, a 200-pound person who could avoid gaining weight by eating 2,000 calories a day may need to eat considerably less than 1,800 daily calories after losing twenty pounds.

Contrary to this common belief, however, metabolism does not have to "slow down" after weight loss in most people, provided muscle mass is maintained and the loss comes from fat. This means, though, that long-term weight loss without exercise is nearly impossible, and that strength-building exercise is needed in addition to aerobic (heart-conditioning) exercise.

While herbal treatments can at least make dealing with the difficult realities of weight maintenance a little easier, they must be used as part of a program of sensible eating and exercise. Herbal formulas should be used with the supervision and help of a skilled herbal practitioner.

Recommendations

❏ Eat minimally processed foods that are rich in fiber and bulk, and drink at least eight glasses of water daily. It is especially important to drink water whenever you are thirsty. Together with eating fiber-rich foods, drinking more water contributes to a feeling of fullness that can last five to six hours after a meal.

❏ To lower total calories consumed, avoid fats but concentrate on "low-energy-density" foods rather than just "low-fat" foods. Fresh foods that are minimally processed and do not require cooking have the lowest energy density. For example, a fresh apple and a dried apple have the same number of calories, but the fresh apple is bulkier and more satisfying. A slice of fat-free apple pie is no more filling than an apple, but it has added sugar and many more calories, and regular apple pie has still more calories from the added fat.

❏ Foods with low glycemic indexes are also important to lose weight. These are carbohydrate-containing foods that are minimally processed and usually rich in fiber. Such foods include whole-grain cereal and bread, fruits, and vegetables. Eating protein at each meal is necessary to maintain body muscle stores while losing body fat. It is best to eat 30 grams of protein at each meal; protein builds muscle and burns fat. Include at least two to three servings of low-fat dairy products in your diet every day. Dairy uniquely seems to control hunger and the desire to eat.

❏ Never reward success in following a diet with food. Instead, make occasional treats a part of your overall eating plan, reducing other foods to compensate for the special food.

❏ For long-term weight loss, get regular aerobic and strength-building exercise. The level of aerobic exercise needed to maintain weight loss for a 150-pound

Overweight: Beneficial Herbs

Herb	Form and Dosage	Comments
Aloe vera	Juice. Take as directed on the label.	Improves digestion and cleanses the digestive tract.
Astragalus[1]	Capsule or tincture. Take as directed on the label.	Increases energy and improves nutrient absorption.
Dandelion[2]	Tincture. Take 10–15 drops in ¼ cup water 3 times daily on an empty stomach.	Gentle diuretic; stops short-term weight gain caused by eating salty foods.
Garcinia cambogia	Citrin. Take as directed on the label.	Keeps fatty acids from being stored as fats.
Maté	Tea bags. Take 1 cup daily.	Stimulates the central nervous system, leading to increased calorie burning.
Wild angelica[3]	Angelica dahurica capsules. Take 500–1,500 mg daily.	Prevents weight gain caused by excess insulin.

Precautions for the use of herbs:

[1]Do not use astragalus if you have a fever.

[2]Do not use dandelion if you have gallstones.

[3]Do not take wild angelica if you are pregnant.

Overweight: Formulas

Formula	Comments
Ledebouriella Decoction That Sagely Unblocks[1]	A traditional Chinese herbal formula that treats "beer barrel" pattern of fat deposits. Reduces both percentage of body fat and total body weight without changes in the number of calories consumed.
Major Bupleurum Decoction[2]	A traditional Chinese herbal formula that treats a constant feeling of fullness. Lowers total cholesterol levels while raising levels of high-density lipoprotein (HDL), the "good," artery-clearing kind.

Precautions for the use of formulas:

[1]Do not use Ledebouriella Decoction That Sagely Unblocks if you are trying to become pregnant or if you are nauseous or vomiting.

[2]Do not use Major Bupleurum Decoction if you have a fever.

(70-kilogram) adult is that which burns off about 2,500 calories a week. This is equivalent to briskly walking three miles a day, every day, year round. After several months of regular exercise and checking with your doctor, begin doing part of your aerobic exercise in the form of sprints. Anaerobic exercise, or exertion that is hard enough to make you slightly out of breath, burns calories thirty-four times as fast as aerobic exercise. This is not necessary if you can exercise for a longer time period, such as an hour a day.

❏ To keep your metabolism from slowing down after you have lost weight by dieting, do muscle-building exercises at least three days a week. The most efficient muscle-building exercises are done with free weights or weight machines, but isometrics—resistance exercises that are performed against a stationary object, such as push-ups—are also effective. Muscle-building uses insulin that otherwise would transport fatty acids into fat cells, and additional muscle mass burns more calories than the same amount of fat tissue.

❏ To avoid gaining weight after quitting smoking, start an exercise program.

❏ Use stevia instead of the sweeteners saccharin and aspartame. For more information about stevia, see *The Stevia Cookbook* by Ray Sahelian and Donna Gates (Avery Publishing Group, 2004).

❏ Move your bowels daily. A clean colon may help you start your weight plan.

Considerations

❏ More so than members of other groups, African-American women tend to experience a metabolism slowdown after weight loss. This means that a woman who has dieted down to 90 percent of what she previously weighed must consume less than 90 percent of the calories she consumed before the diet to maintain that loss. To offset this effect, it is critically important for African-American women to maintain muscle mass through strength training and regular aerobic exercise while dieting.

❏ Artificial sweeteners do not promote weight loss. Saccharin saves calories, but causes weight gain because it stimulates the secretion of insulin, which encourages the deposit of fatty acids into fat cells. In one trial against controls who drank sugar-sweetened drinks with a low-calorie lunch, consumers of saccharin-sweetened drinks who ate the same lunch were more motivated to eat and more preoccupied with food for the rest of the day. Using aspartame decreases appetite, but also causes weight gain. Aspartame hinders protein digestion. If less protein enters the bloodstream from the digestive system, the body tends to store glucose as fat. The net result is that eating less food can result in storing more fat. Other sweeteners are available, such as stevia (Truvia) and sucralose (Splenda), which do not have these side effects.

❏ Overall, fake fats are not helpful in weight-control programs. In a double-blind clinical study (a study in which neither the participants nor the researchers knew which foods contained fat substitutes), children offered a variety of foods prepared with either traditional cooking oils or with fat substitutes consumed almost exactly the same number of calories. Using fat substitutes reduced fat consumption by only 1.3 percent and reduced calorie consumption by only 0.5 percent. And in a double-blind test of the fat-substitute olestra (Olean) involving adult men, researchers found that using fat substitutes did reduce the percent of fat consumed in the total diet. Calories consumed, however, stayed the same.

❏ A study sponsored by the U.S. Department of Agriculture revealed that the trace mineral boron may speed the burning of calories. Raisins and onions are good food sources of boron.

❏ If bumpy fat deposits just beneath the skin pose a problem, *see* CELLULITE.

PAIN, CHRONIC

Pain can be useful as a warning sign, such as the pain from a broken bone signaling the need to seek medical attention. Chronic pain, though, is pain that will not go away, like an alarm that keeps ringing long after the emergency is over. Usually there is an anatomical change in the body resulting from a disease or injury, and repeated attempts to relieve the pain are unsuccessful. But some people suffer chronic pain in the absence of any past injury or evidence of body damage. Consultations with a number of specialists may not determine a physical cause of the pain. Possible causes of chronic pain include disease, spinal injury, injuries in general, cancer, fibromyalgia and fibromyositis, surgery, shingles, postherpetic neuralgia, Raynaud's syndrome, temporomandibular joint disorder, and diabetic neuropathy.

Chronic pain creates its own complications. Chronic anxiety and depression may develop, and lower the threshold at which pain is perceived, compounding the problem. Exhaustion from lack of sleep can lead to poor eating and exercise habits, and secondary, stress-related conditions set in. Drug dependency problems may also develop.

The goal of chronic pain treatment is to ease the pain and help the person learn how to live with it. Herbs supplement other measures used to relieve pain.

Recommendations

❏ Use cat's claw to control chronic pain if the underlying problem is food allergy or inflammatory bowel disease. (*See* Food Allergies *under* ALLERGIES; CROHN'S DISEASE; and IRRITABLE BOWEL SYNDROME.) Take 1,500 milligrams daily in capsule form. Do not use if you are pregnant or nursing, or if you take insulin for diabetes.

Chronic Pain: Beneficial Herbs

Herb	Form and Dosage	Comments
Boswellia	Boswellin capsules. Take 150 mg 3 times daily.	Relieves pain without stomach upset, in same manner as celecoxib (Celebrex).
Cayenne[1]	Capsaicin cream. Apply to affected areas daily or as directed on the label.	Causes temporary skin pain that counteracts chronic pain.
Clematis	Wei ling xian capsules. Take as directed on the label.	Increases the threshold of pain.
Condurango	Tincture. Take ½–1 tsp in ¼ cup water 3 times daily.	Relieves pain and restores appetite.
Echinacea	*Echinacea purpurea* tincture. Take ½–1 tsp in ¼ cup water 3 times daily.	Helps relieve pain in advanced cancer.
Ginger	20 percent gingerol and shagaol tablets. Take 100–200 mg 3 times daily.	Reduces production of pain-causing cytokines.
Kava kava	Fluidextract. (Capsule form is less effective for pain.) Take ½–1 tsp in ¼ cup water 1 hour before bedtime.	Relieves pain and induces sleep. May be combined with passionflower or valerian.
Meadowsweet	Tincture. Take 30–60 drops in ¼ cup water up to 4 times daily.	Relieves stomach pain.
Pau d'arco	Tea (loose), prepared with 1 tsp (1 gm) tea and 1 cup water. (*See* TEAS in Part Three.) Take 1 cup up to 8 times daily.	Analgesic; stimulates immune system to destroy bacteria.
Turmeric	Curcumin. Take 400 mg 3 times daily.	Relieves pain and inflammation.
Willow[2]	Willow bark or salicin capsules or tablets. Take as directed on the label.	Relieves pain.

Precautions for the use of herbs:

[1]Do not apply cayenne to broken skin. Avoid contact with eyes or mouth.

[2]Do not use willow if you are sensitive or allergic to aspirin.

Chronic Pain: Formulas

Formula	Comments
Prepared Aconite Decoction[1]	A traditional Chinese herbal formula used under professional supervision for chronic pain. Acts by raising the threshold of pain to make rest possible.

Precautions for the use of formulas:

[1]Discontinue using Prepared Aconite Decoction if a fever occurs. This formula may cause a loss of sensation in the mouth and tongue.

❑ Consume such soy products as tofu, miso, or soymilk daily. Laboratory experiments have found that supplementing the diet with soy foods reduces activity of the sympathetic nervous system, the system essential to the sensation of pain. Soy foods may be helpful in reducing chronic pain after nerve injury caused by accident, surgery, diabetes, cancer, or fibromyalgia.

❑ If you suffer pain caused by an autoimmune disorder—such as ankylosing spondylitis, lupus, multiple sclerosis, rheumatoid arthritis, scleroderma, or Sjögren's syndrome—reduce your intake of animal foods, and eliminate all polyunsaturated vegetable oils, margarine, vegetable shortening, and products made with partially hydrogenated oils of any kind. Use olive oil as your main fat and increase your consumption of omega-3 fatty acids by eating oily fish (salmon, sardines, and herring); flaxseeds and flax oil are less helpful. Increase your consumption of fruits and vegetables, and purchase organic produce whenever possible. Also, try eliminating foods that may trigger autoimmune reactions. Start by eliminating all dairy products for two months. If that does not help, experiment by eliminating wheat, corn, soy, sugar, and citrus fruits, one group at a time. If you continue to omit whole categories of foods such as dairy, replace lost nutrients with supplements. Do not remove food groups from a child's diet without consulting a pediatrician.

❑ Continue to exercise. Aerobic exercise and strength training, preferably under the supervision of a physical therapist or trainer, may help relieve chronic pain after eight to twelve weeks of conditioning. Exercise levels must be maintained to avoid the return of severe pain.

❑ Take 300 to 600 milligrams of lipoic acid daily to help relieve chronic muscle pain.

❑ Use either hot or cold packs to ease pain, depending on which feels better.

❏ Try to distract your attention from the pain. Watch a movie, play a video game, read a book—whatever focuses your mind elsewhere.

Considerations

❏ Invasive evaluations and surgical interventions for chronic pain should be avoided if possible. Supportive measures for pain relief, such as acupuncture (or acupressure), massage, and relaxation techniques, should be used in addition to painkillers. (For more information on these techniques, see Part Three.) In one study, men with chronic prostatitis and pelvic pain were twice as likely to get relief from pain over ten weeks with acupuncture compared to men who received a fake acupuncture procedure. Acupuncture likely works for other conditions as well.

❏ Taking 100 micrograms of vitamin K may have an analgesic effect for people who have cancer with inoperable carcinomas. Since taking vitamin K may increase the risk of bleeding, consult with a physician before using it to treat cancer pain.

❏ Transcutaneous electrical nerve stimulation (TENS) is a procedure in which a gentle electrical current is applied to the skin. This helps some people find pain relief. Home TENS units are available. (See Appendix B: Resources.)

PANIC ATTACK

See under ANXIETY DISORDER.

PARASITIC INFECTION

Parasitic infections are the most common disease conditions in the world, affecting hundreds of millions of people in developing nations and becoming more prevalent in developed nations as well. With massive immigration, the popularization of imported foods, and the advent of adventure travel to previously seldom-visited locations, parasites are affecting more and more people in North America. Trichomoniasis is the most common parasitic infection in the United States, accounting for an estimated 7.4 million cases per year. Giardia and Cryptosporidium are estimated to cause 2 million and 300,000 infections annually in the United States, respectively. Cryptosporidiosis is the most frequent cause of recreational water-related disease outbreaks in the United States, causing multiple outbreaks each year. There are an estimated 1.5 million new Toxoplasma infections and 400 to 4,000 cases of congenital toxoplasmosis in the United States each year. Toxoplasmosis is the third leading cause of death due to foodborne illnesses.

Unless a person has been to a part of the world where parasitic diseases are widespread, parasites are not likely to be the cause of acute illness (except as mentioned above). The most serious parasites produce symptoms that are hard to ignore, such as the spitting up of blood caused by

tapeworms or liver flukes. Severe abdominal pain, blood in the stool, diarrhea, and weight loss can signal acute problems. For some chronic conditions, on the other hand, parasitic infection can be the missing diagnosis. Amebiasis, for example, is sometimes misdiagnosed as Crohn's disease. Roundworm infection can be mistaken for peptic ulcers. In HIV/AIDS and other immune-deficiency disorders, common parasitic infections that usually create no symptoms can have serious consequences.

Parasitic infections can be caused by a number of different organisms, and most of these disorders can be treated with prescription medicines. (See "The Most Common Parasitic Infections" on page 430.) Herbal treatments fill in the gaps for drug treatment, and are the best way to deal with parasites for which no conventional treatment currently exists.

Recommendations

❏ Have diagnostic work done at a laboratory familiar with parasitic infections, such as a university medical center with an active tropical disease unit. Unless a lab is experienced in looking for parasites, such infections can be easily missed.

❏ Do not use vitamin B supplements in any parasitic infection unless directed to do so by a physician. Although supplemental vitamin B is necessary in the treatment of some parasitic infections, such as fish-borne tapeworms, it may worsen others, such as malaria. Using a good multivitamin with B vitamins is fine, just don't take B complex on its own.

❏ To avoid reinfection, practice good personal hygiene. Wash hands with soap and water before eating or preparing food and after using the toilet, and make sure that children do the same.

❏ Be especially sure to practice good hygiene if pinworms are causing the problem, as these parasites are easily spread. Teach children not to put their hands or other objects in their mouths, keep hands and fingers away from the nose and mouth, and to avoid scratching the affected area. Launder bedding and underwear in hot water and a mild bleach solution.

❏ For the latest information on disease hazards and international travel, log on to the U.S. Centers for Disease Control and Prevention website www.cdc.gov/travel. For in-depth information on food parasites, read Guess What Came to Dinner by Anne Louise Gittleman (Avery Publishing Group, 1993).

❏ Echinacea (Echinacea purpurea) may be good for some cases of leishmaniasis, a tropical disease spread by sandflies that causes a variety of symptoms depending on which part of the body is affected. Leishmaniasis in the mucous membranes requires aggressive treatment, for which echinacea is inadequate.

The Most Common Parasitic Infections

AMEBIASIS

Amebiasis is an infection caused by a tiny parasite (*Entamoeba histolytica*) in the large intestine. The parasite can live in the large intestine without causing disease; or it can invade the colon wall causing colitis, acute dysentery, or chronic diarrhea. The infection may also spread through the blood to the liver and, rarely, to the lungs, brain, or other organs.

Amebiasis is present worldwide, but it is most common in tropical areas where crowded living conditions and poor sanitation exist. Transmission occurs through ingestion of cysts in feces-contaminated food or water, use of human excrement as fertilizer, and person-to-person contact. Cockroaches and houseflies can also spread the cysts. There are an estimated 50 million cases worldwide of amebiasis with nearly 100,000 deaths annually.

Typical symptoms of intestinal amebiasis consist of frequent (3 to 8 semiformed) bowel movements with cramps or colicky abdominal pain. Pain on defecation is common. The diarrhea may contain blood or mucus. Uncomplicated attacks may last up to two weeks, and recurrences are common unless the diagnosis is made and the individual is treated. Spread of the amoeba into the wall of the colon may occur in 8 to 10 percent of cases and to the liver in approximately 1 percent.

Malnutrition and alcoholism predispose a person to more severe disease, as do chemotherapy, steroid treatment for arthritis, and HIV/AIDS infection. Recent travel to a tropical region is a risk factor. In the United States, institutionalized mentally retarded people and male homosexuals are high-risk groups.

CHAGAS' DISEASE

Chagas' disease is a tropical infection that in recent years has spread to the United States, especially to southern Texas from South and Central America. Chagas' disease is caused by a protozoan known as *Trypanosoma cruzi*. The microorganism is spread by insect bite. Once the protozoan infects a human host, it draws nourishment from muscle tissue, especially the heart, causing irregular heartbeats and enlarging the heart muscle. It also attacks the smooth muscles lining the gastrointestinal tract, enlarging it.

The standard treatment for Chagas' disease are the drugs nifurtimox and benznidazole, both of which are effective but have side effects. In rare cases, they may cause acute symptoms, such as anaphylactic shock, and chronic symptoms, such as dermatitis, nausea, and vomiting. Once Chagas' disease reaches the chronic phase, medications aren't effective—at this point there are usually heart-related and digestive-related complications. Herbal treatment may offer some protection against the parasite without these side effects, but speak to your doctor first. Do not delay getting the virus treated early.

GIARDIASIS

Giardiasis is infection with the single-celled protozoan parasite *Giardia lamblia*. It usually comes from water-dwelling animals such as beavers or runoff from fecal matter of domestic animals such as sheep. This extremely infectious microorganism lives in an inactive, cyst stage in contaminated water or feces-contaminated food. One to three weeks after it is swallowed, the parasite attaches itself to the mucous membrane of the intestine. In one to three weeks it causes abdominal pain, bloating, putrid diarrhea, swollen abdomen, nausea, low-grade fever, and headache. Outbreaks of giardiasis are found among backpackers and in day-care centers, prisons, schools, and municipalities with undetected breaks in water mains.

Acute giardiasis usually subsides within two weeks, but the disease can persist for months or even years. Chronic irritation of the lining of the intestine may deplete its ability to produce lactase, the enzyme needed to digest milk sugars. The microorganism itself is covered with a layer of proteins made from the amino acid cysteine.

The configuration of these proteins can change, so that the body's immune cells that "remember" one form of the infection cannot recognize the next form. The giardiasis germ constantly provokes immune reactions without allowing the immune system to overcome the disease; however, most people about 80 percent—recover.

Combination prescription drug treatments are successful in treating giardiasis about 80 percent of the time. In addition, you can consider herbs that contain berberine, such as coptis, which may help slow *Giardia* infections.

MALARIA

Malaria is an ancient disease caused by a blood-borne parasite (sporozoites in humans) that infects and then destroys red blood cells. Malaria is a serious and sometimes fatal disease caused by a parasite that commonly infects a certain type of mosquito that feeds on humans. People who get malaria are typically very sick with high fevers, shaking chills, and flulike illness. About 1,500 cases of malaria are diagnosed in the United States each year. The vast majority of cases in the United States are in travelers and immigrants returning from countries where malaria transmission occurs, many from sub-Saharan Africa and South Asia. Thirty-five countries (thirty in sub-Saharan Africa and five in Asia) account for 98 percent of global malaria deaths. Malaria is the fifth cause of death from infectious diseases worldwide (after respiratory infections, HIV/AIDS, diarrheal diseases, and tuberculosis).

The drug-resistant strain of malaria *Plasmodium falciparum* has become increasingly common. Conventional treatments such as chloroquine (Aralen) and quinine offer no protection against this strain of malaria. Laboratory tests on animals have shown that a group of chemicals known as naphthoquinones in pau d'arco may stop the multiplication of the malaria parasite even when it is resistant to chloroquine and quinine. This has not been shown to be true in humans so make sure that you follow the drug regimen dictated by your doctor.

PINWORMS

Pinworm is a contagious intestinal parasite infestation that occurs commonly in children and is the most common type of intestinal worm infection in the United States. The organism causing pinworm infection is a small whitish worm called *Enterobius vermicularis*. It is visible to the naked eye at about ¼ to ½ inch long. The parasite is found throughout the United States, especially in urban areas and crowded settings and in nontropical areas.

Pinworms are easily spread. Symptoms of pinworm infection include itching of the anal or vaginal area, insomnia, irritability, restlessness, intermittent abdominal pain, and nausea. There may be vaginal irritation or discomfort in young girls, and wearing away of the skin or infection around the anus from constant scratching in people of either sex.

Adult pinworms live in the large intestine, that is, in the cecum and colon. Eggs are laid outside the anus during the night and are spread from person to person from contaminated clothing, articles, and hands. Eggs can also drift and can be swallowed in contaminated food or drink. The eggs hatch in the small intestine and travel to the large intestine where they mature. School-age children (usually aged five to ten years) are most likely at risk for contracting pinworms.

SCHISTOSOMIASIS (SWIMMER'S ITCH)

Schistosomiasis is an infection contracted from contaminated water. The parasite in its infective stages swims freely in open bodies of water. On contact with humans, it burrows into the skin, matures into another larval stage (schistosomula), then migrates to the lungs and liver, where it matures into the adult form. The adult worm then migrates to the anatomic area of its preference, depending on which species is involved. Likely areas include the bladder, rectum, intestines, liver, portal venous system, spleen, or lungs.

The symptoms of schistosomiasis vary with the species of worm. Initial invasion of the skin may cause itching and a rash, known as swimmer's itch. Heavy infestation may cause fever, chills, lymph node enlargement, and liver and spleen enlargement. Urinary symptoms may include frequency, painful urination, and blood in urine. Intestinal symptoms include abdominal pain and diarrhea (which may be bloody).

This is not usually seen in the United States, but is in many tropical and subtropical areas worldwide.

TRICHOMONIASIS

Trichomoniasis is caused by *Trichomonas vaginalis*. This parasite is a single-cell protozoan parasite with a whiplike tail that it uses to propel itself through vaginal and urethral mucus. This sexually transmitted disease is found worldwide. In the United States the highest incidence is in women between the ages of sixteen and thirty-five. Transmission is usually through sexual contact. Women can acquire the disease from infected men and women, whereas men usually only contract it from infected women.

The symptoms of the disease are quite different in men than in women. In men, the infection often is without symptoms (asymptomatic), and clears spontaneously in a few weeks. Symptomatic men may experience a mild urethral itching or discharge, mild burning after urination or ejaculation, and, on occasion, slight discharge from the urethra. Women develop a foamy, foul-smelling, green-white or yellowish vaginal discharge. The volume of discharge may be large. Itching may occur on the vulva, the vagina, and the inner thighs. (*See also* VAGINOSIS.)

Parasitic Infection: Beneficial Herbs

Herb	Form and Dosage	Comments
Agrimony	Tea (loose), prepared with 1½ tsp (1.5 gm) tea and 1 cup water. (*See* TEAS in Part Three.) Take 3 times daily between meals.	Prevents and treats early stages of trichomoniasis infection.
Artemisia	Tea (loose), prepared with 1 tsp (1.5 gm) tea in 1 cup water. (*See* TEAS in Part Three.) Take 1–2 times daily.	Treats drug-resistant malaria and pinworms. (*See under* "The Most Common Parasitic Infections," page 430).
Barberry[1] or coptis[1] or goldenseal[1] or Oregon grape root[1]	Tincture. Take 1½–3 tsp (6–12 ml) in ¼ cup water 3 times daily.	Treats giardiasis and malaria.
Betel nut	Use in the form and dosages recommended by a traditional Chinese medicine practitioner.	Kills pork tapeworm.
Black walnut	Verma-key or Verma-plus from Uni-key. Take as directed on the label.	Purges all forms of parasitic infection, especially worms.
Bromelain[2] with papain	Zymex II from Standard Process Inc. Take as directed on the label.	Digests foodborne parasite eggs and larvae.
Cajueiro	Tincture. Take as directed on the label.	Treats schistosomiasis.
Echinacea	*Echinacea angustifolia* capsules. Take 500 mg every 3 hours until symptoms improve; or *Echinacea purpurea* capsules. Take 2,000 mg every 3 hours until symptoms improve.	Treats trichomoniasis. Treats leishmaniasis of the skin.
Garlic	Oil. Take 2 tsp (8 ml) daily for 4 days.	Treats Chagas' disease.
Ipecac	Syrup. Take as directed on the label.	Stops dehydration in amoebic dysentery; keeps amoebas from lodging in intestinal lining.
Pau d'arco	Tincture. Take as directed on the label.	Treats Chagas' disease, drug-resistant malaria.
Prickly ash	Tea (loose), prepared with 1–4 tsp (1.5–6 gm) and 1 cup water. (*See* TEAS in Part Three.) Take 3 times daily.	Causes pinworms to be eliminated in the stool.
Wolfberry	Tea (loose), prepared with 1 oz (30 gm) and 1½ cups water. (*See* TEAS in Part Three.) Take 2–3 hours before expected onset of fever.	Stops malarial fevers. Also known as lycium.

Precautions for the use of herbs:

[1]Do not use barberry, coptis, goldenseal, or Oregon grape root if you are pregnant or have gallbladder disease. Do not take these herbs with supplemental vitamin B_6 or with protein supplements containing the amino acid histidine. Do not take coptis for longer than two weeks at a time. Do not use goldenseal if you have cardiovascular disease or glaucoma. Do not take Oregon grape root for longer than two weeks at a time.

[2]People who are allergic to pineapple may develop a rash from bromelain. If itching develops, stop using it.

❑ To reduce your chances of contracting fish tapeworm from sushi, always eat the pickled ginger served with it. Ginger contains a potent meat tenderizer, zingibain, that has been shown in laboratory studies to reduce foodborne parasites by dissolving them and their eggs in the human digestive system. If you make sushi at home, be sure to freeze the fish for twenty-four to forty-eight hours to kill tapeworms. Do not use freshwater fish for sushi; rockfish and snapper are the species least likely to contain parasites. If you are fearful of tapeworm, avoid sushi

Parasitic Infection: Formulas

Formula	Comments
Minor Bupleurum Decoction[1]	A traditional Chinese herbal formula that prevents fevers and chills of malaria.

Precautions for the use of formulas:

[1]Do not use Minor Bupleurum Decoction if you have a fever or a skin infection. Taken long term, it can cause headache, dizziness, and bleeding gums. Side effects can be avoided if the formula is taken as a tea.

altogether. If you have a chronic condition that weakens your immune system, such as AIDS, do not eat sushi.

PARKINSON'S DISEASE

Parkinson's disease is a brain disorder that causes shaking and difficulty with walking, movement, and coordination. It affects both men and women, and is one of the most common neurological disorders in older people. This disorder can, however, strike young adults and even children.

Parkinson's disease is caused by progressive deterioration of the nerve cells (for reasons yet unknown) in the part of the brain that controls muscle movement. These cells produce dopamine, one of the neurotransmitters used by nerve cells to transmit impulses, and this deterioration reduces dopamine levels. Insufficient dopamine disturbs the balance between dopamine and other neurotransmitters. Without dopamine, the nerve cells cannot properly transmit messages, resulting in the loss of muscle control.

The symptoms of Parkinson's disease include shaking (tremors); muscle rigidity and stiffness; difficulty in bending the arms and legs; and stooped or slumped-over posture. Tremors are more common when the muscle is at rest. There may be reduced ability to show facial expression, producing a masklike appearance to the face. Loss of fine motor skills, such as difficulty in writing and eating, occurs. Nasal congestion, increased susceptibility to colds and flu, and gastrointestinal problems, especially constipation and heartburn, are common. The disorder may ultimately affect both sides of the body.

Although early loss of mental capacities is uncommon, persons with severe Parkinson's disease may exhibit overall mental deterioration, including dementia and hallucinations. (Dementia also can be a side effect of some of the medications used to treat the disorder.) Milder cases of mental deterioration involve difficulty in adjusting to changes and learning new information.

Medical tests are not specific for Parkinson's disease, but they may be required to rule out other disorders that cause similar symptoms. There is no known cure for this disorder, but early and consistent medical treatment can greatly decrease disability and increase quality of life. Medications control symptoms primarily by controlling the imbalance between neurotransmitters. Herbal treatments, in turn, are used to help control side effects, and act in milder ways to balance neurotransmitter levels.

Herbs to Avoid

❑ Kava kava may interfere with the action of levodopa, an important prescription medication for advanced Parkinson's disease. (For more information regarding this herb, see KAVA KAVA under The Herbs in Part One.)

Recommendations

❑ Eat the right kinds and amounts of protein. Use fava (broad) beans as a protein source, provided you do not have an allergy to them (as do many people of Mediterranean descent). A 3-ounce serving of broad beans contains as much as 250 milligrams of L-dopa. However, this does not substitute for taking levodopa, if you are prescribed levodopa by your doctor. Limit total consumption of protein foods to, at most, four to five servings per day. Protein foods supply an array of amino acids that compete with the amino acid tyrosine for entry into the brain, and tyrosine is essential for the creation of dopamine. Therefore, limiting protein may slow progression of the disease. Sometimes a doctor may tell you not to consume protein around the time that you take levodopa, so make sure you get adequate amounts during the rest of the day.

❑ Take a balanced antioxidant formula. Antioxidants are especially important for maintaining intellectual function and preventing dementia.

❑ Take 200 to 400 international units (IU) of vitamin D daily to help prevent fractures. It is important to avoid extensive exposure to sunlight, usually recommended for the production of vitamin D for people who are on the drug selegiline (Eldepryl). Sunlight exposure accelerates the rate at which the body breaks down this important medication.

❑ Avoid iron and choline supplements. These substances may cause the breakdown of dopamine in the brain. Also avoid iron-rich foods, such as liver and organ meats, but other kinds of meat, poultry, and seafood are fine.

❑ Avoid aluminum and especially manganese compounds, which may accelerate the progression of this

Parkinson's Disease: Beneficial Herbs

Herb	Form and Dosage	Comments
Acerola	Tablets with vitamin C USP. Take as directed on the label.	Superior source of antioxidant vitamin C for the brain.
Ginkgo[1]	Ginkgolide tablets. Take 240 mg in a single dose daily.	May reverse brain damage caused by toxic chemicals.
Milk thistle[2]	Silymarin gelcaps. Take 360 mg daily.	Maintains the brain's supply of the antioxidant glutathione. Lessens constipation and heartburn.
Oligomeric proanthocyanidins (OPCs)	Grapeseed or pine-bark extract tablets. Take 200 mg daily.	Helps prevent blood-vessel changes in the brain that can complicate Parkinson's disease.
Yellow dock	Capsules or tea. Take as directed on the label.	Cleanses the blood and detoxifies the liver.

Precautions for the use of herbs:

[1]Do not take ginkgo if you have a bleeding disorder, or are scheduled for surgery or a dental procedure. Avoid ginkgo if you are taking any type of blood-thinning medication.

[2]Milk thistle may cause mild diarrhea. If this occurs, decrease dose or stop taking it.

disease. Aluminum can leach from aluminum cookware used to prepare acidic foods and is found in some antacids and deodorants. Manganese is included in some multivitamin/mineral preparations, but only in very small amounts.

❑ Get adequate exercise, with the level of activity adjusted to meet the changing energy levels that may occur. Be sure to rest—fatigue can make symptoms worse. A well-thought-out program of rest, exercise, and physiotherapy can significantly improve the symptoms of Parkinson's disease.

Considerations

❑ Creatine, often used by bodybuilders to increase muscle mass, has been shown to be safe and may be of benefit for patients with Parkinson's disease.

❑ Simple aids—such as railings or banisters placed in commonly used areas of the house, special eating utensils, or other devices—may be of great benefit to a person who is experiencing difficulties with daily living activities.

❑ Stress aggravates Parkinson's disease, and relaxation therapy has been found useful in the treatment of this disorder. (See STRESS.) Others have derived benefit from yoga, massage, and tai chi.

❑ Parkinson's disease can cause severe depression. (See DEPRESSION.) In one study, patients with Parkinson's disease who were taking antidepressants had further improvements in depressive symptom scores when they took omega-3 fatty acid supplements. Even patients who were sad but not enough to require antidepressants experienced improvements in depression symptoms with the fish oil alone.

❑ If you have a family history of Parkinson's disease but have not developed the disease, reduce animal fat from your diet. Studies at the University of Washington have found that consumption of high amounts of animal fat

increases the risk for developing this disease. However, heredity is not a significant factor in Parkinson's disease; there is only about a 4 to 6 percent increased risk.

❑ Some people with Parkinson's disease have been found to have high levels of lead in their brains. Chelation therapy may be one way to remove lead from the body.

❑ Iron supplementation appears to be beneficial to some people with Parkinson's disease. The production of tyrosine hydroxylase, an enzyme involved in the production of dopa (the precursor of dopamine), apparently can be stimulated by iron supplementation. However, consult with your physician before taking supplemental iron.

❑ If you are taking levodopa, avoid taking supplements of vitamin B$_6$ (pyridoxine). However, if you are not taking this drug, vitamin B$_6$ can be very beneficial because the production of dopamine depends on the presence of adequate amounts of this vitamin. In fact, B$_6$ was shown to protect against developing Parkinson's disease. Those with the highest intake of B$_6$ had a 30 percent reduced chance of developing the condition. This was a ten-year study with over 5,000 participants.

PELVIC INFLAMMATORY DISEASE

Pelvic inflammatory disease (PID) is an infection of the female reproductive tract. Most cases of PID result from infection with a sexually transmitted disease, such as chlamydia or gonorrhea. PID can also develop after surgical injury to the uterus or insertion of an intrauterine device (IUD) for contraception. According to the Centers for Disease Control and Prevention (CDC), each year in the United States, more than 750,000 women experience an episode of acute PID. Up to 10 to 15 percent of these women may become infertile as a result of PID.

Vaginal discharge is usually the first symptom of PID,

and may be followed by tension in the anal area, fever, nausea, pain along the midline of the abdomen, and vaginal bleeding. Women infected with chlamydia or gonorrhea often experience pain when leaning the trunk to the left or right. PID infections often are so mild that they go undetected until they are discovered as the cause of infertility, which occurs when scar tissue forms in the fallopian tubes.

PID is conventionally treated with antibiotics after the infectious agent is identified. (Surgery may be necessary to remove abscesses.) However, about 20 percent of women treated with standard antibiotics do not respond to treatment. These are the women who may benefit most from herbal treatment.

Recommendations

❑ If you take antibiotics, also include a probiotic supplement such as *Lactobacillus acidophilus* or *Bifidobacterium bifidus* while you are taking the medication and for two weeks afterward. This will help maintain helpful bacteria in the digestive tract. Take the probiotic supplement as far apart in time from the antibiotic as possible. Check expiration dates to make sure the supplement is fresh and the bacteria are live.

❑ Avoid sexual intercourse until you finish all medication and the infection has cleared, unless your doctor recommends otherwise.

Considerations

❑ Researchers in both Japan and the United States have noted that PID that does not respond to antibiotics sometimes can improve after the removal of dental amalgams containing mercury. Dr. Yoshiaki Omura of the Heart Disease Research Foundation has also noted that "purging" the body of mercury compounds—by taking 100 milligrams of dried Chinese parsley (cilantro) four times a day—has a similar, positive effect. Although the science behind these findings is still being examined, these methods pose no risk and may help when other treatments do not. Speak to your dentist regarding filling removal.

Pelvic Inflammatory Disease: Beneficial Herbs

Herb	Form and Dosage	Comments
Barberry[1] or coptis[1] or goldenseal[1] or Oregon grape root[1]	Tincture. Take 20 drops in ¼ cup water 3 times daily.	Fights gonorrhea, as well as giardiasis and trichomoniasis infections that can be misidentified as PID.
Scutellaria[2]	Capsules. Take 250–500 mg 3 times daily.	May treat antibiotic-resistant strains of gonorrhea.

Precautions for the use of herbs:

[1]Do not use barberry, coptis, goldenseal, or Oregon grape root if you are pregnant or have gallbladder disease. Do not take these herbs with supplemental vitamin B_6 or with protein supplements containing the amino acid histidine. Do not take coptis for longer than two weeks at a time. Do not use goldenseal if you have cardiovascular disease or glaucoma. Do not take Oregon grape root for longer than two weeks at a time.

[2]Do not take scutellaria if you have diarrhea.

Pelvic Inflammatory Disease: Formulas

Formula	Comments
Dong Quai and Peony Powder	A traditional Chinese herbal formula used to prevent miscarriage in women who have had PID.
Eight-Ingredient Pill with Rehmannia (Rehmannia-Eight Combination)	A traditional Chinese herbal formula that relaxes the walls of the bladder and increases urination, effectively flushing PID organisms (which have a very short life span) out of the genitourinary tract before they can cause damage.
Gentiana Longdancao Decoction to Drain the Liver	A traditional Chinese herbal formula used to treat PID with fever, especially if there is a shortened menstrual period with unusually dark blood.
Peony and Licorice Decoction[1]	A traditional Chinese herbal formula used to treat PID compounded by abdominal or perianal pain and cramping. Increases estrogen production, and can increase probability of pregnancy.

Precautions for the use of formulas:

[1]Do not use Peony and Licorice Decoction if you have estrogen-sensitive disorders, such as breast cancer, endometriosis, or fibrocystic breasts.

Epimedium may reduce infection in male sexual partners of women with PID by stimulating urination. It also may help with male fertility. Use as directed by the herbalist. Do not use more than directed, since high dosages decrease, rather than increase, frequency of urination, leading to retention of disease-causing microorganisms.

See also GONORRHEA AND CHLAMYDIA.

PEPTIC ULCER

Peptic ulcers are inflamed lesions in the lining of the upper digestive tract—stomach, upper duodenum, and lower esophagus. They occur when the lining is exposed to stomach, or gastric, juices. The major forms of peptic ulcer are duodenal ulcer (intestinal ulcer) and gastric ulcer (stomach ulcer). Men experience ulcers more often than women, by a ratio of two to one.

Normally, the stomach and duodenum (the upper segment of the small intestine) are protected from stomach acid by a layer of mucus. If too much acid is produced, or too little mucus, the acid then starts to break down the body's own tissues. Helicobacter pylori (H. pylori), a bacterium often found in the stomach, is strongly associated with ulcer formation. Other factors involved in ulcer formation include stress, taking certain drugs such as bisphosphonates (Actonel, Fosamax), and the regular use of pain relievers such as ibuprofen (Advil) and naproxen (Aleve). A number of conventional medications are used to treat ulcers. (See under Considerations, page 437.)

The main symptom of peptic ulcer is a burning pain

Peptic Ulcer: Beneficial Herbs

Herb	Form and Dosage	Comments
Herbs That Fight Helicobacter pylori Infection		
Barberry[1] or coptis[1] or goldenseal[1] or Oregon grape root[1]	Capsules. Take 500 mg 3 times daily.	Kills H. pylori.
Cat's claw[2]	Capsules. Take 500 mg 3 times daily.	Prevents reinfection. Stops inflammation, especially from nonsteroidal anti-inflammatory drugs (NSAIDs).
Chamomile	Tea bags. Take 1 cup 3 times daily.	Counteracts H. pylori. Stops inflammation.
Herbs That Ease Ulcer Symptoms		
Aloe[3]	Juice. Take ¼–2 cups daily.	Stops bleeding from ulcers.
Chen-pi[4]	Tea (loose), prepared with 1 tsp (2–3 gm) tea and 1 cup water. (See TEAS in Part Three.) Take 3 times daily before meals.	Relaxes stomach muscles; relieves belching, bloating, and gas. May also be sold as bitter orange peel.
Cinnamon	Tea (loose), prepared with 1 scant tsp (0.5–1 gm) tea and 1 cup water or in 1 cup other tea as flavoring. (See TEAS in Part Three.) Take 3 times daily.	Increases blood circulation to the stomach, which speeds the healing process.
Clove	Oil of cloves. Take 15–20 drops in ¼ cup water 3 times daily.	Relieves gas pressure. Reduces risk of stomach cancer.
Codonopsis	Tea (loose). Prepare and take as recommended by an herbalist.	Slows passage of food through stomach; relieves diarrhea.
Licorice	Deglycyrrhizinated licorice (DGL) tablets. Take 380 mg 2–4 times daily, 20 minutes before meals. Do not substitute whole licorice.	More effective than Tagamet or Zantac in relieving ulcer symptoms. Reduces frequency of vomiting.
Malva	Tea. Prepare and take as directed on the label.	Calms the stomach and reduces intestinal irritation.
Marshmallow root	Powder. Take 1 tsp (2 gm) in 1 cup cold water 3 times daily.	Forms protective layer over stomach lining. May also be sold as althaea.
Rhubarb	Juice or tablets. Take as directed on the label.	Good for treating intestinal bleeding.

Precautions for the use of herbs:

[1]Do not use barberry, coptis, goldenseal, or Oregon grape root if you are pregnant or have gallbladder disease. Do not take these herbs with supplemental vitamin B$_6$ or with protein supplements containing the amino acid histidine. Do not take coptis for longer than two weeks at a time. Do not use goldenseal if you have cardiovascular disease or glaucoma. Do not take Oregon grape root for longer than two weeks at a time.

[2]Do not use cat's claw if you have to take insulin for diabetes. Do not use it if you are pregnant or nursing. Do not give it to a child under age six.

[3]Do not take aloe vera internally if you have diarrhea. Aloe has laxative effects if taken in dosages larger than those recommended. Do not use if you are menstruating, have rectal bleeding, or are taking any kind of diuretic.

[4]Do not use chen-pi if you have bloody stools.

Peptic Ulcer: Formulas

Formula	Comments
Astragalus Decoction to Construct the Middle	A traditional Chinese herbal formula used when pain is spasmodic rather than continuous. Relieves respiratory problems, such as allergies or asthma, occurring at the same time as ulcer attacks.
Calm the Stomach Powder	A traditional Chinese herbal formula that relieves ulcers accompanied by fullness throughout the digestive tract, loss of taste and appetite, loose stool or diarrhea, easy fatigue, nausea and vomiting, belching, and/or acid regurgitation.
Coptis Decoction to Relieve Toxicity[1]	A traditional Chinese herbal formula traditionally used to treat ulcers accompanied by signs of stress. Contains herbs that defend the mucous lining, stop stomach-lining changes caused by alcohol, and act against *Helicobacter pylori*.
Four-Gentlemen Decoction	A traditional Chinese herbal formula used to treat ulcers caused by improper eating habits, excessive consumption of alcohol, excessive deliberation, or overwork.
Ophiopogonis Decoction[2]	A traditional Chinese herbal formula used to treat ulcers accompanied by symptoms of allergy or asthma.
Six-Gentlemen Decoction[3]	A traditional Chinese herbal formula used to treat ulcers accompanied by loss of appetite, nausea, stifling sensation in the chest and over the stomach, and/or vomiting.
Warm the Gallbladder Decoction[4]	A traditional Chinese herbal formula used to treat ulcers accompanied by anxiety, bitter taste in the mouth, dizziness or vertigo, insomnia, nausea or vomiting, palpitations, and slight thirst. May also be sold as Bamboo and Hoelen Decoction.

Precautions for the use of formulas:

[1]Do not use Coptis Decoction to Relieve Toxicity if you are trying to become pregnant.

[2]Do not use Ophiopogonis Decoction if you have a fever.

[3]Do not attempt self-treatment with Six-Gentlemen Decoction unless you have been medically diagnosed with a peptic ulcer. The symptoms treated by this formula can indicate other, serious conditions. Avoid using this formula if you have a fever.

[4]Avoid using Warm the Gallbladder Decoction if you have a fever.

occurring before a meal, about an hour after a meal, or during the night. There may be discomfort in the chest or back. Other symptoms include headache, a choking sensation, itching, and nausea and/or vomiting. Some people find that they eat more when ulcer pain strikes, while others become queasy and lose their appetite.

Ulcer pain can mimic that of a heart attack. Seek immediate medical attention if chest pain radiates to the jaw or arm; is viselike or squeezing in nature; or is accompanied by heartburn, dizziness, nausea, or cold sweats. Used over a period of several months, herbs may relieve other symptoms of peptic ulcer.

Herbs to Avoid

❑ Individuals who have peptic ulcer should avoid gentian. (For more information regarding this herb, *see* GENTIAN *under* The Herbs in Part One.)

Recommendations

❑ For quick relief of pain, drink a large glass of water. This dilutes stomach acids and flushes them out of the stomach. However, avoid water around mealtime, as doing so seems to help reduce recurrence of ulcers as well as reduce the incidence of nausea and vomiting. In a randomized study in people with duodenal ulcers, those who avoided water one hour before and one hour after meals had the most improvement in dyspepsia and nausea and vomiting.

❑ Avoid hot foods and beverages. They may trigger gastric discomfort.

❑ Avoid all niacin (vitamin B$_3$) supplements if you have ever had peptic ulcers.

❑ Drink up to 2 cups of raw cabbage juice daily. Some people have found that raw cabbage juice has a good effect on peptic ulcers. Its healing action may be due to its glutamine content, which could stimulate protein production in the stomach-lining cells that produce mucus. Since cabbage juice can cause flatulence, start with a smaller dosage (½ cup) and work up to a larger dosage as your system becomes accustomed to it.

❑ Use fermented milk products, such as yogurt, rather than skim or whole milk. Fermented milk products may reduce the risk of ulcers.

❑ Drink black or green tea as a beverage. Both kinds of tea contain catechins, which reduce histamine levels and inhibit *H. pylori* in cell studies. Green tea catechins can be taken in supplement form; doses of up to 5,000 milligrams per day may be helpful.

❑ Eat two to three servings of blueberries per week when in season. One of the pigments in blueberries may protect the stomach lining by stimulating the secretion of mucus. This pigment works best when ulcers are caused by alcohol consumption, aspirin, stomach surgery, and stress.

❏ Use oils that are rich in omega-3 fatty acids, which may reduce the production of inflammatory hormones. This means using canola and soy oil in cooking and consuming seafood two to three times a week.

❏ Take bovine colostrum as directed on the label. Bovine colostrum was shown in laboratory studies to cause *H. pylori* bacteria to "clump" so that they cannot infect the lining of the stomach. Avoid salt and sugar, which have been linked to increased stomach acid production.

❏ Avoid fried foods, tea, caffeine, chocolate, animal fats of any kind, and carbonated beverages. Instead of drinking soda, sip distilled water with a bit of lemon juice added.

❏ Bilberry may stop formation of new ulcers induced by alcohol, allergy, nonsteroidal anti-inflammatory drugs (NSAIDs), or stress. Take four to six 60-milligram tablets daily.

Considerations

❏ Conventional treatment for peptic ulcers typically involves antibiotics to kill the *H. pylori* bacterium and other medications to reduce the level of acid in your digestive system to relieve pain and encourage healing. If your peptic ulcer isn't caused by *H. pylori,* you won't need antibiotics. Instead, your doctor may recommend treatments for your specific situation. Treatments for peptic ulcer can include:

• Medications that block acid production and promote healing. Proton pump inhibitors reduce acid by blocking the action of the parts of cells that produce acid. These drugs include the prescription and over-the-counter (OTC) medications omeprazole (Prilosec), lansoprazole (Prevacid), rabeprazole (Aciphex), esomeprazole (Nexium), and pantoprazole (Protonix). Long-term use of proton pump inhibitors, particularly at high doses, may increase your risk of hip, wrist, and spine fracture. Ask your doctor whether a calcium supplement may reduce this risk.

• Medications to reduce acid production. Acid blockers reduce the amount of acid released into your digestive tract, which relieves ulcer pain and encourages healing. Available by prescription or over the counter, acid blockers include the medications ranitidine (Zantac), famotidine (Pepcid), cimetidine (Tagamet), and nizatidine (Axid).

• Antacids that neutralize stomach acid. Your doctor may include an antacid in your drug regimen. Antacids neutralize existing stomach acid and can provide rapid pain relief. Side effects can include constipation or diarrhea, depending on the main ingredients.

• Medications that protect the lining of your stomach and small intestine. In some cases, your doctor may prescribe medications called cytoprotective agents, which help protect the tissues that line your stomach and

small intestine. They include the prescription medications sucralfate (Carafate) and misoprostol (Cytotec).

❏ Regular use of antacids can lead to malabsorption of calcium, diarrhea, constipation, and increased risk of fractures of the wrist, hip, and spine. Some OTC products use aluminum, which can be toxic if it builds up in the body. Some antacids cause constipation or diarrhea but provide rapid relief. Antacids should be used, if at all, on an occasional basis only.

❏ Bismuth is a naturally occurring mineral element that can protect the lining of the stomach and small intestine. The most commonly available form of bismuth is bismuth subsalicylate, better known as Pepto-Bismol. One of the most effective treatments of peptic ulcers is weight loss, if you are overweight. In one study, people who lost weight—whether they took the drug cimetidine (Tagamet; a drug that blocks acid production in the stomach) or not—had relief of symptoms such as pain and had faster healing in the esophagus.

❏ Although chili and red peppers should be avoided in certain other digestive conditions, they can be eaten by people who have peptic ulcers. In fact, eating chili peppers may help prevent ulcers. Two studies at the National University of Singapore found that red pepper protects the lining of the stomach from irritation by aspirin and prevents the formation of ulcers.

❏ With treatment, most peptic ulcers heal; however, it may take eight weeks or longer for complete healing.

❏ People who take cimetidine (Tagamet) or ranitidine (Zantac) for ulcers should be cautious about ingesting alcohol. These drugs can magnify the effects of alcohol on the brain.

❏ *See also* GASTRITIS.

PERIODONTAL DISEASE

Periodontal means "located around a tooth," and periodontal diseases are disorders of the gums or any other structures supporting the teeth. Bleeding from the gums, as shown by blood in the mouth or on the toothbrush after brushing, is a warning sign of periodontal disease. While gum disease can affect children and young adults, it more often occurs among people middle-aged and older. Periodontal disease is the leading cause of adult tooth loss.

Gingivitis is the early stage of periodontal disease. Gingivitis results when plaque—sticky deposits of bacteria, food, and mucus—adhere to the teeth. Plaque accumulations cause the gums to become inflamed and swollen. As the problem develops into periodontitis, pockets of bacteria accumulate and produce more plaque, separating the gums from the teeth. Bacterial growth causes the gums to become red, soft, and shiny. At this stage, the gums bleed easily, but usually there is no pain. Pyorrhea is a more advanced stage of periodontitis. In pyorrhea, the bone beneath the gums begins to erode. Brushing the teeth causes heavy bleeding, and pus may be visible when the gums are pressed. Bad breath may be a problem. In time, the teeth loosen and fall out.

Poor diet and poor dental hygiene contribute to periodontal disease. Other factors include ill-fitting dental appliances, breathing through the mouth, smoking, chronic illness, and excessive alcohol consumption. Herbal treatments soothe inflammation, and may reduce infection risk.

Recommendations

❑ Eat blackberries, blueberries, cherries, elderberries, gooseberries, raspberries, and strawberries. These fruits contain proanthocyanidins, substances that strengthen the walls of cells within gum tissue.

❑ Take 50 milligrams of coenzyme Q_{10} daily. Some studies have indicated that applying Co-Q_{10} directly to the gums may improve periodontal disease, and a similar effect is likely from taking the supplement orally.

❑ To ease sore gums, mix hydrogen peroxide and baking soda to a paste and work this mixture into and under the gums with a toothbrush. Wait a few minutes; then rinse.

❑ Brush with goldenseal powder every day for at least a month. Then change to any brand of toothpaste containing triclosan, such as Colgate Total. Alternate triclosan toothpastes with products such as Nature's Gate, which contains baking soda, sea salt, and vitamin C, all of which reduce inflammation. (This toothpaste can be found in health food stores and online.) Do not stay with the same brand of toothpaste if you experience further gum irritation. Placing several drops of alcohol-free goldenseal extract on a piece of sterile gauze and applying it to the affected area is good for inflammation. You can also add 6 drops of the extract to ½ cup of water and use it as a mouthwash twice a day. Goldenseal is a powerful herbal antibiotic. See your dentist if bleeding persists.

Periodontal Disease: Beneficial Herbs

Herb	Form and Dosage	Comments
Aloe	Gel. Use as directed on the label.	Soothes inflammation.
Clove	Oil. Use 2–3 drops in ¼ cup warm water as a mouthwash 2–3 times daily.	Stops gum pain. Strongly antibacterial.
Goldenseal	Mouthwash. Use as directed on the label. (Do not swallow.)	Antibacterial. Stops bleeding.
Green tea[1]	Catechin extract. Take 240 mg 3 times daily; or tea bag, prepared with 1 cup water. Take 1 cup 3–5 times daily.	Antibacterial. Helps stop conversion of starch into sugar within the mouth.
Scutellaria[2]	Capsules. Take 250–500 mg 3 times daily.	Reverses gingivitis by stimulating collagen growth.
Tea tree	Oil. Rub on gums as directed on the label.	Helps prevent and treat gum disease.
Thyme	Oil. Take as directed on the label.	Natural antiseptic that reduces the level of bacteria in the mouth.
Turmeric	Tincture. Use 1 tsp (4 ml) in ¼ cup warm water as a mouthwash 3 times daily.	Halts action of a gene that creates gum-irritating chemicals.
Witch hazel	Pure tincture. Use 2 tsp (8 ml) in ¼ cup warm water as a mouthwash twice daily.	Stops inflammation by "tanning" the cells lining the gums.

Precautions for the use of herbs:

[1]Green tea contains vitamin K, which can make anticoagulant medications less effective. Consult your health-care professional if you are using them. The caffeine in green tea could cause insomnia, anxiety, upset stomach, nausea, or diarrhea. Do not use green tea in tea form within one hour of taking other medications.

[2]Do not take scutellaria if you have diarrhea.

Periodontal Disease: Formulas

Formula	Comments
Ophiopogonis Decoction[1]	A traditional Chinese herbal formula especially useful for bleeding gums caused by dry mouth. Use as a mouthwash.

Precautions for the use of formulas:

[1]Do not use Ophiopogonis Decoction while gums are actively bleeding or if you have a fever.

❏ As an alternative, try "dry brushing," or brushing without toothpaste. Some dental studies have found that a soft, dry brush seems to scour away built-up bacterial plaque better than a moistened one. To use this method, start with a soft brush (stiff bristles can be softened by running your thumb through them). Brush the inner surfaces of the bottom teeth, then brush the inner top teeth, and finally brush the outer surfaces, upper and lower. The whole process should take about a minute and a half. Finish with a thirty-second brushing with toothpaste. Speak to your dentist before doing this.

❏ Brush your teeth at least twice a day and after each meal and snack. If you can't brush, rinse your mouth out with water and spit it out.

❏ Get in the habit of using dental floss at least once a day. Use unwaxed dental floss if possible, and get it under the gum line to scrape the tooth surface. Have a dental hygienist teach you how to floss properly.

❏ Several times a day, massage the gums with your fingertips. Also stimulate the gums by running the end of a round wooden toothpick under the gum line.

❏ See a dental hygienist twice a year for a thorough cleaning and get treatment for any pockets of infection that are discovered.

❏ Do not smoke, since smoking can slow the healing process.

❏ Use a new toothbrush every month to keep the disease in check, and keep your toothbrush clean between uses. A bacteria-eliminating device for storing your toothbrush between uses is a good investment.

Considerations

❏ Some of the complex carbohydrates in cranberry juice may reduce the risk of gum disease by blocking some bacteria in the mouth from attaching to each other, preventing the formation of dental plaque. The problem with using even unsweetened cranberry juice is that it contains large amounts of sugar. Therefore, use cranberry extract in tablet form, 250 to 500 milligrams three times daily.

❏ Healthy gums are important for healthy hearts. Gum infections force the body to manufacture fibrinogen, which provides a protective coating for gums but also forms a framework on which blood clots may develop. Gum infections also stimulate the immune system into activating cells known as macrophages. These cells fight bacteria in the gums, but they also gather around cholesterol in the lining of arteries, making the development of artery-narrowing plaques more likely. When the statistics are adjusted for such factors as age, sex, diabetes status, total cholesterol, blood pressure, and smoking, people over age thirty-five who have chronic gum disease are nearly twice as likely to have a fatal heart attack or stroke when compared with people who have healthy gums.

❏ Periodontal disease should be treated by a periodontist, a dentist who specializes in this area of dentistry.

❏ Certain illnesses, such as diabetes and several types of blood disorders, create a higher risk for developing gum disease.

❏ See also TOOTHACHE.

PHOBIA

See under ANXIETY DISORDER.

PINKEYE

See Conjunctivitis (Pinkeye) under EYE PROBLEMS.

PINWORMS

See under PARASITIC INFECTION.

PMS

See PREMENSTRUAL SYNDROME (PMS).

PNEUMONIA

See BRONCHITIS AND PNEUMONIA.

PREMENSTRUAL SYNDROME (PMS)

Premenstrual syndrome (PMS) covers a variety of symptoms, both emotional and physical, experienced by many women a week or two before the start of menstruation. Emotional symptoms include depression, apprehension, irritability, mood swings, and changes in sex drive. Physical symptoms include swollen limbs and fingers, acne, backache, breast tenderness, food cravings, water retention, headaches, insomnia, and cramps. Most women find that one symptom, such as depression, predominates, but that there is a great deal of overlap. Many women will have months in which they have no symptoms. Conventional medicine uses different types of drugs to treat the various PMS symptoms. (See under Considerations, page 441.)

One of the causes of PMS is hormonal imbalance in the form of excessive estrogen, the primary female hormone. Hormonal fluctuations lead to fluid retention. PMS is also related to a monthly depletion of the chemical serotonin, which both maintains mood and regulates bodily rhythms and may increase stress and depressive symptoms. Other causes include a poor diet, lack of vitamins and minerals, alcoholism, and eating salty foods that may cause fluid retention.

Herbs to Avoid

❑ Women who have PMS should avoid taking cordyceps, dan shen, fennel, licorice, and peony. (For more information regarding these herbs, *see* individual entries *under* The Herbs in Part One.)

Recommendations

❑ To relieve bloating, increase both intake of high-fiber foods (to prevent constipation) and exercise levels (to sweat out excess fluids).

❑ Take 50 to 100 milligrams of vitamin B_6 (pyridoxine) daily to relieve and prevent premenstrual symptoms. This vitamin is especially important in relieving premenstrual depression. Ask your doctor if you can try vitamin B_6 before trying such antidepressant medications as fluoxetine (Prozac) or sertraline (Paxil). One study found that B vitamins, especially thiamin and riboflavin, from foods such as enriched grains found in breads and cereals, were associated with easing emotional and physical symptoms in women with PMS.

Premenstrual Syndrome: Beneficial Herbs

Herb	Form and Dosage	Comments
Herbs That Relieve Pain		
Asiasarum[1]	Topical massage oil. Apply to the small of the back as needed.	Relieves pain in the small of the back. May also be sold as wild ginger.
Bromelain[2]	Tablets. Take 250 mg 3 times daily, between meals, for 2–3 days.	Relieves spasms of the cervix.
Chamomile	Tea bags. Take 1 cup as desired.	Relieves muscle pain.
Corn silk	Tea bags. Take 1 cup 2–3 times daily.	Relieves fluid retention, muscle cramps, and pain.
Dong quai[3]	*Angelica sinensis* capsules. Take 500–1,000 mg daily for 3–4 months.	Stops cramps.
Motherwort	Tea (loose), prepared with 1 tsp (1.5 gm) tea in 1 cup water. (*See* TEAS in Part Three.) Take 3 times daily until symptoms subside.	Relieves headache; reduces appetite.
Raspberry leaf	Tea bags. Take 1 cup 3 times daily; or bottled tea. Take 1 cup 3 times daily. (Available in health food stores.)	Relieves premenstrual cramps.
Viburnum[4]	Tincture. Take 10–15 drops in ¼ cup water 3 times daily for 2 weeks before start of period for 3–4 months.	Stops premenstrual cramps.
Wild yam (dioscorea)[5]	Tincture. Take 10 drops in ¼ cup water twice daily until symptoms subside.	Stops premenstrual cramps.
Herbs That Ease Other Symptoms		
Birch leaf	Tea bags. Take 1 cup 3 times daily.	Relieves fluid retention and painful urination.
Black cohosh[6]	Capsules. Take as directed on the label for 3–4 months.	Relieves depression and muscle pain.
Dandelion[7]	Tincture. Take 1 tsp–1 tbsp (4–12 ml) in ¼ cup water 3 times daily until symptoms subside.	Relieves bloating and breast tenderness.
Peppermint	Tea. Take as directed on the label.	Helps stabilize mood swings and tone the nervous system.
Unicorn root	Capsules. Take 500 mg 3 times daily for 3–4 months.	Relieves depression during PMS in women not taking oral contraceptives.
Vitex[8]	Capsules. Take 175–225 mg daily for 3–4 months.	Reduces estrogen production, relieving the full range of PMS symptoms. May also be sold as chasteberry.

Precautions for the use of herbs:

[1]Do not take asiasarum internally.

[2]People who are allergic to pineapple may develop a rash from bromelain. If itching develops, stop using it.

[3]Different forms of dong quai have different effects on the uterus; be sure to use the form specified.

[4]Women who are allergic to aspirin should not take viburnum. Viburnum's aspirinlike effect may also aggravate tinnitus (ringing in the ears).

[5]An overdosage of wild yam (dioscorea) can cause nausea. Do not use wild yam products that contain synthetic progesterone.

[6]Do not take black cohosh if you are pregnant or have any type of chronic disease. Black cohosh should not be used by those with liver problems.

[7]Do not use dandelion if you have gallstones.

[8]Vitex has been known to stimulate release of multiple eggs from the ovary, resulting in multiple births.

Premenstrual Syndrome: Formulas

Formula	Comments
Augmented Rambling Powder[1]	A traditional Chinese herbal formula used to treat PMS by lowering estrogen levels. Traditionally used to treat such symptoms as dry mouth, blurry vision, lower abdominal pressure, red eyes, difficult urination, and increased menstrual flow.
Bupleurum and Cinnamon Twig Decoction[2]	A traditional Chinese herbal formula used to treat joint pain and swelling during PMS.
Bupleurum, Cinnamon Twig, and Ginger Decoction[3]	A traditional Chinese herbal formula used to treat sweating, swelling, thirst, and difficult urination during PMS.

Precautions for the use of formulas:

[1]Augmented Rambling Powder should not be used by women who are trying to become pregnant.

[2]Do not use Bupleurum and Cinnamon Twig Decoction if you have a fever.

[3]Do not use Bupleurum, Cinnamon Twig, and Ginger Decoction if you have a fever.

❑ Take 1,200 milligrams of any calcium and 400 milligrams of magnesium supplements daily. PMS seems to result from an imbalance of calcium and magnesium in which magnesium is deficient. However, if you can tolerate dairy, taking two to three servings of dairy products a day will give you ample amounts of these two nutrients.

❑ To stop premenstrual headaches, take 200 to 400 international units (IU) of vitamin D, in addition to calcium supplements. Vitamin D treatment may reduce headache frequency and severity in about two months.

❑ Some women benefit from 400 international units (IU) of vitamin E to ease symptoms such as cramps and breast tenderness.

❑ Take one or two capsules of black currant oil or evening primrose oil three times daily. These supplements provide gamma-linolenic acid (GLA), an anti-inflammatory agent that may also promote healthy skin, hair, and nails. Eating seafood three times a week provides omega-3 fatty acids that affect the hormones in the blood related to menstrual cramps.

❑ Avoid caffeine and chocolate. Although these substances can lift depression, they also stimulate the production of stress hormones. Studies have shown that women who regularly consume caffeine are four times more likely than others to have severe PMS.

❑ Eat little or no refined sugars. Refined sugars also increase magnesium excretion.

❑ Get regular exercise. Walking, even if only one-half to one mile per day, can be very helpful. Exercise increases the oxygen level in the blood, which aids in nutrient absorption and efficient elimination of toxins from the body. It also helps to keep hormone levels more stable.

❑ Get adequate sleep. Try relaxing with deep breathing exercises, yoga, or a massage.

❑ Do not smoke.

Considerations

❑ PMS is not "all in your mind." Secretion of the hormone progesterone during the second half of the menstrual cycle may increase the ability of stress hormones to bind with nerve cells in the brain, producing a stronger response to stress. So far, however, this has only been seen in laboratory studies. (See STRESS.)

❑ Conventional treatments for PMS seek to correct symptoms rather than correct the underlying process. Different types of drugs are used, including antidepressants (relatively low dosages are usually adequate), antianxiety agents, diuretics, and oral contraceptives. For severe PMS or premenstrual dysphoric disorder (PMDD), an injection of medroxyprogesterone acetate (Depo-Provera) can be used to temporarily stop ovulation. However, Depo-Provera may cause an increase in some of the same signs and symptoms experienced with PMS, such as increased appetite, weight gain, headache, and depressed mood.

❑ If depression is a problem, especially if it is accompanied by tension and exhaustion, St. John's wort can help. (See DEPRESSION.) You may also need antidepressants.

❑ Simple dietary manipulations may help with PMS symptoms. Always take a multivitamin with iron and folic acid. Limit caffeine and alcohol, as they cause fluid retention. Eating a diet rich in fruits and vegetables may help reduce fluid buildup, particularly in the legs. In one study, women who used flavonoid extracts had less bloating and felt better after four menstrual cycles. In another study, eating a low-fat diet (20 percent fat versus 40 percent) helped women feel less bloated and they were more interested in having sexual intercourse with their partners. Consuming whole foods, such as whole grains, fruits, and vegetables, rather than refined grain products, juice or dried fruits, and sweet and salty snacks, provides a diet that has a low glycemic index. A low glycemic index diet was associated with improvements in scores that assess

PMS symptoms such as pain, ability to concentrate, and water retention.

❑ Premenstrual food cravings for up to 20 percent more calories than usual are normal in all women. These cravings occur during the ten days after ovulation in which fertilization and implantation could occur, and are part of the body's way of making sure adequate nutrients are provided for a baby. But trying to counteract cravings by dieting during PMS can aggravate stress, since lower blood sugar levels cause higher levels of stress hormones.

❑ Eat a low salt diet and reduce salty food intake, which should reduce bloating and fluid retention.

❑ Women with Crohn's disease or irritable bowel syndrome usually experience more frequent diarrhea in the five days before and during menstruation than at other times. Changing the cycle with oral contraceptives, or stopping the cycle with leuprolide or progesterone, may help prevent bowel flare-ups. (For more information, *see* CROHN'S DISEASE and IRRITABLE BOWEL SYNDROME.)

❑ Wild yam cream, which contains a natural form of the hormone progesterone, has been helpful for many women. You rub the cream into the skin on your chest, inner arms, thighs, and abdomen just after ovulation, and the active ingredient is absorbed through the skin. Speak to a trained health-care professional before using wild yam.

❑ Some women who suffer from PMS have some sort of thyroid dysfunction. (*See* HYPERTHYROIDISM and HYPOTHYROIDISM.)

❑ Fluid retention due to PMS can aggravate a number of disorders. (*See* CARPAL TUNNEL SYNDROME, HIGH BLOOD PRESSURE [HYPERTENSION], OSTEOARTHRITIS, RHEUMATOID ARTHRITIS, and VARICOSE VEINS.)

PROSTATE, ENLARGED

See BENIGN PROSTATIC HYPERTROPHY (BPH); PROSTATE CANCER; PROSTATITIS.

PROSTATE CANCER

Prostate cancer is the most common type of cancer in men. One in every six men in the United States will be diagnosed with the disease. About 63 percent of all cases occur after age sixty-five. Rates are higher among African-Americans than among members of other ethnic groups. (*See under* Considerations, page 444.)

The prostate is a walnut-sized gland that encircles the urethra, the tube through which urine passes. This gland produces the seminal fluid, which forms the bulk of the ejaculate. Both prostate cancer and benign prostate enlargement have the same symptoms: difficulty passing urine, frequent urination and getting up at night to urinate, pain or burning sensation during urination, blood in the urine, and pain in the lower back or pelvis. Such symptoms should always be brought to a doctor's attention.

More prostate cancers are now detected at earlier stages because of prostate-specific antigen (PSA) test. This blood test measures levels of a protein produced by the prostate. Normally, PSA levels are very low, but they rise if a prostate disorder such as benign enlargement, infection, or cancer is present. (See further discussion of PSA testing in Considerations, page 444.)

The exact cause of prostate cancer is unknown, although there is evidence that obesity may play a role in promoting its development. In addition, a genetic predisposition to prostate cancer, being African-American, and age are also possible factors. Once prostate cancer is diagnosed, it is classified into stages, using one of several staging systems, based on how aggressive it is and how far it has spread.

Prostate Cancer: Beneficial Herbs

Herb	Form and Dosage	Comments
Damiana	Capsules or tincture. Take as directed on the label.	Has ability to balance hormone and glandular function.
Milk thistle	Silymarin gelcaps. Take 360 mg daily.	May slow growth of cancers that do not respond to hormone treatment.
Polysaccharide kureha (PSK)	Tablets. Take 6,000 mg daily.	Reduces rate at which prostate cancer spreads to the lungs.
Red wine catechins	Resveratrol tablets. Take 125–250 mg 3 times daily.	Stops cellular processes that cause tumor development and growth.
Saw palmetto and	Capsules. Take 160 mg twice daily.	Controls inflammation caused by prostate cancer. Do not affect the cancer itself.
pygeum and	Capsules. Take 50–100 mg twice daily.	
zinc picolinate	Tablets. Take 50–100 mg twice daily.	
Soy isoflavone concentrate	Tablets. Take 3,000 mg daily.	Slows tumor growth; reduces risk of spread to lungs.
Turmeric	Curcumin. Take 300 mg twice daily, between meals, for 6 months.	Activates p53, a cancer control gene important in 50 percent of cases; slows spread of prostate cancer to bone.

Prostate cancer may spread to the lymph glands, bones, lungs, liver, or bladder.

A number of conventional treatments are used for prostate cancer. Herbal medicine should always be used as part of a medically directed comprehensive treatment plan for this disorder. (*See under* Considerations, page 444.)

Herbs to Avoid

❑ Men who have prostate cancer should avoid the following herbs: American ginseng, cinnamon, cordyceps, ephedra, epimedium, ginseng, sarsaparilla, and Siberian ginseng. Suma (Brazilian ginseng) and horsetail also should be avoided. These herbs contain high amounts of beta-sitosterol, which encourages growth of prostate cancer cells. (For more information regarding these herbs, *see* AMERICAN GINSENG; CINNAMON; CORDYCEPS; EPHEDRA; EPIMEDIUM; GINSENG; HORSETAIL; SARSAPARILLA; and/or SIBERIAN GINSENG *under* The Herbs in Part One.)

Recommendations

❑ Eat at least two servings of cooked tomatoes weekly. Tomatoes are a rich source of lycopene, which at least thirty scientific studies have found to lower prostate cancer risk. In men who have low lycopene levels, prostate cancer is likely to be especially aggressive. Lycopene is nearly four times more readily available to the body from tomato paste than from fresh tomatoes. Since lycopene is fat-soluble, it is better to prepare the tomatoes with a small amount of vegetable oil (pumpkin seed oil would be best), although this is not a license to consume unlimited quantities of any fatty food, such as pizza, as long as it contains some tomatoes. Lycopene is also found in red grapefruit and watermelon, and in smaller quantities in crab and lobster. In one study, men undergoing surgery for advanced prostate cancer who took a supplement of 2 milligrams a day of lycopene had a greater decrease in PSA level after surgery, a reduction in the size of secondary tumors, and better relief from bone pain and lower urinary tract symptoms compared to a group who did not get lycopene.

❑ Take 200 to 800 international units (IU) of vitamin E daily. Vitamin E may activate the cancer-fighting properties of lycopene. You may take vitamin E supplements and get it from dietary sources such as eggs and nuts. In one study, combining selenium, vitamin E, and the herb silymarin enhanced the action of all three on reducing markers of prostate cancer progression—low-density lipoprotein (LDL, or "bad") cholesterol and total cholesterol—in men with advanced prostate cancer following surgery. In addition, the patients felt better compared to a placebo group.

❑ In laboratory studies, vitamin D has been shown to be effective in controlling prostate cancers that are not stimulated by testosterone. Take vitamin D daily as part of a multivitamin.

❑ Eat five to seven weekly servings of foods rich in vitamin A; this includes green leafy vegetables, and orange and yellow fruits and vegetables. Beta-carotene from these foods compensates for low tissue levels of lycopene, and works with vitamin D to slow the proliferation of prostate cancer cells.

❑ Take any supplement containing inositol or inositol hexaphosphate (IP6). Laboratory studies show that inositol inhibits multiplication and growth of some types of prostate cancers.

❑ Take 150 to 200 micrograms of selenium daily. Prostate cancer progresses more rapidly in men with low selenium levels. However, in one study, healthy men taking 200 micrograms of selenium with or without vitamin E (400 IU) for five years did not have a reduced risk of developing prostate cancer.

❑ Drink at least eight glasses of water daily. Dehydration stresses the prostate gland.

❑ Limit animal fat, especially red meat, eggs, and dairy foods. Prostate cancer tends to progress more quickly when animal fat is consumed, but less quickly when omega-3 fatty acids from seafood are consumed.

❑ Avoid cholesterol-lowering products made from concentrated beta-sitosterol. These products contain large amounts of campesterol and stigmasterol, which are associated with an elevated risk of developing prostate cancer and probably should be avoided if cancer is present.

❑ Consume freshly made vegetable and fruit juices daily. Carrot and cabbage juices are good choices.

Prostate Cancer: Formulas

Formula	Comments
Gentiana Longdancao Decoction to Drain the Liver	A traditional Chinese herbal formula that reduces incontinence caused by prostate enlargement or irritation. Treats symptoms that may accompany prostate cancer, including headache, dizziness, hearing loss, bitter taste in the mouth, and emotional distress.
Peony and Licorice Decoction	A traditional Chinese herbal formula that adjusts sex hormone levels to reduce spread of prostate cancer.

❑ Use cold-pressed organic oils such as sesame or olive oil to obtain essential fatty acids.

❑ Eat two to three servings a week of cold-water fish (such as salmon, tuna, or mackerel), or supplement your diet with MaxEPA fish oil. Borage or evening primrose oil may also be helpful.

Considerations

❑ Conventional medicine uses a variety of treatments in prostate cancer. In some elderly men with localized, slow-growing tumors, treatment consists of simply watching the cancer carefully, and treating it if it spreads. For others, various types of surgery may be appropriate, ranging from complete removal of the prostate to removal of tissue through a tube passed up the urethra. While chemotherapy is not often employed, radiation therapy is used to slow the cancer's spread. Sexual dysfunction and incontinence are potential side effects of these therapies. Prostate cancer is often treated with hormonal therapy, which attempts to reduce the effect testosterone has on the prostate. Drugs called luteinizing hormone-releasing hormone (LH-RH) stimulants reduce the concentration of testosterone in the bloodstream to very low levels. However, they also can cause erectile dysfunction (ED), loss of sex drive, hot flashes, loss of muscle and bone mass, and weight gain.

❑ The introduction of the PSA test has led to a jump in prostate cancer diagnoses. The PSA test can detect high levels of PSA, which may indicate the presence of prostate cancer. However, many other conditions, such as an enlarged or inflamed prostate, can also increase PSA levels. Use of the PSA test is controversial. It's important to discuss with your doctor whether you should get a PSA test and what the results may mean.

❑ Your doctor may use other ways of interpreting PSA results before making decisions about ordering a biopsy to test for cancerous tissue. These other methods are intended to improve the accuracy of the PSA test as a screening tool. As with the standard PSA test, there's little clinical evidence that these variations on the PSA screening test improve treatment outcomes or decrease the number of deaths. Researchers continue investigating these strategies to determine whether they provide a measurable benefit. Variations of the PSA test look at PSA velocity, which is the change in PSA levels over time. A rapid rise in PSA may indicate the presence of cancer or an aggressive form of cancer; or percentage of free PSA. PSA circulates in the blood in two forms—either attached to certain blood proteins or unattached (free). If you have a high PSA level but a low percentage of free PSA, it may be more likely that you have prostate cancer.

❑ Another way to find prostate cancer is the digital rectal exam (DRE). If the results of either the PSA or the DRE are abnormal, further testing is needed to see if there is cancer. Since the use of early detection tests for prostate cancer became fairly common, the prostate cancer death rate has dropped. But it isn't yet clear if this drop is a direct result of screening or caused by something else, like improvements in treatment. Neither the PSA test nor the DRE is 100 percent accurate. The PSA test can help spot many prostate cancers early, but another important issue is that it can't tell how dangerous the cancer is. Some prostate cancers grow so slowly that they would likely never cause problems.

❑ For reasons that are not completely understood, non-fat milk products are even more clearly associated with increased risk of prostate cancer than animal fats.

❑ Fats from vegetable oils such as safflower and corn increase prostate cancer risk, according to a study based on nearly 10,000 men.

❑ Diets rich in soy products are associated with lower rates of prostate and other cancers, and genistein, a soy component, may slow prostate cancer not stimulated by testosterone. Soy foods include miso and tofu.

❑ Excess dietary calcium may increase the risk of prostate cancer. This may be because calcium can reduce the levels of vitamin D, which halts the growth of prostate cancer cells. However, it seems that high calcium intake is associated only with low-grade prostate cancer and not more advanced cancer. In fact, low intake of calcium seems to be related to high-grade cancer of the prostate. The exact dosing is not known, but it may be that less than 500 milligrams of dietary calcium a day is too low and more than 1,000 milligrams of calcium is too much.

❑ For unknown reasons, African-American men have the highest incidence rate for prostate cancer in the United States and are more than twice as likely as Caucasian men to die of the disease. Risk of developing the disease is higher for men who have a family history of prostate cancer (father and brother or two brothers who have had the disease). Men at high risk for prostate cancer should take special care both to eat properly and to go for diagnostic tests regularly.

❑ Two articles in *The Journal of the American Medical Association (Jama)* reported that having a vasectomy increases the risk of developing prostate cancer, and that the risk increases with the number of years since the surgery. The overall increase in risk, however, is 1.5 percent. That is, if there is a 10 percent risk of developing prostate cancer for men in a given age group, there is a 10.1 percent risk for men of the same age who have had vasectomies.

❑ Lymphedema is a swelling of the tissues that may follow cancer surgery. (*See* LYMPHEDEMA.)

❑ If the cancer has spread into the capsule of the gland, the standard approach is some form of radiation therapy. Radiation therapy may result in painful urination, loose stools, and ED. It can also adversely affect the bladder and rectum. (For measures to reduce side effects and increase effectiveness of radiation therapy, *see* "Side Effects of Cancer Treatment" *under* CANCER.)

❑ To learn about herbal treatments that may prevent a cancer from developing its own blood supply, *see* CANCER.

❑ *See also* BENIGN PROSTATIC HYPERTROPHY (BPH) and PROSTATITIS.

PROSTATITIS

Prostatitis is an inflammation of the prostate gland. Although it may involve swelling of tissues within the gland, it does not involve an enlargement of the gland itself. As in benign prostate enlargement, however, urinary retention—that is, inability to completely empty the bladder—may occur if the urethra becomes blocked. Prostatitis may be acute or chronic. Prostatitis can be caused by a number of different things. If it's caused by a bacterial infection, it can usually be treated successfully. However, sometimes prostatitis isn't caused by a bacterial infection (only 5 to 10 percent of cases are bacterial) or a cause is never identified. Symptoms include abdominal pain, chills, fever, low back pain, pain with bowel movements, pain with ejaculation, pain or burning with urination (dysuria), perineal pain (pain between the scrotum and the anus), and urinary retention. Additional symptoms that may be associated with acute prostatitis are blood in the urine or semen, testicular pain, and urinary urgency.

Chronic prostatitis may be associated with or follow urinary tract infection (cystitis), urethritis, epididymitis, or acute prostatitis. Prostatitis can affect men of all ages. According to the National Institutes of Health, prostatitis may account for up to 25 percent of all office visits for complaints involving the genital and urinary systems from young and middle-aged men. In fact, chronic prostatitis is the number-one reason men under the age of fifty visit a urologist.

Factors that may set the stage for chronic prostatitis include excessive alcohol intake, perineal injury, and infrequent ejaculation. These factors may cause congestion of the prostate gland, which produces an excellent breeding ground for various bacteria. In chronic prostatitis, inflammation of the prostate gland develops gradually, continues for a prolonged period, and typically has subtle symptoms, especially lower back pain, burning with urination, pain with ejaculation, and pain with bowel movements.

Herbal treatments complement and extend the benefits of antibiotic treatment. Use the herb indicated for specified microorganisms, if known.

Herbs to Avoid

❑ Men who have prostatitis should avoid the following herbs: American ginseng, cinnamon, cordyceps, ephedra, epimedium, sarsaparilla, and Siberian ginseng. Ginseng (*Panax ginseng*, also known as Korean or red ginseng) should be used with caution. (For more information regarding these herbs, *see* AMERICAN GINSENG; CINNAMON; CORDYCEPS; EPHEDRA; EPIMEDIUM; GINSENG; SARSAPARILLA; and SIBERIAN GINSENG *under* The Herbs in Part One.)

Recommendations

❑ Drink from eight to as many as sixteen glasses of water daily. Increasing fluid intake leads to frequent urination, which may flush bacteria from the bladder and decrease urinary symptoms.

❑ Eat blueberries, which contain substances that may keep *Escherichia coli* (*E.coli*) bacteria from attaching to the lining of the prostate.

❑ Avoid fluids that irritate the bladder, such as alcohol, citrus juices, hot or spicy foods, and caffeine.

Prostatitis: Beneficial Herbs

Herb	Form and Dosage	Comments
Bilberry	Tea bags, prepared with 1 cup water. Take 1 cup 1–2 times daily.	Keeps *E. coli* bacteria from attaching to prostate.
Catuaba	Tincture. Take as directed on the label.	Prevents reinfection with *E. coli*; normalizes prostate function.
Scutellaria[1]	Capsules. Take 250–500 mg 3 times daily.	Multipurpose infection fighter; may treat antibiotic-resistant chlamydia strains.
Uva ursi[2]	Capsules. Take 500–1,000 mg 3 times daily.	Fights *E. coli* infection.

Precautions for the use of herbs:

[1]Do not take scutellaria if you have diarrhea.

[2]Uva ursi is more effective if your urine is alkaline. To achieve this effect, avoid meat and take ¼ teaspoon (0.5 gm) of baking soda in ⅓ cup (50 ml) of water with every dose of the herb.

Prostatitis: Formulas

Formula	Comments
Eight Ingredient Pill with Rehmannia (Rehmannia-Eight Combination)	A traditional Chinese herbal formula that relaxes the walls of the bladder and increases urination, effectively flushing prostatitis organisms (which have a very short life span) out of the genitourinary tract before they can cause damage.

❑ Avoid iron supplements. Iron is an essential element for the growth of the bacteria that can cause prostatitis. Furthermore, it is not needed by men in supplement form—adequate amounts can be obtained from the diet.

❑ Take warm tub baths or sitz baths for relief of the perineal and lower back pain associated with acute prostatitis. (*See* SITZ BATHS in Part Three.)

❑ Wash your hands well after a bowel movement and before handling your penis, as this may prevent the potential transfer of *Escherichia coli* (*E. coli*) organisms from the rectal area to the genitourinary tract. In addition, the genitals should be cleaned regularly, and wiping after bowel movements should be done from front to back.

❑ Do not use stimulant laxatives to reduce the discomfort associated with bowel movements. Bulking agents and stool softeners may be useful. (*See* CONSTIPATION.)

❑ If you develop increased thirst, unintentional weight loss, or testicular pain, see a physician.

❑ Avoid exposure to very cold weather.

❑ If your prostate is enlarged, be cautious about using over-the-counter cold or allergy remedies. Many of these products contain ingredients that can inflame the condition and cause urinary retention.

❑ Get regular exercise. Do not ride a bicycle, however, as this may put pressure on the prostate. Walking is good exercise.

Considerations

❑ The first line of medical treatment for prostatitis consists of antibiotic treatment, but sometimes antibiotics are not able to adequately penetrate the prostate tissue. Often, infectious organisms continue to persist in the prostate despite treatment. Once antibiotic treatment has ended, symptoms may recur. Transurethral resection of the prostate (TURP) may be performed if antibiotic therapy is unsuccessful. This surgical treatment, in which prostate tissue is removed via a tube placed up the urethra, usually is not performed on younger men because it carries potential risks for sterility, erectile dysfunction (ED), and incontinence.

❑ Prostate drainage (or prostate massage) may be useful in treating prostatitis. The procedure is identical to a digital rectal exam, but is performed two or three times a week to release bacteria from tiny acini, or sacs, in which they would otherwise grow within the prostate. Drainage can be painful, especially when it is done for the first time, but will become less painful and less uncomfortable the more often it is done. Drainage can be performed by someone other than a doctor, but should only be performed using a human finger in a non-latex glove with a safe lubricant, such as K-Y Brand Jelly. The procedure may temporarily increase burning with urination, as it releases caustic substances produced by the bacteria. However, not all physicians believe that this technique is effective. For more information on this technique, consult the home page of The Prostatitis Foundation at www.prostatitis.org/drainage.html.

❑ Some people believe prostatitis is caused by an inability to process uric acid, a condition that can lead to gout, but this is not a commonly held belief.

❑ *See also* BENIGN PROSTATIC HYPERTROPHY (BPH); BLADDER INFECTION (CYSTITIS); GONORRHEA AND CHLAMYDIA; and PROSTATE CANCER.

PSORIASIS

Psoriasis is a skin disorder marked by well-defined reddish, scaling, elevated lesions. The area of the skin affected by psoriasis can range from a few spots of dandruff-like scaling to widespread lesions over the elbows, knees, torso, and scalp. The disorder follows a pattern of acute flare-ups followed by periods of remission. The disorder may affect people of any age, but it most commonly begins between ages fifteen and thirty-five.

Psoriasis results when skin cells reproduce too rapidly. New skin cells appear so rapidly that dead skin cells cannot be shed, and the accumulated pileup of cells forms the characteristic silvery scales. The speeded-up reproduction results from an imbalance between two chemicals and alters cell division.

About 40 percent of people who have psoriasis come from families in which the disease runs. This indicates that a strong genetic factor is at work in this disorder. In addition, psoriasis is linked to emotional stress, obesity, and smoking. People with infections or compromised immune systems, such as with AIDS, have a higher risk of getting it. Medical treatment of psoriasis does not cure, but can bring a measure of relief (*see under* Considerations, page 448). If using herbal formulas, seek the advice of the dispensing herbalist on a suitable child's dosage.

Recommendations

❑ Eat one or two servings of cold-water fish weekly. Cold-water fish—such as herring, kipper, mackerel, pilchard, salmon, and sardines—contain omega-3 fatty acids, which reduce the frequency and severity of psoriasis outbreaks. If you are taking prescribed Retinol-A to reduce inflammation, the oils found in cold-water fish are especially useful in increasing the drug's effectiveness. Vegetarians and vegans can use vegetarian docosahexaenoic acid (DHA) (such as Neuromins), but these do not contain one of the essential omega-3 fatty acids associated with inflammation, eicosapentaenoic acid (EPA). Thus, taking flax or soy oil may provide enough omega-3s in addition to the DHA. Borage or evening primrose oil also will be helpful.

❑ Eat three total servings of protein foods (one at each meal) and take a complete vitamin B supplement daily. Psoriasis treatment may deplete the body of both protein and folic acid.

❑ Eat fiber-rich foods, and take 5 grams of water-soluble fiber (guar gum, pectin, or psyllium) nightly at bedtime. Components in dietary fiber may bind toxins and promote their excretion with the stool.

❑ People who have type 2 diabetes who also have psoriasis should take 500 micrograms of chromium picolinate daily. Chromium increases the sensitivity of the skin to insulin, which regulates growth processes.

❑ Expose affected skin to between fifteen and twenty minutes of morning or evening sunlight daily. The ultraviolet rays in sunlight help the skin synthesize vitamin D, which slows the cellular processes involved in the

Psoriasis: Beneficial Herbs

Herb	Form and Dosage	Comments
Herbs to Be Applied Externally		
Aloe	Gel. Use as directed on the label.	Relieves inflammation, prevents infection.
Andiroba and/or copaiba	Oil. Use as directed on the label.	Provides quick inflammation relief. Accelerates healing.
Cayenne[1]	Capsaicin cream. Use as directed on the label.	Relieves pain.
Chamomile	Cream. Use as directed on the label.	Relieves inflammation aggravated by allergy.
Lavender	Bath. Add 2 oz (50 gm) of herb to 1 qt (1 L) water and allow to stand overnight. Bathe the affected area.	Relieves pain.
Licorice	Simicort cream. Use as directed on the label.	Extends the length of time that hydrocortisone is effective.
Marshmallow root	Cream. Use as directed on the label.	Forms protective layer against infection.
Herbs to Be Taken Internally		
Barberry[2] or coptis[2] or goldenseal[2] or Oregon grape root[2]	Tablets. Take 250–500 mg 3 times daily.	Prevents formation of toxins in the bowel.
Dong quai	Capsules. Take 500 mg daily.	Reduces inflammation levels when taken at beginning of an outbreak.
Milk thistle[3]	Silymarin gelcaps. Take 120 mg 3 times daily.	Reduces frequency of outbreaks. Maintains liver health.
Psoralea	Capsules. Take as directed on the label. Requires skin exposure to ultraviolet (UV) light.	Natural source of psoralens, active ingredient of methoxsalen (8-MOP, Oxsoralen).
Sarsaparilla	Fluidextract. Take 1–2 tsp (4–8 ml) 3 times daily.	Binds with intestinal toxins so that they exit the body.
Soy isoflavone concentrate	Capsules. Take 3,000 mg daily.	Stops formation of keratin, protein that forms plaques.

Precautions for the use of herbs:

[1]Do not apply cayenne to broken skin. Avoid contact with eyes and mouth.

[2]Do not use barberry, coptis, goldenseal, or Oregon grape root if you are pregnant or have gallbladder disease. Do not take these herbs with supplemental vitamin B_6 or with protein supplements containing the amino acid histidine. Do not take coptis for longer than two weeks at a time. Do not use goldenseal if you have cardiovascular disease or glaucoma. Do not take Oregon grape root for longer than two weeks at a time.

[3]Milk thistle can cause mild diarrhea.

Psoriasis: Formulas

Formula	Comments
Four-Substance Decoction	A traditional Chinese herbal formula used to treat psoriasis in children.
Warming and Clearing Decoction[1]	A traditional Chinese herbal formula traditionally prescribed for chronic skin diseases. Found in laboratory studies to neutralize the white blood cells that destroy affected skin.

Precautions for the use of formulas:

[1]Do not use Warming and Clearing Decoction if you are trying to become pregnant.

multiplication of skin cells. Any ultraviolet (UV) lamp that provides ultraviolet B (UVB) rays is also effective, as is application of vitamin D creams to the skin. If you plan to expose yourself to the sun or use a UV lamp, use sunscreen with an SPF (sun protection factor) of at least 15.

❑ Avoid alcohol. Alcohol is known to significantly worsen psoriasis by increasing absorption of toxins from the intestine.

❑ Eat only lean beef. Eat a diet rich in fruits and vegetables, whole grains, and fish, as these foods don't seem to aggravate psoriasis. Keep a food log to identify foods that trigger psoriasis. Avoid excessive skin dryness. In particular, it is important to avoid detergents and soaps, since detergents activate a chemical that promotes cell reproduction in psoriasis-affected skin. Lubricating the skin with petrolatum, aloe vera, or vegetable oils brings relief without side effects. Keep skin moist, especially in the winter when you may need to lubricate the skin several times a day with lotion.

❑ Eat a diet that is composed of 50 percent raw foods and includes plenty of fruits, grains, and vegetables.

❑ Some people get relief from applying seawater to the affected area with cotton several times a day.

Considerations

❑ Sarsaparilla may be useful in controlling the more chronic form of psoriasis that causes larger plaques.

❑ Smaller outbreaks of psoriasis are treated with a combination of drugs, including steroids, that together dissolve scales and prevent inflammation. Discontinuing the steroids, unfortunately, can bring on a severe flare-up.

❑ Because psoriasis can flare up under stress, it's important to practice relaxation techniques regularly. Regular daily exercise, as well as breathing exercises, guided visualization, hypnosis, massage, and meditation have all been known to help. (*See* STRESS.)

❑ Weight loss has been shown to improve the response to treatments in people with psoriasis. Compared to a group of patients who did not lose weight, those with

moderate to severe psoriasis who lost about 7 percent of their body weight over twenty-four weeks were more likely to have a positive response to treatment with low-dose cyclosporine.

❑ Psoriasis sometimes improves after treatment for celiac disease or food allergies. (*See* CELIAC DISEASE and Food Allergies *under* ALLERGIES.)

❑ If you are experiencing blisters and oozing, or scabby and scaling skin, eczema may be the problem. (*See* ECZEMA.)

❑ Cortisone creams, which discourage skin cells from multiplying, are often prescribed for psoriasis, but long-term use causes the skin to become thin and delicate.

PYORRHEA

See under PERIODONTAL DISEASE.

RADIATION THERAPY, SIDE EFFECTS OF

See "Side Effects of Cancer Treatment" *under* CANCER.

RENAL CELL CARCINOMA

See KIDNEY CANCER (RENAL CELL CARCINOMA).

RESTLESS LEGS SYNDROME

As many as 10 percent of the U.S. population may have restless legs syndrome (RLS). RLS causes one or more symptoms, including cramps or an "antsy" feeling in the legs, jumpiness and leg-thrashing, numbness, painful pins-and-needles sensations, or the feeling that something is crawling under the skin of the leg. Typically, the discomfort is felt deep within the calf, but many RLS sufferers also have discomfort in the arms, and some report discomfort in the trunk and/or genitals. While RLS is often diagnosed after age fifty, symptoms may begin before the age of twenty. The exact cause is unknown, but doctors suspect that it involves a problem due to an imbalance of the brain chemical dopamine.

Restless Legs Syndrome: Beneficial Herbs

Herb	Form and Dosage	Comments
California poppy with corydalis[1]	Corydalis Formula. Take as directed on the label.	Stops muscle spasms; relieves pain; induces sleep.
Kava kava[2]	Kavapyrone tablets. Take 60–120 mg daily.	Relaxes skeletal muscles; sedates the central nervous system.
Passionflower[3]	Tea bags. Take 1 cup 2–3 hours before bedtime.	Induces muscle relaxation and sleepiness.
Rooibos	Tea bags. Take as directed on the label.	Reduces spasms and induces sleep. Also stops generalized inflammation and pain.
Schisandra[4]	Tincture. Take 1 tsp (4 ml) in ¼ cup water 3 times daily.	Increases effectiveness of benzodiazepines (Ativan and Valium), allowing lower drug dosages.
Valerian	Valepotriate tablets. Take 50–100 mg on an empty stomach 1 hour before bedtime.	Sedates muscles; reduces time required to fall asleep.

Precautions for the use of herbs:

[1]Do not use California poppy with corydalis if you are pregnant.

[2]Kava kava increases the effects of alcohol and such psychoactive drugs as sedatives and tranquilizers. Do not use kava kava if you are pregnant or nursing.

[3]Passionflower increases the effects of alcohol and such psychoactive drugs as sedatives and tranquilizers.

[4]Do not use schisandra if you are pregnant or if you have gallstones or blockages of the bile ducts.

Restless Legs Syndrome: Formulas

Formula	Comments
Gastrodia and Uncaria Decoction[1]	A traditional Chinese herbal formula used to increase blood flow to leg muscles, encourage deep sleep, and relax the central nervous system.

Precautions for the use of formulas:

[1]Do not use Gastrodia and Uncaria Decoction if you are trying to become pregnant.

RLS almost always occurs during rest, usually in the evening or at night, and interferes with a good night's sleep, which compounds the problem. Except in severe RLS, mornings are usually symptom-free. The discomfort is usually relieved by physical activity, such as walking, and is sometimes relieved by mental activity, particularly if the activity is engaging or exciting.

Four out of five people with RLS also have periodic limb movements of sleep (PLMS). To relieve tension, the legs involuntarily flex at the knees during sleep, usually about once every ten minutes. These are the movements that constantly interrupt sleep.

Herbs are especially useful when making the transition off a prescription drug (see under Considerations below). This is best done under a doctor's supervision.

Recommendations

❏ Take the recommended dosage of any calcium/magnesium supplement at bedtime. These minerals may calm the nerves.

❏ Eliminate all forms of caffeine from food and drink. Although caffeine will temporarily relieve symptoms, it will cause rebound symptoms when discontinued.

❏ Reduce alcohol intake.

❏ Try to get a good night's sleep. (See INSOMNIA.) Massage, hot baths, or moderate exercise right before bedtime should help to relax you. (See MASSAGE in Part Three.)

❏ Stop smoking, as smoking impairs blood flow to the leg muscles. In at least one case, someone who stopped smoking found complete RLS relief.

❏ If none of these measures helps, have a complete physical. RLS can be a sign of other health problems, such as diabetes, thyroid problems, kidney disease, or arthritis.

Considerations

❏ RLS is not the same as leg cramps. Leg cramps are obvious contractions in the affected muscles at a fixed location. They are relieved more by stretching than by movement. Although they often occur at night, leg cramps are more common in the middle of sleep, rather than at the onset of sleep.

❏ California poppy and corydalis may complement the action of tranquilizers commonly prescribed for RLS. They act in a mild fashion in the same way as levodopa plus carbidopa (Atamet, Sinemet), which is prescribed for severe RLS. Unlike levodopa plus carbidopa, the herbs may not cause "rebound" symptoms when discontinued, nor do they cause stomach upset.

❏ Even slight iron deficiencies, with or without anemia, can aggravate RLS. Iron supplements, taken for a maximum of three months, may reverse borderline cases. The best course of action is to have a blood test for ferritin levels prior to beginning iron supplements, since iron overload disease is possible. Other nutrients such as folic acid and B vitamins may be of help.

❏ Stress can aggravate RLS. (*See* STRESS.)

RETINOPATHY

See DIABETIC RETINOPATHY.

RHEUMATOID ARTHRITIS

Rheumatoid arthritis (RA) is a joint inflammation that causes pain, stiffness, swelling, and deformity, and often limits the joint's range of motion. People with RA may experience weight loss and fever. RA is more common in women than men, often starting between age twenty-five and fifty-five. It usually follows a pattern of flare-ups followed by remissions. Conventional RA treatment uses several types of drugs (*see* Considerations, page 452).

The current theory of the origins of RA is that is occurs when the immune system attacks the synovium, the lining of the membranes that surround the joints. At first there is loss of appetite, fatigue, and vague pain in the muscles and bones. During this stage of the disease, the body produces large numbers of immune-system cells called T cells to fight the infection. Over the course of several weeks, some of these T cells find their way to the lining of a joint called the synovial membrane. The T cells attack cells in the membrane as if they were germs, and the membrane swells until it no longer fits in the joint. The immune system produces chemicals to clean up the dead cells, and the resulting inflammation causes acute pain, and swelling, thickening, and distortion of the joint lining. As the disease progresses, it dissolves a protein called collagen in cartilage, the substance that makes up the synovial membrane, and eventually attacks the bone itself. RA is, in effect, a disease in which the body can turn on the immune system but cannot turn it off.

RA may be a complication of many other autoimmune diseases, such as lupus, psoriasis, Reiter's syndrome (an inflammation of the joints and mucous membranes), or Sjögren's syndrome (an inflammation that dries the mucous membranes). It also may be aggravated by a condition known as "leaky gut," in which the intestines admit inflammatory substances into the bloodstream. These particles could cause an allergic reaction that can compound the symptoms of RA. RA runs in families and increases with age, and smoking can increase the risk.

Herbs to Avoid

❏ People who have RA should not take agrimony or Siberian ginseng. (For more information regarding these herbs, *see* AGRIMONY and SIBERIAN GINSENG *under* The Herbs in Part One.)

Recommendations

❏ Use cat's claw to help control RA symptoms associated with rare causes such as food allergy and inflammatory bowel disease. Take 1,500 milligrams in capsule form daily. People who take insulin for diabetes should not take this herb. Do not use cat's claw if you are pregnant or nursing.

❏ Eat two to three servings of baked, boiled, broiled, or pickled (but not fried) cold-water fish weekly. Herring, mackerel, sardines, and salmon are natural sources of omega-3 fatty acids, which counteract the effects of inflammatory omega-6 fatty acids and greatly reduce symptoms of RA. In addition, you may benefit from 3 grams of fish oil from capsules plus ⅔ tablespoon of olive oil. In one study, people with rheumatoid arthritis who used this combination of oils had less joint pain, stronger grip strength, less morning stiffness, and less fatigue than those who did not get this combination.

❏ Take 30 milligrams of zinc daily. Zinc is essential for the formation of an enzyme that activates omega-3 fatty acids. Preferred forms of zinc for RA are zinc citrate, mono-methionine, or picolinate, which are slightly more readily absorbed by the body than zinc gluconate or sulfate.

❏ Take 2,000 milligrams of pantothenic acid daily. This vitamin may reduce morning stiffness and pain.

❏ Consult your physician about taking supplemental niacinamide (a form of vitamin B₃). This B vitamin has produced some promising results in controlling RA symptoms, but can cause liver damage in some cases. People with RA who use high-dose niacinamide should have their blood tested every three months to monitor for potential liver problems.

❏ Apply moist heat, such as heat packs or moist baths, for twenty minutes one to three times a day to relieve pain and stiffness. Use cold packs to relieve acute pain.

❏ Perform three to ten repetitions of range-of-motion exercises daily, such as flexing the knee back and forth as

Rheumatoid Arthritis: Beneficial Herbs

Herb	Form and Dosage	Comments
Boswellia[1]	Boswellin. Take 150 mg 3 times daily.	Relieves pain in same manner as celecoxib (Celebrex).
Bromelain	Tablets. Take 250 mg 20 minutes before meals 3 times daily.	Blocks formation of kinins, compounds that cause swelling. Relieves pain and inflammation.
and turmeric	Curcumin tablets. Take 400 mg 20 minutes before meals 3 times daily.	
Bupleurum[2]	Solid-extract capsules. Take 200–400 mg 3 times daily.	Enhances effectiveness of cortisone and prednisone treatment; helps prevent their side effects.
Cat's claw[3]	Capsules. Take as directed on the label.	Helps relieve pain.
Cayenne[4]	Capsaicin cream. Use as directed on the label.	Causes temporary skin pain that counteracts joint pain.
Feverfew[5]	Freeze-dried leaf in capsules. Take 25 mg daily and increase to 100 mg daily after 2 weeks.	Relieves fever in joints and reduces pain.
Ginger	20 percent gingerol and shagaol tablets. Take 100–200 mg 3 times daily.	Stops production of inflammatory chemicals.

Precautions for the use of herbs:

[1]Do not use boswellia if you are pregnant.

[2]Bupleurum may occasionally cause mild stomach upset. If this happens, reduce the dose. Do not take bupleurum if you have a fever or are taking antibiotics.

[3]Do not use cat's claw if you have to take insulin for diabetes. Do not use it if you are pregnant or nursing. Do not give it to a child under age six.

[4]Do not apply cayenne to broken skin. Avoid contact with the eyes and mouth.

[5]Do not use feverfew when pregnant or nursing. People who take prescription blood-thinning medications should consult a health-care provider before using feverfew, as the combination can result in internal bleeding. Discontinue use of feverfew if any signs of allergic reactions occur.

Rheumatoid Arthritis: Formulas

Formula	Comments
Ephedra Decoction (Four Emperors Combination)[1]	A traditional Chinese herbal formula used in the early stages of RA to relieve swelling and pain. This formula is appropriate when symptoms are worse in cold weather.
Kidney Chi Pill from the Golden Cabinet[2]	A traditional Chinese herbal formula used to relieve lower back pain and weakness of the lower extremities.
Ledebouriella Decoction that Sagely Unblocks[3]	A traditional Chinese herbal formula for painful, swollen knees.
Prepared Aconite Decoction[4]	A traditional Chinese herbal formula for people with advanced RA whose primary symptom is pain.
Sairei-to	A combination of two traditional Chinese herbal formulas: Five-Ingredient Powder with Poria, which relieves swelling, and Minor Bupleurum Decoction, which regulates the immune system. This combination stimulates natural steroid production and prevents kidney damage.
True Warrior Decoction[5]	A traditional Chinese herbal formula for people with advanced RA whose primary symptom is swelling.

Precautions for the use of formulas:

[1]Do not use Ephedra Decoction if you are nauseous or vomiting.

[2]Discontinue using Kidney Chi Pill from the Golden Cabinet if you develop a fever. This formula may cause a loss of sensation in the mouth and tongue.

[3]Do not use Ledebouriella Decoction That Sagely Unblocks if you are trying to become pregnant. Do not use this formula if you are nauseous or vomiting.

[4]Discontinue using Prepared Aconite Decoction if you develop a fever. This formula may cause a loss of sensation in the mouth and tongue.

[5]Discontinue using True Warrior Decoction if you develop a fever. This formula may cause a loss of sensation in the mouth and tongue.

far as it will go in both directions. Use swimming as your primary form of aerobic exercise—it is easier on the joints than land-based exercise.

❏ In the morning, take a hot shower or a bath to help relieve morning stiffness.

Considerations

❏ Ironically, the very agents most commonly used to treat RA pain, aspirin and other nonsteroidal anti-inflammatory drugs (NSAIDs), increase the "leakiness" of the intestinal lining and accelerate the faulty immune response responsible for this disease. When these agents no longer stop pain, most people with RA are then given steroid drugs such as cortisone. Steroids can be very effective in relieving pain and preventing new attacks. On the other hand, they increase the risk of infection and have a host of other side effects. Newer medications include disease-modifying drugs such as methotrexate (Rheumatrex), which slow the progression of the disease, and TNF-alpha inhibitors such as etanercept (Enbrel), which reduce this inflammatory substance to reduce pain.

❏ S-adenosyl methionine (SAMe), which is helpful for osteoarthritis pain, is not effective for RA.

❏ Some naturopathic physicians note that corn, wheat, beef, dairy products, and vegetables from the nightshade family (eggplant, peppers, potatoes, and tomatoes) aggravate RA. (To learn about food allergies that can aggravate RA, see Food Allergies under ALLERGIES.)

❏ Some herbs have been studied in clinical trials and have been shown to be effective in patients with RA. In one study, devil's claw reduced pain and stiffness and increased function and improved quality of life after eight weeks. In another study, an extract of the Chinese herb *Tripterygium wilfordii Hook F* was shown to improve many parameters on the scoring system used to assess pain and function in RA. after sixteen weeks. In another study, a fermented wheat germ (Avemar) helped improve symptoms such as stiffness when used over the course of a year in patients who did not get relief from standard medicines used for RA.

❏ To learn more about how to deal with chronic pain, see PAIN, CHRONIC.

❏ See also LUPUS; OSTEOARTHRITIS; and PSORIASIS.

RINGWORM

Despite its name, ringworm is a skin condition caused not by a worm but by a fungus. This moldlike fungus, tinea, lives on the outer layers of the nails, scalp, and skin. It is highly contagious, spreading by contaminated floors, shower stalls, and other shared surfaces, including shared bedding. Ringworm is commonly found in children, but may occur in people of all ages.

The telltale sign of ringworm is a ring-shaped rash. The borders of the rash are well defined and advance and spread while the center of the rash heals. Usually the skin is reddened and either darker or lighter than adjoining skin. If the infection is treated promptly, it usually clears up in three to four weeks. If it is not treated, it can cause a chronic rash or hair loss.

Ringworm is generally treated with over-the-counter (OTC) antifungal agents (*see under* Considerations, below). The effectiveness of these treatments is enhanced by the use of antifungal herbs.

Recommendations

❏ Make compresses with 8 to 10 drops of tea tree oil or walnut leaf tincture in 1 pint of water. (*See* COMPRESSES in Part Three.)

❏ Keep affected skin clean and dry. To reduce the risk of reinfection and infection of other family members, wash clothing after each wearing. Do not allow infected children to share bedding, combs, or clothing (including coats, hats, mittens, or scarves).

❏ For ringworm on the scalp, use a shampoo that contains selenium sulfide, such as Selsun Blue. It is necessary to use selenium sulfide shampoo daily for at least a week.

❏ Avoid contact with infected animals. Ringworm produces the same symptoms in animals as in humans, but may not be noticed until it has caused fur loss.

❏ Use a sterile pad and apply colloidal silver to the affected area. Hands and feet can also be soaked in this solution. Colloidal silver is a natural antibiotic that destroys some 650 different microorganisms, but you still may need other treatments.

❏ Apply crushed raw garlic to the affected area and cover it with sterile gauze or a cotton cloth that allows air to penetrate. Do not cover it tightly with adhesive tape or a plastic bandage, which promotes dampness.

Considerations

❏ Such OTC antifungals as clotrimazole (Lotrimin, Mycelex), miconazole (Micatin, Monistat), and terbinafine (Lamisil AT), used once or twice a day for at least two weeks, usually control ringworm and keep it from recurring.

❏ People with diabetes and children with compromised immune systems are at risk for secondary infections, such as cellulitis. If a rash becomes increasingly swollen, red, warm, or tender, or if a fever or swollen glands develop, consult a physician.

❏ Tinea versicolor is a skin infection related to ringworm. This condition appears as a blotchy white discoloration of the skin, which is more noticeable in darker than lighter skin. Tinea versicolor in people with very

Ringworm: Beneficial Herbs

Herb	Form and Dosage	Comments
Pau d'arco[1]	Tincture. Take as directed on the label.	Activates immune system to fight fungi.
Tea tree[2]	Oil. Apply as a cold compress 3 times daily. (*See* COMPRESSES in Part Three.)	Strongly antifungal.
Tolu balsam	Resin. Apply to affected skin daily for 3 weeks.	Antibacterial and antiseptic. Promotes healing.
Walnut leaf	Extract, used to prepare cold compresses. (*See* COMPRESSES in Part Three.)	Stops oozing and exudation.
Wild oregano	Oil. Use as directed on the label.	Powerful antifungal agent that has the ability to destroy even resistant forms of fungi.

Precautions for the use of herbs:

[1]Pau d'arco should not be used by children.

[2]People who are allergic to celery or thyme should not use tea tree oil products. Do not take tea tree oil internally.

light skin may not be visible until the person gets a suntan and the affected areas remain white. Although tinea versicolor produces few symptoms other than discoloration of the skin, it can be very persistent. Normal skin color does not return until the infection is eliminated. Treatment of tinea versicolor is the same as that for ringworm.

❏ The same fungus that causes ringworm also causes athlete's foot. (*See* ATHLETE'S FOOT.)

SCHISTOSOMIASIS

See under PARASITIC INFECTION.

SEIZURE DISORDERS

A seizure is a temporary change in behavior caused by the abnormal firing of neurons (nerve cells) in the brain. This abnormal activity disrupts cell-to-cell communication in the brain. Seizures can result in loss of consciousness, tingling or numbness, unexplained emotions, inattention, loss of speech, a chewing motion with the mouth, and/or staring. Seizures that involve intense, uncontrolled muscle movements are called convulsions.

Seizures can occur for many reasons, including stopping alcohol use after heavy drinking, poisoning, drug reactions, head injury, and fluctuations in blood sugar levels. Genetic factors also may be involved. Often the seizure is an isolated incident. When seizures reoccur because of a problem within the brain itself, the condition is called epilepsy. Epilepsy is usually first diagnosed in childhood or in people over sixty-five years of age.

Scientists believe that epileptic seizures originate in the portion of the brain associated with thinking, the cerebral cortex. There is no known cause of epilepsy in half of the patients, but for the other half it is related to a genetic influence, head trauma, stroke, dementia, diseases such as meningitis, prenatal injury such as poor nutrition, and developmental disorders such as autism.

If seizures occur chronically, a wide variety of antiseizure medications may be used, either singly or in combination (*see under* Considerations, page 454). For the most part, these drugs do not reliably control seizures. Such drugs need to be used with great care, not only because of side effects but also because the range between an ineffective blood level and a toxic one is narrow. Avoiding drastic changes in fluid volume within the body is critical.

Except as otherwise noted, use the herbs and formulas listed here only with guidance from both an herbal practitioner and a neurologist. Formula dosages for children should be discussed with a knowledgeable health-care practitioner. Never discontinue any conventional medication for seizures without a physician's advice.

Herbs to Avoid

❏ People who are taking medication for a seizure disorder should use with caution or avoid entirely any herbs that change fluid balance in the body or stimulate the central nervous system. These herbs include akebia, alisma, aloe, Cornelian cherry, ephedra, green tea, hawthorn, hoelen, Japanese watermelon, lophatherum, maté, mulberry bark, polyporus, and rhubarb root. In addition, children who are subject to seizures should not be given artemisia, eucalyptus, fennel, hyssop, pennyroyal, rosemary, or sage. (For more information regarding these herbs, *see* the individual entries *under* The Herbs in Part One.)

Recommendations

❏ Take at least 1,000 milligrams of a calcium-magnesium supplement daily. Citrate, gluconate, or chelated forms are best. The combination of calcium and magnesium may lessen nervous excitability.

Seizure Disorders: Beneficial Herbs

Herb	Form and Dosage	Comments
Acorus	Use under professional supervision.	Treats absence seizures.
Black cohosh[1]	Capsules, fluidextract, tablets, or tinctures. Take as directed on the label.	Aids in controlling the central nervous system and has a calming effect.
Chinese senega root[2]	Use under professional supervision.	Reduces likelihood of seizure during emotional stress.
Ginger	Capsules. Take 2,000 mg daily.	Protects the liver from side effects of valproic acid (Depakote, Depakene).
Milk thistle[3]	Silymarin gelcaps. Take 240–360 mg daily.	Protects the liver from damage caused by prescription medications.

Precautions for the use of herbs:

[1]Do not take black cohosh if you are pregnant or have any type of chronic disease. Black cohosh should not be used by those with liver problems.

[2]Do not use Chinese senega root if you have gastritis or peptic or duodenal ulcers.

[3]Milk thistle can cause mild diarrhea.

Seizure Disorders: Formulas

Formula	Comments
Bupleurum Plus Dragon Bone and Oyster Shell Decoction[1]	A traditional Chinese herbal formula that is especially useful for controlling partial seizures that result in slurred speech.
Gastrodia and Uncaria Decoction[2]	A traditional Chinese herbal formula used for epilepsy in children.

Precautions for the use of formulas:

[1]Do not take Bupleurum Plus Dragon Bone and Oyster Shell Decoction if you have a fever.

[2]Do not use Gastrodia and Uncaria Decoction if you are trying to become pregnant.

❑ Reduce stress levels as much as possible. Prolonged exposure to stress hormones produces physical changes in the brain that make it less sensitive to the calming effects of calcium. (*See* STRESS.)

❑ Children treated with divalproex sodium (Depakote) should be given L-carnitine supplements to help prevent toxic side effects. The dosage, usually ranging from 100 to 2,000 milligrams daily, should be worked out with the child's physician.

❑ Women of childbearing age who take seizure medications should also take folic acid supplements daily. This lowers the likelihood of birth defects from seizure medication taken before a pregnancy is detected.

❑ Eliminate all stimulants, including coffee, cola, tea, tobacco, and over-the-counter (OTC) medications containing caffeine or dextromethorphan.

❑ Avoid taking zinc lozenges for preventing colds, and do not take supplemental zinc. Research with animals has found that high levels of zinc in the brain lower the threshold at which seizures are triggered. It is safe to take zinc in your multivitamin and in foods.

❑ Anyone who has had a first-time seizure needs a medical evaluation, which may involve brain scans and brainwave tests. Seizures can be symptoms of conditions other than epilepsy.

❑ Eat small meals.

❑ Do not drink large quantities of liquids at once.

❑ Take 2 tablespoons of olive oil daily.

Considerations

❑ Some people with seizure disorders succeed in eliminating medications, but most people who drop medication have another seizure eventually, weeks, months, or years later. People subject to grand mal seizures probably should continue some level of medication on a lifetime basis. The goal of herbal therapy should not be to eliminate prescription drugs entirely, but to control seizures on lower doses and minimize their side effects.

❑ There are some studies that indicate that the amino acid taurine and the hormone melatonin may offer some benefits. Taurine is a sulfur-based amino acid and one of the most abundant in the body, especially in the excitable tissues of the central nervous system. A study reported in the *Journal of Neurology* found that low melatonin levels were associated with uncontrollable seizures.

❑ Children with severe epilepsy that does not respond to drug treatment are sometimes treated successfully with a ketogenic (high-fat) diet. Simply increasing fat in the diet is not enough—following a precise dietary guideline is necessary. For more information on the ketogenic diet, contact the Charlie Foundation to Help Cure Pediatric Epilepsy. (*See* Appendix B: Resources.) Some children are transitioned to a modified Atkins diet, which is less restrictive. However, it is not effective for all children with epilepsy, so discuss using this less restrictive diet with your child's physician first before making the change.

❑ A low glycemic index diet has been shown to reduce seizure frequency in children with epilepsy. In one study, total carbohydrate was limited to 40 to 60 grams a day, and nearly half of the patients had a 50 percent reduction in the number of seizures over twelve months.

❑ Patients with refractory seizures benefited from taking 9.6 grams of fish oil in capsules. Cardiac risk factors such as triglycerides in the blood went down and heart rate was stabilized, both of which are associated with better heart function. Fish oil may be of benefit, but more studies are needed. For now, it is prudent to eat two to three servings of fish a week. Ask your doctor if fish oil capsules are right for you.

❑ In rare cases, seizure disorders in teenagers and young adults are caused by celiac disease. (*See* CELIAC DISEASE.)

SEX DRIVE, DIMINISHED

Lack of interest in sex, even in situations that would normally arouse desire, can affect both men and women. Some people experience this condition all their lives, while others find that their desire for sex diminishes in midlife. A loss of sex drive can cause problems in relationships, especially if sexual activity is infrequent. Or the affected person can continue to have sex, with no loss of performance, in order to please his or her partner. Loss of sexual interest can occur for many reasons, including boredom, childhood or adolescent trauma, depression, and the use of various drugs, including antidepressants, sedatives, tranquilizers, and certain medications used to treat high blood pressure.

Hormonal imbalances, specifically in levels of testosterone, can also cause loss of desire. The adrenal glands on top of the kidneys secrete androstenedione and dehydroepiandrosterone (DHEA), which are converted to active testosterone (and estrogen) in various organs. Changes in testosterone level stimulate sexual desire. When the amount of testosterone reaching the brain fluctuates, the

brain activates a system regulated by the chemical dopamine that creates a surge of energy in the brain. As a result, memory storage centers release images and signals that flood the mind with sexual ideas. The bodies of both men and women produce both estrogen and testosterone, but testosterone is much more abundant in men. Because of this, women are much more sensitive to slight changes in testosterone levels.

Hormone supplementation, both medically directed and self-administered, has been used to help increase sex drive, with varying results. Herbs can be used to help increase testosterone levels. However, herbal treatments are most effective when they are not overused. It may take several weeks to raise testosterone levels, and increased levels then can be maintained for several months. After that, it is desirable to allow hormone levels to fluctuate downward so that the cycle can be repeated.

Herbs to Avoid

❑ People who have diminished sex drive should avoid herbs that increase estrogen production, including dong quai, fennel, hops, licorice, peony, soy isoflavones, and white willow. (For more information regarding these herbs, *see* DONG QUAI; FENNEL SEED; HOPS; LICORICE; PEONY; SOY ISOFLAVONE CONCENTRATE; and WILLOW BARK *under* The Herbs in Part One.)

Recommendations

❑ Experiment with changes in the diet to see if boosting levels of specific amino acids alters the intensity of sexual desire. Try eating foods that contain the amino acid L-arginine, including chocolate, almonds, peanuts, and most other nuts, or take 500 to 2,000 milligrams of supplemental L-arginine daily. In laboratory studies this amino acid spurs production of nitrous oxide, which is essential to erections and increases blood flow to the vagina. (People with herpesvirus infection or shingles should avoid L-arginine. *See* HERPES.) Or you can try L-tyrosine, an amino acid that the brain uses to make dopamine. Taking 100 to 500 milligrams of supplemental L-tyrosine for one week may lift fatigue and increase sex drive. (This amino acid should be avoided by people with melanoma or skin pigmentation problems.) Foods such as chicken, fish, turkey, and whole milk products provide both L-tyrosine and L-phenylalanine, another amino acid that increases dopamine levels and that may enhance sexual interest. In one study, men who took part in a weight-loss program and used amino acid tablets (Master Amino Acid Pattern [MAP]; 10 grams a day) instead of dietary protein were able to lose weight and counterbalance the effects of most weight-loss diets such as hunger, headaches, and loss of libido. The men lost about three pounds a week. Amino acids are short-term substitutes for protein-rich foods during active weight loss. Speak to your doctor before using amino acid in lieu of food to supply protein.

Diminished Sex Drive: Beneficial Herbs

Herb	Form and Dosage	Comments
Herbs That Increase Testosterone Levels		
Avena (also called wild oats)[1]	Tincture. Take as directed on the label.	Increases levels in men only.
Chrysin[1]	Capsules. Take as directed on the label.	Increases levels in men under thirty-five.
Muira puama[1]	Tincture. Take as directed on the label.	Increases levels in men; intensifies erections.
Pine pollen[1]	Micronized in capsules. Take 3,000–4,000 mg daily. (Do not confuse this herb with bee pollen, which is used for benign prostatic hypertrophy [BPH].)	Anecdotally reported to increase levels in women.
Siberian ginseng[1,2]	*Eleutherococcus senticosus* tincture. Take as directed on the label.	Stimulates production in both men and women. Balances dopamine production in the brain.
Stinging nettle root[1]	Capsules or tablets. Take 500–1,000 mg 3 times daily.	Keeps testosterone in active form in both men and women.
Tribulus terrestris[1]	Tribestan. Take as directed on the label.	Increases levels in younger men and women.
Herbs That Increase Sex Drive in General		
Ashwagandha[3]	Capsules. Take 1,000–2,000 mg daily.	Stabilizes male sex drive; prevents premature ejaculation.
Damiana[4]	Tincture. Take as directed on the label.	Increases sexual desire in women.
Ginseng[2,5]	*Panax ginseng* tincture. Take as directed on the label.	Traditionally used to stimulate sexual desire in men over fifty.
Kava kava[6]	Kavapyrone tablets. Take 60–120 mg daily.	Mild relaxant; relieves inhibitions.
Passionflower[7]	Tea bag, prepared with 1 cup water. Take 1 cup 2–6 hours before sexual activity.	Relaxes without decreasing sex drive.
Sarsaparilla	Fluidextract. Take ½–1 tsp (2–4 ml) in ¼ cup water 3 times daily.	Aphrodisiac.
Star anise	Tea bag, prepared with 1 cup water. Take 1 cup 3 times daily.	Stimulates a woman's sex drive during depression.
Yohimbe[8]	Tincture. Take as directed on the label. Do not use tablets.	Aphrodisiac for both sexes. Increases strength of erection.

Precautions for the use of herbs:

[1]Do not use testosterone-stimulating herbs if you have prostate problems.

[2]Avoid Siberian ginseng if you have prostate cancer or an autoimmune disease, such as lupus or rheumatoid arthritis.

[3]Do not use ashwagandha if you are experiencing a period of acute sexual anxiety.

[4]Do not use damiana if you have anemia or a chronic bleeding condition.

[5]The effects of ginseng are canceled out by the use of morphine drugs or cocaine.

[6]Kava kava increases the effects of alcohol and such psychoactive drugs as sedatives and tranquilizers. Do not take this herb if you are pregnant or nursing.

[7]Passionflower increases the effects of alcohol and such psychoactive drugs as sedatives and tranquilizers.

[8]Never take yohimbe and sildenafil (Viagra) within twelve hours of each other. Avoid "yohimbe" tablets, which often do not contain yohimbe. Because yohimbe is a possible monoamine oxidase (MAO) inhibitor, avoid the following substances when using this herb: foods that contain tyramine (chocolate, most French cheeses, liver, organ meats, and red wine), nasal decongestants, and weight-loss aids containing phenylpropanolamine. Avoid high doses of yohimbe, which can result in priapism, a painful erection that requires surgery. (For more information on this herb, *see* YOHIMBE *under* The Herbs in Part One.)

❑ Men who have diabetes should take 30 milligrams of zinc daily. Low zinc levels, which are common among people with diabetes, interfere with the conversion of androstenedione into forms of testosterone that activate sex drive. Zinc may be necessary to regulate the recycling of testosterone by the liver.

❑ Avoid drinking beer. Hops contain compounds very similar to estrogen, and years of use may diminish sex drive in both men and women, as well as induce erectile dysfunction (ED) and feminization of the body in men.

❑ Seek counseling to address any psychological issues you may have.

❑ Have a complete physical examination to ensure that the loss of sex drive is not being caused by an underlying physical disorder. In men, alcoholism, cancer, coronary artery disease, diabetes, high blood pressure, obesity (more than any other factor), and peptic ulcers all contribute to reduced testosterone levels. (*See* ATHEROSCLEROSIS, CANCER, DIABETES, HIGH BLOOD PRESSURE [HYPERTENSION], OVERWEIGHT, and PEPTIC ULCER.)

Considerations

❑ Various hormonal treatments are used to restore sex drive:

• Doctors may recommend testosterone supplementation, especially for men, but also to some extent for women. However, men who begin taking testosterone supplements may experience increased sexual desire at first, but then it diminishes. In both sexes, but especially in women, testosterone supplements must be given within a "therapeutic window" to be effective. In addition, an overdosage of testosterone can result in an increase in body hair and a lowered voice. Other side effects include acne and mood changes in women. The FDA has not approved giving testosterone to women for sexual dysfunction. Women without ovaries may benefit from its use, however.

• Androstenedione, available commercially, can cause a temporary spike in testosterone levels that increases sex drive in both men and women. Taking 100 milligrams of androstenedione daily for one week every two months will not produce side effects and may increase sex drive. Used on a continuing basis, however, it will not increase sexual desire, since the brain will become accustomed to the new, higher levels of testosterone. And in some people, androstenedione will actually decrease sex drive, since this hormone can be converted into either testosterone or estrogen. Moreover, the increased testosterone levels can cause masculinization in women, and shrunken testicles, ED, prostate problems, skin outbreaks, and mood disorders in men. The U.S. Food and Drug Administration (FDA) has issued a warning not to consume products with "andro" in them.

• DHEA has been described as the "Russian roulette" of supplemental hormones used for loss of sexual desire. Although DHEA may in some cases raise testosterone levels and increase desire, it may also increase estrogen levels and decrease sexual desire. Do not use this without consulting a doctor trained in its use.

• Pregnenolone, another hormone, also has unpredictable effects on sexual desire. This commonly available supplement is used by the body to make both estrogen and testosterone, as well as the stress hormones. Although taking pregnenolone makes many people feel mentally sharper and more alert, it has no reliable effect on sexual desire. Consult with a physician before using this, as side effects include stimulating hormone changes that increase the risk of breast and prostate cancers.

❑ In addition to the herbs listed in the table on page 456, women may respond to combinations of the South American herbs abuta, catuaba, chuchuhuasi, damiana, maca, sarsaparilla, and suma (Brazilian ginseng). These herbs are available combined as a tincture under the brand name Jaguara, available from Raintree Nutrition. Men may respond to combinations of cajueiro, catuaba, and muira puama, which is available as Male Potency Plus.

❑ American ginseng (*Panax quinquefolium*) is a less stimulating alternative to regular ginseng. Use the tincture as directed on the label.

❑ Ginkgo stimulates general brain function and may help make other treatments more effective. Take 120 milligrams of ginkgolide extract once a day.

❑ Going to someone trained in herbal medicine has shown to be effective if you are prescribed your own mixture of herbs based on your symptoms and medical history. In one study, postmenopausal women who received individual recommendations for herbs had improvement in menopausal symptoms, including a significant increase in libido.

❑ Oysters have a reputation as an aphrodisiac, and are high in both zinc and tyrosine. They only stimulate sexual desire, however, when the diet is deficient in these nutrients. Do not eat raw oysters if you have a compromised immune system or are pregnant.

❑ In women, the most common cause of testosterone deficiency is estrogen replacement therapy (ERT). One form of ERT, Estratest, provides both estrogen and testosterone. It is available only by prescription. Getting the dose right is critical, as is choosing the most effective way to administer it. In addition, there may be a need to adjust dosage in the first few months of using the drug. (*See also* MENOPAUSE-RELATED PROBLEMS.)

❑ Birth control pills containing estrogen generally decrease desire. A study at Eastern Michigan University found that a single dose of the supplement 4-adiol (4-androstenediol) can increase testosterone levels by 50 percent or more and compensate for the excess estrogen supplied by birth control pills. Since long-term studies of this supplement have not been done, the study recommended that low doses be taken infrequently unless a doctor directs otherwise. This supplement is not to be confused with androstenedione, which should be used sparingly, if at all, or with nor-4-adiol, which can cause vaginal dryness.

❑ Reduced sex drive may occur simultaneously with ED. (*See* ERECTILE DYSFUNCTION.)

SEXUALLY TRANSMITTED DISEASES

See GONORRHEA AND CHLAMYDIA; HIV/AIDS; SYPHILIS. *See also under* HERPESVIRUS INFECTION; WARTS.

SHIN SPLINTS

A shin splint is pain in the shin muscles caused by strenuous exercise, usually after a period of relative inactivity.

Shin Splints: Beneficial Herbs

Herb	Form and Dosage	Comments
Andiroba Arnica[1]	Oil. Massage a few drops over area of fracture. Cream. Apply to affected area 1–2 times daily.	Anti-inflammatory. Prevents the release of pain-causing hormones.

Precautions for the use of herbs:

[1]Do not apply arnica to broken skin or to an open wound, and do not take internally. If you develop a rash, discontinue use. Do not use arnica if you are pregnant.

It is usually caused by running downhill, running on a slanted surface, running in worn-out footwear, and stopping and starting frequently, such as in basketball. There are two kinds of shin splints: anterolateral, which is a type that affects the front and outer part of the muscles in the shin and is caused by a congenital imbalance in the size of the opposite muscles; and posteromedial shin splint, which is a type that affects the back and inner part of the muscles of the shin and is caused by running and/or by wearing inappropriate footwear.

Recommendations

❏ For both kinds of shin splints, try low-impact exercise such as swimming or cycling. Apply ice to the affected area for fifteen to twenty minutes four to eight times a day for several days.

❏ The pain usually subsides as the muscles become accustomed to vigorous exercise. If pain continues, see a physician.

❏ Wear proper shoes and consider arch supports if pain persists.

❏ Consider over-the-counter (OTC) pain relievers such as ibuprofen (Advil) and naproxen sodium (Aleve), and be sure to elevate the shin about the level of the heart, especially at night.

Considerations

❏ See also FRACTURE.

SHINGLES

See under HERPESVIRUS INFECTION.

SINUSITIS

Sinusitis is an inflammation or infection of the sinuses, the open spaces within the facial bones. When the sinus membranes become irritated, they swell, trapping air and secretions. The accumulating fluid may worsen viral symptoms and feed bacteria, which leads to infection. A deviated septum or other obstruction of the nose, such as nasal polyps or tumors, also may trap fluid in the sinus.

Sinusitis symptoms include fever, chills, frontal headache, and nasal congestion with thick discharge, as well as

Sinusitis: Beneficial Herbs

Herbs	Form and Dosage	Comments
Anise	Tea (in bags). Take 1 cup 3 times daily.	Helps break up sinus congestion.
Bromelain[1]	Tablets. Take 250–500 mg 3 times daily, between meals.	Relieves sinus congestion. Extends effect of prescription antibiotics.
Cat's claw[2]	Capsules. Take 500–1,000 mg twice daily.	Stimulates immune defense against bacterial infection. Relieves inflammation.
Elderberry	Sambucol. Take as directed on the label.	Breaks up mucus. Also prevents and treats flu.
Horehound	Tea bag, prepared with 1 cup water. Take 1 cup 1–2 times daily.	Stimulates secretion of fluids to carry away congestion.
Osha	Tincture. Take 10–15 drops in ¼ cup water 3 times daily.	Antibacterial; antiviral.
Wild thyme	Tea bag, prepared with 1 cup water. Take 1 cup up to 4 times daily.	Breaks up congestion. Safe for use by people who have peptic ulcers.

Precautions for the use of herbs:

[1]People who are allergic to pineapple may develop a rash from bromelain. If itching develops, stop using it.

[2]Do not use cat's claw if you have to take insulin for diabetes. Do not use it if you are pregnant or nursing. Do not give it to a child under age six.

pain, redness, swelling, and tenderness over the affected sinuses. There may also be nosebleed, sore throat, and bad breath.

Sinusitis is increased in people with allergies such as hay fever or esophageal reflux. Airborne irritants, such as air pollution and cigarette smoke, also can injure the sinus linings. Sometimes swimming or immersing the head in water may allow bacteria-laden water to enter the sinuses. Chronic, hard-to-treat sinusitis sometimes results from chronic sinus irritation caused by the reflux of stomach acid into the esophagus. Dental complications, viral infection, small growths in the nose, injury to the nasal bones, smoking, and cystic fibrosis also may trigger sinusitis.

Unless otherwise specified, the herb dosages recommended here are for adults. Children under age six should be given one-quarter of the adult dosage. Children between the ages of six and twelve should be given one-half of the adult dosage. Formula dosages for children should be discussed with a knowledgeable health-care practitioner.

Recommendations

❏ Use steam inhalations of eucalyptus oil to relieve clogged sinuses. (See STEAM INHALATIONS in Part Three.)

❏ Drink plenty of fluids to increase moisture in your body. This is especially important in dry climates, and during winter months or air travel. If the air is extremely dry during the winter, use a humidifier to keep the sinus membranes from drying and cracking. Moisture also thins mucus and helps it drain better.

❏ To relieve pain and promote circulation and drainage, place hot, wet cloths over the face several times daily. Use as much heat as you can stand for ten minutes at a time.

❏ Do not smoke, and use an air filter in your home and office.

❏ Practice nasal irrigation once or twice a day, especially if you have an active infection or nasal allergies. Make a saltwater solution by dissolving ¼ teaspoon of salt in a cup of warm water. Pour it into your cupped hand and inhale it into one nostril at a time, while closing the other nostril with your index finger. You may also use a neti pot, a ceramic container with a curved spout that allows you to pour water directly into the nose. Alternatively, you can use squeeze bottles (called Sinus Rinse). Some have derived benefit from saline nasal sprays or sprays with corticosteroids.

❏ If you have both chronic sinusitis and frequent heartburn or indigestion or gastroesophageal reflux disease (GERD), try sleeping on your left, rather than right, side, but certainly keep your head up. The lower esophagus curves slightly to the left as it connects with the stomach. During sleep, the effects of gravity straighten out this curve, raising the potential for stomach acids to spill into the esophagus. The prevalence of reflux of gastric acid is higher in patients with chronic sinusitis who are unresponsive to conventional treatment. This combination of the two conditions is common and often needs medical attention to figure out the best treatments for both conditions.

❏ If you are taking the antibiotic amoxicillin (Amoxil, Augmentin, Polymox, Trimox, Wymox), use *Lactobacillus* supplements or eat yogurt to maintain healthy digestive bacteria. *Lactobacillus* supplements may also help prevent stomach upset during other forms of antibiotic treatment.

❏ Eat a diet consisting of 75 percent raw foods.

❏ Eliminate sugar from your diet and reduce your salt intake.

❏ Use a vaporizer to ease breathing and help clear secretions.

Considerations

❏ Acupuncture can be effective—it can relieve pain and promote sinus drainage within minutes. (See ACUPUNCTURE in Part Three.)

❏ Although it is not known conclusively that increasing levels of glutathione, the body's own antioxidant, enables the body to fight chronic sinusitis, glutathione levels are depleted in people with chronic sinusitis. Supplementation with glutamine and vitamin C, which the body uses to create glutathione, may help.

❏ Using herbal or other decongestants during upper respiratory infections may reduce the risk of developing sinusitis. However, nasal sprays should be used for only two or three days at a time to avoid the risk of "rebound congestion," in which congestion becomes worse when the spray is withdrawn.

❏ People with sinusitis who also have peptic ulcers sometimes overcome both conditions when they are successfully treated for *Helicobacter pylori* infection. (See PEPTIC ULCER.)

❏ When the sinuses of the cheek are inflamed, the underlying cause may be a tooth infection or gum disease. (See PERIODONTAL DISEASE and TOOTHACHE.)

❏ Although uncommon, polyps and benign cysts that retain mucus can develop in the sinuses, especially in the large maxillary or frontal sinuses. Intrusive or malignant growths require surgical removal.

❏ See also ALLERGIES, HALITOSIS (BAD BREATH), and NOSEBLEED.

SJÖGREN'S SYNDROME

See under DRY MOUTH.

SKIN CANCER

This section addresses two major forms of skin cancer: basal cell carcinoma and melanoma.

Basal Cell Carcinoma

Basal cell carcinoma is a type of nonmelanoma skin cancer, and is the most common form of skin cancer in the United States. According to the American Cancer Society, 75 percent of all skin cancers are basal cell carcinomas. Fortunately, it is a relatively benign disease with a very high cure rate. It develops on skin that is exposed to the ultraviolet (UV) light of the sun over a period of years. It can also develop after exposure to arsenic. Basal cell carcinoma is most common on the scalp, face, neck, hands, and forearms. It is most prevalent in fair-skinned people.

Basal cell carcinoma appears as small patches of white, hard skin, usually smaller in diameter than a pencil eraser. These growths almost never break out of the protein capsules that contain them, but may bleed and form scars. Left unattended over a period of years, however, they can eventually invade adjacent soft tissues or spread elsewhere.

Besides basal cell carcinoma, the other most common type of skin cancer is squamous cell carcinoma. Both are highly curable if treated early. However, recurrences are common, and if they are not treated properly, they can spread and damage the deeper layers of the skin and even the bone.

Unless the cancer has spread, conventional treatment consists of surgery, usually done in a dermatologist's office. If the cancer has spread, other options may be available. Melanoma occurs less frequently than basal cell carcinoma but is much more aggressive. Therefore, all suspicious growths should be brought to a doctor's attention. (A complete discussion of melanoma begins on page 461.)

Recommendations

❑ Use topical herbal treatments only while waiting for your scheduled medical removal of the basal cell carcinoma. Natural healing processes set in motion by herbs may remove the cancer, but should not be relied on as the sole treatment.

❑ Take 150 to 200 micrograms of selenium daily. Selenium may reduce the risk that existing basal cell carcinomas will spread to the colon, prostate, or lungs. Or eat one or two Brazil nuts a day. Each nut contains approximately 120 micrograms of selenium.

❑ Use sunscreen, but take 200 to 400 international units (IU) of vitamin D to compensate for the use of sunscreen. Vitamin D helps the body contain basal cell carcinoma, but sunscreens to protect the skin also deprive the skin of the ultraviolet (UV) rays needed to make this vitamin. It is best to avoid direct sunlight as much as possible.

❑ Avoid tanning salons. The ultraviolet-A (UVA) rays they utilize are as dangerous as the sun's rays. Do not be misled by claims to the contrary.

Basal Cell Carcinoma: Beneficial Herbs

Herb	Form and Dosage	Comments
Aloe and	Gel. Apply as directed on the label.	Prevents production of chemicals needed for cancer growth. Has produced remissions
vitamin E	Cream. Apply as directed on the label.	in some people.
Astragalus[1]	Capsules. Take as directed on the label.	Generates anticancer cells in the body and boosts the immune system.
Bloodroot	Salve. Apply as directed on the label.	Irritates skin, causing scar tissue to surround basal cell carcinoma.

Precautions for the use of formulas:

[1]Do not use astragalus if you have a fever or a skin infection.

Basal Cell Carcinoma: Formulas

Formula	Comments
Two-Cured Decoction[1]	A traditional Chinese herbal formula that contains pinellia, which directly inhibits the growth of basal cell carcinoma.

Precautions for the use of formulas:

[1]Do not take Two-Cured Decoction if you have a fever.

❏ Examine your skin regularly. The Skin Cancer Foundation recommends performing a full-body self-examination every month. To do this, you need a full-length mirror, a handheld mirror, and ample lighting. Using the mirrors, look for any changes in any moles or marks on your body. If you find any irregularities, have them evaluated by a dermatologist. If you are fair skinned or have had a lot of sun exposure, it is prudent to see a dermatologist yearly.

❏ Schisandra contains compounds that may prevent skin cancer development after chemical injury, and is especially recommended for people exposed to arsenic compounds. Take 100 milligrams three times daily of the freeze-dried herb. Do not use this herb if you have gallstones or bile-duct blockages.

❏ Turmeric contains curcumin, which has been shown to prevent the development of skin cancer caused by UV light in animal studies. Apply a turmeric poultice three times daily to the affected area. (See POULTICES in Part Three.) This poultice can also be used as a natural sunscreen to prevent UV damage.

Considerations

❏ Actinic keratosis, a precancerous condition caused by excessive exposure to sunlight, may be treated with a skin ointment that contains 5-fluorouracil (Fluoroplex). A coptis compress, applied and removed before applying Fluoroplex, may increase the skin's ability to absorb this drug, but check with your doctor first. (See COMPRESSES in Part Three.)

❏ Non-melanoma skin cancer may increase the risk of bladder cancer. If you have had basal cell carcinoma or squamous cell carcinoma and you are exposed to cigarette smoke and other bladder-cancer risk factors, speak with your physician about testing for bladder cancer. (See BLADDER CANCER.)

❏ To prevent skin cancer, avoid sun exposure. Wear long sleeves and pants, a hat, and sunglasses with UV protection. Use sunscreen on exposed skin, choosing a sunscreen with a sun protection factor (SPF) of at least 15. Apply sunscreen thirty minutes before heading outside. Be sure to protect children's skin with sunscreen, shade, or protective clothing.

❏ With early detection and treatment, most people recover from skin cancer, but regular checkups are advised for the next five years.

Melanoma

Melanoma is an increasingly common form of skin cancer, particularly in the United States, Israel, and Australia. Most people with melanoma are between the ages of forty and sixty-five, and are fair-skinned. Men and women are affected in equal numbers. Melanoma is the most dangerous type of skin cancer. It is the leading cause of death from skin disease.

This form of cancer can lie latent for as long as fifty years after the sunburn that usually triggers it. Scientists believe that repeated exposure to sunlight itself weakens the immune system's ability to search for and destroy melanoma cells. People with weakened immune systems such as those with AIDS are at increased risk. Other possible risk factors include being fair-skinned, living near the equator, having a lot of moles, and family history.

Melanoma can begin as a new growth. Often, though, it appears as a change to an existing mole. Melanomas are asymmetric, and have irregular borders, multiple colors, and a diameter greater than that of a pencil eraser (6 mm). A smaller, more circular skin lesion may be basal cell carcinoma, a much more common and less aggressive form of cancer, covered on page 460. All suspicious growths should be brought to a doctor's attention.

There are four basic types of melanoma: superficial spreading melanoma (SSM), acral lentiginous melanoma, lentigo maligna melanoma, and nodular melanoma. Melanoma is diagnosed by removing and examining the growth. This disease is classified in stages, from I to IV, depending on how thick the growth is and whether it has spread. Melanoma can spread to almost anywhere in the body, but usually spreads to the liver and lungs.

Surgery, chemotherapy, and immunotherapy are all used in melanoma treatment (see page 463). Herbal therapy always should be used as part of a medically directed overall treatment plan for melanoma.

Herbs to Avoid

❏ People who have melanoma should avoid the following herbs: cordyceps, dan shen, fennel, licorice, and peony (estrogen stimulators), and also garlic (insulin stimulator). (For more information regarding these herbs, see CORDYCEPS, DAN SHEN, FENNEL SEED, GARLIC, LICORICE, and/or PEONY under The Herbs in Part One.)

Recommendations

❏ Stay out of the sun to avoid melanoma, but to ensure the body's production of vitamin D, get at least some sun exposure without using sunscreen, at least twenty minutes a day in the early morning or late afternoon.

❏ Consume orange and yellow fruits and vegetables, and green leafy vegetables. These foods provide a source of vitamin A. On the other hand, overconsumption of vitamin A, such as regular doses of cod liver oil, may increase the risk of melanoma development.

❏ Eat a low-fat diet. In one study, patients with non-melanoma skin cancers who were treated for cancer and who ate a diet with 20 percent of the calories from fat had less recurrence of the disease compared to a group that ate a regular diet of about 38 percent fat calories. In addition, during the two-year study, in the low-fat group, there were fewer cases of skin cancer in the last eight months of

Melanoma: Beneficial Herbs

Herb	Form and Dosage	Comments
Aloe	Gel. Apply liberally on skin.	Contains antihistamines that stop production of a growth factor needed by melanoma.
Astragalus[1]	Capsules. Take 500–1,000 mg 3 times daily.	Increases effectiveness of interteukin-2 (IL-2), stimulates production of natural killer (NK) cells.
Cat's claw[2]	Tincture. Take as directed on the label in ½ cup water with 1 tsp lemon juice.	Stimulates NK cell production. Prevents estrogen from binding to cancer cells.
Kudzu	Tablets. Take 10 mg 3 times daily.	Contains daidzein, which stops growth of certain kinds of melanoma.
Lentinan	Powder. Dosage to be determined by health-care provider.	Reduces rate at which melanoma can invade cells outside the skin.
Polysaccharide kureha (PSK)	Tablets. Take 6,000 mg daily.	Reduces rate at which melanoma spreads to the lungs.
Reishi	Tablets. Take 3,000 mg daily.	Stimulates body's production of IL-2.
Siberian ginseng	Pure eleuthero extract. Take as directed on the label in ¼ cup water.	Useful in forms of cancer that respond to immunotherapy.
Soy isoflavone concentrate[3]	Tablets. Take 3,000 mg daily.	Contains daidzein, which stops growth of certain kinds of melanoma.

Precautions for the use of herbs:

[1]Do not use astragalus if you have a fever or a skin infection.

[2]Do not use cat's claw if you have to take insulin for diabetes. Do not use it if you are pregnant or nursing. Do not give it to a child under age six.

[3]If you develop an upset stomach from taking soy isoflavone concentrate, discontinue use and use kudzu instead.

Melanoma: Formulas

Formula	Comments
Augmented Rambling Powder[1]	A traditional Chinese herbal formula that lowers estrogen levels. According to traditional symptom diagnosis, this formula is used to treat melanomas that appear as bright red nodules with elevated borders.
Cinnamon Twig and Poria Pill	A traditional Chinese herbal formula that reduces the amount of estrogen in the bloodstream.

Precautions for the use of formulas:

[1]Do not use Augmented Rambling Powder if you are trying to become pregnant.

the study compared to the first eight months, indicating that the diet takes a while to work. A low-fat diet should be followed throughout life to reduce the risk of skin cancer. Limit animal fat, especially from beef and eggs. On the other hand, omega-3 fatty acids from seafood may be of benefit to make melanoma tumors less aggressive and reduce the risk of their spread.

❏ Take 150 micrograms of selenium daily, preferably in the form of selenomethionine. Laboratory studies show that selenium reduces the spread of melanoma cells.

❏ Take 30 to 780 milligrams of glycine daily. In laboratory studies, dietary glycine inhibits the growth of melanoma tumors in mice. People with kidney or liver disease should not consume high levels of amino acids without consulting a health-care professional.

❏ Avoid diet soft drinks. These beverages contain phenylalanine, which in laboratory tests increases the ability of melanoma cells to spread to other parts of the body.

❏ Never take tyrosine supplements. Like phenylalanine, tyrosine may increase the ability of melanoma cells to spread, based on laboratory tests.

❏ Examine your skin regularly. The Skin Cancer Foundation recommends performing a full-body self-examination every month. To do this, you need a full-length mirror, a handheld mirror, and ample lighting. Using the mirrors, look for any changes in any moles or marks on your body. Be sure to keep a close watch on any moles or other skin lesions and have them checked regularly by a physician.

Considerations

❏ Surgery is the primary conventional treatment for melanoma, especially for small, early tumors. Chemotherapy is also used. Chemotherapy destroys just the cancer cells, limiting its exposure to other parts of the body. Immunotherapy, in which concentrated amounts of the body's own immune-system chemicals are given, is also used. The agents most often employed are interleukin-2 (IL-2) and interferon. Sometimes the hormone melatonin is added to the treatment program, but speak to your doctor first.

❏ Lymphedema is a swelling of the tissues that may follow cancer surgery. (*See* LYMPHEDEMA.)

❏ To reduce side effects and increase the effectiveness of chemotherapy, *see* "Side Effects of Cancer Treatment" *under* CANCER. To learn about herbal treatments that can prevent a cancer from developing its own blood supply, *see* CANCER.

❏ With early detection and treatment, most people recover from skin cancer, but regular checkups are advised for at least the next five years.

❏ Certain medications may make the skin more susceptible to sun damage. These include antibiotics, antidepressants, diuretics, antihistamines, sedatives, estrogen, and acne medications such as tretinoin (Retin-A) and isotretinoin (Accutane). Ask your health-care provider or pharmacist if any medication that you take might have such an effect.

❏ For a more detailed discussion of skin cancer and its treatment, see the discussion in *Prescription for Nutritional Healing*, 5th ed. (Avery, 2010).

SKIN PROBLEMS

See ACNE; ATHLETE'S FOOT; BOIL; BRUISING; BURNS; CANKER SORES (APHTHOUS ULCERS); ECZEMA; HIVES; INSECT BITES; PSORIASIS; RINGWORM; SKIN CANCER; VITILIGO; WRINKLES. *See also under* HERPESVIRUS INFECTION; PARASITIC INFECTION.

SLEEP PROBLEMS

See INSOMNIA; RESTLESS LEGS SYNDROME.

SORE MUSCLES

See MUSCLES, SORE.

SPRAINS AND STRAINS

The difference between a sprain and strain is intensity and location. A sprain is an injury to a ligament, one of the fibrous cords that connect bones. This occurs when a joint is carried through more than its normal range of motion. A strain occurs when the muscle itself is stressed by being expected to bear too much weight or by being stretched too far.

A strain is not a serious injury, but a sprain may involve twisting or wrenching a joint and rupturing its attachments. Damage to supporting blood vessels, ligaments, muscles, nerves, and tendons may be extensive. There may be considerable pain and swelling, with a resulting loss of mobility. The ankles, wrist, thumb, and knees are especially susceptible to sprains.

If a sprain is especially severe, or if there is a chance that a fracture or dislocation has occurred, seek immediate medical attention.

Recommendations

❏ Elevate a sprain, and apply ice for fifteen to twenty minutes. Remove the ice for ten minutes; then reapply. Repeat for two to three hours after the injury occurs, and occasionally throughout the day for several days afterward. Keep the injured area elevated as much as possible.

❏ For back sprain, rest on a firm surface for several hours. Sit in straight-back chairs, and rest on a firm mattress. Avoid further injury by not lifting anything heavy. When lifting, squat rather than stoop and use your legs to support the weight.

❏ If there is significant swelling, call your physician right away or go to a hospital emergency room to have the

Sprains and Strains: Beneficial Herbs

Herb	Form and Dosage	Comments
Arnica[1]	Cream. Apply 1–3 times daily.	Relieves pain and stiffness.
Horse chestnut	Extract gel. Apply to the injured area.	Reduces swelling and inflammation.
Peppermint	Oil. Massage a few drops into the injured area.	Relieves pain.
Tolu balsam	Cream. Apply 1–3 times daily.	Relieves pain and stiffness.

Precautions for the use of herbs:

[1]Do not apply arnica to broken skin or to an open wound, and do not take it internally. If you develop a rash, stop using it. Do not use this herb if you are pregnant.

injury evaluated. Especially with injuries to the wrists and ankles, it is wise to have X-rays taken to make sure that you have not broken any bones.

❏ To prevent sprains and strains, do stretching exercises both before and after exercise and other physical activity.

Considerations

❏ Arnica cream applied before an athletic event may reduce pain and stiffness after exertion.

❏ Ankle sprain may be avoided by use of a disk-shaped device known as a "wobble board." The disk may prevent contractions of the muscles that cause the ankle to roll outward.

❏ Women are at greater risk for knee sprain during the second half of the menstrual cycle. This is probably due to the effect of estrogen on the knee ligaments, although the hormonal mechanism is not fully understood. Women can reduce risk of knee injury by bending their knees and crouching a little when running. This may relieve stress of the quadriceps muscles at the front of the thigh and the ligaments surrounding the knees.

❏ The risk of injury to the muscles and joints is higher in contact sports than other types of activity.

❏ Strains can lead to tendinitis. (*See* TENDINITIS.)

❏ *See also* FRACTURE.

STOMACH CANCER

Stomach cancer is a disease strongly associated with diet. Factors that increase the risk of stomach cancer include eating salty and smoked foods, a diet low in fruits and vegetables, and family history. In addition, the consumption of nitrites in processed or "cured" meats and fish may contribute to the development of stomach cancer. Nitrates are converted to cancer-causing nitrites by bacteria in the stomach, and *Helicobacter pylori* (*H. pylori*) is the bacterium most closely linked to this process. Stomach cancer is found most often among people age fifty-five or older, and is more common among African-Americans than among members of other ethnic groups. Smoking and chronic gastritis increase the risk.

The early symptoms of stomach cancer include a feeling of fullness or discomfort after eating. Weakness, weight loss, indigestion, and vomiting after eating also may occur. Low-level bleeding may cause anemia. In rare instances, the person will vomit blood or pass tarry, black stools. As the cancer spreads it can affect the liver, causing jaundice and abdominal fluid accumulations.

Stomach Cancer: Beneficial Herbs

Herb	Form and Dosage	Comments
Garlic[1]	Enteric-coated tablets. Take at least 900 mg daily for 3–4 weeks.	Contains compounds that prevent spread of cancer to lymph nodes.
Lentinan	Intramuscular injection or powder given by health-care professional.	Has been used successfully to treat stomach cancer.
Maitake[2]	Maitake-D. Take as directed on the label.	Stimulates immune system to act against stomach cancer.

Precautions for the use of herbs:

[1]Garlic counteracts the effects of *Bifidus* and *Lactobacillus* cultures taken as digestive aids. Consult a doctor before using garlic on a regular basis if you are on an anticoagulant drug such as warfarin (Coumadin). Discuss the use of garlic with your doctor before having any type of surgery. Raw garlic can cause heartburn and flatulence.

[2]Do not take maitake if you have multiple sclerosis.

Stomach Cancer: Formulas

Formula	Comments
Coptis Decoction to Relieve Toxicity[1]	A traditional Chinese herbal formula that contains berberine, which prevents cell multiplication in digestive-tract cancers. Protects the stomach lining.

Precautions for the use of formulas:

[1]Do not take Coptis Decoction to Relieve Toxicity if you are trying to become pregnant. Use this formula only after consulting with a traditional Chinese medicine practitioner who has experience in treating stomach cancer.

Because the early symptoms of stomach cancer are so vague and so easily mistaken for those of other digestive problems, this cancer often is not detected until it is has spread beyond the stomach. Surgery is most successful if the cancer is contained within the stomach itself. If the cancer has spread, radiation therapy or chemotherapy may be used.

Herbal medicine should always be used as part of a medically directed overall treatment plan for stomach cancer (see under Considerations below).

Recommendations

❏ Eat a diet high in fruits, vegetables, rice, pasta, and beans, with limited meat products. In a study comparing the diets of unhealthy eaters and a group of healthy eaters, those who ate a diet rich in fruits, vegetables, and dairy products with low consumption of alcohol had a 70 percent lower incidence of cancer. This was true whether people had H. pylori or not. Another study found that the risk of stomach cancer increased in those who ate few vegetables but consumed a lot of meats, particularly poultry, and high-fat dairy. A third study found that those who ate red meat and processed meats such as red-colored cold cuts had an increased risk of stomach cancer almost double to those who did not eat much of these foods. In people with H. pylori, the risk was increased fivefold if these foods were eaten.

❏ Limit your consumption of smoked, barbecued, pickled, or salt-cured foods.

❏ Avoid alcohol and tobacco products.

❏ Shiitake can be used to reduce the risk of stomach cancer in people who cannot tolerate garlic. In laboratory studies, it works by blocking the formation of cancer-causing chemicals from dietary nitrates. Use the fresh or dried mushroom in food, ¼ to ⅓ ounce (6 to 9 grams) daily. Or take one of the following types of shiitake extract three times daily: three 1-gram tablets, ½ tablespoon (7 to 8 milliliters) syrup, or 1 tablespoon (15 milliliters) tincture in 2 tablespoons water, taken in a single sip.

Considerations

❏ A Japanese study found "excellent" results in treating stomach cancer with lentinan, but only in people who had normal protein levels. Amino acid supplementation will help lentinan work better.

❏ Zinc deficiency may be related to stomach cancer, since a lack of zinc reduces the immune system's effectiveness.

❏ Eating two or more servings of fish per week reduces the chances of developing cancer of the stomach or esophagus by 30 to 40 percent. Avoiding deficiencies of vitamin E (by taking 200 international units [IU] per day and eating one or two servings of eggs or nuts weekly) and

selenium (by taking no more than 150 micrograms per day) also reduces the risk of developing stomach cancer, especially in men. In addition, regular consumption of celery, broccoli, and cabbage (preferably raw), and regular use of cloves and the related Indian spice jambul are associated with a reduced risk.

❏ To reduce side effects and increase effectiveness when using chemotherapy or radiation therapy, see "Side Effects of Cancer Treatment" under CANCER. To learn about herbal treatments that can prevent a cancer from developing its own blood supply, see CANCER.

STREP THROAT

Most cases of sore throat are caused by viral infections, and disappear in a few days. However, some are caused by infection with Streptococcus (strep) bacteria, which can take weeks to go away. Strep throat causes pain on swallowing, redness of the throat, swollen tonsils, and tender lymph nodes in the neck. Strep throat cannot be distinguished from viral sore throat just by looking at the throat and tonsils. Fortunately, physicians now have swabs that can immediately test for the presence of strep.

Strep throat, in rare instances, may lead to rheumatic fever, which causes arthritis, fever, and heart inflammation. Therefore, unlike viral infections, strep infections are treated with antibiotics to prevent damage to other organs. Unfortunately, these drugs are not always effective (see under Considerations, page 466).

Strep throat treated with herbal therapies should improve within three days and go away within three weeks. If it does not, it is possible that a more serious secondary infection is present. In that case, see a health-care professional. It is more common in children aged five to fifteen, so they should be checked by a pediatrician.

Unless otherwise specified, the herb dosages recommended here are for adults. Children under age six should be given one-quarter of the adult dosage. Children between the ages of six and twelve should be given one-half of the adult dosage. Formula dosages for children should be discussed with a knowledgeable health-care practitioner.

Recommendations

❏ Take 250 to 500 milligrams of vitamin C four to six times a day. Vitamin C supplementation is thought by some to reduce the risk of rheumatic fever and strep-induced rheumatoid arthritis.

❏ Always take the full course of any prescribed antibiotic. Taking only part of the prescribed medication wipes out the weakest bacteria but leaves stronger bacteria resistant to the antibiotic to multiply. When these resistant bacteria reinfect you or infect someone else, the antibiotic may not work (see under Considerations, page 466).

Strep Throat: Beneficial Herbs

Herb	Form and Dosage	Comments
Barberry[1] or coptis[1] or goldenseal[1] or Oregon grape root[1]	Tincture. Take 15–20 drops in ¼ cup water 3 times daily for 10 days.	Keeps strep from attaching to the lining of the throat.
Echinacea[2]	*E. purpurea* tablets. Take at least 900 mg daily.	Keeps strep from forming colonies in which they multiply rapidly.
Garlic	Oil. Take 3–4 drops in ¼ cup water once daily as gargle.	Relieves difficulty in swallowing.
Ginger	Tea (powdered), prepared with ⅓ tsp (1 gm) tea and 1 cup water. (*See* TEAS in Part Three.) Take 1 cup 3 times daily.	Relieves pain.
Myrrh	Tincture. Take 10–30 drops in ¼ cup water up to 3 times daily.	Soothes throat ulcers. Stops excessive formation of phlegm.

Precautions for the use of herbs:

[1]Do not use barberry, coptis, goldenseal, or Oregon grape root if you are pregnant or have gallbladder disease. Do not take these herbs with supplemental vitamin B_6 or with protein supplements containing the amino acid histidine. Do not take coptis for longer than two weeks at a time. Do not use goldenseal if you have cardiovascular disease or glaucoma. Do not take Oregon grape root for longer than two weeks at a time.

[2]Do not take echinacea for longer than three months. It should not be used by people who are allergic to ragweed. Do not use echinacea if you have an autoimmune disease such as rheumatoid arthritis or lupus. Do not use it if you have a chronic infection such as HIV or tuberculosis.

Strep Throat: Formulas

Formula	Comments
Lonicera and Forsythia Powder	A traditional Chinese herbal formula found in laboratory tests to kill strep. Recommended for strep throat in people who have chronic viral infections, such as HIV. May be sold as Honeysuckle and Forsythia Powder.

❑ If you take antibiotics, also take a probiotic supplement such as *Lactobacillus acidophilus* or *Bifidobacterium bifidus* while you are taking the medication and for two weeks afterward. This will maintain helpful bacteria in the digestive tract and prevent a later yeast infection. Take the probiotic supplement as far apart in time from the antibiotic as possible. Check expiration dates to make sure the supplement is fresh and the bacteria are live.

❑ Change your toothbrush every two to four weeks. Toothbrushes can be a reservoir for repeated strep infection.

❑ Do not give aspirin or any aspirin-containing product to a child who shows symptoms of a viral infection. Aspirin use can result in Reye's syndrome, a potentially serious complication.

Considerations

❑ Antibiotics usually have little effect on the bacteria in the throat itself, and do not always prevent complications. About 20 percent of the time, antibiotics fail to kill off all of the strep bacteria. When antibiotic treatments for strep throat are unsuccessful, it is usually because there is a secondary infection with *Staphylococcus aureus* or *Bacteroides* bacteria. These bacteria shield the strep bacteria by deactivating penicillin. To help penicillin (Bicillin, Pentids, Pen-Vee, Pfizerpen, Veetids, Wycillin) or erythromycin (Eryc, Ilotycin, PCE, Pediamicin, Pediazole) treatment work better, gargle with 10 to 15 drops of oil of cloves mixed with ¼ cup water twice daily, and take 500 milligrams of scutellaria three times daily as long as you are taking antibiotics.

❑ The primary treatment of strep throat is penicillin or amoxicillin, which is better for children. Otherwise, if penicillin allergies are present, you can take a cephalosporin, such as cephalexin (Keflex), erythromycin (E-Mycin), or azithromycin (Zithromax).

❑ Symptom relief can be gotten from ibuprofen (Advil) and acetaminophen.

❑ Chronic hay fever and food allergies keep the lining of the throat irritated and could cause you to be more susceptible to infection. (*See* ALLERGIES.)

STRESS

Stress is a reaction to any event that upsets the body's balance. Stress can have physical causes, such as pain or cold, or emotional causes, such as worry or frustration. (Even pleasure can cause stress!) Chronic stress is implicated in a host of disorders, including addiction, anorexia, anxiety, high blood pressure, and immune deficiency.

The stress response first developed as a way of releasing quick energy when facing physical danger, or what is known as the "fight or flight" response. The pituitary gland, located at the base of the brain, responds to perceived stress by releasing adrenocorticotropic hormone (ACTH). This hormone is circulated to the adrenal glands, which lie on top of the kidneys. The adrenals convert cholesterol and other substances into cortisol, which initiates a series of profound changes in body chemistry.

In the liver, cortisol stimulates release of the body's principal fuel, glucose. Cortisol also short-circuits the immune system's ability to cause inflammation in response to tissue damage. Less inflammation means that muscles can move more freely and there is less pain. In addition, cortisol makes the red blood cells more likely to clot. When there is loss of blood, the release of cortisol is a potentially lifesaving response.

The problem with stress arises when the body cannot turn off the cycle started by ACTH. This situation can be produced by the chronic stress often found in modern life. Ordinarily, cortisol is broken down during sleep, and is replenished every morning. When stress is unremitting, the body goes out of balance. As the excess glucose is burned, it creates toxic free radicals. These free radicals disrupt processes throughout the body, including normal immune function. The blood continues to clot easily, and the blood vessels constrict. This raises blood pressure and weakens artery walls.

Eventually the adrenal glands themselves could "burn out." The immune system weakens, high blood pressure continues, and the chances of having a heart attack increase because of the highly clotable blood. Even fatigue and depression can follow.

The key to dealing with stress is to address short-term symptoms of stress before they become long-term conditions. Short-term stress produces symptoms that include tight muscles, flushing in the face, high blood pressure, high blood sugar levels, striation on the skin, and in women, development of masculine features, such as hair growth on the face. Long-term stress produces symptoms that include fatigue, pale complexion, low blood sugar levels, and, in women, loss of body hair. Since

Stress: Beneficial Herbs

Herb	Form and Dosage	Comments
American ginseng	*Panax quinquefolium* tincture. Take as directed on the label.	Traditionally used to restore health after long periods of illness or stress.
Ashwagandha	Capsules. Take 1,000–2,000 mg daily.	Reduces fatigue during long-term stress.
Bilberry	Tablets or tea. Take as directed on the label.	Prevents destruction, mutation, and premature death of cells throughout the body.
Catnip	Tea. Take as directed on the label.	Effective against stress. Can cause drowsiness.
Cat's claw[1]	Capsules. Take 1,000–1,500 mg daily.	Reduces the production of inflammatory chemicals caused by short-term stress linked to viral infections.
Chamomile	German chamomile (*Matricaria recutita*) tea bag, prepared with 1 cup water. Take 1 cup as desired.	Calming agent for short-term stress.
Ginseng	*Panax ginseng* tincture. Take as directed on the label.	Helps preserve memory. Reduces burden on cardiovascular system during long-term stress.
Lemon balm	Tea bag, prepared with 1 cup water. Take 1 cup as desired.	Reduces pain and tension during short-term stress.
Reishi	Tablets. Take 6,000–9,000 mg daily.	Can reduce emotional outbursts during long-term stress.
Schisandra[2]	Tincture. Take ½ tsp (2 ml) in ¼ cup water 3 times daily.	Treats headache, insomnia, dizziness, and palpitations associated with emotional stress.
Scutellaria[3]	Capsules. Take 1,000–2,000 mg daily.	Stops overproduction of adrenocorticotropic hormone (ACTH).
Siberian ginseng[4]	*Eleutherococcus senticosus* tincture. Take as directed on the label.	Treats difficulty in concentration. Eases stress due to changes in weather or environment.

Precautions for the use of herbs:

[1]Do not use cat's claw if you have to take insulin for diabetes. Do not use it if you are pregnant or nursing. Do not give it to a child under age six.

[2]Do not take schisandra if you are pregnant or if you have gallstones or blockages of the bile ducts.

[3]Do not take scutellaria if you have diarrhea.

[4]Avoid Siberian ginseng if you have prostate cancer or an autoimmune disease, such as lupus or rheumatoid arthritis.

Stress: Formulas

Formula	Comments
Bupleurum Plus Dragon Bone and Oyster Shell Decoction[1]	A traditional Chinese herbal formula used to reduce the rate at which the body produces cortisol in response to stress. This formula is more effective for emotional stress than for physical stresses caused by accident or disease.
Dong Quai and Peony Powder	A traditional Chinese herbal formula used to prevent free-radical cell damage in the brain caused by prolonged stress.
Four-Substance Decoction	A traditional Chinese herbal treatment used to relieve anxiety and depression and to help maintain intellectual sharpness and short-term memory.
Sairei-to	A combination of two traditional Chinese herbal formulas, Five-Ingredient Powder with Poria and Minor Bupleurum Decoction, that is especially helpful in preventing burnout from long-term stress.

Precautions for the use of formulas:

[1]Do not take Bupleurum Plus Dragon Bone and Oyster Shell Decoction if you have a fever.

stress-related symptoms mimic those of various disorders, it is wise to have such symptoms evaluated by a health-care professional. Appropriately chosen herbal remedies offer short-term relief of the symptoms of stress and long-term restoration of hormonal balances upset by stress. The ultimate treatment is to identify and get rid of the stressor.

Recommendations

❑ Use either hops or rooibos to relieve stress-related digestive problems. Take 500 to 1,000 milligrams of freeze-dried hops in capsules three times a day, or drink 1 cup of rooibos tea (in bags) as desired.

❑ Use relaxation techniques to ease the effects of stress. (See RELAXATION TECHNIQUES in Part Three.)

❑ Limit your intake of caffeine. Caffeine contributes to nervousness and can disrupt sleep patterns.

Considerations

❑ Because the symptoms of stress can be caused by other health problems, people do not always recognize that they are under stress. However, since prolonged stress can lead to a variety of disorders, it is important both to recognize that stress exists and to find the root source of stress, such as work problems, family difficulties, money worries, or other lifestyle factors. It is equally important to find ways to either reduce or offset stress with proper rest, engaging recreation, supportive relationships, and appropriate nutrition. For more information about stress-related disorders, see ANGINA; ANXIETY DISORDER; ASTHMA; CHRONIC FATIGUE SYNDROME; CROHN'S DISEASE; DEPRESSION; DIABETES; ECZEMA; FIBROMYALGIA SYNDROME; HEADACHE; HEART ATTACK (MYOCARDIAL INFARCTION); HIGH BLOOD PRESSURE (HYPERTENSION); INSOMNIA; IRRITABLE BOWEL SYNDROME; MIGRAINE; NAUSEA; PSORIASIS; SEIZURE DISORDERS; STROKE; and VOMITING.

❑ Stress may aggravate certain skin disorders, such as psoriasis, by damaging immune cells in the skin. The damage is done by a chemical released when nerve cells respond to stress. (See PSORIASIS and SKIN CANCER.)

❑ Evidence shows that stress makes allergic symptoms more severe. (See ALLERGIES.)

STROKE

Stroke is a neurological injury that occurs when the brain's supply of oxygen is interrupted. Generally, the longer the oxygen supply is cut off, the greater the damage to brain tissue. Most strokes are caused by blood clots blocking the arteries supplying the brain, or by a leak or burst of the blood vessels. Atherosclerosis, in which fatty deposits build up within artery walls, and high blood pressure are both risk factors for stroke.

The nature and persistence of any disability following a stroke depend on where the stroke occurs and how much of the brain is involved. Possible disabilities include speech or swallowing difficulties, paralysis, blurred vision, loss of bladder or bowel control, or mental difficulties. Very brief "mini-strokes," or transient ischemic attacks (TIAs), may produce strokelike effects, or cause a momentary sense of distraction or dizziness.

While strokes cut off circulation within minutes, medical researchers have learned that the resulting damage to brain tissue is often a long-term process. A blood clot can shut down all circulation to a very small part of the brain. Those nerve tissues die, creating an infarct. Surrounding tissues, however, still receive—and adapt to—a minimal amount of oxygen. When natural healing processes reestablish circulation to the surviving brain cells, those cells are suddenly overwhelmed with oxygen. This oxygen produces toxic free radicals, which attack previously undamaged cells and create further damage. As free-radical damage spreads farther and farther from the infarct, outward symptoms become more severe, and new disabilities may appear.

Never use any herbal remedy for the aftereffects of

stroke before medical diagnosis or without consulting a physician. Herbal remedies are only effective for strokes caused by blocked arteries, and can be harmful if used for those caused by blood-vessel rupture. The doctor will perform the necessary brain scans and other tests to determine the cause of the stroke. Always use herbal therapies as part of a medically directed aftercare program for stroke. If acute stroke symptoms occur—sudden numbness, paralysis, blurred vision, or slurred speech—seek immediate medical attention.

Recommendations

❑ Consult your physician about taking high dosages of several B vitamins, including B_6 (pyridoxine), B_{12} (cobalamin), and folic acid. Very high doses (50 to 100 times the Recommended Daily Allowance [RDA]) of these vitamins over a three-month period have been found to significantly reduce levels of homocysteine and thrombomodulin, substances associated with poor blood-vessel health in people who have had strokes. Since high doses of B vitamins can have side effects, seek medical advice before starting a vitamin B supplementation program.

❑ Take 400 international units (IU) of vitamin E daily. Taking vitamin E supplements seems to help the body build up its own protective mechanisms against stroke, perhaps enabling it to reduce the area affected by a stroke.

❑ Especially if you have been diagnosed with atherosclerosis, avoid fatty meals. Five to seven hours after eating a high-fat meal, especially a meal high in beef fat, the production of clotting factors increases severalfold. This raises the acute risk of clot formation and stroke.

❑ Avoid drastic changes in diet when taking prescribed blood-thinning drugs such as warfarin (Coumadin). Be especially careful not to greatly increase consumption of lettuce, broccoli, spinach, or canola or soybean oil. These foods contain vitamin K, which can increase the blood-thinning potential of Coumadin enough to cause bleeding problems.

❑ Avoid taking blue cohosh, dan shen, feverfew, garlic, ginkgo, red yeast (Cholestin), wintergreen oil, or viburnum if you are taking warfarin (Coumadin) after stroke.

❑ If you smoke, quit. Smoking raises blood pressure, which increases the risk of a second stroke.

❑ Maintain high levels of high-density lipoproteins (HDL, or "good" cholesterol), preferably above 42 mg/dL. One study found that men who maintain an HDL level over 42 mg/dL have a risk of death from stroke due to a blocked blood vessel two-thirds that of men with HDL levels below 35. (For information on maintaining healthy cholesterol levels, see HIGH CHOLESTEROL.)

Stroke: Beneficial Herbs

Herb	Form and Dosage	Comments
Dan shen[1]	Use only under professional supervision.	Helps restore self-expression and mobility after stroke.
Ginkgo[2]	Ginkgolide tablets. Take 240 mg once daily.	Preserves blood flow in healthy portions of the brain.
Hawthorn	Capsules. Take 100–250 mg 3 times daily.	Helps preserve blood-vessel integrity after transient ischemic attacks (TIAs) (mini-strokes).
Oligomeric proanthocyanidins (OPCs)	Grapeseed or pine-bark extract tablets. Take 100 mg daily.	Improves blood-vessel strength and flexibility; reduces risk of second stroke.

Precautions for the use of herbs:

[1]Avoid dan shen if you have an estrogen-sensitive disorder, such as breast cancer, endometriosis, or fibrocystic breasts. Dan shen stops fibroid bleeding, but it increases bloodstream estrogen levels. Do not use it on an ongoing basis.

[2]Do not take ginkgo if you have a bleeding disorder, or are scheduled for surgery or a dental procedure. Avoid ginkgo if you are taking any type of blood-thinning medication.

Stroke: Formulas

Formula	Comments
Rhubarb and Moutan Decoction	A traditional Chinese herbal formula successfully used in Japan to help restore self-expression after a stroke.

❏ Exercise regularly. Maintaining good lung function through regular exercise lowers the risk of stroke, even in smokers.

❏ Avoid pressure on the back of the neck. In particular, exercise care in having hair washed with the neck extended or chair tilted backward in hairdressing salons. The head should be guided down gently and supported by towels placed between the neck and the hard surface of the porcelain. This could prevent tears in arteries, which are a major cause of stroke in younger people.

❏ Avoid binge drinking and the use of illicit drugs, especially cocaine. Cocaine intoxication stimulates the production of endothelin, which constricts blood vessels and greatly increases the risk of stroke.

Considerations

❏ If you do not have high blood pressure, have your blood-pressure levels checked at least weekly after stroke. If you have high blood pressure, follow a medically approved treatment program and check your blood pressure daily. (*See* HIGH BLOOD PRESSURE.)

❏ If you have diabetes, reduce your stroke risk by following your diabetes treatment plan. (*See* DIABETES.)

❏ People who have gum disease are at greater risk for stroke. Inflammatory compounds released from the gum infection narrow blood vessels, such as the carotid arteries of the neck. This increases the risk of clot development. (*See* PERIODONTAL DISEASE.)

❏ For post-stroke depressive symptoms, try B vitamins. People who used them after a stroke (folic acid, 2 mg; vitamin B_6, 25 mg; and vitamin B_{12}, 0.5 mg) for up to ten years had fewer depressive symptoms compared to a placebo group. This is an easy, safe, and affordable way to feel better after having a stroke.

❏ About half of all people who have had a stroke are malnourished and 25 percent have low vitamin levels. In one study, people who took fish oil capsules had a lower death rate after a stroke compared to those who did not take fish oil. In another study, taking a multivitamin did not speed up recovery after a stroke but seems prudent in light of the high rate of malnourishment.

❏ *See also* ATHEROSCLEROSIS.

SWEATING, EXCESSIVE

Sweating is a perfectly natural response to certain conditions, especially heat, exercise, strong emotions, or fever. Excessive sweating, known medically as diaphoresis, is a condition of profuse sweating not brought on by these conditions. Excessive sweating occurs when the sympathetic nervous system—the part of the nervous system that is not under conscious control—responds in an exaggerated manner to environmental or emotional conditions.

When excessive sweating occurs in response to social situations, underlying anxiety or depression is usually the root cause, and doctors frequently elect to treat the condition with powerful antidepressants. Excessive sweating can also occur when the chemical balance of the nervous system is upset by hyperthyroidism, menopause, and withdrawal from alcohol or addictive drugs.

Conventional medicine uses several treatments for excessive sweating (*see* Considerations, page 471). Generally, herbal treatments produce very few or no side effects but must be used consistently to control the condition.

Profuse sweating could be a sign of overdose or intoxication with some common household products, including depilatories, eyedrops, insecticides, mouthwash, and pain relievers.

Herbs to Avoid

People who sweat excessively should avoid cinnamon, ephedra, green tea (except decaffeinated), Japanese mint (schizonepeta), juniper berries, kudzu, ledebouriella, lobelia, maté, red cedar, sassafras, and yohimbe. (For more information regarding these herbs, *see* The Herbs in Part One.)

Recommendations

❏ To control body odor, bathe with a soap containing tea tree oil and/or sage.

❏ To help control foot odor, soak the feet in a basin of warm water with 2 tablespoons of baking soda added every night for a month. Epsom salts or alum may be added to the bath. Foot baths should be avoided by people who have diabetes or any form of nerve damage in the feet. (*See* FOOT BATHS in Part Three.) Use shoe inserts or deodorant crystals and try to avoid wearing the same shoes two days in a row. By airing out shoes for twenty-four hours between wearings, you may starve out the bacteria that cause odor. If you wear sandals, be sure to keep the footbed free of any kind of dirty buildup. Smelly sneakers should be discarded.

❏ Replace lost fluids by drinking water. You may also need to replace the electrolytes sodium and potassium to avoid feeling dizzy. These can be obtained from some sports drinks. Canned foods such as soups are rich in sodium and all fruit juices except cranberry juice are rich in potassium.

❏ Take 30 milligrams of zinc daily to replace zinc lost in sweat.

❏ Avoid coffee, tea, and other stimulants. They increase the activity of apocrine sweat glands, special glands in hairy parts of the body that produce strong-smelling, musky secretions.

Excessive Sweating: Beneficial Herbs

Herb	Form and Dosage	Comments
Sage[1]	Tea bag, prepared with 1 cup water. Take 1 cup 1–2 times daily.	Acts on the sympathetic nervous system to stop excessive sweating. (*See under* Recommendations, page 470.)
Schisandra[2]	Capsules. Take 100 mg 3 times daily.	Alternative to antidepressants for excessive sweating due to emotional distress.
Tea tree[3]	Oil. Use 1 tsp in 2 qts water as a foot bath, once daily. (*See* FOOT BATHS in Part Three.)	Controls foot odor accompanying excessive sweating. (*See* Recommendations, page 470.)
Walnut leaf	Extract. Use in a foot bath once daily. (*See* FOOT BATHS in Part Three.) Or use as a hand bath once daily. (*See* HAND BATHS in Part Three.)	Stops excessive sweating by causing skin proteins to form a barrier to sweat.

Precautions for the use of herbs:

[1]Do not use sage if you are pregnant.

[2]Do not use schisandra if you are pregnant or if you have gallstones or blockages of the bile ducts.

[3]People who are allergic to celery or thyme should not use tea tree oil products. Do not take tea tree oil internally.

Excessive Sweating: Formulas

Formula	Comments
Oyster Shell Powder	A traditional Chinese herbal formula used to treat spontaneous sweating and generalized anxiety.
Shih Qua Da Bu Tang	A traditional Chinese herbal formula used to treat spontaneous sweating and flushing of the face.

❏ Avoid highly spiced foods, especially if you live in a warm climate. Peppers act on the nervous system to increase sweating at high air temperatures (but not at low temperatures).

❏ Avoid monosodium glutamate (MSG). This common flavoring ingredient could cause profuse sweating with nausea and vomiting in susceptible individuals.

❏ To the extent possible, avoid environmental stimuli that can trigger the sympathetic nervous system into an alarm response, such as loud music or lots of interruptions at work.

Considerations

❏ Any antiperspirant containing aluminum helps reduce both sweat and bacteria when used on the feet. Foot powders such as Zeasorb do not control odor directly but absorb sweat. Alternatively, a compounding pharmacist can make a foot powder from equal parts of bentonite, fluffy tannic acid, and talc.

❏ A highly effective, if drastic, treatment for excessive sweating of the hands is endoscopic thoracic sympathectomy (ETS). In this twenty-minute outpatient procedure, a surgeon severs the nerves in the chest that stimulate sweat production in the hands and/or face. The procedure is effective but risky, and often nerve and lung problems arise. For these reasons it is rarely used, and only as a last resort.

❏ Another treatment for sweaty palms is a procedure called iontophoresis, the application of low-level electric current to the surface of the skin. This results in a reduced production of sweat in a specific area. There are battery-operated devices available that seem to work quite well. The drawback of the method is that it has to be repeated every week for continued control of the condition.

❏ *See also* ANXIETY DISORDER, DEPRESSION, HYPERTHYROIDISM, and MENOPAUSE-RELATED PROBLEMS.

SWIMMER'S ITCH

See under PARASITIC INFECTION.

SYPHILIS

Syphilis is a highly contagious sexually transmitted disease caused by a corkscrew-shaped microbe, *Treponema pallidum*. In the United States, more than 60 percent of the syphilis cases are among men who have sex with men.

Syphilis has three stages: primary, secondary, and tertiary. The first sign of primary syphilis is a small, usually solitary sore called a chancre that typically appears

Syphilis: Beneficial Herbs

Herb	Form and Dosage	Comments
Astragalus	Capsules or tincture. Take as directed on the label.	Protects the immune system.
Butcher's broom	Ruscogenin tablets. Take 100 mg once daily.	Shrinks swollen lymph glands.
Copaiba	Oil. Apply to lesions daily.	Soothes inflammation; accelerates healing.
Rooibos	Tea bags. Prepare and take as directed on the label.	Stops generalized inflammation and pain.

from ten days to six weeks after exposure. The chancre is firm and has clearly defined borders that are slightly raised. A chancre on the penis is easily visible. However, those that occur on the labia, cervix, anal area, or mouth are frequently unnoticed because they are usually (but not always) painless. There may also be swollen lymph glands.

Even without treatment, the chancre usually heals spontaneously within two months. This is not a sign that the disease is overcome, however, but rather that it has entered the secondary stage. Lesions that look like the original chancre are usually prominent on the palms of the hands and soles of the feet. There may be a generalized rash accompanied by achy muscles and joints, and fever. Wartlike patches may appear on the genitals. Like the chancre, these symptoms also go away. Throughout primary and secondary syphilis the infection continues to be highly contagious.

In tertiary syphilis, the infection may flare up after being dormant for many years. Soft tumors called gummas may form anywhere in the body, and the disease may damage the cardiovascular or nervous systems. At this stage, syphilis is no longer infectious.

Herbal treatment is highly effective in controlling inflammation and swelling, but not the underlying disease, which must be treated with antibiotics.

Recommendations

❏ Always take the full course of any prescribed antibiotic. Taking only part of the prescribed medication wipes out the weakest bacteria but leaves stronger bacteria resistant to the antibiotic to multiply.

❏ To protect the helpful bacteria in your digestive tract, take antibiotics with a probiotic supplement such as *Lactobacillus acidophilus* or *Bifidobacterium bifidus* for two weeks after the antibiotic prescription runs out. Take the probiotic as far apart in time from the antibiotic as possible.

❏ Avoid 5-hydroxy-L-tryptophan (5-HTP) supplements. In laboratory studies, syphilis alters the body's use of the amino acid tryptophan and related chemicals such as 5-HTP so that they form nerve toxins.

❏ Use a latex condom with nonoxynol-9 lubricant for sexual activity of any kind until the infection is gone completely, as syphilis is highly contagious. Be aware, though, that using a condom does not guarantee complete protection. The only form of complete protection is abstinence.

TENDINITIS

Tendinitis is a common result of sports injuries in which a tendon, the connective tissue that attaches muscles to bones, becomes inflamed. The condition usually results from a strain. Although tendinitis most often goes away by itself within two or three weeks, it can become chronic if calcium salts are deposited along the tendon fibers. The tendons most frequently affected by this condition are the Achilles tendon at the back of the ankle, the biceps at the front of the shoulder, the pollicis brevis and longus of the thumb, the upper patella of the knee, and the rotator cuff of the shoulder.

For any serious sports injury, a physician should be consulted immediately. Treatment of tendinitis involves two phases: protection of the tendon from inflammation and further injury, followed by promotion of healing after acute pain and inflammation have resolved. Treatments that stop swelling and pain are useful at first. Later, treatments that prevent breakdown of collagen, the protein that makes up the tendons, and accelerate regeneration of the tendon should be emphasized.

Recommendations

❏ Take citrus bioflavonoids, 500 to 1,000 milligrams three times per day, to possibly slow the breakdown of collagen in tendon tissue.

❏ Rest until the pain goes away. The tendon must be allowed to rest before healing can begin.

❏ Use gentle exercise to strengthen the affected area as pain and inflammation subside. If muscle atrophy has occurred from disuse or prolonged immobility, perform exercises designed to build strength and increase mobility. Consult a physical therapist trained in healing of tendinitis to learn strength and stretching exercises.

❏ To recover from shoulder injuries, use the rest, ice, maintain mobility, and strengthen (RIMS) system. As soon as shoulder pain is felt, apply ice for thirty minutes; then

Tendinitis: Beneficial Herbs

Herb	Form and Dosage	Comments
Bromelain[1]	Tablets. Take 500–750 mg 3 times daily, between meals.	Relieves swelling.
Cayenne[2]	Capsaicin cream. Apply daily over affected areas.	Causes temporary skin pain that counteracts tendinitis pain.
Devil's claw[3]	Enteric-coated capsules. Take 1,500–2,500 mg 3 times daily for up to 3 weeks.	Relieves pain.
Oligomeric proanthocyanidins (OPCs)	Grapeseed or pine-bark extract tablets. Take 50–100 mg 3 times daily.	Accelerates healing. Prevents further injury.
Turmeric	Curcumin. Take 200–400 mg 3 times daily, between meals.	Relieves inflammation. Prevents breakdown of collagen.

Precautions for the use of herbs:

[1]People who are allergic to pineapple may develop a rash from bromelain. If itching develops, stop using it.

[2]Do not apply cayenne to broken skin. Avoid contact with eyes or mouth.

[3]Devil's claw can slow heartbeat. Do not use this herb if you have congestive heart failure.

let the shoulder return to normal warmth over the next fifteen minutes. Continue this cycle for several hours, but be careful not to freeze the skin. Rest the shoulder for the next two days. After the rest period, gradually begin to strengthen the shoulder muscles. Light weight lifting, with an emphasis on a full range of motion, is recommended.

❑ See a doctor if you have severe pain, loss of mobility, or pain that persists for more than two weeks.

Considerations

❑ If over-the-counter (OTC) medications don't work, you may be prescribed a corticosteroid injection, or even surgery.

❑ Transcutaneous electrical nerve stimulation (TENS) is an effective drug-free method of pain control in sports injuries. It involves the use of electricity to stimulate muscle contractions. Home TENS units are available.

❑ Medical-grade dimethyl sulfoxide (DMSO) may reduce pain and accelerate healing. Do not use commercial-grade DMSO, since it may contain impurities that are quickly transported through the skin to the bloodstream. The use of DMSO may produce a taste and odor similar to a combination of garlic and turpentine. This is temporary and is not a cause for concern.

❑ Both acupuncture and shiatsu (also called tui nei), in which acupuncture points are manipulated by finger pressure, may be good for relief of pain. (See ACUPUNCTURE in Part Three.)

❑ In one study, postal workers in Canada who had rotator cuff tendinitis for at least six weeks were given either naturopathic care—consisting of dietary counseling, acupuncture, and Phlogenzym (which is made of bromelain, trypsin, and rutin)—or just physical exercise. Those people in the naturopathic group had less shoulder pain and were less disabled compared to the other group.

❑ It can sometimes be difficult to differentiate between tendinitis and bursitis. Tendinitis typically causes sharp pain on movement, whereas bursitis causes a dull, persistent ache that increases with movement. Both tendinitis and bursitis can cause swelling, but swelling is more prominent in bursitis. (See BURSITIS.)

TINNITUS (RINGING IN THE EARS)

Tinnitus is the sensation of sound in the absence of actual sound. The sounds that may be heard include tinkling, ringing, buzzing, hissing, and roaring noises. These noises may come and go, or they may be persistent. There may also be hearing loss.

Tinnitus may be caused by a loud noise, earwax blockage, ear bone changes, stress or depression, or head or neck injuries. Tinnitus is marked by damage to the inner ear, a fluid-filled structure that contains thousands of hairlike cells known as cilia. These delicate "hairs" help translate sound impulses from the outside into nerve impulses that are sent on to the brain, and are easily damaged by loud noise. Once the cilia are destroyed, they cannot be replaced.

It is necessary to have tinnitus medically evaluated to ensure that the right problem is being treated. If no underlying disorder is found, using herbal remedies over a period of three to four weeks can treat the condition. It is essential, however, to start therapy in the first six to eight weeks after the condition is first noticed, or herbal treatment is not likely to be effective.

Herbs to Avoid

❑ People who have tinnitus should avoid uva ursi, viburnum, white willow, and wintergreen oil. (For more information regarding these herbs, see UVA URSI, WILLOW BARK, and WINTERGREEN under The Herbs in Part One.)

Tinnitus: Beneficial Herbs

Herb	Form and Dosage	Comments
Cordyceps[1]	Extract. Take 25 mg tablets 4 times daily.	Reduces tinnitus caused by fluid accumulation.
Ginkgo[2]	Ginkgolide tablets. Take 240 mg daily in a single dose.	Prevents free-radical damage.

Precautions for the use of herbs:

[1]Do not take cordyceps if you have an estrogen-sensitive disorder, such as breast cancer, endometriosis, or fibroids. Do not take this herb if you have a testosterone-sensitive disorder, such as benign prostate enlargement or prostate cancer.

[2]Do not take ginkgo if you have a bleeding disorder, or are scheduled for surgery or a dental procedure. Avoid ginkgo if you are taking any type of blood-thinning medication.

Tinnitus: Formulas

Formula	Comments
Gentiana Longdancao Decoction to Drain the Liver[1]	A traditional Chinese herbal formula used to treat ringing in the ears or hearing loss accompanied by blurred vision, body aches, dizziness, headache, insomnia, irritability, palpitations, or sensation of heat in the head.
Six-Ingredient Pill with Rehmannia[2]	A traditional Chinese herbal formula used to treat ringing in the ears accompanied by deafness and dizziness, and/or body aches, dry mouth and throat, low-grade fever, and spontaneous sweating.

Precautions for the use of formulas:

[1]Do not use Gentiana Longdancao Decoction to Drain the Liver if you are trying to become pregnant.

[2]Do not use Six-Ingredient Pill with Rehmannia if you have an estrogen-sensitive disorder, such as breast cancer, endometriosis, or fibrocystic breast disease.

Recommendations

❑ Avoid all sources of caffeine, which has been known to be related to tinnitus in some people. This includes chocolate, coffee, colas, and tea.

❑ Salicylates can also cause tinnitus in susceptible individuals. Avoid aspirin in large doses (more than 12 a day) and limit foods that contain salicylates for a month, and see if that helps. Such foods include almonds, apples, apricots, berries, cherries, cucumbers, grapes, nectarines, oranges, peaches, pickles, plums, prunes, raisins, tomatoes, and many kinds of wine. If the tinnitus improves, eliminate these items from the menu completely.

❑ Never listen to loud music through headphones. If someone standing next to you can hear the music in your headphones, it is too loud. When not wearing headphones, keep music volume low enough so that you can hear the telephone or other sounds over the music.

❑ Always wear ear protection when you know you will be exposed to loud noise, especially percussive noise, such as the firing of a gun.

Considerations

❑ Several types of devices, all of which can be worn in or behind the ear, are available to block out tinnitus. Hearing aids can allow the individual to hear sounds from the environment that may compete with the tinnitus. Specialized maskers produce low-level sounds that can reduce or eliminate the perception of tinnitus. Tinnitus retraining therapy (TRT) uses devices that generate white noise—the sort of noise heard between stations on a radio—to help a person learn to ignore or adjust to tinnitus sounds.

❑ Sometimes drugs are prescribed to help reduce the severity of symptoms or complications. These include tricyclic antidepressants such as amitriptyline (Elavil) or alprazolam (Xanax).

❑ In one study, pine bark (pycnogenol) in doses of 100 or 150 milligrams per day resulted in improved systolic and diastolic blood flow velocities. Blood flow to the ears is impaired in tinnitus and these results suggest that pine bark may be an effective way to relieve symptoms in a short period of time.

❑ *See also* MÉNIÈRE'S DISEASE.

TOOTHACHE

Toothache is usually the result of advanced tooth decay. The abscess that causes a toothache begins as a cavity or chip in the hard enamel that covers a tooth. Such openings allow bacteria to infect the center of the tooth, the pulp. As dead tissue, live and dead bacteria, and white blood cells accumulate as pus, the pulp swells. The swelling of the

Toothache: Beneficial Herbs

Herb	Form and Dosage	Comments
Clove[1]	Oil. Apply 2–3 drops to tooth with a cotton swab.	Relieves toothache pain.
Kava kava[2]	Kavapyrone tablets. Take 60–120 mg daily.	Relieves radiating pain. Useful for nighttime toothache pain.
Thyme	Oil. Use as directed on the label.	Natural antiseptic; reduces level of bacteria in the mouth.
Willow bark	Capsules. Take 20–40 mg 3 times daily.	Aspirinlike pain relief without stomach upset or increased risk of bleeding.
Wintergreen	Mouthwash. Use as directed on the label.	Contains concentrated methyl salicylate, an aspirin-like pain reliever.

Precautions for the use of herbs:

[1] Do not swallow oil of cloves.

[2] Kava kava increases the effects of alcohol and psychoactive drugs such as sedatives and tranquilizers. Avoid this herb if you are pregnant or nursing.

pulp against the remaining enamel causes pain. If the root of the tooth dies, the toothache may stop, but the infection remains active and continues to spread and destroy tissue. It may even spread into the bones that support the tooth, causing the tooth to loosen and fall out.

Most tooth decay is caused by inadequate dental hygiene, although tooth decay does run in families and is worsened by diseases that cause dry mouth. It generally takes months or years of decay before a tooth starts to ache.

Saving an infected tooth requires professional dental care. Herbal treatments can be used to reduce pain without the side effects of aspirin or other pain relievers.

Recommendations

❏ To ease pain of toothache or abscess, rinse the affected area with warm salt water, made by stirring ½ teaspoon of salt into 1 cup of warm water.

❏ To treat teething pain in toddlers, blend 1 drop of oil of cloves—no more—in 1 teaspoon of safflower oil. With a fingertip or a cotton swab, massage the mixture onto the child's sore gums.

❏ Do not place aspirin directly over a tooth or the gums. This increases irritation of the tissues and can result in mouth ulcers.

❏ Eat plenty of raw fruits and vegetables, which contain minerals that keep the saliva from becoming too acidic.

❏ Avoid carbonated soft drinks, which may break down calcium in tooth enamel.

❏ Avoid chewable vitamin C tablets, which can erode tooth enamel. Coated vitamin C tablets that are designed to be swallowed do not cause this problem.

❏ Practice oral hygiene after every meal and snack. If you can't brush, just rinse your mouth out with water. Floss at least once daily. This is the only way to remove cavity-causing plaque.

❏ See your dentist for cleanings every six months. People with heartburn or who are taking certain cancer treatments that reduce saliva may have to see the dentist for routine care every three months or even more often than that. You should have a regularly scheduled dental checkup at least once yearly.

❏ Before having root canal work, be sure to inform your dentist if you have ever had a herpes infection. Disturbing the trigeminal nerve in the cheek can reactivate the infection. (*See* HERPESVIRUS INFECTION.)

❏ Call a physician if you have pain upon opening the mouth wide, fever, earache, or loss of hearing, or if the pain is a throbbing pain or if it lasts more than two days. Tooth pain may also result from ear infections, injury to the jaw or mouth, sinusitis, or heart attack. Tooth pain caused by a heart attack usually occurs with neck pain and/or pain that radiates to the shoulder or arm.

❏ Do not smoke.

Considerations

❏ If routine dental work is painful, it is a good idea to see the dentist more often. The routine dental procedures most likely to be painful are probing and scaling for about 25 percent of people who undergo them. These procedures are more likely to be needed when plaque is allowed to accumulate. Pain after scaling and probing usually subsides in two to eight hours. If you have tooth pain the day after a routine cleaning, call your dentist.

❏ A recent clinical study showed that root canal work done with a pulsed laser was significantly less painful one week to three months after the procedure compared with root canal performed with a drill.

❏ To prevent toothache, prevent tooth decay. In particular, it is important to avoid sticky-textured sweets that cling to the surfaces of teeth. Snacking without brushing afterward also promotes tooth decay.

❏ *See also* DRY MOUTH and PERIODONTAL DISEASE.

TRICHOMONIASIS

See under PARASITIC INFECTION.

TUBERCULOSIS

Tuberculosis (TB) is a chronic disease caused by the bacterium *Mycobacterium tuberculosis.* The World Health Organization estimates that one-third of the world's population is currently infected with TB. Rates of tuberculosis have been falling in the United States, but the disease continues to disproportionately affect racial and ethnic minorities, those who are foreign-born, and people infected with HIV.

TB is passed when bacteria are released during coughing, sneezing, and speech. Symptoms include chronic cough with blood in the sputum, fatigue, fever, night sweats, weight loss, and general malaise. In some people, the disease becomes inactive. In others, it takes an active form and can cause severe lung damage. TB also can start tissue damage in the bones, brain, liver, kidneys, and heart.

TB bacteria are first met and engulfed by immune-system cells called macrophages. The bacteria can survive this process, but as long as they are confined to the macrophages, no symptoms occur. Once the macrophage dies and the bacterium escapes, though, the rest of the immune system sends out huge numbers of fresh immune-system cells to destroy the TB. In the process nearby healthy tissues are also destroyed.

Combination antibiotics are needed to control TB. Herbal treatments can help TB, by diluting the side effects of standard treatment. Always consult a physician before taking any herbal treatment for TB.

Herbs to Avoid

❏ People who have TB infection should avoid the following immune-stimulant herbs: American ginseng, ginseng, ligustrum, psoralea, saw palmetto, and Solomon's seal. (For more information regarding these herbs, *see* the individual entries *under* The Herbs in Part One.)

Recommendations

❏ Continue taking all prescribed medications even if you feel well. Medical treatment is essential to avoid spreading TB to family members and friends. (Members of your household may have to take medication even if they test negative for the disease.) Continued treatment is also necessary to avoid drug resistance (*see under* Considerations, page 477).

❏ To ensure adequate supplies of vitamin D, which suppresses the growth of TB bacteria in cell line studies, take 400 to at most 1,000 milligrams of vitamin D supplements daily.

❏ Limit iron-rich foods and only use iron in supplements if prescribed by your doctor to treat anemia. Stored iron may increase the rate at which TB bacteria multiply. Excessive dietary fat may aggravate TB.

❏ Avoid foods containing the amino acid arginine, which accelerate the growth of TB bacteria in cell line studies. Foods that contain arginine include chocolate, almonds, peanuts, and most other nuts.

❏ Avoid stress. (*See* STRESS.)

❏ Get adequate rest and fresh air, preferably in a dry climate.

Tuberculosis: Beneficial Herbs

Herb	Form and Dosage	Comments
Bletilla	Use under professional supervision.	Reduces sputum production, coughing, and spitting and coughing of blood.
Cardamom or fennel seed[1]	Tincture. Take 10 drops in ¼ cup water 3 times daily. Tea bags. Take 1 cup 3 times daily.	Increases effectiveness of streptomycin against TB.
Coptis[2]	Capsules. Take no more than 250 mg daily for 3 months.	Reduces coughing and spitting of blood; mildly antibacterial.
Lentinan	Injection or powder. Use under professional supervision.	Acts against drug-resistant TB. Reduces likelihood of spreading disease to others.
Siberian ginseng[3]	*Eleuterococcus senticosus* tincture. Take as directed on label.	Suppresses multiplication of TB bacteria.

Precautions for the use of herbs:

[1]Do not use fennel seed if you have an estrogen-sensitive disorder, such as breast cancer, endometriosis, or fibrocystic breast disease.

[2]Do not take coptis for longer than two weeks at a time. Do not use it if you are pregnant or have gallbladder disease. Do not take this herb with supplemental vitamin B$_6$ or with protein supplements containing the amino acid histidine.

[3]Do not take Siberian ginseng if you have prostate cancer or an autoimmune disease, such as lupus or rheumatoid arthritis.

Tuberculosis: Formulas

Formula	Comments
Minor Bupleurum Decoction plus Tonify the Middle and Augment the Chi Decoction	Two traditional Chinese herbal formulas that when combined enable people to take multiple forms of chemotherapy simultaneously. Especially helpful for people who also have either HIV or hepatitis B.
Ophiopogonis Decoction[1]	A traditional Chinese herbal formula traditionally used for coughing and spitting of saliva, dry and uncomfortable sensation in the throat, dry mouth, red tongue, shortness of breath, and wheezing.

Precautions for the use of formulas:

[1]Do not take Ophiopogonis Decoction if you have a fever.

Considerations

❑ TB is usually treated with a number of antibiotics at once. In a small number of people—especially in those who start, but do not finish, a course of treatment—the germ could become resistant to antibiotics. Recently new drugs have been developed, so now there are several choices, including isoniazid (Tubizid), rifampin (Rifadin), ethambutol (Myambutol), and pyrazinamide.

❑ People who have TB should not use cortisone preparations unless prescribed by a physician. Cortisone suppresses immune function and makes the infection more difficult to treat.

❑ Wasting is often present with TB. In one study, patients who took a nutritional supplement rich in calories and protein in addition to meals showed an increase in body weight and muscle mass compared to a group of patients with TB who did not take the supplements. These patients were also stronger with the supplements according to a test of grip strength. If you are losing weight and feel weak, it is useful to find supplements that taste good and that you can use on a regular basis.

❑ In another study, people with TB who used multivitamins had greater weight gain than those who did not. Those who just took a zinc supplement derived no benefit from it. It is fine to include zinc in your multivitamin, however.

❑ *See also* COUGH and HIV/AIDS.

VAGINOSIS

Bacterial vaginosis, previously known as nonspecific vaginitis, is an infection that can develop when the *Gardnerella* bacteria that normally live in the vagina grow unchecked. Ordinarily, this kind of bacteria has to compete with beneficial bacteria such as *Lactobacillus*. When the population of beneficial bacteria diminishes, *Gardnerella* are free to overrun the vagina. No one knows for sure why this overgrowth occurs; yet the main causes are having multiple sex partners or a new sex partner, and douching. Other possible causes of this overgrowth include intrauterine device (IUD) use, being African-American, and a natural lack of *Lactobacillus* bacteria. An antibiotic called metronidazole (Flagyl) is the standard treatment.

Gardnerella overgrowth can cause a thin vaginal discharge or, sometimes, a fishy smell. Other symptoms of vaginosis include a burning sensation, itching, irritation, and redness. A Pap smear will show large numbers of "clue" cells, which have a fuzzy appearance under the microscope due to the large numbers of bacteria attached to them. It is important to treat vaginosis to prevent the bacteria from getting into the uterus or fallopian tubes. It is important to treat vaginosis to avoid pelvic inflammatory disease (PID) after hysterectomy. In pregnant women, vaginosis can lead to low infant birth weight or premature delivery. Particularly during pregnancy, acute, severe symptoms require medical attention. Herbs as preventative therapies, however, are appropriate for long-term care.

Recommendations

❑ Barberry, coptis, goldenseal, or Oregon grape root can be used in a douche. Place 1 tablespoon (10 milliliters) of tincture in 1 cup of warm water. Use as a douche once or twice daily. (*See* DOUCHES in Part Three.) Sometimes douching leads to an overgrowth of anaerobic bacteria that can cause vaginosis. Speak to your doctor before douching with these herbs.

❑ Restore helpful *Lactobacillus* bacteria by taking one or two capsules of acidophilus after meals, unless the label directs otherwise. Additionally, you can place liquid acidophilus culture directly in the vagina with a rubber bulb syringe, or place a capsule in the vagina. Be sure to check the expiration date on any acidophilus product to make sure that you are using live bacteria. If *Lactobacillus* is not readily available, eat at least one serving of yogurt daily. *Lactobacillus* capsules are available for intravaginal use. In one study, the Nugent scoring system was used to assess improvement in symptoms in more than 400 women who used capsules, and the women felt that their symptoms were relieved.

❑ Avoid sugar, fruit, and foods made with yeast, including alcohol, aged cheeses, dried fruit, fermented foods,

Vaginosis: Beneficial Herbs

Herb	Form and Dosage	Comments
Aloe vera	Gel. Apply to the vagina or add to warm water to use as a douche. (*See* DOUCHES in Part Three.)	Helpful for infections and itching.
Barberry[1] or coptis[1] or Oregon grape root[1]	Cream. Apply to vagina; and/or tincture. Take 20 drops in ¼ cup water 3 times daily.	Activates immune system. Useful if there is blood in the urine. (*See* under Recommendations, page 477.)
Calendula	Cream. Apply to vagina.	An antibacterial and anti-inflammatory.
Garlic[2]	Raw garlic. Eat 1–2 cloves with food daily.	Antibacterial; also fights yeast infections.
Goldenseal[3]	Suppositories. Use as directed on the label; or extract. Add to warm water and use as a douche. (*See* DOUCHES in Part Three.)	Useful for all types of infections.
Pau d'arco	Capsules. Take as directed on the label; or tea. Prepare and use as directed on the label. Or as an extract, add to warm water to make a douche. (*See* DOUCHES in Part Three.)	Contains natural antibiotic agents; has a healing effect.
Sangre de drago	Tincture. Place 1½ tbsp (15–20 ml) of tincture in 1 cup warm water. Use as a douche 1–2 times daily. (*See* DOUCHES in Part Three.)	Keeps bacteria from "rooting" in lining of the vagina.
Tea tree[4]	Oil. Place 1½ tbsp (15–20 ml) of oil in 1 cup warm water. Use as a douche 1–2 times daily. (*See* DOUCHES in Part Three.)	Kills *Gardnerella* and other microbes that cause vaginal irritation.

Precautions for the use of herbs:

[1]Do not use barberry, coptis, or Oregon grape root if you are pregnant or have gallbladder disease. Do not take these herbs with supplemental vitamin B6 or with protein supplements containing the amino acid histidine. Do not take coptis for longer than two weeks at a time. Do not take Oregon grape root for longer than two weeks at a time.

[2]Garlic counteracts the effects of *Bifidus* and *Lactobacillus* cultures taken as digestive aids. Consult a doctor before using garlic on a regular basis if you are on an anticoagulant drug such as warfarin (Coumadin). Discuss the use of garlic with your doctor before having any type of surgery. Raw garlic can cause heartburn and flatulence.

[3]Do not take goldenseal internally on a daily basis for more than one week at a time. Do not use it during pregnancy or if you are breastfeeding, and use with caution if you are allergic to ragweed. If you have a history of cardiovascular disease, gallbladder disease, diabetes, or glaucoma, use it only under a doctor's supervision.

[4]People who are allergic to celery or thyme should not use tea tree oil products. Do not take tea tree oil internally.

soy sauce, and vinegar. Also, you may get benefit from avoiding grains containing gluten, such as barley, oats, rye, and wheat.

❏ Avoid organ meats and iron supplements, unless prescribed by your doctor. Iron is essential for *Gardnerella* to grow and multiply.

❏ Avoid tight clothing, and wear white cotton underwear, which absorbs moisture and allows air circulation. Change into dry clothing as soon as possible after swimming.

Considerations

❏ The standard medical treatment for vaginosis is metronidazole (Flagyl). The problem is that Flagyl is not free of side effects. Women who drink alcohol while taking this drug can develop nausea and vomiting. Even the tiny amount of alcohol in a spoon of cough syrup is enough to cause vomiting. Simply avoid alcohol while using this treatment.

❏ If you take the prescription blood-thinner warfarin (Coumadin), you should consult with your doctor before using over-the-counter (OTC) vaginal miconazole products. Miconazole (Monistat) is an antifungal drug found in some creams and suppositories. Bleeding or bruising may occur if warfarin and vaginal miconazole are used together.

❏ Calendula with vitamin A is available as a vaginal suppository. Do not use this until you speak to your doctor.

❏ *See also* BLADDER INFECTION (CYSTITIS), PELVIC INFLAMMATORY DISEASE, and YEAST INFECTION (YEAST VAGINITIS).

VARICOSE VEINS

Varicose veins are swollen, twisted, blue veins close to the surface of the skin. Although varicose veins can occur in people of both sexes and of all ages, they most frequently occur in women thirty to fifty years old.

All leg veins contain one-way flap valves that help blood travel upward on its return to the heart. When one or more of these valves "leaks," some blood is able to flow back down in the wrong direction. This blood overfills and dilates branches of veins underlying the skin. Tiny capillaries also become overfilled, producing multiple spider veins and purple discoloration. Varicose veins are seen most often on the back of the calf or on the inside of the leg between the ankle and the groin. The farther away the vein is from the heart, the harder the heart has to work to overcome the force of gravity, and the more likely the vein is to become varicose.

The valve weakness that causes varicose veins may be inherited, but more often it is the result of physical stress on the veins. Usually that stress is a combination of standing or sitting in one place, obesity, and/or pregnancy. Also, lack of exercise and habitually sitting in a cross-legged position may be contributing factors. Usually varicose veins are primarily a cosmetic problem, although they can throb, swell, and feel heavy. When veins fail to supply tissues with needed oxygen, however, there can be a chronic itch, and even eczema and leg sores. The leg muscles become easily fatigued since they are poorly supplied with oxygen, and muscle spasms and cramping may result. Restlessness in the legs may also occur. Wounded varicose veins are slow to heal.

Conventional treatment for varicose veins consists of injections or surgery (*see under* Considerations). Herbal treatments are among the effective nonsurgical therapies, usually producing noticeable results in three to six months.

Herbs to Avoid

❏ People who have varicose veins should not apply arnica, balsam of Peru, black mustard, camphor, capsaicin, chaparral, comfrey, tolu balsam, or white mustard to the skin over the affected veins. (For more information regarding these herbs, *see* the individual entries *under* The Herbs in Part One.)

Recommendations

❏ Try to avoid becoming constipated, as this may contribute to varicose veins. (*See* CONSTIPATION.)

❏ Maintain a healthy weight. If you are overweight, *see* OVERWEIGHT.

❏ Take regular walks. Walking improves leg and vein strength. Additionally, exercise your legs. From a seated position, rotate your feet at the ankles, turning them first clockwise, then counterclockwise, in a circular motion. Next, extend your legs forward and point your toes to the ceiling, then to the floor. Then lift your feet off the floor and gently bend your legs back and forth at the knees.

❏ Elevate your legs while you are resting.

❏ Stop and take short walks every hour during long car rides.

❏ Get up and move every thirty minutes to an hour when you are in a situation where you are seated for long periods of time and when you are traveling by air. Reserve an aisle seat for such situations.

❏ Avoid standing or sitting for prolonged periods. If your job or activity requires standing, shift your weight from one leg to the other every few minutes.

Varicose Veins: Beneficial Herbs

Herb	Form and Dosage	Comments
Bromelain[1]	Tablets. Take as directed on the label.	Reduces risk of blood-clot formation.
Butcher's broom	Ruscogenin tablets. Take 100 mg once daily.	Particularly effective for burning and itching.
Cayenne	Cream or capsules. Apply to affected area or take as directed on the label.	Relieves pain and inflammation; expands blood vessels, reducing stress on the capillaries.
Gotu kola[2]	Liposome tablets or capsules. Take 60–120 mg daily.	Stabilizes tissues supporting veins; increases oxygen transport. Must be used continuously for 3–4 weeks before results are seen.
Hawthorn	Solid capsules. Take 150–250 mg 3 times daily.	Strengthens fragile veins; increases tone of muscles supporting veins.
Horse chestnut[3]	Aescin tablets. Take up to 150 mg daily.	Relieves swelling and inflammation. Makes blood vessels more elastic (*see under* Considerations).
Oligomeric proanthocyanidins (OPCs)	Grapeseed or pine-bark extract tablets. Take 100 mg daily.	Improves blood-vessel strength and flexibility.
White oak bark	Tea. Prepare as directed on the label and use to bathe the affected area 3 times daily. Also use the tea to make compresses. (*See* COMPRESSES in Part Three.)	Helps stimulate blood flow.
Witch hazel[4]	Tincture. Take ½–1 tsp (2–4 ml) in ¼ cup water 3 times daily.	Increases tone of veins and "shrinks" varicose veins.

Precautions for the use of herbs:

[1]People who are allergic to pineapple may develop a rash from bromelain. If itching develops, stop using it.

[2]Do not take gotu kola if you are trying to become pregnant.

[3]Do not take horse chestnut internally if you are trying to become pregnant.

[4]Witch hazel tincture is the only effective form of witch hazel for varicose veins.

❑ Avoid wearing clothing or undergarments that are tight or that constrict your waist, groin, or legs.

❑ Do not smoke. Smoking just two cigarettes releases enough toxic substances to begin destroying cells in the linings of veins.

❑ If varicose veins become swollen, red, tender, or warm to the touch, or if they are accompanied by a rash or sores on the leg or near the ankle, or if they cause circulation problems in the feet, see your doctor. And be aware that chest pain after surgical procedures for varicose veins, including sclerotherapy, is a medical emergency. However, this is rare, as the procedure does not require anesthesia.

Considerations

❑ The supplement Varicosin from PhytoPharmica, which combines butcher's broom, gotu kola, and horse chestnut extract, may be substituted for any of its individual herbs.

❑ Being at a normal weight is a good way to reduce the risk of varicose veins. In an Italian study of 104 women, those who were obese according to their body mass index (BMI) had a sixfold increased likelihood of getting varicose veins.

❑ Surgical treatment for varicose veins may be necessary when there is tissue damage. Veins are "stripped" by cutting above and below the affected vein and then pulling the vein out with a wire. There is also a procedure known as sclerotherapy, in which the vein is injected with a solution that fuses the walls together, blocking the vein. Once the vein is blocked, of course, circulation is disrupted, and the procedure itself causes bruises that may take as long as six weeks to heal. Laser surgeries are done to close off smaller varicose veins and spider veins. No incisions or needles are needed.

❑ Support hose (compression stockings) are preferable to half-leg stockings, which do not exert as much pressure along the entire length of the leg. Wearing compression stockings could reduce the size of varicose veins approximately 20 percent over three months of daily use. The disadvantages of compression stockings are that they are expensive, hard to put on, and uncomfortable to wear. One clinical study has found that compression stockings are about as equally effective in controlling varicose veins as the regular use of horse chestnut extract. In another study, patients experienced less leg pain and less swelling using horse chestnut. Using compression stockings may be necessary when the doctor has diagnosed a more serious condition called chronic venous insufficiency, a condition that can cause blood clots and tissue damage.

❑ Varicose veins in men are a risk factor for both heart disease and intermittent claudication, a condition in which leg circulation becomes impaired. For more information, see HEART ATTACK (MYOCARDIAL INFARCTION) and INTERMITTENT CLAUDICATION.

❑ Hemorrhoids are inflamed veins that occur in the anus. (See HEMORRHOIDS.)

VISION, BLURRED

See under EYE PROBLEMS.

VITILIGO

Vitiligo, also known as leukoderma, is a skin disorder in which patches of skin lose their pigmentation. Usually, fading skin color begins around the orifices, especially the mouth, nostrils, and ears, and spreads to progressively wider areas. Vitiligo also may start on the wrists, fingers, or toes. It can cause premature graying or whitening of the hair, eyelashes, eyebrows, or beard. People with dark skin may notice a loss of color inside their mouths.

There is little or no inflammation or irritation, but affected skin is more subject to sunburn or melanoma. The change in appearance caused by vitiligo affects emotional and psychological well-being, and is especially difficult for children and adolescents.

The current understanding of vitiligo is that there is a literal bleaching of the skin by naturally produced hydrogen peroxide. The overproduction of hydrogen peroxide, in turn, is due to an overproduction of monoamine oxidase in the skin, the same chemical that is associated with depression in the brain. This mind-body connection explains why vitiligo frequently begins after a period of emotional stress. Stress to the immune system also can precipitate vitiligo outbreaks; people can develop antibodies that destroy melanocytes (pigment-producing skin cells). Some people have reported that a single event, such as sunburn or an emotional shock, triggered the condition. Other rare causes include Addison's disease, pernicious anemia, alopecia areata, and autoimmune problems. Heredity also plays a role in this condition.

Treatment for vitiligo takes a long time—usually six to eighteen months. Each person responds differently to treatment, and no single medicine or herbal treatment works the same for everyone. Although vitiligo makes the skin more sensitive to sunburn, some drug and herbal treatments for vitiligo (except cortisone and herbal creams) require exposing affected skin to ultraviolet (UV) light for short periods under a doctor's supervision.

Unless otherwise specified, the herb dosages recommended here are for adults. Children under age six should be given one-quarter of the adult dosage. Children between the ages of six and twelve should be given one-half of the adult dosage. Formula dosages for children should be discussed with a knowledgeable health-care practitioner.

Recommendations

❑ If you are using certain drugs, such as topical corticosteroids, your doctor may recommend that you get fifteen to twenty minutes of exposure to UV lamplight daily. Take 1,000 milligrams for children to 3,000 milligrams for adults of L-phenylalanine. The combination of UV light and L-phenylalanine may help correct vitiligo in children. In studies with adults, L-phenylalanine supplementation alone has shown more modest results, but the use of both supplements and UV light may provide better results.

❑ Try using the face cream GH-3 (Gerovital), available at some health food stores and online; it sometimes reverses depigmentation. It should be used by adults only.

Considerations

❑ Makeup, stains, and self-tanning lotions are available to camouflage depigmented skin. Brands of cosmetics for vitiligo include Chromelin, Clinique, Dermablend, Fashion Fair, Lydia O'Leary, and Vitadye. These products are available at cosmetic counters or from Beautipharm Biocosmetics. (*See* Appendix B: Resources.)

❑ Depigmentation therapy involves fading the rest of the skin on the body to match the already white areas. The drug monobenzylether of hydroquinone (Benoquin) is applied twice a day to healthy skin until it matches vitiligo-affected areas. Since the drug can be transferred to other people, people using Benoquin must avoid skin-to-skin contact with others for at least two hours after applying the drug.

❑ Surgical treatments are available, including autologous skin grafts where your own skin is removed and put on the affected area of the skin. In addition, other procedures may be tried, such as blister grafting and tattooing, using a special surgical instrument.

❑ People with vitiligo must check moles carefully for signs of melanoma. (*See* Melanoma *under* SKIN CANCER.)

❑ Tinea versicolor is a skin infection similar to ringworm that produces blotchy white patches. (*See* RINGWORM.)

❑ The National Vitiligo Foundation can provide further information about vitiligo and refer people to local chapters that have support groups for patients, families, and physicians. (*See* Appendix B: Resources.)

VOMITING

Vomiting is the ejection of stomach contents up through the esophagus and out of the body. It is a defense mechanism that protects the body against harmful substances. Vomiting is usually accompanied by nausea.

Common causes of vomiting are alcohol intoxication, bulimia, chemotherapy, food allergies, food poisoning, medications, migraine headaches, morning sickness during

Vitiligo: Beneficial Herbs

Herb	Form and Dosage	Comments
Dong quai	*Angelica sinensis* capsules. Take 500–1,000 mg per day. Use when depigmentation first occurs.	Inhibits the formation of skin-attacking antibodies.
Khella[1]	Khellin tablets. Take 120–160 mg daily.	Stimulates repigmentation by increasing sensitivity of remaining melanocytes to sunlight.
Licorice	Simicort cream. Alternate with prescribed cortisone cream for vitiligo in children.	Extends the active period of prescribed cortisone creams.
Picrorrhiza	Use as directed on the label.	An Indian herb that has been shown to reduce the number and size of unpigmented skin patches.
Psoralea	Capsules. Take as directed on the label.	Restores immune balance to skin, slowly correcting vitiligo.
St. John's wort	Cream. Apply to affected area for 3–4 months.	Increases tanning response of vitiligo-affected skin to sunlight. Also reduces stress and anxiety.

Precautions for the use of herbs:

[1]Do not take khella if you are taking blood-thinning medication.

Vitiligo: Formulas

Formula	Comments
Astragalus Decoction to Construct the Middle	A traditional Chinese herbal formula that is gentle enough for use in treating children's vitiligo.
Shih Qua Da Bu Tang	A traditional Chinese herbal formula traditionally used to treat loss of skin color. This formula has been shown in several clinical studies to balance and enhance immune function.

pregnancy, seasickness or motion sickness, viral infections, and chemical poisoning. Usually the best course of action for vomiting is to correct its underlying cause. However, when vomiting is the only or primary symptom, herbal treatments may be helpful. Vomiting that occurs with pain and tenderness in the lower right abdomen can be a sign of appendicitis. In that case, seek immediate medical attention.

Unless otherwise specified, the herb dosages recommended here are for adults. Children under age six should be given one-quarter of the adult dosage. Children between the ages of six and twelve should be given one-half of the adult dosage. Formula dosages for children should be discussed with a knowledgeable health-care practitioner. Vomiting of blood always requires medical treatment.

Recommendations

❏ Take acorus to control vomiting during drug withdrawal. This herb should be used under professional supervision only.

❏ Replace fluids lost by vomiting. Whatever the cause, it is important to take in as much fluid as possible without upsetting the stomach any further. Sip clear fluids such as water, ginger ale, fruit juices, or Gatorade. Do not drink much at any one time, and slowly work back to a normal diet.

❏ Call a doctor if any of the following conditions exist: inability to retain any fluids for twelve hours or more for adults, or eight hours or more for children; headache and stiff neck; signs of dehydration (*see under* Considerations, below); bleeding (bloody or black vomit); or lethargy or marked irritability in a young child.

Considerations

❏ Dehydration is the biggest concern in most episodes of vomiting. Signs of dehydration are increased thirst, infrequent urination or dark-yellow urine, dry mouth, eyes that appear sunken, and skin that has lost its normal elasticity. The rate with which dehydration takes place depends on the size of the person, the frequency of the vomiting, and whether or not there is also diarrhea. Infants with frequent vomiting and diarrhea are at the greatest risk for dehydration, and need immediate medical attention.

❏ For ways to relieve vomiting related to specific conditions, *see* "Side Effects of Cancer Treatment" *under* CANCER; MORNING SICKNESS; and MOTION SICKNESS. *See also* ALLERGIES; HANGOVER; MIGRAINE; NAUSEA; and PARASITIC INFECTION.

WARTS

Warts are small, benign skin growths. Warts are contagious and may also spread from one part of the body to another. Warts are usually painless, and often disappear within one or two years. Some warts, however, persist for years or return even after surgical removal.

Vomiting: Beneficial Herbs

Herb	Form and Dosage	Comments
Codonopsis	Tincture. Use under professional supervision.	Treats vomiting with anorexia and diarrhea.
Fennel seed[1]	Tea bag, prepared with 1 cup water. Take 1 cup up to 3 times daily.	Stops vomiting with mild abdominal pain, indigestion, or acid regurgitation.
Ginger	Tea bag, prepared with 1 cup water. Take 1 cup up to 5 times daily.	Stops vomiting and nausea.
Scutellaria[2]	Tincture. Take 1–1½ tsp (4–6 ml) in ¼ cup water 3 times daily.	Helps control vomiting.

Precautions for the use of herbs:

[1]Do not take fennel seed if you have an estrogen-sensitive disorder, such as endometriosis, fibrocystic breasts, or fibroids.

[2]Do not take scutellaria if you have diarrhea.

Vomiting: Formulas

Formula	Comments
Five-Ingredient Powder with Poria	A traditional Chinese herbal formula used to control vomiting by reducing fluid in the digestive tract and stimulating urination. This formula is most useful when vomiting occurs immediately after drinking water or electrolyte drinks such as Gatorade.

Common warts can appear anywhere, but are usually found on the face (usually in groups), fingers, knees, elbows, forearms, scalp, and the skin around the nails. They are usually less than one-half inch (one centimeter) in diameter, round, and colored brown, gray, or yellow. Common warts can be spread if they are bitten, trimmed, picked, or touched. Shaving can spread warts on the face. Filiform warts are small, thin, long warts that appear on the eyelids, face, lips, or neck. You can get warts from others if you touch a towel or other object that someone with the virus has touched. Biting your nails if you have warts on your fingers can cause them to spread to other areas on your fingertips.

Genital warts occur singly or in clusters as bumpy, rough growths on and near the sex organs. Genital warts, like all warts, are caused by human papillomavirus (HPV), which is contagious and which increases risk of bladder and cervical cancer in women and penile and rectal cancer in men.

Plantar warts, found on the bottom of the feet, have a soft center surrounded by rough rings, and a rough, corrugated surface. They may contain little black dots, which are bits of coagulated blood. Because the entire weight of the body is placed on the feet every day, plantar warts often become inflamed and painful. Like genital warts, they are caused by HPV. Plantar **warts do not tend to** spread to other parts of the body.

Not technically a wart, skin tags, also called acrochordons, are small, soft, flesh-colored growths of excess tissue that hang from the skin. They usually occur in clusters on the armpits, eyelids, groin, neck, and other body folds. Skin tags stay the same size and color. Though harmless, they can be annoying, especially when they become irritated by clothing.

A number of conventional treatments are available for warts. Herbal treatments work more slowly, but are inexpensive and painless. For best results, use herbal treatments with the nutritional and other recommendations made here.

Recommendations

❏ Try vitamin E. Dr. Earl Mindell recommends treating warts with 400 international units (IU) of vitamin E orally each day and also applying a vitamin E cream.

❏ Avoid pork products. Pork intake is associated with the growth of warts and tumors caused by HPV, and abstinence from fried pork has brought about regression of genital warts.

❏ People who have genital warts should avoid alcohol. Consuming five or more drinks per week doubles the risk of genital warts.

❏ To remove common warts, try this remedy: Crush a garlic clove and apply the garlic directly on the wart, avoiding the surrounding skin. Cover it with a bandage and leave it in place for twenty-four hours. Blisters should then form, and the wart should fall off in about a week. Be certain, however, that it is a wart, and not some other type of growth.

Considerations

❏ Doctors use several methods to remove warts. They remove genital warts through surgery, freezing with liquid nitrogen, laser removal, and a procedure called curettage and electrodessication, or scraping away the skin and

Warts: Beneficial Herbs

Herb	Form and Dosage	Comments
Aloe vera[1]	Gel. Place a small dab on the wart 2 or 3 times daily until the wart is gone.	Aloe has antiviral and antibacterial properties.
Astragalus[2]	Capsules. Take as directed on the label.	Protects the immune system, which is important in warding off warts.
Black walnut	Extract. Use as directed on the label.	Has healing properties especially useful in treating mouth and throat warts.
Bloodroot	Bloodroot paste from Alpha Omega Labs. Apply as directed on the label and cover with a bandage.	Especially useful for skin tags; can be used for warts elsewhere except genitals.
Bromelain[3]	Tablets. Take 1,000–2,000 mg 3 times daily, between meals, until warts disappear.	Activates immune system, provides enzymes that dissolve warts.
Comfrey[4]	Allantoin cream. Apply as directed on the label and cover with a bandage.	Treats skin tags, plus common, flat, and filiform warts.

Precautions for the use of herbs:

[1]Do not take aloe vera internally if you have diarrhea. Aloe has laxative effects if taken in dosages larger than those recommended. Do not use if you are menstruating, have rectal bleeding, or are taking any kind of diuretic.

[2]Do not use astragalus if you have a fever or a skin infection.

[3]People who are allergic to pineapple may develop a rash from bromelain. If itching develops, stop using it.

[4]Comfrey is recommended for external use only. Do not use comfrey if you are pregnant. Avoid contact with unaffected skin; allantoin may cause skin irritation. Wash your hands after application. Be especially careful not to rub your eyes if there is any residue on your hands.

then destroying the warts with a heated electric needle. Doctors remove plantar warts with acid, liquid nitrogen, or curettage and desiccation. They remove skin tags with liquid nitrogen. Other treatments include immunotherapy with imiquimod (Aldara), bleomycin (Blenoxane) to kill the virus, and retinoids from vitamin A to disrupt the warts' skin cell growth.

❏ Condoms do not always prevent the spread of genital warts. They cannot prevent infection when the warts are on the scrotum or vulva.

❏ Women who have been diagnosed with genital warts should have a vaginal and cervical Pap smear every six months, as the warts are associated with an increased risk of cervical cancer.

❏ It is best to see a dermatologist to have skin tags removed. It takes only a few minutes in the doctor's office. It is also good to see a physician to remove any wart that seems irritated.

❏ *See also* CERVICAL CANCER.

WEIGHT PROBLEMS

See OVERWEIGHT.

WOUNDS

See BURNS; CUTS, SCRAPES, AND ABRASIONS.

WRINKLES

Wrinkles are visible creases in the skin. Wrinkles form as the skin loses its collagen, a protein that allows the skin to retain fluids that support a smooth, supple contour. As the collagen-filled elastic tissues underlying the skin are increasingly damaged, wrinkles deepen and become more prominent.

Although wrinkling is a normal part of aging, exposure to ultraviolet (UV) light and free radicals accelerates the process. Frequent exposure to sunshine results in premature skin wrinkling and increased pigmentation, called liver spots. Exposure to cigarette smoke means exposure to toxic free radicals that also contribute to wrinkling. In women, smoking exacerbates skin wrinkling that occurs after menopause, canceling out the anti-wrinkling effects of estrogen treatment. Other factors that can lead to premature wrinkling include poor diet and nutrition, poor muscle tone, habitual facial expressions, stress, excess sun exposure, and heredity.

Herbal treatments cannot stop the aging process, but they may slow it down. Herbal antioxidants in skin creams stop the free-radical processes that destroy collagen. Herbal sources of alpha-hydroxy acids could stimulate the production of hyaluronic acid, the body's natural agent for moisturizing and restoring suppleness to the skin. Together with stronger treatments such as tretinoin (Retin-A), these therapies may soften existing wrinkles and prevent new wrinkles from forming.

Recommendations

❏ Never intentionally expose your skin to midday sun. Between 9 A.M. and 3 P.M., always use sunscreen to avoid skin damage. However, to get adequate vitamin D, which is important to numerous bodily processes, take a multivitamin with vitamin D.

❏ Take 100 to 300 milligrams of coenzyme Q_{10} (Co-Q_{10}) daily. There is some scientific evidence that this supplement can act as an antioxidant and energizer that may slow many of the detrimental effects of sunlight exposure.

❏ Take 1,000 milligrams of chondroitin sulfate daily for premature wrinkling of the skin (wrinkles that appear before age thirty-five). In laboratory studies, chondroitin stimulates the growth of skin cells and accelerates metabolic processes that help the skin retain moisture.

Wrinkles: Beneficial Herbs

Herb	Form and Dosage	Comments
Acerola	Tablets with vitamin C USP. Take as directed on the label.	Contains mineral salts that complement alpha-hydroxy acids in rejuvenating skin.
Aloe	Gel containing 1–3 percent alpha-hydroxy acids. Apply daily for 8–16 weeks.	Most potent natural source of alpha-hydroxy acids.
Calendula	Cream. Apply as directed on the label.	Stimulates growth of skin cells. Soothes sun-damaged skin and protects it from infection.
Comfrey[1]	Allantoin cream. Apply as directed on the label.	Stops reddening and irritation of the skin around wrinkles.
Green tea	Cream. Apply daily as directed on the label.	Prevents free-radical damage to skin.
Witch hazel	Cream (glycine base). Apply as directed on the label.	Natural astringent that tones the skin.

Precautions for the use of herbs:

[1]Comfrey is recommended for external use only. Do not use comfrey if you are pregnant. Avoid contact with unaffected skin; allantoin may cause skin irritation. Wash your hands after application. Be especially careful not to rub your eyes if there is any residue on your hands.

❏ Drink eight glasses of water daily. Adequate hydration helps maintain skin tone.

❏ Use natural oils rather than harsh soaps and cold creams to remove dirt and makeup.

❏ Avoid alcohol-based toning solutions. These can dry and chap the skin.

❏ Get regular exercise, and treat high blood pressure and other circulatory disorders. Like other organs, the skin receives its nourishment through the bloodstream. Exercise increases circulation to the skin.

❏ Do not smoke. Smoking intensifies sunlight damage to the skin.

Considerations

❏ Moisturizers work by trapping moisture in the skin and building a protective barrier against toxins. Not all moisturizers, however, can prevent wrinkles. Only those containing sunscreens with a sun protection factor (SPF) of at least 15 help to prevent wrinkles. Some ingredients to look for in skin-care products are allantoin, alpha-hydroxy acids, aloe vera, arnica, burdock, calendula, chamomile, comfrey, cucumber, essential fatty acids, ginkgo, glycerine, ivy, liposomes, panthenol, retinoic acid, sage, witch hazel, and yarrow.

YEAST INFECTION (YEAST VAGINITIS)

The human body is normally host to a great variety of bacteria and fungi that play neutral or even helpful roles in normal bodily functions. A yeast infection occurs when one of these organisms, the yeast *Candida albicans,* grows out of control. The resulting overgrowth is known as candidiasis. *C. albicans* only becomes a problem when the "good" bacteria that normally keep it in check, such as *Lactobacillus acidophilus,* become weakened. Candida infection may take the form of athlete's foot and jock itch. Systemic candidiasis is an overgrowth of candida throughout the body. In the most severe cases, candida can travel throughout the body, causing a type of blood poisoning called candida septicemia. Candidiasis affects both women and men. It is rarely transmitted sexually. It is most common in babies (an infected mother may pass it on to her newborn) and people with compromised immune systems.

Because candidiasis can affect many areas of the body at once, it can cause a variety of disorders and symptoms. In the mouth, *C. albicans* can produce thrush, or white plaques in the mouth and throat. In women, it is one of the sources of vaginitis, which produces itching, burning, and a sticky white or yellow discharge. Yeast infections may develop in the urethra or sinuses. The growth of *C. albicans* is spurred by several factors. Broad-spectrum antibiotics can kill off the good bacteria that keep the yeast under control. Taking corticosteroid drugs has been linked to *C. albicans* overgrowth. *C. albicans* is more common with high blood sugar levels associated with diabetes. And yeast can overgrow if the immune system does not function as it should, especially in people with HIV infection or AIDS and other diseases that affect the immune system. *C. albicans* overgrowth is also associated with being sexually active and may occur in women who are using high-dose estrogen birth control pills or are pregnant.

Conventional medicine uses various antifungal agents (*see under* Considerations, below). Except for barberry and related herbs, which should not be used for more than two weeks at a time, it may be necessary to take herbs for as long as six months to control yeast overgrowth.

Recommendations

❏ Take *Lactobacillus* probiotic supplements daily. These friendly bacteria grow to form a protective lining over the digestive tract that keeps yeast colonies from forming. Be sure to check expiration dates on the package. For vaginal infections, place the probiotic capsules in the vagina before going to bed every other night for two weeks, if your physician recommends this.

❏ Take 1,000 to 2,000 milligrams of caprylic acid daily with meals. This naturally occurring fatty acid has been shown to have antifungal properties for the treatment of yeast infection in laboratory studies. Since caprylic acid is readily absorbed by the intestines, it is necessary to take a timed-release or enteric-coated form so that the supplement is released gradually throughout the entire digestive tract.

❏ Avoid refined sugar, honey, maple syrup, and fruit juices. Also avoid chewing gums flavored with xylitol, which may aggravate thrush.

❏ Avoid antibiotics, steroids, and birth control pills unless medically directed to take them.

Considerations

❏ Several different antifungal agents are used to treat yeast infections. Topical creams include butoconazole (Gynazole) and miconazole (Monistat), some of which are now available without prescription. Nystatin (Bio-statin, Mycostatin, Nilstat) is relatively safe because it is not absorbed from the gastrointestinal tract. Stronger agents include fluconazole (Diflucan), itraconazole (Sporanox), and ketoconazole (Nizoral). Use of ketoconazole should be avoided, if possible, since this drug can be toxic to the liver. If ketoconazole is called for, its use should be supervised by an infectious disease specialist.

❏ If you take the prescription blood-thinner warfarin (Coumadin), you should consult your doctor before using over-the-counter vaginal miconazole products. Miconazole is an antifungal drug found in some creams and suppositories used to treat vaginal yeast infection. Bleeding or bruising may occur if warfarin and vaginal miconazole are used together.

Yeast Infection: Beneficial Herbs

Herb	Form and Dosage	Comments
Aloe vera[1]	Juice. Take as directed on the label.	Boosts the ability of white blood cells to kill yeast cells.
Barberry[2] or coptis[2] or goldenseal[2] or Oregon grape root[2]	Tincture. Take 1½–3 tsp (6–12 ml) in ¼ cup water 3 times daily.	Antifungal. Prevents diarrhea.
Cinnamon	Oil. Take 15–20 drops in ¼ cup water 3 times daily (gargle and swallow for thrush).	Treats thrush and fluconazole-resistant yeast infections.
Echinacea[3]	*Echinacea purpurea* capsules. Take 1,000 mg 3 times daily.	Stimulates production of macrophages, which destroy yeast cells.
Garlic[4]	Enteric-coated allicin tablets. Take as directed on the label.	Antifungal action stronger than nystatin (Bio-statin, Mycostatin).
Jatobá	Tincture. Take as directed on the label.	Useful when other herbal treatments fail.
Lavender	Fresh herb. Prepare a bath with 2 oz (50 gm) herb steeped in 1 qt water overnight and bathe affected area.	Treats yeast infections of the skin.
Olive leaf	Extract with oleuropein. Use as directed on the label.	Powerful healer of microbial infections.
Oregano[5] or peppermint[5] or rosemary[5] or thyme[5]	Enteric-coated oil capsules. Take 200–400 mg twice daily between meals.	Strong antifungal agents.
Pau d'arco	Capsules. Take as directed on the label.	Stimulates immune system to destroy yeast cells.
Reishi	Tablets. Take 3,000 mg daily.	Stops inflammatory processes.

Precautions for the use of herbs:

[1]Do not take aloe vera internally if you have diarrhea. Aloe has laxative effects if taken in dosages larger than those recommended. Do not use if you are menstruating, have rectal bleeding, or are taking any kind of diuretic.

[2]Do not use barberry, coptis, goldenseal, or Oregon grape root if you are pregnant or have gallbladder disease. Do not take these herbs with supplemental vitamin B_6 or with protein supplements containing the amino acid histidine. Do not take coptis for longer than two weeks at a time. Do not use goldenseal if you have cardiovascular disease or glaucoma. Do not take Oregon grape root for longer than two weeks at a time.

[3]Do not take echinacea for longer than three months. It should not be used by people who are allergic to ragweed. Do not use echinacea if you have an autoimmune disease such as rheumatoid arthritis or lupus. Do not use it if you have a chronic infection such as HIV or tuberculosis.

[4]Garlic counteracts the effects of *Bifidus* and *Lactobacillus* cultures taken as digestive aids. Consult a doctor before using garlic on a regular basis if you are on an anticoagulant drug such as warfarin (Coumadin). Discuss the use of garlic with your doctor before having any type of surgery. Raw garlic can cause heartburn and flatulence.

[5]Oregano, peppermint, rosemary, or thyme must be taken in capsule form to avoid heartburn.

Yeast Infection: Formulas

Formula	Comments
Gentiana Longdancao Decoction to Drain the Liver[1]	A traditional Chinese herbal formula used to treat inflammation of the urinary tract caused by yeast infection.

Precautions for the use of formulas:

[1]Do not use Gentiana Longdancao Decoction to Drain the Liver if you are trying to become pregnant.

❏ In otherwise healthy people, high sugar consumption has very little effect on the growth of yeast. Only when the balance of yeast and other naturally occurring bacteria is upset by antibiotic treatment or injury to the immune system does yeast overgrowth become a problem.

❏ While yeast overgrowth in the mucous membranes lining the gastrointestinal tract, throat, nose, urethra, and vagina are relatively common, yeast infections of the blood and inner organs are extremely rare. If a breast-fed baby develops oral thrush or a nursing mother develops a thrush infection of the nipples, both the mother and the baby should be treated to eradicate the infection, even if only one of them seems to be affected.

❏ Vaginal infections can be caused by bacteria. (*See* VAGINOSIS.)

PART THREE

Techniques of
Herbal Healing

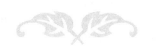

Introduction

Part One of this book defined the principles and materials of targeting herbal healing. Part Two offered an A-to-Z listing of medical conditions that can be managed with these herbs and formulas. In Part Three, you will find instructions that will help you to implement the various methods of natural healing mentioned in Part Two.

The entries in this section explain and show how to prepare the various types of herbal treatments; how to use foot baths, hand baths, sitz baths, and skin washes; and how to be an informed consumer of the services of acupuncturists and massage therapists. There are also entries explaining how to improve your health through aromatherapy, bowel retraining, estrogen-reducing diet, Kegel exercises, and more. When you become familiar with the techniques and procedures described here, you will be fully equipped to achieve maximum health through complementary and alternative health care, and herbal healing.

ACUPUNCTURE

In acupuncture, thin, sterile needles are inserted into the skin at specific points on the body to relieve pain and improve health. This technique has been part of the healthcare system of China and East Asia for at least 2,500 years. The general theory of acupuncture is based on the premise that energy flows through the body along pathways called meridians, each of which is linked to a specific organ. Disruptions, or imbalances, in the flow of energy are believed to be responsible for disease. The purpose of acupuncture is to restore health by correcting these imbalances. The combinations of points at which the needles are inserted correspond to the combination of symptoms noted by the acupuncturist.

Once dismissed as unscientific, acupuncture is slowly finding a scientific basis. For example, in laboratory studies Chinese scientists have measured increases in blood flow to the brain during acupuncture treatments; Japanese scientists have found that acupuncture regulates the production of stress hormones; and in Europe, it was found that acupuncture produces changes in receptor sites in the brain that respond to opiates and endorphins, chemicals in the brain that elevate mood. These scientific discoveries and others like them are beginning to explain the advantages of acupuncture in controlling pain.

The FDA estimates that 3.1 million adults and 150,000 children visit acupuncturists in the United States each year. The National Institutes of Health has confirmed that acupuncture is an effective treatment for many ailments, including chemotherapy-related nausea and vomiting, nausea from pregnancy, and dental pain, and is an acceptable alternative for treating asthma, lower back pain, carpal tunnel syndrome, fibromyalgia, headache, menstrual cramps, and tennis elbow. It is also beneficial in stroke rehabilitation.

In an acupuncture session, which lasts from thirty minutes to one hour, the practitioner, known as an acupuncturist, may ask you a series of questions to get to know more about you. Usually, he or she will take your pulse from different areas of your body to determine the location of the imbalances in energy flow. Before inserting the needles, the practitioner may lightly massage the target area. You may not even feel the needles as they are inserted. Other times, you may feel a sensation like an electric shock upon insertion, but this will be no more severe than touching a doorknob after walking across a carpet on a winter day. The experience varies greatly but is nothing to fear.

The incidence of adverse effects resulting from acupuncture treatments is lower than that of many drugs or other accepted medical procedures used for the same problems. For example, musculoskeletal conditions, such as fibromyalgia, myofascial pain, and tennis elbow are disorders for which acupuncture may be beneficial. These painful conditions are often treated with anti-inflammatory medications, such as aspirin or ibuprofen, or with steroid injections. These medical interventions have potentially harmful side effects but are still widely used and are considered acceptable treatments.

Complications of acupuncture include infections from inadequately sterilized needles or punctured organs. With each visit, a practitioner should use a new set of disposable needles taken from a sealed package. The affected skin sites should be swabbed with alcohol or another disinfectant. Possible side effects from an acupuncture session include dizziness, temporary low blood pressure, and increased perspiration. These also can occur during routine drawing of blood or injections of medications. Among untrained acupuncturists, other complications are possible, but are still uncommon. The most serious complications, such as damage to connective tissues and even collapsed lungs, can occur when acupuncture is improperly performed on infants, and for that reason, acupuncture treatment is not recommended for children under six years of age.

The benefits of acupuncture treatment can be achieved without the use of needles through the practice of shiatsu, also known as acupressure. Shiatsu, which can be performed on children, is recommended for the treatment of back pain and headache and for people who have strong aversions to needles. It is also appropriate when the pain of muscle spasms or fibromyalgia is so intense that only brief contact with the skin can be tolerated. Ask your child's pediatrician before allowing any of these procedures to be done on your child.

More information on acupuncture is available from the American Association of Acupuncture and Oriental Medicine (AAAOM). (*See* Appendix B: Resources.)

AROMATHERAPY

Aromatherapy is the use of pure essential oils extracted from fragrant plants to help relieve a variety of health problems. Traditional uses of aromatherapy include assisting breathing and loosening mucous secretions; healing minor cuts and insect bites; promoting relaxation and sleep; reducing pain; relieving digestive problems; and soothing muscle aches and pains. Relatively new to the United States, aromatherapy has been used for thousands of years in other parts of the world, especially in the Middle East. The modern practice of aromatherapy developed primarily in the 1930s in Europe and made its way to the United States in the 1950s. Although aromatherapists specialize in this type of therapy, you can reap the benefits of aromatherapy on your own with some knowledge of essential oils.

Essential oils are concentrated extracts commercially prepared from various parts of a plant, which may include the blossoms, leaves, or roots. Most essential oils evaporate easily, making them highly fragrant but also making them potentially flammable. Because they are so concentrated, essential oils typically need to be diluted with water or carrier (or base) oil before use. They may be used singly, or some may be used in combination to produce complementary effects.

In aromatherapy, essential oils can be used either by applying them to the skin or by inhaling them through the nose. When applied to the skin, essential oils are absorbed into the body. Some oils have physical effects, such as relieving swelling. They may also have anti-infection properties when the pure essential oils are put in products, such as cleansing creams and shampoos, where they may kill external bacteria. When inhaled, the aromatic molecules of the essential oils are thought to stimulate the olfactory nerve. This sends messages to the brain's limbic system, the part of the brain that controls memory and emotion. Researchers believe that when the limbic system is stimulated, it can positively affect the nervous, endocrine, and immune systems. Inhalation of essential oils can also impact the respiratory system directly. For instance, when the essential oils from eucalyptus leaf are inhaled, they can help clear the sinuses and respiratory tract and, thereby, could help fight upper respiratory infections.

Scientific Evidence Supporting Aromatherapy

Until very recently, medical scientists tended to scoff at the idea of aromatherapy, but recent research confirms that it has a direct effect on the human brain. Scientists at the University of Miami School of Medicine used electroencephalogram (EEG) measurements to confirm aromatherapy's direct effects on the brain. They found that aromatherapy with lavender causes the brain to produce more beta waves, increasing relaxation, lifting depression, and, interestingly, enabling test participants to solve math problems more accurately. They also found that aromatherapy with rosemary causes the brain to produce fewer alpha and beta waves, suggesting increased alertness, but without increased anxiety.

Other scientific studies are beginning to show how aromatherapy affects the endocrine and immune systems. For example, research at Kurume University School of Medicine in Japan found that aromatherapy with lemon oil helps to restore the immune systems of laboratory animals during stress. However, in a study using aromatherapy with lemon and lavender, neither worked to reduce markers of stress, though lemon scent had a positive effect on mood. Researchers at the University of Alaska at Fairbanks found that aromatherapy with lavender oil accelerates recovery of the cardiovascular system after aerobic workouts; and in a study at the University of Pittsburgh, researchers found that pleasant aromas reduce the craving for cigarettes in smokers trying to quit. Other clinical studies have shown that aromatherapy can help limit hair loss, improve the mental function of people with Alzheimer's disease, and even accelerate recovery from coronary bypass surgery. Neroli oil helped people about to undergo a colonoscopy. Systolic blood pressure was lower in this group compared to a group who inhaled safflower oil fumes.

Applying Essential Oils to the Skin

Before applying essential oil to skin, *always* dilute the oil first. A carrier (or base) oil can be used for this purpose. Use a pure, unperfumed vegetable oil, such as soybean, olive, or almond oil. Chemicals in synthetic oils may interfere with the properties of the essential oil and with your body's absorption of the oil. If you do not wish to use a carrier oil, add the essential oil to an unperfumed, vegetable-based lotion or skin cream.

Adults generally should use essential oils diluted to three parts per hundred. For instance, for 1 cup (48 teaspoons) of carrier oil, add about 1 teaspoon of essential oil. Children and people with sensitive skin should use a dilution half as strong, about ½ teaspoon of essential oil per 1 cup of carrier oil. The scented carrier oil then can be massaged into the skin over the affected area. Be sure to wash your hands thoroughly after coming in contact with the oil before touching your eyes, as some oils can cause burning or stinging.

Essential oils also can be applied to the skin by mixing 4 to 10 drops of the oil with 1 quart of warm or cool water, soaking a cloth in the water, and then applying the cloth as a compress, or by adding about 6 drops of the oil to a tub of warm water and soaking in the bath for at least fifteen minutes. (*See* COMPRESSES.)

Inhaling Essential Oils

The simplest way to inhale an essential oil is to sniff the undiluted oil itself. Do not allow the liquid to get into your nose. Instead, sniff the air above the oil, as you might when smelling the scent of a perfume. There are many other ways to inhale essential oils, including the following:

- Place one drop of oil on your pillowcase to smell its scent as you sleep.
- Burn a store-bought wax candle scented with an essential oil. Note that adding your own essential oil to a flame is a fire hazard.
- Use a diffuser, a device that uses heat to disperse scented molecules of essential oil into the air.
- Spray the oil into the air. For air-freshening water sprays, add 3 drops of essential oil to a pint-sized spray bottle full of water.

Precautions for Using Essential Oils

When using essential oils, start slowly, gradually adding just enough oil to achieve the level of aroma you desire. Essential oils are usually sold in small bottles with droppers so that you can add the oil drop by drop. The concentration of essential oils may vary depending on the brand you choose.

Avoid prolonged use of the same essential oil, that is, for more than one hour per day, or daily for more than one month at a time. Prolonged use can result in developing an allergic reaction to the oil, skin reactions, or even mild toxic reactions in the liver.

Do not ingest drinks made from essential oils unless you are working with a skilled aromatherapy practitioner. Overdose of essential oils may cause agitation, convulsions, drowsiness, nausea, or vomiting. Pregnant women and children under age three should not ingest essential oils. In almost all cases, essential oils should be used externally, yet some flower essences may be used internally as directed on the label.

If you buy a prepared product that claims to be aromatherapeutic, read the label to be sure the product actually contains essential oil. Some products are made with artificial fragrances rather than herbal oils. Artificial fragrances should never be used in diffusers. Candles that contain manufactured fragrances can cause headaches.

BOWEL RETRAINING

Bowel retraining is a program for producing regular bowel movements. It can be used with other therapies for treating fecal incontinence, a condition in which a person experiences uncontrollable bowel movements. Bowel retraining also can be useful by itself for treating chronic constipation. The therapies most notably used in conjunction with bowel retraining for fecal incontinence are Kegel exercises, which are meant to strengthen the pelvic floor muscles, and/or biofeedback, a therapy that uses monitoring equipment to measure biological reactions to various techniques to create a desired response. (*See* KEGEL EXERCISES and/or RELAXATION TECHNIQUES.)

Within a few weeks of beginning a bowel-retraining program, most people can achieve regular bowel movements. Before beginning this program, however, it is necessary that you receive a thorough physical examination to identify the cause of the fecal incontinence and treat any correctable disorders, such as a fecal impaction (accumulation of hard stool blocking bowel movement) or infectious diarrhea.

The key to bowel retraining is setting aside the same time each day for daily bowel movements and sticking to that time. It is very important to be consistent in the time of day that bowel training is performed, as consistency is crucial for the success of a bowel-retraining program. The best time for a bowel movement is twenty to forty-five minutes after eating a meal, since food stimulates bowel activity.

If necessary, it is possible to stimulate bowel movements by drinking warm prune juice, herbal tea, or fruit nectar. Also, bowel movements may be encouraged by digital stimulation, which is performed by inserting a lubricated finger (olive oil or vitamin E oil works well) into the anus and moving it in a circular motion. Be sure your nails are not sharp or jagged, as this can cause irritation. This method stimulates the lower bowel until the sphincter relaxes. The process may require anywhere from one to two minutes. If digital stimulation does not produce a bowel movement within twenty minutes after performing the exercise, the procedure may be repeated. Digital stimulation should be performed every day until a pattern of regular bowel movements is established. Using a glycerin suppository, such as Dulcolax, or a small enema may also stimulate bowel movements.

After stimulation has been performed, assume a normal posture for bowel movement. If you are confined to bed, use a bedpan in as close to a sitting position as possible or, if you are unable to sit, use a left-side lying position. Try to ensure privacy as much as possible. Also, some people find that reading while sitting on the commode helps them relax and aids in bowel evacuation. Try to contract the abdominal muscles and bear down while expelling the stool. Some people find it helpful to bend forward while bearing down, as this increases the abdominal pressure and helps evacuate the bowel.

As part of a bowel-retraining program and as a permanent lifestyle change, the diet should be modified to include adequate fiber and fluid intake to promote regular, soft, bulky stools. Add high-fiber foods to the diet, including whole wheat grains, fresh vegetables, and beans. Additionally, psyllium products can be used to add bulk to the stools. Drink eight to ten 8-ounce glasses, or 2 to 3 liters, of fluid each day unless you have a medical condition that requires you to restrict your fluid intake, such as kidney or heart disease.

COMPRESSES

A compress is a cloth or a piece of cotton soaked in an herb solution, which is then applied to the skin. Compresses may be applied cold or hot. A cold compress is known as a wrap, and a hot compress is known as a fomentation. Cold compresses are traditionally used to relieve conditions such as fever, skin inflammation, headache, sore throat, and inflamed gums after oral surgery. Hot and cold compresses are used for conditions such as muscle pain, breast engorgement, arthritic swelling, colds, and flu. In one study, postnatal women with breast engorgement used hot and cold compresses and had a significant decrease in breast size and pain. People with back pain related to muscle issues seem to benefit from using a cold pack several times a day for 20 minutes for the first two to three days. Afterward, heat should be applied (such as a heating lamp or hot pad) for brief periods to relax muscles and increase blood flow. Avoid sleeping on a heating pad, which can cause burns. Compresses can also be as simple as a cool wet towel on the forehead to relieve a headache or cold tea bags placed over the eyelids to relieve tired eyes. (Be careful with certain herbal extracts over the eyes, as some may cause burning or stinging.)

To make a cold compress, dip a piece of cotton gauze or a cotton ball in a cold herbal tea or a mixture made with a dropperful of herb tincture in ¼ cup, or 60 milliliters, of water, except as otherwise noted in Part Two. (*See* TEAS and/or TINCTURES.) Place the soaked cotton between two layers of clean cloth and apply to the affected area. Hold the cloth in place with a long cloth strip or a clean scarf; do not cover the compress with plastic. When the compress warms to body temperature, add a few more drops of the tea or tincture mixture to the cotton and reapply. Cold compresses may be left in place overnight.

To make a hot compress, soak a clean towel in hot herbal tea and apply as hot as possible to the affected area. When the compress has cooled to body temperature, the process is repeated and the compress is reapplied as desired. Most of the teas used for compresses can be made from tea bags. For loose teas, specific amounts are given in the appropriate Part Two entries.

CREAMS

See OINTMENTS.

DOUCHES

Douches are used to clean the vagina such as after monthly periods and to get rid of odor. Some suggest douches will kill sexually transmitted disease and end pregnancy, but they won't do either of these. Prepared with herbal solutions, douches may help soothe the vagina. To prepare the solution for an herbal douche, place the recommended quantity of tincture in 1 quart of warm water, or 1 tablespoon of the herb in 1 quart of *boiling* water. (Using boiling water kills any bacteria that may have adhered to the surface of the herb.) Douches prepared with tinctures may be used as soon as the water is cool enough; otherwise, allow the herb-and-water mixture to stand in a covered container overnight, strain, and use at room temperature. (*See* TINCTURES.)

Overfrequent douching with baking soda, Betadine, and prepared commercial douches has been linked to increased risk of *Chlamydia* infection, ectopic pregnancy, and pelvic inflammatory disease (PID). Risk of infection and complications increase with the use of commercial douches because they disrupt the normal balance of beneficial bacteria and the microorganisms that cause infection. The right balance keeps an acidic environment, which reduces the chances of developing a bacterial infection or yeast infection. The antiseptic chemicals in herbal douches may spare more of the protective bacteria and could be safer to use than commercial products; however, even herbal douches should be used only when needed and are not for preventive use. It is important to allow the vagina to generate protective mucus, which captures disease-causing microorganisms. Overfrequent douching can hinder this production.

After using any herbal douche, place *acidophilus* or *Lactobacillus* suppositories in the vagina, or douche again with two *acidophilus* or *Lactobacillus* capsules emptied into a pint of warm water, thus regenerating protective bacteria. Alkalinity is increased when the diet minimizes meat and emphasizes fresh vegetables, and when herbal douches are alternated with douches made with 1 teaspoon of vinegar per quart of water.

Do not use douches if you have a bacterial infection; when a vaginal discharge smells bad or is thick, white or yellowish-green; when there is burning or redness, pain upon urination, or pain during sex. For these conditions, see a physician for treatment. The American College of Obstetrics and Gynecology suggests that women should avoid douching completely because women who douche have an increased risk of vaginal infections, bacterial vaginosis, sexually transmitted infections, and pelvic inflammatory disease (PID). However, if you choose to douche, the Water Works device was found to be superior to over-the-counter devices for reducing vaginal odor in the absence of an infection based on a group of 100 women.

ESTROGEN-REDUCING DIET

A proper diet could reduce lifetime exposure to estrogen, which in turn may reduce the risk of a variety of disorders, including breast cancer, endometriosis, and fibrocystic breast disease. Both proper nutrition and reduced estrogen exposure are important considerations for a person who has or has had an estrogen-influenced disorder. You can reduce your lifetime exposure to estrogen by making the following dietary changes:

• *Reduce your overall calorie intake.* Reducing calorie consumption increases levels of a hormone called SHBG (sex hormone binding globulin), which keeps estrogen from stimulating the growth of healthy and cancerous cells in the breast. Scientists believe that calorie reduction has the same effect on other estrogen-influenced disorders. Calorie reduction is not recommended, however, during chemotherapy or radiation treatment. To reduce calories, avoid eating so-called empty calorie foods, which do not provide any nutrition. Such foods include salty snacks, sugared beverages, and sweets such as pastries and candies.

• *Eat more whole grains, legumes, and berries, and more fiber-rich foods in general.* Fiber increases the rate at which estrogen is excreted from the body. Also, some experts believe that simply adding fiber to the diet can reduce the risk of breast cancer.

Fiber in the intestine keeps excreted estrogen by-products from being reassembled by bacteria and reabsorbed into the bloodstream. Because the effects of estrogen are cumulative, the benefits of fiber are also cumulative—eating fiber-rich foods confers lifetime reduction of breast cancer risk. For this effect, it is necessary to eat at least 25 grams of fiber daily, which is difficult without eating high-fiber cereals. If high-fiber cereal is unpalatable, mix it with regular cereal. Use skim milk in your cereal rather than whole milk to reduce fat consumption.

• *Reduce your fat consumption but do not completely exclude healthy fats from your diet.* Low-fat diets do not decrease estrogen production but do increase estrogen excretion through the urine. Low-fat diets also tend to include a lot of fruits and vegetables, many of which contain compounds that protect against cancer.

Note, however, that some kinds of fat are cancer protective. Omega-3 essential fatty acids from fish oils have been shown to reduce the risk of breast cancer. Eating two to three servings a week of salmon, sardines, or other cold-water fish, or taking fish-oil capsules confers this benefit. In laboratory studies, cancer cells grown in the same test tube as healthy cells without essential fatty acids overtake the healthy cells. However, when essential fatty acids are added to the medium, healthy cells overtake the cancer cells. Limit your intake of vegetable oils rich in omega-6s, such as corn, safflower, and sunflower oils, which work against the omega-3 oils. Better oils to include in the diet are canola and olive oils.

• *If you are overweight, lose weight.* Gradual weight loss after menopause reverses the effects of estrogen overexposure.

• *Use acidophilus supplements.* While the liver breaks down estrogen before sending it to the digestive tract for elimination, bacteria in the intestines can turn these breakdown products back into estrogen. Small amounts of the hormone can then be reabsorbed through the intestinal wall. Taking *Lactobacillus acidophilus* supplements daily can provide your body with the beneficial microbes that could potentially compete with the estrogen-forming bacteria.

FOOT BATHS

Herbal foot baths are used to treat excessive sweating of the feet and athlete's foot. To make a foot bath, place 1 ounce of the recommended herb in 2 quarts of water—unless otherwise specified in Part Two—which has just been boiled and removed from the source of heat. Allow the mixture to stand for one hour; then strain. Making sure the herbal mixture is lukewarm, pour it into an empty basin or tub. Immerse the feet in the herbal solution for ten to fifteen minutes one to two times daily until symptoms improve.

People who have diabetes and those with congestive heart failure or nerve damage to the feet should not use foot baths unless they can confirm that the foot bath solution is cooler than 108°F (43°C) with a thermometer and they check with their doctor. In addition, foot baths should be avoided by those who have open wounds on the feet or varicose veins.

HAND BATHS

Herbal hand baths are used to treat excessive sweating and skin infections of the hands. To make a hand bath, place 1 ounce of the recommended herb in 2 quarts of water—unless otherwise specified in Part Two—that has just been boiled and removed from the source of heat. Allow the mixture to stand for one hour; then strain. Making sure the herbal mixture is lukewarm, pour it into an empty basin or tub. Immerse the hands in the herbal solution for ten to fifteen minutes one to two times daily until symptoms improve.

People who have diabetes and those with nerve damage to the hands should not use hand baths unless they can confirm that the hand bath solution is cooler than 108°F (43°C) with a thermometer and they check with their doctor. Hand baths should be avoided if there are open wounds on the hands.

KEGEL EXERCISES

Kegel exercises are performed to strengthen the muscles that support the urethra, bladder, uterus, and rectum. Also known as pelvic floor exercises, these exercises are good for controlling incontinence resulting from childbirth, urinary stress, urge, and prostate surgery. Doctors at Connecticut Children's Medical Center have found that 90 percent of children who wet the bed and 100 percent of children who have trouble controlling urination during the day improve after approximately six months of performing the exercises with the help of a biofeedback computer game. In another study, using Kegel exercises alone or Kegels with biofeedback reduced episodic urinary incontinence and urinary tract infections in older women.

Strengthening and restoring muscle tone is the main principle behind Kegel exercises. This improves the ure-thral and/or rectal sphincter function. The success of Kegel exercises depends on proper technique and adher-ence to a regular exercise program.

The first step in learning how to perform Kegel exer-cises is to identify the pelvic floor muscles. To do so, try stopping the flow of urine midstream. The muscles used to do this are the pelvic floor muscles. Continue this until you feel sure you can contract the correct muscles with-out having to urinate. For women, another approach to help locate the correct muscles is to use a vaginal cone, a weighted device inserted into the vagina. The woman then contracts her pelvic floor muscles to hold the cone in place. People who are unsure whether or not they have located the correct muscles may consult a doctor, nurse, or physi-cal therapist who can assist them in locating the proper group of muscles. Also, biofeedback is sometimes recom-mended for people who cannot locate the correct muscles. (See Biofeedback under RELAXATION TECHNIQUES.)

Once you have learned which muscles are involved, you are ready to perform the exercise: Make sure your bladder is empty and then begin tightening your pelvic floor muscles. Start by holding the muscles in for three to five seconds and gradually work up to ten seconds. Then, relax for a count of ten. Repeat this up to ten times, three to four times throughout the day. Increasing the frequency of the exercise can cause more harm than good. Too much exercise can wear out the muscles and cause more urine leakage. A certain indication of overexercise is intense pain in the muscles of the anal sphincter.

Although Kegel exercises can be performed at any time and in any place, the best results occur if they are per-formed on a schedule at the same time and place each day. Many people report that performing the exercise five min-utes before they get up in the morning and five minutes before they go to sleep at night is a helpful routine. Note that it may take eight to twelve weeks before any improve-ment is noticed.

MASSAGE

Massage is the therapeutic manipulation of the soft tissues of the body. Every form of massage therapy includes some form of kneading, pressing, or stroking with the use of pressure and movement, no matter how slight the touch or how often it is used. Although the health benefits of massage are limited in scientific terms, massage is most often employed as a unique way of communicating with-out words, sharing energy, enjoying pleasurable relax-ation, and experiencing peace of mind.

Medical literature contains nearly 10,000 studies on the health benefits of massage. Massage therapy has been used successfully to treat conditions as diverse as acne,

anxiety (by reducing blood pressure and heart rate), pain associated with end-stage cancer, chronic neck pain, and constipation. In a review of forty-nine articles on the use of various treatments for low back pain, massage was one of several (along with biofeedback and acupuncture) that helped with pain management. People with chronic consti-pation may also derive benefit from abdominal massage. A massage seems to work by stimulating peristalsis (move-ment of stool in the GI tract), decreasing colonic transit time, and increasing the frequency of bowel movements, thereby reducing discomfort and pain. Other bodywork systems include acupressure, reflexology, Reiki, shiatsu, and sports, Swedish, Traeger, and tui nei massage.

The best way to find a massage therapist in your area is to get a referral from someone you know who has a massage therapist, or from a health professional who is knowledge-able about forms of complementary and alternative health care. Since there are many styles of massage, you may want to shop around to find someone who practices the style of massage most suited to your needs. You may need to try a few different massage therapists before finding one who is right for you. Side effects are rare, but caution is needed for people with bleeding disorders, fractures or open heal-ing wounds, and cancer. Women who are pregnant should consult their obstetrician before having a massage.

Whenever you are interviewing a massage therapist, you should feel comfortable asking if he or she has gradu-ated from an accredited school or has been approved by a reputable accrediting agency such as the Commission for Massage Training Accreditation (COMTA). It is also proper to ask whether the therapist is licensed in your state or is nationally certified by the National Certifica-tion Board for Therapeutic Massage and Bodywork. More information on massage is available from The American Massage Therapy Association (AMTA). (See Appendix B: Resources.)

OINTMENTS

Herbal ointments, also known as liniments and salves, are semisolid preparations of herbs that, when applied, hold the herbs close to the skin for maximum absorption of their anti-inflammatory or antibacterial ingredients. In a cell study, Ficus infectoria, F. religiosa, and piper betel ointments were effective at killing drug-resistant strains of the common bacterium Pseudomonas. In another study, a cream made with aloe vera reduced pain and increased healing time in patients who received it compared to those who didn't after a hemorrhoidectomy. The patients who got the aloe vera also used fewer analgesics to control pain after surgery over a four-week period. Ointments are a convenient way to apply essential oils, which would oth-erwise evaporate shortly after being applied to the skin. Herbal creams are ointments used specifically to moistur-ize the skin.

Traditionally, herbal ointments are made by mixing

herbs in a base of lard, or animal fat. Lard was a useful base for ointments because its fatty structure is very similar to human skin. Most users of herbs today, however, prefer to use beeswax and vegetable oil in homemade ointments.

To make a base for an ointment, combine beeswax and vegetable oil, preferably olive oil, in a ratio of ¼ cup of melted beeswax for each cup of vegetable oil at room temperature. Add powdered dried herbs (purchased as powders or ground with kitchen mortar and pestle) in a ratio of 1 ounce for each cup of beeswax-oil base. If using more than one herb in an ointment, use equal quantities of each herb to total approximately 1 ounce per cup. Essential oils are also useful in ointments. (See AROMATHERAPY for a discussion of essential oils.) They should be added to the base in a ratio of 1 teaspoon of essential oil per cup of base.

Keep homemade ointments in jars in the refrigerator. Be sure to label them so that they are not mistaken for food. If the ointment is not easy to spread, add more oil until it reaches the desired consistency. If the ointment is runny, add more melted beeswax until it reaches the desired consistency. Never expose homemade ointments to high heat to prevent the essential oils from evaporating.

PLASTERS

A plaster is a thick, moist, warm herbal paste placed between two layers of cloth or in a cloth pouch. A plaster is similar to a poultice, except that the herbal paste is not applied directly to the skin. (See POULTICES.) Therefore, plasters are applied when the herbs being used are potentially irritating to the skin. Although plasters are most frequently used in the treatment of respiratory congestion, they can be useful in the treatment of conditions as diverse as skin infections, irritable bowel syndrome, and high blood pressure. In addition, plasters promote blood circulation, relax muscle spasms, and relieve pain. In one study in which an herbal plaster was used in children with mental retardation, the children showed better socialization and improved mental development when the plaster was used along with other alternative practices, including acupuncture. A Chinese prickly ash plaster, available commercially as Tian He Gu Tong from traditional Chinese medicine practitioners and in Chinese herb shops, is used to treat pain resulting from arthritic spurs, frozen shoulder, back strain, lumbar muscle strain, stiff neck, and rheumatoid arthritis. Other common herbs used in plasters include white flower oil, Zheng Gu Shui, and Guanjie Zhitong Gao.

Since plasters do not touch the skin, they act through the release of volatile oils stored in the herb. For this reason, it is necessary to grind the (usually dried) herb *immediately before* making the plaster to release its healing ingredients. Grinding the herb releases "pockets" of enzymes that activate the essential oils. Once ground, mix approximately ¼ cup (2 ounces) of the herb in just enough lukewarm water to make a thick slurry; do not use hot water, as it may deactivate the enzymes. Take care not to get the powder under your fingernails or in your eyes. Place the slurry between several layers of clean cloth, such as cheesecloth or muslin, and put the plaster over the affected area of the body.

Most of the herbs used in plasters generate a strong burning sensation as part of the healing process. This sensation is a sign that the volatile oils of the herb have entered the deeper layers of the skin. The plaster should be left on the skin only until the burning sensation begins—usually within five minutes—and *must* be removed within fifteen minutes to avoid skin injury.

Mustard seed plasters and prickly ash plasters should not be applied to any part of the body where there is insufficient blood circulation. Do not place these plasters on varicose veins. People who have circulatory problems should not use any type of plaster.

POULTICES

A poultice is a thick, moist, warm herbal paste applied to the skin to relieve pain, inflammation, swelling, or muscle spasms. Poultices are commonly made with dried, powdered herbs to which hot water is added, but they also can be made with fresh herbs, especially plantain.

To make a poultice from dried herbs, place a steamer, heat-proof colander, strainer, or sieve over a pot of rapidly boiling water. Layer ¼ cup (2 ounces) of the recommended herb in the steamer or other utensil, reduce the heat to a simmering temperature, and cover the pot. Allow the steam to thoroughly penetrate and wilt the herbs. Or, if you do not have a utensil in which to steam the herbs, mix the powdered or crushed herb with just enough hot water to make a thick paste. Some people add all-purpose flour to thicken the mixture.

After about five minutes, spread the softened and warmed herbs on a clean white, loosely woven cloth, such as cheesecloth or gauze; fold one layer of the cloth over the herb, and apply to the affected area. To hold in the heat, cover the poultice with a towel or woolen cloth. The poultice should remain in place for at least twenty minutes and may be left on as long as overnight, but should remain covered. You may wish to oil the skin first to protect it and make removing the poultice easier.

To make a pulped poultice from fresh herbs, place the herbs between two layers of a clean white cloth twice the size of the affected area. Using a rolling pin (if you do not have a rolling pin, use a quart-sized bottle of water with the lid closed tightly), roll over the herbs in the cloth until they are finely crushed and the cloth is dampened with moisture from the herbs. Apply the dampened cloth to the affected area of the body. You can also place the fresh herbs in a food processor and mix with a small amount of hot water. To trap the juices and hold the fresh poultice in place, overwrap it well with a towel or woolen cloth. Like a poultice made from dried herbs, a pulped compress can remain in place overnight if covered.

The use of poultices as a source of lasting moist heat is often overlooked. Poultices made of hayflower, which is used for its heat-storage properties, radiate moist heat as much as five times longer than a hot water bottle. It is important to remember, however, that the herbs can be used only once for this purpose. St. John's wort in a poultice may help with joint pain and stiffness, mullein may help with chest congestion, and for skin problems you can use chickweed or calendula. Some herbs should not be put in a poultice, such as arnica, mustard, and capsicum, but can be used in a compress. In addition, there have been cases reported of phytodermatitis erupting from a poultice of *Ranunculus arvensis* when it was used for treatment of joint pain (osteoarthritis). The skin irritations resembled a burn injury and had to be treated with topical antibiotics and daily wound dressings.

RELAXATION TECHNIQUES

Relaxation techniques can be performed regularly to enhance your well-being and promote an overall state of physical and mental relaxation, no matter what your current state of health. Children as well as adults can practice relaxation techniques. The techniques that have been clinically shown to improve the health conditions covered in this book are discussed below. You should note that willingness to take time for yourself is the best predictor of successful relaxation. Which method of relaxation you choose is less important than spending time enjoying it.

The term "relaxation response" was coined by Dr. Herbert Benson of Harvard Medical School. It is a technique used to help people reduce stress, decrease oxygen consumption, lower blood pressure, and slow heart rate. The procedure involves finding a quiet place where you are comfortable to sit and close your eyes and focus on a word, phrase, or prayer. Breathe slowly and naturally, inhaling through your nose. Pause for a few seconds and exhale through your mouth. Repeat the exercise for ten to twenty minutes per day, at least three to four times a week. For those with mental health issues, this therapy will help increase awareness and enable you to recognize signs of tension. Eventually you should be able to use this exercise to relax and improve your concentration. One study used relaxation response techniques in patients with high blood pressure who were using medications to control it. The group that used the relaxation response exercise along with changes in lifestyle was four times more likely to not have to use medications to control blood pressure.

Biofeedback

Biofeedback is a technology for learning relaxation. The basic idea of biofeedback is that once a conscious awareness of an involuntary function is developed, it is possible to learn to change it. An example of this principle is the use of biofeedback to warm cold hands.

Skin temperature in the hands is determined by the flow of blood through the arteries into them. The autonomic, or unconscious, nervous system regulates this blood flow. It can stimulate the sympathetic nerves in the hand to constrict the arteries, reducing blood flow and lowering temperature, or it can stimulate the parasympathetic nerves in the hand to relax the arteries, increasing blood flow and raising temperature. Without a biofeedback device, the conscious mind does not know how to regulate the nerve functions that control the flow of blood. In a biofeedback setup, however, it is possible to connect temperature sensors to the fingers. By watching or listening to temperature readouts, the person learns to consciously control the constriction or relaxation of the arteries and thereby control the temperature of the hands.

Biofeedback is most commonly used to redirect the balance of the autonomic nervous system away from sympathetic functions (the body's response to stress) and toward parasympathetic functions (the body's maintenance functions). Reducing the activity of the sympathetic nervous system lowers blood pressure and improves digestive function. Biofeedback is used to relieve muscle tension in conditions such as tension headaches and bruxism, involuntary grinding of the teeth at night, as well as heart problems, chronic pain, constipation, irritable bowel syndrome (IBS), incontinence, and Raynaud's disease (a disorder of the blood vessels that may result in cold hands and/or feet). Biofeedback works best in people whose tension causes bodily complaints. It is also attractive to children who enjoy machines with beeps, dials, and lights. It is noninvasive, may eliminate the need for certain drugs, and allows people to take charge of their health. Biofeedback can help with many health problems in 10 to 50 sessions of 30 to 60 minutes each.

Breathing

Breathing influences body, mind, and mood. Breathing is a natural relaxation technique for which changes are needed only if the rate of breathing is too fast. The average rate of breathing while at rest is approximately twelve to fourteen times a minute. Breathing faster than this normal rate causes the body to hyperventilate—that is, to take quick, shallow breaths from the top of the chest. These sharply reduce the level of carbon dioxide in the blood, causing the arteries, including the carotid artery going to the brain, to constrict, thus reducing the flow of blood throughout the body.

When this occurs, no matter how much oxygen is taken into the lungs, the brain and body will experience a shortage of oxygen. The lack of sufficient oxygen switches on the sympathetic nervous system—the "fight or flight" reflex. This may cause anxiety and tension. It may also reduce the ability to think clearly and tends to put the mind at the mercy of obsessive thoughts and images.

Fortunately, poor breathing habits are easy to correct. Simply paying attention to breathing without doing anything to change it initiates relaxation. When dwelling on upsetting thoughts, focusing on your breathing instead will decrease anxiety.

Deep-Breathing Exercises

Shallow or poor breathing could contribute to some disorders. We need to learn to breathe deeply, and from the abdomen rather than from the chest, which produces short and shallow breathing. Learning this technique helps you to breathe in more oxygen, which passes through the lungs and is absorbed into the bloodstream. Oxygen is needed for cellular respiration, cell metabolism, and proper brain function. If you breathe too shallowly, the body may not eliminate sufficient carbon dioxide for good health. Proper breathing techniques may increase lung capacity; increase energy levels; and could help to relieve anxiety, asthma symptoms, insomnia, and stress.

To practice deep breathing, do the following: Slowly breathe in through your nose and from your abdomen as deeply as you can and hold the breath for a count of ten. Place your tongue between your front teeth and the roof of your mouth, and slowly breathe out through your mouth. Do this for five minutes three times daily. Choose an environment with fresh air when doing this exercise, not a place with a lot of traffic or pollution.

The rationale for keeping the tongue against the ridge of the teeth is found in yoga philosophy. Yoga describes two energy circuits in the body, one negative and one positive. These begin and end at the tip of the tongue and the ridge of the teeth. Putting those structures in contact is thought to complete a circuit, keeping the energy of the breath in the body instead of allowing it to dissipate. Whether or not this position completes a literal energy circuit, the effect of doing the exercise following the instructions above is induced relaxation. The cycle breaths may induce a temporary feeling of lightheadedness; this is normal.

If you want to relax quickly—say, if you are under tension or stress, or are having an anxiety attack—place your arms down along the sides of your body. As you are inhaling deeply, stretch your arms up and out as if to form a V shape. Then exhale slowly through your mouth and bring your arms back down to your sides. This is a stretching and breathing exercise at the same time. Repeat this as many times as is comfortable every hour until you feel relief.

Advanced Breathing Exercises

Advanced breathing exercises, such as pranayama yoga, Gurdjieff exercises, and Liangong Shi Ba Fa, are not recommended for self-instruction. To avoid injury to the diaphragm, you must achieve deep relaxation before using these techniques. For training in advanced breathing methods, consult a teaching center near you.

Exercise

Exercise induces relaxation and lowers stress by giving the conscious mind a respite from anxiety. Moderate to heavy exercise generates endorphins, morphinelike chemicals that relax the brain to relieve anxiety. Different kinds of exercise may produce different effects. The rhythm of aerobic exercises such as biking or swimming, for example, may induce greater relaxation than an activity that lacks rhythm, such as lifting weights.

If the mind is not given a chance to rest, however, exercise does not induce relaxation. For example, studying for an exam while riding an exercise bike could cancel out the relaxing effects of exercise. Rest also is essential to avoid muscle injury. For this reason, it is important to do a warm-up routine to relax the muscles before working out to relax the mind. The three main warm-up methods are discussed below, but only the third is recommended. Exercise also will increase lung capacity and improve breathing.

Ballistic Stretching

Ballistic stretching is the most time-honored approach to preparing muscles for a workout. In this method, the muscles are bounced a little to push joints into a greater range of motion. Although this method is standard for activities as diverse as ballet, football, and tae kwon do, it is not recommended. Ballistic stretching can cause microscopic muscle tears and actually shorten muscles.

Static Stretching

Athletic trainers frequently recommend this method. In this yogalike method, the muscles are allowed to elongate on their own against the force of gravity while the exerciser helps them by breathing carefully. However, static stretching increases the risk of injury to the knees.

Proprioceptive Neuromuscular Facilitation

Proprioceptive neuromuscular facilitation (PNF) consists of contracting a targeted muscle as tightly as possible without causing pain for five seconds and then relaxing it with a static stretch. The muscle will be more relaxed than if static stretching were begun immediately.

In the same way that it is important not to strain muscles during exercise for relaxation, it is important not to "tax" the immune system during heavy exercise. (For more information, see "Siberian Ginseng Goes to the Gym" under SIBERIAN GINSENG in Part One.)

Meditation

Meditation is directed concentration. It is a process of putting attention on a chosen object of thought, which may be the breath, a phrase or word repeated silently, a memorized inspirational passage, or a mental image. Researchers have documented immediate benefits of meditation in decreased heart and respiratory rate, increased blood flow, lowered blood pressure, and other measurements of a relaxation response. In addition, it has helped people with allergies, anxiety disorders, asthma, binge eating, cancer, depression, fatigue, heart disease, pain, sleep problems, and substance abuse. Emotional benefits include gaining a new perspective, managing stress, increasing self-awareness, focusing on the present, and reducing negative emotions.

Although some forms of meditation are complicated, many are not. It is important for beginners to remember that meditation is not necessarily focused concentration—it is usually not possible to stop all extraneous thoughts. It is helpful to remember that meditation is a *process* of putting attention on the chosen object of thought.

Meditation can be learned from books, instructional tapes, meditation classes, and meditation retreats. Most people should be able to find a form of meditation that makes them feel comfortable and does not interfere with their personal belief system. Whatever form of meditation is chosen, however, daily practice over a period of months is necessary before major changes in health are observed.

Progressive Relaxation

Progressive relaxation is a method of releasing tension in the muscles. Extensively studied in clinics in the United States, Britain, Korea, and Japan, this technique has been useful in treating headaches, insomnia, drug withdrawal, and premature labor. Some suggest that progressive relaxation techniques are useful in managing obsessive compulsive (OCD) symptoms. However, in one study, it was not as good a treatment for adults with OCD compared to acceptance and commitment therapy, another treatment for this condition. Although the OCD patients who received progressive relaxation therapy did experience reduced OCD symptoms and less depression, the acceptance and commitment therapy group had better results.

Although there are many variations of progressive relaxation, a simple method is to begin by lying on your back in a comfortable position. Take a series of deep slow breaths and then focus awareness on different parts of the body in turn, becoming aware of muscular tension and then releasing it. One way to do this is to tense a muscle deliberately and then relax it. The muscle is held tight to a count of four and then relaxed until comfort is felt.

Start with the front of the body, tensing and relaxing the muscles of the toes, feet, lower legs, thighs, and abdomen, and then moving on to the chest, neck, jaw, and upper face. Tensing and releasing can be repeated several times until relaxation is felt. Repeat the process going down the back of the body, tensing and relaxing the muscles of the back of the neck, back, hips, thighs, calves, and ankles. Finally, lie still with your eyes closed, concentrating on breathing and enjoying relaxation.

Progressive relaxation is easy to learn without a teacher, but it is enjoyable to follow spoken instructions from someone with a pleasant voice. Mastering the technique usually takes about two weeks of daily practice. Progressive

relaxation also can be practiced from a seated position at work—but beware of excessive relaxation (such as falling out of your chair). Using progressive relaxation with the breathing techniques discussed on pages 496 and 497 intensifies its effect.

Progressive relaxation also is effective for children eight years old and older, especially in relieving tension headaches. To learn the technique, children may require four to six one-hour sessions with a parent or teacher over the course of a month. The effects of progressive relaxation are greater the longer it is practiced, especially if done for one-half hour each week for six months.

Visualization

Visualization, also known as guided imagery, is a practice of concentration on images held in the mind's eye. Visualization works with the connection between the visual cortex at the back of the head and the involuntary nervous system. When this part of the brain is not engaged by input from the eyes, it seems to be able to influence physical and emotional states. There is considerable scientific evidence that visualization can affect health. Visualization can be learned from books, self-help tapes, or from instructors, especially psychologists and hypnotherapists who specialize in it.

Yoga

The term *yoga* originally meant "to join together." The practice of yoga is widely used to harmonize body, mind, and spirit. Although there are a number of different types of yoga, all involve coordinated patterns of breathing and movement.

Yoga is an excellent form of relaxation as well as a means of nonaerobic body conditioning. It is successfully used to improve health in ways as varied as reducing stress from academic exams, easing insomnia, reducing the risk of heart attack, lowering cholesterol and triglyceride levels, boosting immune function, increasing manual dexterity, lifting depression, and increasing the cardiovascular conditioning effects of aerobic workouts. But since yoga requires commitment to a formal practice, it is best done with a teacher, at least in the beginning.

SITZ BATHS

A sitz bath is a treatment in which you sit either in plain water or in an herbal solution. Sitz baths are used to treat anal fissures and hemorrhoids. In a group of more than 100 people with first time, acute anal fissures, those who used sitz baths plus a high intake of unprocessed bran had less pain and more healed fissures after three weeks than those who received Lignocaine ointment or hydrocortisone ointment. Sitz baths are easy to use and inexpensive and bring about quick relief to people with anal fissures. To make a sitz bath, place 1 ounce of the recommended herb in

2 quarts of water that have just been boiled and removed from the source of heat. Allow the mixture to stand for one hour; then strain. Making sure the herbal mixture is lukewarm, pour it into a tub to which just enough water has been added to reach portions of the body to be bathed. Use water that is slightly on the hot side but not so hot that it is unbearable. Immerse the affected area for fifteen to twenty minutes once or twice daily; you may need to refill the bath to keep the water warm enough.

For external hemorrhoids, taking a sitz bath in plain, warm water to relieve irritation and pain can be helpful. Fill a bathtub with enough water to cover up to the middle of the abdomen. Use water that is about 120°F. If the water is uncomfortably hot, try using a cold compress on your forehead to cool you down while you're soaking. (People who have congestive heart failure should avoid hot baths.) Stay in the bath for twenty to forty minutes, and finish by splashing the area with cool water or taking a quick cold shower.

SKIN WASHES

Skin washes are used to relieve skin inflammation and excessive sweating. To make a skin wash, prepare an herbal tea or a mixture made with a dropperful of herb tincture in ¼ cup, or 60 milliliters, of warm water. (See TEAS and/or TINCTURES.) Bathe the affected area with a cloth, or immerse it in a washbasin filled with the mixture. To reduce inflammation, you can make the wash by adding 5 to 10 drops of essential oil to 1 quart of lukewarm water. (See AROMATHERAPY for a discussion of essential oils.)

For acne, dip a clean soft cotton cloth in the lukewarm herbal infusion and wash the infected area with light, circular motions. The herb acts on diseased skin, and light rubbing increases blood flow to the area. This differs from a compress in that the compress is placed against the skin without rubbing. (See COMPRESSES.)

STEAM INHALATIONS

Steam inhalations are a combination of steam and herbal antiseptic ingredients that can help clear up colds, hay fever, and perhaps sinusitis. To make a steam inhalation, pour 1 quart of water that has just been boiled into a large bowl, add 5 to 10 drops of essential oil, and stir well. (See AROMATHERAPY for a discussion of essential oils.) If essential oil is not available, make an infusion by brewing 1 ounce (30 grams) of the recommended herb in 1 quart of hot water for fifteen minutes.

Lean over the bowl without getting too close, and cover your head and the bowl with a large towel. Keeping your eyes closed, inhale the steam for about ten minutes or until the preparation cools. After a steam inhalation, it is advisable to stay in a warm room for at least thirty minutes to allow air passages to adjust and mucus to clear.

SYRUPS

Syrups are sweetened liquids used to relieve coughing or to mask the flavor of an herbal tincture. To make syrup, combine 1 pound (450 grams) of sugar and 1 cup (250 milliliters) of water in a saucepan. Stirring constantly, bring the mixture to a boil and then simmer until all the sugar crystals are dissolved. Let the syrup cool and store in a dark bottle in the refrigerator. Add the syrup to tinctures as needed to make them palatable. (See TINCTURES.)

Cough syrups are made by combining tinctures of any of the herbs recommended for cough in a ratio of one part tincture to two parts syrup. Take the same number of tablespoons of syrup as teaspoons recommended for the tincture. For example, if a remedy calls for 1 teaspoon of tincture, take 1 tablespoon of the syrup. For children, be sure to use glycerin-based tinctures rather than alcohol-based tinctures, but do not use either before consulting the child's pediatrician. Cough syrups should be stored in the refrigerator, properly labeled, and can be used for up to three months.

TEAS

Teas are the traditional means of preparing herbs for health. For practical purposes, the term *tea* is synonymous with decoction, which is any liquid preparation of a medicinal herb made with boiling water. Almost all herbs can be taken as teas; exceptions to this rule are noted in the descriptions of each herb in Part One.

The easiest way to prepare an herbal tea is to use a tea bag. Simply bring a cup of water to boiling, and place the water and the tea bag in a porcelain teapot or cup, preferably covered. Allow the water and tea bag to stand for about five to ten minutes. Remove the tea bag and drink the tea or use the tea as part of one of the suggested remedies in this book.

Tea bags offer many advantages, but also have certain disadvantages. The major advantage of using tea bags is that it is not necessary to measure the herb. Also, the herbs in bagged teas are more finely ground than the herbs in loose teas, and therefore release more water-soluble healing ingredients into the tea. However, not all the healing ingredients in herbs are water soluble, which is one of the disadvantages of using tea bags. The healing properties of some herbs are in their essential oils, which are released when the herb is ground or crushed. Therefore, the oil "glands" in the herb must be broken just before the tea is made. If the herb is ground to fill a tea bag without making lumps, the volatile oils are released into the air at the factory, not when the tea is prepared. Also, bagged teas cannot be inspected for the presence of foreign matter.

To make teas from loose herbs, always use a nonmetallic pot, although the water can be boiled in a metal kettle (stainless steel is best) before being poured into the brewing vessel. Do not use a metallic tea ball for brewing medicinal herbs. Metals, particularly aluminum and iron, could leach out of metallic and aluminum-coated utensils and could cause unknown chemical reactions with the herbs. The pot must have a tight-fitting lid and be clean. Place the recommended amount of the herb in the teapot, cover with 1 cup of water (use good-quality bottled water) that has been brought to a boil, and allow to stand for five to ten minutes with the cover on. Strain and drink.

Chinese herbal teas are always prepared from custom-made combinations of loose herbs. They are heated on the stove rather than brewed in a pot. If the amount of water to be used is not specified, the rule is to cover the herbs with about 1 inch of water before heating. Usually this is 1 to 1¼ cups of water for every ounce of herbs. Before beginning this process, allow the herbs to soak in the water for ten to fifteen minutes. The rule for heating Chinese herbal teas is "start fast, end slow." Bring the water to a boil, using high heat, and then simmer. Most formulas are heated for between twenty and thirty minutes, and then taken in the number of doses prescribed by an herbalist.

It is important not to lift the lid of the pot too often during the tea-making process, since many herbs contain aromatic oils that can escape if they are boiled in an open pot. If the tea is overcooked or burned, discard the herbs. Never add water to cook again.

In making teas from herbs dispensed by a Chinese pharmacy or practitioner of traditional Chinese medicine (TCM), certain herbs and other healing substances require special handling. Some, such as "dragon bone," should be boiled for thirty to forty-five minutes to ensure that its active ingredients enter the tea. Other herbs, such as peppermint, are added at the end of the tea-making process, approximately five minutes before the water is taken off the heat. These herbs contain aromatic oils that may escape during a long boil. Ginseng, because of its expense, is usually boiled separately to obtain maximum effect. It may be sliced thin and then boiled in a double-boiler for two to three hours to ensure that all the active ingredients are released.

TINCTURES

Tinctures are made by soaking an herb in alcohol. This causes the active constituents of the plant to dissolve, and gives tinctures a stronger action than teas or infusions. Tinctures are simple to use and can be kept for up to two years.

To make a tincture, place the herb in a large, clean glass (not plastic) jar, preferably one that is dark. For every one part of herb, add five parts of vodka or rum. Usually, 200 to 300 grams (6 to 10 ounces) of herb is enough to make 1 quart (1 liter) of tincture. Make sure that the herb is completely covered. Close and label the jar. Shake well for one to two minutes; then allow the herbs and alcohol to stand in a cool dark place for two weeks.

After the herbs have soaked in the alcohol for two weeks, strain the liquid through muslin or a winepress. Once the liquid has been extracted, discard the leftover herbs. Pour the tincture into clean dark bottles using a funnel. When the bottles are full, stopper with a cork or screw top and label the bottles.

Alcohol tinctures should be avoided by children and pregnant women, and by anyone who has gastritis or peptic ulcers. To remove the alcohol from a tincture, place the dose of tincture in a small glass of water that has just been taken off the boil. Allow the mixture to stand for five minutes. This allows the alcohol to evaporate. To make alcohol-free tinctures for children's use, substitute the vodka or rum with glycerol or natural cider vinegar and follow the directions above, but check with the child's pediatrician first.

Never use industrial alcohol, methylated spirits (methyl alcohol), or rubbing alcohol (isopropyl alcohol) in the preparation of tinctures.

References

The recommendations in this book have been based on the authority of some 2,000 published studies in medical journals and scientific reviews. In addition, for almost every herb and health problem entry we have consulted *The Complete German Commission E Monographs* and the *PDR for Herbal Medicines*.

PART ONE: UNDERSTANDING HERBAL HEALING

Principles of Herbal Treatment

Aboelsoud N.H., "Herbal Medicine in Ancient Egypt," *Journal of Medicinal Plants Research* 42 (2010): 82–86.

Angell, M., and J.P. Kassirer, "Alternative Medicine—the Risks of Untested and Unregulated Remedies," *The New England Journal of Medicine* 339 (1998): 839–841.

Blumenthal M., "Herb Sales Down in Mainstream Market," *HerbalGram* 66 (2005): 63.

Blumenthal, M., senior ed., Werner R. Busse, Alicia Goldberg, Joerg Gruenwald, et al., eds., *The Complete German Commission E Monographs: Therapeutic Guide to Herbal Medicines*, trans. Sigrid Klein and Robert S. Rister, foreword by Varro E. Tyler (Boston, MA: Integrative Medicine Communications, 1998).

"Dangerous Supplements," *Consumer Reports*, September 2010: 16–23.

Druss, B.G., and R.A. Rosenheck, "Association Between Use of Unconventional Therapies and Conventional Medical Services," *Journal of the American Medical Association* 282(7) (1999): 651–656.

Gebo, K.A., J.A. Fleishman, R. Conviser, et al., "Contemporary Costs of HIV Healthcare in the HAART Era," *AIDS* 24 (2010): 2705–2715.

Gruenwald J., T. Brendler, and C. Jaenicke, *PDR for Herbal Medicine*, 4th ed. (Montvale, NJ: Thompson Healthcare, Inc., 2007).

"Homeopathy," http://www.amfoundation.org/homeopathinfo.htm.

Lazarou, J., "Incidence of Adverse Drug Reactions in Hospitalized Patients: A Meta-Analysis of Prospective Studies," *Journal of the American Medical Association* 279 (1998): 1200–1205.

The Herbs

Acerola

Càceres, M., B. López, X. Juárez, et al., "Plants Used in Guatemala for the Treatment of Dermatophytic Infections. 2. Evaluation of Antifungal Activity of Seven American Plants," *Journal of Ethnopharmacology* 40(3) (December 1993): 207–213.

Leme, J., Jr., H. Fonseca, and J.N. Nogueira, "Variation of Ascorbic Acid and Beta-Carotene Content in Lyophilized Cherry from the West Indies," *Archivos Latinoamericanos de Nutrición* [*Latin American Archives of Nutrition*] 23(2) (June 1973): 207–215.

Taylor, L., *Wealth of the Rainforest* (Austin, TX: Raintree Marketing Group, 1997), p. 18.

Agrimony

Swanston-Flatt, S.K., C. Day, C.J. Bailey, et al., "Traditional Plant Treatments for Diabetes. Studies in Normal and Streptozotocin Diabetic Mice," *Diabetologia* 33(8) (August 1990): 462–464.

Alfalfa

Crellin, J.K., and J. Philpott, *A Reference Guide to Medicinal Plants: Herbal Medicine Past and Present* (Durham, NC: Duke University Press, 1990), pp. 45–46.

Malinow, M.R., "Alfalfa," *Atherosclerosis* 30 (1973): 27–43.

Molgaard, J., H. von Schenck, A.G. Olsson, et al., "Alfalfa Seeds Lower Low Density Lipoprotein Cholesterol and Apolipoprotein B Concentrations in Patients with Type II Hyperlipoproteinemia," *Atherosclerosis* 65 (1987): 173–179.

Roberts, J.L., and J.A. Hayashi, "Exacerbation of SLE Associated with Alfalfa Ingestion," *The New England Journal of Medicine* 308 (1983): 1381.

Zhao, W.S., Y.Q. Zhang, L.J. Ren, et al., "Immunopotentiating Effects of Polysaccharides Isolated from Medicago Sativa L.," *Chung-Kuo Yao Li Hsueh Pao* [*Acta Pharmacologica Sinica*] 14(3) (May 1993): 273–276.

Aloe

Agarwal, O.P., "Prevention of Atheromatous Heart Disease," *Angiology* 36 (1985): 485–492.

Brusick, D., and U. Mengs, "Assessment of the Genotoxic Risk from Laxative Senna Products," *Environmental and Molecular Mutagenesis* 29(1) (1997): 1–9.

Chung, J.H., J.C. Cheong, J.Y. Lee, et al., "Acceleration of the Alcohol Oxidation Rate in Rats with Aloin, a Quinone Derivative of Aloe," *Biochemical Pharmacology* 52(9) (8 November 1996): 1461–1468.

Danhof, I., "Potential Reversal of Chronological and Photo-Aging of the Skin by Topical Application of Natural Substances," *Phytotherapy Research* 7 (1993): S53–S56.

Davis, R.H., W.L. Parker, and D.P. Murdoch, "Aloe Vera as a Biologically Active Vehicle for Hydrocortisone Acetate," *Journal of the American Podiatric Medical Association* 81(1) (January 1991): 1–9.

Desai, K.N., H. Wei, and C.A. Lamartiniere, "The Preventive and Therapeutic Potential of the Squalene-Containing Compound, Roidex, on Tumor Promotion and Regression," *Cancer Letters* 101(1) (19 March 1996): 93–96.

Egger, S.F., G.S. Brown, L.S. Kelsey, et al., "Hematopoietic Augmentation by a Beta-(1,4)-Linked Mannan," *Cancer Immunology and Immunotherapy* 43(4) (December 1996): 195–205.

Fulton, J.E., Jr., "The Stimulation of Postdermabrasion Wound Healing with Stabilized Aloe Vera Gel-Polyethylene Oxide Dressing," *Journal of Dermatologic Surgery and Oncology* 16(5) (May 1990): 460–467.

Ghannam, N., M. Kingston, I.A. Al-Meshall, et al., "The Antidiabetic Activity of Aloes: Preliminary Clinical and Experimental Observations," *Hormone Research* 24 (1986): 288–294.

Gribel, N.V., and V.G. Pashinskii, "Antimetastatic Properties of Aloe Juice," *Voprosy Onkologii* [*Questions in Oncology*] 32(12) (1986): 38–40.

Hutter, J.A., M. Salman, W.B. Stavinoha, et al., "Anti-Inflammatory C-Glucosyl Chromone from *Aloe Barbadensis*," *Journal of Natural Products* 59(5) (May 1996): 541–543.

Imanishi, K., "Aloctin A, An Active Substance of *Aloe arborescens* Miller, as an Immunomodulator," *Phytotherapy Research* 7 (Spring 1993): S20–S23.

Imanishi, K., T. Ishiguro, H. Saito, and I. Suzuki, "Pharmacological Studies on a Plant Lectin, Aloctin A. I. Growth Inhibition of Mouse Methylcholanthrene-Induced Fibrosarcoma (Meth A) in Ascites Form by Aloctin A," *Experientia*, 37 (1981): 1186–1187.

Karaca, K., J.M. Sharma, and R. Nordgren, "Nitric Oxide Production by Chicken Macrophages Activated by Acemannan, a Complex Carbohydrate Extracted from Aloe Vera," *International Journal of Immunopharmacology* 17(3) (March 1995): 183–188.

Kim, H.S., and B.M. Lee, "Inhibition of Benzoapyrene-DNA Adduct Formation by *Aloe Barbadensis* Miller," *Carcinogenesis* 18(4) (April 1997): 771–776.

Langmead, L., R. M. Feakins, S. Goldthorpe, et al., "Randomized, Double-Blind, Placebo-Controlled Trial of the Aloe Vera Gel for Active Ulcerative Colitis," *Alimentation Pharmacology Therapy* 19(7) (2004): 739–47.

Odes, H.S., and Z. Madar, "A Double-Blind Trial of a Celandin, Aloe Vera and Psyllium Laxative Preparation in Adult Patients with Constipation," *Digestion* 49(2) (1991): 65–71.

Roberts, D.B., and E.L. Travis, "Acemannan-Containing Wound Dressing Gel Reduces Radiation-Induced Skin Reactions in C3H Mice," *International Journal of Radiation Oncology, Biology, and Physics* 32(4) (15 July 1995): 1047–1052.

Saito, H., K. Imanishi, and S. Okabe, "Effects of Aloe Extract, Aloctin A, on Gastric Secretion and on Experimental Gastric Lesions in Rats," *Yakugaku Zasshi* [*Journal of the Pharmaceutical Society of Japan*] 109 (1989): 335–339.

Saito, H., K. Imanishi, and I. Suzuki, "Pharmacological Studies on a Plant Lectin, Aloctin A. II. Inhibitory Effect of Aloctin A on Experimental Models of Inflammation in Rats," *Japanese Journal of Pharmacology* 32 (1982): 139–142.

Sakai, K., Y. Saitoh, C. Ikawa, et al., "Effect of Water Extracts of Aloe and Some Herbs in Decreasing Blood Ethanol Concentration in Rats. II," *Chemical and Pharmaceutical Bulletin* 37(1) (January 1989): 155–159.

Sakai, R., "Epidemiologic Survey on Lung Cancer with Respect to Cigarette Smoking and Plant Diet," *Japanese Journal of Cancer Research* 80(6) (June 1989): 513–520.

Siegers, C.P., E. Von Hertzberg-Lottin, M. Otte, et al., "Anthranoid Laxative Abuse—a Risk for Colorectal Cancer?" *Gut* 34(8) (August 1993): 1099–1101.

Suzuki, I., H. Saito, S. Inoue, et al., "Purification and Characterization of Two Lectins from *Aloe arborescens* Mill.," *Journal of Biochemistry* 85 (1979): 163–171.

Sydiskis, R.J., D.G. Owen, J.L. Lohr, et al., "Inactivation of Enveloped Viruses by Anthraquinones Extracted from Plants," *Antimicrobial Agents and Chemotherapy* 35(12) (December 1991): 2463–2466.

Syed, T.A., M. Afral, A.S. Ashfaq, et al., "Management of Genital Herpes in Men with 0.5% Aloe Vera Extract in a Hydrophilic Cream: A Placebo-Controlled Double-Blind Study," *The Journal of Dermatological Treatment* 8 (1997): 99–102.

Syed, T.A., S.A. Ahmad, A.H. Holt, et al., "Management of Psoriasis with Aloe Vera Extract in a Hydrophilic Cream, a Placebo-Controlled, Double-Blind Study,"

Tropical Medicine and International Health 1(4) (August 1996): 505–509.

Visuthikosol, V., B. Chowchuen, Y. Sukwanarat, et al., "Effect of Aloe Vera Gel to Healing of Burn Wound: A Clinical and Histologic Study," *Journal of the Medical Association of Thailand* 78(8) (August 1995): 403–409.

Womble, D., and J.H. Helderman, "Enhancement of Allo-Responsiveness of Human Lymphocytes by Acemannan (Carrisyn)," *International Journal of Immunopharmacology* 10(8) (1988): 967–974.

Yagi, T., K. Yamauchi, and S. Kuwano, "The Synergistic Purgative Action of Aloe-Emodin Anthrone and Rhein Anthrone in Mice, Synergism in Large Intestinal Propulsion and Water Secretion," *Journal of Pharmacy and Pharmacology* 49(1) (January 1997): 22–25.

Zawahry, M.E., M.R. Hegazy, and M. Heial, "Use of Aloe in Treating Leg Ulcers and Dermatoses," *International Journal of Dermatology* 12 (1973): 69–73.

Zhang, L., and I.R. Tizard, "Activation of a Mouse Macrophage Cell Line by Acemannan, the Major Carbohydrate Fraction from Aloe Vera Gel," *Immunopharmacology* 35(2) (November 1996): 119–128.

American Ginseng

Benishin, C.G., R. Lee, L.C. Wang, et al., "Effects of Ginsenoside Rb1 on Central Cholinergic Metabolism," *Pharmacology* 42(4) (1991): 223–229.

Chen, X., S.J. Yang, L. Chen, et al., "The Effects of Panax Quinquefolium Saponin (PQS) and Its Monomer Ginsenoside on Heart," *Chung-Kuo Chung Yao Tsa Chih* [*China Journal of Chinese Materica Medica*] 19(10) (October 1994): 617–620.

Huang, Kee C., and Kee Chang, eds., *The Pharmacology of Chinese Herbs* (Boca Raton, FL: CRC Press, 1992), p. 35.

Wang, W.K., H.L. Chen, T.L. Hsu, et al., "Alteration of Pulse in Human Subjects by Three Chinese Herbs," *American Journal of Chinese Medicine* 22(2) (1994): 197–203.

Andiroba

Ando, H., A. Ryu, A. Hashimoto, et al., "Linoleic Acid and Alpha-Linolenic Acid Lightens Ultraviolet-Induced Hyperpigmentation of the Skin," *Archives of Dermatological Research* 290(7) (July 1998): 375–381.

Steinert, P.M., S.Y. Kim, S.I. Chung, et al., "The Transglutaminase 1 Enzyme Is Variably Acylated by Myristate and Palmitate During Differentiation in Epidermal Keratinocytes," *Journal of Biological Chemistry* 271(4) (18 October 1996): 26242–26250.

Andrographis

Basak, A., S. Cooper, A.G. Roberge, et al., "Inhibition of Proprotein Covertases-1, -7 and Furin by Diterpines of *Andrographis paniculata* and their Succinoyl Esters," *Biochemistry Journal* 338 (Part1) (15 February 1999): 107–113.

Bone, K., "*Andrographis paniculata*," *British Journal of Phytotherapy* 5 (2001): 107–113.

Caceres, D.D., J.L. Haricke, R.A. Burgos, and G.K. Wilkman, "Prevention of Common Colds with *Andrographis paniculata* Dried Extract: A Pilot Double-Blind Trial," *Phytomedicine* 4(2) (1997): 101–104.

Chang, R.S., L. Ding, G.Q. Chen, et al., "Dehydroandographolide Succinic Acid Monoester as an Inhibitor Against the Human Immunodeficiency Virus," *Proceedings of the Society for Experimental Biology and Medicine* 197(1) (May 1991): 59–66.

Melchior, J., S. Palm, and G. Wikman, "Controlled Study of Standardized *Andrographis paniculata* Extract in the Common Cold—A Pilot Trial," *Phytomedicine* 3(4) (1996/97): 315–318.

Paracelsian, Inc., "Preliminary Results of Safety Study Show Androvir Is Well Tolerated," Press Release, 12 December 1996.

Zhang, Y.Z., J.Z. Tang, and Y.J. Zhang, "Study of *Andrographis paniculata* Extracts on Antiplatelet Aggregation and Release Reaction and Its Mechanism," *Chung-Kuo Chung Hsi I Chieh Ho Tsa Chih* [*Chinese Journal of Modern Developments in Traditional Medicine*] 14(1) (January 1994): 28–30, 34, 35.

Anise

Bruneton, Jean N., *Pharmacognosy, Phytochemistry, Medicinal Plants* (Paris, France: Lavoisier Publishing, 1995), p. 444.

Arjuna

Bharani, A., A. Ganbuly, and K.D. Bhargava, "Salutary Effect of *Terminalia arjuna* in Patients with Severe Refractory Heart Failure," *International Journal of Cardiology* 49(3) (May 1995): 191–199.

Dwivedi, S., and M.P. Agarwal, "Antianginal and Cardioprotective Effects of *Terminalia arjuna,* an Indigenous Drug, in Coronary Artery Disease," *Journal of the Association of Physicians of India* 42(4) (April 1994): 287–289.

Lalla, J.K., S.Y. Nandedkar, M.H. Paranjape, et al., "Clinical Trials of Ayurvedic Formulations in the Treatment of Acne Vulgaris," *Journal of Ethnopharmacology* 78(1) (November 2001): 99–101.

Pettie, G.R., M.S. Hoard, D.L. Doubek, et al., "Antineoplastic Agents 338. The Cancer Cell Growth Inhibitory. Constituents of *Terminalia arjuna* (Combretaceae)," *Journal of Ethnopharmacology* 53(2) (August 1996): 57–63.

Singh, B.B., S.P. Vinjamury, C. Der-Martirosian, et al., "Ayurvedic and Collateral Herbal Treatments for Hyperlipidemia: A Systematic Review of Randomized Controlled Trials and Quasi-Experimental Designs," *Alternative Therapy* 13(4) (2007): 22–28.

Arnicia

Hart, O., M.A. Muller, G. Lewith, et al., "Double-Blind, Placebo-Controlled Randomized Clinical Trial of Homeopathic Arnica C30 for Pain and Infection After Total Abdominal Hysterectomy," *Journal of the Royal Society of Medicine* 5(5) (1997): 73–78.

Robertson, A., R. Suryanarayanan, A. Banerjee, "Homeopathic *Arnica montana* for Post-Tonsillectomy Analgesia: A Randomized Placebo Control Trial," *Homeopathy* 96(1) (2007): 17–21.

Schroder, H., W. Losche, H. Strobach, et al., "Helenalin and 11-Alpha,13-Dihydrohelenalin, Two Constituents from *Arnica montana* L., Inhibit Human Platelet Function via Thiol-Dependent Pathways," *Thrombosis Research* 57(6) (15 March 1990): 839–845.

Tveiten, D., S. Bruseth, C.F. Borchgrevink, and K. Lohne, "Effect of Arnica D 30 During Hard Physical Exertion. A Double-Blind Randomized Trial During the Oslo Marathon 1990," *Tidsskrift for den Norske Lægeforening* [*Norwegian Physicians' Journal*] 111(30) (10 December 1991): 3630–3631.

Wagner, H., A. Proksch, I. Riess-Maurer, et al., "Immunostimulatory Effects of Polysaccharides (Heteroglycans) of Higher Plants," *Arzneimittel-forschung* [*Medication Research*] 35(7) (1985): 1069–1075.

Wichtl, Max, ed., *Herbal Drugs and Phytopharmaceuticals: A Handbook for Practice on a Scientific Basis*, trans. Norman Grainger Bisset (Boca Raton, FL: MedPharm Scientific Publishers, 1995), p. 85.

Artemisia

"Differentiations to UTI Protocol," *Protocol Journal of Botanical Medicine* 1(1) (Summer 1995): 135.

Huang, Kee C., and Kee Chang, eds., *The Pharmacology of Chinese Herbs* (Boca Raton, FL: CRC Press, 1992), p. 344.

Asafoetida

Bordia, A., and S.K. Arora, "The Effect of Essential Oil (Active Principle) of Asafoetida on Alimentary Lipemia," *Indian Journal of Medical Research* 63 (1975): 707–711.

Bradley, P.R., *British Herbal Compendium* (Dorset, England: British Herbal Medical Association, 1992), p. 25.

Ashwagandha

Devi, P.U., "*Withania somnifera* Dunal (Ashwagandha): Potential Plant Source of a Promising Drug for Cancer Chemotherapy and Radiosensitization," *Indian Journal of Experimental Biology* 34(10) (October 1996): 927–932.

Schliebs, R., A. Liebmann, S.K. Bhattacharya, et al., "Systemic Administration of Defined Extracts from *Withania somnifera* (Indian Ginseng) and Shilajit Differentially Affects Cholinergic but Not Glutamatergic and GABAergic Markers in Rat Brain," *Neurochemistry International* 30(2) (February 1997): 181–190.

Sodhi, Verender, "Ashwagandha for Rejuvenation," New Editions Health World, cited in Landis, R. *Herbal Defense* (New York, NY: Warner Books, 1997), p. 378.

Wurtman, Robert J., et al., "Choline Metabolism in Cholinergic Neurons: Implications for the Pathogenesis of Neurodegenerative Diseases," in *Advances in Neurology* 51: *Alzheimer's Disease*, ed. Judith Wurtman (New York, NY: Raven Press, 1990), pp. 117–125.

Yarnell, E., and K. Abascal, "Botanical Medicine for Thyroid Regulation," *Alternative & Complementary Therapy* (June 2009): 107–112.

Ziauddin, M., N. Phansalkar, P. Patki, et al., "Studies on the Immunomodulatory Effects of Ashwagandha," *Journal of Ethnopharmacology* 50(2) (February 1996): 69–76.

Astragalus

Bensky, Dan, and Andrew Gamble, compilers, *Chinese Herbal Medicine: Materia Medica*, rev. ed. (Seattle, WA: Eastland Press, 1993), p. 320.

Cha, R.J., D.W. Zeng, and Q.S. Chang, "Non-Surgical Treatment of Small Cell Lung Cancer with Chemo-Radio-Immunotherapy and Traditional Chinese Medicine," *Chung-Hua Nei Ko Tsa Chih* [*Chinese Journal of Internal Medicine*] 33(7) (July 1994): 462–466.

Chang, H.M., and P.P.H. But, *Pharmacology and Applications of Chinese Materia Medica*, vol. 2 (Teaneck, NJ: World Scientific Publishing, 1987), pp. 1041–1046.

Chen, L.X., J.Z. Liao, and W.Q. Guo, "Effects of *Astragalus membranaceus* on Left Ventricular Function and Oxygen Free Radical in Acute Myocardial Infarction Patients and Mechanism of Its Cardiotonic Action," *Chung-Kuo Chung Hsi I Chieh Ho Tsa Chih* [*Chinese Journal of Modern Developments in Traditional Medicine*] 15(3) (March 1995): 141–143.

Chen, Y.C., "Experimental Studies on the Effects of *Danggui Buxue* Decoction on IL-2 Production of

Blood-Deficient Mice," *Chung-Kuo Chung Yao Tsa Chih* [*China Journal of Chinese Materia Medica*] 19(12) (December 1994): 739–741, 763.

Chu, D.T., J.R. Lin, and W. Wong, "The In Vitro Potentiation of LAK Cell Cytotoxicity in Cancer and AIDS Patients Induced by F3—a Fractionated Extract of *Astragalus membranaceus*," *Chung-Hua Chung Liu Tsa Chih* [*Chinese Journal of Oncology*] 16(3) (May 1994): 167–171.

Deng, C.Q., J.W. Ge, and Q. Wang, "Comparison of Effect of *Astragalus membranaceus* and *Huoxuefang* on Thromboxane, Prostacyclin and Adenosine Cyclic Monophosphate in Cerebral Reperfusion Injury in Rabbits," *Chung-Kuo Chung Hsi I Chieh Ho Tsa Chih* [*Chinese Journal of Modern Developments in Traditional Medicine*] 15(3) (March 1995): 165–167.

Guo, Q., T.Q. Peng, and Y.Z. Yang, "Effect of *Astragalus membranaceus* on Ca2+ Influx and Coxsackie Virus B3 RNA Replication in Cultured Neonatal Rat Heart Cells," *Chung-Kuo Chung Hsi I Chieh Ho Tsa Chih* [*Chinese Journal of Modern Developments in Traditional Medicine*] 15(8) (August 1995): 483–485.

Hong, C.Y., J. Ku, and P. Wu, "*Astragalus membranaceus* Stimulates Human Sperm Motility in Vitro," *American Journal of Chinese Medicine* 20(3–4) (1992): 289–294.

Huang, W.M., J. Yan, and J. Xu, "Clinical and Experimental Study on Inhibitory Effect of Sanhuang Mixture on Platelet Aggregation," *Chung-Kuo Chung Hsi I Chieh Ho Tsa Chih* [*Chinese Journal of Modern Developments in Traditional Medicine*] 15(8) (August 1995): 465–467.

Jin, R., L.L. Wan, and T. Mitsuishi, "Effects of *Shi-ka-ron* and Chinese Herbs in Mice Treated with Anti-tumor Agent Mitomycin C," *Chung-Kuo Chung Hsi I Chieh Ho Tsa Chih* [*Chinese Journal of Modern Developments in Traditional Medicine*] 15(2) (February 1995): 101–103.

Jingzi, L.I., Y.U. Kei, L.I. Ningjur, et al., "*Astragalus mongholicus* and *Angelica sinensis* Compound Alleviates Nephrotic Hyperlipidemia in Rats," *Clinical Medicine Journal* 113(4) (2000): 310–314.

Li, S.Q., R.X. Yuan, and H. Gao, "Clinical Observation on the Treatment of Ischemic Heart Disease with *Astragalus membranaceus*," *Chung-Kuo Chung Hsi I Chieh Ho Tsa Chih* [*Chinese Journal of Modern Developments in Traditional Medicine*] 15(2) (February 1995): 77–80.

Liang, H., Z. Wang, F. Tian, and B. Geng, "Effects of Astragalus Polysaccharides and Ginsenosides of Ginseng Stems and Leaves on Lymphocytes Membrane Fluidity and Lipid Peroxidation in Traumatized Mice," *Chung-Kuo Chung Yao Tsa Chih* [*China Journal of Chinese Materia Medica*] 20(9) (September 1995): 558–560, inside back cover.

Liang, H., Y. Zhang, and B. Geng, "The Effect of Astragalus Polysaccharides (APS) on Cell Mediated Immunity (CMI) in Burned Mice," *Chung-Hua Cheng Hsing Shao Shang Wai Ko Tsa Chih* [*Chinese Journal of Plastic Surgery and Burns*] 10(2) (March 1994): 138–141.

Lin, L., H. Zhang, Q. Gao, and J. Ma, "A Clinical Study on Treatment of Vascular Complications of Diabetes with the Sugar-Reducing and Pulse-Invigorating Capsule," *Journal of Traditional Chinese Medicine* (English-language version) 14(1) (March 1994): 3–9.

Luo, H.M., R.H. Dai, and Y. Li, "Nuclear Cardiology Study on Effective Ingredients of *Astragalus membranaceus* in Treating Heart Failure," *Chung-Kuo Chung Hsi I Chieh Ho Tsa Chih* [*Chinese Journal of Modern Developments in Traditional Medicine*] 15(12) (December 1995): 707–709.

McCulloch, M., C. See, X.J. Shu, et al., "Astragalus-Based Chinese Herbs and Plantinum-Based Chemotherapy for Advanced Non-Small-Cell Lung Cancer: Meta-Analysis of Randomized Trials," *Journal of Clinical Oncology* 24 (2006): 419–430.

Shi, H.M., R.H. Dai, and W.H. Fan, "Intervention of Lidocaine and *Astragalus membranaceus* on Ventricular Late Potentials," *Chung-Kuo Chung Hsi I Chieh Ho Tsa Chih* [*Chinese Journal of Modern Developments in Traditional Medicine*] 14(10) (October 1994): 598–600.

Taixiang, W., A.J. Munro, L. Guanjian, and G.J. Liu, "Chinese Medical Herbs for Chemotherapy Side Effects in Colorectal Cancer Patients," Cochrane Database of Systematic Reviews 2005, Issue 1. Art. No.: CD004540. DOI: 10.1002/14651858.CD004540.pub2.

Tang, W., and G. Eisenbrand, *Chinese Drugs of Plant Origin: Chemistry, Pharmacology, and Use in Traditional and Modern Medicine* (Berlin, Germany: Springer Verlag, 1992), p. 196.

Tu, L.H., D.R. Huang, R.Q. Zhang, et al., "Regulatory Action of *Astragalus* Saponins and *Buzhong Yiqi* Compound on Synthesis of Nicotinic Acetylcholine Receptor Antibody in Vitro for Myasthenia Gravis," *Chinese Medical Journal* 107(4) (April 1994): 300–303.

Wagner, H., A. Proksch, I. Riess-Maurer, et al., "Immunostimulatory Effects of Polysaccharides (Heteroglycans) of Higher Plants," *Arzneimittel-forschung* [*Medication Research*] 35 (1985): 1069–1075.

Weng, X.S., "Treatment of Leukopenia with Pure Astragalus Preparation: An Analysis of 115 Leukopenic Cases," *Chung-Kuo Chung Hsi I Chieh Ho Tsa Chih* [*Chinese Journal of Modern Developments in Traditional Medicine*] 15(8) (August 1995): 462–464.

Yan, H.J., "Clinical and Experimental Study of the Effect of *Kang Er Xin-i* on Viral Myocarditis," *Chung-Kuo Chung Hsi I Chieh Ho Tsa Chih* [*Chinese Journal of Modern*

Developments in Traditional Medicine] 11(8) (August 1991): 452, 468–470.

Zhao, X.Z., "Effects of *Astragalus membranaceus* and *Tripterygium hypoglancum* on Natural Killer Cell Activity of Peripheral Blood Mononuclear in Systemic Lupus Erythematosus," *Chung-Kuo Chung Hsi I Chieh Ho Tsa Chih* [*Chinese Journal of Modern Developments in Traditional Medicine*] 12(11) (November 1992): 645, 669–671.

Avena (Oat Extract)

Weiss, R.F., *Herbal Medicine* (Beaconsfield, England: Beaconsfield Publishers Ltd., 1988), p. 286.

Barberry

Bensky, Dan, and Andrew Gamble, compilers, *Chinese Herbal Medicine: Materia Medica*, rev. ed. (Seattle, WA: Eastland Press, 1993), p. 79.

Franzblau, S.G., and C. Cross, "Comparative in Vitro Antimicrobial Activity of Chinese Medicinal Herbs," *Journal of Ethnopharmacology* 15(3) (March 1986): 279–288.

Gupta, R.S., and V.P. Dixit, "Testicular Cell Population Dynamics Following Palmitine Hydroxide Treatment in Male Dogs," *Journal of Ethnopharmacology* 25(2) (April 1989): 151–157.

Huang, Y.X., "Treatment of Osteomyelitis of the Fingers by Steeping in a Coptis Decoction," *Chung-Kuo Chung Hsi I Chieh Ho Tsa Chih* [*Chinese Journal of Modern Developments in Traditional Medicine*] 5(10) (October 1985): 579.

Kaneda, Y., T. Tanaka, and T. Saw, "Effects of Berberine, a Plant Alkaloid, on the Growth of Anaerobic Protozoa in Axenic Culture," *Tokai Journal of Experimental and Clinical Medicine* 15(6) (November 1990): 417–423.

Kumazawa, Y., A. Itaake, M. Fukumoto, et al., "Activation of Peritoneal Macrophages by Berberine-Type Alkaloids in Terms of Induction of Cytostatic Activity," *International Journal of Immunopharmacology* 6 (1984): 587–592.

Mahajan, V.M., A. Sharma, and A. Rattan, "Antimycotic Activity of Berberine Sulphate: An Alkaloid from an Indian Medicinal Herb," *Sabouradia* 20 (1982): 79–81.

Mitscher, L.A., "Plant-Derived Antibiotics," in *Antibiotics, Journal of Chromatography* (Library) 15, ed. M.J. Weinstein and G.H. Wagman (New York, NY: Plenum Press, 1978), pp. 363–477.

Sabir, M., and N. Bhide, "Study of Some Pharmacologic Actions of Berberine," *Indian Journal of Pharmacy* 15 (1971): 111–132.

Zhang, L., L.W. Yang, and L.J. Yang, "Relation Between *Helicobacter pylori* and Pathogenesis of Chronic Atrophic Gastritis and the Research of Its Prevention and Treatment," *Chung-Kuo Chung Hsi I Chieh Ho Tsa Chih*

[*Chinese Journal of Modern Developments in Traditional Medicine*] 12(9) (September 1992): 515–516.

Bilberry

Allen, F.M., "Blueberry Leaf Extract: Physiologic and Clinical Properties in Relation to Carbohydrate Metabolism," *Journal of the American Medical Association* 89 (1927): 1577–1581.

Cignarella, A., M. Nastasi, E. Cavalli, and L. Puglisi, "Novel Lipid-Lowering Properties of *Vaccinium myrtillus* L. Leaves, a Traditional Antidiabetic Treatment, in Several Models of Rat Dyslipidaemia: A Comparison with Ciprofibrate," *Thrombosis Research* 84(5) (1 December 1996): 311–322.

Morazzoni, P., S. Livio, A. Scilingo, and S. Malandrino, "*Vaccinium myrtillus* Anthocyanosides Pharmacokinetics in Rats," *Arzneimittel-forschung* [*Medication Research*] 41(2) (February 1991): 128–131.

Morazzoni, P., and M.J. Magistretti, "Activity of Myrtocian, an Anthocyanoside Complex from *Vaccinium myrtillus* (VMA), on Platelet Aggregation and Adhesiveness," *Fitoterapia* [*Phytotherapy*] 61 (1990): 13–21.

Ofek, I., J. Goldhar, D. Zafrini, et al., "Anti-*Escherichia Coli* Adhesion Activity of Cranberry and Blueberry Juices," *The New England Journal of Medicine* 327 (1991): 1599.

Wichtl, Max, ed., *Herbal Drugs and Phytopharmaceuticals: A Handbook for Practice on a Scientific Basis,* trans. Norman Grainger Bisset (Boca Raton, FL: MedPharm Scientific Publishers, 1995), p. 349.

Birch

Hänsel, R., and H. Haas, *Therapie mit Phytopharmaka* (Berlin, Germany: Springer-Verlag, 1983).

Tang, J.J., J.G. Li, W. Qi, et al., "Inhibition of SREBP by a Small Molecule, Betulin, Improves Hyperlipidemia and Insulin Resistance and Reduces Atherosclerotic Plaques," *Cell Metabolism* (January 5, 2010). DOI: 10.1016/j.cmet.2010.12.004.

Wichtl, Max, ed., *Herbal Drugs and Phytopharmaceuticals: A Handbook for Practice on a Scientific Basis,* trans. Norman Grainger Bisset (Boca Raton, FL: MedPharm Scientific Publishers, 1995), p. 107.

Bitter Melon

Bever, B.O., and G.R. Zahnd, "Plants with Oral Hypoglycemic Action," *Quarterly Journal of Crude Drug Research* 17 (1979): 139–196.

Bourinbaiar, A.S., and S. Lee-Huang, "The Activity of Plant-Derived Antiretroviral Proteins MAP30 and GAP31 against Herpes Simplex Virus in Vitro,"

Biochemical and Biophysical Research Communications 219(3) (February 1996): 923–929.

Cakici, I., C. Hurmoglu, B. Tunctan, et al., "Hypoglycaemic Effect of *Momordica Charantia* Extracts in Normoglycaemic or Cyproheptadine-Induced Hyperglycaemic Mice," *Journal of Ethnopharmacology* 44(2) (October 1994): 117–121.

John, A.J., R. Cherian, H.S. Subhash, et al., "Evaluation of the Efficacy of Bitter Gourd (*Momordica charantia*) as an Oral Hypoglycemic Agent—A Randomized Controlled Clinical Trial," *Indian Journal of Physiology and Pharmacology* 47(3) (2003): 363–365.

Pongnikorn, S., D. Fongmoon, W. Kasinrerk, et al., "Effect of Bitter Melon (*Momordica charantia* Linn) on Level and Function of Natural Killer Cells in Cervical Cancer Patients with Radiotherapy," *Journal of the Medical Association of Thailand* 86(1) (January 2003): 61–68.

Tennekoon, K.H., S. Jeevathayaparan, P. Angunawala, et al., "Effect of *Momordica Charantia* on Key Hepatic Enzymes," *Journal of Ethnopharmacology* 44(2) (October 1994): 93–97.

Welihinda, J., G. Arvidson, E. Gylfe, et al., "The Insulin-Releasing Activity of the Tropical Plant *Momordica Charantia*," *Acta Biologica et Medica Germanica* 41(12) (1982): 1229–1240.

Bitter Orange

Bensky, Dan, and Andrew Gamble, compilers, *Chinese Herbal Medicine: Materia Medica*, rev. ed. (Seattle, WA: Eastland Press, 1993), p. 235.

Hosoda, K., M. Noguchi, Y.P. Chen, et al., "Studies on the Preparation and Evaluation of Kijitsu, the Immature Citrus Fruits. IV. Biological Activities of Immature Fruits of Different Citrus Species," *Yakugaku Zasshi* [*Journal of the Pharmaceutical Society of Japan*] 111(3) (March 1991): 188–192.

Black Cohosh

Bruneton, Jean N., *Pharmacognosy, Phytochemistry, Medicinal Plants* (Paris, France: Lavoisier Publishing, 1995), pp. 296–297.

Düker, E.M., L. Kopanski, H. Jarry, et al., "Effects of Extracts from *Cimicifuga Racemosa* on Gonadotropin Release in Menopausal Women and Ovariectomized Rats," *Planta Medica* 57(5) (October 1991): 420–424.

Lehmann-Willenbrock, E., and H.H. Riedel, "Clinical and Endocrinologic Studies of the Treatment of Ovarian Insufficiency Manifestations Following Hysterectomy with Intact Adnexa," *Zentralblatt für Gynakologie* [*International Journal of Gynecology*] 110(10) (1988): 611–618.

Zepelin, H.H., H. Meden, K. Kostev, et al., "Isopropanolic Black Cohosh Extract and Recurrence-free Survival After Breast Cancer," *International Journal of Clinical Pharmacology Therapy* 45(3) (2007): 143–154.

Zheng, R.L., and H. Zhang, "Effects of Ferulic Acid on Fertile and Asthenozoospermic Infertile Human Sperm Motility, Viability, Lipid Peroxidation, and Cyclic Nucleotides," *Free Radical Biology and Medicine* 22(4) (1997): 581–586.

Boswellia

Gupta, I., et al., "Effects of Gum Resin of *Boswellia Serrata* in Patients with Chronic Colitis," *Planta Medica* 67 (2001): 391–395.

Holtmeier, W., et al., "Randomized, Placebo-Controlled, Double-Blind Trial of *Boswellia serrata* in Maintaining Remission of Crohn's Disease: Good Safety Profile but Lack of Efficacy," *Inflammatory Bowel Diseases* 17 (February 2011): 573–582.

Kulkani, R.R., P.S. Patki, V.P. Jog, et al., "Treatment of Osteoarthritis with a Herbomineral Formulation: A Double-Blind, Placebo-Controlled, Cross-Over Study," *Journal of Ethnopharmacology* 33 (1991): 91–95.

Reddy, C.K., G. Chandrakasan, and S.C. Dhar, "Studies on the Metabolism of Glycosaminoglycans Under the Influence of New Herbal Anti-Inflammatory Agents," *Biochemical Pharmacology* 20 (1989): 3527–3534.

Brahmi

Kidd, P.M., "A Review of Nutrients and Botanicals in the Integrative Management of Cognitive Dysfunction," *Alternative Medicine Review* 4(3) (June 1999): 144–161.

Rao, A.B., P. Sisodia, and P.B. Sattur, "Lysosomal Membrane Stabilization by Anti-Inflammatory Drugs," *Indian Journal of Experimental Biology* 27(12) (December 1989): 1097–1098.

Shukia, B., N.K. Khanna, and J.L. Godhwani, "Effect of Brahmi Rasayan on the Central Nervous System," *Journal of Ethnopharmacology* 21(1) (September–October 1987): 65–74.

Singh, H.K., and B.N. Dhawan, "Effect of *Bacopa monniera* Linn. (brahmi) Extract on Avoidance Responses in Rat," *Journal of Ethnopharmacology* 5(2) (March 1982): 205–214.

Bromelain

Desser, L., et al., "Oral Therapy with Proteolytic Enzymes Decreases Excessive TGF-Beta Levels in Human Blood," *Cancer Chemotherapy and Pharmacology* 47(supplement) (2001): S10–S15.

Heinicke, R.M., I. Van Der Wal, and M. Yokoyama, "Effect of Bromelain (Ananase) on Human Platelet Aggregation," *Experientia* 28 (1972): 844–845.

Helms, S., A.L. Miller, "Natural Treatment of Chronic Rhinosinusitis," *Alternative Medicine Review* 11(3) (2006): 196–207.

Hunter, R.G., G.W. Henry, and R.M. Henicke, "The Action of Papain and Bromelain on the Uterus," *American Journal of Obstetrics and Gynecology* 73 (1957): 867–880.

Klein, G., et al., "Efficacy and Tolerance of an Oral Enzyme Combination in Painful Osteoarthritis of the Hip. A Double-Blind, Randomised Study Comparing Oral Enzymes with Non-Steroidal Anti-Inflammatory Drugs," *Clinical and Experimental Rheumatology* 24(1) (2006): 25–30.

Murray, Michael T., and Joseph E. Pizzorno, *Encyclopedia of Natural Medicine,* 2d. ed. (Rocklin, CA: Prima Publishing, 1997), p. 191.

Bupleurum

Bone, K., "Bupleurum: A Natural Steroid Effect," *Canadian Journal of Herbalism* (Early Winter 1996): 22–41.

Hiai, S., H. Yokoyama, T. Nagasawa, and H. Oura, "Stimulation of the Pituitary-Adrenocortical Axis by Saikosaponin of *Bupleuri radix,*" *Chemical Pharmaceutical Bulletin* 29 (1981): 495–499.

Huang, Kee C., and Kee Chang, eds., *The Pharmacology of Chinese Herbs* (Boca Raton, FL: CRC Press, 1992), p. 152.

Johnson, L., "Hepatitis C: The Quiet Epidemic," *Herbs for Health* (March/April 2000): 50–55.

Sung, C.K., G.H. Kang, S.S. Yoon, et al., "Glycosidases That Convert Natural Glycosides to Bioactive Compounds," in *Saponins Used in Traditional and Modern Medicine,* Advances in Experimental Medicine and Biology, 404, ed. George R. Waller and Kazuo Yamasaki (New York, NY: Kluwer Academic Publishers, 1996), p. 28.

Yamamoto, M., A. Kumagai, and Y. Yokoyama, "Structure and Actions of Saikosaponins Isolated from *Bupleurum falcatum* L.," *Arzneimittel-forschung* [*Medication Research*] 25 (1975): 1021–1040.

Burdock

Bensky, Dan, and Andrew Gamble, compilers, *Chinese Herbal Medicine: Materia Medica,* rev. ed. (Seattle, WA: Eastland Press, 1993), p. 42.

Lin, C.C., J.M. Lu, J.J. Yang, et al., "Anti-Inflammatory and Radical Scavenge Effects of *Arctium Lappa,*" *American Journal of Chinese Medicine* 24 (1996): 127-137.

Morita, T., K. Ebihara, and S. Kiriyama, "Dietary Fiber and Fat-Derivatives Prevent Mineral Oil Toxicity in Rats by the Same Mechanism," *Journal of Nutrition* 123(9) (September 1993): 1575–1585.

Nose, M., T. Fujimoto, T. Takeda, et al., "Structural Transformation of Lignan Compounds in Rat Gastrointestinal Tract," *Planta Medica* 58(6) (December 1992): 520–523.

Pizzorno, Joseph E., and Michael T. Murray, *A Textbook of Natural Medicine* (Seattle, WA: John Bastyr College Publications, 1985), IV: Food A1.

Butcher's Broom

Berg, D., "Venous Tone Varicose Veins in Pregnancy," *Fortschritte der Medizin* [*Advances in Medicine*] 110(3) (30 January 1992): 67–68, 71–72.

Cluzan, R.V., F. Alliot, S. Ghabboun, and M. Pascot, "Treatment of Secondary Lymphedema of the Upper Limb with CYCLO 3 FORT," *Lymphology* 29(1) (March 1996): 29–35.

Facino, R.M., M. Carini, R. Stefani, et al., "Anti-Elastase and Anti-Hyaluronidase Activities of Saponins and Sapogenins from *Hedera helix, Aesculus hippocastanum,* and *Ruscus aculeatus*: Factors Contributing to their Efficacy in the Treatment of Venous Insufficiency," *Archiv der Pharmazie* [*Archives of Pharmacology*] 328(10) (October 1995): 720–724.

Rudofsky, G., "Improving Venous Tone and Capillary Sealing. Effect of a Combination of Ruscus Extract and Hesperidine Methyl Chalcone in Healthy Probands in Heat Stress," *Fortschritte der Medizin* [*Advances in Medicine*] 107(19) (June 30, 1989): 52, 55–58.

Cajueiro

Franca, F., E.L. Lago, and P.D. Marsden, "Plants Used in the Treatment of Leishmanial Ulcers Due to *Leishmania (Viannia) Braziliensis* in an Endemic Area of Bah'a, Brazil," *Revista da Sociedade Brasileira de Medicina Tropical* [*Journal of the Brazilian Society of Tropical Medicine*] 29(3) (May–June 1996): 229–232.

George, J., and R. Kuttan, "Mutagenic, Carcinogenic and Cocarcinogenic Activity of Cashew Nut Shell Liquid," *Cancer Letters* 112(1) (15 January 1997): 11–16.

Jurberg, P., O. Sarquis, J.A. Dos Santos, and R. da C. Ferreira, "Effect of Niclosamide (Bayluscide WP 70), *Anacardium occidentale* Hexane Extract and *Euphorbia splendens* Latex on Behavior of *Biomphalaria glabrata* (Say, 1818), Under Laboratory Conditions," *Memorias do Instituto Oswaldo Cruz* 90(2) (March–April 1995): 191–194.

Kubo, I., I. Kinst-Hori, and Y. Yokokawa, "Tyrosinase Inhibitors from *Anacardium occidentale* Fruits," *Journal of Natural Products* 57(4) (April 1994): 545–551.

Swanston-Flatt, S.K., C. Day, P.R. Flatt, et al., "Glycaemic Effects of Traditional European Plant Treatments for Diabetes. Studies in Normal and Streptozotocin Diabetic Mice," *Diabetes Research* 10(2) (February 1989): 69–73.

Calendula

Chakurski, I., M. Matev, G. Stefanov, et al., "Treatment of Duodenal Ulcers and Gastroduodenitis with an Herbal Combination of *Symphitum officinalis* and *Calendula officinalis* with and without Antacids," *Vnutreshni Bolesti* [*Internal Disorders*] 20(6) (1981): 44–47.

Duke, J.A., "Pot Marigold," *Alternative and Complementary Therapy* 14(3) (June 2008): 109–115.

Dumenil, G., R. Chemli, C. Balansard, et al., "Evaluation of Antibacterial Properties of Marigold Flowers (*Calendula officinalis* L.) and Mother Homeopathic Tinctures of *C. officinalis* L. and *C. Arvensis* L.," *Annales pharmaçeutiques Françaises* [*French Annals of Pharmaceutics*] 38 (1980): 493.

Garg, S., and S.N. Sharma, "Development of Medicated Aerosol Dressings of Chlorhexidine Acetate with Hemostatics," *Pharmazie* 47(12) (December 1992): 924–926.

Mozherenkov, V.P., and L.F. Shubina, "Treatment of Chronic Conjunctivitis with *Calendula*," *Meditsinskaia Sestra* [*Nurse*] 35(4) (April 1976): 33–34.

Pommier, P., F. Gomez, M.P. Sunyach, et al., "Phase III Randomized Trial of *Calendula officinalis* Compared with Trolamine for the Prevention of Acute Dermatitis During Irradiation for Breast Cancer," *Journal of Clinical Oncology* 22 (2004): 1447–1453.

Shipochliev, T., A. Dimitrov, and E. Aleksandrova, "Anti-Inflammatory Action of a Group of Plant Extracts," *Veterinarno-Meditsinski Nauki* [*Veterinary-Medical Sciences*] 18(6) (1981): 87–94.

Ulbricht, C. (ed), E. Basch, S. Bent, et al., "Marigold (*Calendula officinalis* L.): An Evidence-Based Systematic Review by the Natural Standard Research Collaboration," *Journal of Herbal Pharmacotherapy* 6(3/4) (2006): 135–159.

Wagner, H., A. Proksch, I. Riess-Maurer, et al., "Immunostimulatory Effects of Polysaccharides (Heteroglycans) of Higher Plants," *Arzneimittel-forschung* [*Medication Research*] 35(7) (1985): 1069–1075.

California Poppy

Hanus, M., J. Lafton, and M. Mathieu, "Double-Blind, Randomised, Placebo-Controlled Study to Evaluate the Efficacy and Safety of a Fixed Combination Containing Two Plant Extracts (*Crataegus oxyacantha* and *Eschscholtzia californica*) and Magnesium in Mild-to-Moderate Anxiety Disorders," *Current Medical Research and Opinion*, 20(1) (January 2004): 63–71.

Rolland, A., J. Fleurentin, M.C. Lanhers, et al., "Behavioural Effects of the American Traditional Plant *Eschscholzia californica*: Sedative and Anxiolytic Properties," *Planta Medica* 57(3) (June 1991): 212–216.

Cardamom

Bensky, Dan, and Andrew Gamble, compilers, *Chinese Herbal Medicine: Materia Medica,* rev. ed. (Seattle, WA: Eastland Press, 1993), p. 218.

Dharmananda, Subhuti, *Chinese Herbology: A Professional Training Program* (Portland, OR: Institute for Traditional Medicine and Preventive Health Care, 1992), p. 177.

Catnip

Osterhoudt, K.C., S.K. Lee, J.M. Callahan, et al., "Catnip and the Alteration of Human Consciousness," *Veterinary & Human Toxicology* 39(6) (December 1997): 373–375.

Panizzi, L., G. Flamini, P.L. Cioni, and I. Morelli, "Composition and Antimicrobial Properties of Essential Oils of Four Mediterranean Lamiaceae," *Journal of Ethnopharmacology* 39(3) (August 1993): 167–170.

Cat's Claw

Aquino, R., V. De Feo, F. De Simone, et al., "Plant Metabolites. New Compounds and Anti-Inflammatory Activity of *Uncaria tomentosa*," *Journal of Natural Products* 54(2) (March–April 1991): 453–459.

Keplinger, K., "Composition Allowing for Modifying the Growth of Living Cells: Preparation and Utilization," *Internationale Veröffentlichungsdatum* WO 82/01130 (15 April 1982).

Keplinger, K., G. Laus, M. Wurm, et al., "*Uncaria tomentosa* (Willd.) DC.—Ethnomedicinal Use and New Pharmacological, Toxicological and Botanical Results," *Journal of Ethnopharmacology* 64(1) (January 1999): 23–24.

Der Krallendorn Tee (Innsbruck, Austria: Immodal Pharmaka), brochure.

Krallendorn, Uncaria tomentosa (Willd.) DC Root Extract: Information for Physicians and Dispensing Chemists, 3d ed. (Volders, Austria: Immodal Pharmaka GmbH, September 1995), pamphlet.

Rizzi, R., F. Re, A. Bianchi, et al., "Mutagenic and Antimutagenic Activities of *Uncaria tomentosa* and Its Extracts," *Journal of Ethnopharmacology* 38(1) (January 1993): 63–77.

Catuaba

Keplinger, K., "Composition Allowing for Modifying the Growth of Living Cells: Preparation and Utilization," *Internationale Veröffentlichungsdatum* WO 82/01130 (15 April 1982).

Manabe, H., H. Sakagami, H. Ishizone, et al., "Effects of Catuaba Extracts on Microbial and HIV Infection," *Vivo* 6(2) (March–April 1992): 161–165.

Cayenne

Ahuja, K.D., I.K. Robertson, D.P. Geragherty, et al., "Effects of Chili Consumption on Postprandial Glucose, Insulin, and Energy Metabolism," *American Journal of Clinical Nutrition* 84(1) (2006): 63–69.

Chang, A.B., P.D. Phelan, S.M. Sawyer, et al., "Cough Sensitivity in Children with Asthma, Recurrent Cough, and Cystic Fibrosis," *Archives of Diseases in Childhood* 77(4) (1997): 331–334.

Cichewicz, R.H., and P.A. Thorpe, "The Antimicrobial Properties of Chile Peppers (*Capsicum* Species) and Their Uses in Mayan Medicine," *Journal of Ethnopharmacology* 52(2) (June 1996): 61–70.

Ellison, N., C.L. Loprinzi, J. Kugler, et al., "Phase III Placebo-Controlled Trial of Capsaicin Cream in the Management of Surgical Neuropathic Pain in Cancer Patients," *Journal of Clinical Oncology* 15(8) (1997): 2974–2980.

Espinosa-Aguirre, J.J., R.E. Reyes, J. Rubio, et al., "Mutagenic Activity of Urban Air Samples and Its Modulation by Chili Extracts," *Mutation Research* 303(2) (October 1993): 55–61.

Gagnier, J.J., M. van Tulder, B. Berman, et al., "Herbal Medicine for Low Back Pain (Review)," Cochrane Database of Systematic Reviews 2006, Issue 2. Art. No. CD004504. DOI 10.1002/14651858.CD004504.pub3.

McCarthy, G.M., and D.J. McCarty, "Effect of Topical Capsaicin in the Therapy of Painful Osteoarthritis of the Hands," *Journal of Rheumatology* 19(4) (1992): 604–607.

Murray, Michael T., and Joseph E. Pizzorno, *Encyclopedia of Natural Medicine*, 2d. ed. (Rocklin, CA: Prima Publishing, 1997), p. 419.

Pellicer, F., O. Picazo, B. Gomez-Tagle, and O.I. De La Roldan, "Capsaicin or Feeding with Red Peppers During Gestation Changes the Thermonociceptive Response of Rat Offspring," *Physiology and Behavior* 60(2) (August 1996): 435–438.

Zhang, Z., S.M. Hamilton, C. Stewart, et al., "Inhibition of Liver Microsomal Cytochrome P450 Activity and Metabolism of the Tobacco-Specific Nitrosamine NNK by Capsaicin and Ellagic Acid," *Anticancer Research* 13(6A) (November–December 1993): 2341–2346.

Zhang, Z., H. Huynh, and R.W. Teel, "Effects of Orally Administered Capsaicin, the Principal Component of Capsicum Fruits, on the in Vitro Metabolism of the Tobacco-Specific Nitrosamine NNK in Hamster Lung and Liver Microsomes," *Anticancer Research* 17(2A) (March–April 1997): 1093–1098.

Chamomile

Bradley, P.R., ed., *British Herbal Compendium* (Bournemouth, England: British Herbal Medicine Association, 1992), p. 155.

Carle, R., and O. Isaac, "Die Kamille—Wirkung und Wirksamkeit. Ein Kommentar zur Monographie Matricariae Flos (Kamillenblüten)," *Zeitschrift für Phytotherapie* [*Phytotherapy Journal*] 8 (1987): 67–77.

Fidler, P., et al., "Prospective Evaluation of a Chamomile Mouthwash for Prevention of 5-FU-Induced Oral Mucositis," *Cancer* 77 (1997): 522–525.

Gerritsen, M.F., W.W. Carley, G.E. Ranges, et al., "Flavonids Inhibit Cytokine-Induced Endoethlial Cell Adhesion Protein Gene Expression," *American Journal of Pathology* 147 (1995): 278–292.

Glowania, H.J., C. Raulin, and M. Swoboda, "Effect of Chamomile on Wound Healing—a Clinical Double-Blind Study," *Zeitschrift für Hautkrankheiten* [*Journal for Skin Diseases*] 62(17) (1 September 1987): 1262, 1267–1271.

Mazokopakis, E.E., G.E. Vrentzos, J.A. Papadakis, et al., "Wild Chamomile (*Matricaria recutita* L.) Mouthwashes in Methotrexate-Induced Oral Mucositis," *Phytomedicine* 12 (2005): 25–27.

Miller, T., U. Wittstock, U. Lindequist, and E. Teuscher, "Effects of Some Components of the Essential Oil of Chamomile, *Chamomilla Recutita,* on Histamine Release from Rat Mast Cells," *Planta Medica* 62(1) (1 February 1996): 60–61.

Rekka, E.A., A.O. Kourounakis, and P.N. Kourounakis, "Investigation of the Effect of Chamazulene on Lipid Peroxidation and Free Radical Processes," *Research Communications in Molecular Pathology and Pharmacology* 92(3) (June 1996): 361–364.

Safayhi, H., J. Sabieraj, E.R. Sailer, and H.P. Ammon, "Chamazulene: An Antioxidant-Type Inhibitor of Leukotriene B4 Formation," *Planta Medica* 60(5) (October 1994): 410–413.

Segal, R., and L. Pilote, "Warfarin Interaction with *Matricaria Chamomilla,*" *Canadian Medical Association Journal* 174 (2006): 1281–1286.

Szelenyi, I., O. Isaac, and K. Thiemer, "Pharmacological Experiments with Compounds of Chamomile. III. Experimental Studies of the Ulcerprotective Effect of Chamomile," *Planta Medica* 35(3) (March 1979): 8–27.

Wagner, H., A. Proksch, I. Riess-Maurer, et al., "Immunostimulating Polysaccharides (Heteroglycans) of Higher Plants," *Arzneimittel-forschung* [*Medication Research*] 35 (1985): 1069–1075.

Wichtl, Max, ed., *Herbal Drugs and Phytopharmaceuticals: A Handbook for Practice on a Scientific Basis*, trans. Norman Grainger Bisset (Boca Raton, FL: MedPharm Scientific Publishers, 1995), p. 323.

Yamada, K., T. Miura, Y. Mimaki, and Y. Sashida, "Effect of Inhalation of Chamomile Oil Vapour on Plasma ACTH Level in Ovariectomized-Rat Under Restriction Stress," *Biological and Pharmaceutical Bulletin* 19(9) (September 1996): 1244–1246.

Chanca Piedra

Maxwell, Nicole, *Witch-Doctor's Apprentice: Hunting for Medicinal Herbs in the Amazon* (New York, NY: Citadel Press, 1990), pp. 363–381.

Shimizu, M., S. Horie, S. Terashima, et al., "Studies on Aldose Reductase Inhibitors from Natural Products. II. Active Components of a Paraguayan Crude Drug 'Para-parai mi,' *Phyllanthus niruri*," *Chemical and Pharmaceutical Bulletin* 37(9) (September 1989): 2531–2532.

Srividya, N., and S. Periwal, "Diuretic, Hypotensive and Hypoglycaemic Effect of *Phyllanthus amarus*," *Indian Journal of Experimental Biology* 33(11) (November 1995): 861–864.

Ueno, H., S. Horie, Y. Nishi, et al., "Chemical and Pharmaceutical Studies on Medicinal Plants in Paraguay. Geraniin, an Angiotensin-Converting Enzyme Inhibitor from 'Paraparai mi,' *Phyllanthus niruri*," *Journal of Natural Products* 51(2) (March–April 1988): 357–359.

Chaparral

Gordon, D.W., et al., "Chaparral Ingestion. The Broadening Spectrum of Liver Injury Caused by Herbal Medications," *Journal of the American Medical Association* 273 (1995): 489-490.

Granados, H., and R. Cardenas, "Biliary Calculi in the Golden Hamster. XXXVII. The Prophylactic Action of the Creosote Bush (*Larrea tridentata*) in Pigmented Cholelithiasis Produced by Vitamin A," *Revista De Gastroenterologia De México* [*Mexican Journal of Gastroenterology*] 59(1) (January–March 1994): 31–35.

Leonforte, J.F., "Contact Dermatitis from *Larrea* (Creosote Bush)," *Journal of the American Academy of Dermatology* 14(2, Part 1) (February 1986): 202–207.

Sheikh, N.M., R.M. Philen, and L.A. Love, "Chaparral-Associated Hepatotoxicity," *Archives of Internal Medicine* 157(8) (28 April 1977): 913–919.

Chen-Pi (Bitter Orange Peel)

Bruneton, Jean N., *Pharmacognosy, Phytochemistry, Medicinal Plants* (Paris, France: Lavoisier Publishing, 1995), pp. 280–281.

Chinese Senega Root

Yoshikawa, M., and J. Yamahara, "Inhibitory Effect of Oleanene-Type Triterpene Oligoglycosides on Ethanol Absorption: The Structure-Activity Relationships," in *Saponins Used in Traditional and Modern Medicine*, Advances in Experimental Medicine and Biology 404, ed. George R. Waller and Kazuo Yamasaki (New York, NY: Kluwer Academic Publishers, 1996), pp. 207–218.

Chiretta

Saxena, A.M., P.S. Murthy, and S.K. Mukherjee, "Mode of Action of Three Structurally Different Hypoglycemic Agents: A Comparative Study," *Indian Journal of Experimental Biology* 34(4) (April 1996): 351–355.

Sekar, B.C., B. Mukherjee, R.B. Chakravarti, and S.K. Mukherjee, "Effect of Different Fractions of *Swertia chirayita* on the Blood Sugar Level of Albino Rats," *Journal of Ethnopharmacology* 21(2) (November 1987): 175–181.

Cinnamon

Ling, J., and W.Y. Liu, "Cytotoxicity of Two New Ribosome-Inactivating Proteins, Cinnamomin and Camphorin, to Carcinoma Cells," *Cell Biochemistry and Function* 14(3) (September 1996): 157–161.

Okano, K., M. Iwai, Y. Iga, and K. Yokoyama, "Antiulcerogenic Compounds Isolated from Chinese Cinnamon," *Planta Medica* 55(3) (June 1989): 245–248.

Osawa, K., T. Matsumoto, H. Yasuda, et al., "The Inhibitory Effect of Plant Extracts on the Collagenolytic Activity and Cytotoxicity of Human Gingival Fibroblasts by *Porphyromonas gingivalis* Crude Enzyme," *Bulletin of Tokyo Dental College* 32(1) (February 1991): 1–7.

Quale, J.M., D. Landman, M.M. Zaman, et al., "In Vitro Activity of *Cinnamomum zeylanicum* Against Azole Resistant and Sensitive *Candida* Species and a Pilot Study of Cinnamon for Oral Candidiasis," *American Journal of Chinese Medicine* 24(2) (1996): 103–109.

Singh, H.B., M. Srivastava, A.B. Singh, and A.K. Srivastava, "Cinnamon Bark Oil, a Potent Fungitoxicant Against Fungi Causing Respiratory Tract Mycoses," *Allergy* 50(12) (December 1995): 995–999.

Yu, S.M., T.S. Wu, and C.M. Teng, "Pharmacological Characterization of Cinnamophilin, a Novel Dual Inhibitor of Thromboxane Synthase and Thromboxane A2 Receptor," *British Journal of Pharmacology* 111(3) (March 1994): 906–912.

Cloves

Bensky, Dan, and Andrew Gamble, compilers, *Chinese Herbal Medicine: Materia Medica,* rev. ed. (Seattle, WA: Eastland Press, 1993), p. 306.

Huang, Kee C., and Kee Chang, eds., *The Pharmacology of Chinese Herbs* (Boca Raton, FL: CRC Press, 1992), p. 39

Kurokawa, M., K. Nagasaka, T. Hirabayashi, et al., "Efficacy of Traditional Herbal Medicines in Combination with Acyclovir Against Herpes Simplex Virus Type 1 Infection in Vitro and in Vivo," *Antiviral Research* 27(1–2) (May 1995): 19–37.

Schattner, P., and D. Randerson, "Tiger Balm as a Treatment of Tension Headache: A Clinical Trial in General Practice," *Australian Family Physician* 25(2) (1996): 216–222.

Codonopsis

Chen, Y.R., J.H. Yen, C.C. Lin, et al., "The Effects of Chinese Herbs on Improving Survival and Inhibiting Anti-DS DNA Antibody Production in Lupus Mice," *American Journal of Chinese Medicine* 21(3–4) (1993): 257–262.

Wang, Z.T., Q. Du, G.J. Xu, et al., "Investigations on the Protective Action of *Codonopsis Pilosula (Dangshen)* Extract on Experimentally-Induced Gastric Ulcer in Rats," *General Pharmacology* 28(3) (March 1997): 469–473.

Coix

Hidaka, Y., T. Kaneda, N. Amino, and K. Miyai, "Chinese Medicine, Coix Seeds Increase Peripheral Cytotoxic T and NK Cells," *Biotherapy* 5(3) (1992): 201–203.

Kaneda, T., Y. Hidaka, T. Kashiwai, et al., "Effect of Coix Seed on the Changes in Peripheral Lymphocyte Subsets," *Rinsho Byori* [*Journal of Clinical Pathology*] 40(2) (February 1992): 179–181.

Coleus

Bauer, K., F. Dietersdorfer, K. Sertl, et al., "Pharmacodynamic Effects of Inhaled Dry Powder Formulations of Fenterol and Colforsin in Asthma," *Clinical Pharmacological Therapies* 53(1) (January 1993): 76–83.

Busse, W.W., and S.D. Lantis, "Impaired H2 Histamine Granulocyte Response in Active Atopic Eczema," *Journal of Investigational Dermatology* 73(2) (August 1979): 184–187.

"Coleus forskohlii," *Alternative Medical Review* 11(1) (monograph) (March 2006): 47–51.

Henderson, S., B. Magu, C. Rasmussen, et al., "Effect of *Coleus forskohlii* Supplementation on Body Composition and Hematological Profiles in Mildly Overweight Women," *Journal of the International Society of Sports Nutrition* 2(2) (2005): 54–62.

Marone, G., M. Columbo, M. Triggianai, et al., "Forskolin Inhibits the Release of Histamine from Human Basophils and Mast Cells," *Agents and Actions* 18 (1986): 96–99.

Schlepper, M., J. Thormann, P. Kremer, et al., "Present Use of Positive Inotropic Drugs in Heart Failure," *Journal of Cardiovascular Pharmacology* 14 (Supplement 1) (1989): S9–S19.

Schlepper, M., J. Thormann, and V. Mitrovic, "Cardiovascular Effects of Forskolin and Phosphodiesterase-III Inhibitors," *Basic Research in Cardiology* 84 (Supplement 1) (1989): 197–212.

Snow, J.M., *"Coleus forskohlii Wild. (Lamiaceae),"* *The Protocol Journal of Botanical Medicine* (Autumn 1995): 39–42.

Whitfield, J.F., P. Morley, G.E. Willick, et al., "Stimulation of Femoral Trabecular Bone Growth in Ovarietomized Rats by Human Parathyroid Hormone (hPTH)-(1–30) NH(2)," *Calciferous Tissue International* 65(2) (August 1999): 143–147.

Yousif, M.H., and O. Thulesius, "Forskolin Reverse Tachyphylaxis to the Bronchodilator Effects of Salbutamol: An In-Vitro Study on Isolated Guinea-Pig Trachea," *Journal of Pharmaceutics and Pharmacology* 51(2) (February 1999): 181–186.

Coltsfoot

Bensky, Dan, and Andrew Gamble, compilers, *Chinese Herbal Medicine: Materia Medica,* rev. ed. (Seattle, WA: Eastland Press, 1993), p. 201.

Wiedenfeld, Helmut, personal correspondence, 6 April 1996.

Comfrey

Betz, J.M., R.M. Eppley, W.C. Taylor, and D. Andrzejewski, "Determination of Pyrrolizidine Alkaloids in Commercial Comfrey Products (*Symphytum* Spp.)," *Journal of Pharmaceutical Sciences* 83(5) (May 1994): 649–653.

Couet, C.E., C. Crews, and A.B. Hanley, "Analysis, Separation, and Bioassay of Pyrrolizidine Alkaloids from Comfrey (*Symphytum officinale*)," *Natural Toxins* 4(4) (1996): 163–167.

Grube, B., J. Grünwald, L. Krug, et al., "Efficacy of a Comfrey Root (*Symphyti offic. radix*) Extract Ointment in the Treatment of Patients with Painful Osteoarthritis of the Knee: Results of a Double-Blind, Randomised, Bicenter, Placebo-Controlled Trial," *Phytomedicine* 14(1) (2007): 10.

Kucera, M., J. Kalal, and Z. Polesna, "Effects of Symphytum Ointment on Muscular and Functional Locomotor Disturbances," *Advances in Therapy* 17(4) (2000): 204–210.

Copaiba

Basile, A.C., J.A. Sertie, P.C. Freitas, and A.C. Zanini, "Anti-Inflammatory Activity of Oleoresin from Brazilian *Copaifera*," *Journal of Ethnopharmacology* 22(1) (January 1988): 101–109.

Coptis

Chang, K.S., "Down-Regulation of C-Ki-Ras2 Gene Expression Associated with Morphologic Differentiation in Human Embryonal Carcinoma Cells Treated with Berberine," *Taiwan I Hsueh Hui Tsa Chih* [*Journal of the Taiwan Medical Association*] 90(1) (1991): 10–14.

Chang, K.S.S., C. Gao, and L.C. Wang, "Berberine-Induced Morphologic Differentiation and Down-Regulation of C-Ki-Ras2 Protooncogene Expression in Human Teratocarcinoma Cells," *Cancer Letters* 55(2) (1990): 103–108.

Chi, C.W., Y.F. Chang, T.W. Chao, et al., "Flowcytometric Analysis of the Effect of Berberine on the Expression of Glucocorticoid Receptors in Human Hepatoma HepG2 Cells," *Life Sciences* 54(26) (1994): 2099–2107.

Head, K.A., "Natural Approaches to Prevention and Treatment of Infections of the Lower Urinary Tract," *Alternative Medicine Review* 13(3) (2008): 227–244.

Namba, T., K. Sekiya, A. Toshinal, et al., "Study on Baths with Crude Drug. II.: The Effects of Coptidis Rhizoma Extracts as Skin Permeation Enhancer," *Yakugaku Zasshi* [*Journal of the Pharmaceutical Society of Japan*] 115(8) (August 1995): 618–625.

Shen, Z.F., and M.Z. Xie, "Determination of Berberine in Biological Specimen by High Performance TLC and Fluoro-Densitometric Method," *Yao Hsueh Hsueh Pao* [*Acta Pharmaceutica Sinica*] 28(7) (1993): 532–536.

Song, L.C., K.Z. Chen, and J.Y. Zhu, "The Effect of *Coptis Chinensis* on Lipid Peroxidation and Antioxidase Activity in Rats," *Chung-Kuo Chung Hsi I Chieh Ho Tsa Chih* [*Chinese Journal of Modern Developments in Traditional Medicine*] 12(7) (July 1992): 390, 421–423.

Yin, J., H. Xing, and J. Ye, "Efficacy of Berberine in Patients with Type 2 Diabetes Mellitus," *Metabolism Clinical Experimental* 57 (2008): 712–717.

Cordyceps

Furuya, T., et al., "N6-(2-Hydroxyethyl)adenosine, a Biologically Active Compound from Cultured Mycelia of *Cordyceps* and *Isaria* Species," *Phytochemistry* 22 (1983): 2509–2511.

Hobbs, Christopher, and Michael Miovic, eds., *Medicinal Mushrooms: An Exploration of Tradition, Healing, and Culture,* 2d. ed. (Santa Cruz, CA: Botanica Press, 1995), p. 82.

Naoki, T., et al., "Pharmacological Studies on *Cordyceps Sinensis* from China," *Fifth Mycological Congress Abstracts,* Vancouver, BC, Canada, 14–21 August 1994.

Xu, F., et al., "Amelioration of Cyclosporin Nephrotoxicity by *Cordyceps Sinensis* in Kidney-Transplanted Recipients," *Nephrology, Dialysis, and Transplantation* 10 (1995): 142–143.

Xu, N., and B. Zhang, "Effect of Cordyceps on Plasma Lipids in Normal, Stressed, and Hyperlipemic Rats," *Abstracts of Chinese Medicines* 2 (1987): 317.

Zhu, J.S., et al., "The Scientific Rediscovery of a Precious Ancient Chinese Herbal Regime: *Cordyceps Sinensis.* Part I," *Journal of Alternative and Complementary Medicine* 4 (1998): 289–303.

Zhuang, J., and H. Chen, "Treatment of Tinnitus with Cordyceps Infusion: A Report of 23 Cases," *Abstracts of Chinese Medicines* 1 (1990): 66.

Corn Silk

Wichtl, Max, ed., *Herbal Drugs and Phytopharmaceuticals: A Handbook for Practice on a Scientific Basis,* trans. Norman Grainger Bisset (Boca Raton, FL: MedPharm Scientific Publishers, 1995), pp. 311–312.

Corydalis

Huang, Kee C., and Kee Chang, eds., *The Pharmacology of Chinese Herbs* (Boca Raton, FL: CRC Press, 1992), p. 142.

Kubo, M., H. Matsuda, K. Tokuoka, et al., "Studies of Anti-Cataract Drugs from Natural Sources. I. Effects of a Methanolic Extract and the Alkaloidal Components from Corydalis Tuber on in Vitro Aldose Reductase Activity," *Biological and Pharmaceutical Bulletin* 17(3) (March 1994): 458–459.

Reimeier, C., I. Schneider, W. Schneider, et al., "Effects of Ethanolic Extracts from *Eschscholtzia Californica* and *Corydalis Cava* on Dimerization and Oxidation of Enkephalins," *Arzneimittel-forschung* [*Medication Research*] 45(2) (February 1995): 132–136.

Damiana

Balch, James F., and Phyllis A. Balch, *Prescription for Nutritional Healing,* 2d. ed. (Garden City Park, NY: Avery Publishing Group, 1996), p. 68.

Taylor, L., *Male Plus Amazon Formula for Men: Technical Report* (Austin, TX: Raintree Marketing, 1996).

Waynberg, J., "Male Sexual Asthenia Interest in a Traditional Plant-Derived Medication 'Testor-Plus,'" (Austin, TX: Raintree Marketing, 1999).

Dan Shen

Huang, Kee C., and Kee Chang, eds., *The Pharmacology of Chinese Herbs* (Boca Raton, FL: CRC Press, 1992), p. 82.

Li, W., C.H. Zhou, and Q.L. Lu, "Effects of Chinese Materia Medica in Activating Blood Stimulating Menstrual Flow on the Endocrine Function of Ovary-Uterus and Its Mechanisms," *Chung-Kuo Chung Hsi I Chieh Ho Tsa Chih* [*Chinese Journal of Modern Developments in Traditional Medicine*] 12(30) (1992): 165–168.

Liu, J., G. Hua, W. Liu, et al., "The Effect of IH764–3 on Fibroblast Proliferation and Function," *Chinese Medical Science Journal* 7(3) (September 1992): 142–147.

Shanghai Hospital Team, *Chinese Medical Journal* 11 (1976): 68.

Wang, D., T.J. Girard, T.P. Kasten, et al., "Inhibitory Activity of Unsaturated Fatty Acids and Anacardic Acids Toward Soluble Tissue Factor—Factor VIIa Complex," *Journal of Natural Products* 61(110) (November 1998): 1352–1355.

Winston, D., "Eclectic Specific Condition Review: Uterine Fibroids," *Protocol Journal of Botanical Medicine* 1(4) (Spring 1996): 211.

Wu, Y.J., C.Y. Hong, S.J. Lin, et al., "Increase of Vitamin E Content in LDL and Reduction of Atherosclerosis in Cholesterol-Fed Rabbits by a Water-Soluble Antioxidant-Rich Fraction of Salvia Miltiorrhiza," *Arteriosclerosis, Thrombosis, and Vascular Biology* 18(3) (March 1998): 481–486.

Zhao, B., W. Jiang, Y. Zhao, et al., "Scavenging Effects of *Salvia Miltiorrhiza* on Free Radicals and Its Protections for Myocardial Mitochondrial Membranes from Ischemia-Reperfusion Injury," *Biochemistry and Molecular Biology International* 38(6) (May 1996): 1171–1182.

Zhou, X.M., Z.Y. Lu, and D.W. Wang, "Experimental Study of *Salvia Miltiorrhiza* on Prevention of Restenosis After Angioplasty," *Chung-Kuo Chung Hsi I Chieh Ho Tsa Chih* [*Chinese Journal of Modern Developments in Traditional Medicine*] 16(8) (August 1996): 480–482.

Dandelion

Chakurski, I., M. Matev, A. Koichev, et al., "Treatment of Chronic Colitis with an Herbal Combination of *Taraxacum officinale, Hypericum perforatum, Melissa officinalis, Calendula officinalis* and *Foeniculum vulgare*," *Vnutreshni Bolesti* [*Internal Disorders*] 20(6) (1981): 51–54.

Faber, K., "The Dandelion—*Taraxacum officinale* Weber," *Pharmazie* 13 (1958): 423–435.

Racz-Kotilla, E., G. Racz, and A. Solomon, "The Action of *Taraxacum officinale* Extracts on the Body Weight and Diuresis of Laboratory Animals," *Planta Medica* 26(3) (November 1974): 212–217.

Swanston-Flatt, S.K., C. Day, P.R. Flatt, et al., "Glycaemic Effects of Traditional European Plant Treatments for Diabetes. Studies in Normal and Streptozotocin Diabetic Mice," *Diabetes Research* 10(2) (February 1988): 69–73.

Zhu, M., P.Y. Wong, and R.C. Li, "Effects of *Taraxacum mongolicum* on the Bioavailability and Disposition of Ciprofloxacin in Rats," *Journal of Pharmacological Science* 88(6) (June 1999): 632–634.

Devil's Claw

Circosta, C., F. Occhiuto, S. Ragusa, et al., "A Drug Used in Traditional Medicine: *Harpagophytum procumbens* DC. II. Cardiovascular Activity," *Journal of Ethnopharmacology* 11(3) (August 1984): 259–274.

Dienstleistung Phytopharmaka Rheda-Widenbrück (no title listed), *Wiener medizinischer Wochenschrift* 149(8–10) (1999): 254–257.

Lanhers, M.C., J. Fleurentin, F. Mortier, et al., "Anti-Inflammatory and Analgesic Effects of an Aqueous Extract of *Harpagophytum procumbens*," *Planta Medica* 58(2) (April 1992): 117–123.

Moussard, C., D. Alber, M.M. Toubin, et al., "A Drug Used in Traditional Medicine, *Harpagophytum procumbens*: No Evidence for NSAID-Like Effect on Whole Blood Eicosanoid Production in Humans," *Prostaglandins, Leukotrienes, and Essential Fatty Acids* 46(4) (August 1992): 283–286.

Soulimani, R., C. Younos, F. Mortier, and C. Derrieu, "The Role of Stomachal Digestion on the Pharmacological Activity of Plant Extracts, Using as an Example Extracts of *Harpagophytum procumbens*," *Canadian Journal of Physiology and Pharmacology* 72(12) (December 1994): 1532–1536.

Wegener, T., and N.P. Lupke, "Treatment of Patients with Arthrosis of Hip or Knee with an Aqueous Extract of Devil's Claw (*Harpagophytum procumbens* DC.)," *Phytotherapy Research* 17(10) (December 2003): 1165–1172.

Dong Quai

Carlassare, F., F. Baccichetti, F. Bordin, and L. Anselmo, "Psoralen Photosensitization of L 1210 Leukaemia Cells: An Approach to a New Combined Therapy," *Zeitschrift für Naturforschung* [*Journal of Biosciences*], 33(1–2) (January–February 1978): 92–95.

Chang, H.M., and P.P.H. But, *Pharmacology and Applications of Chinese Materia Medica*, vol. 1 (Singapore: World Scientific Publishing, 1986), p. 446.

Hickey, M., S.R. Davis, and D.W. Sturdee, "Treatment of Menopausal Symptoms: What Shall We Do Now?" *Lancet* 366(9683) (2005): 409-421.

Hirata, J.D., L.M. Swiersz, B. Zell, et al., "Does Dong Quai Have Estrogenic Effects in Postmenopausal Women? A Double-Blind, Placebo-Controlled Trial," *Fertility and Sterility* 68(6) (December 1997): 981–986.

Huang, Kee C., and Kee Chang, eds., *The Pharmacology of Chinese Herbs* (Boca Raton, FL: CRC Press, 1992), p. 248.

Lau, C.B., et al., "Use of Dong Quai (*Angelica Sinensis*) to Treat Peri- or Postmenopausal Symptoms in Women with Breast Cancer: Is it Appropriate?" *Menopause* 12(6) (2005): 734–740.

Newton, K.M., S.D. Reed, A.Z. LaCroix, et al., "Treatment of Vasomotor Symptoms of Menopause with Black Cohosh, Multibotanicals, Soy, Hormone Therapy, or Placebo: A Randomized Trial," *Annals of Internal Medicine* 145(2) (2006): 869–879.

Page, R.L., II, and J.D. Lawrence, "Potential of Warfarin by Dong Quai," *Pharmacotherapy* 19(7) (July 1999): 870–876.

Raman, A., Z.X. Lin, E. Sviderskaya, and D. Kowalska, "Investigation of the Effect of *Angelica Sinensis* Root Extract on the Proliferation of Melanocytes in Culture," *Journal of Ethnopharmacology* 54(2–3) (November 1996): 165–170.

Rotem, C., and B. Kaplan, "Phyto-Female Complex for the Relief of Hot Flushes, Night Sweats and Quality of Sleep: Randomized, Controlled, Double-Blind Pilot Study," *Gynecological Endocrinology* 23(2) (2007): 117–122.

Scott, B.C., J. Butler, B. Halliwell, and O.I. Aruoma, "Evaluation of the Antioxidant Actions of Ferulic Acid and Catechins," *Free Radical Research Communications* 19(4) (1993): 241–253.

Wang, C.C., L.G. Chen, and L.L. Yang, "Inducible Nitric Oxide Synthase Inhibitor of the Chinese Herb I. *Saposhnikovia Divaricata* (Turcz.) *Schischk,*" *Cancer Letters* 145(1–2) (18 October 1999): 151–157.

Wang, S.R., Z.Q. Guo, and L.Z. Liao, "Experimental Study on Effects of 18 Kinds of Chinese Herbal Medicine for Synthesis of Thromboxane A2 and PGI2," *Chung-Kuo Chung Hsi I Chieh Ho Tsa Chih* [*Chinese Journal of Modern Developments in Traditional Medicine*] 13(3) (March 1993): 134, 167–170.

Zheng, R.L., and H. Zhang, "Effects of Ferulic Acid on Fertile and Asthenozoospermic Infertile Human Sperm Motility, Viability, Lipid Peroxidation, and Cyclic Nucleotides," *Free Radical Biology and Medicine* 22(4) (1997): 581–586.

Echinacea

Barrett, B.P., R.L. Brown, K. Locken, et al., "Treatment of the Common Cold with Unrefined Echinacea," *Annals of Internal Medicine* 137(12) (2002): 939–946.

Bauer, R., and H. Wagner, "Echinacea Species as Potential Immunostimulatory Drugs," in Economic and Medicinal Plant Research, 5, ed. H. Wagner, Hiroshi Hikino, and Norman R. Farnsworth (London, England: Academic Press, 1994), pp. 289–292.

Brinkeborn, R.M., D.V. Shah, and F.H. Degenring, "Echinaforce and Other Echinacea Fresh Plant Preparations in the Treatment of the Common Cold. A Randomized, Placebo Controlled, Double-Blind Clinical Trial," *Phytomedicine* 6(1) (March 1999): 1–6.

Caruso, T.J., and J.M. Gwaltney, "Treatment of the Common Cold with Echinacea: A Structured Review," *Journal of Clinical Infectious Diseases* 40(6) (2005): 807–810.

Facino, R.M., M. Carini, G. Aldini, et al., "Direct Characterization of Caffeoyl Esters with Antihyaluronidase Activity in Crude Extracts from *Echinacea angustifolia* Roots by Fast Atom Bombardment Tandem Mass Spectrometry," *Farmaco* 48(10) (October 1993): 1447–1461.

Facino, R.M., M. Carini, G. Aldini, et al., "Echinacoside and Caffeoyl Conjugates Protect Collagen from Free Radical-Induced Degradation: A Potential Use of Echinacea Extracts in the Prevention of Skin Photodamage," *Planta Medica* 61(6) (December 1995): 510–614.

Goel, V., R. Lovlin, R. Bartion, et al., "Efficacy of a Standardized Echinacea Preparation (Echinilin) for the Treatment of the Common Cold: A Randomized, Double-Blind, Placebo-Controlled Trial," *Journal of Clinical Pharmacy and Therapeutics* 29(1) (2004): 75–83.

Grimm, W., and H.H. Müller, "A Randomized Controlled Trial of the Effect of Fluid Extract of *Echinacea purpurea* on the Incidence and Severity of Colds and Respiratory Infections," *American Journal of Medicine,* 106(2) (February 1999): 138–143.

Kuhn, O., untitled article, *Arzneimittel-forschung* [*Medication Research*] 3 (1953): 194–200.

Lersch, C., M. Zeuner, A. Bauer, et al., "Stimulation of the Immune Response in Outpatients with Hepatocellular Carcinomas by Low Doses of Cyclophosphamide (LDCY), *Echinacea purpurea* Extracts (Echinacin) and Thymostimulin," *Archiv für Geschwulstforschung* [*Archives of Tumor Research*] 60(5) (1990): 379–383.

Lersch, C., M. Zeuner, A. Bauer, et al., "Nonspecific Immunostimulation with Low Doses of Cyclophosphamide (LDCY), Thymostimulin, and *Echinacea purpurea* Extracts (Echinacin) in Patients with Far Advanced

Colorectal Cancers: Preliminary Results," *Cancer Investigation* 10(5) (1992): 343–348.

Linde, K., B. Barrett, K. Wölkart, et al., "Echinacea for Preventing and Treating the Common Cold," Cochrane Database of Systematic Reviews 2006, Issue 1. Art. No.: CD000530. DOI: 10.1002/14651858.CD000530.pub2.

Luettig, B., C. Steinmuller, G.E. Gifford, et al., "Macrophage Activation by the Polysaccharide Arabinogalactan Isolated from Plant Cell Cultures of *Echinacea Purpurea*," *Journal of the National Cancer Institute* 81(9) (3 May 1989): 669–675.

Melchart, D., K. Linde, F. Worku, et al., "Immunomodulation with Echinacea—A Systematic Review of Controlled Clinical Trials," *Phytomedicine* 1 (1994): 245–254.

Melchart, D., E. Walther, K. Linde, et al., "Echinacea Root Extracts for the Prevention of Upper Respiratory Tract Infections: A Double-Blind, Placebo-Controlled Randomized Trial," *Archives of Family Medicine* 7(6) (November–December 1998): 541–545.

Mengs, U., C.B. Clare, and J.A. Piley, "Toxicity of *Echinacea purpurea*: Acute, Subacute and Genotoxicity Studies," *Arzneimittel-forschung* [*Medication Research*] 41(11) (1991): 20, 1076–1081.

Rehman, J., J.M. Dillow, S.M. Carter, et al., "Increased Production of Antigen-Specific Immunoglobulins G and M Following In Vivo Treatment with the Medical Plants *Echinacea angustifolia* and *Hydrastis canadensis*," *Immunology Letters* 68(2–3) (1 June 1999) 391–395.

See, D.M., N. Broumand, L. Sahl, and J.G. Tilles, "In Vitro Effects of Echinacea and Ginseng on Natural Killer and Antibody-Dependent Cell Cytotoxicity in Healthy Subjects and Chronic Fatigue Syndrome or Acquired Immunodeficiency Syndrome Patients," *Immunopharmacology* 35(3) (January 1997): 229–235.

Sperber, S.J., L.P. Shah, R.D. Gilbert, et al., "*Echinacea purpurea* for Prevention of Experimental Rhinovirus Colds," *Clinical Infectious Diseases* 38(10) (2004): 1367–1371.

Turner, R.B., D.K. Riker, and J.D. Gangerni, "Ineffectiveness of Echinacea for Prevention of Experimental Rhinovirus Colds," *Antimicrobial Agents and Chemotherapy* 44(6) (2000): 1708–1709.

Vestweber, A.M., J. Beuth, H.L. Ko, et al., "In Vitro Activity of *Mercurius cyanatus* Complex Against Relevant Pathogenic Bacterial Isolates," *Arzneimittel-forschung* [*Medication Research*] 45(9) (September 1995): 1018–1020.

Vonau, B., S. Chard, S. Mandalia, et al., "Does the Extract of the Plant *Echinacea purpurea* Influence the Clinical Course of Recurrent Genital Herpes?" *International Journal of STD & AIDS* 12 (2001): 154–158.

Weber, W., J.A. Taylor, A.V. Stoep, et al., "*Echinacea purpurea* for Prevention of Upper Respiratory Tract Infections in Children," *Journal of Alternative & Complementary Medicine* 11(6) (2005): 1021–1026.

Wildfeuer, A., and D. Mayerhofer, "The Effects of Plant Preparations on Cellular Functions in Body Defense," *Arzneimittel-forschung* [*Medication Research*] 44(3) (March 1994): 361–366.

Yale, S.Y., and K. Liu, "*Echinacea purpurea* Therapy for the Treatment of the Common Cold: A Randomized, Double-Blind, Placebo-Controlled Clinical Trial," *Archives of Internal Medicine* 164 (2004): 1237–1241.

Elderberry

Baum, L.G., and J.C. Paulson, "Sialylogiosaccharides of the Respiratory Epithelium in the Selection of Human Influenza Virus Receptor Specificity," *Acta Histochemica* 40 (supplement) (1990): 35–38.

Bergner, P., "Elderberry (*Sambucus nigra, canadensis*)," *Medical Herbalism* 8(4) (Winter 1996–1997): 11–12.

Zakay-Rones, Z., E. Thom, T. Wollan, et al., "Randomized Study of the Efficacy and Safety of Oral Elderberry Extract in the Treatment of Influenza A and B Virus Infections," *Journal of International Medical Research* 32(2) (2004): 132–140.

Zakay-Rones, Z., N. Varsano, M. Zlotnik, et al., "Inhibition of Several Strains of Influenza Virus in Vitro and Reduction of Symptoms by an Elderberry Extract (*Sambucus nigra* L.) During an Outbreak of Influenza B in Panama," *Journal of Alternative and Complementary Medicine* 1(40) (1995): 361–369.

Elecampane

Seth, S.D., M. Maulki, C.K. Katiyar, and S.K. Maulik, "Role of Lipistat in Protection Against Isoproterenol Induced Myocardial Necrosis in Rats: A Biochemical and Histopathological Study," *Indian Journal of Physiology and Pharmacology* 42(1) (January 1998): 101–106.

Tripathi, Y.B., P. Tripathi, and B.N. Upadhyay, "Assessment of the Adrenergic Beta-Blocking Activity of Inula Racemosa," *Journal of Ethnopharmacology* 23(1) (May–June 1988): 3–9.

Epimedium

Huang, Kee C., and Kee Chang, eds., *The Pharmacology of Chinese Herbs* (Boca Raton, FL: CRC Press, 1992), p. 91.

Iinuma, M., T. Tanaka, N. Sakakibara, et al., "Phagocytic Activity of Leaves of Epimedium Species on Mouse Reticuloendothelial System," *Yakugaku Zasshi* [*Journal of the Pharmaceutical Society of Japan*] 110(3) (March 1990): 179–185.

Zhang, G., L. Qin, and Y. Shi, "Epimedium-Derived Phytoestrogen Flavonoids Exert Beneficial Effect on Preventing Bone Loss in Late Postmenopausal Women: A 24-month Randomized, Double-Blind and Placebo-Controlled Trial," *Journal of Bone and Mineral Research* 22(7) (2007): 1072–1079.

Espinheira Santa

Kuo, Y.H., M.L. King, C.F. Chen, et al., "Two New Macrolide Sesquiterpene Pyridine Alkaloids from *Maytenus emarginata*: Emarginatine G and the Cytotoxic Emarginatine F," *Journal of Natural Products* 57(2) (February 1994): 263–269.

Nozaki, H., Y. Matsuura, S. Hirono, et al., "Antitumor Agents, 116. Cytotoxic Triterpenes from *Maytenus diversifolia*," *Journal of Natural Products* 53(4) (July–August 1990): 1039–1041.

Oliveira, M.G., M.G. Monteiro, C. Macaubas, et al., "Pharmacologic and Toxicologic Effects of Two *Maytenus* Species in Laboratory Animals," *Journal of Ethnopharmacology* 34(1) (August 1991): 29–41.

Sekar, K.V., A.T. Sneden, and F.A. Flores, "Mayteine and 6-Benzoyl-6-Deacetylmayteine from *Maytenus krukovit*," *Planta Medica* 61(4) (August 1995): 390.

Sneden, A.T., and G.L. Beemsterboer, "Normaytansine, a New Antileukemic Ansa Macrolide from *Maytenus buchananii*," *Journal of Natural Products* 43(5) (September–October 1980): 637–640.

Souza-Formigoni, M.L., M.G. Oliveira, M.G. Monteiro, et al., "Antiulcerogenic Effects of Two *Maytenus* Species in Laboratory Animals," *Journal of Ethnopharmacology* 34(1) (August 1991): 21–27.

Eucalyptus

Burkhard, P.R., K. Burkhardt, C.A. Haenggeli, and T. Landis, "Plant-Induced Seizures: Reappearance of an Old Problem," *Journal of Neurology* 246(8) (August 1999): 667–670.

Gardulf, A., I. Wohlfart, and R. Gustafson, "A Prospective Cross-Over Field Trial Shows Protection of Lemon Eucalyptus Extract Against Tick Bites," *Journal of Medical Entomology* 41(6) (2004): 1064–1067.

Kehrl, W., U. Sonnemann, and U. Dethlefsen, "Therapy for Acute Nonpurulent Rhinosinusitis with Cineole: Results of a Double-Blind, Randomized, Placebo-Controlled Trial," *Laryngoscope* 114(4) (2004): 738–742.

Sato, S., N. Yoshinuma, K. Ito, et al., "The Inhibitory Effect of Funoran and Eucalyptus Extract-Containing Chewing Gum on Plaque Formation," *Journal of Oral Science* 40(3) (1998): 115–117.

Shahi, S.K., A.C. Shukla, A.K. Bajaj, et al., "Broad Spectrum Herbal Therapy Against Superficial Fungal Infections," *Skin Pharmacology and Applied Skin Physiology* 13 (2004): 60–64.

Tibballs, J., "Clinical Effects and Management of Eucalyptus Oil Ingestion in Infants and Young Children," *The Medical Journal of Australia* 163 (August 1985): 177–180.

Warnke, P.H., et al., "Antibacterial Essential Oils in Malodorous Cancer Patients: Clinical Observations in 30 Patients," *Phytomedicine* 13(7) (July 2006): 463–467.

Eyebright

Harkiss, K.J., and P. Timmins, "Studies in the Scrophulariaceae. 8. Phytochemical Investigation of *Euphrasia officinalis*," *Planta Medica* 23(4) (June 1973): 342–347.

Li, Y., K. Metori, K. Koike, et al., "Improvement in the Turnover Rate of the Stratum Corneum in False Aged Model Rats by the Administration of Geniposidic Acid in Eucommia Ulmoides Olvier Leaf," *Biological Pharmacology Bulletin* 22(6) (June 1999): 582–585.

Recio, M.C., R.M. Ginger, S. Manez, and J.L. Rios, "Structural Considerations on the Iridoids as Anti-Inflammatory Agents," *Planta Medica* 60(3) (June 1994): 232–234.

Fennel Seed

Bensky, Dan, and Andrew Gamble, compilers, *Chinese Herbal Medicine: Materia Medica*, rev. ed. (Seattle, WA: Eastland Press, 1993), p. 307.

Fenugreek

Bhardwaj, P.K., D.J. Dasgupta, B.S. Prashar, and S.S. Kaushal, "Control of Hyperglycaemia and Hyperlipidaemia by Plant Product," *Journal of the Association of Physicians of India* 42(1) (January 1994): 33–35.

Broca, C., R. Gross, P. Petit, et al., "4-Hydroxyisoleucine: Experimental Evidence of Its Insulinotropic and Antidiabetic Properties," *American Journal of Physiology* 277 (4, Part 1) (October 1999): E617–E623.

Raghuram, T.C., and R.D. Sharma, "Effect of Fenugreek Seeds on Intravenous Glucose in Non-Insulin Dependent Diabetic Patients," *Phytotherapy Research* 8 (1994): 83–86.

Sambaiah, K., and K. Srinivasan, "Influence of Spices and Spice Principles on Hepatic Mixed Function Oxygenase System in Rats," *Indian Journal of Biochemistry and Biophysics* 26(4) (August 1989): 254–258.

Sharma, R.D., T.C. Raghuram, and N.S. Rao, "Effect of Fenugreek Seeds on Blood Glucose and Serum Lipids in Type I Diabetes," *European Journal of Clinical Nutrition* 44(4) (April 1990): 301–306.

Sharma, R.D., et al., "Hypolipidaemic Effect of Fenugreek Seeds: A Chronic Study in Non-Insulin Dependent Diabetic Patients," *Phytotherapy Research* 10 (1996): 332–334.

Stark, A., and Z. Madar, "The Effect of an Ethanol Extract Derived from Fenugreek (*Trigonella foenum-graecum*) on Bile Acid Absorption and Cholesterol Levels in Rats," *British Journal of Nutrition* 69(1) (January 1993): 277–287.

Feverfew

Diener, H., V. Pfaffenrath, J. Schnitker, et al., "Efficacy and Safety of 6.25 mg t.i.d. Feverfew C02-extract (MIG-99) in Migraine Prevention—A Randomized, Double-Blind, Multicentre, Placebo-Controlled Study," *Cephalalgia* 25 (2005): 1031–1041.

Johnson, E.S., N.P. Kadam, D.M. Hylands, et al., "Efficacy of Feverfew as Prophylactic Treatment of Migraine," *British Medical Journal* 291 (6495) (August 1985): 569–573.

Maizels, M., A. Blumenfeld, and R. Burchette, "A Combination of Riboflavin, Magnesium, and Feverfew for Migraine Prophylaxis: A Randomized Trial," *Headache* 44(9) (2004): 885–890.

Murphy, J.J., S. Heptinstall, and J.R. Mitchell, "Randomised Double-Blind Placebo-Controlled Trial of Feverfew in Migraine Prevention," *Lancet* 2(8604) (23 July 1988): 189–192.

O'Neill, L.A., M.L. Barrett, and G.P. Lewis, "Extracts of Feverfew Inhibit Mitogen-Induced Human Peripheral Blood Mononuclear Cell Proliferation and Cytokine Mediated Responses: A Cytotoxic Effect," *British Journal of Clinical Pharmacology* 23(1) (January 1987): 81–83.

Pattrick, M., S. Heptinstall, and M. Doherty, "Feverfew in Rheumatoid Arthritis: A Double Blind, Placebo Controled Study," *Annals of Rheumatic Disease* 48(7) (July 1989): 547–549.

Pittler, M.H., and E. Ernst, "Feverfew for Preventing Migraine," Cochrane Database of Systematic Reviews 2004, Issue 1. Art. No.: CD 002286. DOI: 10.1002/14651858.CD002286.pub2.

Sumner, H., U. Salan, D.W. Knight, and J.R. Hoult, "Inhibitor of 5-Lipoxygenase and Cyclo-Oxygenase in Leukocytes by Feverfew. Involvement of Sesquiterpene Lactones and Other Components," *Biochemical Pharmacology* 43(11) (9 June 1992): 2313–2320.

Williams, C.A., J.B. Harborne, H. Geiger, and J.R. Hoult, "The Flavonoids of *Tanacetum parthenium* and *T. vulgare* and Their Anti-Inflammatory Properties," *Phytochemistry* 51(3) (June 1999): 417–423.

Fritillaria

Huang, Kee C., and Kee Chang, eds., *The Pharmacology of Chinese Herbs* (Boca Raton, FL: CRC Press, 1992), p. 217.

Lee, G.I., J.Y. Ha, K.R. Min, et al., "Inhibitory Effects of Oriental Herbal Medicines on IL-8 Induction in Lipopolysaccharide-Activated Rat Macrophages," *Planta Medica* 61(1) (February 1995): 26–30.

Garlic

Augusti, K.T., and M.E. Benaim, "Effect of Essential Oil of Onion (Allyl Propyl Disulphide) on Blood Glucose, Free Fatty Acid, and Insulin Levels of Normal Subjects," *Chemical Abstracts* 83(22) (1975): 593.

Bordia, A., S.K. Verma, and K.C. Srivastava, "Effect of Garlic on Platelet Aggregation in Humans: A Study in Healthy Subjects and Patients with Coronary Artery Disease," *Prostaglandins, Leukotrienes, and Essential Fatty Acids* 55(3) (September 1996): 201–205.

Brosche, T., and N. Platt, "Knoblauchtherapie und zellulaere Immunabwehr in Alter [Garlic Therapy and Cellular Immunocompetence in the Elderly]," *Zeitschrift für Phytotherapie* [*Phytotherapy Journal*] 15 (1994): 23–24.

Budoff, M., "Aged Garlic Extract Retards Progression of Coronary Artery Calcification," *Journal of Nutrition* 136 (2006): 741S–744S.

Chander, J., S. Maini, S. Subrahmanyan, and A. Handa, "Otomycosis—a Clinico-Mycological Study and Efficacy of Mercurochrome in Its Treatment," *Mycopathologia* 135(1) (1996): 9–12.

Chang, H.M., and P.P.H. But, *Pharmacology and Applications of Chinese Materia Medica*, vol. 1 (Singapore: World Scientific Publishing, 1986), p. 90.

Chung, J.G., G.W. Chen, L.T. Wu, et al., "Effects of Garlic Compounds Diallyl Sulfide and Diallyl Disulfide on Arylamine N-Acetyltransferase Activity in Strains of *Helicobacter Pylori* from Peptic Ulcer Patients," *American Journal of Chinese Medicine* 26(3-4) (1998): 353–364.

Feng, Z.H., G.M. Zhang, T.L. Hao, et al., "Effect of Diallyl Trisulfide on the Activation of T-Cell and Macrophage-Mediated Cytotoxicity," *Journal of Tongji Medical University* 14 (1994): 142–147.

Fleischauer, A.T., C. Poole, and L. Arab, "Garlic Consumption and Cancer Prevention: Meta-Analyses of Colorectal and Stomach Cancers," *American Journal of Clinical Nutrition* 72(4) (2000): 1047–1052.

Ishikawa, K., R. Naganawa, H. Yoshida, et al., "Antimutagenic Effects of Ajoene, an Organosulfur Compound Derived from Garlic," *Bioscience, Biotechnology, and Biochemistry* 60(12) (December 1996): 2086–2088.

Jaiswal, S.K., and A. Bordia, "Radio-Protective Effect of Garlic *Allium sativum* Linn. in Albino Rats," *Indian Journal of Medical Sciences* 50(7) (July 1996): 231–233.

Koch, H.P., and L.D. Lawson, *Garlic: The Science and Therapeutic Application of Allium sativum L. and Related Species,* 2d ed. (Baltimore, MD: Williams and Wilkins, 1996), p. 177.

Koscielny, J., D. Klussendorf, R. Latza, et al., "The Anti-atherosclerotic Effect of *Allium sativum*," *Atherosclerosis* 144(1) (May 1999): 237–249.

Martin, N., L. Bardisa, C. Pantoja, et al., "Involvement of Calcium in the Cardiac Depressant Actions of a Garlic Dialysate," *Journal of Ethnopharmacology* 55(2) (January 1997): 113–118.

Milner, J.A., "Garlic: Its Anticarcinogenic and Antitumorigenic Properties," *Nutrition Reviews* 54(11, Part 2) (November 1996): S82–S86.

Nok, A.J., S. Williams, and P.C. Onyenekwe, "*Allium sativum*-Induced Death of African Trypanosomes," *Parasitology Research*, 82(7) (1996): 634–637.

Polasa, K., and K. Krishnaswamy, "Reduction of Urinary Mutagen Excretion in Rats Fed Garlic," *Cancer Letters*, 114(1–2) (19 March 1997): 185–186.

Rivlin, R., M. Budoff, H. Amagase, et al., "Significance of Garlic and Its Constituents in Cancer and Cardiovascular Disease," *Journal of Nutrition* 136 (2006): preface.

Romano, E.L., R.F. Montano, B. Brito, et al., "Effects of Ajoene on Lymphocyte and Macrophage Membrane-Dependent Functions," *Immunopharmacology and Immunotoxicology* 19(1) (February 1997): 15–36.

Schaffer, E.M., J.Z. Liu, and J.A. Milner, "Garlic Powder and Allyl Sulfur Compounds Enhance the Ability of Dietary Selenite to Inhibit 7,12-Dimethylbenz[a]-anthracene-Induced Mammary DNA Adducts," *Nutrition and Cancer* 27(2) (1997): 162–168.

Sigounas, G., J. Hooker, A. Anagnostou, and M. Steiner, "S-Allylmercaptocysteine Inhibits Cell Proliferation and Reduces the Viability of Erythroleukemia, Breast, and Prostate Cancer Cell Lines," *Nutrition and Cancer* 27(2) (1997): 186–191.

Silagy, C.A., and H.A. Neil, "Garlic as a Lipid Lowering-Agent: A Meta-Analysis," *Journal of the Royal College of Physicians* (London) 28(1) (1994): 39–45.

Sivam, G.P., J.W. Lampe, B. Ulness, et al., "*Helicobacter pylori*—in Vitro Susceptibility to Garlic (*Allium sativum*) Extract," *Nutrition and Cancer* 27(2) (1997): 118–121.

Sobenin, I.A., V.V. Prianishnikov, L.M. Kunnova, et al., "Reduction of Cardiovascular Risk in Primary Prophylaxy of Coronary Heart Disease," *Klinicheskaia Meditsina* [*Clinical Medicine*] 83(4) (2005): 52–55.

Tanaka, S., K. Haruma, M. Yoshihara, et al., "Aged Garlic Extract Has Potential Suppressive Effect on Colorectal Adenomas in Humans," *Journal of Nutrition* 136 (2006): 821S–826S.

Villar, R., M.T. Alvarino, and R. Flores, "Inhibition by Ajoene of Protein Tyrosine Phosphatase Activity in Human Platelets," *Biochimica et Biophysica Acta,* 1337(2) (8 February 1997): 233–240.

Weiss, N., et al., "Aged Garlic Extract Improves Homocysteine-Induced Endothelial Dysfunction in Macro- and Microcirculation," *Journal of Nutrition* 136 (2006): 750S–754S.

Gentian

Zhang, J.Q., and Y.P. Zhou, "Inhibition of Aldose Reductase from Rat Lens by Some Chinese Herbs and Their Components," *Chung-Kuo Chung Yao Tsa Chih* [*China Journal of Chinese Materia Medica*] 14(9) (September 1989): 557–559, 576.

Ginger

Adewunmi, C.O., B.O. Oguntimein, and P. Furu, "Molluscicidal and Antischistosomal Activities of *Zingiber officinale*," *Planta Medica* 56(4) (August 1990): 374–376.

Ahmed, R.S., and S.B. Sharma, "Biochemical Studies on Combined Effects of Garlic (*Allium sativum* Linn) and Ginger (*Zingiber officinale* Rosc.) in Albino Rats," *Indian Journal of Experimental Biology* 35(8) (1997): 841–843.

Bliddal, H., A. Rosetzsky, P. Schlichting, et al., "A Randomized, Placebo-Controlled, Cross-Over Study of Ginger Extracts and Ibuprofen in Osteoarthritis," *Osteoarthritis and Cartilage* 8 (2000): 9–12.

Bordia, A., S.K. Verma, and K.C. Srivastava, "Effect of Ginger (*Zingiber officinale* Rosc.) and Fenugreek (*Trigonella foenumgraecum* L.) on Blood Lipids, Blood Sugar, and Platelet Aggregation in Patients with Coronary Artery Disease," *Prostaglandins, Leukotrienes, and Essential Fatty Acids* 56(5) (1997): 379–384.

Chang, C.P., J.Y. Chang, F.Y. Wang, and J.G. Chang, "The Effect of Chinese Medicinal Herb Zingiberis Rhizoma Extract on Cytokine Secretion by Human Peripheral Blood Mononuclear Cells," *Journal of Ethnopharmacology* 48(1) (11 August 1995): 13–19.

Chrubasik, S., et al., "*Zingiberis Rhizoma*: A Comprehensive Review on the Ginger Effect and Efficacy Profiles," *Phytomedicine* 12 (2005): 684–701.

Denyer, C.V., P. Jackson, D.M. Loakes, et al., "Isolation of Antirhinoviral Sesquiterpenes from Ginger (*Zingiber officinale*)," *Journal of Natural Products* 57(5) (May 1994): 658–662.

Fulder, S., and M. Tenne, "Ginger as an Anti-Nausea Remedy in Pregnancy: The Issue of Safety," *HerbalGram* 38 (Fall 1996): 49.

Goto, C., S. Kasuya, K. Koga, et al., "Lethal Efficacy of Extract from *Zingiber officinale* (traditional Chinese Medicine) or [6]-Shogaol and [6]-Gingerol in Anisakis Larvae in Vitro," *Parasitology Research* 76(8) (1990): 653–656.

Grontbved, A., T. Braks, J. Kambskard, and E. Hentzer, "Ginger Root Against Seasickness: A Controlled Trial on the Open Sea," *Acta Otolaryngolica* 105 (1988): 45–49.

Janssen, P.L., S. Meyboom, W.A. Van Staveren, et al., "Consumption of Ginger (*Zingiber officinale* Roscoe) Does Not Affect Ex Vivo Platelet Thromboxane Production in Humans," *European Journal of Clinical Nutrition* 50(11) (November 1996): 772–774.

Kawakishi, S., Y. Morimitsu, and T. Osawa, "Chemistry of Ginger Components and Inhibitory Factors of the Arachidonic Acid Cascade," in *Food Phytochemicals for Cancer Prevention II: Teas, Spices, and Herbs*, ed. Chi-Tang Ho, Toshihiko Osawa, Mou-Tuan Huang, and Robert E. Rosen (Washington, DC: American Chemical Society, 1994), pp. 244–249.

Kiuchi, F., "Nematocidal Activity of Some Anthelmintics, Traditional Medicines, and Spices by New Assay Method Using Larvae of Toxocara Canis," *Yakugaku Zasshi* [*Journal of the Pharmaceutical Society of Japan*] 43(4) (1989): 279–287.

Manusirivithaya, S., M. Sripramote, S. Tagjitgamol, et al., "Antiemetic Effect of Ginger in Gynecologic Oncology Patients Receiving Cisplatin," *International Journal of Gynecological Cancer* 14(6) (2004): 1063–1069.

Meyer, K., J. Schwartz, D. Crater, and B. Keyes, "*Zingiber officinale* (Ginger) Used to Prevent 8-MOP Associated Nausea," *Dermatology Nursing* 7(4) (August 1995): 242–244.

Minematsu, S., M. Taki, M. Watanabe, et al., "Effects of Shosaiko-to-go-keishikashakuyaku-to (TJ-960) on the Valproic Acid Induced Anomalies of Rat Fetuses," *Nippon Yakurigaku Zasshi* [*Folia Pharmacologica Japonica*] 96(5) (November 1990): 265–273.

Mowrey, D., and D. Clayson, "Motion Sickness, Ginger, and Psychophysics," *Lancet* 8 (1982): 655–657.

Sharma, J.N., K.C. Srivastava, and E.K. Gan, "Suppressive Effects of Eugenol and Ginger Oil on Arthritic Rats," *Pharmacology* 49(5) (November 1994): 314–318.

Srivastava, K.C., "Effects of Aqueous Extracts of Onion, Garlic and Ginger on Platelet Aggregation and Metabolism of Arachidonic Acid in the Blood Vascular System: In Vitro Study," *Prostaglandins in Medicine*, 13 (1984): 227–235.

Srivastava, K.C., and T. Mustafa, "Ginger (*Zingiber officinale*) in Rheumatism and Musculoskeletal Disorders," *Medical Hypotheses* 39(4) (December 1992): 342–348.

Tanabe, M., Y.D. Chen, K. Saito, and Y. Kano, "Cholesterol Biosynthesis Inhibitory Component from *Zingiber officinale* Roscoe," *Chemical and Pharmaceutical Bulletin* 41(4) (April 1993): 710–713.

Verma, S.K., J. Singh, R. Khamesra, and A. Bordia, "Effect of Ginger on Platelet Aggregation in Man," *Indian Journal of Medical Research* 98 (October 1993): 240–242.

Vogel, H.C.A., *The Nature Doctor* (New Canaan, CT: Keats Publishing, 1991), p. 446.

Vutyavanich, T., T. Kraisarin, and R. Ruangsri, "Ginger for Nausea and Vomiting in Pregnancy: Randomized, Double-Masked, Placebo-Controlled Trial," *Obstetrics and Gynecology* 97(4) (2001): 577–582.

Wu, H., D.J. Ye, Y.A. Zhao, and S.L. Wang, "Effect of Different Preparations of Ginger on Blood Coagulation Time in Mice," *Chung-Kuo Chung Yao Tsa Chih* [*China Journal of Chinese Materia Medica*] 18(3) (March 1993): 147–149, 190.

Ginkgo Biloba

Barabasz, A., and M. Barabasz, "Attention Deficit Hyperactivity Disorder: Neurological Basis and Treatment Alternatives," *Journal of Neurotherapy* 1 (1985): 1–10.

Brochet, B., P. Guinot, J.M. Orgogozo, et al., "Double Blind Placebo Controlled Multicentre Study of Ginkgolide B in Treatment of Acute Exacerbations of Multiple Sclerosis," *Journal of Neurology, Neurosurgery, and Psychiatry* 38(3) (March 1995): 360–362.

Brochet, B., J.M. Orgogozo, P. Guinot, et al., "Pilot Study of Ginkgolide B, a PAF-Acether Specific Inhibitor in the Treatment of Acute Outbreaks of Multiple Sclerosis," *Revue Neurologique* (Paris) 148(4) (1992): 299–301.

Burns, N.R., J. Bryan, and T. Nettlebeck, "*Ginkgo biloba*: No Robust Effect on Cognitive Abilities or Mood in Healthy Young or Older Adults," *Human Psychopharmacology Clinical Experiments* 21 (2006): 27–37.

Cohen, A.J., and B.J. Bartik, "*Ginkgo biloba* for Antidepressant-Induced Sexual Dysfunction," *Sex and Marital Therapy* 24(2) (April 1998): 139–143.

Coles, R., "Trial of an Extract of Ginkgo biloba (EGB) for Tinnitus and Hearing Loss," *Clinical Otolaryngology* 13 (1988): 501–504.

Doly, M., M.T. Droy-Lefaix, and P. Braquet,"Oxidative Stress in Diabetic Retina," *EXS* 62 (1992): 299–307.

Elsabagh, S., D.E. Hartley, and S.E. File, "Limited Cognitive Benefits in Stage +2 Postmenopausal Women After 6 Weeks of Treatment with Ginkgo Biloba," *Journal of Psychopharmacology* (2005): 173–181.

Fünfgeld, E.W., "A Natural and Broad Spectrum Nootropic Substance for Treatment of SDAT—*Ginkgo biloba* Extract," *Progress in Clinical and Biological Research* 317 (1989): 1247–1260.

Guinot, P., E. Caffrey, R. Lambe, and A. Darragh, "Tanakan Inhibits Platelet-Activating Aggregation in Healthy Male Volunteers," *Haemostasis* 19 (1986): 219–223.

Haase, J., P. Halama, and R. Horr, "Effectiveness of Brief Infusions with *Ginkgo biloba* Special Extract EGb 761 in Dementia of the Vascular and Alzheimer Type," *Zeitschrift für Gerontologie und Geriatrie* [*Journal of Gerontology and Geriatrics*] 29(4) (July–August 1996): 302–309.

Hasenorhl, R.U., C.H. Nichau, C.H. Frisch, M.A. De Sourza Silva, J.P. Huston, C.M. Mattern, and R. Hacker, "Anxiolytic-Like Effect of Combined Extracts of *Zingiber officinale* and *Ginkgo biloba* in the Elevated Plus-Maze," *Pharmacology, Biochemistry and Behavior* 53(20) (February 1996): 271–275.

Hauns, B., B. Häring, S. Hohler, et al., "Phase II Study of Combined 5-Fluorouracil/Ginkgo Biloba Extract (GBE 761 ONC) Therapy in 5-Fluorouracil Pretreated Patients with Advanced Colorectal Cancer," *Phytotherapy Research* 15 (2001): 34–38.

Hemmer, R., and O. Tzavellas, "On Cerebral Effect of Plant Preparation from *Ginkgo biloba*," *Arzneimittel-forschung* [*Medication Research*] 17(4) (April 1967): 491–493.

Hofferberth, B., "The Efficacy of EGb 761 in Patients with Senile Dementia of the Alzheimer Type, a Double Blind, Placebo-Controlled Study on Different Levels of Investigation," *Human Psychopharmacology* 9 (1994): 215–222.

Hoffmann, F., C. Beck, A. Schutz, and P. Offermann, "Ginkgo Extract EGb 761 (tenobin)/HAES versus Naftidrofuryl (Dusodril)/HAES. A Randomized Study of Therapy of Sudden Deafness," *Laryngo-Rhino-Otologie* 73(3) (March 1994): 149–152.

Horsch, S., and C. Walther, "*Ginkgo biloba* Special Extract EGb 761 in the Treatment of Peripheral Arterial Occlusive Disease (PAOD)—A Review Based on Randomized, Controlled Studies," *International Journal of Clinical Pharmacology and Therapeutics* 42(2) (2004): 63–67.

Howat, D.W., N. Chand, P. Braquet, and D.A. Willoughby, "An Investigation into the Possible Involvement of Platelet-Activating Factor in Experimental Allergic Encephalomyelitis in Rats," *Agents and Actions* 27(3–4) (June 1989): 473–476.

Itil, T., "Natural Substances in Psychiatry," *Psychopharmacology Bulletin* 31 (1995): 147–158.

Johnson, S.K., B.J. Diamond, S. Rausch, et al., "The Effect of *Ginkgo biloba* on Functional Measures in Multiple Sclerosis: A Pilot Randomized Controlled Trial," *Explore* 2 (2006): 19–24.

Knighton, D.R., T.K. Hunt, H. Scheuenstuhl, et al., "Oxygen Tension Regulates the Expression of Angiogenesis Factor by Macrophages," *Science* 221 (1983): 1283–1285.

Koc, R.K., H. Akdemir, A. Kurtsoy, et al., "Lipid Peroxidation in Experimental Spinal Cord Injury. Comparison of Treatment with *Ginkgo biloba*, TRH, and Methylprednisolone," *Research in Experimental Medicine* 195(2) (1995): 117–123.

Koltai, M., D. Hosford, P. Guinot, et. al., "PAF: A Review of Its Effects, Antagonists, and Possible Future Clinical Implication. Part II," *Drugs* 42 (1991): 174–204.

Lanthony, P., and J.P. Cosson, "The Course of Color Vision in Early Diabetic Retinopathy Treated with *Ginkgo biloba* Extract. A Preliminary Double-Blind Versus Placebo Study," *Journal Français d'Ophthalmologie* [*French Journal of Ophthalmology*] 11(10) (February 1995): 671–674.

Larocca, L.M., M. Guistacchini, N. Maggiano, et al., "Growth-Inhibitory Effect of Quercetin and Presence of Type II Estrogen Binding Sites in Primary Human Transitional Cell Carcinomas," *Journal of Urology* 1523(3) (1994): 1029–1033.

Larocca, L.M., L. Teofili, G. Leone, et al., "Antiproliferative Activity of Quercetin on Normal Bone Marrow and Leukaemic Progenitors," *British Journal of Haematology* 79(4) (1991): 562–566.

Le Bars, P.L., F.M. Velasco, J.M. Ferguson, et al., "Influence of the Severity of Cognitive Impairment on the Effect of the *Ginkgo biloba* Extract EGb 761 in Alzheimer's Disease," *Neuropsychobiology* 45 (2002): 19–26.

Lingaerde, O., A.R. Foreland, and A. Magnusson, "Can Winter Depression be Prevented by *Ginkgo biloba* Extract? A Placebo-Controlled Trial," *Acta Psychiatrica Scandanavica* 100 (1999): 62–66.

Matsukawa, Y., M. Yoshida, T. Sakai, et al., "The Effect of Quercetin and Other Flavonoids on Cell Cycle Progression Growth of Human Gastric Cancer Cells," *Planta Medica* 56 (1990): 677–678.

Mazza, M., A. Capuano, P. Bria, et al., "Ginkgo Biloba and Donepezil: A Comparison in the Treatment of Alzheimer's Dementia in a Randomized Placebo-Controlled Double-Blind Study," *European Journal of Neurology* 13 (2008): 981–985.

Meyer, B., "Etude Multicentrique Randomisee a Double Insu Face Au Placebo Du Tratiement Des Acouphenes Par L'extrait De Ginkgo Biloba," *Presse Med* 15 (1986): 1562–1564.

Moongkarndi, P., A. Srivattana, N. Bunyapraphatsara, et al., "Cytotoxicity Assay of Hispidulin and Quercetin Using Chlorimetric Technique," *Warasan Phesetchasat* 18(2) (1991): 25–31.

Moulton, P.L., L.N. Boyko, J.L. Fitzpatrick, et al., "The Effect of *Ginkgo biloba* on Memory in Healthy Male Volunteers," *Physiology & Behavior* 73 (2001): 659–665.

Ni, Y., B. Zhao, J. Hour, and W. Xin, "Preventive Effect of Ginkgo Biloba Extract on Apoptosis in Rat Cerebellar Neuronal Cells Induced by Hydroxyl Radicals," *Neuroscience Letters* 214(2–3) (23 August 1996): 115–118.

Paick, J.S., and J.H. Lee, "An Experimental Study of the Effect of *Ginkgo biloba* Extract on Human and Rabbit Corpus Cavernosum Tissue," *Journal of Urology* 156(5) (November 1996): 1876–1880.

Punkt, K., A. Unger, K. Welt, et al., "Hypoxia-Dependent Changes of Enzyme Activities in Different Fibre Types of Rat Soleus and Extensor Digitorum Longus Muscles. A Cytophotometrical Study," *Acta Histochemica* 98(3) (July 1996): 255–269.

Ranelletti, F.O., R. Ricci, L.M. Larocca, et al., "Growth-Inhibitory Effect of Quercetin and Presence of Type-II Estrogen Binding Sites in Human Colon-Cancer Cell Lines and Primary Colorectal Tumors," *International Journal of Cancer* 50(3) (1992): 486–492.

Reisser, C.H., and H. Weidauer, "*Ginkgo biloba* Extract EGb 761 or Pentoxifylline for the Treatment of Sudden Deafness: A Randomized, Reference-Controlled, Double-Blind Study," *Acta Otolaryngologica* (Stockholm) 121 (2001): 579–584.

Rejali, D., A. Sivakumar, and N. Balaji, "*Ginkgo biloba* Does Not Benefit Patients with Tinnitus: A Randomized, Placebo-Controlled, Double-Blind Trial and Meta-Analysis of Randomized Trials," *Clinical Otolaryngology and Allied Sciences* 29(3) (2004): 226–231.

Rong, Y., Z. Geng, and B.H. Lau, "*Ginkgo biloba* Attenuates Oxidative Stress in Macrophages and Endothelial Cells," *Free Radical Biology and Medicine* 20(1) (1996): 121–127.

Rowin, J., and S.L. Lewis, "Spontaneous Bilateral Subdural Hematomas Associated with Chronic *Ginkgo biloba* Ingestion," *Neurology* 46(6) (June 1996): 1775–1776.

Scambia, G., F.O. Ranelletti, P.P. Benedetti, et al., "Quercetin Potentiates the Effect of Adriamycin in a Multidrug-Resistant MCF-7 Human Breast-Cancer Cell Line; P-Glycoprotein as a Possible Target," *Cancer Chemotherapy and Pharmacology* 28(4) (1991): 255–258.

Scambia, G., F.O. Ranelletti, P.B. Panici, et al., "Inhibitory Effect of Quercetin on OVCA 433 Cells and Presence of Type II Oestrogen Binding Sites in Primary Ovarian Tumours and Cultured Cells," *British Journal of Cancer* 62(6) (1990): 942–946.

Schubert, H., and P. Halama, "Depressive Episode Primarily Unresponsive to Therapy in Elderly Patients: Efficacy of *Ginkgo biloba* Extract (EGb 761) in Combination with Antidepressants," *Geriatrische Forschung* 3 (1993): 45–53.

Seif-El-Nasr, M., and A.A. El-Fattah, "Lipid Peroxide, Phospholipids, Glutathione Levels and Superoxide Dismutase Activity in Rat Brain After Ischaemia: Effect of Ginkgo Biloba Extract," *Pharmacological Research* 32(5) (November 1995): 273–278.

Sohn, M., and R. Sikora, "*Ginkgo biloba* Extract in the Therapy of Erectile Dysfunction," *Journal of Urology* 141 (1991): 188A.

Solomon, P.R., F. Adams, A. Silver, et al., "Ginkgo for Memory Enhancement: A Randomized Controlled Trial," *Journal of the American Medical Association* 288(7) (2002): 835–840.

Wei, Y.Q., X. Zhao, Y. Kariya, et al., "Induction of Apoptosis by Quercetin Involvement of Heat Shock Protein," *Cancer Research*, 54(18) (1994): 4952–4957.

Winston, D., "Eclectic Specific Condition Review: Cataracts," *Protocol Journal of Botanical Medicine* 2(2) (1997): 39.

Yan, L.J., M.T. Droy-Lefaix, and L. Packer, "*Ginkgo biloba* Extract (EGb 761) Protects Human Low Density Lipoproteins Against Oxidative Modification Mediated by Copper," *Biochemical and Biophysical Research Communications* 212(2) (17 July 1995): 360–366.

Zeng, X., M. Liu, Y. Tang, et al., "Ginkgo biloba for Acute Ischaemic Stroke," *Cochrane Database of Systematic Reviews* 2005, Issue 4. Art. No.: CD003691. DOI: 10.1002/14651858.CD003691.pub2.

Zhang, X.Y., D.F. Zhou, L.Y. Cao, et al., "The Effects of *Ginkgo biloba* Extract Added to Haloperidol on Peripheral T-cell Subsets in Drug-Free Schizophrenia: A Double-Blind, Placebo-Controlled Trial," *Psychopharmacology* 188(1) (2006): 12–17.

Zhang, X.Y., D.F. Zhou, P.Y. Zhang, et al., "A Double-Blind, Placebo-Controlled Trial of Extract of *Ginkgo biloba* Added to Haloperidol in Treatment-Resistant Patients with Schizophrenia," *Journal of Clinical Psychiatry* 62 (2001): 878–883.

Ginseng

Allen, J.D., J. McLung, A.G. Nelson, et al., "Ginseng Supplementation Does Not Enhance Healthy Young Adults' Peak Aerobic Exercise Performance," *Journal of the American College of Nutrition* 17(5) (1998): 462–466.

Cha, R.J., D.W. Zeng, and Q.S. Chang, "Non-Surgical Treatment of Small Cell Lung Cancer with Chemo-Radio-Immunotherapy and Traditional Chinese Medicine," *Chung-Hua Nei Ko Tsa Chih* [*Chinese Journal of Internal Medicine*] 33(7) (July 1994): 462–466.

Chen, X., and T.J. Lee, "Ginsenosides-Induced Nitric Oxide-Mediated Relaxation of the Rabbit Corpus Cavernosum," *British Journal of Pharmacology* 115(1) (May 1995): 15–18.

Choi, Y.D., K.H. Rha, and H.K. Choi, "In Vitro and in Vivo Experimental Effect of Korean Red Ginseng on Erection," *Journal of Urology* 162(4) (October 1999): 1508–1511.

Ding, D.Z., T.K. Shen, and Y.A. Cui, "Effects of Red Ginseng on Congestive Heart Failure and Its Mechanism," *Chung-Kuo Chung Hsi I Chieh Ho Tsa Chih* [*Chinese Journal of Modern Developments in Traditional Medicine*] 15(6) (1995): 325–327.

Han, M.Q., J.X. Liu, and H. Gao, "Effects of 24 Chinese Medicinal Herbs on Nucleic Acid, Protein and Cell Cycle of Human Lung Adenocarcinoma Cell," *Chung-Kuo Chung Hsi I Chieh Ho Tsa Chih* [*Chinese Journal of Modern Developments in Traditional Medicine*] 15(3) (1995): 147–149.

Hiai, S., K. Yokoyama, H. Oura, and S. Yano, "Features of Ginseng Saponin-Induced Corticosterone Secretion," *Endocronologica Japonica* 26(6) (1979): 661.

Huang, Kee C., and Kee Chang, eds., *The Pharmacology of Chinese Herbs* (Boca Raton, FL: CRC Press, 1992), p. 43.

Kang, S.Y., V.B. Schini-Kerth, and N.D. Kim, "Ginsenosides of the Protopanaxatriol Group Cause Endothelium-Dependent Relaxation in the Rat Aorta," *Life Sciences* 56(19) (1995): 1577–1586.

Kim, H.S., J.G. Kang, and K.W. Oh, "Inhibition by Ginseng Total Saponin of the Development of Morphine Reverse Tolerance and Dopamine Receptor Supersensitivity in Mice," *General Pharmacology* 26(5) (September 1995): 1071–1076.

Kim, H.S., J.G. Kang, H.M. Rheu, et al., "Blockade by Ginseng Total Saponin of the Development of Methamphetamine Reverse Tolerance and Dopamine Receptor Supersensitivity in Mice," *Planta Medica* 61(1) (February 1995): 22–25.

Kim, H.S., J.G. Kang, Y.H. Seong, et al., "Blockade by Ginseng Total Saponin of the Development of Cocaine-Induced Reverse Tolerance and Dopamine Receptor Supersensitivity in Mice," *Pharmacology, Biochemistry, and Behavior* 50(1) (January 1995): 23–27.

Kim, H.S., and K.S. Kim, "Inhibitory Effects of Ginseng Total Saponin on Nicotine-Induced Hyperactivity, Reverse Tolerance and Dopamine Receptor Supersensitivity," *Behavior and Brain Research* 103(1) (August 1999): 55–61.

Kim, S.H., C.K. Cho, S.Y. Yoo, et al., "In Vivo Radioprotective Activity of *Panax ginseng* and Diethyldithiocarbamate," *Vivo* 7(5) (September–October 1993): 467–470.

Kiyohara, H., M. Hirano, X.G. Wen, et al., "Characterisation of an Anti-Ulcer Pectic Polysaccharide from Leaves of *Panax ginseng* C.A. Meyer," *Carbohydrate Research* 263(1) (3 October 1994): 89–101.

Lee, S.J., J.H. Sung, S.J. Lee, et al., "Antitumor Activity of a Novel Ginseng Saponin Metabolite in Human Pulmonary Adenocarcinoma Cells Resistant to Cisplatin," *Cancer Letters* 44(1) (20 September 1999): 39–43.

Lee, Y.S., I.S. Chung, I.R. Lee, et al., "Activation of Multiple Effector Pathways of Immune System by the Antineoplastic Immunostimulator Acidic Polysaccharide Ginsan Isolated from *Panax ginseng*," *Anticancer Research* 17(1A) (January–February 1997): 323–331.

Matsunaga, H., M. Katano, T. Saita, et al., "Potentiation of Cytotoxicity of Mitomycin C by a Polyacetylenic Alcohol, Panaxytriol," *Cancer Chemotherapy and Pharmacology* 33(4) (1994): 291–297.

Nguyen, T.T., K. Matsumoto, K. Yamasaki, et al., "Crude Saponin Extracted from Vietnamese Ginseng and Major Constituent Majonoside-R2 Attenuate the Psychological Stress- and Foot-Shock Stress-Induced Antinociception in Mice," *Pharmacology, Biochemistry, and Behavior* 52(2) (1995): 427–432.

Nishiyama, N., Y.L. Wang, and H. Saito, "Beneficial Effects of S-113m, a Novel Herbal Prescription, on Learning Impairment Model in Mice," *Biological and Pharmaceutical Bulletin* 18(11) (November 1995): 1498–1503.

Okamura, N., K. Kobayashi, A. Akaike, and A. Yagi, "Protective Effect of Ginseng Saponins Against Impaired Brain Growth in Neonatal Rats Exposed to Ethanol," *Biological and Pharmaceutical Bulletin* 17(2) (1994): 270–274.

Park, H.J., J.H. Lee, Y.B. Song, and K.H. Park, "Effects of Dietary Supplementation of Lipophilic Fraction from *Panax ginseng* on CGMP and CAMP in Rat Platelets and on Blood Coagulation," *Biological and Pharmaceutical Bulletin* 19(11) (November 1996): 1434–1439.

Reay, J.L., D.O. Kennedy, and A.B. Scholey, "Effects of *Panax ginseng*, Consumed with and Without Glucose, on Blood Glucose Levels and Cognitive Performance During Sustained 'Mentally Demanding' Tasks," *Journal of Psychopharmacology* 20(6) (2006): 771–781.

Reay, J.L., D.O. Kennedy, and A.B. Scholey, "Single Doses of *Panax ginseng* (G115) Reduce Blood Glucose Levels and Improve Cognitive Performance During Sustained Mental Activity," *Journal of Psychopharmacology* 19(4) (2005): 357–365.

Rim, B.M., "Ultrastructural Studies on the Effects of Korean *Panax ginseng* on the Theca Interna of Rat Ovary," *American Journal of Chinese Medicine* 7(4) (Winter 1979): 333–344.

Rosenfeld, M.S., "Evaluation of the Efficacy of a Standardized Ginseng Extract in Patients with Psychophysical Asthenia and Neurological Disorders," *La Semana Médica* [*Medical Week*] 173 (1989): 148–154.

Salvati, G., G. Genovesi, L. Marcellini, et al., "Effects of *Panax ginseng* C.A. Meyer Saponins on Male Fertility," *Panminerva Medica* 38(4) (December 1996): 249–254.

Sato, K., M. Mochizuki, I. Saiki, et al., "Inhibition of Tumor Angiogenesis and Metastasis by a Saponin of *Panax ginseng,* Ginsenoside-Rb2," *Biological and Pharmaceutical Bulletin* 17(5) (May 1994): 635–639.

See, D.M., N. Broumand, L. Sahl, and J.G. Tilles, "In Vitro Effects of Echinacea and Ginseng on Natural Killer and Antibody-Dependent Cell Cytotoxity in Healthy Subjects and Chronic Fatigue Syndrome or Acquired Immunodeficiency Syndrome Patients," *Immunopharmacology* 35(3) (January 1997): 229–235.

Siegel, R.K., "Ginseng Abuse Syndrome: Problems with the Panacea," *Journal of the American Medical Association* 241(1979): 1614–1615.

Sorenson, H., and J. Sonne, "A Double-Masked Study of the Effects of Ginseng on Cognitive Functions," *Current Therapeutic Research* 57 (1996): 959–968.

Sotaniemi, E.A., E. Haapakoski, and A. Rautio, "Ginseng Therapy in Non-Insulin-Dependent Diabetic Patients," *Diabetes Care* 18(10) (October 1995): 1373–1375.

Sung, J., K.H. Han, J.H. Zo, et al., "Effects of Red Ginseng Upon Vascular Endothelial Function in Patients with Essential Hypertension," *American Journal of Chinese Medicine* 28(2) (2000): 205–216.

Toh, H.T., "Improved Isolated Heart Contractility and Mitochondrial Oxidation After Chronic Treatment with *Panax ginseng* in Rats," *American Journal of Chinese Medicine* 22(3–4) (1994): 275–284.

Yi, R.L., W. Li, and X.Z. Hao, "Differentiation Effect of Ginsenosides on Human Acute Non-Lymphocytic Leukemic Cells in 58 Patients," *Chung-Kuo Chung Hsi I Chieh Ho Tsa Chih* [*Chinese Journal of Modern Developments in Traditional Medicine*] 13(12) (December 1993): 708, 722–724.

Yun, T.K., and S.Y. Choi, "Preventive Effect of Ginseng Intake Against Various Human Cancers, a Case-Control Study on 1987 Pairs," *Cancer Epidemiology, Biomarkers, and Prevention* 4(4) (June 1995): 401–408.

Zhang, Y.G., and T.P. Liu, "Influences of Ginsenosides Rb1 and Rg1 on Reversible Focal Brain Ischemia in Rats," *Chung-Kuo Yao Li Hsueh Pao* [*Acta Pharmacologica Sinica*] 17(1) (January 1996): 44–48.

Goldenseal

Kong, W., J. Wei, P. Abidi, et al., "Berberine Is a Novel Cholesterol-Lowering Drug Working Through a Unique Mechanism Distinct From Statins," *Nature Medicine* 10(12) (2004): 1344–1351.

Zhang, R.X., D.V. Dougherty, and M.L. Rosenblum, "Laboratory Studies of Berberine Used Alone and in Combination with 1,3-bis(2-chloroethyl)-1-Nitrosourea to Treat Malignant Brain Tumors," *Chinese Medical Journal* (Engl) 103(8) (1990): 658–665.

Gotu Kola

Cesarone, M.R., G. Laurora, M.T. De Sanctis, et al., "The Microcirculatory Activity of *Centella asiatica* in Venous Insufficiency. A Double-Blind Study," *Minerva Cardioangiologica* 42(6) (June 1994): 299–304.

Grimaldi, R., F. De Ponti, L. D'Angelo, et al., "Pharmacokinetics of the Total Triterpenic Fraction of *Centella asiatica* After Single and Multiple Administrations to Healthy Volunteers. A New Assay for Asiatic Acid," *Journal of Ethnopharmacology* 28(2) (February 1990): 235–241.

Montecchio, G.P., A. Samaden, S. Carbone, et al., "*Centella asiatica* Triterpenic Fraction (CATTF) Reduces the Number of Circulating Endothelial Cells in Subjects with Post Phlebitic Syndrome," *Haematologica* 76(3) (May–June 1991): 256–259.

Murray, Michael T., and Joseph E. Pizzorno, *Encyclopedia of Natural Medicine,* 2d. ed. (Rocklin, CA: Prima Publishing, 1997), p. 201.

Nalini, K., A.R. Aroor, K.S. Karanth, et al., "Effect of *Centella asiatica* Fresh Leaf Aqueous Extract on Learning and Memory and Biogenic Amine Turnover in Albino Rats," *Fitoterapia* 46 (1992): 330–335.

Sastravha, G., G. Gassmann, P. Sangtherapitikul, et al., "Adjunctive Periodontal Treatment with *Centella asiatica* and *Punica granatum* Extracts in Supportive Periodontal Therapy," *Journal of the International Academy of Periodontology* 7(3) (2005): 70–79.

Sharma, R., A.N. Jaiswal, S. Kumar, et al., "Role of Brahmi (*Centella asiatica*) in Educable Mentally Retarded Children," *Journal of Research and Education in Indian Medicine* 4 (1985): 55–57.

Green Tea

Bruneton, Jean N., *Pharmacognosy, Phytochemistry, Medicinal Plants* (Paris, France: Lavoisier Publishing, 1995), p. 886.

Chiu, A.E., J.L. Chan, D.G. Kern, et al., "Double-Blinded, Placebo-Controlled Trial of Green Tea Extracts in the Clinical and Histologic Appearance of Photoaging Skin," *Dermatologic Surgery* 31(7) (Part 2) (2005): 855–860.

Fukino, Y., M. Shimbo, N. Aoki, et al., "Randomized Controlled Trial for an Effect of Green Tea Consumption on Insulin Resistance and Inflammation Markers," *Journal of Nutritional Science and Vitaminology* 51(5) (2005): 335–342.

Hara, Y., "Prophylactic Functions of Tea Polyphenols," in *Food Phytochemicals for Cancer Prevention II: Teas, Spices, and Herbs*, ed. Chi-Tang Ho, Toshihiko Osawa, Mou-Tuan Huang, and Robert E. Rosen (Washington, DC: American Chemical Society, 1994), pp. 36, 39, 43, 44–45, 47.

Honda, M., F. Nanjo, and Y. Hara, "Inhibition of Saccharide Digestive Enzymes by Tea Polyphenols," in *Food Phytochemicals for Cancer Prevention II: Teas, Spices, and Herbs*, ed. Chi-Tang Ho, Toshihiko Osawa, Mou-Tuan Huang, and Robert E. Rosen (Washington, DC: American Chemical Society, 1994), pp. 83–89.

Huang, Kee C., and Kee Chang, eds., *The Pharmacology of Chinese Herbs* (Boca Raton, FL: CRC Press, 1992), p. 168.

Iso, H., C. Date, W. K. Wakai, et al., "The Relationship Between Green Tea and Total Caffeine Intake and Risk for Self-Reported Type 2 Diabetes Among Japanese Adults," *Annals of Internal Medicine* 144(8) (2006): 554–562.

Kim, M., N. Hagiwara, S.J. Smith, et al., "Preventive Effect of Green Tea Polyphenols on Colon Carcinogenesis," in *Food Phytochemicals for Cancer Prevention II: Teas, Spices, and Herbs*, ed. Chi-Tang Ho, Toshihiko Osawa, Mou-Tuan Huang, and Robert E. Rosen (Washington, DC: American Chemical Society, 1994), pp. 51–55.

Kinae, N., K. Shimoi, S. Masumoria, et al., "Suppression of the Formation of Advanced Glycosylation Products by Tea Extracts," in *Food Phytochemicals for Cancer Prevention II: Teas, Spices, and Herbs*, ed. Chi-Tang Ho, Toshihiko Osawa, Mou-Tuan Huang, and Robert E. Rosen (Washington, DC: American Chemical Society, 1994), pp. 68–75.

Kuriyama, S., T. Shimazu, K. Ohmori, et al., "Green Tea Consumption and Mortality Due to Cardiovascular Disease, Cancer, and All Causes in Japan: The Ohsaki Study," *Journal of the American Medical Association* 296(10) (2006): 1255–1265.

Nakachi, K., K. Suemasu, K. Suga, et al., "Influence of Drinking Green Tea on Breast Cancer Malignancy Among Japanese Patients," *Japanese Journal of Cancer Research* 89(3) (1998): 254–261.

Nanjo, F., Y. Hara, and Y. Kikuchi, "Effects of Tea Polyphenols on Blood Rheology in Rats Fed a High-Fat Diet," in *Food Phytochemicals for Cancer Prevention II: Teas, Spices, and Herbs*, ed. Chi-Tang Ho, Toshihiko Osawa, Mou-Tuan Huang, and Robert E. Rosen (Washington, DC: American Chemical Society, 1994), pp. 76–82.

Shimamura, T., "Inhibition of Influenza Virus Infection by Tea Polyphenols," in *Food Phytochemicals for Cancer Prevention II: Teas, Spices, and Herbs*, ed. Chi-Tang Ho, Toshihiko Osawa, Mou-Tuan Huang, and Robert E. Rosen (Washington, DC: American Chemical Society, 1994), pp. 101–104.

Terada, A., H. Hara, S. Nakajyo, et al., *Microbial Ecology in Health and Disease* 6 (1993): 3–9.

Guggul

Beg, M., K.C. Singhal, and S. Afzaal, "A Study of Effect of Guggulsterone of Hyperlipidemia of Secondary Glomerulopathy," *Indian Journal of Physiology and Pharmacology* 40(3) (July 1996): 237–240.

Dalvi, S.S., V.K. Nayak, S.M. Pohujani, et al., "Effect of Gugulipid on Bioavailability of Diltiazem and Propranolol," *Journal of the Association of Physicians of India* 42(6) (June 1994): 454–455.

Nityananad, S., J.S. Srivastava, and O.P. Asthana, "Clinical Trials with Gugulipid. A New Hypolipidaemic Agent," *Journal of the Association of Physicians of India* 37(5) (May 1989): 323–328.

Sheela, C.G., and K.T. Augusti, "Effects of S-Allyl Cysteine Sulfoxide Isolated from *Allium sativum* Linn. and Guggulipid on Some Enzymes and Fecal Excretions of Bile Acids and Sterols in Cholesterol-Fed Rats," *Indian Journal of Experimental Biology* 33(10) (October 1995): 749–751.

Singh, R.B., M.A. Niaz, and S. Ghosh, "Hypolipidemic and Antioxidant Effects of *Commiphora mukul* as an Adjunct to Dietary Therapy in Patients with Hypercholesterolemia," *Cardiovascular Drugs and Therapy* 8 (1994): 659–664.

Singh, V., S. Kaul, R. Chander, and N.K. Kapoor, "Stimulation of Low-Density Lipoprotein Receptor Activity in Liver Membrane of Guggulsterone-Treated Rats," *Pharmacology Research* 22(1) (January–February 1990): 37–44.

Szapary, P.O., M.L. Wolfe, L.T. Bloedon, et al., "Guggulipid for the Treatment of Hypercholesterolemia: A Randomized Controlled Trial," *Journal of the American Medical Association* 290 (2003): 765–772.

Thappa, D.M., and J. Dogra, "Nodulocystic Acne: Oral Gugulipid Versus Tetracycline," *Journal of Dermatology* 21(10) (October 1994): 729–731.

Hawthorn

Bahorun, T., B. Gressier, F. Trotin, et al., "Oxygen Species Scavenging Activity of Phenolic Extracts from Hawthorn Fresh Plant Organs and Pharmaceutical Preparations," *Arzneimittel-forschung* [*Medication Research*] 46(110) (November 1996): 1086–1089.

Blumenthal, Mark, senior ed., Werner R. Busse, Alicia Goldberg, Joerg Gruenwald, et al., eds., *The Complete German Commission E Monographs: Therapeutic Guide to Herbal Medicines,* trans. Sigrid Klein and Robert S. Rister, foreword by Varro E. Tyler (Boston, MA: Integrative Medicine Communications, 1998), pp. 142–144.

Degenring, F.H., A. Sutera, M. Weber, et al., "A Randomised Double Blind Placebo Controlled Clinical Trial of a Standardised Extract of Fresh Crataegus Berries (Crataegisan) in the Treatment of Patients with Congestive Heart Failure NYHA II," *Phytomedicine* 10(5) (2003): 363–369.

Della Loggia, R., A. Tubaro, and C. Redaelli, "Evaluation of the Activity on the Mouse CNS of Several Plant Extracts and a Combination of Them," *Rivista di Neuroligia* [*Journal of Neurology*] 51(5) (September–October 1981): 297–310.

Hanus, M., J. Lafon, and M. Mathieu, "Double-Blind, Randomised, Placebo-Controlled Study to Evaluate the Efficacy and Safety of a Fixed Combination Containing Two Plant Extracts (*Crataegus oxyacantha* and *Eschscholtzia californica*) and Magnesium in Mild-to-Moderate Anxiety Disorders," *Current Medical Research and Opinion* 20(1) (2004): 63–71.

Havsteen, B., "Flavonoids, a Class of Natural Products of High Pharmacological Potency," *Biochemical Pharmacology* 32 (1982): 1141–1148.

He, G., "Effect of the Prevention and Treatment of Atherosclerosis of a Mixture of Hawthorn and Motherwort," *Chung-Kuo Chung Hsi I Chieh Ho Tsa Chih* [*Chinese Journal of Modern Developments in Traditional Medicine*] 10(6) (June 1990): 361, 326.

Kuhnau, J., "The Flavonoids, a Class of Semi-Essential Food Components: Their Role in Human Nutrition," *World Review of Nutrition and Dietetics* 24 (1976): 117–191.

Leuchtgens, H., "Crataegus Special Extract WS 1442 in NYHA II Heart Failure: A Placebo-Controlled Randomized Double-Blind Study," *Fortschritte der Medizin* [*Advances in Medicine*] 111(20–21) (20 July 1993): 352–354.

Petkov, E., N. Nikolov, and P. Uzunov, "Inhibitory Effect of Some Flavonoids and Flavonoid Mixtures on Cyclic AMP Phosphodiesterase Activity of Rat Heart," *Planta Medica* 43 (1981): 183–186.

Petkov, V., "Plants and Hypotensive, Antiatheromatous and Coronarodilatating Action," *American Journal of Chinese Medicine* 7(3) (1979): 197–236.

Pourrat, H., "Anthocyanidin Drugs in Vascular Disease," *Plant Medicinal Phytotherapy* 11 (1977): 143–151.

Rajendran, S., P.D. Deepalakshmi, K. Parasakthy, et al., "Effect of Tincture of Crataegus on the LDL-Receptor Activity of Hepatic Plasma Membrane of Rats Fed an Atherogenic Diet," *Atherosclerosis* 123 (1–2) (June 1996): 235–241.

Rakotoarison, D.A., B. Gressier, F. Trotin, et al., "Antioxidant Activities of Polyphenolic Extracts from Flowers, in Vitro Callus and Cell Suspension Cultures of *Crataegus monogyna*," *Pharmazie* 52(1) (January 1997): 60–64.

Saenz, M.T., M.C. Ahumada, and M.D. Garcia, "Extracts from Viscum and Crataegus Are Cytotoxic Against Larynx Cancer Cells," *Zeitschrift für Naturforschung* [*Journal of Biosciences*] 52(1–2) (January–February 1997): 42–44.

Schmidt, U., et al., "Efficacy of the Hawthorn Preparation in 78 Patients with Chronic Congestive Heart Failure Defined as NYHA Functional Class II," *Phytomedicine* 1 (1994): 17–23.

Schussler, M., J. Holzl, and U. Fricke, "Myocardial Effects of Flavonoids from *Crataegus* Species," *Arzneimittelforschung* [*Medication Research*] 45(8) (August 1995): 842–845.

Shanthi, S., K. Parasakthy, P.D. Deepalakshmi, and S.N. Devaraj, "Hypolipidemic Activity of Tincture of Crataegus in Rats," *Indian Journal of Biochemistry and Biophysics* 31(2) (April 1994): 143–146.

Vibes, J., B. Lasserre, J. Gleye, and C. Declume, "Inhibition of Thromboxane A2 Biosynthesis in Vitro by the Main Components of *Crataegus oxycantha* (Hawthorn) Flower Heads," *Prostaglandins, Leukotrienes, and Essential Fatty Acids* 50(4) (April 1994): 175–176.

Ho She Wu

Kimura, Y., H. Ohminani, H. Okuda, et al., "Effects of Stilbene Components of Roots of *Polygonum* Spp. on Liver Injury in Peroxidized Oil-Fed Rats," *Planta Medica* 49 (1983): 51–54.

Mei, M.Z., Q.Q. Zhuang, G.Z. Liu, and W.J. Xie, "Rapid Screening Method for Hypocholesterolemic Agents," *Chung-Kuo Yao Li Hsueh Pao* [*Acta Pharmacologica Sinica*] 14 (1979): 8–11.

Hoelen

Ding, X., "Effects of Poriatin on Mouse Peritoneal Macrophages," *Zhongguo Y'lxue Kexueyuan* 9 (1987): 433–438.

Hattori, T., K. Hayashi, T. Nagao, et al., "Studies on Anti-nephritic Effects of Plant Components (3): Effect of Pachyman, a Main Component of Poria Cocos Wolf on Original-Type Anti-GBM Nephritis in Rats and Its Mechanisms," *Japanese Journal of Pharmacology* 59(1) (May 1992): 89–96.

Wang, G., "Effect of Poriatin on Mouse Immune System," *South China Journal of Antibiotica* 17 (1992): 42–47.

Yu, S.J., and J. Tseng, "Fu-Ling, a Chinese Herbal Drug, Modulates Cytokine Secretion by Human Peripheral Blood Monocytes," *International Journal of Immunopharmacology* 18(1) (January 1996): 37–44.

Hops

Heyerick, A., S. Vervarcke, H. Depypere, et al., "A First Prospective, Randomized, Double-Blind, Placebo-Controlled Study on the Use of a Standardized Hop Extract to Alleviate Menopausal Discomforts," *Maturitas* 54(2) (2006): 164–175.

Milligan, S.R., J.C. Kalita, A. Heyerick, et al., "Identification of a Potent Phytoestrogen in Hops (*Humulus lupulus* L.) and Beer," *Journal of Clinical Endocrinology and Metabolism* 84(6) (June 1999): 2249–2252.

Morin, C.M., U. Koetter, C. Bastien, et al., "Valerian-Hops Combination and Diphenhydramine for Treating Insomnia: A Randomized, Placebo-Controlled Clinical Trial," *Sleep* 28(1) (2005): 1465–1471.

Horehound

Roman-Ramos, R., F. Alarcon-Aguilar, A. Lara-Lemus, and J.L. Flores-Saenz, "Hypoglycemic Effect of Plants Used in Mexico as Antidiabetics," *Archives of Medical Research* 23(1) (Spring 1992): 59–64.

Horse Chestnut

Annoni, F., A. Mauri, F. Marincola, and L.F. Resele, "Venotonic Activity of Aescin on the Human Saphenous Vein," *Arzneimittel-forschung* [*Medication Research*] 29 (1979): 672–675.

Leach, M.J., J. Pincombe, and G. Foster, "Clinical Efficacy of Horsechestnut Seed Extract in the Treatment of Venous Ulceration," *Journal of Wound Care* 15(4) (2006): 159–167.

Pittler, M.H., and E. Ernst, "Horse Chestnut Seed Extract for Chronic Venous Insufficiency," Cochrane Database of Systematic Reviews 2006, Issue 1. Art. No. CD003230. DOI 10.1002/14651858.CD003230.pub3.

Iporuru

Ogungbamila, F.O., and G. Samuelsson, "Smooth Muscle Relaxing Flavonoids from *Alchornea cordifolia*," *Acta Pharmaceutica Nordica* 2(6) (1990): 421–422.

Raymond-Hamet Goutarel, R., "Are the Stimulant Effects of *Alchornea Floribunda* Mueller Arg. in Men Due to Yohimbine?" *Comptes rendus hebdomadaires des seances de l'Academie des Sciences. Serie D: Sciences naturelles* [*Weekly Reports of Sessions of the Academy of Sciences. Series D: Natural Sciences*] 261(16) (18 October 1965): 3223–3224.

Jambul

Achrekar, S., G.S. Kaklij, M.S. Pote, and S.M. Kelkar, "Hypoglycemic Activity of *Eugenia jambolana* and *Ficus bengalensis*: Mechanism of Action," *In Vivo* 5(2) (March–April 1991): 143–147.

Balanehru, S., and B. Nagarajan, "Intervention of Adriamycin-Induced Free Radical Damage," *Biochemistry International* 28(4) (December 1992): 735–744.

Balanehru, S., and B. Nagarajan, "Protective Effect of Oleanolic Acid and Ursolic Acid Against Lipid Peroxidation," *Biochemistry International* 24(5) (July 1991): 981–990.

Chirvan-Nia, P., and A.R. Ratsimamanga, "Regression of Cataract and Hyperglycemia in Diabetic Sand Rats (*Psammomys obesus*) Having Received an Extract of *Eugenia Jambolana* Lamarck," *Comptes rendus hebdomadaires des seances de l'Academie des Sciences. Serie D: Sciences naturelles* [*Weekly Reports of Sessions of the Academy of Sciences. Series D: Natural Sciences*] 274(2) (10 January 1972): 254–257.

Zheng, G.Q., P.M. Kenney, J. Zhang, and L.K. Lam, "Chemoprevention of Benzo[a]pyrene-Induced Forestomach Cancer in Mice by Natural Phthalides from Celery Seed Oil," *Nutrition and Cancer* 19(1) (1993): 77–86.

Kava Kava

Geier, F.P., and T. Konstaninowicz, "Kava Treatment in Patients with Anxiety," *Phytotherapy Research* 18(4) (2004): 297–300.

Klohs, M.W., F. Keller, R.E. Wiliams, et al., "A Chemical and Pharmacological Investigation of Piper Methysticum Forst," *Journal of Medicine, Pharmacology, and Chemistry* 1 (1959): 95–103.

Lehrl, S., "Clinical Efficacy of Kava Extract WS 1490 in Sleep Disturbances Associated with Anxiety Disorders: Results of a Multicenter, Randomized, Placebo-Controlled, Double-Blind Clinical Trial," *Journal of Affective Disorders* 78(2–3) (2004): 101–110.

Kelp

Grauffle, V., B. Kloareg, S. Mabeau, et al., "New Natural Polysaccharides with Potent Antithrombic Activity, Fucans from Brown Algae," *Biomaterials* 10(6) (1989): 363–368.

REFERENCES

Konno, N., H. Makita, K. Yuri, et al., "Association Between Dietary Iodine Intake and Prevalence of Subclinical Hypothyroidism in the Coastal Regions of Japan," *Journal of Clinical Endocrinology and Metabolism* 78(2) (February 1994): 393–397.

Long, A., "Vitamin B$_{12}$ for Vegans," *British Medical Journal* 2(6080) (16 July 1977): 192.

Sakata, T., "A Very-Low-Calorie Conventional Japanese Diet: Its Implications for Prevention of Obesity," *Obesity Research* 3 (Supplement 2) (September 1995): 233S–239S.

Teas, J., "The Dietary Intake of Laminaria, a Brown Seaweed, and Breast Cancer Prevention," *Nutrition and Cancer* 4(3) (1983): 217–222.

Tyler, Varro E., *The Honest Herbal: A Sensible Guide to the Use of Herbs and Related Remedies*, 3d ed. (New York, NY: Pharmaceutical Products Press, 1993), p. 190.

Khella

Duarte, J., F. Perez-Vizcaino, A.I. Torres, et al., "Vasodilator Effects of Visnagin in Isolated Rat Vascular Smooth Muscle," *European Journal of Pharmacology* 286(2) (14 November 1995): 115–122.

Harvengt, C., and J.P. Desager, "HDL-Cholesterol Increase in Normolipaemic Subjects on Khellin: A Pilot Study," *International Journal of Clinical Pharmacology Research* 3(5) (1983): 363–366.

Rauwald, H.W., O. Brehm, and K.P. Odenthal, "The Involvement of a Ca2+ Channel Blocking Mode of Action in the Pharmacology of *Ammi visnaga* Fruits," *Planta Medica* 60(2) (April 1994): 101–105.

Kudzu

Adlercreutz, H., "Diet, Breast Cancer and Sex Hormone Metabolism," *Annals of the New York Academy of Sciences* 595 (1990): 281.

Bruneton, Jean N., *Pharmacognosy, Phytochemistry, Medicinal Plants* (Paris: Lavoisier Publishing, 1995), pp. 296–297, 298.

Han, R., "Highlight on the Studies of Anticancer Drugs Derived from Plants from China," *Stem Cells* 12(1) (1994): 53–63.

Jing, Y., and R. Han, "Differentiation of B16 Melanoma Cells Induced by Daidzein," *Chinese Journal of Pharmacology and Toxicology* 6(4) (1993): 278–280.

Jing, Y., K. Nakaya, and R. Han, "Differentiation of Promyeloctic Leukemia Cells HL-60 Induced by Daidzen in Vitro and in Vivo," *Anticancer Research* 13(4) (1993): 1049–1054.

Lukas, S.E., D. Penetar, J. Berko, et al., "An Extract of the Chinese Herbal Root Kudzu Reduces Alcohol

Drinking by Heavy Drinkers in a Naturalistic Setting," *Alcoholism, Clinical Experimental Research* 29(5) (2005): 756–762.

Woo, J., E. Lau, S.C. Ho, et al., "Comparison of *Pueraria Lobata* with Hormone Replacement Therapy in Treating the Adverse Health Consequences of Menopause" *Menopause* 10(4) (2003): 352–361.

Xie, C.I., R.C. Lin, V. Antony, et al., "Daidzin, an Antioxidant Isoflavonoid, Decreases Blood Alcohol Levels and Shortens Sleep Time Induced by Ethanol Intoxication," *Alcoholism, Clinical and Experimental Research* 18(6) (December 1994): 1443–1447.

Lavender

Akhondzadeh, S., L. Kashani, A. Fotouhi, et al., "Comparison of *Lavandula angustifolia* Mill. Tincture and Imipramine in the Treatment of Mild to Moderate Depression: A Double-Blind, Randomized Trial," *Progress in Neuropsychopharmacology & Biological Psychiatry* 27 (2003): 123–127.

Buchbauer, G., L. Jirovetz, W. Jager, et al., "Aromatherapy: Evidence for Sedative Effects of the Essential Oil of Lavender After Inhalation," *Zeitschrift für Naturforschung* [*Journal of Biosciences*] Section C 46(11–12) (November–December 1991): 1067–1072.

Duke, James A., *The Green Pharmacy* (Emmaus, PA: Rodale Press, 1997), p. 105.

Holmes, C., V. Hopkins, C. Hensford, et al., "Lavender Oil as a Treatment for Agitated Behaviour in Severe Dementia: A Placebo-Controlled Study," *International Journal of Geriatric Psychiatry* 17 (2002): 305–308.

Larrondo, J.V., M. Agut, and M.A. Calvo-Torras, "Antimicrobial Activity of Essences from Labiates," *Microbios* 82(332) (1995): 171–172.

Lin, P.W., W.C. Chan, B.F. Ng, et al., "Efficacy of Aromatherapy (*Lavandula angustifolia*) as an Intervention for Agitated Behaviours in Chinese Older Persons with Dementia: A Cross-Over Randomized Trial," *International Journal of Geriatric Psychiatry* 22(5) (May 2007): 405–410.

Shimizu, M., H. Shogawa, T. Matsuzawa, et al., "Anti-Inflammatory Constituents of Topically Applied Crude Drugs. IV. Constituents and Anti-Inflammatory Effect of Paraguayan Crude Drug 'Alhucema' (*Lavandula latifolia* Vill.)," *Chemical and Pharmaceutical Bulletin* 38(8) (August 1990): 2283–2284.

Shubina, L.P., S.A. Siurin, and V.M. Savchenko, "Inhalations of Essential Oils in the Combined Treatment of Patients with Chronic Bronchitis," *Vrachebnoe Delo* [*Doctors' Concerns*] 5 (May 1990): 66–67.

Soden, K., K. Vincent, S. Craske, et al., "A Randomized Controlled Trial of Aromatherapy Massage in a Hospice Setting," *Palliative Medicine* 18 (2004): 87–92.

Lemon Balm

Akhondzadeh, S., M. Noroozian, M. Mohammadi, et al., "*Melissa officinalis* Extract in the Treatment of Patients with Mild to Moderate Alzheimer's Disease: A Double-Blind, Randomised and Placebo-Controlled Trial," *Journal of Neurology, Neurosurgery, and Psychiatry* 74 (2003): 863–866.

Dimitrova, Z., B. Dimov, N. Manolova, et al., "Antiherpes Effect of *Melissa officinalis* L. Extracts," *Acta Microbiologica Bulgarica* 29 (1993): 65–72.

Forster, H.B., H. Niklas, and S. Lutz, "Antispasmodic Effect of Some Medicinal Plants," *Planta Medica* 40 (1980): 309–319.

Kennedy, D.O., W. Little, C.F. Haskell, et al., "Anxiolytic Effects of a Combination of *Melissa officinalis* and *Valeriana officinalis* During Laboratory Induced Stress," *Phytotherapy Research* 20(2) (February 2006): 96–102.

Larrondo, J.V., M. Agut, and M.A. Calvo-Torras, "Antimicrobial Activity of Essences from Labiates," *Microbios* 82(332) (1995): 171–172.

Soulimani, R., J. Fleurentin, F. Mortier, et al., "Neurotropic Action of the Hydroalcoholic Extract of *Melissa officinalis* in the Mouse," *Planta Medica* 57(2) (April 1991): 105–109.

Wöbling, R.H., and K. Leonhardt, "Local Therapy of Herpes Simplex with Dried Extract from *Melissa officinalis*," *Phytomedicine* 1 (1994): 25–31.

Lentinan

Aoki, T., "Lentinan," in *Immune Modulation Agents and their Mechanisms,* ed. R.L. Fenichel and M.A. Chirigos (New York, NY: Marcel Dekker, 1984), pp. 62–77.

Kanai, K., and E. Kondo, "Immunomodulating Activity of Lentinan as Demonstrated by Frequency Limitation Effect on Post-Chemotherapy Relapse in Experimental Mouse Tuberculosis," in *Manipulation of Host Defence Mechanisms,* ed. by T. Aoki (Amsterdam: Excerpta Medica, 1981), p. 50.

Kosaka, A., M. Kuzoka, K. Yamafuji, et al., "Synergistic Effect of Lentinan and Surgical Endocrine Therapy on the Growth of DMBA-Induced Mammary Tumors of Rats and of Recurrent Human Breast Cancer," *International Congress Series—Excerpta Medica* 690 (1985): 138–150.

Maeda, Y.Y., G. Chihara, and K. Ishimura, "Unique Increase of Serum Protein Components and Action of Antitumour Polysaccharides," *Nature* 252(5480) (15 November 1974): 250–252.

Mashiko, H., J. Satoh, H. Hatayama, and H. Kitamura, "A Case of Advanced Gastric Cancer with Liver Metastasis Completely Responding to a Combined Immunochemotherapy with UFT, Mitomycin C and Lentinan," *Gan to Kagaku Ryoho* [*Japanese Journal of Cancer and Chemotherapy*] 19(5) (May 1992): 715–718.

Moriyama, M., et al., "Anti-Tumor Effect of Polysaccharide Lentinan on Transplanted Ascites Hepatoma-134 in C3H/He Mice," in *Manipulation of Host Defence Mechanisms,* ed. T. Aoki (Amsterdam: Excerpta Medica, 1981).

Oka, M., et al., "Immunological Analysis and Clinical Effects of Intra-abdominal and Intrapleural Injection of Lentinan for Malignant Ascites and Pleural Effusion," *Biotherapy* 5 (1992): 107–112.

Shimuzu, T., et al., "A Combination of Regional Chemotherapy and Systemic Immunotherapy for the Treatment of Inoperable Gastric Cancer," in *Manipulation of Host Defence Mechanisms,* ed. T. Aoki (Amsterdam: Excerpta Medica, 1981).

Taguchi, T., et al., "Phase I and II Studies of Lentinan," in *Manipulation of Host Defence Mechanisms,* ed. T. Aoki (Amsterdam: Excerpta Medica, 1981).

Togami, M., I. Takeuchi, F. Imaizume, and M. Kawakami, "Studies on *Basidiomycetes*. I. Antitumor Polysaccharide from Bagasse Medium on Which Mycelia of *Lentinus Edodes* (Berk.) Sing. Had Been Grown," *Chemical Pharmacology Bulletin* 30(4) (April 1982): 1134–1140.

Usuda, Y., et al., "Drug-Resistant Pulmonary Tuberculosis Treated with Lentinan," in *Manipulation of Host Defence Mechanisms,* ed. T. Aoki (Amsterdam: Excerpta Medica, 1981), p. 50.

Yamasaki, K., S. Sone, T. Yamashita, and T. Ogura, "Synergistic Induction of Lymphokine (IL-2)-Activated Killer Activity by IL-2 and the Polysaccharide Lentinan, and Therapy of Spontaneous Pulmonary Metastases," *Cancer Immunology and Immunotherapy* 29(2) (1989): 87–92.

Ying, Jianzhe, and Mao Xiaolan, *Icons of Medicinal Fungi from China* (Beijing: Science Press, 1987).

Licorice

Abe, Y., T. Ueda, T. Kato, and Y. Kohli, "Effectiveness of Interferon, Glycyrrhizin Combination Therapy in Patients with Chronic Hepatitis C," *Nippon Rinsho* [*Japanese Journal of Clinical Medicine*] 52(7) (July 1994): 1817–1822.

Baschetti, R., "Chronic Fatigue Syndrome and Liquorice," *New Zealand Medical Journal* 108(1002) (28 June 1995): 259.

Baschetti, R., "Chronic Fatigue Syndrome and Neurally Mediated Hypotension," *Journal of the American Medical Association* 275 (1996): 359.

Bianchi, P.G., M. Petrillo, M. Lazzaroni, et al., "Comparison of Pirenzepine and Carbenoxolone in the Treatment of Chronic Gastric Ulcer: A Double-Blind Endoscopic Trial," *Hepatogastroenterology* 32 (1985): 293–295.

Chen, M.F., F. Shimada, H. Kato, et al., "Effect of Glycyrrhizin on the Pharmacokinetics of Prednisolone Following Low Dosage of Prednisolone Hemisuccinate," *Endocronologica Japonica* 37(3) (June 1990): 331–341.

Cinatl, J., B. Morgenstern, G. Bauer, et al., "Glycyrrhizin, an Active Component of Liquorice Roots, and Replication of SARS-Associated Coronavirus," *Lancet* 361(9374) (2003): 2045–2046.

Demitrack, M.A., "Evidence for Impaired Activation of the Hypothalamic-Pituitary-Adrenal Axis in Patients with Chronic Fatigue Syndrome," *Journal of Clinical Endocrinology and Metabolism* 73 (1991): 1224–1234.

Kassir, Z.A., "Endoscopic Controlled Trial of Four Drug Regimens in the Treatment of Chronic Duodenal Ulceration," *Irish Medical Journal* 78 (1985): 153–156.

Madisch, A., et al., "Treatment of Functional Dyspepsia with an Herbal Preparation: A Double-Blind, Randomized, Placebo-Controlled, Multicenter Trial," *Digestion* 69 (2004): 45–52.

Miyake, K., T. Tango, Y. Ota, et al., "Efficacy of Stronger Neo-Minophagen C Compared Between Two Doses Administered Three Times a Week on Patients with Chronic Viral Hepatitis," *Journal of Gastroenterolgy and Hepatology* 17(11) (2002): 1198–1204.

Mori, K., "Effects of Glycyrrhizin (SNMC: Stronger Neo-Minophagen C) in Hemophilia Patients with HIV-1 Infection," *Tohoku Journal of Experimental Medicine* 162 (1990): 183–193.

Murray, Michael T., and Joseph E. Pizzorno, *Encyclopedia of Natural Medicine,* 2d. ed. (Rocklin, CA: Prima Publishing, 1997), p. 522.

Nagai, T., and H. Yamada, "In Vivo Anti-Influenza Virus Activity of Kampo (Japanese Herbal) Medicine 'Shoseiryu-to' and Its Mode of Action," *International Journal of Immunopharmacology* 16(8) (August 1994): 605–613.

Numazaki, K., M. Umetsu, and S. Chiba, "Effects of Glycyrrhizin in Children with Liver Dysfunction Associated with Cytomegalovirus Infection," *Tohoku Journal of Experimental Medicine* 172 (1994): 147–153.

Plyasunova, O.A., "Inhibition of HIV Reproduction in Cell Cultures by Glycyrrhizic Acid," *International Conference on AIDS* 8 (1992): 31.

Schambelan, M., "Licorice Ingestion and Blood Pressure Regulating Hormones," *Steroids* 59(2) (February 1994): 127–130.

Shibata, S., "Antitumor-Promoting and Anti-Inflammatory Activities of Licorice Principles and their Modified Compounds," in *Food Phytochemicals for Cancer Prevention II: Teas, Spices, and Herbs,* ed. Chi-Tang Ho, Toshihiko Osawa, Mou-Tuan Huang, and Robert E. Rosen (Washington, DC: American Chemical Society, 1994), p. 310.

Sigurjonsdottir, H.A., K. Manhem, M. Axelson, et al., "Subjects with Essential Hypertension Are More Sensitive to the Inhibition of 11 Beta-HSD by Liquorice," *Journal of Human Hypertension* 17(2) (2003): 125–131.

Tajiri, H., K. Kozaiwa, Y. Ozaki, et al., "Effect of Shosaiko-to (xiao-chai-hu-tang) on HBeAg Clearance in Children with Chronic Hepatitis B Virus Infection and with Sustained Liver Disease," *American Journal of Chinese Medicine* 19(2) (1991): 121–129.

Takahara, T., A. Watanabe, and K. Shiraki, "Effects of Glycyrrhizin on Hepatitis B Surface Antigen, a Biochemical and Morphological Study," *Journal of Hepatology* 21(4) (October 1994): 601–609.

Takeuchi, T., O. Nishii, T. Okamura, and T. Yaginuma, "Effects of Paeoniflorin, Glycyrrhizin, and Glycyrrhetic Acid on Ovarian Androgen Production," *American Journal of Chinese Medicine* 19(1) (1991): 73–78.

Tangri, K.K., P.K. Seth, S.S. Parmar, and K.P. Bhargava, "Biochemical Study of Anti-Inflammatory and Anti-Arthritic Properties of Glycyrrhetic Acid," *Biochemical Pharmacology* 14(8) (August 1965): 1277–1281.

Tewari, S.N., and A.K. Wilson, "Deglycyrrhizinated Liquorice in Duodenal Ulcer," *Practitioner* 210 (1972): 820–825.

Wang, Z.Y., R. Agarwal, Z.C. Zhou, et al., "Inhibition of Mutagenicity in *Salmonella typhimurium* and Skin Tumor Initiating and Tumor Promoting Activities in Sencar Mice by Glycyrrhetinic Acid: Comparison of the 18-a and 18-b Steroisomers," *Carcinogenesis* 12(2) (February 1991): 187–192.

Westman, E.C., "Does Smokeless Tobacco Cause Hypertension?" *Southern Medical Journal* 88(7) (July 1995): 716–720.

Wichtl, Max, ed., *Herbal Drugs and Phytopharmaceuticals: A Handbook for Practice on a Scientific Basis,* trans. Norman Grainger Bisset (Boca Raton, FL: MedPharm Scientific Publishers, 1995), p. 303.

Maitake

Finkelstein, M.P., S. Aynehchi, A.A. Samadi, et al., "Chemosensitization of Carmustine with Maitake Beta-Glucan on Androgen-Independent Prostatic Cancer Cells: Involvement of Glyoxalase I," *The Journal of Alternative and Complementary Medicine* 8 (2002): 573–380.

Hobbs, Christopher, and Michael Miovic, eds., *Medicinal Mushrooms: An Exploration of Tradition, Healing, and Culture*, 2d. ed. (Santa Cruz, CA: Botanica Press, 1995), p. 114.

Miller, D., Clinical Protocol Submitted to the NIH Scientific Director, Cancer Treatment Research Foundation, Arlington Heights, IL, 1994.

Mori, K., et al., "Antitumor Activities of Edible Mushrooms by Oral Administration," in *Cultivating Edible Fungi*, ed. P.J. Wuest, D.J. Royse, and R.B. Beelman (Amsterdam: Elsevier, 1987), pp. 1–6.

Nakai, R., H. Masui, H. Horio, and M. Ohtsuru, "Effect of Maitake (*Grifola Frondosa*) Water Extract on Inhibition of Adipocyte Conversion of C3H10T1/2B2C1 Cells," *Journal of Nutritional Science and Vitaminology* (Tokyo) 45(3) (June 1999): 385–389.

Nanba, H., "Activity of Maitake D-Fraction to Prevent Cancer Growth and Metastasis," *Journal of Naturopathic Medicine* (1994), Cited in *Medicinal Mushrooms: An Exploration of Tradition, Healing, and Culture*, 2d. ed., ed. Christopher Hobbs and Michael Miovic (Santa Cruz, CA: Botanica Press, 1995), p. 229.

Nanba, H., "Maitake D-Fraction Healing and Preventing Potentials for Cancer," *Townsend Letter for Doctors & Patients* (February–March 1996): 84–85.

Nouza, K., and H. Krejcova, "Pathogenesis and Therapy of Multiple Sclerosis," *Bratislavsky Lekarske L'sty* [*Bratislava Medical Journal*] 98(4) (April 1997): 199–203.

Shimaoka, I., et al., "Preparation of Therapeutic Metal-Bound Proteins from Mushrooms," *Chemical Abstracts* 114 (1993): 3250–3240.

Squillacote, D., M. Martínez, and W. Sheremata, "Natural Alpha Interferon for Multiple Sclerosis: Results of Three Preliminary Studies," *Journal of International Medical Research* 24 (1996): 246–257.

Won, S.J., M.T. Lin, and W.L. Wu, "*Ganoderma Tsugae* Mycelium Enhances Splenic Natural Killer Cell Activity and Serum Interferon Production in Mice," *Japanese Journal of Pharmacology* 59(2) (June 1992): 171–176.

Yang, D.A., S.Q. Li, and X.T. Li, "Prophylactic Effects of Zhuling and BCG on Postoperative Recurrence of Bladder Cancer," *Chung-Hua Wai Ko Tsa Chih* [*Chinese Journal of Surgery*] 32(7) (July 1994): 433–434.

Marshmallow Root

Franz, G., "Polysaccharides in Pharmacy: Current Applications and Future Concepts," *Planta Medica* 55 (1989): 493–497.

Tomoda, M., S. Noriko, T. Oshima., et al., "Hypoglycemic Activity of Twenty Plant Mucilages and Three Modified Products," *Planta Medica* 53 (1987): 8–12.

Wichtl, Max, ed., *Herbal Drugs and Phytopharmaceuticals: A Handbook for Practice on a Scientific Basis*, trans. Norman Grainger Bisset (Boca Raton, FL: MedPharm Scientific Publishers, 1995), p. 66.

Maté

De Stefani, E., L. Fierro, P. Correa, et al., "Maté Drinking and Risk of Lung Cancer in Males: A Case-Control Study from Uruguay," *Cancer Epidemiological Biomarkers Preview* 5(7) (July 1996): 515–519.

Gugliucci, A., and A.J. Stahl, "Low Density Lipoprotein Oxidation Is Inhibited by Extracts of *Ilex paraguariensis*," *Biochemistry and Molecular Biology International* 35(1) (January 1995): 47–56.

Pintos, J., et al., "Maté, Coffee, and Tea Consumption and Risk of Cancers of the Upper Aerodigestive Tract in Southern Brazil," *Epidemiology* 5 (1994): 583–590.

Tenorio Sanz, M.D., and M.E. Torija Isasa, "Mineral Elements in Maté Herb," *Archivos Latinamericanos de Nutrición* [*Latin American Archives of Nutrition*] 41(3) (September 1991): 441–454.

Milk Thistle

Albrecht, M., "Therapy of Toxic Liver Pathologies with Legalon," *Zeitschrift für Klinische Medizin* [*Journal of Clinical Medicine*] 47(2) (1992): 87–92.

Allain, H., S. Schuck, S. Lebreton, et al., "Aminotransferase Levels and Silymarin in De Novo Tacrine-Treated Patients with Alzheimer's Disease," *Dementia and Other Geriatric Cognitive Disorders* 10(3) (May–June 1999): 181–185.

Bokemeyer, C., L.M. Fels, T. Dunn, et al., "Silibinin Protects Against Cisplatin-Induced Nephrotoxicity without Compromising Cisplatin or Ifosfamide Anti-Tumour Activity," *British Journal of Cancer* 74(12) (December 1996): 2036–2041.

Dehmlow, C., J. Erhard, and H. De Groot, "Inhibition of Kupffer Cell Functions as an Explanation for the Hepatoprotective Properties of Silibinin," *Hepatology* 23(4) (April 1996): 749–754.

Ferenci, P., B. Dragosics, H. Dittrich, et al., "Randomisierte Kontrollierte Studie Über Die Silymarin-Therapie

Bei Patienten Mit Leberzirrhose," *Journal of Hepatology* 9 (1989): 105–113.

Grossmann, M., R. Hoermann, M. Weiss, et al., "Spontaneous Regression of Hepatocellular Carcinoma," *American Journal of Gastroenterology* 90(9) (September 1995): 1500–1503.

Locher, R., P.M. Stuer, R. Weyhenmeyer, and W. Vetter, "Inhibitory Action of Silibinin Low Density Lipoprotein Oxidation," *Arzneimittel-forschung* [*Medication Research*] 48(3) (March 1998): 236–239.

Scambia, G., R. De Vincenzo, F.O. Ranelletti, et al., "Antiproliferative Effect of Silybin on Gynaecological Malignancies: Synergism with Cisplatin and Doxorubicin," *European Journal of Cancer* 32A(5) (May 1996): 877–882.

Schreiber, M., and S. Trojan, "Protective Effect of Flavonoids and Tocopherol in High Altitude Hypoxia in the Rat: Comparison with Ascorbic Acid," *Ceskoslovenska Fysiologie* [*Czechoslovak Physiology*] 47(2) (June 1998): 51–52.

Schriewer, H., U. Kramer, G. Rutkowski, and K.J. Borgis, "Influence of Silybin-Dihemisuccinate on Fatty Acid Synthesis in Rat Liver," *Arzneimittel-forschung* [*Medication Research*] 29(3) (1979): 524–526.

Skottova, N., V. Krecman, D. Walterova, et al., "Effect of Silymarin on Serum Cholesterol Levels in Rats," *Acta Universitatis Palackianae Olomucensis Facultatis Medicae* 141 (1998): 87–89.

Sonnebichler, J., and I. Zetl, "Specific Binding of a Flavonolignane Derivative to an Estradiol Receptor," *Progress in Clinical Biological Research* 280 (1988): 369–374.

Soto, C.P., B.L. Perez, L.P. Favari, and J.L. Reyes, "Prevention of Alloxan-Induced Diabetes Mellitus in the Rat by Silymarin," *Comprehensive Biochemistry and Physiology. C. Pharmacology, Toxicology, and Endocrinology* 119(2) (February 1998): 125–129.

Velussi, M., A.M. Cernigoi, A. De Monte, et al., "Long-Term (12 Months) Treatment with an Anti-Oxidant Drug (silymarin) Is Effective on Hyperinsulinemia, Exogenous Insulin Need and Malondialdehyde Levels in Cirrhotic Diabetic Patients," *Journal of Hepatology* 26(4) (April 1997): 871–879.

Vojtisek, B., B. Hronova, J. Hamrik, and B. Jankova, "Milk Thistle (*Silybum marianum* (L.) Gaertn.) in the Feed of Ketotic Cows," *Veterinarni Medicina* 36(6) (June 1991): 321–330.

Wagner, H., "Antihepatotoxic Flavonoids," in *Plant Flavonoids in Biology and Medicine: Biochemical, Pharmacological, and Structure-Activity Relationships,* ed. Vivian Cody, Elliot Middleton, and Jeffrey B. Harborne (New York, NY: Alan R. Liss, 1986), pp. 545–558.

Zi, X., and R. Agarwal, "Silibinin Decreases Prostate-Specific Antigen with Cell Growth Inhibition via G1 Arrest, Leading to Differentiation of Prostate Carcinoma Cells: Implications for Prostate Cancer Intervention," *Proceedings of the National Academy of Sciences of the USA* 96(13) (22 June 1999): 7490–7495.

Zi, X., D.K. Feyes, and R. Agarwal, "Anticarcinogenic Effect of a Flavonoid Antioxidant, Silymarin, in Human Breast Cancer Cells MDA-MB 468: Induction of GI Arrest Through an Increase in Cip1/p21 Concomitant with a Decrease in Kinase Activity of Cyclin-Dependent Kinases and Associated Cyclins," *Clinical Cancer Research* 4(4) (April 1998): 1055–1064.

Mistletoe

Antony, S., R. Kuttan, and G. Kuttan, "Effect of *Viscum album* in the Inhibition of Lung Metastasis in Mice Induced by B16F10 Melanoma Cells," *Journal of Experimental and Clinical Cancer Research* 16(2) (June 1997): 159–162.

Ernst, E., K. Schmidt, and M. Steuer-Vogt, "Mistletoe for Cancer? A Systematic Review of Randomised Clinical Trials," *International Journal of Cancer* 107(2) (2003): 262–267.

Grossarth-Maticek, R., et al., "Use of Iscador, an Extract of European Mistletoe (*Viscum album*), in Cancer Treatment: Prospective Nonrandomized and Randomized Matched-Pair Studies Nested within a Cohort Study," *Alternative Therapies in Health and Medicine* 7 (2001): 57–78.

Heiny, B.M., V. Albrecht, J. Beuth, "Correlation of Immune Cell Activities and Beta-Endorphin Release in Breast Carcinoma Patients Treated with Galactose-Specific Lectin Standardized Mistletoe Extract," *Anticancer Research* 18 (1998): 583–586.

Kovacs, E., T. Hajto, and K. Hostanska, "Improvement of DNA Repair in Lymphocytes of Breast Cancer Patients Treated with *Viscum album* Extract (Iscador)," *European Journal of Cancer* 27(12) (1991): 1672–1676.

Kuttan, G., and R. Kuttan, "Reduction of Leukopenia in Mice by *Viscum album* Administration During Radiation and Chemotherapy," *Tumori* 79(1) (28 February 1993): 74–76.

Mueller, E.A., and F.A. Anderer, "Chemical Specificity of Effector Cell/Tumor Cell Bridging by a *Viscum album* Rhamnogalacturonan Enhancing Cytotoxicity of Human NK Cells," *Immunopharmacology* 19(1) (January 1991): 69–77.

Nikolai, G., P. Friedl, M. Werner, and K.S. Zanker, "Donor-Dependent and Dose-Dependent Variation in the Induction of T Lymphocyte Locomotion in a Three-Dimensional Collagen Matrix System by a Mistletoe

Preparation (Iscador)," *Anticancer Drugs* 8 (Supplement 1) (April 1997): S61–S64.

Steuer-Vogt, M.K., et al., "The Effect of an Adjuvant Mistletoe Treatment Programme in Resected Head and Neck Cancer Patients: A Randomised Controlled Clinical Trial," *European Journal of Cancer* 37 (2001): 23–31.

Timoshenko, A.V., K. Kayser, P. Drings, et al., "Modulation of Lectin-Triggered Superoxide Release from Neutrophils of Tumor Patients with and without Chemotherapy," *Anticancer Research* 13(5C) (September 1993): 1782–1792.

Zhu, H.G., T.M. Zollner, A. Klein-Franke, et al., "Enhancement of MHC-Unrestricted Cytotoxic Activity of Human CD56+ CD3- Natural Killer (NK) Cells and CD3+ T Cells by Rhamnogalacturonan: Target Cell Specificity and Activity Against NK-Insensitive Targets," *Journal of Cancer Research and Clinical Oncology* 120(7) (1994): 383–388.

Morinda

Cui, C., M. Yang, Z. Yao, et al., "Antidepressant Active Constituents in the Roots of *Morinda officinalis* How.," *Chung-Kuo Chung Yao Tsa Chih* [*China Journal of Chinese Materia Medica*] 20(1) (January 1995): 36–39.

Langford, J., A. Doughty, M. Wang, et al., "Effects of *Morinda citrifolia* on Quality of Life and Auditory Function in Postmenopausal Women," *Journal of Alternative and Complementary Medicine* 10(5) (2004): 747–739.

Millonig, G., S. Stadimann, and W. Vogel, "Herbal Hepatotoxicity: Acute Hepatitis Caused by a Noni Preparation (*Morinda citrifolia*)," *European Journal of Gastroenterology and Hepatology* 17 (2005): 445–447.

Motherwort

Blumenthal, Mark, senior ed., Werner R. Busse, Alicia Goldberg, Joerg Gruenwald, et al., eds., *The Complete German Commission E Monographs: Therapeutic Guide to Herbal Medicines,* trans. Sigrid Klein and Robert S. Rister, foreword by Varro E. Tyler (Boston, MA: Integrative Medicine Communications, 1998), p. 172.

Muira Puama

Waynberg, J., "Aphrodisiacs: Contribution to the Clinical Validation of the Traditional Use of *Ptychopetalum guyana*," Paper presented at the First International Congress on Ethnopharmacology, Strasbourg, France, 5–9 June 1990.

Myrrh

Malhortra, S.C., and M.M.S. Ahuja, "Comparative Hypolipidaemic Effectiveness of Gum Guggulu (*Commiphora mukul*) Fraction 'A,' Ethyl-p-chlorophenoxyisobutyrate and Ciba-13437-Su," *Indian Journal of Medical Research* 59 (1971): 1621–1632.

Wichtl, Max, ed., *Herbal Drugs and Phytopharmaceuticals: A Handbook for Practice on a Scientific Basis,* trans. Norman Grainger Bisset (Boca Raton, FL: MedPharm Scientific Publishers, 1995), p. 346.

Oligomeric Proanthocyanidins (OPCs)

Carper, Jean, *Miracle Cures* (New York, NY: HarperCollins, 1997), pp. 233–234.

Corbe, C., "Light Vision and Chorioretinal Circulation: Study of the Effect of Procyanidolic Oligomers," *Journal française d'opthamologie* [*French Journal of Ophthalmology*] 11(5) (1988): 453–460.

Delacroix, P., "A Double Blind Study of Endotelon in Chronic Venous Insufficiency," *La Revue de Médicine* [*Review of Medicine*] 27–28 (31 August–7 September 1981).

Masquelier, J., "Stabilisation Du Collagene Par Les Oligomeres Procyanidoliques," *Acta Therapeutica* 7 (1981): 101–105.

Robert, L., "The Effect of Procyanidolic Oligomers on Vascular Permeability," *Pathologie et Biologie* [*Pathology and Biology*] (Paris) 38(6) (1990): 608–616.

Ryan, J., et al., "An Examination of the Effects of the Antioxidant Pycnogenol on Cognitive Performance, Serum Lipid Profile, Endocrinological and Oxidative Stress Biomarkers in an Elderly Population," *Journal of Psychopharmacology* 22(5) (2008): 553–562.

Tenenbaum, S., et al., "An Experimental Comparison of Pycnogenol and Methylphenidate in Adults with Attention-Deficit Hyperactivity Disorder (ADHD)," *Journal of Attention Disorders* 6(2) (2002): 49–60.

Osha

Beck, J.J., and F.R. Stermitz, "Addition of Methyl Thioglycolate and Benzylamine to (Z)-Ligustilide, a Bioactive Unsaturated Lactone Constituent of Several Herbal Medicines. An Improved Synthesis of (Z)-Ligustilide," *Journal of Natural Products* 58(7) (July 1995): 1047–1055.

Papain

Beuth, J., et al., "Impact of Complementary Oral Enzyme Application on the Postoperative Treatment Results of Breast Cancer Patients—Results of an Epidemiolgical Multicentre Retrolective Cohort Study," *Cancer Chemotherapy and Pharmacology* 47(suppl.) (2001): S45–S54.

Billigmann, P., "Enzyme Therapy—an Alternative in Treatment of Herpes Zoster: A Controlled Study of 1932 Patients," *Fortschritte der Medizin* [*Advances in Medicine*] 113(4) (10 February 1995): 43–48.

Chabot, J.A., W.Y. Tasi, R.L. Fine, et al., "Pancreatic Proteolytic Enzyme Therapy Compared with Gemcitabine-Based Chemotherapy for the Treatment of Pancreatic Cancer," *Journal of Clinical Oncology* 12 (2010): 2058–63; Epub August 17, 2009.

Gujral, M.S., et al., "Efficacy of Hydrolytic Enzymes in Preventing Radiation Therapy-Induced Side Effects in Patients with Head and Neck Cancers," *Cancer Chemotherapy and Pharmacology* 47(supplement) (2001): S23–S28.

Messer, M., C.M. Anderson, and L. Hubbard, "Studies on the Mechanism of Destruction of the Toxic Action of Wheat Gluten in Coeliac Disease by Crude Papain," *Gut* 5 (1964): 295–303.

Messer, N.M., and P.E. Baume, "Oral Papain in Gluten Intolerance," *Lancet* II (1976): 1022.

Smirnov, V.E., P.M. Lavreshin, L.E. Vartanov, et al., "Diagnosis and Treatment of Acute Paraproctitis," *Khirurgiia* [*Surgery*] (Moscow) 2 (1995): 21–23.

Passionflower

Akhondzadeh, S., et al., "Passionflower in the Treatment of Generalized Anxiety: A Pilot Double-Blind Randomized Controlled Trial with Oxazepam," *Journal of Clinical Pharmacology and Therapeutics* 26 (2001): 363–367.

Akhondzadeh, S., et al., "Passionflower in the Treatment of Opiates Withdrawal: A Double-Blind Randomized Controlled Trial," *Journal of Clinical Pharmacology and Therapeutics* 26 (2001): 369–373.

Campbell, D.R., and M.S. Kurzer, "Flavonoid Inhibition of Aromatase Enzyme Activity in Human Preadipocytes," *Journal of Steroid Biochemistry and Molecular Biology* 46(3) (September 1993): 381–388.

Capasso, A., S. Piacenta, C. Pizza, et al., "Flavonoids Reduce Morphine Withdrawal In-Vitro," *Journal of Pharmacy and Pharmacology* 50(5) (May 1998): 561–564.

Herrera, M.D., A. Zarzuelo, J. Jimenez, et al., "Effects of Flavonoids on Rat Aortic Smooth Muscle Contractility: Structure-Activity Relationships," *General Pharmacology* 27(2) (March 1996): 273–277.

Kniper, G.G., J.G. Lemen, B. Carlsson, et al., "Interaction of Estrogenic Chemicals and Phytoestrogens with Estrogen Receptor Beta," *Endocrinology* 139(10) (October 1998): 4252–4263.

Mak, P., F.D. Cruz, and S. Chen, "A Yeast Screen System for Aromatase Inhibitor and Ligands for Androgen Receptor: Yeast Cells Transformed with Aromatase and Androgen Receptor," *Environmental Health Perspectives* 107(11) (November 1999): 855–860.

Medina, J.H., A.C. Paladini, C. Wolfman, et al., "Chrysin (5,7-di-OH-Flavone), a Naturally Occurring Ligand for Benzodiazepine Receptors, with Anticonvulsant Properties," *Biochemical Pharmacology* 40(10) (15 November 1990): 2227–2231.

Movafegh, A., et al., "Preoperative Oral *Passiflora incarnata* Reduces Anxiety in Ambulatory Surgery Patients: A Double-Blind, Placebo-Controlled Study," *Anesthesia and Analgesia* 106(6) (June 2008): 1728–1732.

Paladini, A.C., M. Marder, H. Viola, et al., "Flavonoids and the Central Nervous System: From Forgotten Factors to Potent Anxiolytic Compounds," *Journal of Pharmacy and Pharmacology* 51(5) (May 1999): 519–526.

Soulimani, R., C. Younos, S. Jarmouni, et al., "Behavioural Effects of *Passiflora incarnata* L. and Its Indole Alkaloid and Flavonoid Derivatives and Maltol in the Mouse," *Journal of Ethnopharmacology* 57(1) (June 1997): 11–20.

Speroni, E., and A. Minghetti, "Neuropharmacological Activity of Extracts from *Passiflora incarnata*," *Planta Medica* 54(6) (December 1988): 488–491.

Walle, U.K., A. Galijatovic, and T. Wallte, "Transports of the Flavonoid Chrysin and Its Conjugated Metabolites by the Human Intestinal Cell Line Caco-2," *Biochemical Pharmacology* 53(3) (1 August 1999): 431–438.

Yin, F., A.E. Ciuliano, and A.J. Van Herle, "Growth Inhibitory Effects of Flavonoids in Human Thyroid Cancer Cell Lines," *Thyroid* 9(4) (April 1999): 369–376.

Pau D'Arco

Austin, F.G., "*Schistosoma mansoni* Chemoprophylaxis with Dietary Lapachol," *American Journal of Tropical Medicine and Hygiene* 23(3) (May 1974): 412–419.

Block, J.B., et al., "Early Clinical Studies with Lapachol," *Cancer Chemotherapy Reports* 4 (1974): 27–28.

Carvalho, L.H., E.M. Rocha, D.S. Raslan, et al., "In Vitro Activity of Natural and Synthetic Naphthoquinones Against Erythrocytic Stages of Plasmodium Falciparum," *Brazilian Journal of Medical and Biological Research* 21(3) (1988): 485–487.

Goel, R.K., N.K. Pathak, M. Biswas, et al., "Effect of Lapachol, a Naphthoquinone Isolated from Tectona Grandis, on Experimental Peptic Ulcer and Gastric Secretion," *Journal of Pharmacy and Pharmacology* 39(2) (February 1987): 138–140.

Grüne, U., *Sobre o Princípio Antidiabético de Pedro-hume-caá, Myrcia multiflora* (Lam.) DC (Rio De Janiero: Federal University of Rio De Janiero, 1979); cited in Kenneth Jones, *Pau D'arco: Immune Power from the Rain Forest* (Rochester, VT: Healing Arts Press, 1995), p. 111.

Kreher, B., et al., "New Furanonapthoquinones and Other Constituents of *Tabebuia avellanedae* and Their Immunostimulating Activities in Vitro," *Planta Medica* 54(6) (1988): 562.

Montbriand, M.J., "An Overview of Alternative Therapies Chosen by Patients with Cancer," *Oncology Nursing Forum* 21(9) (1994): 1547–1554.

Peppermint

Cappello, G., M. Spezzaferro, L. Grossi, et al., "Peppermint Oil (Mintoil) in the Treatment of Irritable Bowel Syndrome: A Prospective Double Blind Placebo-Controlled Randomized Trial," *Digestive and Liver Disease* 39(6) (2007): 530–536.

Dew, M.J., "Peppermint Oil for the Irritable Bowel Syndrome: A Multicentre Trial," *British Journal of Clinical Practice* 38 (1984): 394–398.

Gobel, H., "Effectiveness of Oleum Menthae Pipertae and Paracetamol in Therapy of Headache of the Tension Type," *Nervenarzt* [*Neurologist*] 67(8) (1996): 672–681.

Grigoleit, H.G., and P. Grigoleit, "Peppermint Oil in Irritable Bowel Syndrome," *Phytomedicine* 12(8) (2006): 601–616.

Leicester, R., "Peppermint Oil to Reduce Colonic Spasm During Endoscopy," *Lancet* II (1982): 989.

May, B., H. Kuntz, M. Kieser, et al., "Efficacy of a Fixed Peppermint Oil/Caraway Oil Combination in Non-Ulcer Dyspepsia," *Arzneimittelforschung* 46 (1996): 1149–1153.

Somerville, K.W., W.R. Ellis, B.H. Whitten, et al., "Stones in the Common Bile Duct: Experience with Medical Dissolution Therapy," *Postgraduate Medical Journal* 61 (1985): 313–316.

Tassou, C.C., E.H. Drosinos, and G.J. Nychas, "Effects of Essential Oil from Mint (*Mentha piperita*) on *Salmonella enteritidis* and *Listeria Monocytogenes* in Model Food Systems at 4 Degrees and 10 Degrees C," *Journal of Applied Bacteriology* 78(6) (January 1995): 593–600.

Pollen

Bevzo, V.V., and N.P. Grygor'eva, "Effect of Bee Pollen Extract on Glutathione System Activity in Mice Liver Under X-Ray Irradiation," *Ukrainskii Biokhimskii Zhurnal* [*Ukrainian Journal of Biochemistry*] 69(4) (July–August 1997): 115–117.

Rugendorff, E.W., W. Weidner, L. Ebeling, et al., "Results of Treatment with Pollen Extract (Cernilton) in Chronic Prostatitis and Prostatodynia," *British Journal of Urology* 71 (1993): 433–438.

Prickly Ash

Adesany, S.A., and A. Sofowora, "Phytochemical Investigation of Candidate Plants for the Management of Sickle Cell Anaemia," in *Proceedings of the Phytochemical Society of Europe* 37: *Phytochemistry of Plants Used in Traditional Medicine*, ed. K. Hostettmann, A. Marston, M. Maillard, and M. Hamburger (Oxford, England: Clarendon Press, 1995), pp. 189–204.

Bensky, Dan, and Andrew Gamble, compilers, *Chinese Herbal Medicine: Materia Medica*, rev. ed. (Seattle, WA: Eastland Press, 1993), p. 305.

Cichewicz, R.H., and P.A. Thorpe, "The Antimicrobial Properties of Chile Peppers (*Capsicum* Species) and Their Uses in Mayan Medicine," *Journal of Ethnopharmacology* 52(2) (June 1996): 61–70.

Prunella

Tabba, H.D., R.S. Chang, and K.M. Smith, "Isolation, Purification, and Partial Characterization of Prunellin, an Anti-HIV Component from Aqueous Extracts of *Prunella vulgaris*," *Antiviral Research* 11(5–6) (June 1989): 263–273.

Yamasaki, K., T. Otake, H. Mori, et al., "Screening Test of Crude Drugs Extract on Anti-HIV Activity," *Yakugaku Zasshi* [*Journal of the Pharmaceutical Society of Japan*] 113(11) (November 1993): 818–824.

Yao, X.J., M.A. Wainberg, and M.A. Parniak, "Mechanism of Inhibition of HIV-1 Infection in Vitro by Purified Extract of *Prunella vulgaris*," *Virology* 187(1) (March 1992): 56–62.

Yarnell, E., and K. Abascal, "Herbs for Treating Herpes Simplex Infections," *Alternative & Complementary Therapies* 11(2) (April 2005): 83–88.

Zheng, M., "Experimental Study of 472 Herbs with Antiviral Action Against the Herpes Simplex Virus," *Chung-Kuo Chung Hsi I Chieh Ho Tsa Chih* [*Chinese Journal of Modern Developments in Traditional Medicine*] 10(1) (January 1990): 39–41.

PSK

Ebina, T., and K. Murata, "Antitumor Effect of PSK at a Distant Site: Tumor-Specific Immunity and Combination with Other Chemotherapeutic Agents," *Japanese Journal of Cancer Research* 83(7) (July 1992): 775–782.

Ebina, T., and K. Murata, "Antitumor Effect of Intratumoral Administration of a Coriolus Preparation, PSK: Inhibition of Tumor Invasion in Vitro," *Gan to Kagaku Ryoho* [*Japanese Journal of Cancer and Chemotherapy*] 21(13) (September 1994): 2241–2243.

Fisher, M., and L.X. Yang, "Anticancer Effects and Mechanisms of Polysaccharide-K (PSK): Implications of Cancer Immunotherapy," *Anticancer Research* 22(3) (May–June 2002): 1737–1754.

Fukushima, M., "The Overuse of Drugs in Japan," *Nature* 342 (1989): 850–851.

Furuta, M., and H. Niibe, "Effect of Krestin (PSK) as Adjuvant Treatment on the Prognosis After Radical Radiotherapy in Patients with Non-Small Cell Lung Cancer," *Anticancer Research* 13(5C) (September–October 1993): 1815–1820.

Harada, M., K. Matsunaga, Y. Oguchi, et al., "Oral Administration of PSK Can Improve the Impaired Anti-Tumor CD4+ T-Cell Response in Gut-Associated Lymphoid Tissue (GALT) of Specific-Pathogen-Free Mice," *International Journal of Cancer* 70(3) (27 January 1997): 362–372.

Katsumatsu, T., "The Radiation-Sensitizing Effect of PSK in Treatment of Cervical Cancer Patients," in *Immunomodulation by Microbial Products and Related Synthetic Compounds*, ed. Y. Yamamura (Amsterdam: Excerpta Medica 1982), pp. 463–466.

Kawa, K., S. Konishi, G. Tsujino, et al., "Effects of Biological Response Modifiers on Childhood ALL Being in Remission After Chemotherapy," *Biomedicine and Pharmacotherapy* 45(2–3) (1991): 113–116.

Kikuchi, Y., I. Kizawa, K. Oomori, et al., "Effects of PSK on Interleukin-2 Production by Peripheral Lymphocytes of Patients with Advanced Ovarian Carcinoma During Chemotherapy," *Japanese Journal of Cancer Research* 79(1) (January 1988): 125–130.

Matsunaga, K., M. Ohhara, Y. Oguchi, et al., "Antimetastatic Effect of PSK, a Protein-Bound Polysaccharide, Against the B16-BL6 Mouse Melanoma," *Invasion and Metastasis* 16(1) (1996): 27–38.

Mickey, D.D., P.S. Bencuya, and K. Foulkes, "Effects of the Immunomodulator PSK on Growth of Human Prostate Adenocarcinoma in Immunodeficient Mice," *International Journal of Immunopharmacology* 11(7) (1989): 829–838.

Nishiwaki, Y., K. Furuse, M. Fukuoka, et al., "A Randomized Controlled Study of PSK Combined Immuno-Chemotherapy for Adenocarcinoma of the Lung,"

Gan to Kagaku Ryoho [*Japanese Journal of Cancer and Chemotherapy*] 17(1) (January 1990): 131–136.

Sugiyama, Y., S. Saji, K. Miya, et al., "Locoregional Therapy for Liver Metastases of Colorectal Cancer," *Gan to Kagaku Ryoho* [*Japanese Journal of Cancer and Chemotherapy*] 23(11) (September 1996): 1433–1436.

Takashima, S., Y. Kinami, and I. Miyazaki, "Clinical Effect of Postoperative Adjuvant Immunochemotherapy with the FT-207 Suppository and PSK in Colorectal Cancer Patients," *Gan to Kagaku Ryoho* [*Japanese Journal of Cancer and Chemotherapy*] 15(8) (August 1988): 2229–2236.

Torisu, M., A. Uchiyama, T. Goya, et al., "Eighteen-Year Experience of Cancer Immunotherapies—Evaluation of Their Therapeutic Benefits and Future," *Nippon Geka Gakkai Zasshi* [*Journal of Japan Surgical Society*] 92(9) (September 1991): 1212–1216.

Ueno, Y., Y. Kohgo, S. Sakamaki, et al., "Immunochemotherapy in B-16-Melanoma-Cell-Transplanted Mice with Combinations of Interleukin-2, Cyclophosphamide, and PSK," *Oncology* 51(3) (May–June 1994): 296–302.

Yuan, C., Z. Mei, S. Liu, et al., "PSK Protects Macrophages from Lipoperoxide Accumulation and Foam Cell Formation Caused by Oxidatively Modified Low-Density Lipoprotein," *Atherosclerosis* 124(2) (1 August 1996): 171–181.

Psoralea

Bensky, Dan, and Andrew Gamble, compilers, *Chinese Herbal Medicine: Materia Medica,* rev. ed. (Seattle, WA: Eastland Press, 1993), p. 345.

Boik, John, *Cancer and Natural Medicine: A Textbook of Basic Science and Clinical Research* (Princeton, MN: Oregon Medical Press, 1995), pp. 217–218.

Psyllium

Heckers, H., and D. Zielinsky, "Fecal Composition and Colonic Function Due to Dietary Variables. Results of a Long-Term Study in Healthy Young Men Consuming 10 Different Diets," *Motility* (Lisbon) (1984): 24–29.

Kecmanovic, D., M. Pavlov, and M. Ceranic, "*Plantago ovata* (Laxomucil) After Hemorrhoidectomy," *Acta Chirurgica Lugoslavica* 51(3) (2004): 121–123.

Moreyra, A.E., A.C. Wilson, and A. Koraym, "Effect of Combining Psyllium Fiber with Simvastatin in Lowering Cholesterol," *Archives of Internal Medicine* 165(1) (2005): 1161–1166.

Perez-Miranda, M., A. Gomez-Cedenilla, and T. Leon-Colombo, "Effect of Fiber Supplements on Internal

Bleeding Hemorrhoids," *Hepatogastroenterology* 43(12) (1996): 1504–1507.

Prior, A., and P.J. Whorwell, "Double-Blind Study of Ispaghula in Irritable Bowel Syndrome," *Gut* 28 (1987): 1510–1513.

Ziai, S.A., B. Larijani, S. Akhoondzadeh, et al., "Psyllium Decreased Serum Glucose and Glycosylated Hemoglobin Significantly in Diabetic Outpatients," *Journal of Ethnopharmacology* 102(2) (2005): 202–207.

Pygeum

Bruneton, Jean, *Pharmacognosy, Phytochemistry, Medicinal Plants* (Paris, France: Lavoisier Publishing, 1995), p. 142.

Ishani, A., R. MacDonald, D. Nelson, et al., "*Pygeum africanum* for the Treatment of Patients with Benign Prostatic Hyperplasia: A Systematic Review and Quantitative Meta-Analysis," *American Journal of Medicine* 109(8) (December 2000): 654–664.

Paubert-Braquet, M., A. Cave, R. Hocquemiller, et al., "Effect of *Pygeum africanum* Extract on A23187-Stimulated Production of Lipoxygenase Metabolites from Human Polymorphonuclear Cells," *Journal of Lipid Mediators and Cell Signalling* 9(3) (May 1994): 285–290.

Yablonsky, F., V. Nicolas, J.P. Riffaud, et al., "Antiproliferative Effect of *Pygeum africanum* Extract on Rat Prostatic Fibroblasts," *Journal of Urology* 157(6) (June 1997): 2381–2387.

Quercetin

Beatty, E., et al., "Effect of Dietary Quercetin on Oxidative DNA Damage in Healthy Human Subjects," *British Journal of Nutrition* 84 (2000): 919–925.

Bindoli, A., M. Valente, and L. Cavallini, "Inhibitory Action of Quercetin on Xanthine Oxidase and Xanthine Dehydrogenase Activity," *Pharmaceutical Research Communications* 17 (1985): 831–839.

Busse, W.W., D.E. Kopp, and E. Middleton, "Flavonoid Modulation of Human Neutrophil Function," *Journal of Allergy and Clinical Immunology* 73 (1984): 801–809.

Caprioli, J., S. Kitano, and J.E. Morgan, "Hyperthermia and Hypoxia Increase Tolerance of Retinal Ganglion Cells to Anoxia and Excitotoxicity," *Investigative Ophthalmology and Visual Science* 37(12) (November 1996): 2376–2381.

Edwards, R.L., T. Lyon, S.E. Litwin, et al., "Quercetin Reduces Blood Pressure in Hypertensive Subjects," *Journal of Nutrition* 137(11) (November 2007): 2405–2411.

Elia, G., and M.G. Santor, "Regulation of Heat Shock Protein Synthesis by Quercetin in Human Erythroleukemia Cells," *Biochemical Journal* 300 (Part 1) (1994): 201–209.

Ferry, D.R., A. Smith, J. Malkhandi, et al., "Phase I Clinical Trial of the Flavonoid Quercetin: Pharmacokinetics and Evidence for in Vivo Tyrosine Kinase Inhibition," *Clinical Cancer Research* 2(4) (April 1996): 659–668.

Hollman, P.C., M. V.d. Gaag, M.J. Mengelers, et al., "Absorption and Disposition Kinetics of the Dietary Antioxidant Quercetin in Man," *Free Radical Biology and Medicine* 21(5) (1996): 703–707.

Kim, S.J., M.H. Lim, I.K. Chun, et al., "Effects of Flavonoids of *Ginkgo biloba* on Proliferation of Human Skin Fibroblast," *Skin Pharmacology* 10(4) (1997): 200–205.

Koishi, M., N. Hosokawa, M. Sato, et al., "Quercetin, an Inhibitor of Heat Shock Protein Synthesis, Inhibits the Acquisiton of Thermotolerance in a Human Colon Carcinoma Cell Lines," *Japanese Journal of Cancer Research* 83(11) (1992): 1216–1222.

Kowolik, M.J., K.F. Muir, and I.T. MacPhee, "Disodium Cromoglycate and the Treatment of Recurrent Aphthous Ulceration," *British Dental Journal* 144 (1978): 384–389.

Kuo, S.M., "Antiproliferative Potency of Structurally Distinct Dietary Flavonoids on Human Colon Cancer Cells," *Cancer Letters* 110(1–2) (20 December 1996): 41–48.

Leuti, M., and M. Vignali, "Influence of Bromelain on Penetration of Antibiotics in Uterus, Salpinx and Ovary," *Drugs Under Experimental Clinical Research* 4 (1978): 45–48.

Monro, J., J. Brostoff, C. Carini, et al., "Food Allergy in Migraine," *Lancet* 88 (1980): 865–869.

Murray, Michael T., and Joseph E. Pizzorno, *Encyclopedia of Natural Medicine,* 2d. ed. (Rocklin, CA: Prima Publishing, 1997), pp. 314–315.

Otsuka, H., M. Inaba, T. Fujikura, et al., "Histochemical and Functional Characteristics of Metachromatic Cells in the Nasal Epithelium in Allergic Rhinitis: Studies of Nasal Scrapings and Their Dispersed Cells," *Journal of Allergy and Clinical Immunology* 96(4) (October 1995): 528–536.

Slobodianik, G.I., "The Effect of Activated Anthracite with Quercetin on Interstitial Relations During Skin Healing," *Likar'ska Sprava* 2 (March–April 1998): 128–130.

Slobodianyk, H.I., "The Characteristics of Peripheral Nervous System Regeneration in Skin Wounds by the Use of Antioxidant-Bound Charcoal Sorbent," *Klinicheskii Khirgurii* [*Clinical Surgery*] 9–10 (1998): 58–60.

So, F.V., N. Guthrie, A.F. Chambers, et al., "Inhibition of Human Breast Cancer Cell Proliferation and Delay of Mammary Tumorgenesis by Flavonoids and Citrus Juices," *Nutrition and Cancer* 26(2) (1996): 167–181.

Steerenberg, P.A., J. Garssen, P. Dortant, et al., "Protection of UV-Induced Suppression of Skin Contact Hypersensitivity: A Common Feature of Flavonoids After Oral Administration?" *Photochemistry and Photobiology* 67(4) (April 1998): 456–461.

Weber, G., F. Shen, N. Prajda, et al., "Increased Signal Transduction Activity and Down-Regulation in Human Cancer Cells," *Anticancer Research* 16(6A) (November–December 1996): 3271–3282.

Yoshimoto, T., M. Furukawa, S. Yamamoto, et al., "Flavonoids: Potent Inhibitors of Arachidonate 5-Lipoxygenase," *Biochemistry and Biophysics Research Communications* 116 (1983): 612–618.

Raspberry Leaf

Duggal, M.S., K.J. Toumba, M.A. Pollard, et al., "The Acidogenic Potential of Herbal Baby Drinks," *British Dental Journal* 180(3) (1996): 98–103.

McFarlin, B.L., M.H. Gibson, J. O'Rear, et al., "A National Survey of Herbal Preparation Use by Nurse-Midwives for Labor Stimulation. Review of the Literature and Recommendations for Practice," *Nurse Midwifery* 44(3) (May–June 1999): 205–216.

Ozaki, Y., and J.P. Ma, "Inhibitory Effects of Tetramethylpyrazine and Ferulic Acid on Spontaneous Movement of Rat Uterus in Situ," *Chemical Pharmacology Bulletin* 38(6) (1990): 1620–1623.

Red Wine Catechins

Arima, N., I.K. Matsushita, H. Obata, et al., "NF-KappaB Involvement in the Activation of Primary Adult T-Cell Leukemia Cells and Its Clinical Implications," *Experimental Hematology* 27(7) (July 1999): 1168–1175.

Casper, R.F., M. Quesne, I.M. Rogers, et al., "Resveratrol Has Antagonist Activity on the Aryl Hydrocarbon Receptor: Implications for Prevention of Dioxin Toxicity," *Molecular Pharmacology* 56(4) (October 1999): 784–790.

Chun, Y.J., M.Y. Kim, and F.P. Guengerich, "Resveratrol Is a Selective Human Cytochrome P450 1A1 Inhibitor," *Biochemistry and Biophysics Research Communications* 262(1) (19 August 1999): 20–24.

Ciolino, H.P., and G.C. Yeh, "Inhibition of Aryl-Hydrocarbon-Induced Cytochrome P-450 1A1 Enzyme Activity and CYP1A1 Expression by Resveratrol," *Molecular Pharmacology* 56(4) (October 1999): 760–767.

Hsieh, T.C., and J.M. Wu, "Differential Effects on Growth, Cell Cycle Arrest, and Induction of Apoptosis by Resveratrol in Human Prostate Cancer Cell Lines," *Experimental Cell Research* 249(1) (25 May 1999): 109–115.

Huang, C., W.Y. Ma, A. Goranson, et al., "Resveratrol Suppresses Cell Transformation and Induces Apoptosis Through a P53-Dependent Pathway," *Carcinogenesis* 20(2) (February 1999): 237–242.

Jang, M., L. Cai, G.O. Udeani, et al., "Cancer Chemopreventive Activity of Resveratrol, a Natural Product Derived from Grapes," *Science* 275(5297) (10 January 1997): 218–220.

Lu, R., and G. Serrero, "Resveratrol, a Natural Product Derived from Grape, Exhibits Antiestrogenic Activity and Inhibits the Growth of Human Breast Cancer Cells," *Journal of Cellular Physiology* 179(3) (June 1999): 297–304.

Ronzio, B., "Polyphenols as Anti-Inflammatory Agents," *Journal of Naturopathic Medicine* 9(1) (2000): 44–50.

Tsai, S.H., S.Y. Lin-Shiau, and J.K. Lin, "Suppression of Nitric Oxide Synthase and the Down-Regulation of the Activation of NFkappaB in Macrophages by Resveratrol," *British Journal of Pharmacology* 126(3) (February 1999): 673–680.

Reishi

Chang, H.M., and P.P.H. But, *Pharmacology and Applications of Chinese Materia Medica*, vol. 1 (Singapore: World Scientific Company, 1987), pp. 144–146.

Chan, W.K., C.C. Cheung, H.K. Law, et al., "*Ganoderma lucidum* Polysaccharides Can Induce Human Monocytic Leukemia Cells into Dendritic Cells with Immuno-Stimulatory Function," *Journal of Hematology and Oncology* 1(1) (2008): 9.

Gao, Y., et al., "Effects of Ganopoly (*Ganoderma lucidum* Polysaccharide Extract) on the Immune Functions in Advanced-Stage Cancer Patients," *Immunobiological Investigations* 32(3) (2003): 201–215.

Haak-Frendscho, M., K. Kino, T. Sone, et al., "Ling Zhi-8: A Novel T-Cell Mitogen Induces Cytokine Production and Upregulation of ICAM-1 Expression," *Cellular Immunology* 150(1) (1993): 101–113.

Hobbs, Christopher, and Michael Miovic, eds., *Medicinal Mushrooms: An Exploration of Tradition, Healing, and Culture*, 2d. ed. (Santa Cruz, CA: Botanica Press, 1995), p. 104.

Kohda, H., W. Tokumoto, K. Sakamoto, et al., "The Biologically Active Constituents of *Ganoderma lucidum* (Fr.) Karst. Histamine Release-Inhibitory Triterpenes," *Chemical Pharmacy Bulletin* 33 (1985): 1367–1374.

Lei, L., and Z. Lin, "Effects of Ganoderma Polysaccharides on the Activity of DNA Polymerase a in Spleen Cells Stimulated by Alloantigens in Mice in Vitro," *Beijing Yike Daxue Xuebao* [*Journal of Beijing Medical University*] 23 (1991): 329–333.

Matsumoto, K-Osai, *The Mysterious Reishi Mushroom* (Santa Barbara, CA: Woodbridge Press, 1979).

Noguchi, M., et al., "Randomized Clinical Trial of an Ethanol Extract of *Ganoderma lucidum* in Men with Lower Urinary Tract Symptoms," *Asian Journal of Andrology* 10(5) (September 2008): 777–785.

Toth, J.O., et al., "Les Acides Ganoderques T à Z: Triterpenes Cytotoxiques de *Ganoderma lucidum* (Polyporacée)," *Tetrahedron Letters* 24 (1983): 1081–1084.

Wachtel-Galor, S., Y.T. Szeto, B. Tomlinson, et al., "*Ganoderma lucidum* ('Lingzhi'); Acute and Short-Term Biomarker Response to Supplementation," *International Journal of Food Sciences and Nutrition* 55(1) (2004): 75–83.

Zhang, L.X., H. Mong, and X.B. Zhou, "Effect of Japanese *Ganoderma lucidum* (GL) Planted in Japan on the Production of Interleukin-2 from Murine Splenocytes," *Chung-Kuo Chung Hsi I Chieh Ho Tsa Chih* [*Chinese Journal of Modern Developments in Traditional Medicine*] 10(11) (1993): 672–674.

Rooibos

Duke, James A., *The Green Pharmacy* (Emmaus, PA: Rodale Press, 1997), pp. 277, 298.

Erikson, L., "Rooibos Tea: Research into Antioxidant and Antimutagenic Properties," *Herbalgram* 59 (2003): 34–45.

Hesseling, P.B., J.F. Klopper, and P.D. Van Heerden, "The Effect of Rooibos Tea on Iron Absorption," *South African Medical Journal* 55(16) (14 April 1979): 631–632.

Nakano, M., Y. Itoh, T. Mizuno, et al., "Polysaccharide from *Aspalathus linearis* with Strong Anti-HIV Activity," *Bioscience, Biotechnology, and Biochemistry* 61(2) (February 1997): 267–271.

Nakano, M., H. Nakashima, and Y. Itoh, "Anti-Human Immunodeficiency Virus Activity of Oligosaccharides from Rooibos Tea (*Aspalathus linearis*) Extracts in Vitro," *Leukemia* 11 (Supplement 3) (April 1997): 128–130.

Rosemary

Bruneton, Jean N., *Pharmacognosy, Phytochemistry, Medicinal Plants* (Paris, France: Lavoisier Publishing, 1995), p. 220.

Duke, J.A., "Rosemary, the Herb of Remembrance for Alzheimer's Disease," *Alternative and Complementary Therapy* (December 2007): 287–290.

Foster, H.B., H. Niklas, and S. Lutz, "Antispasmodic Effects of Some Medicinal Plants," *Planta Medica* 40 (1980): 309–319.

Kennedy, D.O., and A.B. Scholey, "The Psychopharmacology of European Herbs with Cognition-Enhancing Properties," *Current Pharmaceutical Design* 12 (35) (2006): 4613–4623.

Sangre de Drago

DiCesare, D., H.L. DuPont, J.J. Mathewson, et al., "A Double Blind, Randomized, Placebo-Controlled Study of SP-303 (Provir) in the Symptomatic Treatment of Acute Diarrhea Among Travelers to Jamaica and Mexico," *American Journal of Gastroenterology* 97(10) (2002): 2585–2588.

Duke, James A., and Rodolfo Vasquez Martinez, *Amazonian Ethnobotanical Dictionary* (Boca Raton, FL: CRC Press, 1994).

Holodniy, M., J. Koch, M. Mistal, et al., "A Double Blind, Randomized, Placebo-Controlled Phase II Study to Assess the Safety and Efficacy of Orally Administered SP-303 for the Symptomatic Treatment of Diarrhea in Patients with AIDS," *American Journal of Gastroenterology* 94(11) (1999): 3267–3273.

Jones, K., "Review of Sangre de Drago (*Croton lechleri*)—A South American Tree Sap in the Treatment of Diarrhea, Inflammation, Insect Bites, Viral Infections, and Wounds: Traditional Uses to Clinical Research," *Journal of Alternative and Complementary Medicine* 9(6) (2003): 877–896.

Maxwell, Nicole, *Witch Doctor's Apprentice: Hunting for Medicinal Plants in the Amazon*, 3d. ed. (New York, NY: Citadel Press, 1990).

Meijia, K., and R. Reng, *Plantas Medicinales de Uso Popular en la Amazonia Peruana* (Lima, Peru: AECI and IIAP, 1995), p. 75.

Orozco-Topete, R., J. Sierra-Madero, C. Cano-Dominguez, et al., "Safety and Efficacy of Virend for Topical Treatment of Genital and Anal Herpes Simplex Lesions in Patients with AIDS," *Antiviral Research* 35 (1997): 91–103.

Phillipson, J.D., "A Matter of Some Sensitivity," *Phytochemistry* 38(6) (April 1995): 1319–1343.

Pieters, L., T. De Bruyne, M. Claeys, et al., "Isolation of a Dihydrobenzofuran Lignan from South American Dragon's Blood (*Croton* Spp.) as an Inhibitor of Cell Proliferation," *Journal of Natural Products* 56(6) (June 1993).

Vaisberg, A.J., M. Milla, M.C. Planas, et al., "Taspine Is the Cicatrizant Principle in Sangre de Grado Extracted from *Croton lechleri*," *Planta Medica* 55(2) (1989): 140–143.

Sarsaparilla

Harnischfeger, G., and H. Stolze, "Simlax Species—Sarsaparille," in *Bewährte Pflanzendrogen in Wissenschaft und Medizin* (Bad Homburg, Germany: Notamed Verlag, 1983), pp. 216–225.

Li, G.S., W.L. Jiang, X.D. Yue, et al., "Effect of Astilbin on Experimental Diabetic Nephropathy In Vivo and In Vitro," *Planta Medica* (June 16, 2009).

Rollier, R., "Treatment of Lepromatous Leprosy by a Combination of DDS and Sarsaparilla (*Smilax ornata*)," *International Journal of Leprosy* 27 (1959): 328–340.

Thurmon, F.M., "The Treatment of Psoriasis with a Sarsaparilla Compound," *The New England Journal of Medicine* 227 (1942): 128–133.

Saw Palmetto

Anceschi, R., M. Bisi, N. Ghidini, et al., "*Serenoa repens* (Permixon) Reduces Intra- and Postoperative Complications of Surgical Treatments of Benign Prostatic Hyperplasia," *Minerva Urologica e Nephrologica* [*The Italian Journal of Urology and Nephrology*] 62(3) (September 2010): 219–223.

Bent, S., C. Shinohara, K. Neuhaus, et al., "Saw Palmetto for Benign Prostatic Hyperplasia," *New England Journal of Medicine* 354(6) (2006): 557–566.

Boccafoschi, C., "Confronto Fra Estratto di Serenoa Repens e Placebo Mediate Prova Clinica Controllata in Pazienti con Adnomatosi Prostatica," *Urologia* 50 (1983): 1257–1268.

Breu, W., M. Hagenlocher, K. Redl, et al., "Anti-Inflammatory Activity of Sabal Fruit Extracts Prepared with Supercritical Carbon Dioxide: In Vitro Antagonists of Cyclooxygenase and 5-Lipoxygenase Metabolism," *Arzneimittel-forschung* [*Medication Research*] 42(4) (1992): 547–551.

Carilla, E., M. Briley, F. Fauran, et al., "Binding of Permixon, a New Treatment for Prostatic Benign Hyperplasia, to the Cytosolic Androgen Receptor in Rat Prostate," *Journal of Steroid Biochemistry* 20 (1984): 521–523.

Champault, A., "Double Blind Trial of an Extract of the Plant *Serenoa repens* in Benign Prostate Hyperplasia," *British Journal of Clinical Pharmacology* 18 (1984): 461–462.

Chevallier, Andrew, *Encyclopedia of Medicinal Plants* (London, England: DK Publishing, 1996), p. 127.

Debruyne, F., G. Koch, P. Boyle, et al., "Comparison of a Phytotherapeutic Agent (Permixon) with an Alpha-Blocker (Tamsulosin) in the Treatment of Benign Prostatic Hyperplasia: A 1-Year Randomized International Study," *European Urology* 41 (2002): 497–507.

Giannarini, G., and R. Autorino, "*Serenoa repens* Associated with Urtica dioica (ProstaMEV) and Curcumin and Quercetin (FlogMEV) Extracts are Able to Improve the Efficacy of Prulifloxacin in Bacterial Prostatitis Patients: Results from a Prospective Randomised Study," *International Journal of Antimicrobial Agents* 33(6) (June 2009): 549–553.

Graedon, J., and T. Graedon, *The People's Pharmacy Guide to Home and Herbal Remedies* (New York, NY: St. Martin's Press, 1999), p. 359.

Preuss, H.G., C. Marcusen, J. Regan, et al., "Randomized Trial of a Combination of Natural Products (Cernitin, Saw Palmetto, B-Sitosterol, Vitamin E) on Symptoms of Benign Prostatic Hyperplasia (BPH)," *International Urology and Nephrology* 33(2) (2001): 217–225.

Sciarra, F., "Sex Steroids and Epidermal Growth Factor in Benign Prostatic Hyperplasia (BPH)," *Annals of the Academy of Sciences* 761 (1995): 66–78.

Tolino, A., A. Petrone, F. Sarnacchiaro, et al., "Finasteride in the Treatment of Hirsutism: New Therapeutic Perspectives," *Fertility and Sterility* 66(1) (July 1996): 61–65.

Ulbricht, C., E. Basch, S. Bent, et al., "Evidence-Based Systematic Review of Saw Palmetto by the Natural Standard Research Collaboration," *Journal of the Society for Integrative Oncology* 4(4) (2006): 170–186.

Vahlensieck, W., Jr., "Benigne Prostatahyperplasie—Behandlung Mit Sabalfruchtextrakt," *Fortschrift für Medizin* [*Advances in Medicine*] 111 (1993): 323–326.

Schisandra

Bensky, Dan, and Andrew Gamble, compilers, *Chinese Herbal Medicine: Materia Medica*, rev. ed. (Seattle, WA: Eastland Press, 1993), p. 378.

Chen, Y.Y., and Y.Q. Yang, "Studies on the SGPT-Lowering Active Component of the Fruits of *Schisandra rubriflora* Rhed Et Wils," *Yao Hsueh Hsueh Pao* [*Acta Pharmaceutica Sinica*] 17(4) (April 1982): 312–313.

Ko, K.M., S.P. Ip, M.K. Poon, et al., "Effect of a Lignan-Enriched Fructus Schisandrae Extract on Hepatic Glutathione Status in Rats: Protection Against Carbon Tetra-chloride Toxicity," *Planta Medica* 61(2) (April 1995): 134–137.

Kubo, S., Y. Ohkura, Y. Mizoguchi, et al., "Effect of Gomisin A (TJN-101) on Liver Regeneration," *Planta Medica* 58(6) (December 1992): 489–492.

Lin, T.J., "Antioxidant Mechanism of Schizandrin and Tanshinonatic Acid and Their Effects on the Protection of Cardiotoxic Action of Adriamycin," *Sheng Li Ko Hsueh Chin Chan* [*Progress in Physiology*] 22(4) (October 1991): 342–345.

Lin, T.J., and G.T. Liu, "Effect of Schisanhenol on the Anti-tumor Activity of Adriamycin," *Biochemistry and Biophysics Research Communications* 178(1) (15 July 1991): 207–212.

Lin, T.J., G.T. Liu, Y. Pan, et al., "Protection by Schisanhenol Against Adriamycin Toxicity in Rat Heart Mitochondria," *Biochemical Pharmacology* 42(9) (9 October 1991): 1805–1810.

Nomura, M., Y. Ohtaki, T. Hida, et al., "Inhibition of Early 3-Methyl-4-Dimethylaminoazobenzene-Induced Hepatocarcinogenesis by Gomisin A in Rats," *Anticancer Research* 14(5A) (1994): 1967–1971.

Ohkura, Y., Y. Mizoguchi, S. Morisawa, et al., "Effect of Gomisin A (TJN-101) on the Arachidonic Acid Cascade in Macrophages," *Japanese Journal of Pharmacology* 52(2) (February 1990): 331–336.

Ohkura, Y., Y. Mizoguchi, and Y. Sakagami, "Inhibitory Effect of TJN-101 ((+)-(6S,7S,R-Biar)-5,6,7,8-Tetrahydro-1,2,3,12-Tetramethoxy-6,7-Dimethyl-10,11-ethylenedioxy-6-Dibenzo[a,c]cyclooctenol) on Immunologically Induced Liver Injuries," *Japanese Journal of Pharmacology* 44(2) (June 1987): 179–185.

Panossian, A., and G. Wikman, "Pharmacology of *Schisandra chinensis* Bail: An Overview of Russian Research and Uses in Medicine," *Journal of Ethnopharmacology* 118(2) (July 23, 2008): 183–212.

Song, W., "Quality of *Schisandra incarnata* Stapf.," *Chung-Kuo Chung Yao Tsa Chih* [*China Journal of Chinese Materia Medica*] 16(4) (April 1991): 204–206, 253.

Takeda, S., I. Arai, M. Hasegawa, et al., "Effect of Gomisin A (TJN-101), a Lignan Compound Isolated from Schisandra Fruits, on Liver Function in Rats," *Nippon Yakurigaku Zasshi* [*Folia Pharmacologica Japonica*] 91(4) (April 1988): 237–244.

Upton, R., ed., "Schisandra Berry (*Schisandra chinensis*): Analytical, Quality Control and Therapeutic Monograph," *American Herbal Pharmacopoeia and Therapeutic Compendium* (1999): Santa Cruz, Calif., 1–25.

Yasukawa, K., Y. Ikeya, H. Mitsuhashi, et al., "Gomisin A Inhibits Tumor Promotion by 12-O-Tetradecanoylphorbol-13-Acetate in Two-Stage Carcinogenesis in Mouse Skin," *Oncology* 49(1) (1992): 68–71.

Schizonepeta

Ding, A.W., H. Wu, L.D. Kong, et al., "Research on Hemostatic Mechanism of Extracts from Carbonized *Schizonepeta tenuifolia* Brig.," *Chung-Kuo Chung Yao Tsa Chih* [*China Journal of Chinese Materia Medica*] 18(10) (October 1993): 598–600.

Huang, Kee C., and Kee Chang, eds., *The Pharmacology of Chinese Herbs* (Boca Raton, FL: CRC Press, 1992), p. 153.

Scutellaria

Bensky, Dan, and Andrew Gamble, compilers, *Chinese Herbal Medicine: Materia Medica*, rev. ed. (Seattle, WA: Eastland Press, 1993), pp. 76, 77.

Chung, C.P., J.B. Park, and K.H. Bae, "Pharmacological Effects of Methanolic Extract from the Root of *Scutellaria baicalensis* and Its Flavonoids on Human Gingival Fibroblast," *Planta Medica* 61(2) (April 1995): 150–153.

Costarella, L., "Naturopathic Condition Review: Asthma," *Protocol Journal of Botanical Medicine* 1(2) (Autumn 1995): 103.

Gao, J., A. Sanchez-Medina, B.A. Pendry, et al., "Validation of a HPLC Method for Flavonoid Biomarkers in Skullcap (Scutellaria) and Its Use to Illustrate Wide Variability in the Quality of Commercial Tinctures," *Journal of Pharmacy and Pharmaceutical Sciences* 11(1) (2008): 77–87.

Gao, D., K. Sakurai, J. Chen, et al., "Protection by Baicalein Against Ascorbic Acid-Induced Lipid Peroxidation of Rat Liver Microsomes," *Research Communications in Molecular Pathology and Pharmacology* 90(1) (October 1995): 103–114.

Huang, H.C., H.R. Wang, and L.M. Hsieh, "Antiproliferative Effect of Baicalein, a Flavonoid from a Chinese Herb, on Vascular Smooth Muscle Cell," *European Journal of Pharmacol3ogy* 251(1) (4 January 1994): 91–93.

Kim, K.W., U.H. Jin, D.I. Kim, et al., "Antiproliferative Effect of *Scutellaria barbata* D. Don, on Cultured Human Uterine Leiomyoma Cells by Down-Regulation of the Expression of Bcl-2 Protein," *Phytotherapy Research* 22(5) (May 2008): 583–590.

Konoshima, T., M. Kokumai, M. Kozuka, et al., "Studies on Inhibitors of Skin Tumor Promotion. XI. Inhibitory Effects of Flavonoids from *Scutellaria baicalensis* on Epstein-Barr Virus Activation and Their Anti-Tumor-Promoting Activities," *Chemical and Pharmaceutical Bulletin* 40(2) (February 1992): 531–533.

Kyo, R., N. Nakahta, I. Sakakibara, et al., "Effects of Sho-saiko, To, San'o-shashin-to and *Scutellariae radix* on Intracellular Ca2+ Mobilization in C6 Rat Glioma Cells," *Biological Pharmacology Bulletin* 21(10) (October 1998): 1067–1071.

Murray, Michael T., and Joseph E. Pizzorno, *Encyclopedia of Natural Medicine*, 2d. ed. (Rocklin, CA: Prima Publishing, 1997), p. 153.

Nagai, T., Y. Miyaichi, T. Tomimori, et al., "Inhibition of Influenza Virus Sialidase and Anti-Influenza Virus Activity by Plant Flavonoids," *Chemical and Pharmaceutical Bulletin* 38(5) (May 1990): 1329–1332.

Nagai, T., Y. Suzuki, T. Tomimori, et al., "Antiviral Activity of Plant Flavonoid, 5,7,4'-Trihydroxy-8-Methoxyflavone, from the Roots of *Scutellaria baicalensis* Against Influenza A (H3N2) and B Viruses," *Biological and Pharmaceutical Bulletin* 18(2) (February 1995): 295–299.

Powell, C.B., P. Fung, J. Jackson, et al., "Aqueous Extract of Herba *Scutellaria barbatae,* A Chinese Herb Used for Ovarian Cancer, Induces Apoptosis of Ovarian Cancer Cell Lines," *Gynecologic and Oncology* 91(2) (2003): 332–340.

Razina, T.G., S.N. Udintsev, T.P. Prishchep, et al., "Enhancement of the Selectivity of the Action of the Cytostatics Cyclophosphane and 5-Fluorouracil by Using an Extract of the Baikal Skullcap in an Experiment," *Voprosy Onkologii* [*Cancer Questions*] 33(2) (1987): 80–84.

Rugo, H., E. Shtivelman, A. Perez, et al., "Phase I Trial and Antitumor Effects of BZL101 for Patients with Advanced Breast Cancer," *Breast Cancer Research and Treatment* 105(1) (September, 2007): 17–28.

Udintsev, S.N., S.G. Krylova, and O.N. Konovalova, "Correction by Natural Adaptogens of Hormonal-Metabolic Status Disorders in Rats During the Development of Adaptation Syndrome Using Functional Tests with Dexamethasone and ACTH," *Builletin Eksperimentalnii Biologii i Medizina* [*Bulletin of Experimental Biology and Medicine*] 112(12) (December 1991): 599–601.

Wolfman, P., and D.L. Hoffman, "An Investigation into the Efficacy of *Scutellaria lateriflora* in Healthy Volunteers," *Alternative Therapies in Health and Medicine* 9(2) (2003): 74–78.

Wong, B.Y., B.H. Lau, T. Yamasaki, et al., "Inhibition of Dexamethasone-Induced Cytochrome P450-Mediated Mutagenicity and Metabolism of Aflatoxin B1 by Chinese Medicinal Herbs," *European Journal of Cancer Prevention* 2(4) (July 1993): 351–356.

Wong, B.Y., et al., "*Oldenlandia diffusa* and *Scutellaria barbata* Augment Macrophage Oxidative Burst and Inhibit Tumor Growth," *Cancer Biotherapy and Radiopharmaceuticals* 11(1) (1996): 51–56.

Yang, D., D. Michel, F. Bevalot, et al., "Antifungal Activity in Vitro of *Scutellaria baicalensis* Georgi Upon Cutaneous and Ungual Pathogenic Fungi," *Annales Pharmaceutiques Françaises* [*French Annals of Pharmaceutics*] 53(3) (1995): 138–141.

Yang, T., et al., "Inhibitory Activity on Aldose Reductase and Lipid Peroxidation by Components of Four Chinese Medicinal Herbs," *Chinese Biochemical Journal* 8(1) (1992): 169–173.

Ye, F., L. Xui, J. Yi, et al., "Anticancer Activity of *Scutellaria baicalensis* and Its Potential Mechanism," *Journal of Alternative and Complementary Medicine* 8(5) (2002): 567–572.

Zhang, H., and J. Huang, "Preliminary Study of Traditional Chinese Medicine Treatment of Minimal Brain Dysfunction: Analysis of 100 Cases," *Chung-Kuo Chung Hsi I Chieh Ho Tsa Chih* [*Chinese Journal of Modern Developments in Traditional Medicine*] 10(5) (May 1990): 260, 278–279.

Shepherd's Purse

Kuroda, K., and K. Takagi, "Physiologically Active Substance in *Capsella bursa-pastoris,*" *Nature* 220(168) (16 November 1968): 707–708.

Wichtl, Max, ed., *Herbal Drugs and Phytopharmaceuticals: A Handbook for Practice on a Scientific Basis,* trans. Norman Grainger Bisset (Boca Raton, FL: MedPharm Scientific Publishers, 1995), p. 113.

Shiitake

deVere, R.W., et al., "Effects of a Mushroom Mycelium Extract on the Treatment of Prostate Cancer," *Urology* 60(4) (2002): 640–644.

Gordon, M., B. Bihari, E. Goosby, et al., "A Placebo-Controlled Trial of the Immune Modulator, Lentinan, in HIV-Positive Patients: A Phase I/II Trial," *Journal of Medicine* 29(5–6) (1998): 305–330.

Hobbs, Christopher, and Michael Miovic, eds., *Medicinal Mushrooms: An Exploration of Tradition, Healing, and Culture,* 2d. ed. (Santa Cruz, CA: Botanica Press, 1995), p. 104.

Kimoto, M., et al., "Effects of Shiitake Mushroom on Plasma and Liver Lipid Contents in Rats," *Eiyo to Shokuryo* 29 (1976): 275–281.

Ngai, P.H., and T.B. Ng, "Lentin, a Novel and Potent Antifungal Protein from Shiitake Mushroom with Inhibitory Effects on Activity of Human Immunodeficiency Virus-1 Reverse Transcriptase and Proliferation of Leukemia Cells," *Life Sciences* 73(6) (November 14, 2003): 3363–3374.

Okamoto, T., R. Kodoi, Y. Nonaka, et al., "Lentinan from Shiitake Mushroom (*Lentinus edodes*) Suppresses Expression of Cytochrome P450 1A Subfamily in the Mouse Liver," *Biofactors* 21(1–4) (2004): 407–409.

Szuki, K., H. Tanaka, H. Sugawara, et al., "Chronic Hypersensitivity Pneumonitis Induced by Shiitake

Mushroom Spores Associated with Lung Cancer," *Internal Medicine* 40(11) (2001): 1132–1135.

Siberian Ginseng

Barenboim, G.M., and N.B. Koslova, "Eleutherococcus Extract as an Agent Increasing the Biological Resistance of Man Exposed to Unfavorable Factors," in *Eleutherococcus: Strategy of the Use and New Fundamental Data* (Moscow: MedExport, not dated).

Cicero, A.F., G. Derosa, R. Brillante, et al., "Effects of Siberian Ginseng (*Eleutherococcus senticosus* maxium.) on Elderly Quality of Life: A Randomzied Clinical Trial," *Archives of Gerontology and Geriatrics* 9 (Supplement) (2004): 69–73.

Hartz, A.J., S. Bentler, R. Noyes, et al., "Randomized Controlled Trial of Siberian Ginseng for Chronic Fatigue," *Psychological Medicine* 34 (2004): 51–61.

Jung, C.H., H. Jung, Y.C. Shin, et al., "*Eleutherococcus senticosus* Extract Attenuates LPS-Induced iNOS Expression Through the Inhibition of AKt and JNK Pathways in Murine Macrophage," *Journal of Ethnopharmacology* 113(1) (August 15, 2007): 183–187.

Lee, Y.J., H.Y. Chung, H.K. Kwak, et al., "The Effects of *A. senticosus* Supplementation on Serum Lipid Profiles, Biomarkers of Oxidative Stress, and Lymphocyte DNA Damage in Postmenopausal Women," *Biochemical and Biophysical Research Communications* 375(1) (October 10, 2008): 44–48.

Mar, S., personal communication, 5 June 1996.

Murray, Michael T., *Healing Power of Herbs* (Rocklin, CA: Prima Publishing, 1991), p. 56.

Wagner, H., "Immunostimulants from Medicinal Plants," in *Advances in Chinese Medicinal Materials Research,* ed. H.M. Chang, W. Yeung, W. Tso, and A. Koo (Singapore: World Scientific, 1985).

Wagner, H., A. Proksch, I. Riess-Maurer, et al., "Immunostimulatory Effects of Polysaccharides (Heteroglycans) of Higher Plants," *Arzneimittel-forschung* [*Medication Research*] 35(7) (1985): 1069–1075.

Siberian Ginseng Goes to the Gym

Dowling, E.A., D.R. Redondo, J.D. Branch, et al., "Effect of *Eleutherococcus senticosus* on Maximal and Submaximal Exercise Performance," *Medicine and Science in Sports and Medicine* 28(4) (April 1996): 482–489.

Kalashnikov, B.N., "The Effect of Long-Term Prophylactic Administration of *Eleutherococcus* on Morbidity Among Coal Miners in the Far North," *Tesisi Dokladov Vsyesoyuznii Konferenz po Adaptatzii Chegovyeka k Razduchnii Geografichyeskiim, Klimatichyeskim i Proizbochestbinim Faktori* (Novosibirsk, Russia: USSR Academy of Medical Sciences, Far Eastern Division, 1977), pp. 43–44.

Mar, S., personal communication, 26 May 1996.

Murano, S., and R.R. Lo Russo, "Experiencia con ARM 229," *Prensa Medícinales de Argentina* 71 (1984): 178–183.

Pieralisi, G., P. Ripari, and L. Vecchiet, "Effects of S/a Standardized Ginseng Extract Combined with Dimethylaminoethanol Bitartrate, Vitamins, Minerals, and Trace Elements on Physical Performance During Exercise," *Clinical Therapeutics* 13 (1991): 373–382.

Slippery Elm

Beveridge, R.J., J.F. Stoddard, W.A. Szarek, et al., "Some Structural Features of the Mucilage from the Bark of *Ulmus fulva* (Slippery Elm Mucilage)," *Carbohydrate Research* 9 (1969): 429–439.

Karn, H., and M.J. Moore, "The Use of the Herbal Remedy ESSIAC in an Outpatient Cancer Population," *Proceeding ASCO* 16 (1997): 71.

Locock, R.A., "Essiac," *Canadian Pharmacy Journal* 130 (1997): 18–20.

Snow Fungus

Gao, Q., et al., "Polysaccharides and the Antitumor Activity of *Tremella fuciformis*," *Tianran Chanwu Yanjiu Yu Kaifa* 3 (1991): 43–48.

Hobbs, Christopher, and Michael Miovic, eds., *Medicinal Mushrooms: An Exploration of Tradition, Healing, and Culture,* 2d. ed. (Santa Cruz, CA: Botanica Press, 1995), p. 168.

Liu, S.H., et al., "Inhibition Effect of *Tremella fuciformis* Berk. Preparation (TFB) on Growth of Transplanted Mouse Tumor Cells," *Zhong Guo Zhong Liu Lin Chuang* 21 (1994): 68–70.

Ma, L., and Z. Lin, "Effect of *Tremella* Polysaccharide on IL-2 Production by Mouse Splenocytes," *Yao Xue Xue Bao* [*Acta Pharmaceutica Sinica*] 27(1) (1992): 1–4.

Wang, Z.C., S. Yang, L.X. Li, et al., "Studies on the Effects of *Tremella fuciformis* Bark Preparations on Immunity and Blood Formation in Rhesus Monkeys," *Journal of Traditional Chinese Medicine* 3(1) (March 1983): 13–16.

Yang, J., et al., "Stimulatory Effect and Kinetics of Carboxymethylpachymaran on the Induction of Interferon by Lymphoblastoid Cell Culture," *Chinese Journal of Microbiology and Immunology* 6 (1987): 157–159.

Zheng, L., et al., "Effects of *Ling Zhi* on the Production of Interleukin-2 from Immunopharmacological Study

(5)," *The Research on Ganoderma lucidum, Part One* (Shanghai, China: Shanghai Medical University Press, 1993), pp. 259–265.

Soy Isoflavone Concentrate

Adlercreutz, H., Y. Mousavia, and K. Höckerstedt, "Diet and Breast Cancer," *Acta Oncologica* 31(2) (1992): 175–181.

Baum, J.A., H. Teng, J.W. Erdman, et al., "Long-Term Intake of Soy Protein Improves Blood Lipid Profiles and Increases Mononuclear Cell Low-Density-Lipoprotein Receptor Messenger RNA in Hypercholesterolemic, Postmenopausal Women," *Amercian Journal of Clinical Nutrition* 68(3) (1998): 545–551.

Bowen, R., S. Barnes, and H. Wei, "Antipromotional Effect of the Soybean Isoflavone Genistein," *Proceedings of the American Association for Cancer Research* 34 (1991): 555.

Bruneton, Jean N., *Pharmacognosy, Phytochemistry, Medicinal Plants* (Paris, France: Lavoisier Publishing, 1995), pp. 296–297.

Crouse, J.R., III, T. Morgan, J.G. Terry, et al., "A Randomized Trial Comparing the Effect of Casein with That of Soy Protein Containing Varying Amounts of Isoflavones on Plasma Concentrations of Lipids and Lipoproteins," *Archives of Internal Medicine* 159(17) (27 September 1999): 2070–2076.

File, S., N. Jarrett, and E. Fluck, "Eating Soya Improves Human Memory," *Psychopharmacology* 157(4) (2001): 430–436.

Fotsis, T., M. Pepper, H. Adlercreutz, et al., "Genistein, a Dietary-Derived Inhibitor of in Vitro Angiogenesis," *Proceedings of the National Academy of Sciences of the USA* 90 (1993): 2690–2694.

Hall, W.L., N.L. Formanuik, D. Harnpanich, et al., "A Meal Enriched with Soy Isoflavones Increases Nitric Oxide-Mediated Vasodilation in Healthy Postmenopausal Women," *Journal of Nutrition* 138 (2008): 1288–1292.

Han, R., "Highlight on the Studies of Anticancer Drugs Derived from Plants from China," *Stem Cells* 12(1) (1994): 53–63.

Jing, Y., and R. Han, "Differentiation of B16 Melanoma Cells Induced by Daidzein," *Chinese Journal of Pharmacology and Toxicology* 6(4) (1993): 278–280.

Jing, Y., K. Nakaya, and R. Han, "Differentiation of Promyelocytic Leukemia Cells HL-60 Induced by Daidzein in Vitro and in Vivo," *Anticancer Research* 13(4) (1993): 1049–1054.

Kok, L., S. Kreijkamp-Kaspers, D.E. Grobbee, et al., "A Randomized, Placebo-Controlled Trial on the Effects of Soy Protein Containing Isoflavones on Quality of Life in Postmenopausal Women," *Journal of North American Menopause* 12(1) (2005): 56–62.

Komine, M., I.M. Freedberg, and M. Blumenberg, "Regulation of Epidermal Expression of Keratin K17 in Inflammatory Skin Diseases," *Journal of Investigative Dermatology* 107(4) (October 1996): 569–575.

Kreijkamp-Kaspers, S., L. Kok, D.E. Grobbee, et al., "Effect of Soy Protein Containing Isoflavones on Cognitive Function, Bone Mineral Density, and Plasma Lipids in Postmenopausal Women. A Randomized Controlled Trial," *Journal of the American Medical Association* 292(1) (2004): 65–74.

Kritz-Silverstein, D., D. Von Muhlen, E. Barrett-Connor, et al., "Isoflavones and Cognitive Function in Older Women: The Soy and Postmenopausal Health in Aging (SOPHIA) Study," *Menopause* 10(3) (2003): 196–202.

Lian, F., Y. Li, M. Bhuiyan, et al., "p53-Independent Apoptosis Induced by Genistein in Lung Cancer Cells," *Nutrition and Cancer* 33(2) (1999): 125–131.

Ma, Y., D. Chiriboga, B.C. Olendzki, et al., "Effect of Soy Protein Containing Isoflavones on Blood Lipids in Moderately Hypercholesterolemic Adults: A Randomized Controlled Trial," *Journal of the American College of Nutrition* 24(4) (2005): 275–285.

Mori, M., T. Aizawa, M. Tokoro, et al., "Soy Isoflavone Tablets Reduce Osteoporosis Risk Factors and Obesity in Middle-Aged Japanese Women," *Clinical and Experimental Pharmacology & Physiology* 31 (2004): S44–S46.

Nelson, H.D., K.K. Vesco, E. Haney, et al., "Nonhormonal Therapies for Menopausal Hot Flashes: Systematic Review and Meta-Analysis," *Journal of the American Medical Association* 295(1) (2006): 2057–2071.

Ohta, H., S. Komukai, K. Makita, et al., "Effects of 1-Year Ipriflavone Treatment on Lumbar Bone Mineral Density and Bone Metabolic Markers in Postmenopausal Women with Low Bone Mass," *Hormone Research* 51(4) (1999): 178–183.

Panno, M.L., M. Salerno, V. Pezzi, et al., "Effect of Oestradiol and Insulin on the Proliferative Pattern and on Oestrogen and Progesterone Receptor Contents in MCF-7 Cells," *Journal of Cancer Research and Clinical Oncology* 122(12) (1996): 745–749.

Rivas, M., R. Garay, J.P. Escanero, et al., "Soy Milk Lowers Blood Pressure in Men and Women with Mild to Moderate Essential Hypertension," *Journal of Nutrition* 132(7) (2002): 1900–1902.

Schabath, M., L.M. Hernandez, X. Wu, et al., "Dietary Phytoestrogens and Lung Cancer Risk," *Journal of the American Medical Association* 294(12) (September 2005): 1493–1504.

Scheiber, M.D., and R.W. Rebar, "Isoflavones and Post-menopausal Bone Health: A Viable Alternative to Estrogen Therapy?" *Menopause* 6(3) (Fall 1999): 233–241.

Shu, X.O., Y. Zheng, H. Cai, et al., "Soy Food Intake and Breast Cancer Survival," *Journal of the American Medical Association* 302(22) (2009): 2437–2443.

Teede, H.J., D. Giannopoulos, F.S. Dalais, et al., "Randomised, Controlled, Cross-Over Trial of Soy Protein with Isoflavones on Blood Pressure and Arterial Function in Hypertensive Subjects," *Journal of the American College of Nutrition* 25(6) (2006): 533–540.

Van Patten, C.L., et al., "Effect of Soy Phytoestrogens on Hot Flashes in Postmenopausal Women with Breast Cancer: A Randomized, Controlled Clinical Trial," *Journal of Clinical Oncology* 20 (2002): 1449–1455.

Watanabe, T., K. Kondo, and M. Oishi, "Induction of in Vitro Differentiation of Mouse Erytholeukemia Cells by Genistein, and Inhibitor of Tyrosine Protein Kinases," *Cancer Research* 51 (1991): 764–768.

Welshons, W.V., C.S. Murphy, R. Koch, et al., "Stimulation of Breast Cancer Cells in Vitro by the Environmental Estrogen Enterolactone and the Phytoestrogen Equol," *Breast Cancer Research and Treatment* 10 (1987): 169–175.

Soy Lecithin

Holford, N.H., and K. Peace, "The Effect of Tacrine and Lechithin in Alzheimer's Disease: A Population Pharmacodynamic Analysis of Five Clinical Trials," *European Journal of Clinical Pharmacology* 47(1) (1994): 17–23.

Kobayashi, K., M. Han, S. Watarai, et al., "Availability of Liposomes as Drug Carriers to the Brain," *Acta Medica Okayama* 50(2) (April 1996): 67–72.

Tong, X.W., and Q.M. Xue, "Alterations of Serum Phospholipids in Patients with Multiple Sclerosis," *Chinese Medical Journal* 106(9) (September 1993): 650–654.

St. John's Wort

Aizenmann, B.E., "Antibiotic Preparations from *Hypericum perforatum*," *Mikrobiologicheskii Zhyurnal* [*Journal of Microbiology*] 31 (1969): 128–133.

Couldwell, W.T., R. Gopalakrishna, D.R. Hinton, et al., "Hypericin: A Potential Antiglioma Therapy," *Neurosurgery* 35 (1994): 705–710.

Davidson, J.T., and K.M. Connor, "St. John's Wort in Generalized Anxiety Disorder: Three Case Reports (Letter)," *Journal of Clinical Psychopharmacology* 21(6) (2001): 635–636.

De Smet, P.A., and W.A. Nolen, "St. John's Wort as an Antidepressant," *British Medical Journal* 313 (1996): 241–247.

Demisch, L., J. Nispel, T. Sielaff, et al., "Influence of Subchronic Hyperforat Administration on Melatonin Production," *Pharmacopsychiatry* (1991), cited in *HerbalGram* 40 (1997): 30.

Griffin, W.S., O. Yeralan, J.G. Sheng, et al., "Overexpression of the Neurotrophic Cytokine S100 Beta in Human Temporal Lobe Epilepsy," *Journal of Neurochemistry* 65(1) (July 1995): 228–233.

Gulick, R.M., V. McAuliffe, J. Holden-Wiltse, et al., "Phase I Studies of Hypericin, the Active Compound in St. John's Wort, as an Antiretroviral Agent in HIV-Infected Adults, AIDS Clinical Trials Group Protocols 150 and 258," *Annals of Internal Medicine* 130(6) (16 March 1999): 510–514.

Hahn, G., "*Hypericum perforatum* (St. John's Wort)—a Medicinal Herb Used in Antiquity and Still of Interest Today," *Journal of Naturopathic Medicine* 3 (1994): 94–96.

Kasper, S., I.G. Anghelescu, A. Szegedi, et al., "Superior Efficacy of St. John's Wort Extract WS 5570 Compared to Placebo in Patients with Major Depression: A Randomized, Double-Blind, Placebo-Controlled, Multi-Center Trial," *BMC Medicine* 4 (2006): 14.

Kim, H.L., J. Streltzer, and D. Goebert, "St. John's Wort for Depression: A Meta-Analysis of Well-Defined Clinical Trials," *Journal of Nervous and Mental Disease* 187(9) (1999): 532–539.

Linde, K., G. Ramirez, C.D. Mulrow, et al., "St. John's Wort for Depression—an Overview and Meta-Analysis of Randomised Clinical Trials," *British Medical Journal* 313(7052) (3 August 1996): 253–258.

Melzer, R., U. Fricke, and J. Holzl, "Vasoactive Properties of Procyanidins from *Hypericum perforatum* L. in Isolated Porcine Coronary Arteries," *Arzneimittel-forschung* [*Medication Research*] 41(5) (May 1991): 481–483.

Müller, W.E., and R. Rossol, "Effects of Hypericum Extract on the Expression of Serotonin Receptors," *Journal of Geriatric Psychiatry and Neurology* 7 (Supplement 1) (October 1994): S63–S64.

Rao, S.G., et al., "Calendula and Hypericum: Two Homeopathic Drugs Promoting Wound Healing in Rats," *Fitoterapia* 6 (1991): 508–510.

Saljic, J., "Ointment for the Treatment of Burns," *Chemical Abstracts* 1977–1997 (1975).

Sarrell, E.M., H.A. Cohen, and E. Kahan, "Naturopathic Treatment for Ear Pain in Children," *Pediatrics* 111(5) (2003): e574–e579.

Schempp, C.M., S. Hezel, and J.C. Simon, "Topical Treatment of Atopic Dermatitis with Hypericum Cream: A Randomised, Placebo-Controlled, Double-Blind

Half-Side Comparison Study," *Der Hautarzt* 54(3) (2003): 248–253.

Schulz, H., and M. Jobert, "Effects of Hypericum Extract on the Sleep EEG in Older Volunteers," *Journal of Geriatric Psychiatry and Neurology* 7 (Supplement 1) (October 1994): S39–S43.

Shelton, R.C., M.B. Keller, A. Gelenberg, et al., "Effectiveness of St. John's Wort in Major Depression: A Randomized Contolled Trial," *Journal of the American Medical Association* 285(15) (2001): 1978–1986.

Suzuki, O., Y. Katsumata, M. Oya, et al., "Inhibition of Monoamine Oxidase by Hypericin," *Planta Medica* 50 (1984): 272–274.

Szegedi, A., R. Kohnen, A. Dienel, et al., "Acute Treatment of Moderate to Severe Depression with Hypericum Extract WS 5570 (St. John's Wort): Randomised Controlled Double-Blind Non-inferiority Trial Versus Paroxetine," *British Medical Journal* 330(7490) (2005): 503.

Thiele, B., I. Brink, and M. Ploch, "Modulation of Cytokine Expression by Hypericum Extract," *Journal of Geriatric Psychiatry and Neurology* 7 (Supplement 1) (1994): S60–S62.

Upton, R., ed., "American Herbal Pharmacopoeia and Therapeutic Compendium: St. John's Wort (*Hypericum perforatum*), Quality Control, Analytical and Therapeutic Monograph," *HerbalGram* 40 (1997): 18.

Stinging Nettle Leaf

Obertreis, B., K. Giller, T. Teucher, et al., "Anti-Inflammatory Effect of *Urtica dioica* Folia Extract in Comparison to Caffeic Malic Acid," *Arzneimittel-forschung* [*Medication Research*] 46(1) (January 1996): 52–56.

Teucher, T., B. Obertreis, T. Ruttkowski, et al., "Cytokine Secretion in Whole Blood of Healthy Subjects Following Oral Administration of *Urtica dioica* L. Plant Extract," *Arzneimittel-forschung* [*Medication Research*] 46(9) (September 1996): 906–910.

Stinging Nettle Root

Chrubasik, S., W. Enderlein, R. Bauer, et al., "Evidence for the Antirheumatic Effectiveness of Stewed Herba *Urticae dioicae* in Acute Arthritis: A Pilot Study," *Phytomedicine* 4 (1997): 105–108.

Entzian, P., J. Barth, U. Schumacher, et al., "Effect of Lectins on the Number of Glucocorticoid Receptor Sites," in *Lectins—Biology, Biochemistry, Clinical Biochemistry*, ed. T.C. Bog-Hansen and D.L.J. Freed (St. Louis, MO: Sigma Chemical Company, 1988), pp. 111–115.

Mittman, P., "Randomized, Double-Blind Study of Freeze-Dried *Urtica dioica* in the Treatment of Allergic Rhinitis," *Planta Medica* 56(1) (February 1990): 44–47.

Musette, P., A. Galelli, H. Chabre, et al., "*Urtica dioica* Agglutinin, a V Beta 8.3-Specific Superantigen, Prevents the Development of the Systemic Lupus Erythematosus-Like Pathology of MRL Lpr/lpr Mice," *European Journal of Immunology* 26(8) (August 1996): 1707–1711.

Obertreis, B., K. Giller, T. Teucher, et al., "Anti-Inflammatory Effect of *Urtica dioica* Folia Extract in Comparison to Caffeic Malic Acid," *Arzneimittel-forschung* [*Medication Research*] 46(1) (January 1996): 52–56.

Safarinejad, M.R., "*Urtica dioica* for Treatment of Benign Prostatic Hyperplasia: A Prospective, Randomized, Double-Blind, Placebo-Controlled, Crossover Study," *Journal of Herbal Pharmacotherapy* 5 (2005): 1–11.

Schneider, T., H. Rübben, "Stinging Nettle Root Extract (*Bazoton uno*) in Long Term Treatment of Benign Prostatic Syndrome (BPS). Results of a Randomized, Double-Blind, Placebo-Controlled Multicenter Study after 12 Months," *Der Urologe* A 43(3) (2004): 302–306.

Schottner, M., D. Gansser, and G. Spiteller, "Lignans from the Roots of *Urtica dioica* and Their Metabolites Bind to Human Sex Hormone Binding Globulin (SHBG)," *Planta Medica* 63(6) (December 1997): 529–532.

Wagner, H., F. Willer, and R. Samtleben, "Lektine und Polysaccharide—die Hauptwirprinzipien von *Urtica dioica* Wurzeln," in *Benigne Prostathyperplasie*, 4th ed., ed. G. Boos (Frankfurt, Germany: PMI Verlagsgruppe, 1994), pp. 115–122.

Tea Tree Oil

Bassett, I.B., D.L. Pannowitz, and R.S. Barnetson, "A Comparative Study of Tea-Tree Oil Versus Benzoylperoxide in the Treatment of Acne," *Medical Journal of Australia* 153(8) (15 October 1990): 455–458.

Buck, D.S., D.M. Nidorf, and J.G. Addino, "Comparison of Two Topical Preparations for the Treatment of Onychomycosis: *Melaleuca alternifolia* (Tea Tree) Oil and Clotrimazole," *Journal of Family Practice* 38(6) (June 1994): 601–605.

Carson, C.F., B.D. Cookson, H.D. Farrelly, et al., "Susceptibility of Methicillin-Resistant *Staphylococcus aureus* to the Essential Oil of *Melaleuca alternifolia*," *Journal of Antimicrobial Chemotherapy* 35(3) (March 1995): 421–424.

Enshaieh, S., A. Jooya, A.H. Siadat, et al., "The Efficacy of 5% Topical Tea Tree Oil Gel in Mild to Moderate Acne Vulgaris: A Randomized, Double-Blind, Placebo-Controlled Study," *Indian Journal of Dermatology, Venereology and Leprology* 73(1) (2007): 22–25.

Koh, K.J., A.L. Pearce, G. Marshman, et al., "Tea Tree Oil Reduces Histamine-Induced Skin Inflammation," *British Journal of Dermatology* 147 (2002): 1212–1217.

Magiin, P.J., J. Adams, G.S. Heading, et al., "Complementary and Alternative Medicine Therapies in Acne, Psoriasis, and Atopic Eczema: Results of a Qualitative Study of Patients' Experiences and Perceptions," *Journal of Alternative and Complementary Medicine* 12(5) (2006): 451–457.

Nenoff, P., U.F. Haustein, and W. Brandt, "Antifungal Activity of the Essential Oil of *Melaleuca alternifolia* (Tea Tree Oil) Against Pathogenic Fungi in Vitro," *Skin Pharmacology* 9(6) (1996): 388–394.

Pena, E.F., "*Maleleuca alternifolia* Oil: Its Use for Trichomonal Vaginitis and Other Vaginal Infections," *Obstetrics and Gynecology* 19 (1962): 793–795.

Tong, M.M., P.M. Altman, and R.S. Barnetson, "Tea Tree Oil in the Treatment of Tinea Pedis," *Australian Journal of Dermatology* 33(3) (1992): 145–149.

Thyme

Basch, E., C. Ulbricht, P. Hammerness, et al., "Thyme (*Thymus vulgaris* L.), Thymol," *Journal of Herbal Pharmacotherapy* 4(1) (2004): 49–67.

Hammer, K.A., C.F. Carson, and T.V. Riley, "Antimicrobial Activity of Essential Oils and Other Plant Extracts,"*Journal of Applied Microbiology* 86(6) (June 1999): 985–990.

Wichtl, Max, ed., *Herbal Drugs and Phytopharmaceuticals: A Handbook for Practice on a Scientific Basis*, trans. Norman Grainger Bisset (Boca Raton, FL: MedPharm Scientific Publishers, 1995), p. 494.

Tilden Flower

Duquénois, P.A., "Rétrospective sur les hydolats de tilleul, narcisse. Bourrache et primevère," *Quarterly Journal of Crude Drug Research* 15 (1977): 203–211.

Glasl, H., and U. Becerk, "Flavonol-O-Glycoside: Photometrische Gehaltsbestimmung," *Deutsche Apotheke Zeitung* [*German Pharmacy News*] 124 (1984): 2147–2152.

Kanschat, H., and C. Lander, "Welche Aussagerkraft besitzt die Quellungzahl (AZ) als Wertbestimmungsmethode bei Tiliae Flos DAB 8?" *Pharmakozeutischer Zeitung* [*Pharmaceutical News*] 129 (1984): 370–373.

Tolu Balsam

Koh, W.S., S.Y. Yoon, B.M. Kwon, et al., "Cinnamaldehyde Inhibits Lymphocyte Proliferation and Modulates T-Cell Differentiation," *International Journal of Immunopharmacology* 20(11) (November 1998): 643–660.

Sarau, H.M., J.J. Foley, D.B. Schmidt, et al., "In Vitro and in Vivo Pharmacological Characterization of SB 201993, an Eicosanoid-Like LTB4 Receptor Antagonist with Anti-Inflammatory Activity," *Prostaglandins, Leukotrienes, and Essential Fatty Acids* 61(1) (July 1999): 55–64.

Turmeric

Arora, R., N. Basu, V. Kapoor, et al., "Anti-Inflammatory Studies on *Curcuma longa* (Turmeric)," *Indian Journal of Medical Research* 59 (1971): 1289–1295.

Babu, P.S., and K. Srinivasan, "Influence of Dietary Curcumin and Cholesterol on the Progression of Experimentally Induced Diabetes in Albino Rat," *Molecular and Cellular Biochemistry* 152(1) (8 November 1995): 13–21.

Baum, L., S.K. Cheung, V.C. Mok, et al., "Curcumin Effects on Blood Lipid Profile in a 6-Month Human Study," *Pharmacological Research* 56(6) (December 2007): 509–514.

Belcaro, G., M.R. Cesarone, M. Dugall, et al., "Product-Evaluation Registry of Meriva, a Curcumin-Phosphatidylcholine Complex, For the Complementary Management of Osteoarthritis," *PanMinerva Medica* 52(Supplement 1) (2010): 55–62.

Camoirano, A., R.M. Balansky, C. Bennicelli, et al., "Experimental Databases on Inhibition of the Bacterial Mutagenicity of 4-Nitroquinoline 1-Oxide and Cigarette Smoke," *Mutation Research* 317(2) (April 1994): 89–109.

Chan, M.M., "Inhibition of Tumor Necrosis Factor by Curcumin, a Phytochemical," *Biochemical Pharmacology* 49(11) (26 May 1995): 1551–1556.

Chan, T.A., P.J. Morin, B. Vogelstein, et al., "Mechanisms Underlying Nonsteroidal Anti-Inflammatory Drug-Mediated Apoptosis," *Proceedings of the National Academy of Sciences of the USA* 95(2) (20 January 1998): 681–686.

Chandra, D., and S. Gupta, "Anti-Inflammatory and Anti-Arthritic Activity of Volatile Oil of *Curcuma longa* (Haldi)," *Indian Journal of Medical Research* 60 (1972): 138–142.

Chen, Y.C., T.C. Kuo, S.Y. Lin-Shiau, et al., "Induction of HSP70 Gene Expression by Modulation of Ca(+2) Ion and Cellular P53 Protein by Curcumin in Colorectal Carcinoma Cells," *Molecular Carcinogenesis* 17(4) (December 1996): 224–234.

Dikshit, M., L. Rastogi, R. Shukla, et al., "Prevention of Ischaemia-Induced Biochemical Changes by Curcumin and Quinidine in the Cat Heart," *Indian Journal of Medical Research* 101 (January 1995): 31–35.

Firozi, P.F., V.S. Aboobaker, and R.K. Bhattacharya, "Action of Curcumin on the Cytochrome P450-System Catalyzing the Activation of Aflatoxin B1," *Chemico-Biological Interactions* 100(1) (8 March 1996): 41–51.

Hanai, H., T. Iida, K. Takeuchi, et al., "Curcumin Maintenance Therapy for Ulcerative Colitis: Randomized, Multicenter, Double-Blind, Placebo-Controlled Study," *Clinical Gastroenterology and Hepatology* 4(12) (2006): 1502–1506.

Huang, M.T., W. Ma, P. Yen, et al., "Inhibitory Effects of Topical Application of Low Doses of Curcumin on 12-O-Tetradecanoylphorbol-13-Acetate-Induced Tumor Promotion and Oxidized DNA Bases in Mouse Epidermis," *Carcinogenesis* 18(1) (January 1997): 83–88.

Hussain, M.S., and N. Chandrasekhara, "Biliary Proteins from Hepatic Bile of Rats Fed Curcumin or Capsaicin Inhibit Cholesterol Crystal Nucleation in Supersaturated Model Bile," *Indian Journal of Biochemistry and Biophysics* 31(5) (October 1994): 407–412.

Iersel, M.L., J.P. Ploemen, I. Struik, et al., "Inhibition of Glutathione S-Transferase Activity in Human Melanoma Cells by Alpha, Beta-Unsaturated Carbonyl Derivatives. Effects of Acrolein, Cinnamaldehyde, Citral, Crotonaldehyde, Curcumin, Ethacrynic Acid, and Trans-2-Hexenal," *Chemico-Biological Interactions* 102(2) (21 October 1996): 117–132.

Ishizaki, C., T. Oguro, T. Yoshida, et al., "Enhancing Effect of Ultraviolet A on Ornithine Decarboxylase Induction and Dermatitis Evoked by 12-o-Tetradecanoylphorbol-13-Acetate and Its Inhibition by Curcumin in Mouse Skin," *Dermatology* 193(4) (1996): 311–317.

James, J.S., "Curcumin: Clinical Trial Finds No Antiviral Effect," *AIDS Treatment News* 241 (1996): 1.

Jiang, M.C., H.F. Yang-Yen, J.J. Yen, et al., "Curcumin Induces Apoptosis in Immortalized NIH 3T3 and Malignant Cancer Cell Lines," *Nutrition and Cancer* 26(1) (1996): 111–120.

Kawamori, T., et al., "Chemopreventive Effect of Curcumin, A Naturally Occurring Anti-Inflammatory Agent, During the Promotion/Progression Stages of Colon Cancer," *Cancer Research* 59 (1999): 597–601.

Kawashima, H., K. Akimoto, N. Shirasaka, et al., "Inhibitory Effects of Alkyl Gallate and Its Derivatives on Fatty Acid Desaturation," *Biochimica et Biophysica Acta* 1299(1) (5 Janaury 1996): 34–38.

Kuo, M.L., T.S. Huang, and J.K. Lin, "Curcumin, An Antioxidant and Anti-Tumor Promoter, Induces Apoptosis in Human Leukemia Cells," *Biochimica et Biophysica Acta* 1317(2) (15 November 1996): 95–100.

Kuptniratsaikul, V., S. Thanakhumtorn, P. Chinswangwatanakul, et al., "Efficacy and Safety of *Curcuma domestica* Extracts in Patients with Knee Osteoarthritis," *Journal of Alternative and Complementary Medicine* 15(8) (August 2009): 891–897.

Leri, A., Y. Liu, A. Malhotra, et al., "Pacing-Induced Heart Failure in Dogs Enhances the Expression of P53 and P53-Dependent Genes in Ventricular Myocytes," *Circulation* 97(2) (20 January 1998): 194–203.

Li, J.K., et al., "Mechanisms of Cancer Chemoprevention by Curcumin," *Proceedings of the National Science Council of the Republic of China* B 25 (2001): 59–66.

Mazumder, A., S. Wang, N. Neamati, et al., "Antiretroviral Agents as Inhibitors of Both Human Immunodeficiency Virus Type 1 Integrase and Protease," *Journal of Medicinal Chemistry* 39(13) (21 June 1996): 2472–2481.

Mehta, K., et al., "Antiproliferation Effect of Curcumin (diferuloylmethane) Against Human Breast Tumor Cell Lines," *Anticancer Drugs* 8 (1997): 470–481.

Menon, L.G., R. Kuttan, and G. Kuttan, "Inhibition of Lung Metastasis in Mice Induced by B16F10 Melanoma Cells by Polyphenolic Compounds," *Cancer Letters* 95(1–2) (16 August 1995): 221–225.

Nagabhushan, M., and S.V. Bhide, "Curcumin as an Inhibitor of Cancer," *Journal of the American College of Nutritionists* 11 (1992): 192–198.

Nirmala, C., and R. Puvanakrishnan, "Protective Role of Curcumin Against Isoproterenol Induced Myocardial Infarction in Rats," *Molecular and Cellular Biochemistry* 159(2) (21 June 1996): 85–93.

Oetari, S., M. Sudibyo, J.N. Commandeur, et al., "Effects of Curcumin on Cytochrome P450 and Glutathione S-Transferase Activities in Rat Liver," *Biochemical Pharmacology* 51(1) (12 January 1996): 39–45.

Patel, K., and K. Srinivasan, "Influence of Dietary Spices or Their Active Principles on Digestive Enzymes of Small Intestinal Mucosa in Rats," *International Journal of Food Sciences and Nutrition* 47(1) (January 1996): 55–59.

Rao, C.V., et al., "Chemoprevention of Colon Carcinogenesis by Dietary Curcumin, A Naturally Occurring Plant Phenolic Compound," *Cancer Research* 55 (1995): 259–266.

Sreejayan, N., and M.N. Rao, "Curcuminoids as Potent Inhibitors of Lipid Peroxidation," *Journal of Pharmacy and Pharmacology* 46(12) (December 1994): 1013–1016.

Sreejayan, N., and M.N. Rao, "Nitric Oxide Scavenging by Curcuminoids," *Journal of Pharmacy and Pharmacology* 49(1) (January 1997): 105–107.

Srivastava, K.C., A. Bordia, and S.K. Verma, "Curcumin, a Major Component of Food Spice Turmeric (*Curcuma longa*) Inhibits Aggregation and Alters Eicosanoid Metabolism in Human Blood Platelets," *Prostaglandins, Leukotrienes, and Essential Fatty Acids* 52(4) (April 1995): 223–227.

Sui, Z., R. Salto, J. Li, et al., "Inhibition of the HIV-1 and HIV-2 Proteases by Curcumin and Curcumin Boron Complexes," *Bioorganic and Medicinal Chemistry* 1(6) (December 1993): 415–422.

Tanaka, T., H. Makita, M. Ohnishi, et al., "Chemoprevention of 4-Nitroquinoline 1-Oxide-Induced Oral Carcinogenesis by Dietary Curcumin and Hesperidin—Comparison with the Protective Effect of Beta-Carotene," *Cancer Research* 54(17) (1 September 1994): 4653–4659.

Thresiamma, K.C., J. George, and R. Kuttan, "Protective Effect of Curcumin, Ellagic Acid and Bixin on Radiation Induced Toxicity," *Indian Journal of Experimental Biology* 34(9) (September 1996): 845–847.

Venkatesan, N., and G. Chandrakasan, "Modulation of Cyclophosphamide-Induced Early Lung Injury by Curcumin, an Anti-Inflammatory Antioxidant," *Molecular and Cellular Biochemistry* 142(1) (12 January 1995): 79–87.

Watanabe, A., A. Takeshita, S. Kitano, et al., "CD14-Mediated Signal Pathway of *Porphyromonas gingivalis* Lipopolysaccharide in Human Gingival Fibroblasts," *Infection and Immunity* 64(11) (November 1996): 4488–4494.

Yasni, S., K. Yoshiie, H. Oda, et al., "Dietary *Curcuma xanthorrhiza* Roxb. Increases Mitogenic Responses of Splenic Lymphocytes in Rats, and Alters Populations of the Lymphocytes in Mice," *Journal of Nutritional Science and Vitaminology* 39(4) (August 1993): 345–354.

Uva Ursi

Beaux, D., J. Fleurentin, and F. Mortier, "Effect of Extracts of *Orthosiphon stamineus* Benth, *Hieracium pilosella* L., *Sambucus nigra* L., and *Arctostaphylos uva-ursi* (L.) Spreng. In Rats," *Phytotherapy Research* 13(3) (May 1999): 222–225.

Chevallier, Andrew, *Encyclopedia of Medicinal Plants* (London: DK Publishing, 1996), p. 168.

Duke, James A., *The Green Pharmacy* (Emmaus, PA: Rodale Press, 1997), p. 423.

Frohne, V., "Untersuchungen zur Frage der Harndesifizierenden Wirkungen von Barentraubenblatt-Extracten," *Planta Medica* 18 (1970): 1–25.

Larsson, B., A. Jonasson, and S. Fianu, "Prophylactic Effect of UVA-E in Women with Recurrent Cystitis: A Preliminary Report," *Current Therapeutic Research, Clinical and Experimental* 53(4) (1993): 441–443.

Valerian

Francis, A.J., and R.J. Dempster, "Effect of Valerian, *Valeriana edulis*, on Sleep Difficulties in Children with Intellectual Deficits: Randomised Trial," *Phytomedicine* 9 (2002): 273–279.

Jacobs, B., et al., "An Internet-Based Randomized, Placebo-Controlled Trial of Kava and Valerian for Anxiety and Insomnia," *Medicine* 84(4) (July 2005): 197–207.

Leathwood, P.D., and F. Chauffard, "Aqueous Extract of Valerian Reduces Latency to Fall Asleep in Man," *Planta Medica* 54 (1985): 144–148.

Leathwood, P., F. Chauffard, E. Heck, et al., "Aqueous Extract of Valerian Root (*Valeriana officinalis* L.) Improves Sleep Quality in Man," *Pharmacology and Biochemistry of Behavior* 17 (1982): 65–71.

Miyasaka, L.S., A.N. Atallah, and B.G. Soares, "Valerian for Anxiety Disorders," *Cochrane Database of Systematic Reviews* 2006, Issue 4. Art. No. CD004515. DOI: 10.1002/14651858.CD004515.pub2.

Panijel, M., "Die Behandlung mittelschwerer Angstzustände," *Therapiewoche* 41 (1985): 4659–4668.

Schulz, H., C. Stolz, and J. Müller, "The Effect of Valerian Extract on Sleep Polygraphy in Poor Sleepers: A Pilot Study," *Pharmacopsychiatry* 27(4) (1994): 147–151.

Varuna

Malini, M.M., R. Baskar, and P. Varalakshmi, "Effect of Lupeol, a Pentacyclic Triterpene, on Urinary Enzymes in Hyperoxaluric Rats," *Japanese Journal of Medical Science and Biology* 48(5–6) (October–December 1995): 211–220.

Varalakshmi, P., Y. Shamila, and E. Latha, "Effect of *Crataeva nurvala* in Experimental Urolithiasis," *Journal of Ethnopharmacology* 28(3) (March 1990): 313–321.

Vitex

Bhargava, S.K., "Antiandrogenic Effects of a Flavonoid-Rich Fraction of Vitex Negundo Seeds: A Histological and Biochemical Study in Dogs," *Journal of Ethnopharmacology* 27(3) (December 1989): 327–339.

Cahill, D.J., R. Fox, P.G. Wardel, et al., "Multiple Follicular Development Associated with Herbal Medicine," *Human Reproduction* 9(8) (August 1994): 1469–1470.

Hobbs, C., and M. Amster, "Naturopathic Specific Condition Review: Premenstrual Syndrome," *Protocol Journal of Botanical Medicine* 1(4) (Spring 1996): 168–173.

Jarry, H., S. Leonhardt, C. Gorkow, et al., "In Vitro Prolactin but Not LH and FSH Release Is Inhibited by Compounds in Extracts of *Agnus castus*: Direct Evidence for a Dopaminergic Principle by the Dopamine Receptor Assay," *Experimental and Clinical Endocrinology* 102(6) (1994): 448–454.

Miliewicz, A., E. Gejdel, H. Sworen, et al., "*Vitex agnus castus* Extract in the Treatment of Luteal Phase Defects Due to Latent Hyperprolactinemia: Results of a Randomized Placebo-Controlled Double-Blind Study," *Arzneimittel-forschung* [*Medication Research*] 43(7) (July 1993): 752–756.

Okuyama, E., S. Fujimori, M. Yamazaki, et al., "Pharmacologically Active Components of Viticis Fructus (*Vitex rotundifolia*). II. The Components Having Analgesic Effects," *Chemical Pharmacology Bulletin* 46(4) (1998): 655–662.

Prilepskaya, V.N., A.V. Ledina, A.V. Tagiyeva, et al., "*Vitex agnus castus*: Successful Treatment of Moderate to Severe Premenstrual Syndrome," *Maturitas* 55S (2006): S55–S63.

Schellenberg, R., "Treatment for the Premenstrual Syndrome with Agnus Castus Fruit Extract: Prospective, Randomised, Placebo Controlled Study," *British Medical Journal* 322(7279) (2001): 134–137.

Wild Angelica

Kimura, Y., H. Ohminami, H. Arichi, et al., "Effects of Various Coumarins from Roots *Angelica dahurica* on Actions of Adrenaline, ACTH, and Insulin in Fat Cells," *Planta Medica* 45 (1982): 183–187.

Wild Yam (Dioscorea)

Araghiniknam, M.S., T. Chung, C. Nelson-White, et al., "Antioxidant Activity of Dioscorea and Dehydroepiandrosterone (DHEA) in Older Humans," *Life Sciences* (1996): 147–157.

Iwu, M.M., C.O. Okunji, G.O. Ohiaeri, et al., "Hypoglycaemic Activity of Dioscoretine from Tubers of *Dioscorea Dumetorum* in Normal and Alloxan Diabetic Rabbits," *Planta Medica* 56(3) (June 1990): 264–267.

Komesaroff, P.A., C.V. Black, V. Cable, et al., "Effects of Wild Yam Extract on Menopausal Symptoms, Lipids, and Sex Hormones in Healthy Menopausal Women," *Climacteric* 4 (2001): 144–150.

Undie, A.S., and P.I. Akubue, "Pharmacological Evaluation of *Dioscorea Dumetorum* Tuber Used in Traditional Antidiabetic Therapy," *Journal of Ethnopharmacology* 15(2) (February 1986): 133–144.

Vasiukova, N.I., V.A. Paseshnichenko, M.A. Davydova, and G.I. Chalenko, "Fungiotoxic Properties of Steroid Saponins from the Rhizomes of Deltoid Dioscorea," *Prikladnaya Biokhimiya i Mikrobiologiya* [*Applied Biochemistry and Microbiology*] 13(2) (March–April 1977): 172–176.

Willow Bark

Chevallier, Andrew, *Encyclopedia of the Medicinal Plants* (London: DK Publishing, 1996), p. 128.

Chrubasik, S., et al., "Treatment of Low Back Pain Exacerbations with Willow Bark Extract: A Randomized Double-Blind Study," *American Journal of Medicine* 109 (2000): 14.

Mills, S.Y., R.K. Jacoby, M. Chacksfield, et al., "Effect of a Proprietary Herbal Medicine on the Relief of Chronic Arthritic Pain: A Double-Blind Study," *British Journal of Rheumatology* 35(9) (1996): 874–878.

Pentz, R., et al., "Bioverfübarkeit von Salicylsäure und Coffein aus einem phytoanalgetischen Kombinationspräparat," *Deutsche Apotheke Zeitung* [*German Pharmacy News*] 10 (1989): 92–96.

Schmid, B., et al., "Efficacy and Tolerability of a Standardized Willow Bark Extract in Patients with Osteoarthritis: Randomized, Placebo-Controlled, Double Blind Clinical Trial," *Phytotherapy Research* 15 (2001): 344–350.

Senahayake, F., K. Piggott, and J.M. Hamilton-Miller, "A Pilot Study of Salix SST (Saliva-Stimulating Lozenges) Post-Irradiation Xerostomia," *Current Medical Research and Opinion* 14(3) (1998): 155–159.

Steinegger, E., and H. Hövel, "Analytische und biologische Untersuchungen an Salicaceen-Wirkstoffen, insbesodere an Salicin. II. Biologische Untersuchungen," *Pharmaca Acta Helvetica* 47 (1972): 232–234.

Wintergreen

Murray, Michael T., and Joseph E. Pizzorno, *Encyclopedia of Natural Medicine*, 2d ed. (Rocklin, CA: Prima Publishing, 1997), p. 77.

Ziment, I., "Complementary and Alternative Medicine Therapies for Chronic Obstructive Pulmonary Disease," *Focus on Alternative and Complementary Therapies* 8(4) (2003): 385–391.

Witch Hazel

Hughes-Formella, B.J., K. Bohnsack, F. Rippke, et al., "Anti-Inflammatory Effect of Hamamelis Lotion in a UVB Erythema Test," *Dermatology* 196(3) (1998): 316–322.

Korting, H.C., M. Schafer-Koring, H. Hart, et al., "Anti-Inflammatory Activity of Hamamelis Distillate Applied Topically to the Skin. Influence of Vehicle and Dose," *European Journal of Clinical Pharmacology* 44(4) (1993): 315–318.

Tyler, Varro E., *Herbs of Choice: Therapeutic Use of Phytomedicinals* (New York, NY: Pharmaceutical Products Press, 1994).

Yarrow

Goldberg, A.S., E.C. Mueller, E. Eigen, et al., "Isolation of the Anti-Inflammatory Principles from *Achillea millefo-*

lium (Compositae)," *Journal of Pharmacological Science* 58 (1969): 938–941.

Huseini, H.F., S.M. Alavian, R. Heshmat, et al., "The Efficacy of Liv-52 on Liver Cirrhotic Patients: A Randomized, Double-Blind, Placebo-Controlled First Approach," *Phytomedicine* 12(9) (2005): 619–624.

Lietava, J., "Medicinal Plants in a Middle Paleolithic Grave Shanidar IV," *Journal of Ethnopharmacology* 35(3) (January 1992): 263–266.

Loggia, R., W. Kubelka, and C. Franz, "Sesquiterpenelactones of *Achillea setacea* with Antiphlogistic Activity," *Planta Medica* 57(5) (October 1991): 444–446.

Montanari, T., J.E. De Carvalho, and H. Dolder, "Antispermatogenic Effect of *Achillea millefolium* L. in Mice," *Contraception* 58(5) (November 1998): 309–313.

Muller-Jakic, B., W. Breu, A. Probstle, et al., "In Vitro Inhibition of Cyclooxygenase and 5-Lipoxygenase by Alkamides from *Echinacea* and *Achillea* Species," *Planta Medica* 60(1) (February 1994): 37–40.

Wichtl, Max, ed., *Herbal Drugs and Phytopharmaceuticals: A Handbook for Practice on a Scientific Basis*, trans. Norman Grainger Bisset (Boca Raton, FL: MedPharm Scientific Publishers, 1995), p. 343.

Zeylstra, H., "Just Yarrow?" *British Journal of Phytotherapy* 4(4) (Winter 1997): 184–189.

Yohimbe

Betz, J.M., K.D. White, and A. Der Marderosian, "Gas Chromatographic Determination of Yohimbine in Commercial Yohimbe Products," *Journal of AOAC International* 78(5) (1995): 1189–1194.

Clark, J.T., E.R. Smith, and J.M. Davidson, "Evidence for the Modulation of Sexual Behavior by Alpha-Adenoceptors in Male Rats," *Neuroendocrinology* (Switzerland) 41(1) (1985): 36–43.

Clark, J.T., E.R. Smith, and J.M. Davidson, "Testosterone Is Not Required for the Enhancement of Sexual Motivation by Yohimbine," *Physiology and Behavior* 35(4) (1985): 517–521.

Ernst, E., and M.H. Pittler, "Yohimbine for Erectile Dysfunction: A Systematic Review and Meta-Analysis of Randomized Clinical Trials," *Journal of Urology* 159(2) (February 1998): 433–436.

Grasing, K., M.G. Sturgill, R.C. Rosen, et al., "Effects of Yohimbine on Autonomic Measures Are Determined by Individual Values for Area Under the Concentration-Time Curve," *Journal of Clinical Pharmacology* 36(9) (1996): 814–822.

Hollander, E., and A. McCarley, "Yohimbine Treatment of Sexual Side Effects Induced by Serotonin Reuptake Blockers," *Journal of Clinical Psychiatry* 53(6) (June 1992): 207–209.

Jacobsen, F.M., "Fluoxetine-Induced Sexual Dysfunction and Open Trial of Yohimbine," *Journal of Clinical Psychiatry* 53(4) (April 1992): 119–122.

Kunelius, P., J. Häkkinen, and O. Lukkarinen, "Is High-Dose Yohimbine Hydrochloride Effective in the Treatment of Mixed-Type Impotence? A Prospective, Randomized, Controlled, Double-Blind Crossover Study," *Urology* 49 (1997): 441–444.

Morales, A., M. Condra, J.A. Owen, et al., "Is Yohimbine Effective in the Treatment of Organic Impotence? Results of a Controlled Trial," *Journal of Urology* 137(6) (June 1987): 1168–1172.

Morgenthaler, John, and Dan Joy, *Better Sex Through Chemistry* (Petaluma, CA: Smart Publications, 1995), pp. 127–129.

Ostojic, S.M., "Yohimbine: The Effects on Body Composition and Exercise Performance in Soccer Players," *Research in Sports Medicine* 14(4) (2006): 289–299.

Yonazawa, A., S. Kawamura, R. Ando, et al., "Chronic Clonidine Treatment and Its Termination: Effects on Penile Erection and Ejaculation in the Dog," *Life Sciences* 51(25) (1992): 1999–2007.

THE FORMULAS

Introduction

Hosoya, E., and Y. Yamamura, "Recent Advances in the Pharmacology of Kampo (Japanese Herbal) Medicines," *Excerpta Medica* (1988), cited by H. Bacowsky, personal communication with author, 20 October 1993.

Zhou, J., "Composite Recipe of Chinese Medicine, the Natural Combination of Chemicals and Mechanism of Multi-Target Action," *Chung-Kuo Chung Hsi I Chieh Ho Tsa Chih* [*Chinese Journal of Modern Developments in Traditional Medicine*] 18 (1998): 67.

Alzium

Costarella, L., "Naturopathic Condition Review: Asthma," *Protocol Journal of Botanical Medicine* 1(2) (Autumn 1995): 103.

Espinosa-Aguirre, J.J., R.E. Reyes, J. Rubio, et al., "Mutagenic Activity of Urban Air Samples and Its Modulation by Chili Extracts," *Mutation Research* 303(2) (October 1993): 55–61.

Gao, D., K. Sakurai, J. Chen, et al., "Protection by Baicalein Against Ascorbic Acid-Induced Lipid Peroxidation of Rat Liver Microsomes," *Research Communications in*

Molecular Pathology and Pharmacology 90(1) (October 1995): 103–114.

Konoshima, T., M. Kokumai, M. Kozuka, et al., "Studies on Inhibitors of Skin Tumor Promotion. XI. Inhibitory Effects of Flavonoids from *Scutellaria baicalensis* on Epstein-Barr Virus Activation and Their Anti-Tumor-Promoting Activities," *Chemical and Pharmaceutical Bulletin* 40(2) (February 1992): 531–533.

Lersch, C., M. Zeuner, A. Bauer, et al., "Stimulation of the Immune Response in Outpatients with Hepatocellular Carcinomas by Low Doses of Cyclophosphamide (LDCY), *Echinacea purpurea* Extracts (Echinacin) and Thymostimulin," *Archiv für Geschwulstforschung* [*Archives of Tumor Research*] 60(5) (1990): 379–383.

Lersch, C., M. Zeuner, A. Bauer, et al., "Nonspecific Immunostimulation with Low Doses of Cyclophosphamide (LDCY), Thymostimulin, and *Echinacea purpurea* Extracts (Echinacin) in Patients with Far Advanced Colorectal Cancers: Preliminary Results," *Cancer Investigation* 10(5) (1992): 343–348.

Razina, T.G., S.N. Udintsev, T.P. Prishchep, et al., "Enhancement of the Selectivity of the Action of the Cytostatics Cyclophosphane and 5-Fluorouracil by Using an Extract of the Baikal Skullcap in an Experiment," *Voprosy Onkologii* [*Cancer Questions*] 33(2) (1987): 80–84.

Zhang, Z., S.M. Hamilton, C. Stewart, et al., "Inhibition of Liver Microsomal Cytochrome P450 Activity and Metabolism of the Tobacco-Specific Nitrosamine NNK by Capsaicin and Ellagic Acid," *Anticancer Research* 13(6A) (November–December 1993): 2341–2346.

Zhang, Z., H. Huynh, and R.W. Teel, "Effects of Orally Administered Capsaicin, the Principal Component of Capsicum Fruits, on the in Vitro Metabolism of the Tobacco-Specific Nitrosamine NNK in Hamster Lung and Liver Microsomes," *Anticancer Research* 17(2A) (March–April 1997): 1093–1098.

Arrest Wheezing Decoction

Couet, C.E., C. Crews, and A.B. Hanley, "Analysis, Separation, and Bioassay of Pyrrolizidine Alkaloids from Comfrey (*Symphytum officinale*)," *Natural Toxins* 4(4) (1996): 163–167.

Fruehauf, H., "Commonly Used Chinese Herb Formulas for the Treatment of Mental Disorders," *Journal of Chinese Medicine* 48 (May 1985): 21

Huang, Kee C., and Kee Chang, eds., *The Pharmacology of Chinese Herbs* (Boca Raton, FL: CRC Press, 1992), p. 196.

Ryu, J.H., Y.S. Jeong, and D.H. Sohn, "A New Bisabolene Epoxide from *Tussilago farfara*, and Inhibition of Nitric Oxide Synthesis in LPS-Activated Macrophages,"

Journal of Natural Products 62(10) (October 1999): 1437–1438.

Sperl, W., H. Stuppner, I. Gassner, et al., "Reversible Hepatic Veno-Occlusive Disease in an Infant after Consumption of Pyrrolizidine-Containing Herbal Tea," *European Journal of Pediatrics* 154(2) (February 1995): 112–116.

Zaacks, S.M., L. Klein, C.D. Tan, et al., "Hypersensitivity Myocarditis Associated with Ephedra Use," *Journal of Toxicology and Clinical Toxicology* 37(4) (1999): 485–489.

Astragalus Decoction to Construct the Middle

Chen, Y.C., "Experimental Studies on the Effects of Danggui Buxue Decoction of IL-2 Production of Blood-Deficient Mice," *Chung-Kuo Chung Yao Tsa Chih* [*China Journal of Chinese Materia Medica*] 19(12) (December 1994): 739–741, 763.

Hayakawa, T., Y. Kase, K. Saito, et al., "Effects of Daikenchu-to on Intestinal Obstruction Following Laparotomy," *Journal of Smooth Muscle Research* 35(2) (April 1999): 47–54.

Nagano, T., H. Itoh, and M. Takeyama, "Effect of Daikenchu-to on Levels of 3 Brain-Gut Peptides (Motilin, Gastrin and Somatostain) in Human Plasma," *Biological Pharmacology Bulletin* 22(10) (October 1999): 1131–1133.

Yan, M., H. Song, N. Xie, et al., "Changes of Intestinal Flora in Senile Mouse Models and the Antagonistic Acitivty of the Root of *Astragalus membraceus* (Fisch) Bge.," *Chung-Kuo Chung Yao Tsa Chih* [*China Journal of Chinese Materia Medica*] 20(10) (October 1995): 624–626, inside back cover.

Augmented Rambling Powder

Boik, John, *Cancer and Natural Medicine: A Textbook of Basic Science and Clinical Research* (Princeton, MN: Oregon Medical Press, 1995), p. 253.

Sato, T., H. Yamaguichi, T. Fujii, et al., "Inhibitory Effect of Various Traditional Chinese Medicines on Rabbit Platelet Phospholipase A2 in Vitro and Suppressive Effect of Toki-syakuyaku-san on Increased Aggregability in Hypercholesterolemic Rabbit Ex Vivo," *Yakugaku Zasshi* [*Journal of the Pharmaceutical Society of Japan*] 109(11) (November 1989): 869–876.

Biota Seed Pill to Nourish the Heart

Han, B.H., H.O. Yang, Y.H. Kang, et al., "In Vitro Platelet-Activating Factor Receptor Binding Inhibitory Activity of Pinusolide Derivatives: A Structure-Activity Study," *Journal of Medicinal Chemistry* 41(14) (2 July 1998): 2626–2630.

Kim, K.A., T.C. Moon, S.W. Lee, et al., "Pinusolide from the Leaves of *Biota orientalis* as Potent Platelet Activating Factor Antagonist," *Planta Medica* 65(10) (February 1999): 39–42.

Nishiyama, N., P.J. Chu, and H. Saito, "Beneficial Effects of Biota, a Traditional Chinese Herbal Medicine on Learning Impairment Induced by Basal Forebrain-Lesion in Mice," *Biological Pharmacology Bulletin* 18(110) (November 1995): 1513–1517.

Bupleurum and Cinnamon Twig Decoction

Chang, C.P., J.Y. Chang, F.Y. Wang, et al., "The Effect of Chinese Medicinal Herb *Zingiberis rhizoma* Extract on Cytokine Secretion by Human Peripheral Blood Mononuclear Cells," *Journal of Ethnopharmacology* 48(1) (11 August 1995): 13–19.

Hiai, S., H. Yokoyama, T. Nagasawa, et al., "Stimulation of the Pituitary-Adrenocortical Axis by Saikosaponin of Bupleuri Radix," *Chemical Pharmaceutical Bulletin* 29 (1981): 495–499.

Huang, Kee C., and Kee Chang, eds., *The Pharmacology of Chinese Herbs* (Boca Raton, FL: CRC Press, 1992), p. 196.

Saifutdinov, R.R., and V.A. Khazanov, "The Effect of an Extract of Baikal Skullcap on Succinic Acid Oxidation by the Brain Mitochondria in Rats with Hypoxia," *Ekspirimentii I Klinikicheskii Farmacologii* [*Experimental and Clinical Pharmacology*] 61(5) (September–October 1998): 27–29.

Sung, C.K., G.H. Kang, S.S. Yoon, et al., "Glycoidases That Convert Natural Glycosides to Bioactive Compounds," in *Saponins Used in Traditional and Modern Medicine,* Advances in Experimental Medicine and Biology 404, ed. George R. Waller and Kazuo Yamasaki (New York, NY: Kluwer Academic Publishers, 1996), p. 24.

Yamamoto, M., A. Kumagai, and Y. Yokoyama, "Structure and Actions of Saikosaponins Isolated from *Bupleurum falcatum* L.," *Arzneimittel-forschung* [*Medication Research*] 25 (1975): 1021–1040.

Yu, S.M., T.S. Wu, and C.M. Teng, "Pharmacological Characterization of Cinnamophilin, a Novel Dual Inhibitor of Thromboxane Synthase and Thromboxane A2 Receptor," *British Journal of Pharmacology* 111(3) (March 1994): 906–912.

Bupleurum Plus Dragon Bone and Oyster Shell Decoction

Fushitani, S., K. Tsuchiya, K. Minakuchi, et al., "Studies on Attenuation of Post-Ischemic Brain Injury by Kampo Medicines—Inhibitory Effects of Free Radical Production," *Yakugaku Zasshi* [*Journal of the Pharmaceutical Society of Japan*] 114(6) (June 1994): 388–394.

Tsumura, Akira, *Kampo: How the Japanese Updated Traditional Herbal Medicine* (Tokyo: Japan Publications, 1991), pp. 67–68.

Calm the Stomach Powder

Bensky, Dan, and Andrew Gamble, compilers, *Chinese Herbal Medicine: Materia Medica,* rev. ed. (Seattle, WA: Eastland Press, 1993), pp. 73, 235, 322.

Huang, Kee C., and Kee Chang, eds., *The Pharmacology of Chinese Herbs* (Boca Raton, FL: CRC Press, 1992), p. 174.

Murray, Michael T., and Joseph E. Pizzorno, *Encyclopedia of Natural Medicine,* 2d. ed. (Rocklin, CA: Prima Publishing, 1997), p. 522.

Cinnamon Twig and Poria Pill

Fushitani, S., K. Tsuchiya, K. Minakuchi, et al., "Studies on Attenuation of Post-Ischemic Brain Injury by Kampo Medicines—Inhibitory Effects on Free Radical Production. I.," *Yakugaku Zasshi* [*Journal of the Pharmaceutical Society of Japan*] 114(6) (June 1994): 388–394.

Ishikawa, H., M. Ohashi, K. Hayakawa, et al., "Effects of *Guizhi-fuling-wan* on Male Infertility with Varicocele," *American Journal of Chinese Medicine* 24(3–4) (1996): 372–331.

Mori, T., S. Sakamoto, T. Singitripop, et al., "Suppression of Spontaneous Development of Uterine Adenomyosis by a Chinese Herbal Medicine, *Keishi-Bukuryo-gan,* in Mice," *Planta Medica* 59(4) (August 1993): 308–311.

Sakamoto, S., H. Kudo, T. Kawasaki, et al., "Effect of a Chinese Herbal Medicine, *Keishi-Bukuryo-gan,* on the Gonadal System of Rats," *Journal of Ethnopharmacology* 23(2–3) (July–August 1998): 151–158.

Sheng, F.Y., A. Ohta, and M. Yamaguchi, "Inhibition of Collagen Production by Traditional Chinese Herbal Medicine in Scleroderma Fibroblast Cultures," *Internal Medicine* 33(8) (August 1994): 466–471.

Coptis Decoction to Relieve Toxicity

Chang, K.S., "Down-Regulation of C-Ki-Ras2 Gene Expression Associated with Morphologic Differentiation in Human Embryonal Carcinoma Cells Treated with Berberine," *Taiwan I Hsueh Hui Tsa Chih* [*Journal of the Taiwan Medical Association*] 90(1) (1991): 10–14.

Chang, K.S.S., C. Gao, and L.C. Wang, "Berberine-Induced Morphologic Differentiation and Down-Regulation of C-Ki-Ras2 Protooncogene Expression in Human Teratocarcinoma Cells," *Cancer Letters* 55(2) (1990): 103–108.

Fushitani, S., K. Tsuchiya, K. Minakuchi, et al., "Studies on Attenuation of Post-Ischemic Brain Injury by

Kampo Medicines—Inhibitory Effects of Free Radical Production," *Yakugaku Zasshi* [*Journal of the Pharmaceutical Society of Japan*] 114(6) (June 1994): 388–394.

Higaki, S., M. Nakamura, M. Morohashi, et al., "Activity of Eleven Kampo Formulations and Eight Kampo Crude Drugs Against Propionibacterium Acnes Isolated from Acne Patients: Retrospective Evaluation in 1990 and 1995," *Journal of Dermatology* 23(12) (December 1996): 871–875.

Mori, M., E. Hojo, and K. Takano, "Action of *Oren-geodku-to* on Platelet Aggregation in Vitro," *American Journal of Chinese Medicine* 19(2) (1991): 131–143.

Takase, H., O. Inoue, Y. Saito, et al., "Roles of Sulfhydryl Compounds in the Gastric Mucosal Protection of the Herb Drugs Composing *Oren-gedoku-to* (a Traditional Herbal Medicine)," *Japanese Journal of Pharmacology* 56(4) (August 1991): 433–439.

Zhang, L., L.W. Yang, and L.J. Yang, "Relation Between *Helicobacter pylori* and Pathogenesis of Chronic Atrophic Gastritis and the Research of Its Prevention and Treatment," *Chung-Kuo Chung Hsi I Chieh Ho Tsa Chih* [*Chinese Journal of Modern Developments in Traditional Medicine*] 12(9) (September 1992): 515–516, 521–523.

Zhang, Qingcai, and Hong-Yen Hsu, *AIDS and Chinese Medicine: Applications of the Oldest Medicine to the Newest Disease* (New Canaan, CT: Keats Publishing, 1995), p. 107.

Dong Quai and Peony Powder

Benesova, M., and L. Benes, "Effect of Kampo Preparations on Peptidase Activity after Damage by Free Radicals," *Ceskoslovenska Farmacie* [*Czechoslovak Pharmacy*] 41(7–8) (1992): 246–249.

Imai, A., S. Horibe, S. Fuseya, et al., "Possible Evidence That the Herbal Medicine *Shakuyaku-kanzo-to* Decreases Prostaglandin Levels through Suppressing Arachidonate Turnover in Endometrium," *Journal of Medicine* 26(3–4) (1995): 163–174.

Takahashi, K., and M. Kitao, "Effect of TJ-68 (*Shakuyaku-kanzo-to*) on Polycystic Ovarian Disease," *International Journal of Fertility and Menopausal Studies* 39(2) (March–April 1994): 69–76.

Usuki, S., "Effects of *Hachimijiogan, Tokishakuyakusan, Keishibukuryogan, Ninjinto* and *Unkeito* on Estrogen and Progesterone Secretion in Preovulatory Follicles Incubated in Vitro," *American Journal of Chinese Medicine* 19(1) (1991): 65–71.

Eight-Ingredient Pill with Rehmannia

Hidaka, S., Y. Okamoto, K. Nakajima, et al., "Preventive Effects of Traditional Chinese (Kampo) Medicines on Experimental Osteoporosis Induced by Ovariectomy in Rats," *Calciferous Tissues International* 61(3) (September 1997): 239–246.

Hirawa, N., Y. Uehara, Y. Kawabata, et al., "*Hachimi-jio-gan* Extract Protects the Kidney from Hypertensive Injury in Dahl Salt-Sensitive Rat," *American Journal of Chinese Medicine* 24(3–4) (1996): 241–254.

Hirokawa, S., M. Nose, S. Amagaya, et al., "Protective Effect of *Hachimi-jio-gan,* an Oriental Herbal Medicinal Mixture, Against Cerebral Anoxia," *Journal of Ethnopharmacology* 40(3) (December 1993): 201–206.

Huang, Kee C., and Kee Chang, eds., *The Pharmacology of Chinese Herbs* (Boca Raton, FL: CRC Press, 1992), p. 105.

Kamei, A., T. Hisada, and S. Iwata, "The Evaluation of Therapeutic Efficacy of *Hachimi-jio-gan* (Traditional Chinese Medicine) to Rat Galactosemic Cataract," *Journal of Ocular Pharmacology* 3(3) (Fall 1987): 239–248.

Kamei, A., T. Hisada, and S. Iwata, "The Evaluation of Therapeutic Efficacy of *Hachimi-jio-gan* (Traditional Chinese Medicine) to Mouse Hereditary Cataract," *Journal of Ocular Pharmacology* 4(4) (Winter 1988): 311–319.

Sakamoto, S., H. Kudo, T. Kawasaki, et al., "Effect of *Ba-wei-di-huang-wan* (*hachimi-jio-gan*) on Thymidine Kinase and Its Isozyme Activities in the Prostate Glands in Rats," *American Journal of Traditional Chinese Medicine* 16(1–2) (1988): 29–36.

Shoji, M., H. Sato, Y. Hirai, et al., "Pharmacological Effects of *Gosha-jinki-gan-ryo* Extract, Effects on Experimental Diabetes," *Nippon Yakurigaku Zasshi* [*Folia Pharmacologica Japonica*] 99(3) (March 1992): 143–152.

Ephedra Decoction

Huang, Kee C., and Kee Chang, eds., *The Pharmacology of Chinese Herbs* (Boca Raton, FL: CRC Press, 1992), p. 145.

Ikeda, Y., T. Oyama, and M. Taki, "Effect of Processed *Aconiti tuber* on Catecholamine and Indoleamine Contents in Brain in Rats," *Acta Anaesthesiologica Belgica* 45(3) (1994): 113–118.

Naito, K., M. Ishihara, Y. Senoh, et al., "Seasonal Variations of Nasal Resistance in Allergic Rhinitis and Environmental Pollen Counts. II. Efficacy of Preseasonal Therapy," *Auris, Nasus, Larynx* 20(1) (1993): 31–38.

Ozaki, Y., "Studies on Anti-Inflammatory Effect of Japanese Oriental Medicines (Kampo Medicines) Used to Treat Inflammatory Diseases," *Biological and Pharmaceutical Bulletin* 18(4) (April 1995): 559–562.

Wang, C.M., S. Ohta, and M. Shinota, "Studies on Chemical Protectors Against Radiation. XXVII. Survival Effects of Methanol Extracts of Various Chinese

Traditional Medicines on Radiation Injury," *Yakugaku Zasshi* [*Journal of the Pharmaceutical Society of Japan*] 109(12) (December 1989): 949–953.

Wang, C.M., S. Ohta, and M. Shinoda, "Studies of Chemical Protectors Against Radiation. XXIX. Protective Effects of Methanol Extracts of Various Chinese Traditional Medicines on Skin Injury Induced by X-Irradiation," *Yakugaku Zasshi* [*Journal of the Pharmaceutical Society of Japan*] 110 (3) (March 1990): 218–224.

Essiac

Kupchan, S.M., and A. Karim, "Tumor Inhibitors: Aloe Emodin: Antileukemic Principle Isolated from *Rhamnus frangula* L.," *Lloydia* 39 (1976): 223–224.

Moss, Ralph W., *Herbs Against Cancer* (Brooklyn, NY: Equinox Press, 1998), p. 134.

Shimizu, J., N. Yamada, K. Nakamura, et al., "Effects of Different Types of Dietary Fiber Preparations Isolated from Bamboo Shoots, Edible Burdock, Apple and Corn on Fecal Steroid Profiles of Rats," *Journal of Nutritional Science and Vitaminology* (Tokyo) 42(6) (December 1996): 527–539.

Walker, W.M., "The Anticancer Components of Essiac," *Townsend Letter for Doctors and Patients* 173 (December 1997): 76–82.

Zava, D.T., C.M. Dollbaum, and M. Blen, "Estrogen and Progestin Bioactivity of Foods, Herbs, and Spices," *Proceedings of the Society for Experimental Biology and Medicine* 217(3) (March 1998): 369–378.

Zhang, L., and M.C. Hung, "Sensitization of HER-2/neu-Overexpressing Non-Small Cell Lung Cancer Cells to Chemotherapeutic Drugs by Tyrosine Kinase Inhibitor Emodin," *Oncogene* 12(3) (1 February 1996): 571–576.

Zhang, L., Y.K. Lau, W. Xia, et al., "Tyrosine Kinase Inhibitor Emodin Suppresses Growth of HER-2/neu-Overexpressing Breast Cancer Cells in Athymic Mice and Sensitizes These Cells to the Inhibitory Effect of Paclitaxel," *Clinical Cancer Research* 5(2) (February 1999): 343–353.

Five-Accumulation Powder

Chang, C.P., J.Y. Chang, F.Y. Wang, et al., "The Effect of Chinese Medicinal Herb *Zingiberis rhizoma* Extract on Cytokine Secretion by Human Peripheral Blood Mononuclear Cells," *Journal of Ethnopharmacology* 48(1) (11 August 1995): 13–19.

Okano, K., M. Iwai, Y. Iga, et al., "Antiulcerogenic Compounds Isolated from Chinese Cinnamon," *Planta Medica* 55(3) (June 1989): 245–248.

Five-Ingredient Powder with Poria

Bensky, Dan, and Andrew Gamble, compilers, *Chinese Herbal Medicine: Materia Medica*, rev. ed. (Seattle, WA: Eastland Press, 1993), p. 322.

Guandong Medical Journal Editorial Department, "Clinical Observation of Curative Effects of *Wu Long San* for Treatment of Glaucoma," *Guandong Medical Journal* 3(2) (1982): 40.

Hattori, T., K. Hayashi, T. Nagao, et al., "Studies on Antinephritic Effects of Plant Components (3): Effect of Pachyman, a Main Component of Poria Cocos Wolf on Original-Type Anti-GBM Nephritis in Rats and Its Mechanisms," *Japanese Journal of Pharmacology* 59(1) (May 1992): 89–96.

Hattori, T., and S. Shindo, "Effects of *Sairei-to* (TJ-114) on the Expression of Adhesion Molecule in Anti-GBM Nephritic Rats," *Nippon Jinzo Gakkai Shi* [*Japanese Journal of Nephrology*] 37(7) (July 1995): 373–383.

Okano, K., M. Iwai, Y. Iga, et al., "Antiulcerogenic Compounds Isolated from Chinese Cinnamon," *Planta Medica* 55(3) (June 1989): 245–248.

Rangelov, A., D. Toreva, and M. Pisanets, "Cholagogic and Choleretic Activity of Products from the High Fungus Polyporus Squamosus in Test Animals," *Folia Medica* 32(1) (1990): 36–44.

Shimizu, N., S. Ohtsu, M. Tomoda, et al., "A Glucan with Immunological Activities from the Tuber of *Alisma orientale*," *Biological and Pharmaceutical Bulletin* 17(12) (December 1994): 1666–1668.

Four-Gentlemen Decoction

Hiai, S., K. Yokoyama, H. Oura, et al., "Features of Ginseng Saponin-Induced Corticosterone Secretion," *Endocronologica Japonica* 26(6) (1979): 661.

Kiyohara, H., M. Hirano, X.G. Wen, et al., "Characterisation of an Anti-Ulcer Pectic Polysaccharide from Leaves of *Panax ginseng* C.A. Meyer," *Carbohydrate Research* 263(1) (3 October 1994): 89–101.

Murray, Michael T., and Joseph E. Pizzorno, *Encyclopedia of Natural Medicine*, 2nd ed. (Rocklin, CA: Prima Publishing, 1997), p. 522.

Nguyen, T.T., K. Matsumoto, K. Yamasaki, et al., "Crude Saponin Extracted from Vietnamese Ginseng and Major Constituent Majonoside-R2 Attenuate the Psychological Stress- and Foot-Shock Stress-Induced Antinociception in Mice," *Pharmacology, Biochemistry and Behavior* 52(2) (1995): 427–432.

Yu, S.J., and J. Tseng, "Fu-Ling, a Chinese Herbal Drug, Modulates Cytokine Secretion by Human Peripheral

Blood Monocytes," *International Journal of Immunopharmacology* 18(1) (January 1996): 37–44.

Four-Substance Decoction

Chang, H.M., and P.P.H. But, *Pharmacology and Applications of Chinese Materia Medica*, vol. 1 (Singapore: World Scientific Publishing, 1986), p. 446.

Raman, A., Z.X. Lin, E.K. Sviderskaya, et al., "Investigation of the Effect of *Angelica sinensis* Root Extract on the Proliferation of Melanocytes in Culture," *Journal of Ethnopharmacology* 54(2–3) (November 1996): 165–170.

Wang, C.C., L.G. Chen, and L.L. Yang, "Inducible Nitric Oxide Synthase Inhibitor of the Chinese Herb I. *Saposhnikovia divaricata* (Turcz.) Schischk.," *Cancer Letters* 145(1–2) (18 October 1999): 151–157.

Wang, S.R., Z.Q. Guo, and L.Z. Liao, "Experimental Study on Effects of 18 Kinds of Chinese Herbal Medicine for Synthesis of Thromboxane A2 and PGI2," *Chung-Kuo Chung Hsi I Chieh Ho Tsa Chih* [*Chinese Journal of Modern Developments in Traditional Medicine*] 13(3) (March 1993): 134, 167–170.

Frigid Extremities Decoction

Ikeda, Y., T. Oyama, and M. Taki, "Effect of Processed *Aconiti tuber* on Catecholamine and Indoleamine Contents in Brain in Rats," *Acta Anaesthesiologica Belgica* 45(3) (1994): 113–118.

Frigid Extremities Powder

Hiai, S., H. Yokoyama, T. Nagasawa, et al., "Stimulation of the Pituitary-Adrenocortical Axis by Saikosaponin of Bupleuri Radix," *Chemical Pharmaceutical Bulletin* 29 (1981): 495–499.

Hosoda, K., M. Noguchi, Y.P. Chen, et al., "Studies on the Preparation and Evaluation of Kijitsu, the Immature Citrus Fruits. IV. Biological Activities of Immature Fruits of Different Citrus Species," *Yakugaku Zasshi* [*Journal of the Pharmaceutical Society of Japan*] 111(3) (March 1991): 188–192.

Murray, Michael T., and Joseph E. Pizzorno, *Encyclopedia of Natural Medicine*, 2d. ed. (Rocklin, CA: Prima Publishing, 1997), p. 522.

Yamamoto, M., A. Kumagai, and Y. Yokoyama, "Structure and Actions of Saikosaponins Isolated from *Bupleurum falcatum* L.," *Arzneimittel-forschung* [*Medication Research*] 25 (1975): 1021–1040.

Yang, D.G., "Comparison of Pre- and Post-Treatment Hepatohistology with Heavy Dosge of *Paeonia rubra* on Liver Fibrosis Due to Chronic Active Hepatitis,"

Chung Kuo Chung Hsi I Chieh Ho Tsa Chih [*Chinese Journal of Modern Developments in Traditional Medicine*] 14(4) (April 1994): 195, 207–209.

Gastrodia and Uncaria Decoction

Huang, J.H., "Comparison Studies on Pharmacological Properties of Injectio Gastrodia Elata, Gastrodin-Free Fraction and Gastrodin," *Chung-Kuo I Hsueh Ko Hsueh Yuan Hsueh Pao* [*Acta Academiae Medicinae Sinicae*] 11(2) (April 1989): 147–150.

Liu, J., and A. Mori , "Antioxidant and Free Radical Scavenging Activities of *Gastrodia elata* Bl. and *Uncaria rhynchophylla* (Miq.) Jacks," *Neuropharmacology* 31(12) (December 1992): 1287–1298.

Gentiana Longdancao Decoction to Drain the Liver

Bensky, Dan, and Andrew Gamble, compilers, *Chinese Herbal Medicine: Materia Medica*, rev. ed. (Seattle, WA: Eastland Press, 1993), p. 76.

Huang, Kee C., and Kee Chang, eds., *The Pharmacology of Chinese Herbs* (Boca Raton, FL: CRC Press, 1992), pp. 152, 203.

Shimizu, N., S. Ohtsu, M. Tomoda, et al., "A Glucan with Immunological Activities from the Tuber of *Alisma orientale*," *Biological and Pharmaceutical Bulletin* 17(12) (December 1994): 1666–1668.

Tsen, T.T., "Pharmacological Studies on the Components of *Akebia longeracemosa*, Especially on the Chemical and Pharmacological Properties of Akebia Saponins," *Shikoku Igaku Zasshi* 29 (1973): 65–83.

Udintsev, S.N., S.G. Krylova, and O.N. Konovalova, "Correction by Natural Adaptogens of Hormonal-Metabolic Status Disorders in Rats During the Development of Adaptation Syndrome Using Functional Tests with Dexamethasone and ACTH," *Builletin Eksperimentalnii Biologii I Medizina* 112(12) (December 1991): 599–601.

Yamahra, J., Y. Takagi, T. Sawada, et al., "Effects of Crude Drugs on Congestive Edema," *Chemical Pharmacy Bulletin* 27 (1979): 1464–1468.

Yamasaki, K., K. Kajimura, M. Nakano, et al., "Effects of Preparations of Chinese Medicinal Prescriptions on Digestive Enzymes in Vitro and in Vivo," *Biological Pharmacology Bulletin* 21(2) (February 1998): 133–139.

Yang, D., D. Michel, F. Bevalot, et al., "Antifungal Activity in Vitro of *Scutellaria baicalensis* Georgi upon Cutaneous and Ungual Pathogenic Fungi," *Annales Pharmaceutiques Françaises* 53(3) (1995): 138–141.

Ginseng Decoction to Nourish the Nutritive Chi

Zhou, N.N., S. Nakai, T. Kawakita, et al., "Combined Treatment of Autoimmune MRL/MP-lpr/lpr Mice with an Herbal Medicine, *Ren-shen-yang-rong-tang* (Japanese Name, *Ninjin-youei-to*) Plus Suboptimal Dosage of Prednisolone," *International Journal of Immunopharmacology* 16(10) (October 1994): 845–854.

Hochu-ekki-to

Cho, J.M., N. Sato, and K. Kikuchi, "Prophylactic Anti-Tumor Effect of *Hochu-ekki-to* (TJ-41) by Enhancing Natural Killer Cell Activity," *In Vivo* 5(4) (July–August 1991): 389–391.

Ikeda, S., M. Kaneko, Y. Kumazawa, et al., "Protective Activities of a Chinese Medicine, *Hochu-ekki-to,* to Impairment of Hematopoietic Organs and to Microbial Infection," *Yakugaku Zasshi* [*Journal of the Pharmaceutical Society of Japan*] 110(9) (September 1990): 682–687.

Kuroiwa, A., S. Liou, H. Yan, et al., "Effect of a Traditional Japanese Herbal Medicine, *Hochu-ekki-to* (*Bu-Zhong-Yi-Qi Tang*) on Immunity in Elderly Persons," *International Immunopharmacology* 4(2) (2004): 317–324.

Sudo, K., K. Honda, M. Taki, et al., "Effects of TJ-41 (*Tsumura Hochu-ekki-to*) on Spermatogenic Disorders in Mice Under Current Treatment with Adriamycin," *Nippon Yakurigaku Zasshi—Folia Pharmacologica Japonica* 92(4) (October 1988): 251–61.

Yoshida, H., T. Tanifuji, H. Sakurai, et al., "Clinical Effects of Chinese Herbal Medicine (*hochu-ekki-to*) on Infertile Men," *Hinyokika Kiyo—Acta Urologica Japonica* 32 (2) (February 1986): 297–302.

Honey-Fried Licorice Decoction

Baschetti, R., "Chronic Fatigue Syndrome and Liquorice," *New Zealand Medical Journal* 108(1002) (28 June 1995): 259.

Bensky, Dan, and Andrew Gamble, compilers, *Chinese Herbal Medicine: Materia Medica,* rev. ed. (Seattle, WA: Eastland Press, 1993), pp. 69, 333.

Chang, C.P., J.Y. Chang, F.Y. Wang, et al., "The Effect of Chinese Medicinal Herb *Zingiberis rhizoma* Extract on Cytokine Secretion by Human Peripheral Blood Mononuclear Cells," *Journal of Ethnopharmacology* 48(1) (11 August 1995): 13–19.

Demitrack, M.A., "Evidence for Impaired Activation of the Hypothalamic-Pituitary-Adrenal Axis in Patients with Chronic Fatigue Syndrome," *Journal of Clinical Endocrinology and Metabolism* 73 (1991): 1224–1234.

Hiai, S., K. Yokoyama, H. Oura, et al., "Features of Ginseng Saponin-Induced Corticosterone Secretion," *Endocronologica Japonica* 26(6) (1979): 661.

Huang, Kee C., and Kee Chang, eds., *The Pharmacology of Chinese Herbs* (Boca Raton, FL: CRC Press, 1992), pp. 92, 261.

Kiyohara, H., M. Hirano, X.G. Wen, et al., "Characterisation of an Anti-Ulcer Pectic Polysaccharide from Leaves of *Panax ginseng* C.A. Meyer," *Carbohydrate Research* 263(1) (3 October 1994): 89–101.

Nguyen, T.T., K. Matsumoto, K. Yamasaki, et al., "Crude Saponin Extracted from Vietnamese Ginseng and Major Constituent Majonoside-R2 Attenuate the Psychological Stress- and Foot-Shock Stress-Induced Antinociception in Mice," *Pharmacology, Biochemistry, and Behavior* 52(2) (1995): 427–432.

Tangri, K.K., P.K. Seth, S.S. Parmar, et al., "Biochemical Study of Anti-Inflammatory and Anti-Arthritic Properties of Glycyrrhetic Acid," *Biochemical Pharmacology* 14(8) (August 1965): 1277–1281.

Yao, G.S., Y.J. Li, X.Q. Chang, et al., "Vitamin C Content in Vegetables and Fruits in the Shenyang (China) Market During Four Season," *Acta Nutritica Sinica* 5 (1983): 373–379.

Yu, S.J., and J. Tseng, "*Fu-Ling,* a Chinese Herbal Drug, Modulates Cytokine Secretion by Human Peripheral Blood Monocytes," *International Journal of Immunopharmacology* 18(1) (January 1996): 37–44.

Yu, S.M., T.S. Wu, and C.M. Teng, "Pharmacological Characterization of Cinnamophilin, a Novel Dual Inhibitor of Thromboxane Synthase and Thromboxane A2 Receptor," *British Journal of Pharmacology* 111(3) (March 1994): 906–912.

Hoxsey Formula

Chung, J.G., L.T. Wu, C.B. Chu, et al., "Effects of Berberine on Arylamine N-Acetyltransferase Activity in Human Bladder Tumour Cells," *Food and Chemical Toxicology* 37(4) (April 1999): 319–326.

Fukuda, K., Y. Hibiya, M. Mutoh, et al., "Inhibition of Activator Protein 1 Activity by Berberine in Human Hepatoma Cells," *Planta Medica* 65(4) (May 1999): 381–383.

Fukuda, K., Y. Hibiya, M. Mutoh, et al., "Inhibition by Berberine of Cyclooxygenase-2 Transcriptional Activity in Human Colon Cancer Cells," *Journal of Ethnopharmacology* 66(2) (August 1999): 227–233.

Kuo, C.L., C.C. Chou, and B.Y. Yung, "Berberine Complexes with DNA in the Berberine-Induced Apoptosis in Human Leukemic HL-60 Cells," *Cancer Letters* 93(2) (13 July 1995): 193–200.

Lin, H.L., T.Y. Liu, W.Y. Lui, et al., "Up-Regulation of Multidrug Resistance Transporter Expression by

Berberine in Human and Murine Hepatoma Cells," *Cancer* 85(9) (1 May 1999): 1937–1942.

Lin, H.L., T.Y. Liu, C.W. Wu, et al., "Berberine Modulates Expression of Mdr 1 Gene Product and the Responses of Digestive Tract Cells to Paclitaxel," *British Journal of Cancer* 81(3) (October 1999): 416–422.

Sanders, M.M., A.A. Liu, T.K. Li, et al., "Selective Cytotoxicity of Topoisomerase-Directed Protoberberines Against Gliobastoma Cells," *Biochemical Pharmacology* 56(9) (1 November 1998): 1157–1166.

Shimizu, J., N. Yamada, K. Nakamura, et al., "Effects of Different Types of Dietary Fiber Preparations Isolated from Bamboo Shoots, Edible Burdock, Apple and Corn on Fecal Steroid Profiles of Rats," *Journal of Nutritional Science and Vitaminology* (Tokyo) 42(6) (December 1996): 527–539.

Wang, Z.Y., R. Agarwal, Z.C. Zhou, et al., "Inhibition of Mutagenicity in *Salmonella typhimurium* and Skin Tumor Initiating and Tumor Promoting Activities in Sencar Mice by Glycyrrhetinic Acid: Comparison of the 18-a and 18-b Steroisomers," *Carcinogenesis* 12(2) (February 1991): 187–192.

Wu, S.N., H.S. Yu, C.R. Jan, et al., "Inhibitory Effects of Berberine on Voltage- and Calcium-Activated Potassium Currents in Human Myeloma Cells," *Life Sciences* 62(25) (1998): 2283–2294.

Zava, D.T., C.M. Dollbaum, and M. Blen, "Estrogen and Progestin Bioactivity of Foods, Herbs, and Spices," *Proceedings of the Society for Experimental Biology and Medicine* 217(3) (March 1998): 369–378.

Zhang, L., and M.C. Hung, "Sensitization of HER-2/neu-Overexpressing Non-Small Cell Lung Cancer Cells to Chemotherapeutic Drugs by Tyrosine Kinase Inhibitor Emodin," *Oncogene* 12(3) (1 February 1996): 571–576.

Zhang, L., Y.K. Lau, W. Xia, et al., "Tyrosine Kinase Inhibitor Emodin Suppresses Growth of HER-2/neu-Overexpressing Breast Cancer Cells in Athymic Mice and Sensitizes these Cells to the Inhibitory Effect of Paclitaxel," *Clinical Cancer Research* 5(2) (February 1999): 343–353.

Kidney Chi Pill from the Golden Cabinet

Ikeda, Y., T. Oyama, and M. Taki, "Effect of Processed *Aconiti tuber* on Catecholamine and Indoleamine Contents in Brain in Rats," *Acta Anaesthesiologica Belgica* 45(3) (1994): 113–118.

Kudzu Decoction

Nagasaka, K., M. Kurokawa, M. Imakita, et al., "Efficacy of *Kakkon-to,* a Traditional Herbal Medicine, in Herpes

Simplex Virus Type 1 Infection in Mice," *Journal of Medical Virology* 46(1) (May 1995): 28–34.

Ledebouriella Decoction That Sagely Unblocks

Bensky, Dan, and Andrew Gamble, compilers, *Chinese Herbal Medicine: Materia Medica,* rev. ed. (Seattle, WA: Eastland Press, 1993), p. 33.

Takamura, S., J. Yoshida, and S. Suzuki, "Effect of an Extract Prepared from *Dai-bofu-to* on Morphine Withdrawal Responses," *Nippon Yakurigaku Zasshi* [*Folia Pharmacologica Japonica*] 105(2) (February 1995): 87–95.

Yoshida, T., N. Sakane, Y. Wakabayashi, et al., "Thermogenic, Anti-Obesity Effects of *Bofu-tsusho-san* in MSG-Obese Mice," *International Journal of Obesity and Related Metabolic Disorders* 19(10) (October 1995): 717–722.

Licorice, Wheat, and Jujube Decoction

Paroli, E., "Opioid Peptides from Food (the Exorphins)," *World Review of Nutrition and Dietetics* 55 (1988): 58–97.

Winston, D., "Eclectic Specific Condition Review: Depression," *Protocol Journal of Botanical Medicine* 2(1) (Spring 1997): 72.

Major Bupleurum Decoction

"Effects of Chinese Herbal Drugs on Serum Lipids, Lipoproteins and Apolipoproteins in Mild to Moderate Essential Hypertensive Patients," *Journal of Human Hypertension* 6(5) (October 1992): 393–395.

Fushitani, S., K. Minakuchi, K. Tsuchiya, et al., "Studies on Attenuation of Post-Ischemic Brain Injury by Kampo Medicines—Inhibitory Effects of Free Radical Production," *Yakugaku Zasshi* [*Journal of the Pharmaceutical Society of Japan*] 115(8) (August 1995): 611–617.

Goto, M., M. Hayashi, T. Todoroki, et al., "Effects of Traditional Chinese Medicines (*Dai-saiko-to, Sho-saiko-to* and *Hachimi-zio-to*) on Spontaneously Diabetic Rat (WBN/Kob) with Experimentally Induced Lipid and Mineral Disorders," *Nippon Yakurigaku Zasshi—Folia Pharmacologica Japonica* 100(4) (October 1992): 353–358.

Saku, K., K. Hirata, B. Zhang, et al., "The Inhibitory Effects of *Dai-chai-hu-tang* (*dai-saiko-to*) Extract on Supersaturated Bile Formation in Cholesterol Gallstone Disease [letter]," *American Journal of Gastroenterology* 91(4) (April 1996): 828–830.

Major Construct the Middle Decoction

Hayakawa, T., Y. Kase, K. Saito, et al., "Effects of *Dai-kenchu-to* on Intestinal Obstruction Following Laparotomy," *Journal of Smooth Muscle Research* 35(2) (April 1999): 47–54.

Nagano, T., H. Itoh, and M. Takeyama, "Effect of *Dai-ken-chu-to* on Levels of 3 Brain-Gut Peptides (Motilin, Gastrin and Somatostain) in Human Plasma," *Biological Pharmacology Bulletin* 22(10) (October 1999): 1131–1133.

Minor Bluegreen Dragon Decoction

Ikeda, K., D.Z. Wu, M. Ishigaki, et al., "Inhibitory Effects of *Sho-seiryu-to* on Acetylcholine-Induced Responses in Nasal Gland Acinar Cells," *American Journal of Chinese Medicine* 22(2) (1994): 191–196.

"Japan's Health Ministry Confirms Efficacy of Another of Tsumura's Kampo Drugs," *Kampo Today* 2(1) (February 1997): 3.

Nagai, T. and H. Yamada, "In Vivo Anti-Influenza Virus Activity of Kampo (Japanese Herbal) Medicine 'Sho-seiryu-to' and Its Mode of Action," *International Journal of Immunopharmacology* 16(8) (August 1994): 605–613.

Sakaguchi, M., A. Iizuka, M. Yuzurihara, et al., "Pharmacological Characteristics of *Sho-seiryu-to*, an Antiallergic Kampo Medicine without Effects on Histamine H1receptors and Muscarinic Cholinergic System in the Brain," *Methods and Findings in Experimental and Clinical Pharmacology* 18(1) (January–February 1996): 41–47.

Minor Bupleurum Decoction

Inoue, M., Y. Kikuta, Y. Nagatsu, et al., "Response of Liver to Glucocorticoid Is Altered by Administration of *Sho-saiko-to* (Kampo Medicine)," *Chemical and Pharmaceutical Bulletin* 38(2) (February 1990): 418–421.

Nakagawa, A., T. Yamaguchi, T. Tako, et al., "Five Cases of Drug-Induced Pneumonitis Due to *Sho-saiko-to* or Interferon-Alpha or Both," *Nippon Kyobu Shikkan Gakkai Zasshi* 33(120) (December 1995): 1361–1366.

Oka, H. et al., "Prospective Study of Chemoprevention of Hepatocellular Carcinoma with *Sho-saiko-to* (TJ-9)," *Cancer* 76 (1995): 743–749.

Ono, K., H. Nakane, M. Fukushima, et al., "Differential Inhibition of the Activities of Reverse Transcriptase and Various Cellular DNA Polymerases by a Traditional Kampo Drug, *Sho-saiko-to*," *Biomedicine and Pharmacotherapy* 44(1) (1990): 13–16.

Sakamoto, S., N. Muroi, M. Matsuda, et al., "Suppression by Kampo Medicines in Preneoplastic Mammary Hyperplastic Alveolar Nodules of SHN Virgin Mice," *Planta Medica* 59(5) (October 1993): 425–427.

Satomi, N., A. Sakurai, F. Iimura, et al., "Japanese Modified Traditional Chinese Medicines as Preventive Drugs of the Side Effects Induced by Tumor Necrosis Factor and Lipopolysaccharide," *Molecular Biotherapy* 1(3) (1989): 155–162.

Yamamoto, S., H. Oka, T. Kanno, et al., "Controlled Prospective Trial to Evaluate *Syosakiko-to* in Preventing Hepatocellular Carcinoma in Patients with Cirrhosis of the Liver," *Gan to Kagaku Ryoho* [*Japanese Journal of Cancer and Chemotherapy*] 16 (4, Part 2–2) (April 1989): 1519–1524.

Yamaoka, Y., T. Kawakita, M. Kaneko, et al., "A Polysaccharide Fraction of *Sho-saiko-to* Active in Augmentation of Natural Killer Activity by Oral Administration," *Biological and Pharmaceutical Bulletin* 18(6) (1995): 846–849.

Yamashiki, M., Y. Kosaka, A. Nishimura, et al., "Efficacy of an Herbal Medicine 'Sho-saiko-to' on the Improvement of Impaired Cytokine Production or Peripheral Blood Mononuclear Cells in Patients with Chronic Viral Hepatitis," *Journal of Clinical and Laboratory Immunology* 37(3) (1992): 111–121.

Yamashiki, M., A. Nishimura, T. Noboria, et al., "In Vitro Effects of *Sho-saiko-to* on Production of Granulocyte Colony-Stimulating Factor by Mononuclear Cells from Patients with Chronic Hepatitis C," *International Journal of Immunopharmacology* 19(7) (July 1997): 381–385.

Yoshida, K., H. Mizukawa, A. Honmura, et al., "The Effect of *Sho-saiko-to* on Concentration of Vitamin E in Serum and on Granuloma Formation in Carrigeenan Cotton Pellet-Induced Granuloma Rats," *American Journal of Chinese Medicine* 22(2) (1994): 183–189.

Zhou, N.N., S. Nakai, T. Kawakita, et al., "Combined Treatment of Autoimmune MRL/MP-lpr/lpr Mice with an Herbal Medicine, *Ren-shen-yang-rong-tang* (Japanese Name, *Ninjin-youei-to*) Plus Suboptimal Dosage of Prednisolone," *International Journal of Immunopharmacology* 16(10) (October 1994): 845–854.

Ophiopogonis Decoction

Miyata, T., J. Fuchikami, H. Kai, et al., "Antitussive Effects of *Bakumondo-to* and Codeine in Bronchitic Guinea-Pigs," *Nippon Kyobu Shikkan Gakkai Zasshi* [*Japanese Journal of Thoracic Diseases*] 27(10) (October 1989): 1157–1162.

Ohno, S., T. Suzuki, and Y. Dohi, "The Effect of *Bakumondo-to* on Salivary Secretion in Sjögren's Syndrome," *Ryumachi* [*Rheumatism*] 30(1) (February 1990): 10–16.

Tamaoki, J., A. Chiyotani, K. Takeyama, et al., "Potentiation of Beta-Adrenergic Function *Saiboku-to* and *Bakumondo-to* in Canine Bronchial Smooth Muscle," *Japanese Journal of Pharmacology* 62(2) (June 1993): 155–159.

Oyster Shell Powder

Paroli, E., "Opioid Peptides from Food (the Exorphins)," *World Review of Nutrition and Dietetics* 55 (1988): 58–97.

Zhao, X.Z., "Effects of *Astragalus membranaceus* and *Tripterygium hypoglancum* on Natural Killer Cell Activity of Peripheral Blood Mononuclear in Systemic Lupus Erythematosus," *Chung-Kuo Chung Hsi I Chieh Ho Tsa Chih* [*Chinese Journal of Modern Developments in Traditional Medicine*] 12(11) (November 1992): 645, 669–671.

Peony and Licorice Decoction

Kato, T., and R. Okamoto, "Effect of *Shakuyaku-kanzo-to* on Serum Estrogen Levels and Adrenal Gland Cells in Ovariectomized Rats," *Nippon Sanka Fujinka Gakkai Zasshi* 44(4) (1992): 433–439.

Sakamoto, K., and K. Wakabayashi, "Inhibitory Effect of Glycyrrhetinic Acid on Testosterone Production in Rat Gonads," *Endocrinologia Japonica* 35(2) (April 1988): 333–342.

Takahashi, K., and M. Kitao, "Effect of TJ-68 (*shakuyaku-kanzo-to*) on Polycystic Ovarian Disease," *International Journal of Fertility and Menopausal Studies* 39(2) (March–April 1994): 69–76.

Pinellia Decoction to Drain the Epigastrium

Kase, Y., T. Hayakawa, S. Takeda, et al., "Pharmacological Studies on Antidiarrheal Effects of *Hange-shashin-to*," *Biological and Pharmaceutical Bulletin* 19(10) (October 1996): 1367–1370.

Suzuki, M., T. Nikaido, and T. Ohmoto, "The Study of Chinese Herbal Medicinal Prescription with Enzyme Inhibitory Activity. V. The Study of *Hange-shashin-to, Kanzo-shashin-to, Shokyo-shashin-to* with Adenosine 3′,5′-Cyclic Monophosphate Phosphodiesterase," *Yakugaku Zasshi* [*Journal of the Pharmaceutical Society of Japan*] 111(11) (November 1991): 695–701.

Wang, C.M., S. Ohta, and M. Shinoda, "Studies of Chemical Protectors Against Radiation. XXIX. Protective Effects of Methanol Extracts of Various Chinese Traditional Medicines on Skin Injury Induced by X-Irradiation," *Yakugaku Zasshi* [*Journal of the Pharmaceutical Society of Japan*] 110 (3) (March 1990): 218–224.

Pinellia and Magnolia Bark Decoction

Bensky, Dan, and Andrew Gamble, compilers, *Chinese Herbal Medicine: Materia Medica*, rev. ed. (Seattle, WA: Eastland Press, 1993), p. 73.

Huang, Kee C., and Kee Chang, eds., *The Pharmacology of Chinese Herbs* (Boca Raton, FL: CRC Press, 1992), p. 196.

Polyporus Decoction

Sugaya, K., O. Nishizawa, H. Noto, et al., "Effects of Tsumura *Chorei-to* and Tsumura *Chorei-to-go-shimotsu-to* on Patients with Urethral Syndrome," *Hinyokika Kiyo* [*Acta Urologica Japonica*] 38(6) (June 1992): 731–735.

Prepared Aconite Decoction

Bensky, Dan, and Andrew Gamble, compilers, *Chinese Herbal Medicine: Materia Medica*, rev. ed. (Seattle, WA: Eastland Press, 1993), p. 322.

Hiai, S., K. Yokoyama, H. Oura, et al., "Features of Ginseng Saponin-Induced Corticosterone Secretion," *Endocronologica Japonica* 26(6) (1979): 661.

Ikeda, Y., T. Oyama, and M. Taki, "Effect of Processed *Aconiti tuber* on Catecholamine and Indoleamine Contents in Brain in Rats," *Acta Anaesthesiologica Belgica* 45(3) (1994): 113–118.

Kim, H.S., and K.S. Kim, "Inhibitory Effects of Ginseng Total Saponin on Nicotine-Induced Hyperactivity, Reverse Tolerance and Dopamine Receptor Supersensitivity," *Behavior and Brain Research* 103(1) (August 1999): 55–61.

Kiyohara, H., M. Hirano, X.G. Wen, et al., "Characterisation of an Anti-Ulcer Pectic Polysaccharide from Leaves of *Panax ginseng* C.A. Meyer," *Carbohydrate Research* 263(1) (3 October 1994): 89–101.

Nguyen, T.T., K. Matsumoto, K. Yamasaki, et al., "Crude Saponin Extracted from Vietnamese Ginseng and Major Constituent Majonoside-R2 Attenuate the Psychological Stress- and Foot-Shock Stress-Induced Antinociception in Mice," *Pharmacology, Biochemistry and Behavior* 52(2) (1995): 427–432.

Yang, D.G., "Comparison of Pre- and Post-Treatment Hepatohistology with Heavy Dosge of *Paeonia rubra* on Liver Fibrosis Due to Chronic Active Hepatitis," *Chung Kuo Chung Hsi I Chieh Ho Tsa Chih* [*Chinese Journal of Modern Developments in Traditional Medicine*] 14(4) (April 1994): 195, 207–209.

Robert's Formula

Bivol, G.K., "Gastric Secretory Function in Peptic Ulcer in Youth and the Effect on It of Diet Therapy," *Voprosii Pitanskii* 4 (July–August 1977): 57–63.

Kuhn, O., untitled article, *Arzneimittel-forschung* [*Medication Research*] 3 (1953): 194–200.

Murray, Michael T., and Joseph E. Pizzorno, *Encyclopedia of Natural Medicine*, 2d. ed. (Rocklin, CA: Prima Publishing, 1997), p. 598.

Wichtl, Max, ed., *Herbal Drugs and Phytopharmaceuticals: A Handbook for Practice on a Scientific Basis*, trans. Norman Grainger Bisset (Boca Raton, FL: MedPharm Scientific Publishers, 1995), p. 66.

Sairei-to

Borigini, M.J., M.J. Egger, H.J. Williams, et al., "TJ-114 (*Sairei-to*), An Herbal Medicine in Rheumatoid Arthritis," *Journal of Clinical Rheumatology* 2(6) (December 1996): 309–316.

Fujii, T., Y. Hamai, S. Kozuma, et al., "Effects of *Sairei-to* and *Tokishakuyaku-san* on Cytokine Release from Peripheral Blood Mononuclear Cells Upon Recognition of HLA-G Protein in Treatment of Recurrent Abortion," *Methods and Findings in Experimental and Clinical Pharmacology* 21(4) (May 1999): 261–264.

Sakai, A., Z. Kondo, K. Kamei, et al., "Induction of Ovulation by *Sairei-to* for Polycystic Ovary Syndrome Patients," *Endocrinology Journal* 46(1) (February 1999): 217–220.

Sugiura, Y., Y. Ohashi, and Y. Nakai, "Roxythromycin Prevents Endotoxin-Induced Otitis Media with Effusion in the Guinea Pig," *Acta Otolaryngologica Supplement* (Stockholm) 531 (1997): 39–51.

Tozawa, K., H. Akita, H. Yamamoto, et al., "Clinical Efficacy of *Sairei-to* in Prevention of Recurrence of Urethral Stenosis: Report of Two Cases," *Hinyokika Kiyo* 44(1) (January 1998): 49–51.

Tozawa, F., I. Dobashi, N. Horiba, et al., "*Saireito* (a Chinese Herbal Drug) Decreases Inhibitory Effect of Prednisolone and Accelerates the Recovery of Rat Hypothalamic-Pituitary-Adrenal Axis," *Endocrinology Journal* 45(1) (February 1998): 69–74.

Yamashiki, M., A. Nishimura, T. Noboria, et al., "In Vitro Effects of *Sho-saiko-to* on Production of Granulocyte Colony-Stimulating Factor by Mononuclear Cells from Patients with Chronic Hepatitis C," *International Journal of Immunopharmacology* 19(7) (July 1997): 381–385.

Yano, H., S. Hiraki, and S. Hayasaka, "Effects of *Kakkon-to* and *Sairei-to* on Experimental Elevation of Aqueous Flare in Pigmented Rabbits," *Japanese Journal of Ophthalmology* 43(4) (July–August 1999): 279–284.

Yoshikawa, N., H. Ito, Y. Takekoshi, et al., "Standard Versus Long-Term Prednisolone with *Sairei-to* for Initial Therapy in Childhood Steroid-Responsive Nephrotic Syndrome: A Prospective Controlled Study," *Nippon Jinzo Gakkai Shi* 49(8) (November 1998): 587–590.

Seven-Treasure Pill for Beautiful Whiskers

Chang, H.M., and P.P.H. But, *Pharmacology and Applications of Chinese Materia Medica*, vol. 1 (Singapore: World Scientific Publishing, 1986), p. 446.

Hoffmann, R., E. Wenzel, A. Huth, et al., "Growth Factor MRNA Levels in Alopecia Areata Before and After Treatment with the Contact Allergen Diphenylcyclopropenone," *Acta Dermato-Venereologica* 76(1) (January 1996): 17–20.

Wang, S.R., Z.Q. Guo, and J.Z. Liao, "Experimental Study on Effects of 18 Kinds of Chinese Herbal Medicine for Synthesis of Thromboxane A2 and PGI2," *Chung-Kuo Chung Hsi I Chieh Ho Tsa Chih* [*Chinese Journal of Modern Developments in Traditional Medicine*] 13(3) (March 1993): 134, 167–170.

Shih Qua Da Bu Tang

Amato, P., et al., "Estrogenic Activity of Herbs Commonly Used as Remedies for Menopausal Symptoms," *Menopause* 9(2) (March–April 2002): 145–150.

Chang, H.M., and P.P.H. But, *Pharmacology and Applications of Chinese Materia Medica*, vol. 1 (Singapore: World Scientific Publishing, 1986), p. 446.

Ohnishi, Y., R. Yasumizu, and S. Ikehara, "Preventative Effect of TJ-48 on Recovery from Radiation Injury," *Gan to Kagaku Ryoho* [*Japanese Journal of Cancer and Chemotherapy*] 16 (4, Part 2–2) (April 1989): 1494–1499.

Satoh, H., et al., "Japanese Herbal Medicine in Patients with Advanced Lung Cancer: Prolongation of Survival," *Journal of Alternative and Complementary Medicine* 8(2) (2002): 107–108.

Wang, S.R., Z.Q. Guo, and J.Z. Liao, "Experimental Study on Effects of 18 Kinds of Chinese Herbal Medicine for Synthesis of Thromboxane A2 and PGI2," *Chung-Kuo Chung Hsi I Chieh Ho Tsa Chih* [*Chinese Journal of Modern Developments in Traditional Medicine*] 13(3) (March 1993): 134, 167–170.

Zee-Cheng, R.K., "*Shi-quan-da-bu-tang* (Ten Significant Tonic Decoction), SQT: A Potent Chinese Biological Response Modifier in Cancer Immunotherapy, Potentiation and Detoxification of Anticancer Drugs," *Methods and Findings in Experimental and Clinical Pharmacology* 14(9) (November 1992): 725–736.

Zhang, Qingcai, and Hong-Yen Hsu, *AIDS and Chinese Medicine: Applications of the Oldest Medicine to the Newest Disease* (New Canaan, CT: Keats Publishing, 1995), p. 30.

Six-Ingredient Pill with Rehmannia

Cai, B., and T. Jiang, "Study on Preventive and Curative Effects of Liu We Di Huang Tang on Tumors," *Journal of Traditional Chinese Medicine* 14(3) (September 1994): 207–211.

Chen, J., "Liu Wei Di Huang Wan (Six-Ingredient Pill with Rehmannia) Traditional Use, Pharmacological Effects and Clinical Research," Lotus Institute of Medicine, November 2008.

Naeser, Margaret A., *Outline Guide to Chinese Herbal Patent Medicines in Pill Form with Sample Pictures of the Boxes: An Introduction to Chinese Herbal Medicines*, 2d. ed. (Boston, MA: Boston Chinese Medicine, 1996), p. 292.

Yu, S.J., and J. Tseng, "Fu-Ling, a Chinese Herbal Drug, Modulates Cytokine Secretion by Human Peripheral Blood Monocytes," *International Journal of Immunopharmacology* 18(1) (January 1996): 37–44.

Triphala

Chawla, Y.K., P. Dubey, R. Singh, et al., "Treatment of Dyspepsia with Amalaki (*Emblica officinalis* Linn.)—an Ayurvedic Drug," *Indian Journal of Medical Research* 76 (Supplement) (December 1982): 95–98.

Thakur, C.P., B. Thakur, S. Singh, et al., "The Ayurvedic Medicines Haritaki, Amala and Bahira Reduce Cholesterol-Induced Atherosclerosis in Rabbits," *International Journal of Cardiology* 21(2) (November 1988): 167–175.

True Man's Decoction to Nourish the Organs

Chen, J., "Zhen Ren Yang Zang Tang (True Man's Decoction for Nourishing the Organs)," Lotus Institute of Medicine, April 2008.

Tachikawa, E., K. Kudo, K. Harada, et al., "Effects of Ginseng Saponins on Responses Induced by Various Receptor Stimuli," *European Journal of Pharmacology* 369(1) (12 March 1999): 23–32.

True Warrior Decoction

Chang, C.P., J.Y. Chang, F.Y. Wang, et al., "The Effect of Chinese Medicinal Herb *Zingiberis rhizoma* Extract on Cytokine Secretion by Human Peripheral Blood Mononuclear Cells," *Journal of Ethnopharmacology* 48(1) (11 August 1995): 13–19.

Ikeda, Y., T. Oyama, and M. Taki, "Effect of Processed *Aconiti tuber* on Catecholamine and Indoleamine Contents in Brain in Rats," *Acta Anaesthesiologica Belgica* 45(3) (1994): 113–118.

Yang, D.G., "Comparison of Pre- and Post-Treatment Hepatohistology with Heavy Dosage of *Paeonia rubra* on Liver Fibrosis Due to Chronic Active Hepatitis," *Chung Kuo Chung Hsi I Chieh Ho Tsa Chih* [*Chinese Journal of Modern Developments in Traditional Medicine*] 14(4) (April 1994): 195, 207–209.

Warm the Gallbladder Decoction

Chang, C.P., J.Y. Chang, F.Y. Wang, et al., "The Effect of Chinese Medicinal Herb *Zingiberis rhizoma* Extract on Cytokine Secretion by Human Peripheral Blood Mononuclear Cells," *Journal of Ethnopharmacology* 48(1) (11 August 1995): 13–19.

Murray, Michael T., and Joseph E. Pizzorno, *Encyclopedia of Natural Medicine*, 2d. ed. (Rocklin, CA: Prima Publishing, 1997), p. 522.

Sato, T., M. Matsuhashi, and O. Iida, "Fungi Isolated from Diseased Medicinal Plants," *Eisei Shikenjo Hokoku* [*Bulletin of National Institute of Hygienic Sciences*] 110 (1992): 60–66.

Tang, W., and Gerhard Eisenbrand, *Chinese Drugs of Plant Origin: Chemistry, Pharmacology, and Use in Traditional and Modern Medicine* (New York, NY: Springer-Verlag, 1992), p. 350.

Yu, S.J., and J. Tseng, "Fu-Ling, a Chinese Herbal Drug, Modulates Cytokine Secretion by Human Peripheral Blood Monocytes," *International Journal of Immunopharmacology* 18(1) (January 1996): 37–44.

Warm the Menses Decoction

Hidaka, S., Y. Okamoto, K. Nakajima, et al., "Preventive Effects of Traditional Chinese (Kampo) Medicines on Experimental Osteoporosis Induced by Ovariectomy in Rats," *Calciferous Tissue International* 61(3) (September 1997): 239–246.

Okamoto, Y., S. Hidaka, Y. Yamada, et al., "Thermal Analysis of Bones from Ovariectomized Rats," *Journal of Biomedical Material Research* 41(2) (August 1998): 221–226.

Ushiroyama, T., S. Tsubokura, A. Ikeda, et al., "The Effect of *Unkei-to* on Pituitary Gonadotropin Secretion and Ovulation in Anovulatory Cycles of Young Women," *American Journal of Chinese Medicine* 23(3–4) (1995): 223–230.

White Tiger Decoction

Nakashima, N., I. Kimura, M. Kimura, et al., "Isolation of Pseudoprototimosaponin AIII from Rhizomes of Anemarrhena Asphodeloides and Its Hypoglycemic Activity in Streptozotocin-Induced Diabetic Mice," *Journal of Natural Products* 56(3) (March 1993): 345–350.

Yogaraj Guggulu

Beg, M., K.C. Singhal, and S. Afzaal, "A Study of Effect of Guggulsterone of Hyperlipidemia of Secondary Glomerulopathy," *Indian Journal of Physiology and Pharmacology* 40(3) (July 1996): 237–240.

PART TWO: HERBAL PRESCRIPTIONS FOR COMMON HEALTH PROBLEMS

Acne

Epinette, W.W., M.C. Greist, and I.I. Ozols, "The Role of Cosmetics in Postadolescent Acne," *Cutis* 29(5) (May 1982): 500–504.

Goulden, V., S.M. Clark, and W.J. Cunliffe, "Post-Adolescent Acne: A Review of Clinical Features,"

British Journal of Dermatology 136(1) (January 1997): 66–70.

Griffith, R., D. DeLong, and J. Nelson, "Relation of Arginine-Lysine Antagonism to Herpes Simplex Growth in Tissue Culture," *Chemotherapy* 27 (1981): 209–213.

Heffernan, M.P., M.M. Nelson, and M.J. Anadkat, "A Pilot Study of the Safety and Efficacy of Picolinic Acid Gel in the Treatment of Acne Vulgaris," *The British Journal of Dermatology* 156(3) (2007): 548–552.

Michaelson, G., L. Juhlin, and K. Ljunghall, "A Double-Blind Study of the Effect of Zinc and Oxytetracycline in Acne Vulgaris," *British Journal of Dermatology* 97 (1977): 561–565.

Morrow, G.L., and R.L. Abbott, "Minocycline-Induced Scleral, Dental, and Dermal Pigmentation," *American Journal of Ophthalmology* 125(3) (March 1998): 396–397.

Sansone, G., and R. Reisner, "Differential Rates of Conversion of Testosterone to Dihydrotestosterone in Acne and Normal Human Skin—A Possible Pathogenic Factor in Acne," *Journal of Investigational Dermatology* 56 (1971): 366–372.

Schavone, F., R. Rietschel, D. Squotas, et al., "Elevated Free Testosterone Levels in Women with Acne," *Archives of Dermatology* 119 (1982): 799–802.

AIDS

Roederer, M., F.J. Staa, M. Anderson, et al., "Disregulation of Leukocyte Glutathione in AIDS," *Annals of the New York Academy of Sciences* 677 (20 March 1993): 113–125.

Alcoholism

Caballeria, J., A. Gimenez, H. Andreu, et al., "Zinc Administration Improves Gastric Alcohol Dehydrogenase Activity and First-Pass Metabolism in Alcohol-Fed Rats," *Alcoholism in Clinical and Experimental Research* 21(9) (December 1997): 1619–1622.

Cahill-Morasco, R., R.S. Hoffman, and L.R. Goldfrank, "The Effects of Nutrition on Plasma Cholinesterase Activity and Cocaine Toxicity in Mice," *Journal of Toxicology and Clinical Toxicology* 36(7) (1998): 667–672.

Cruz-Coke, R., "Genetics and Alcoholism," *Neurobehavioral Toxicology and Teratology* 5 (1983): 179–180.

Kampov-Polevoy, A.B., J.C. Garbutt, C.E. Davis, et al., "Preference for Higher Sugar Concentrations and Tridimensional Personality Questionnaire Scores in Alcoholic and Nonalcoholic Men," *Alcoholism in Clinical and Experimental Research* 22(3) (May 1998): 610–614.

Lieber, C.S., "Alcohol, Liver, and Nutrition," *Journal of the American College of Nutrition* 10 (1991): 602–632.

Rubenstein, E., and D. Federman, *Scientific American Textbook of Medicine* (New York, NY: Scientific American, 1985), pp. 13–14.

Severus, W.E., B. Ahrens, and A.L. Stoll, "Omega-3 Fatty Acids: The Missing Link?" *Archives of General Psychiatry* 56(4) (April 1999): 380–381.

Tipton, K.F., G.T.M. Heneman, and J.M. McCrodden, "Metabolic and Nutritional Aspects of Alcohol," *Biochemical Society Transactions* 11 (1983): 59–61.

Vannucchi, H., and F.S. Moreno, "Interaction of Niacin and Zinc Metabolism in Patients with Alcoholic Pellagra," *The American Journal of Clinical Nutrition* 50(2) (1989): 364–369.

Allergies, Food

McGovern, J.J., "Correlation of Clinical Food Allergy Symptoms with Serial Pharmacological and Immunological Changes in the Patient's Plasma," *Annals of Allergy* 44 (1980): 57.

Schnappinger, M., S. Sausenthaler, J. Linseisen, et al., "Fish Consumption, Allergic Sensitisation and Allergic Disease in Adults," *Annals of Nutrition and Metabolism* 54(1) (2009): 67–74.

Trevino, R.J., "Immunological Mechanisms in the Production of Food Sensitivities," *Laryngoscope* 91 (1981): 1913.

Allergies, Respiratory

Cingi, C., M. Conk-Dalay, H. Cakli, et al., "The Effects of Spirulina on Allergic Rhinitis," *European Archives of Otorhinolaryngology* 265(10) (October 2008): 1219–1223.

Hansen, O., "A Psychosomatic Theory of Allergic Sensitization; Allergy as a Quasi-Conditioned Reaction," *Zeitschrift für psychosomatischer Medizin und Psychoanalyse* [*Journal for Psychosomatic Medicine and Psychoanalysis*] 27(2) (April–June 1981): 143–160.

Michel, F.B., "Psychology of the Allergic Patient," *Allergy* 49 (18) (Supplement) (1994): 28–30.

Nesse, Randolph M., and George C. Williams, *Why We Get Sick: The New Science of Darwinian Medicine* (New York, NY: Random House, 1994), p. 169.

Xiao, J.Z., S. Kondo, N. Yanagisawa, et al., "Clinical Efficacy of Probiotic *Bifidobacterium longum* for the Treatment of Symptoms of Japanese Cedar Pollen Allergy in Subjects Evaluated in an Environmental Exposure Unit," *Allergology International* 56(1) (2007): 67–75.

Alzheimer's Disease

Chandra, R.K., "Effect of Vitamin and Trace-Element Supplementation on Cognitive Function in Elderly Subjects," *Nutrition* 17(9) (September 2001): 709–712.

Frolich, L., and P. Riederer, "Free Radical Mechanisms in Dementia of the Alzheimer's Type and the Potential for Antioxidative Treatment," *Drug Research* 45(1) (1995): 3A, 443–446.

Gandy, S.E., R. Bhasin, V. Ramabhadran, et al., "Alzheimer B/A4-Amyloid Precursor Protein: Evidence for Putative Amyloidogenic Fragment," *Journal of Neurochemistry* 548 (1992): 383–386.

Roberts, H.J., "Allopathic Specific Condition Review: Alzheimer's Disease," *Protocol Journal of Botanical Medicine* 2(1) (1997): 94.

Samieri, C., C. Feart, L. Letenneur, et al., "Low Plasma Eicosapentaenoic Acid and Depressive Symptomatology Are Independent Predictors of Dementia Risk," *American Journal of Clinical Nutrition* 88(3) (September 2008): 714–721.

Schaefer, E.J., V. Bongard, A.S. Beiser, et al., "Plasma Phosphatidylcholine Docosahexaenoic Acid Content and Risk of Dementia and Alzheimer Disease: The Framingham Heart Study," *Archives of Neurology* 63(11) (November 2006): 1545–1550.

Alzheimer's Disease and Ginkgo, the Memory Herb

Andrieu, S., S. Gillette, K. Amouyal, et al., "Association of Alzheimer's Disease Onset with Ginkgo Biloba and Other Symptomatic Cognitive Treatments in a Population of Women Aged 75 Years and Older from the EPIDOS Study," *Journal of Gerontology. Series A, Biological Sciences and Medical Sciences,* 58 (4) (April 2003): 372–377.

DeFeudis, F.V., ed., *Ginkgo biloba Extract (EGb 761): Pharmacological Activities and Clinical Activities* (Amsterdam: Elsevier, 1991).

Kanowski, S., W.M. Herrmann, K. Stephan, et al., "Proof of the Efficacy of the Ginkgo Biloba Special Extract EGb 761 in Patients Suffering from Mild to Moderate Primary Degenerative Dementia of the Alzheimer Type of Multi-Infarct Dementia," *Phytomedicine* 4 (1997): 3–13.

Le Bars, P.L., M.M. Katz, N. Berman, et al., "A Placebo-Controlled, Double-Blind, Randomized Trial of an Extract of Ginkgo Biloba for Dementia," *Journal of the American Medical Association* 278 (22 October 1997): 1327–1332.

Snitz, B.E., E.S. O'Meara, M.C. Carlson, et al., "Ginkgo Biloba for Preventing Cognitive Decline in Older Adults: A Randomized Trial," *Journal of the American Medical Association* 302 (24) (December 2003): 2663–2673.

Stone, M.B., M.A. Vaughan, C.D. Ingersoll, et al., "A Single Dose of Ginkgo Biloba Does Not Affect Soleus Motoneuron Pool Excitability," *Journal of Strength and Conditioning Research* 17 (August 2003): 587–590.

Anemia

Adosj, A.A., S.A. Esrey, T.W. Gyorkos, et al., "Effect of Consumption of Food Cooked in Iron Pots on Iron Status and Growth of Young Children: A Randomised Trial," *Lancet* 353(9154) (27 February 1999): 712–716.

Liu, D.Y., Z.G. Chen, H.Q. Lei, et al., "Investigation of the Amount of Dissolved Iron in Food Cooked in Chinese Iron Pots and Estimation of Daily Iron Intake," *Biomedical and Environmental Science* 3(3) (September 1990): 276–280.

Looker, A.C., P.R. Dallman, M.D. Carroll, et al., "Prevalence of Iron Deficiency in the United States," *Journal of the American Medical Association* 277(12) (26 March 1997): 973–976.

Van Dokkum, W., "Significance of Iron Bioavailability for Iron Recommendations," *Biological Trace Element Research* 35(1) (October 1992): 1–11.

Vogelzang, N.J., W. Breitbart, and D. Cella, "Patient, Caregiver, and Oncologist Perceptions of Cancer-Related Fatigue: Results of a Tripart Assessment Survey: The Fatigue Coalition," *Seminars in Hematology* 34(3) (Supplement 2) (July 1997): 4–12.

Angina

Biasucci, L.M., G. Liuzzo, G. Fantuzzi, et al., "Increasing Levels of Interleukin (IL)-1Ra and IL-6 During the First 2 Days of Hospitalization in Unstable Angina Are Associated with Increased Risk of In-Hospital Coronary Events," *Circulation* 99(16) (27 April 1999): 2079–2084.

Buckland, G., C.A. González, A. Agudo, et al., "Adherence to the Mediterranean Diet and Risk of Coronary Heart Disease in the Spanish EPIC Cohort Study," *American Journal of Epidemiology* 170(2) (December 2009): 1518–1529.

Galan, P., E. Kesse-Guyot, S. Czernichow, et al., "Effects of B Vitamins and Omega 3 Fatty Acids on Cardiovascular Diseases: A Randomised Placebo Controlled Trial," *British Medical Journal* (November 29, 2010). DOI: 10.1136/bmj.c6273.

Ito, K., H. Akita, K. Kanazawa, et al., "Comparison of Effects of Ascorbic Acid on Endothelium-Dependent Vasodilation in Patients with Chronic Congestive Heart Failure Secondary to Idiopathic Dilated Cardiomyopathy Versus Patients with Effort Angina Pectoris Secondary to Coronary Artery Disease," *American Journal of Cardiology* 82(6) (15 September 1998): 762–767.

Kabat-Zinn, J., "An Outpatient Program in Behavioral Medicine for Chronic Pain Patients Based on the Practice of Mindfulness Meditation: Theoretical Considerations and Preliminary Results," *General Hospital Psychiatry* 4(1) (April 1982): 33–47.

Kearney, M.T., A.J. Cowley, and I.A. Macdonald, "Triglycerides and Postprandial Angina," *Circulation* 98(17) (27 October 1998): 1827.

Lonn, E., J. Bosch, S. Yusuf, et al., "Effects of Long-Term Vitamin E Supplementation on Cardiovascular Events and Cancer: A Randomized Controlled Trial," *Journal of the American Medical Association* 293(11) (March 2005): 1338–1347.

Meyers, D.G., D. Strickland, P.A. Maloley, et al., "Possible Association of a Reduction in Cardiovascular Events with Blood Donation," *Heart* 78(2) (August 1997): 188–193.

Steinberg, D., S. Parthasarathy, T.E. Carew, et al., "Beyond Cholesterol: Modification of the Low-Density Lipoprotein That Increase Its Atherogenicity," *The New England Journal of Medicine* 320 (1989): 915–924.

Angina: Is Surgery Necessary?

CASS Principal Investigators and Their Associates, "Coronary Artery Surgery (CASS): A Randomized Trial of Coronary Artery Bypass Surgery," *Circulation* 68 (1983): 939–950.

CASS Principal Investigators and Their Associates, "Myocardial Infarction and Mortality in the Coronary Artery Surgery Study (CASS) Randomized Trial," *The New England Journal of Medicine* 310 (1984): 750–758.

Graboys, T.D., et al., "Results of a Second-Opinion Program for Coronary Artery Bypass Surgery," *Journal of the American Medical Association* 258 (1987): 1611–1614.

Graboys, T.D., et al., "Results of a Second-Opinion Program for Coronary Artery Bypass Surgery," *Journal of the American Medical Association* 268 (1992): 2537–2540.

Ankles, Swollen

Diehm, C., H.J. Trampisch, S. Lange, et al., "Comparison of Leg Compression Stocking and Oral Horse-Chestnut Seed Extract Therapy in Patients with Chronic Venous Insufficiency," *Lancet* 347(8997) (3 February 1996): 292–294.

Anxiety Disorder

Buydens-Branchey, L., M. Branchey, "n-3 Polyunsaturated Fatty Acids Decrease Anxiety Feelings in a Population of Substance Abusers," *Journal of Clinical Psychopharmacology* 26(6) (December 2006): 661–665.

De Felipe, C., J.F. Herrero, J.A. O'Brien, et al., "Altered Nociception, Analgesia and Aggression in Mice Lacking the Receptor for Substance P," *Nature* 392 (26 March 1998): 394–397.

Garvin, A.W., K.F. Koltyn, and W.P. Morgan, "Influence of Acute Physical Activity and Relaxation on State Anxiety and Blood Lactate in Untrained College Males," *International Journal of Sports Medicine* 18(6) (August 1997): 470–476.

Gorman, J.M., D. Battista, R.R. Goetz, et al., "A Comparison of Sodium Bicarbonate and Sodium Lactate Infusion in the Induction of Panic Attacks," *Archives of General Psychiatry* 46(2) (February 1989): 145–150.

Kalman, D.S., S. Feldman, R. Feldman, et al., "Effect of a Proprietary Magnolia and Phellodendron Extract on Stress Levels in Healthy Women: A Pilot, Double-Blind, Placebo-Controlled Clinical Trial," *Nutrition Journal* 21 (April 2008): 7–11.

Murray, Michael T., and Joseph E. Pizzorno, *Encyclopedia of Natural Medicine,* 2d. ed. (Rocklin, CA: Prima Publishing, 1997), p. 252.

Raglin, J.S., and M. Wilson, "State Anxiety Following 20 Minutes of Bicycle Ergometer Exercise at Selected Intensities," *International Journal of Sports Medicine* 17(6) (August 1996): 467–471.

Reed, J., K.E. Berg, R. Latin, et al., "Affective Responses of Physically Active and Sedentary Individuals During and After Moderate Aerobic Exercise," *Journal of Sports Medicine and Physical Fitness* 38(3) (September 1998): 272–278.

Rudin, D.O., "The Major Psychoses and Neuroses as Omega-3 Essential Fatty Acid Deficiency Syndrome: Substrate Pellagra," *Biological Psychiatry* 16 (1981): 837–850.

Schiffer, F., "Affect Changes Observed with Right Versus Left Lateral Visual Field Stimulation in Psychotherapy Patients: Possible Physiological, Psychological, and Therapeutic Implications," *Comprehensive Psychiatry* 38(5) (September–October 1997): 289–295.

Shannahoff-Khalsa, D.S., and L.R. Beckett, "Clinical Case Report: Efficacy of Yogic Techniques in the Treatment of Obsessive Compulsive Disorders," *International Journal of Neuroscience* 85(1–2) (March 1996): 1–17.

Asthma

Akiyama, K., T. Shida, H. Yasueda, et al., "Atopic Asthma Caused by *Candida albicans* Acid Protease: Case Reports," *Allergy* 49 (1994): 778–781.

Baker, J.C., W.S. Tunnicliffe, R.C. Duncanson, et al., "Dietary Antioxidants and Magnesium in Type 1 Brittle Asthma: A Case Control Study," *Thorax* 54(2) (February 199 9): 115–118.

Benard, A., P. Desreumeaux, D. Huglo, et al., "Increased Intestinal Permeability in Bronchial Asthma," *Journal of Allergy and Clinical Immunology* 97 (1996): 1173–1178.

Biltagi, M.A., A.A. Baset, M. Bassiouny, et al., "Omega-3 Fatty Acids, Vitamin C and Zinc Supplementation in Asthmatic Children: A Randomized Self-Controlled Study," *Acta Paediatrica* 98(4) (April 2009): 737–742.

Bircher, A.J., G. Van Melle, E. Haller, et al., "IgE to Food Allergens Are Highly Prevalent in Patients Allergic to Pollens, with and without Symptoms of Food Allergy," *Clinical and Experimental Allergy* 24(4) (1994): 367–374.

Bray, G.W., "The Hypochlorhydria of Asthma in Childhood," *Quarterly Journal of Medicine* 24 (1931): 181–197.

Broughtonk, K.S., et al., "Reduced Asthma Symptoms with Omega-3 Fatty Acid Ingestion Are Related to 5-Series Leukotriene Production," *American Journal of Clinical Nutrition* 65 (1997): 1011–1017.

Bucca, C., G. Rolla, W. Arossa, et al., "Effect of Ascorbic Acid on Increased Bronchial Responsiveness During Upper Airway Infection," *Respiration* 55(4) (1989): 214–219.

Businco, L., P. Falconieri, P. Giampietro, et al., "Food Allergy and Asthma," *Pediatric Pulmonology* 11 (Supplement) (1995): 59–60.

Covar, R., M. Gleason, B. Macomber, et al., "Impact of a Novel Nutritional Formula on Asthma Control and Biomarkers of Allergic Airway Inflammation in Children," *Clinical and Experimental Allergy* 40(8) (August 2010): 1163–1174.

Eiserich, J.P., A. Van Der Vliet, G.J. Handelman, et al., "Dietary Antioxidants and Cigarette Smoke-Induced Biomolecular Damage: A Complex Interaction," *American Journal of Clinical Nutrition* 62(6) (Supplement) (December 1995): 1490S–1500S.

El-Serag, H.B., and A. Sonnenberg, "Comorbid Occurrence of Laryngeal or Pulmonary Disease with Esophagitis in United States Military Veterans," *Gastroenterology* 113(3) (September 1997): 755–760.

Field, T., T. Henteleff, M. Hernandez-Reif, et al., "Children with Asthma Have Improved Pulmonary Functions after Massage Therapy," *Journal of Pediatrics* 132(5) (May 1998): 854–858.

Gergen, P.J., J.A. Fowler, K.R. Maurer, et al., "The Burden of Environmental Tobacco Smoke Exposure on the Respiratory Health of Children 2 Months Through 5 Years of Age in the United States: Third National Health and Nutrition Examination Survey, 1988 to 1994," *Pediatrics* 101(2) (February 1998): E8.

Grievink, L., H.A. Smit, M.C. Ocke, et al., "Dietary Intake of Antioxidant (Pro)-Vitamins, Respiratory Symptoms and Pulmonary Function: The MORGEN Study," *Thorax* 53(3) (March 1998): 166–171.

Hodge, L., et al., "Consumption of Oily Fish and Childhood Asthma Risk," *Medical Journal of Australia* 164 (1989): 137–140.

Kaliner, M., and R. Lemanske, "Rhinitis and Asthma," *Journal of the American Medical Association* 268 (1992): 2807–2829.

Maneechotesuwan, K., S. Supawita, K. Kasetsinsombat, et al., "Sputum Indoleamine-2,3-dioxygenase Activity Is Increased in Asthmatic Airways by Using Inhaled Corticosteroids," *Journal of Allergy and Clinical Immunology* 12(1) (January 2008): 43–50.

Marrades, R.M., J. Roca, J.A. Barbera, et al., "Nebulized Glutathione Induces Bronchoconstriction in Patients with Mild Asthma," *American Journal of Respiratory Critical Care in Medicine* 156 (2, Part 1) (August 1997): 425–430.

Odent, M.R., E.E. Culpin, and T. Kimmel, "Pertussis Vaccination and Asthma: Is There a Link?" *Journal of the American Medical Association* 272 (1994): 592–593.

Oehling, A., "Importance of Food Allergy in Childhood Asthma," *Allergology and Immunopathology Supplement* 9 (1981): 71–73.

Ogle, K.A., and J.D. Bullocks, "Children with Allergic Rhinitis and/or Bronchial Asthma Treated with Elimination Diet: A Five-Year Follow-Up," *Annals of Allergy* 44 (1980): 273–278.

Onorato, J., N. Merland, C. Terral, et al., "Placebo-Controlled Double-Blind Food Challenge in Asthma," *Journal of Allergy and Clinical Immunology* 78(6) (December 1986): 1139–1146.

Reynolds, R.D., and C.L. Natta, "Depressed Plasma Pyriodoxal Phosphate Concentrations in Adult Asthmatics," *American Journal of Clinical Nutrition* 41 (1985): 684–688.

Sontag, S., *Medical Tribune* (5 June 1997).

Tan, Y., and C. Collins-Williams, "Aspirin-Induced Asthma in Children," *Annals of Allergy* 48 (1982): 1–5.

Unge, G., J. Grubbstrom, P. Olsson, et al., "Effect of Dietary Tryptophan Restriction on Clinical Symptoms in Patients with Endogenous Asthma," *Allergy* 38 (1983): 211–212.

Vanderhoek, J.Y., S.L. Ekborg, and J.M. Bailey, "Nonsteroidal Anti-Inflammatory Drugs Stimulate 15-Lipoxygenase/Leukotriene Pathway in Human Polymorphonuclear Leukocytes," *Journal of Allergy and Clinical Immunology* 74 (1984): 412–417.

Atherosclerosis

Bao, B., A.S. Prasad, F.W. Beck, et al., "Zinc Decreases C-Reactive Protein, Lipid Peroxidation, and Inflammatory Cytokines in Elderly Subjects: A Potential Implication of Zinc as an Atheroprotective Agent," *American Journal of Clinical Nutrition* 91(6) (June 2010): 1634–1641.

Birnie, D.H., E.R. Holme, I.C. McKay, et al., "Association Between Antibodies to Heat Shock Protein 65 and Coronary Atherosclerosis. Possible Mechanism of Action of *Helicobacter pylori* and Other Bacterial Infections in Increasing Cardiovascular Risk," *European Heart Journal* 18 (March 1998): 387–394.

Cawood, A.L., R. Ding, F.L. Napper, et al., "Eicosapentaenoic Acid (EPA) from Highly Concentrated n-3 Fatty Acid Ethyl Esters Is Incorporated into Advanced Atherosclerotic Plaques and Higher Plaque EPA Is Associated with Decreased Plaque Inflammation and Increased Stability," *Atherosclerosis* 212(1) (September 2010): 252–259.

Cuevas, A.M., V.L. Irribarra, O.A. Castillo, et al., "Isolated Soy Protein Improves Endothelial Function in Postmenopausal Hypercholesterolemic Women," *European Journal of Clinical Nutrition* 57(8) (August 2003): 889–894.

Davidson, M., C.C. Kuo, J.P. Middaugh, et al., "Confirmed Previous Infection with *Chlamydia pneumoniae* (TWAR) and Its Presence in Early Coronary Atherosclerosis," *Circulation* 98 (18 August 1998): 628–633.

Devaraj, S., S. Mathur, A. Basu, et al., "A Dose-Response Study on the Effects of Purified Lycopene Supplementation on Biomarkers of Oxidative Stress," *Journal of the American College of Nutrition* 27(2) (2008): 267–273.

Dubuisson, J.T., L.E. Wagenknecht, R.B. D'Agostino, Jr., et al., "Association of Hormone Replacement Therapy and Carotid Wall Thickness in Women with and without Diabetes," *Diabetes Care* 21(11) (November 1998): 1790–1796.

Folts, J.D., B. Begollie, D. Shanmuganayagam, et al., "Inhibition of Platelet Activity with Red Wine and Grape Products," *Biofactors* 6(4) (1997): 411–414.

Furlong, C.E., et al., "Paraoxonase May Protect Against Heart Disease," *Nature* 394 (1998): 284–287.

Goldman, I.L., M. Kopelberg, J.E. Debaene, et al., "Antiplatelet Activity in Onion (*Allium cepa*) Is Sulfur Dependent," *Thrombosis and Haemostasis* 76(3) (September 1996): 450–452.

Howard, G., L.E. Wagenknecht, G.L. Burke, et al., "Cigarette Smoking and Progression of Atherosclerosis: The Atherosclerosis Risk in Communities (ARIC) Study," *Journal of the American Medical Association* 279 (14 January 1998): 119–124.

Kiechl, S., J. Willeit, G. Rungger, et al., "Alcohol Consumption and Atherosclerosis: What Is the Relation? Prospective Results from the Bruneck Study," *Stroke* 29 (1998): 900–907.

Matthews, K.A., J.F. Owens, L.H. Kuller, et al., "Are Hostility and Anxiety Associated with Carotid Atherosclerosis in Healthy Postmenopausal Women?" *Psychosomatic Medicine* 60(5) (September–October 1998): 633–638.

Nagao, T., T. Hase, and I. Tokimitsu, "A Green Tea Extract High in Catechins Reduces Body Fat and Cardiovascular Risks in Humans," *Obesity* 15(6) (June 2007): 1437–1483.

Radcliffe, J.D., and D.M. Czajka-Narins, "Partial Replacement of Dietary Casein with Soy Protein Isolate Can Reduce the Severity of Retinoid-Induced Hypertriglyceridemia," *Plant Foods in Human Nutrition* 52(2) (1998): 97–108.

Staprans, I., X.M. Pan, J.H. Rapp, et al., "Oxidized Cholesterol in the Diet Accelerates the Development of Aortic Atherosclerosis in Cholesterol-Fed Rabbits," *Arteriosclerosis, Thrombosis and Vascular Biology* 18 (June 1998): 1881–1887.

Watson, K.E., M.L. Abrolat, L.L. Malone, et al., "Active Serum Vitamin D Levels Are Inversely Correlated with Coronary Calcification," *Circulation* 96 (September 1997): 1755–1760.

Wolf, A., C. Zalpour, G. Theilmeier, et al., "Dietary L-Arginine Supplementation Normalizes Platelet Aggregation in Hypercholesterolemic Humans," *Journal of the American College of Cardiology* 29(3) (March 1997): 279–285.

Athlete's Foot

Klein, P.A., R.A. Clark, and N.H. Nicol, "Acute Infection with *Trichophyton rubrum* Associated with Flares of Atopic Dermatitis," *Cutis* 63(3) (March 1999): 171–172.

Ninomiya, J., M. Ide, Y. Ito, et al., "Experimental Penetration of *Trichophyton mentagrophytes* into Human Stratum Corneum," *Mycopathologia* 141(3) (1998): 153–157.

Tanuma, H., M. Doi, A. Yaguchi, et al., "Efficacy of Oral Fluconazole in Tinea Pedis of the Hyperkeratotic Type: Stratum Corneum Levels," *Mycoses* 41(3–4) (March–April 1998): 153–162.

Attention Deficit Disorder/Attention Deficit Hyperactivity Disorder (ADD/ADHD)

Arnsten, A.F., J.C. Steer, and R.D. Hunt, "The Contribution of Alpha 2-Noradrenergic Mechanisms of Prefrontal Corticol Cognitive Function. Potential Significance for Attention-Deficit Hyperactivity Disorder," *Archives of General Psychiatry* 53(5) (May 1996): 448–455.

Barabasz, A., and M. Barabasz, "Attention Deficit Hyperactivity Disorder: Neurological Basis and Treatment Alternatives," *Journal of Neurotherapy* 1 (1985): 1–10.

Carskadon, M.A., and C. Acebo, "Parental Reports of Seasonal Mood and Behavior Changes in Children," *Journal of the American Academy of Childhood and Adolescent Psychiatry* 32(2) (March 1993): 264–269.

Chervin, R.D., J.E. Dillon, C. Bassetti, et al., "Symptoms of Sleep Disorders, Inattention, and Hyperactivity in Children," *Sleep* 20(12) (December 1997): 1185–1192.

Egger, J., A. Stolla, and L.M. McEwen, "Controlled Trial of Hyposensitisation in Children with Food-Induced Hyperkinetic Syndrome," *Lancet* 339(8802) (9 May 1992): 1150–1153.

Girardi, N.L., F.S. Shaywitz, B.A. Shaywitz, et al., "Blunted Catecholamine Responses After Glucose Ingestion in Children with Attention Deficit Disorder," *Pediatrics Research* 4 (October 1995): 539–542.

Haskell, C.F., D.O. Kennedy, K.A. Wesnes, et al., "A Double-Blind, Placebo-Controlled, Multi-Dose Evaluation of the Acute Behavioural Effects of Guaraná in Humans," *Journal of Psychopharmacology* 21(1) (2007): 65–70.

Huss, M., A. Völp, and M. Stauss-Grabo, "Supplementation of Polyunsaturated Fatty Acids, Magnesium and Zinc in Children Seeking Medical Advice For Attention-Deficit/Hperactivity Problems—An Observational Cohort Study," *Lipids in Heath and Disease* 24 (September 2010): 105.

Langseth, L., and J. Dowd, "Glucose Tolerance and Hyperkinesis," *Food and Cosmetic Toxicology* 16 (1978): 129–133.

Lombard, Jay, and Carl Germano, *The Brain Wellness Plan: Breakthrough Medical, Nutritional and Immune-Boosting Therapies* (New York, NY: Kensington Books, 1997), pp. 152–153.

Mefford, I.N., and W.Z. Potter, "A Neuroanatomical and Biochemical Basis for Attention Deficit Disorder with Hyperactivity in Children: A Defect in Tonic Adrenal Mediated Inhibition of Locus Ceruleus Stimulation," *Medical Hypotheses* 29(1) (May 1989): 33–42.

Picchietti, D.L., S.J. England, A.S. Walters, et al., "Periodic Limb Movement Disorder and Restless Legs Syndrome in Children with Attention-Deficit Hyperactivity Disorder," *Journal of Child Neurology* 13(12) (December 1998): 588–594.

Rowe, S.K., and K.J. Rowe, "Synthetic Food Coloring and Behavior: A Dose Response Effect in a Double-Blind, Placebo-Controlled, Repeated-Measures Study," *Journal of Pediatrics* 125(Pt 1) (November 1994): 691–698.

Weber, W., A. Vander-Stoep, R.L. McCarty, et al., "*Hypericum perforatum* (St. John's Wort) for Attention-Deficit/ Hyperactivity Disorder in Children and Adolescents: A Randomized Controlled Trial," *Journal of the American Medical Association* 299(22) (June 2008): 2633–2631.

Zanette, G., C. Bonato, A. Polo, et al., "Long-Lasting Depression of Motor-Evoked Potentials to Transcranial Magnetic Stimulation Following Exercise," *Experimental Brain Research* 107(1) (1995): 80–86.

Bed-Wetting

Cleper, R., M. Davidovitz, R. Halevi, et al., "Renal Functional Reserve after Acute Poststreptococcal Glomerulonephritis," *Pediatric Nephrology* 11(40) (August 1997): 473–476.

Egger, J., C.H. Carter, J.F. Soothill, et al., "Effect of Diet Treatment on Enuresis in Children with Migraine or Hyperkinetic Behavior," *Clinical Pediatrics* (Philadelphia) 31(5) (May 1992): 302–307.

Eiberg, H., "Total Genome Scan Analysis in a Single Extended Family for Primary Nocturnal Enuresis: Evidence for a New Locus (ENUR3) for Primary Nocturnal Enuresis on Chromosome 22q1," *European Urologist* 33 (Supplement 3) (1998): 34–36.

Eller, D.A., Y.L. Homsy, P.F. Austin, et al., "Spot Urine Osmolality, Age, and Bladder Capacity as Predictors of Response to Desmopressin in Nocturnal Enuresis," *Scandinavian Journal of Urology and Nephrology* 183(Supplement) (1997): 41–45.

Hansen, A., B. Hansen, and T.L. Dahm, "Urinary Tract Infection, Day Wetting and Other Voiding Symptoms in Seven- to Eight-Year-Old Danish Children," *Acta Paediatrica* 86(12) (December 1997): 1345–1349.

Hunsballe, J.M., T.K. Hansen, S. Rittig, et al., "The Efficacy of DDAVP Is Related to the Circadian Rhythm of Urine Output in Patients with Persisting Nocturnal Enuresis," *Clinical Endocrinology* (Oxford) 49(6) (December 1998): 793–801.

Kruse, S., A.L. Hellstrom, and K. Hjalmas, "Daytime Bladder Dysfunction in Therapy-Resistant Nocturnal Enuresis: A Pilot Study in Urotherapy," *Scandinavian Journal of Urology and Nephrology* 33(1) (February 1999): 49–52.

Rona, R.J., L. Li, and S. Chinn, "Determinants of Nocturnal Enuresis in England and Scotland in the 90's," *Development and Medical Child Neurology* 39(10) (October 1997): 677–681.

Wieting, J.M., D.D. Dykstra, M.P. Ruggiero, et al., "Central Nervous System Ischemia after Varicella Infection and Desmopressin Therapy for Enuresis," *Journal of the American Osteopathic Association* 97(5) (May 1997): 293–295.

Bell's Palsy

Adour, K.K., J.M. Ruboyianes, P.G. Von Doersten, et al., "Bell's Palsy Treatment with Acyclovir and Prednisone Compared with Prednisone Alone: A Double-Blind, Randomized, Controlled Trial," *Annals of Otology, Rhinology, and Laryngology* 105 (1996): 371–378.

Diego Sastre, J.I., and M.P. Prim Espada, "Use of Acyclovir in Idiopathic Acute Facial Paralysis," *Acta Otorrinolaringológica de España* 50(2) (March 1999): 121–124.

Ohye, R.G., and E.A. Altenberger, "Bell's Palsy," *American Family Physician* 40 (1989): 159–166.

Xing, W., S. Yang, and X. Guo, "Treating Old Facial Nerve Paralysis of 260 Cases with the Acupuncture Treatment Skill of Pause and Regress in Six Parts," *Chen Tzu Yen Chiu* 19(2) (1994): 8–10.

Benign Prostatic Hypertrophy (BPH)

Roehrborn, C.G., J.E. Oesterling, S. Auerbach, et al., "The Hytrin Community Assessment Trial Study: A One-Year Study of Terazosin Versus Placebo in the Treatment of Men with Symptomatic Benign Prostatic Hyperplasia," *Urology* 47(2) (February 1996): 159–168.

Bladder Cancer

Alvares, A.P., "Interactions Between Environmental Chemicals and Drug Biotransformation in Man," *Clinical Pharmacokinetics* 3 (1978): 462.

Augustsson, K., K. Skog, M. Jagerstad, et al., "Dietary Heterocyclic Amines and Cancer of the Colon, Rectum, Bladder, and Kidney: A Population-Based Study," *Lancet* 353(9154) (27 February 1999): 703–707.

Baud, E., P.P. Catilina, and Y.J. Bignon, "Tracking the Gatekeeper Gene in the Stages of Carcinogenesis in the Bladder," *Bulletin du Cancer* 84(10) (October 1997): 971–975.

Bernardini, S., G.L. Adessi, C. Billerey, et al., "Immunohistochemical Detection of p53 Protein Overexpression Versus Gene Sequencing in Urinary Bladder Carcinomas," *Journal of Urology* 162(4) (October 1999): 1496–1501.

Bloom, N., "Cherry Hamburgers Lower in Suspected Carcinogens," press release, American Chemical Society, 7 November 1998.

Boik, John, *Cancer and Natural Medicine: A Textbook of Basic Science and Clinical Research* (Princeton, MN: Oregon Medical Press, 1995), p. 237.

Campbell, A., and T. Jack, "Acute Reactions to Mega Ascorbic Acid Therapy in Malignant Disease," *Scottish Medical Journal* 24 (1979): 151–153.

Den Otter, W., Z. Dobrowolski, A. Bugajski, et al., "Intravesical Interleukin-2 in T1 Papillary Bladder Carcinoma: Regression of Marker Lesion in 8 of 10 Patients," *Journal of Urology* 159(4) (April 1998): 1183–1186.

Isselbacher, K.J., E. Braunwald, J. Wilson, et al., eds. *Harrison's Principles of Internal Medicine,* 13th ed. (New York, NY: McGraw-Hill, 1995), p. 1338.

Kawamoto, K., H. Enokida, T. Gotanda, et al., "p16INK4a and p14ARF Methylation as a Potential Biomarker for Human Bladder Cancer," *Biochemical and Biophysical Research Communication,* 339(3) (January 2006): 790–796.

Larocca, L.M., M. Giustacchini, N. Maggiano, et al., "Growth-Inhibitory Effect of Quercetin and Presence of Type II Estrogen Binding Sites in Primary Human Transitional Cell Carcinomas," *Journal of Urology* 152(3) (1994): 1029–1033.

Michaud, D.S., D. Spiegelman, S.K. Clinton, et al., "Fruit and Vegetable Intake and Incidence of Bladder Cancer in a Male Prospective Cohort," *Journal of the National Cancer Institute* 90 (1998): 1072–1079, 1028–1029.

Michaud, D.S., D. Spiegelman, S.K. Clinton, et al., "Fluid Intake and the Risk of Bladder Cancer in Men," *The New England Journal of Medicine* 340(18) (6 May 1999): 1390.

Nowicky, J.W., G. Manolakis, D. Meijer, et al., "Ukrain Both as an Anticancer and Immunoregulatory Agent," *Drugs in Clinical and Experimental Research* (18) (supplement) (1992): 51–54.

Ornish, D., J. Lin, J. Daubenmier, et al., "Increased Telomerase Activity and Comprehensive Lifestyle Changes: A Pilot Study," *Lancet Oncology* 9(11) (November 2008): 1048–1057.

Schabath, M.B., H.B. Grossman, G.L. Delclos, et al., "Dietary Carotenoids and Genetic Instability Modify Bladder Cancer Risk," *Journal of Nutrition* 134(2) (December 2004): 3362–3369.

Yeager, R.T., A. DeVries, D.F. Jarrard, et al., "Overcoming Cellular Senescence in Human Cancer Pathogenesis," *Genes and Development* 12(2) (15 January 1998): 163–174.

Bladder Infection (Cystitis)

Lidefelt, K.J., L. Bollgren, and C.E. Nord, "Changes in Periurethral Microflora after Antimicrobial Drugs," *Archives of Disease in Childhood* 66 (1991): 683–685.

Murray, Michael T., and Joseph E. Pizzorno, *Encyclopedia of Natural Medicine,* 2d. ed. (Rocklin, CA: Prima Publishing, 1997), p. 285.

Palaszynski, S., J. Pinkner, S. Leath, et al., "Systemic Immunization with Conserved Pilus-Associated Adhesins Protects Against Mucosal Infections," *Developmental Biology* 92 (1998): 117–122.

Reid, G., A.W. Bruce, and R.L. Cook, "Effect on Urogenital Flora of Antibiotic Therapy of Urinary Tract Infection," *Scandinavian Journal of Infectious Disease* 22 (1990): 43–47.

Boil

Murray, Michael T., and Joseph E. Pizzorno, *Encyclopedia of Natural Medicine,* 2d. ed. (Rocklin, CA: Prima Publishing, 1997), p. 292.

Bone Cancer

Joshua, S.E., S. MacCallum, and J. Gibson, "Role of Alpha Interferon in Multiple Myeloma," *Blood Review* 11(4) (December 1997): 191–200.

Salmon, S.E., J.J. Crowley, S.P. Balcerzak, et al., "Interferon Versus Interferon Plus Prednisone Remission Maintenance Therapy for Multiple Myeloma: A Southwest Oncology Group Study," *Journal of Clinical Oncology* 16(3) (March 1998): 896–900.

Vacca, A., D. Ribatti, M. Iurlaro, et al., "Human Lymphoblastoid Cells Produce Extracellular Matrix-Degrading Enzymes and Induce Endothelial Cell Proliferation, Migration, Morphogenesis, and Angiogenesis," *International Journal of Clinical Laboratory Research* 28(1) (1998): 55–68.

Breast Cancer

Brain, K., P. Norman, J. Gray, et al., "Anxiety and Adherence to Breast Self-Examination in Women with a Family History of Breast Cancer," *Psychosomatic Medicine* 61(2) (March–April 1999): 181–187.

Deng, G., H. Lin, A. Seidman, et al., "A Phase I/II Trial of a Polysaccharide Extract from *Grifola frondosa* (Maitake mushroom) in Breast Cancer Patients: Immunological Effect," *Journal of Cancer Research and Clinical Oncology* 135(9) (September 2009): 1215–1221.

Dziaman, T., T. Huzarski, D. Gackowski, et al., "Selenium Supplementation Reduced Oxidative DNA Damage in Adnexectomized BRCA1 Mutations Carriers," *Cancer Epidemiology, Biomarkers and Prevention* 18(11) (November 2009): 2923–2928.

Fan, S., J. Wang, R. Yuan, et al., "BRCA1 Inhibition of Estrogen Receptor Signaling in Transfected Cells," *Science* 284(5418) (21 May 1999): 1354–1356.

Frampton, R., S.A. Omond, and J.A. Eisman, "Inhibition of Human Cancer Cell Growth by 1,25-Dihydroxyvitamin D3 Metabolites," *Cancer Research* 43 (1983): 4443–4447.

Hurd, C., N. Khattree, S. Dinda, et al., "Regulation of Tumor Suppressor Proteins, P53 and Retinoblastoma, by Estrogen and Antiestrogens in Breast Cancer Cells," *Oncogene* 15(3) (18 August 1997): 991–995.

Ip, C., "Attenuation of the Anticarcinogenic Action of Selenium by Vitamin E Deficiency," *Cancer Letters* 25 (1985): 325–331.

Jacobs, E.T., C.A. Thomson, S.W. Flatt, et al., "Vitamin D and Breast Cancer Recurrence in the Women's Healthy Eating and Living (WHEL) Study," *American Journal of Clinical Nutrition* 93(1) (January 2011): 108–117.

London, R.S., G.S. Sundaram, M. Schultz, et al., "Endocrine Parameters and Alpha-Tocopherol Therapy of Patients with Mammary Dysplasia," *Cancer Research* 41 (1981): 3811–3813.

Loret De Mola, J.R., "Endometrial Changes with Chronic Tamoxifen Use," *Current Opinion in Obstetrics and Gynecology* 9(3) (June 1997): 160–164.

Michnovicz, J.J., and H.L. Bradlow, "Altered Estrogen Metabolism and Excretion in Humans Following Consumption of Indole-3-Carbinol," *Nutrition and Cancer* 1 (1991): 59–66.

Morabia, A., M. Bernstein, J. Ruiz, et al., "Relation of Smoking to Breast Cancer by Estrogen Receptor Status," *International Journal of Cancer* 75(3) (January 1998): 339–342.

Potischan, N., et al., "Breast Cancer and Dietary Plasma Concentrations of Carotenoids and Vitamin A," *American Journal of Clinical Nutrition* 52 (1990): 909–915.

Ramesha, A., N. Rao, A. Rao, et al., "Chemoprevention of 7,12-Dimethylbenz(a)anthracene-Induced Mammary Carcinogenesis in Rats by the Combined Actions of Selenium, Magnesium, Ascorbic Acid, and Retinyl Acetate," *Japanese Journal of Cancer Research* 81 (1980): 1239–1246.

Santamaria, L.A., and A.B. Santamaria, "Cancer Chemoprevention by Supplemental Carotenoids and Synergism with Retinol in Mastodynia Treatment," *Medical Oncology and Tumor Pharmacotherapy* 7 (1990): 53–67.

Sergeev, I.N., Y.P. Arkhapchev, and V.B. Spirichev, "Ascorbic Acid Effects on Vitamin D Hormone Metabolism and Binding in Guinea Pigs," *Journal of Nutrition* 120(10) (October 1990): 1185–1190.

Stendell-Hollis, N.R., C.A. Thomson, P.A. Thompson, et al., "Green Tea Improves Metabolic Biomarkers, Not Weight or Body Composition: A Pilot Study in Overweight Breast Cancer Survivors," *Journal of Human Nutrition and Dietetics* 23(6) (December 2010): 590–600.

Stevens, J., M.W. Plankey, D.F. Williamson, et al., "The Body Mass Index-Mortality Relationship in White and African American Women," *Obesity Research* 6(4) (July 1998): 268–277.

Thomson, C.A., A.T. Stopeck, J.W. Bea, et al., "Changes in Body Weight and Metabolic Indexes in Overweight

Breast Cancer Survivors Enrolled in a Randomized Trial of Low-Fat vs. Reduced Carbohydrate Diets," *Nutrition and Cancer* 62(8) (November 2010): 1142–1152.

Wilson, S.T., D.E. Blask, and A.M. Lemus-Wilson, "Melatonin Augments the Sensitivity of MCF-7 Human Breast Cancer Cells to Tamoxifen in Vitro," *Journal of Clinical Endocrinology and Metabolism* 75(2) (August 1992): 669–670.

Yamaguchi, Y., Y. Hirooka, I. Konishi, et al., "Studies on Recurrent Breast Cancer—Clinicopathological Factors and P53, P21Cip1/Waf1 and Cyclin D1 Protein Expression," *Gan to Kagaku Ryoho* [*Japanese Journal of Cancer and Chemotherapy*] 26(5) (April 1999): 673–677.

Yong, C., S. Xiao-Ou, G. Yu-Tnag, et al., "Association of Ginseng Use with Survival and Quality of Life Among Breast Cancer Patients," *American Journal of Epidemiology* 163(7) (February 2006): 645–653.

Zhang, S., D.J. Hunter, S.E. Hankinson, et al., "A Prospective Study of Folate Intake and the Risk of Breast Cancer," *Journal of the American Medical Association* 281 (3 May 1999): 1632–1637.

Breast Cancer in Men

Sloan, B.S., L.S. Rickman, E.M. Blau, et al., "Schistosomiasis Masquerading as Carcinoma of the Breast," *Southern Medical Journal* 89(3) (March 1996): 345–347.

Wolf, D.A., S. Wang, M.A. Panzica, et al., "Expression of a Highly Conserved Oncofetal Gene, TA1/E16, in Human Colon Carcinoma and Other Primary Cancers: Homology to *Schistosoma mansoni* Amino Acid Permease and Caenorhabditis Elegans Gene Products," *Cancer Research* 56(21) (1 November 1996): 5012–5022.

Bronchitis and Pneumonia

"Childhood Trauma and Adult Illness," *Journal of Psychosocial Nursing and Mental Health Services* 36(9) (September 1998): 10–11.

Gonzales, R., and M. Sande, "What Will It Take to Stop Physicians from Prescribing Antibiotics in Acute Bronchitis?" *Lancet* 345 (1995): 665.

La Vecchia, C., A. Decarli, and R. Pagano, "Vegetable Consumption and Risk of Chronic Disease," *Epidemiology* 9(2) (March 1998): 208–210.

Murray, Michael T., and Joseph E. Pizzorno, *Encyclopedia of Natural Medicine,* 2d. ed. (Rocklin, CA: Prima Publishing, 1997), p. 295.

Orr, P.H., K. Scherer, A. Macdonald, et al., "Randomized Placebo-Controlled Trials of Antibiotics for Acute Bronchitis: A Critical Review of the Literature," *Journal of Family Practice* 36(5) (May 1993): 507–512.

Scannapieco, F.A., G.D. Papandonatos, and R.G. Dunford, "Associations Between Oral Conditions and Respiratory Disease in a National Sample Survey Population," *Annals of Periodontology* 3(1) (July 1998): 251–256.

Cancer

Basu, A., and V. Imrhan, "Tomatoes Versus Lycopene in Oxidative Stress and Carcinogenesis: Conclusions From Clinical Trials," *European Journal of Clinical Nutrition* 61 (2007): 295–303.

Ostermann, T., C. Raak, and A. Büssing, "Survival of Cancer Patients Treated with Mistletoe Extract (Iscador): A Systemic Literature Review," *BioMed Central* 9 (2009): 451–460.

Wu, T.H., T.Y. Chiu, J.S. Tsai, et al., "Effectiveness of Taiwanese Traditional Herbal Diet for Pain Management in Terminal Cancer Patients," *Asia Pacific Journal of Clinical Nutrition* 17(1) (2008): 17–22.

Canker Sores (Aphthous Ulcers)

Hay, K.D., and P.C. Reade, "The Use of An Elimination Diet in the Treatment of Recurrent Aphthous Ulceration of the Oral Cavity," *Oral Surgery* 57 (1984): 504–507.

Healy, C.M., M. Paterson, S. Joyston-Bechal, et al., "The Effect of a Sodium Lauryl Sulfate-Free Dentifrice on Patients with Recurrent Oral Ulceration," *Oral Disease* 5(1) (January 1999): 39–43.

Wilson, C.W.M., "Food Sensitivities, Taste Changes, Aphthous Ulcers, and Atopic Symptoms in Allergic Disease," *Annals of Allergy* 44 (1980): 302–307.

Carpal Tunnel Syndrome

Folkers, K., and J. Ellis, "Successful Therapy with Vitamin B_6 and Vitamin B_2 of the Carpal Tunnel Syndrome and Need for Determination of the RDAs for Vitamin B_6 and B_2 Disease States," *Annals of the New York Academy of Sciences* 585 (1990): 295–301.

Folkers, K.A., A. Walniuk, and S. Vadhanavkit, "Enzymology of the Response of Carpal Tunnel Syndrome to Riboflavin and to Combined Riboflavin and Pyridoxine," *Proceedings of the National Academy of Sciences* 81 (1984): 7067–7078.

Garfinke, M.S., A. Singhal, W.A. Katz, et al., "Yoga-Based Intervention for Carpal Tunnel Syndrome: A Randomized Trial," *Journal of the American Medical Association* 280(18) (11 November 1998): 1601–1603.

Cataracts

Bouton, S., "Vitamin C and the Aging Eye," *Archives of Internal Medicine* 63 (1939): 930–945.

Chylack, L.T., Jr., "Cataracts and Inhaled Corticosteroids," *The New England Journal of Medicine* 337 (1997): 8–14, 46–48.

Cumming, R.G., and P. Mitchell, "Medications and Cataract: The Blue Mountains Eye Study," *Ophthalmology* 105(9) (September 1998): 1751–1758.

Lu, M., A. Taylor, L.T. Chylack, et al., "Dietary Fat Intake and Early Age-Related Lens Opacities," *American Journal of Clinical Nutrition* 81(4) (April 2005): 773–779.

Moeller, S.M., R. Voland, L. Tinker, et al., "Associations Between Age-Related Nuclear Cataract and Lutein and Zeaxanthin in the Diet and Serum in the Carotenoids in the Age-Related Eye Disease Study, an Ancillary Study of the Women's Health Initiative," *Archive of Ophthalmology* 126(3) (March 2008): 354–364.

Olmedilla, B., F. Granado, S. Southon, et al., "Serum Concentrations of Carotenoids and Vitamins A, E, and C in Control Subjects from Five European Countries," *British Journal of Nutrition* 85(2) (February 2001): 227–238.

Rathbun, W., and S. Hanson, "Glutathione Metabolic Pathway as a Scavenging System in the Lens," *Ophthalmology Research* 11 (1979): 172–176.

Taylor, A., "Cataract: Relationship Between Nutrition and Oxidation," *Journal of the American College of Nutritionists* 12 (1993): 138–146.

Celiac Disease

Carbonnel, F., L. Grollet-Bioui, J.C. Brouet, et al., "Are Complicated Forms of Celiac Disease Cryptic T-Cell Lymphomas?" *Blood* 92(10) (15 November 1998): 3879–3886.

Carroccio, A., G. Iacono, G. Montalto, et al., "Pancreatic Enzyme Therapy in Childhood Celiac Disease: A Double-Blind Prospective Randomized Study," *Digestive Diseases and Sciences* 40(12) (December 1995): 2555–2560.

Dohan, F.C., and J.C. Gasberger, "Relapsed Schizophrenics: Earlier Discharge from the Hospital after Cereal-Free, Milk-Free Diet," *American Journal of Psychiatry* 130(6) (1973): 685–688.

Kapur, G., A.K. Patwari, S. Narayan, et al., "Iron Supplementation in Children with Celiac Disease," *Indian Journal of Pediatrics* 70(12) (December 2003): 955–958.

Cellulite

Draelos, Z.D., and K.D. Marenus, "Cellulite: Etiology and Purported Treatment," *Dermatological Surgery* 23(12) (December 1997): 1177–1181.

Knoblock, K., B. Joest, and P.M. Vogt, "Cellulite and Extracorporeal Shockwave Therapy (CelluShock-2009)—A Randomized Trial," *BMC Women's Health* 10 (October 2010): 29.

Kullick, M.I., "Evaluation of a Non-Invasive, Dual-Wavelength, Laser-Suction and Massage Device for the Regional Treatment of Cellulite," *Plastic and Reconstruction Surgery* 125(6) (June 2010): 1788–1796.

Rosenbaum, M., V. Prieto, J. Hellmer, et al., "An Exploratory Investigation of the Morphology and Biochemistry of Cellulite," *Plastic and Reconstructive Surgery* 101(7) (June 1998): 1934–1939.

Winter, M.L., "Post-Pregnancy Body Contouring Using a Combined Radiofrequency, Infrared Light and Tissue Manipulation Device," *Journal of Cosmetic and Laser Therapy* 11(4) (December 2009): 229–235.

Cervical Cancer

Apgar, B.S., and G. Brotzman, "HPV Testing in the Evaluation of the Minimally Abnormal Papanicolaou Smear," *American Family Physician* 59(10) (15 May 1999): 2794–2801.

Bedikian, A.Y., et al., "Prospective Evaluation of Thymosin Fraction V Immunotherapy in Patients with Non-Small-Cell Lung Cancer Receiving Vindesine, Doxorubicin, and Cisplatin (VAP) Chemotherapy," *American Journal of Clinical Oncology* 7 (1984): 399–404.

Boik, John, *Cancer and Natural Medicine: A Textbook of Basic Science and Clinical Research* (Princeton, MN: Oregon Medical Press, 1995), p. 235.

Butterworth, C.E., Jr., K.D. Hatch, M. Macaluso, et al., "Folate Deficiency and Cervical Dysplasia," *Journal of the American Medical Association* 267(4) (22–29 January 1992): 528–533.

Cho, H., M.K. Kim, J.K. Lee, et al., "Relationship of Serum Antioxidant Micronutrients and Sociodemographic Factors to Cervical Neoplasia: A Case-Control Study," *Clinical Chemistry and Laboratory Medicine* 47(8) (2009): 1005–1012.

Cobb, N., and R.E. Paisano, "Patterns of Cancer Mortality Among Native Americans," *Cancer* 83(11) (December 1998): 2377–2383.

Colombo, A., F. Landoni, G. Cormio, et al., "Concurrent Carboplatin-5FU and Radiotherapy Compared to Radiotherapy Alone in Locally Advanced Cervical Carcinoma: A Case-Control Study," *Tumori* 83(6) (November 1997): 895–899.

Creek, K.E., G. Geslani, A. Batova, et al., "Progressive Loss of Sensitivity to Growth Control by Retinoic Acid and Transforming Growth Factor-Beta at Late Stages of Human Papillomavirus Type 16–Initiated Transformation of Human Keratinocytes," *Advances in Experimental Medicine and Biology* 375 (1995): 117–135.

Dillner, J., M. Lehtinene, T. Bjorge, et al., "Prospective Seroepidemiologic Study of Human Papillomavirus Infection as a Risk Factor for Invasive Cervical Cancer," *Journal of the National Cancer Institute* 89(17) (September 1997): 1293–1299.

Giuliano, A.R., M. Papenfuss, M. Nour, et al., "Antioxidant Nutrients: Associations with Persistent Human Papillomavirus Infection," *Cancer Epidemiology, Biomarkers, and Prevention* 6(11) (November 1997): 917–923.

Goodman, M.T., N. Kiviat, K. McDuffie, et al., "The Association of Plasma Micronutrients with the Risk of Cervical Dysplasia in Hawaii," *Cancer Epidemiology, Biomarkers and Prevention* 7(6) (June 1998): 537–544.

Hurd, C., N. Khattree, S. Dinda, et al., "Regulation of Tumor Suppresser Proteins, P53 and Retinoblastoma, by Estrogen and Antiestrogens in Breast Cancer Cells," *Oncogene* 15(3) (18 August 1997): 991–995.

Lu, X., T. Toki, I. Konishi, et al., "Expression of P21WAF1/C1P1 in Adenocarcinoma of the Uterine Cervix: A Possible Immunohistochemical Marker of a Favorable Prognosis," *Cancer* 82(120) (15 June 1993): 2409–2417.

Mallmann, P., and D. Krebs, "The Effect of Immunotherapy with Thymopentin on the Parameters of Cellular Immunity and the Clinical Course of Gynecologic Tumor Patients," *Onkologie* 3 (1989): 15–21.

Martens, J.E., F. Smedts, B. Ter Harmsel, et al., "Glutathione S-Transferase Pi Is Expressed in (Pre) Neoplastic Lesions of the Human Uterine Cervix Irrespective of Their Degree of Severity," *Anticancer Research* 17(6D) (November 1997): 4305–4309.

Prabhu, N.S., K. Somasundaram, K. Satyamoorthy, et al., "P73, Unlike P53, Suppresses Growth and Induces Apoptosis of Human Papillomavirus E6-Expressing Cancer Cells," *International Journal of Oncology* 13(1) (July 1998): 5–9.

Prokopczyk, B., J.E. Cox, D. Hoffmann, et al., "Identification of Tobacco-Specific Carcinogen in the Cervical Mucus of Smokers and Nonsmokers," *Journal of the National Cancer Institute* 89(12) (18 June 1998): 868–873.

Rock, C.L., A. Moskowitz, B. Huizar, et al., "High Vegetable and Fruit Diet Intervention in Premenopausal Women with Cervical Intraepithelial Neoplasia," *Journal of the American Dietetic Association* 101(10) (October 2001): 1167–1174.

Roy, M., and M. Plante, "Pregnancies after Radical Vaginal Trachelectomy for Early-Stage Cervical Cancer," *American Journal of Obstetrics and Gynecology* 179(6, Part 1) (December 1998): 1491–1496.

Verreault, R., J. Chu, M. Mandelson, et al., "A Case-Control Study of Diet and Invasive Cervical Cancer," *International Journal of Cancer* 43(6) (15 June 1989): 1050–1054.

Von Knebel Doeberitz, M., D. Spitkovsky, and R. Ridder, "Interactions Between Steroid Hormones and Viral Oncogenes in the Pathogenesis of Cervical Cancer," *Verhandlungen der deutscher Gesellschaft für Pathologie* 81 (1997): 233–239.

Chemotherapy Side Effects

Matsuzaki, T., I. Kato, T. Yokokura, et al., "Augmentation of Antitumor Activity of *Lactobacillus casei* YIT 8018 (LC 9018) in Combination with Various Antitumor Drugs," *Gan to Kgaku Ryoho* [*Cancer and Chemotherapy*] 11 (1984): 445–451.

Chronic Fatigue Syndrome

Ablashi, D.V., P.H. Levine, C. De Vinci, et al., "Use of Anti HHV-6 Transfer Factor for the Treatment of Two Patients with Chronic Fatigue Syndrome (CFS): Two Case Reports," *Biotherapy* 9(1–3) (1996): 81–86.

Baschetti, R., "Chronic Fatigue Syndrome and Liquorice," *New Zealand Medical Journal* 108(1002) (28 June 1995): 259.

Baschetti, R., "Chronic Fatigue Syndrome and Neurally Mediated Hypotension," *Journal of the American Medical Association* 275 (1996): 359.

Clague, J.E., R.H. Edwards, and M.J. Jackson, "Intravenous Magnesium Loading in Chronic Fatigue Syndrome," *Lancet* 340(8811) (11 July 1992): 124–125.

Demitrack, M.A., "Evidence for Impaired Activation of the Hypothalamic-Pituitary-Adrenal Axis in Patients with Chronic Fatigue Syndrome," *Journal of Clinical Endocrinology and Metabolism* 73 (1991): 1224–1234.

Fiatarone, M.A., J.E. Morley, E.T. Bloom, et al., "The Effect of Exercise on Natural Killer Cells Activity in Young and Old Subjects," *Journal of Gerontology* 44(2) (March 1989): M37–M45.

Gray, J.B., and A.M. Martinovic, "Eicosanoids and Essential Fatty Acid Modulation in Chronic Disease and the Chronic Fatigue Syndrome," *Medical Hypotheses* 43(1) (July 1994): 31–42.

Hobday, R.A., S. Thomas, T.S. O'Donovan, et al., "Dietary Intervention in Chronic Fatigue Syndrome," *Journal of Human Nutrition and Dietetics* 21(2) (April 2008): 141–149.

Isselbacher, K.J., E. Braunwald, J. Wilson, et al., eds., *Harrison's Principles of Internal Medicine,* 13th ed. (New York, NY: McGraw-Hill, 1995), pp. 2398–2400.

Levine, P.H., "The Use of Transfer Factors in Chronic Fatigue Syndrome: Prospects and Problems," *Biotherapy* 9(1–3) (1996): 77–79.

Lombard, Jay, and Carl Germano, *The Brain Wellness Plan* (New York, NY: Kensington Press, 1998), p. 177.

Makinnon, LT., "Exercise and Natural Killer Cells: What Is Their Relationship?" *Sports Medicine* 7 (1989): 141–149.

Xusheng, S., X. Yugi, and X. Yunjian, "Determination of E-Rosette-Forming Lymphocytes in Aged Subjects with Tai Chi Quan Exercise," *International Journal of Sports Medicine* 10 (1989): 217–219.

Cirrhosis of the Liver

Cadranel, J.F., V. Di Martino, and B. Devergie, "Grapefruit Juice for the Pruritus of Cholestatic Liver Disease," *Annals of Internal Medicine* 126(11) (1 June 1997): 920–921.

Das, I., R.E. Burch, and H.K.J. Hahn, "Effects of Zinc Deficiency on Ethanol Metabolism and Alcohol and Aldehyde Dehydrogenase Activities," *Journal of Laboratory and Clinical Medicine* 104 (1984): 610–617.

Floreani, A., I. Carderi, F. Ferrara, et al., "A 4-year Treatment with Clodronate Plus Calcium and Vitamin D Supplements Does Not Improve Bone Mass in Primary Biliary Cirrhosis," *Digestive and Liver Diseases* 39(6) (June 2007).

He, K., K.R. Iyer, R.N. Hayes, et al., "Inactivation of Cytochrome P450 3A4 by Bergamottin, a Component of Grapefruit Juice," *Chemical Research in Toxicology* 11(40) (April 1998): 252–259.

Lieber, C.S., "Alcohol, Liver, and Nutrition," *Journal of the American College of Nutrition* 10 (1991): 602–632.

Lieber, C.S., "Ethanol Metabolism, Cirrhosis and Alcoholism," *Clinica Chimica Acta* 257(1) (January 1997): 59–84.

Lieber, C.S., "Role of Oxidative Stress and Antioxidant Therapy in Alcoholic and Nonalcoholic Liver Disease," *Advances in Pharmacology* 38 (1997): 601–628.

Malaguarnera, M., M.P. Gargante, G. Malaguarnera, et al., "*Bifidobacterium* Combined with Fructo-Oligosaccharide Versus Lactulose in the Treatment of Patients with Hepatic Encelphalopathy," *European Journal of Gastroenterology and Hepatology* 22(2) (February 2010): 199–206.

Matsuoka, M., M.Y. Zhang, and H. Tsukamoto, "Sensitization of Hepatic Lipocytes by High-Fat Diet to Stimulatory Effects of Kupffer Cell-Derived Factors: Implication in Alcoholic Liver Fibrogenesis," *Hepatology* 11(2) (February 1990): 173–182.

Takeshita, S., T. Ichikawa, K. Nakao, et al., "A Snack Enriched with Oral Branched-Chain Amino Acids

Prevents a Fall in Albumin in Patients with Liver Cirrhosis Undergoing Chemoembolization for Hepatocellular Carcinoma," *Nutrition Research* 29(2) (February 2009): 89–93.

Yunice, A.A., and R.D. Lindeman, "Effect of Ascorbic Acid and Zinc Sulphate on Ethanol Toxicity and Metabolism," *Proceedings of the Society for Experimental Biology in Medicine* 154 (1977): 146–150.

Colic

Arikan, D., H. Alp, S. Gözüm, et al., "Effectiveness of Massage, Sucrose Solution, Herbal Tea, or Hydrolysed Formula in the Treatment of Infantile Colic," *Journal of Clinical Nursing* 17(13) (July 2008): 1754–1761.

Bruneton, Jean N., *Pharmacognosy, Phytochemistry, Medicinal Plants* (Paris: Lavoisier Publishing, 1995), p. 444.

Hill, D.J., N. Roy, R.G. Heine, et al., "Effect of a Low-Allergen Maternal Diet on Colic Among Breastfed Infants: A Randomized, Controlled Trial," *Pediatrics* 116(5) (November 2005): e709–e715.

Savino, F., E. Pelle, E. Palumeri, et al., "*Lactobacillus reuteri* (American Type Culture Collection Strain 55730) Versus Simethicone in the Treatment of Infantile Colic: A Prospective Randomized Study," *Pediatrics* 119(1) (January 2007): e124–e130.

Colorectal Cancer

Ahearn, T.U., M.L. McCullough, W.D. Flanders, et al., "A Randomized Clinical Trial of the Effects of Supplemental Calcium and Vitamin D_3 on Markers of Their Metabolism in Normal Mucosa of Colorectal Adenoma Patients," *Cancer Research* 71(2) (January 2011): 413–423.

Anti, M., F. Armelao, G. Marra, et al., "Effects of Different Doses of Fish Oil on Rectal Cell Proliferation in Patients with Sporadic Colonic Adenomas," *Gastroenterology* 107(6) (December 1994): 1709–1718.

Das, U.N., N. Madhavi, G. Sravan Kumar, et al., "Can Tumour Cell Drug Resistance Be Reversed by Essential Fatty Acids and their Metabolites?" *Prostaglandins, Leukotrienes, and Essential Fatty Acids* 58(1) (January 1998): 39–54.

Davis, C.D., and Y. Feng, "Dietary Copper, Manganese and Iron Affect the Formation of Aberrant Crypts in Colon of Rats Administered 3,2'-Dimethyl-4-Aminobipheny," *Journal of Nutrition* 129(5) (May 1999): 1060–1067.

Garland, C.F., F.C. Garland, and E.D. Gorham, "Can Colon Cancer Incidence and Death Rates Be Reduced with Calcium and Vitamin D?" *American Journal of Clinical Nutrition* 54 (1991): 193S–201S.

Honda, T., I. Kai, and G. Ohi, "Fat and Dietary Fiber Intake and Colon Cancer Mortality: A Chronological Comparison Between Japan and the United States," *Nutrition and Cancer* 33(1) (1999): 95–99.

Jenab, M., H.B. Bueno-de-Mesquita, P. Ferrari, et al., "Association between Pre-Diagnostic Circulating Vitamin D Concentration and Risk of Colorectal Cancer in European Populations: A Nested Case-Control Study," *British Medical Journal* (January 2011). DOI: 10.1136/bmj .b5500.

Sansbury, L.B., K. Wanke, P.S. Albert, et al., "The Effect of Strict Adherence to a High-Fiber, High-Fruit and Vegetable, and Low-Fat Eating Pattern on Adenoma Recurrence," *American Journal of Epidemiology* 170(5) (September 2009).

Sergeev, I.N., Y.P. Arkhapchev, and V.B. Spirichev, "Ascorbic Acid Effects on Vitamin D Hormone Metabolism and Binding in Guinea Pigs," *Journal of Nutrition* 120(10) (October 1990): 1185–1190.

Tang, R., J.Y. Wang, S.K. Lo, et al., "Physical Activity, Water Intake and Risk of Colorectal Cancer in Taiwan: A Hospital-Based Case-Control Study," *International Journal of Cancer* 82(4) (12 August 1999): 484–489.

Waddell, W., and R. Loughry, "Sulindac for Polyposis of the Colon," *Journal of Surgical Oncology* 24 (1983): 83–87.

Willett, W.C., M.J. Stampfer, G.A. Colditz, et al., "Relation of Meat, Fat, and Fiber Intake to the Risk of Colon Cancer in a Prospective Study Among Women," *The New England Journal of Medicine* 323(24) (13 December 1990): 1664–1672.

Common Cold

Barrett, B., R. Brown, D. Rakel, et al., "Echinacea for Treating the Common Cold: A Randomized Trial," *Annals of Internal Medicine* 153 (December 2010): 769–777.

Rowe, C.A., M.P. Nantz, J.F. Bukowski, et al., "Specific Formulation of *Camellia sinensis* Prevents Cold and Flu Symptoms and Enhances Gamma, Delta T Cell Function: A Randomized, Double-Blind, Placebo-Controlled Study," *Journal of the American College of Nutriton* 26(5) (2007): 445–452.

Schoop, R., P. Klein, A. Suter, et al., "Echinacea in the Prevention of Induced Rhinovirus Colds: A Meta-Analysis," *Clinical Therapeutics* 28(2) (2006): 174–183.

Yale, S.H., and K. Liu, "*Echinacea purpurea* Therapy for the Treatment of the Common Cold: A Randomized, Double-Blind, Placebo-Controlled Trial," *Archives of Internal Medicine* 164 (2004): 1237–1241.

Congestive Heart Failure

Almoznino-Sarafian, D., S. Berman, A. Mor, et al., "Magnesium and C-reactive Protein in Heart Failure: An Anti-Inflammatory Effect of Magnesium Administration?" *European Journal of Nutrition* 46(4) (June 2007): 230–237.

Andrews, R., P. Greenhaff, S. Curtis, et al., "The Effect of Dietary Creatine Supplementation on Skeletal Muscle Metabolism in Congestive Heart Failure," *European Heart Journal* 19(4) (April 1998): 617–622.

CoQ$_{10}$ Drug Surveillance Investigators, "Italian Multicenter Study on the Safety and Efficacy of Coenzyme Q$_{10}$ as Adjunctive Therapy in Heart Failure," *Molecular Aspects of Medicine* 15 (Supplement) (1994): S287–S294.

Costello, R.B., P.B. Moser-Veillon, and R. Bianco, "Magnesium Supplementation in Patients with Congestive Heart Failure," *Journal of the American College of Nutritionists* 16(1) (February 1997): 22–31.

Douban, S., M.A. Brodsky, D.D. Whang, et al., "Significance of Magnesium in Congestive Heart Failure," *American Heart Journal* 132(3) (September 1996): 664–671.

Fernandes, J.S., et al., "Therapeutic Effect of a Magnesium Salt in Patients Suffering from Mitral Valvular Prolapse and Latent Tetany," *Magnesium* 4 (1985): 283–289.

Ferrari, R., and F. De Giuli, "The Propionyl-L-Carnitine Hypothesis: An Alternative Approach to Treating Heart Failure," *Journal of Cardiac Failure* 3(3) (September 1997): 217–224.

Frustaci, A., N. Magnavita, C. Chimenti, et al., "Marked Elevation of Myocardial Trace Elements in Idiopathic Dilated Cardiomyopathy Compared with Secondary Cardiac Dysfunction," *Journal of the American College of Cardiology* 33(6) (May 1999): 1578–1583.

Galland, L.D., S.M. Baker, and R.K. McLellan, "Magnesium Deficiency in the Pathogenesis of Mitral Valve Prolapse," *Magnesium* 5 (1986): 165–174.

Kanaya, Y., M. Nakamura, N. Kobayashi, et al., "Effect of L-Arginine on Lower Limb Vasodilator Reserve and Exercise Capacity in Patients with Chronic Heart Failure," *Heart* 81(5) (May 1999): 512–517.

Kawasaki, N., J.D. Lee, H. Shimizu, et al., "Long-Term L-Carnitine Treatment Prolongs the Survival in Rats with Adriamycin-Induced Heart Failure," *Journal of Cardiac Failure* 2(4) (December 1996): 293–299.

Keuthe, F., A. Krack, B.M. Richartz, et al., "Creatine Supplementation Improves Muscle Strength in Patients with Congestive Heart Failure," *Die Pharmazie* 61(3) (March 2006): 218–222.

Schleithoff, S.S., A. Zittermann, G. Tenderich, et al., "Vitamin D Supplementation Improves Cytokine Profiles in Patients with Congestive Heart Failure: A Double-Blind, Randomized, Placebo-Controlled Trial," *American Journal of Clinical Nutrition* 83(4) (April 2006): 754–759.

Schleithoff, S.S., A. Zittermann, G. Tenderich, et al., "Combined Calcium and Vitamin D Supplementation Is Not Superior to Calcium Supplementation Alone in Improving Disturbed Bone Metabolism in Patients with Congestive Heart Failure," *European Journal of Clinical Nutrition* 62(12) (December 2008): 1388–1394.

Shimon, I., S. Almog, Z. Vered, et al., "Improved Left Ventricular Function after Thiamine Supplementation in Patients with Congestive Heart Failure Receiving Long-Term Furosemide Therapy," *American Journal of Medicine* 98(5) (May 1995): 485–490.

Struthers, A.D., "Aldosterone Escape During Angiotensin-Converting Enzyme Inhibitor Therapy in Chronic Heart Failure," *Journal of Cardiac Failure* 2(1) (March 1996): 47–54.

Waiser, B., R.M. Giordano, and C.L. Stebbins, "Supplementation With Omega-3 Polyunsaturated Fatty Acids Augments Brachial Artery Dilation and Blood Flow During Forearm Contraction," *European Journal of Applied Physiology* 97(3) (June 2006): 347–354.

Constipation

Akao, T., Q.M. Che, K. Kobashi, et al., "A Purgative Action of Barbaloin Is Induced by *Eubacterium* Sp. Strain BAR, a Human Intestinal Anaerobe, Capable of Transforming Barbaloin to Aloe-Emodin Anthrone," *Biological and Pharmaceutical Bulletin* 19(1) (January 1996): 136–138.

Bub, S., J. Brinckmann, G. Cicconetti, et al., "Efficacy of an Herbal Dietary Supplement (Smooth Move) in the Management of Constipation in Nursing Home Residents: A Randomized, Double-Blind, Placebo-Controlled Study," *Journal of the American Medical Directors Association* 7(9) (November 2006): 556–561.

Del Piano, M., S. Carmagnola, A. Anderloni, et al., "The Use of Probiotics in Healthy Volunteers with Evacuation Disorders and Hard Stools: A Double-Blind, Randomized, Placebo-Controlled Study," *Journal of Clinical Gastroenterology* 44 (supplement 1) (September 2010): S30–S34.

Jacobs, E.J., and E. White, "Constipation, Laxative Use, and Colon Cancer Among Middle-Aged Adults," *Epidemiology* 9 (July 1998): 371–372, 385–391.

Meshkinpour, H., S. Selod, H. Movahedi, et al., "Effects of Regular Exercise in Management of Chronic Idiopathic Constipation," *Digestive Diseases and Sciences* 43 (1998): 2379–2383.

Shah, N., K. Lindley, and P. Milla, "Cow's Milk and Chronic Constipation in Children," *The New England Journal of Medicine* 340(11) (18 March 1999): 891–892.

Sturtzel, B., A. Dietrich, K.H. Wagner, et al., "The Status of Vitamins B_6, B_{12}, Folate, and of Homocysteine in Geriatric Home Residents Receiving Laxatives or Dietary Fiber," *Journal of Nutrition, Health and Aging,* 14(3) (March 2010): 219–223.

Taubman, B., and M. Buzby, "Overflow Encopresis and Stool Toileting Refusal During Toilet Training: A Prospective Study on the Effect of Therapeutic Efficacy," *Pediatrics* 99 (November 1997): 54–58.

Cough

Bucca, C., G. Rolla, W. Arossa, et al., "Effect of Ascorbic Acid on Increased Bronchial Responsiveness During Upper Airway Infection," *Respiration* 55(4) (1989): 214–219.

Burr, M.L., H.R. Anderson, J.B. Austin, et al., "Respiratory Symptoms and Home Environment in Children: A National Survey," *Thorax* 54(1) (January 1999): 27–32.

Grievink, L., H.A. Smit, M.C. Ocke, et al., "Dietary Intake of Antioxidant (Pro)-Vitamins, Respiratory Symptoms and Pulmonary Function: The MORGEN Study," *Thorax* 53(3) (March 1998): 166–171.

Van Bever, H.P., M.H. Wieringa, J.J. Weyler, et al., "Croup and Recurrent Croup: Their Association with Asthma and Allergy: An Epidemiological Study on 5–8-Year-Old Children," *European Journal of Pediatrics* 158(3) (March 1999): 253–257.

Crohn's Disease

Belluzzi, A., C. Brignola, M. Campieri, et al., "Effect of An Enteric-Coated Fish-Oil Preparation on Relapses in Crohn's Disease," *The New England Journal of Medicine* 334(24) (13 June 1996): 1557–1560.

Bentz, S., M. Hausmann, H. Pbierger, et al., "Clinical Relevance of IgG Antibodies Against Food Antigens in Crohn's Disease: A Double-Blind Cross-Over Diet Intervention Study," *Digestion* 81(4) (2010): 252–264.

Caprilli, R., G. Taddei, and A. Viscido, "In Favour of Prophylactic Treatment for Post-Operative Recurrence in Crohn's Disease," *Italian Journal of Gastroenterology and Hepatology* 30(2) (April 1998): 219–225.

Darroch, D.J., R.M. Barnes, and J. Dawson, "Circulating Antibodies to *Saccharomyces cerevisiae* (Bakers'/Brewers' Yeast) in Gastrointestinal Disease," *Journal of Clinical Pathology* 51(1) (January 1999): 47–53.

Feagan, B.G., W.J. Sandborn, U. Mittmann, et al., "Omega-3 Free Fatty Acids for the Maintenance of

Remission in Crohn Disease: The EPIC Randomized Controlled Trial," *Journal of the American Medical Association* 299(14) (April 2008): 1690–1696.

Fujimori, S., A. Tatsuguchi, K. Gudis, et al., "High Dose Probiotic and Prebiotic Cotherapy For Remission Induction of Active Crohn's Disease," *Journal of Gastroenterology & Hepatology* 22(8) (August 2007): 1199–1204.

Garcia Vilela, E., M. De Lourdes De Abreu de Ferrari, H. Oswaldo Da Gama Torres, et al., "Influence of *Saccharomyces boulardii* on the Intestinal Permeability of Patients with Crohn's Disease in Remission," *Scandanavian Journal of Gastroenterolgy* 43(7) (2008): 842–848.

Hillier, K., R. Jewell, L. Dorrell, et al., "Incorporation of Fatty Acids from Fish Oil and Olive Oil into Colonic Mucosal Lipids and Effects upon Eicosanoid Synthesis in Inflammatory Bowel Disease," *Gut* 32(10) (October 1991): 1151–1155.

Kumari, M., N.B. Khazai, T.R. Ziegler, et al., "Vitamin D-Mediated Calcium Absorption in Patients with Clinically Stable Crohn's Disease: A Pilot Study," *Molecular Nutrition & Food Research* 54(8) (August 2010): 1085–1091.

Lorenz-Meyer, H., P. Bauer, C. Nicolay, et al., "Omega-3 Fatty Acids and Low Carbohydrate Diet for Maintenance of Remission in Crohn's Disease: A Randomized Controlled Multicenter Trial. Study Group Members (German Crohn's Disease Study Group)," *Scandinavian Journal of Gastroenterology* 31(8) (August 1996): 778–785.

Dandruff

Fälth-Magnusson, K., and N.I. Kjellman, "Development of Atopic Disease in Babies Whose Mothers Were Receiving Exclusion Diet During Pregnancy—A Randomized Study," *Journal of Allergy and Clinical Immunology* 80(6) (December 1987): 868–875.

Depression

Abou-Saleh, M.T., and A. Coppen, "The Biology of Folate in Depression: Implications for Nutritional Hypotheses of Psychoses," *Journal of Psychiatric Research* 20(2) (1982): 91–101.

Agargun, M.Y., E.E. Algun, R. Skeroglu, et al., "Low Cholesterol Level in Patients with Panic Disorder: The Association with Major Depression," *Journal of Affective Disorders* 50(1) (July 1998): 29–32.

Alpert, J.E., G. Papakostas, D. Mischoulon, et al., "S-adenosyl-L-methionine (SAMe) as an Adjunct for Resistant Major Depressive Disorder: An Open Trial Following Partial or Nonresponse to Selective Serotonin Reuptake Inhibitors or Veniafaxine," *Journal of Clinical Psychopharmacology* 24(6) (December 2004): 661–664.

American Psychiatric Association, *Diagnostic and Statistical Manual of Mental Disorders,* 4th ed. (Washington, DC: American Psychiatric Association, 1994), p. 199.

Bell, I.R., J.S. Edman, F.D. Morrow, et al., "B Complex Vitamin Patterns in Geriatric and Young Adult in Patients with Major Depression," *Journal of the American Geriatric Society* 39(3) (March 1991): 252–257.

Blair, J., C. Morar, C. Hamon, et al., "Tetrahydrobiopterin Metabolism in Depression," *Lancet* 1 (1984): 163.

Delgado, P.L., C.S. Charney, L.H. Price, et al., "Neuroendocrine and Behavioral Effects of Dietary Tryptophan Restriction in Healthy Subjects," *Life Science* 45 (1990): 2323–2332.

Fuller, R.W., "The Involvement of Serotonin in Regulation of Pituitary Adrenal Cortical Function," *Frontiers of Neuroendocrinology* 13 (1992): 250–270.

Huszti, Z., H. Prast, M.H. Tran, et al., "Glial Cells Participate in Histamine Inactivation in Vivo," *Naunyn-Schmiedebergs Archives of Pharmacology* 357(1) (January 1998): 49–53.

Kasper, S., M. Gastpar, W.E. Müller, et al., "Efficacy of St. John's Wort Extract WS 5570 in Acute Treatment of Mild Depression: A Reanalysis of Data from Controlled Clinical Trials," *European Archives of Psychiatry and Clinical Neuroscience* 285(1) (February 2008): 59–63.

Krikorian, R., J.C. Eliassen, E.L. Boespflug, et al., "Improved Cognitive-Cerebral Function in Older Adults with Chromium Supplementation," *Nutritional Neuroscience* 13(3) (June 2010): 116–122.

Leeming, R., J. Harpey, S. Brown, et al., "Tetrahydrofolate and Hydroxycobalamin in the Management of Dihydropteridine Reductase Deficiency," *Journal of Mental Deficiency Research* 26 (1982): 21–25.

Luo, H., F. Meng, Y. Jia, et al., "Clinical Research on the Therapeutic Effect of the Electro-Acupuncture Treatment in Patients with Depression," *Psychiatry and Clinical Neuroscience* 52 (supplement) (December 1998): S338–S340.

Maes, M., A. Christophe, J. Delanghe, et al., "Lowered Omega-3 Polyunsaturated Fatty Acids in Serum Phospholipids and Choesteryl Esters of Depressed Patients," *Psychiatry Research* 85(3) (22 March 1999): 275–291.

Maes, M., et al., "The Relationship Between the Viability of L-Tryptophan to the Brain: The Spontaneous HPA Axis Activity and the HPA Axis Response to Dexamethasone in Depressed Patients," *Amino Acids* 1 (1991): 57–65.

Marshall, R.D., and C. J. Douglas, "Phenylpropanolamine-Induced Psychosis. Potential Predisposing Factors,"

General Hospital Psychiatry 16(5) (September 1994): 358–360.

Matsushima, K., R. Schmidt-Kastner, M.J. Hogan, et al., "Cortical Spreading Depression Activates Trophic Factor Expression in Neurons and Astrocytes and Protects Against Subsequent Focal Brain Ischemia," *Brain Research* 807(1–2) (5 October 1998): 47–60.

Rondanelli, M., A. Giacosa, A. Opizzi, et al., "Effect of Omega-3 Fatty Acids Supplementation on Depressive Symptoms and on Health-Related Quality of Life in the Treatment of Elderly Women with Depression: A Double-Blind, Placebo-Controlled, Randomized Clinical Trial," *Journal of the American College of Nutrition* 29(1) (February 2010): 55–64.

Shippy R.A., D. Mendez, K. Jones, et al., "S-adenosylmethione (SAMe) for the Treatment of Depression in People living with HIV/AIDS," *BioMed Central Psychiatry* 11(4) (November 2004): 38.

Suarez, C., "Relations of Trait Depression and Anxiety to Low Lipid and Lipoprotein Concentrations in Healthy Young Adult Women," *Psychosomatic Medicine* 61(3) (May–June 1999): 273–279.

Diabetes

Aljabri, K.S., S.A. Bokhari, and M.J. Khan, "Glycemic Changes After Vitamin D Supplementation in Patients with Type 1 Diabetes Mellitus and Vitamin D Deficiency," *Annals of Saudi Medicine* 30(6) (November–December 2010): 454–458.

Grant, S.J., A. Bensoussan, D. Chang, et al., "Chinese Herbal Medicines for People with Impaired Glucose Tolerance or Impaired Fasting Blood Glucose," Cochrane Database of Systematic Reviews 2009, Issue 4. Art No.: CD 006690. DOI: 10.1002/14651856.CD006690.pub2.

Huseini, H.F., B. Larijani, R. Heshmat, et al., "The Efficacy of *Silybum Marianum* (L.) *Gaertn.* (Silymarin) in the Treatment of Type II Diabetes: A Randomized, Double-Blind, Placebo-Controlled, Clinical Trial," *Phytotherapy Research* 20 (2006): 1036–1039.

Hussain, S.A., "Silymarin as an Adjunct to Glibenclamide Therapy Improves Long-Term and Postprandial Glycemic Control and Body Mass Index in Type 2 Diabetes," *Journal of Medicinal Food* 10(3) (2007): 543–547.

Matsumoto, J., "Vanadate, Molybdate and Tungstate for Orthomolecular Medicine," *Medical Hypotheses* 43(3) (September 1994): 177–182.

Okamura, F., A. Tahsiro, A. Utsumi, et al., "Insulin Resistance in Patients with Depression and Its Changes in the Clinical Course of Depression: A Report on Three Cases Using the Minimal Model Analysis," *Internal Medicine* 38(3) (March 1999): 257–260.

Shidfar, F., M. Aghasi, M. Vafa, et al., "Effects of Combination of Zinc and Vitamin A Supplementation on Serum Fasting Blood Sugar, Insulin, Apoprotein B and Apoprotein A-1 in Patients with Type 1 Diabetes," *International Journal of Food Sciences and Nutrition* 61(12) (November 2010): 182–191.

Sievenpiper, J.L., M.K. Sung, M. Di Buono, et al., "Korean Red Ginseng Rootlets Decrease Acute Postprandial Glycemia: Results from Sequential Preparation- and Dose-Finding Studies," *Journal of the American College of Nutrition* 25(2) (2006): 100–107.

Solomon, T.P., J.M. Haus, K.R. Kelly, et al., "A Low-Glycemic Index Diet Combined with Exercise Reduces Insulin Resistance, Postprandial Hyperinsulinemia, and Glucose-Dependent Insulinotropic Polypeptide Responses in Obese, Prediabetic Humans," *American Journal of Clinical Nutrition* 92(6) (December 2010): 1359–1368.

Stirban, A., S. Nandrean, C. Gotting, et al., "Effects of n-3 Fatty Acids on Macro- and Microvascular Function in Subjects with Type 2 Diabetes Mellitus," *American Journal of Clinical Nutrition* 91(3) (March 2010): 808–813.

Suzuki, Y., H. Kadowaki, M. Taniyama, et al., "Insulin Edema in Diabetes Mellitus Associated with the 3243 Mitochondrial TRNA(Leu(UUR)) Mutation: Case Reports," *Diabetes Research and Clinical Practice* 29(2) (August 1995): 137–142.

Wickenberg, J., S.L. Ingemansson, and J. Hlebowicz, "Effects of *Curcuma longa* (Turmeric) on Postprandial Plasma Glucose and Insulin in Healthy Subjects," *Nutrition Journal* 12 (9) (October 2010): 43.

Diabetic Retinopathy

Barnett, N.L., and N. Osborne, "Redistribution of GABA Immunoreactivity Following Central Retinal Artery Occlusion," *Brain Research* 677(2) (24 April 1995): 337–240.

Cox, B.D., and W.J. Butterfield, "Vitamin C Supplements and Diabetic Cutaneous Capillary Fragility," *British Medical Journal* (July 1995): 205.

Gerstein, H.C., "Preventive Medicine in a Diabetes Clinic: An Opportunity to Make a Difference," *Lancet* 353(9153) (20 February 1999): 606–608.

MacLeod, K.M., A.E. Gold, and B.M. Frier, "Tight Glucose Control and Diabetic Complications," *Lancet* 342(8871) (4 September 1993): 617–618.

Mayer-Davis, E.J., R.A. Bell, B.A. Reboussin, et al., "Antioxidant Nutrient Intake and Diabetic Retinopathy: The San Luis Valley Diabetes Study," *Ophthalmology* 105(12) (December 1998): 2264–2270.

Wang, Q., D.G. Dills, R. Klein, et al., "Does Insulin-Like Growth Factor I Predict Incidence and Progression of

Diabetic Retinopathy?" *Diabetes* 44(2) (February 1995): 161–164.

Williams, G., and G.V. Gill, "Eating Disorders and Diabetic Complications," *The New England Journal of Medicine* 336(26) (26 June 1997): 1905–1906.

Diaper Rash

Berg, R.W., M.C. Milligan, and F.C. Sarbaugy, "Association of Skin Wetness and pH with Diaper Dermatitis," *Pediatric Dermatology* 11(1) (March 1994): 18–20.

Hunt, L., P. Fleming, and J. Golding, "Does the Supine Sleeping Position Have Any Adverse Effects on the Child? I. Health in the First Six Weeks," *Pediatrics* 100(1) (July 1997): E11.

Patrizi, A., I. Neri, S. Marzaduri, et al., "Pigmented and Hyperkeratotic Napkin Dermatitis: A Liquid Detergent Irritant Dermatitis," *Dermatology* 193(1) (1996): 36–40.

Philipp, R., A. Hughes, and J. Golding, "Getting to the Bottom of Nappy Rash. ALSPAC Survey Team. Avon Longitudinal Study of Pregnancy and Childhood," *British Journal of General Practice* 47(421) (August 1997): 493–497.

Pierard-Franchimont, C., C. Letawe, and E.G. Pierard, "Tribological and Mycological Consequences of the Use of a Miconazole Nitrate-Containing Paste for the Prevention of Diaper Dermatitis: An Open Pilot Study," *European Journal of Pediatrics* 155(9) (September 1996): 756–758.

Reid, G., C. Tieszer, and D. Lam, "Influence of *Lactobacilli* on the Adhesion of *Staphylococcus aureus* and *Candida albicans* to Fibers and Epithelial Walls," *Journal of Industrial Microbiology* 15(3) (September 1995): 248–253.

Diarrhea

Chandler, D.S., and T.L. Mynott, "Bromelain Protects Piglets from Diarrhoea Caused by Oral Challenge with K88 Positive Enterotoxigenic *Escherichia coli*," *Gut* 43(2) (1998): 196–202.

Costa F.R., R.V. Lacorte, M.A. Lima, et al., "Life Quality of Postsurgical Patients with Colorectal Cancer After Supplemented Diet with *Agaricus sylvaticus* Fungus," *Nutrición Hospitalaria* [*Nutrition Hospital*] 25(4) (July-August 2010): 586–596.

Rabbani, G.H., T. Teka, S.K. Saha, et al., "Green Banana and Pectin Improve Small Intestinal Permeability and Reduce Fluid Loss in Bangladeshi Children with Persistent Diarrhea," *Digestive Diseases and Sciences* 49(3) (March 2004): 475–484.

Scariati, P.D., L.M. Grummer-Strawn, and S.B. Fein, "A Longitudinal Analysis of Infant Morbidity and the

Extent of Breastfeeding in the United States," *Pediatrics* 99 (June 1997): E6.

Speissbach, K., "Milk for Children with Diarrhea," *Pediatric News* 14 (September 1997).

Dry Mouth

Blom, M., S. Kopp, and T. Lundeberg, "Prognostic Value of the Pilocarpine Test to Identify Patients Who May Obtain Long-Term Relief from Xerostomia by Acupuncture Treatment," *Archives of Otolaryngology and Head and Neck Surgery* 125(5) (May 1999): 561–566.

Singh, M., P.C. Stark, C.A. Palmer, et al., "Effect of Omega-3 and Vitamin E Supplementation on Dry Mouth in Patients with Sjögren's Syndrome," *Special Care in Dentistry* 30(6) (November–December 2010): 225–229.

Ear Infection

Batchelder, H.J., "Allopathic Specific Condition Review: Otitis Media," *Protocol Journal of Botanical Medicine* 2(2) (1997): 95.

Cantekin, E.I., T.W. McGuire, and T.L. Griffith, "Antimicrobial Therapy for Otitis Media with Effusion," *Journal of the American Medical Association* 266(23) (18 December 1991): 3309–3317.

Froom, J., L. Culpepper, M. Jacobs, et al., "Antimicrobials for Acute Otitis Media? A Review from the International Primary Care Network," *British Medical Journal* 315(7100) (12 July 1997): 98–102.

Job, A., M. Raynal, and P. Rondet, "Hearing Loss and Use of Personal Stereos in Young Adults with Antecedents of Otitis Media," *Lancet* 353(9146) (2 January 1999): 35.

Klein, J.O., "Role of Nontypeable *Haemophilus influenzae* in Pediatric Respiratory Tract Infections," *Pediatric Infectious Disease Journal* 16(2) (supplement) (February 1997): S5–S8.

Kleinman, L.C., J. Kosecoff, R.W. Dubois, et al., "The Medical Appropriateness of Tympanostomy Tubes Proposed for Children Younger Than 16 Years in the United States," *Journal of the American Medical Association* 271(16) (27 April 1994): 1250–1255.

Lagace, E., "Xylitol for Prevention of Acute Otitis Media," *Journal of Family Practice* 48(2) (February 1999): 89.

Nsouli, T.M., S.M. Nsouli, R.E. Linde, et al., "Role of Food Allergy in Serous Otitis Media," *Annals of Allergy* 73(3) (September 1994): 215–219.

Saarinen, U.M., E. Savilahti, and P. Arjomaa, "Increased IgM-Type Betalactoglobulin Antibodies in Children with Recurrent Otitis Media," *Allergy* 38(3) (November 1983): 571–576.

Witsell, D.L, C.G. Garrett, W.G. Yarbrough, et al., "Effect of *Lactobacillus acidophilus* on Antibiotic-Associated Gastrointestinal Morbidity: A Prospective Randomized Trial," *Journal of Otolaryngology* 24(4) (August 1995): 230–233.

Eczema

Ewig, C.I., A.C. Gibbs, C. Ashcroft, and T.J. David, "Failure of Oral Zinc Supplementation in Atopic Eczema," *European Journal of Clinical Nutrition* 45(10) (October 1991): 507–510.

Filipiak, B., A. Zutavern, S. Koletzko, et al., "Solid Food Introduction in Relation to Eczema: Results from a Four-Year Prospective Birth Cohort Study," *Journal of Pediatrics* 151(4) (October 2007): 352–358.

Gfesser, M., D. Abeck, J. Rugemer, et al., "The Early Phase of Epidermal Barrier Regeneration Is Faster in Patients with Atopic Eczema," *Dermatology* 195(4) (1997): 332–336.

Horneff, G., C. Schou, and V. Wahn, "Diagnostic Significance of in Vitro T-Cell Proliferative Responses to House-Dust Mite Der P 1 in Children with Dust-Mite Allergy," *Allergy* 51(11) (November 1996): 842–846.

Isselbacher, K.J., E. Braunwald, J. Wilson, et al., eds., *Harrison's Principles of Internal Medicine*, 13th ed. (New York, NY: McGraw-Hill, 1995), p. 275.

Koch, C., S. Dölle, M. Metzger, et al., "Docosahexaenoic acid (DHA) Supplementation in Atopic Eczema: A Randomized, Double-Blind, Controlled Trial," *British Journal of Dermatology* 158(4) (April 2008): 786–792.

Miyake, Y., S. Sasaki, and K. Tanaka, "Maternal Fat Consumption During Pregnancy and Risk of Wheeze and Eczema in Japanese Infants Aged 16–24 Months: The Osaka Maternal and Child Health Study," *Thorax* 64(9) (September 2009): 815–821.

Nielsen, G.D., U. Soderberg, P.J. Jorgensen, et al., "Absorption and Retention of Nickel from Drinking Water in Relation to Food Intake and Nickel Sensitivity," *Toxicology and Applied Pharmacology* 154(1) (January 1999): 67–75.

Saarinen, U.M., and M. Kajosaari, "Breast Feeding as Prophylaxis Against Atopic Disease: Prospective Follow-Up Study Until 17 Years Old," *Lancet* 346(8982) (21 October 1995): 1065–1069.

Sampson, H.A., and S.M. Scanlon, "Natural History of Food Hypersensitivity in Children with Atopic Dermatitis," *Journal of Pediatrics* 115 (1993): 23–27.

Savolainen, J., K. Lammintausta, K. Kalimo, et al., "*Candida albicans* and Atopic Dermatitis," *Clinical Experience in Allergy* 23(4) (April 1993): 332–339.

Sharma, A.D., "Disulfiram and Low Nickel Diet in the Management of Hand Eczema: A Clinical Study," *Indian Journal of Dermatology, Venereology and Leprology* 72(2) (March–April 2006): 113–118.

Theoharides, T.C., L.K. Singh, W. Boucher, et al., "Corticotropin-Releasing Hormone Induces Skin Mast Cell Degranulation and Increased Vascular Permeability, a Possible Explanation for Its Proinflammatory Effects," *Endocrinology* 139(1) (January 1998): 403–413.

Endometrial Cancer

Adlercreutz, H., H. Markkanen, and S. Watanabe, "Plasma Concentrations of Phyto-Estrogens in Japanese Men," *Lancet* 342(8881) (13 November 1993): 1209–1210.

Adlercreutz, H., Y. Mousavi, J. Clark, et al., "Dietary Phyto-estrogens and Cancer: In Vitro and in Vivo Studies," *Journal of Steroid Biochemistry and Molecular Biology* 41(3–8) (1992): 331–337.

Duncan, A.M., B.E. Merz, X. Xu, et al., "Soy Isoflavones Exert Modest Hormonal Effects in Premenopausal Women," *Journal of Clinical Endocrinology and Metabolism* 84(1) (January 1999) 192–197.

Levi, F., S. Franceschi, E. Negri, et al., "Dietary Factors and the Risk of Endometrial Cancer," *Cancer* 71(11) (1 June 1993): 3575–3581.

Lucenteforte, E., R. Talamini, M. Montella, et al., "Macronutrients, Fatty Acids and Cholesterol Intake and Endometrial Cancer," *Annals of Oncology* 19(1) (January 2008): 168–172.

Mallmann, P., and D. Krebs, "The Effect of Immunotherapy with Thymopentin on the Parameters of Cellular Immunity and the Clinical Course of Gynecologic Cancer Patients," *Onkologie* 3 (1989): 15–21.

Olson, S.H., J.E. Vena, J.P. Dorn, et al., "Exercise, Occupational Activity, and Risk of Endometrial Cancer," *Annals of Epidemiology* 7(1) (January 1997): 46–53.

Endometriosis

Carpenter, S.E., B. Tjaden, J.A. Rock, et al., "The Effect of Regular Exercise on Women Receiving Danazol for Treatment of Endometriosis," *International Journal of Gynaecology and Obstetrics* 49(3) (June 1995): 299–304.

Covens, A.L., P. Christopher, and R.F. Casper, "The Effect of Dietary Supplementation with Fish Oil Fatty Acids on Surgically Induced Endometriosis in the Rabbit," *Fertility and Sterility* 49(4) (April 1998): 698–703.

Fleming, R.M., "What Effect, If Any, Does Soy Protein Have on Breast Tissue?" *Integrative Cancer Therapies* 2(3) (September 2003): 225–228.

Grodstein, F., M.B. Goldman, L. Ryan, et al., "Relation of Female Infertility to Consumption of Caffeinated Beverages," *American Journal of Epidemiology* 137(12) (15 June 1993): 1353–1360.

Mier-Cabrera, J., T. Aburto-Soto, S. Burrola-Mendez, "Women with Endometriosis Improved Their Peripheral Antioxidant Markers After the Application of a High Antioxidant Diet," *Reproductive Biology and Endocrinology* 7 (28 May 2009): 54.

Misao, R., J. Fujimoto, Y. Nakanishi, et al., "Expression of Estrogen and Progesterone Receptors and their MRNAs in Ovarian Endometriosis," *Gynecological Endocrinology* 10(5) (October 1996): 303–310.

Erectile Dysfunction

Cormio, L., M. De Siai, F. Lorusso, et al., "Oral L-Citrulline Supplementation Improves Erection Hardness in Men with Mild Erectile Dysfunction," *Urology* 77(1) (January 2011): 119–122.

de Andrade, E., A.A. de Mesquita, J.A. Claro, et al., "Study of the Efficacy of Korean Red Ginseng in the Treatment of Erectile Dysfunction," *Asian Journal of Andrology* 9(2) (2007): 241–244.

Grasing, K., M.G. Sturgill, R.C. Rosen, et al., "Effects of Yohimbine on Autonomic Measures Are Determined by Individual Values for Area Under the Concentration-Time Curve," *Journal of Clinical Pharmacology* 36(9) (1996): 814–822.

Langford, H.G., R.W. Rockhold, S. Wasertheil-Smoller, et al., "Effect of Weight Loss on Thiazide Produced Erectile Problems in Men," *Transactions of the American Clinical Association* 101 (1989): 190–194.

Lau, B.H., and E.W. Lau, "Kyo-Green Improves Sexual Dysfunction in Men and Women," *Medical Science Monitor* 9(2) (February 2003): P112–118.

Melman, A., and J.C. Gingell, "The Epidemiology and Pathophysiology of Erectile Dysfunction," *Journal of Urology* 161(1) (January 1999): 5–11.

Fibrocystic Breasts

Guo, C., W. Zhang, S. Zheng, et al., "Clinical Observation on Efficacy of Electro-Acupuncture Therapy in Hyperplasia of Mammary Glands and Its Effect on Immunological Function," *Journal of Traditional Chinese Medicine* 16(4) (December 1996): 281–287.

Isselbacher, K.J., E. Braunwald, J. Wilson, et al., eds., *Harrison's Principles of Internal Medicine,* 13th ed. (New York, NY: McGraw-Hill, 1995), p. 1841.

Levinson, W., and P.M. Dunn, "Nonassociation of Caffeine and Fibrocystic Breast Disease," *Archives of Internal Medicine* 146(9) (September 1986): 1773–1775.

Noble, L.S., K. Takayama, K.M. Zeitoun, et al., "Prostaglandin E2 Stimulates Aromatase Expression in Endometriosis-Derived Stromal Cells," *Journal of Clinical Endocrinology and Metabolism* 82(2) (February 1997): 600–606.

Parazzini, F., C. LaVecchia, R. Riundi, et al., "Methylxanthine, Alcohol-Free Diet and Fibrocystic Breast Disease: A Factorial Clinical Trial," *Surgery* 99(5) (May 1986): 576–581.

Pasquali, D., A. Bellastella, A. Valente, et al., "Retinoic Acid Receptors Alpha, Beta and Gamma, and Cellular Retinol Binding Protein-I Expression in Breast Fibrocystic Disease and Cancer," *European Journal of Endocrinology* 137(4) (October 1997): 410–414.

Rock, C.L., G.A. Saxe, M.T. Ruffin, IV, et al., "Carotenoids, Vitamin A, and Estrogen Receptor Status in Breast Cancer," *Nutrition and Cancer* 25(3) (1996): 281–296.

Vobecky, J., A. Simard, J.S. Vobecky, et al., "Nutritional Profile of Women with Fibrocystic Breast Disease," *International Journal of Epidemiology* 22(6) (December 1993): 989–999.

Fibroids, Uterine (Uterine Myomas)

The Boston Women's Health Book Collective, *The New Our Bodies, Ourselves: A Book by and for Women* (New York, NY: Simon and Schuster Touchstone Books, 1992), p. 597.

Govan, Alasdair D.T., *Gynecology Illustrated,* 4th ed. (New York, NY: Churchhill-Livingstone, 1993), pp. 242–243.

Kaminski, B.T., and J. Rzempoluch, "Evaluation of the Influence of Certain Epidemiologic Factors on Development of Uterine Myomas," *Wiadomosci Lekarskie* 46 (15–16) (August 1993): 592–596.

Viville, B., D.S. Charnock-Jones, A.M. Sharkey, et al., "Distribution of the A and B Forms of the Progesterone Receptor Messenger Ribonucleic Acid and Protein in Uterine Leiomyomata and Adjacent Myometrium," *Human Reproduction* 12(4) (April 1997): 815–822.

Fibromyalgia Syndrome

Azad, K.A., M.N. Alam, S.A. Hag, et al., "Vegetarian Diet in the Treatment of Fibromyalgia," *Bangladesh Medical Research Council Bulletin* 26(2) (August 2000): 41–47.

Di Benedetto, P., L.G. Iona, and V. Zidarich, "Clinical Evaluation of S-Adenosyl-L-Methionine Versus Transcutaneous Nerve Stimulation in Primary Fibromyalgia," *Current Therapeutic Research* 53 (1993): 222–229.

Donaldson, M.S., N. Speight, and S. Loomis, "Fibromyalgia Syndrome Improved Using a Mostly Raw Vegetarian

Diet: An Observational Study," *BMC Complementary and Alternative Medicine* 1 (September 2001): 7.

"Is Fibromyalgia Caused by a Glycolysis Impairment?" *Nutrition Reviews* 52(7) (July 1994): 248–250.

Jacobsen, S., B. Danneskiold-Samsoe, and R.B. Andersen, "Oral S-Adenosylmethionine in Primary Fibromyalgia: Double-Blind Clinical Evaluation," *Scandinavian Journal of Rheumatology* 20(4) (1991): 294–302.

Merchant, R.E., and C.A. Andre, "A Review of Recent Clinical Trials of the Nutritional Supplement *Chlorella pyrenoidosa* in the Treatment of Fibromyalgia, Hypertension, and Ulcerative Colitis," *Alternative Therapies in Health and Medicine* 7(3) (May–June 2001): 79–91.

Michalsen, A., M. Riegert, R. Lüdtke, et al., "Mediterranean Diet or Extended Fasting's Influence on Changing the Intestinal Microflora, Immunoglobulin A Secretion and Clinical Outcome in Patients with Rheumatoid Arthritis and Fibromyalgia: An Observational Study," *BMC Complementary and Alternative Medicine* 5 (December 2005): 22.

Sprott, H., S. Franke, H. Kluge, et al., "Pain Treatment of Fibromyalgia by Acupuncture," *Rheumatology International* 18(10) (1998): 35–36.

Tavoni, A., G. Jeracitano, and G. Cirigliano, "Evaluation of S-Adenosylmethionine in Secondary Fibromyalgia: A Double-Blind Study," *Clinical Experience in Rheumatology* 16(1) (January–February 1998): 106–107.

Tavoni, A., C. Vitali, S. Bombardieri, et al., "Evaluation of S-Adenosylmethionine in Primary Fibromyalgia: A Double-Blind Crossover Study," *American Journal of Medicine* 83(5A) (20 November 1987): 107–110.

Volkmann, H., J. Norregaard, S. Jacobsen, et al., "Double-Blind, Placebo-Controlled Cross-Over Study of Intravenous S-Adenosyl-L-Methionine in Patients with Fibromyalgia," *Scandinavian Journal of Rheumatology* 26(3) (1997): 206–211.

White, K.P., and M. Harth, "An Analytical Review of 24 Controlled Clinical Trials for Fibromyalgia Syndrome (FMS)," *Pain* 64 (1996): 211–219.

Food Poisoning

Centers for Disease Control, "Aldibarb as a Cause of Food Poisoning—Louisiana, 1998," *Journal of the American Medical Association* 281(21) (2 June 1999): 1979–1980.

Fracture

Chevalley, T., P. Hoffmeyer, J.P. Bonjour, et al., "Early Serum IGF-I Response to Oral Protein Supplements in Elderly Women with a Recent Hip Fracture," *Clinical Nutrition* 29(1) (February 2010): 78–83.

Feskanich, D., P. Weber, W.C. Willett, et al., "Vitamin K Intake and Hip Fractures in Women: A Prospective Study," *American Journal of Clinical Nutrition* 69(1) (January 1999): 74–79.

Larsen, H.M., and I.L. Hansen, "Effect of Specific Training on Menstruation and Bone Strength," *Ugeskrift for Læger* [*Weekly Journal for Physicians*] 160(33) (10 August 1998): 4762–4767.

McTiernan, A., J. Wactawski-Wende, L. Wu, et al., "Low-Fat, Increased Fruit, Vegetable, and Grain Dietary Pattern, Fractures, and Bone Mineral Density: The Women's Health Initiative Dietary Modification Trial," *American Journal of Clincial Nutrition* 89(6) (June 2009): 1864–1876.

Melhus, H., K. Michaelsson, A. Kindmark, et al., "Excessive Dietary Intake of Vitamin A Is Associated with Reduced Bone Mineral Density and Increased Risk for Hip Fracture," *Annals of Internal Medicine* 129(10) (15 November 1998): 770–778.

Munger, R.G., J.R. Cerhan, and B.C. Chiu, "Prospective Study of Dietary Protein Intake and Risk of Hip Fracture in Postmenopausal Women," *American Journal of Clinical Nutrition* 69(1) (January 1999): 147–152.

Nieves, J.W., K. Melsop, M. Curtis, et al., "Nutritional Factors That Influence Change in Bone Density and Stress Fracture Risk Among Young Female Cross-Country Runners," *PM & R* 2(8) (August 2010): 740–750.

Reginster, J.Y., L. Meurmans, B. Zegels, et al., "The Effect of Sodium Monofluorophosphate Plus Calcium on Vertebral Fracture Rate in Postmenopausal Women with Moderate Osteoporosis: A Randomized, Controlled Trial," *Annals of Internal Medicine* 129 (1998): 1–8.

Seelig, M.S., "Vitamin D—Risk vs. Benefit," *Journal of the American College of Nutrition* 2(2) (1983): 109–110.

Thomas, M.K., D.M. Lloyd-Jones, R.I. Thadhani, et al., "Hypovitaminosis D in Medical Inpatients," *The New England Journal of Medicine* 338(12) (19 March 1998): 777–783.

Gallstones

Breneman, J.C., "Allergy Elimination Diet as the Most Effective Gallbladder Diet," *Annals of Allergy* 26 (1986): 83.

Heaton, K.W., P.M. Emmett, C.L. Symes, et al., "An Explanation for Gallstones in Normal-Weight Women: Slow Intestinal Transit," *Lancet* 341 (1993): 8–10.

Jonkers, I.J., A.H. Smelt, H.M. Princen, et al., "Fish Oil Increases Bile Acid Synthesis in Male Patients with Hypertriglyceridemia," *Journal of Nutrition* 136(4) (April 2006): 987–991.

Méndez-Sánchez, N., V. González, P. Aguayo, et al., "Fish Oil (n-3) Polyunsaturated Fatty Acids Beneficially

Affect Biliary Cholesterol Nucleation Time in Obese Women Losing Weight," *Journal of Nutrition* 131(9) (September 2001): 2300–2303.

Pixley, F., and J. Mann, "Dietary Factors in the Aetiology of Gall Stones: A Case Control Study," *Gut* 29 (1988): 1511–1515.

Wudel, L.J., J.K. Wright, J.P. Debelak, et al., "Prevention of Gallstone Formation in Morbidly Obese Patients Undergoing Rapid Weight Loss: Results of a Randomized Controlled Pilot Study," *Journal of Surgical Research* 102(1) (January 2002): 50–56.

Gastritis

Inoue, M., K. Tajima, S. Kobayashi, et al., "Protective Factor Against Progression from Atrophic Gastritis to Gastric Cancer—Data from a Cohort Study in Japan," *International Journal of Cancer* 66(30) (3 May 1996): 309–314.

Miki, K., Y. Urita, F. Ishikawa, et al., "Effect of *Bifidobacterium bifidum* Fermented Milk on *Helicobacter pylori* and Serum Pepsinogen Levels in Humans," *Journal of Dairy Science* 90(6) (June 2009): 2630–2640.

Moses, F.M., "Gastrointestinal Bleeding and the Athlete," *American Journal of Gastroenterology* 88(8) (August 1993): 1157–1159.

Pedrosa, M.C., B.B. Golner, B.R. Goldin, et al., "Survival of Yogurt-Containing Organisms and *Lactobacillus gasseri* (ADH) and Their Effect on Bacterial Enzyme Activity in the Gastrointestinal Tract of Healthy and Hypochlorhydric Elderly Subjects," *American Journal of Clinical Nutrition* 61(2) (February 1995): 353–359.

Saltzman, J.R., and R.M. Russell, "The Aging Gut. Nutritional Issues," *Gastroenterological Clinics of North America* 27(2) (June 1998): 309–324.

Tsubono, Y., S. Okubo, M. Hayashi, et al., "A Randomized Controlled Trial for Chemoprevention of Gastric Cancer in High-Risk Japanese Population; Study Design, Feasibility and Protocol Modification," *Japanese Journal of Cancer Research* 88(4) (April 1997): 344–349.

Yanaka, A., J.W. Fahey, A. Fukumoto, et al., "Dietary Sulforaphane-Rich Broccoli Sprouts Reduce Colonization and Attenuate Gastritis in *Helicobacter pylori*-Infected Mice and Humans," *Cancer Prevention Research* (Philadelphia) 2(4) (April 2009): 353–360.

Glaucoma

Coleman, A.L., K.L. Stone, G. Kodjebacheva, et al., "Glaucoma Risk and the Consumption of Fruits and Vegetables Among Older Women in the Study of Osteoporotic Fractures," *American Journal of Ophthalmology* 145(6) (June 2008): 1081–1089.

Gaspar, A.Z., P. Gasser, and J. Flammer, "The Influence of Magnesium on Visual Field and Peripheral Vasospasms in Glaucoma," *Ophthalmologica* 209 (1995):11–13.

Higginbotham, E.J., H.A. Kilimanjaro, J.T. Wilensky, et al., "The Effect of Caffeine on Intraocular Pressure in Glaucoma Patients," *Ophthalmology* 96(5) (May 1989): 624–626.

Stewart, W.C., "The Effect of Lifestyle on the Relative Risk to Develop Open-Angle Glaucoma," *Current Opinion in Ophthalmology* 6(2) (April 1995): 3–9.

Strömland, K., and M.D. Pinazo-Durán, "Optic Nerve Hypoplasia: Comparative Effects in Children and Rats Exposed to Alcohol During Pregnancy," *Teratology* 50(2) (August 1994): 100–111.

Gout

Blau, L.W., "Cherry Diet Control for Gout and Arthritis," *Texas Reports on Biology and Medicine* 8 (1950): 309–311.

Choi, H.K., M.A. De Vera, and E. Krishnan, "Gout and the Risk of Type 2 Diabetes Among Men with a High Cardiovascular Risk Profile," *Rheumatology* (Oxford) 47(10) (October 2008): 1567–1570.

Kuhnau, J., "The Flavonoids: A Class of Semi-Essential Food Components: Their Role in Human Nutrition," *World Review of Nutrition and Dietetics* 24 (1976): 117–119.

Hair Loss

Grüber, D.M., M.O. Sator, E.M. Kokoschka, et al., "Thymopentin in Alopecia Areata," *Acta Medica Austriaca* 25(1) (1998): 33–35.

Hoffmann, R., E. Wenzel, A. Huth, et al., "Growth Factor MRNA Levels in Alopecia Areata Before and After Treatment with the Contact Allergen Diphenylcyclopropenone," *Acta Dermato-Venereologica* 76(1) (January 1996): 17–20.

Nabaie, L., S. Kavand, R.M. Robati, et al., "Androgenic Alopecia and Insulin Resistance: Are They Really Related?" *Clinical and Experimental Dermatology* 34(6) (August 2009): 694–697.

Sharma, V.K., "Pulsed Administration of Corticosteroids in the Treatment of Alopecia Areata," *International Journal of Dermatology* 35(2) (February 1996): 133–136.

Signorello, L.B., J. Wuu, C.C. Hsieh, et al., "Hormones and Hair Patterning in Men: A Role for Insulin-Like Growth Factor I?" *Journal of the American Academy of Dermatology* 40(2, Part 1) (February 1999): 200–203.

Halitosis (Bad Breath)

Amir, E., R. Shimonov, and M. Rosenberg, "Halitosis in Children," *Journal of Pediatrics* 134(3) (March 1999): 338–343.

Ierardi, E., A. Amoruso, T. La Notte, "Halitosis and *Helicobacter pylori*: A Possible Relationship," *Digestive Science* 43(12) (December 1998): 2733–2777.

Senol, M., and P. Fireman, "Body Odor in Dermatologic Diagnosis," *Cutis* 63(2) (February 1999): 107–111.

Suarez, F., J. Springfield, J. Furne, et al., "Differentiation of Mouth Versus Gut as Site of Origin of Odoriferous Breath Gases after Garlic Ingestion," *American Journal of Physiology* 276(2, Part 1) (February 1999): G425–G430.

Hangover

Peng, G.S., Y.C. Chen, T.P. Tsao, et al., "Pharmacokinetic and Pharmacodynamic Basis for Partial Protection Against Alcoholism in Asians, Heterozygous for the Variant ALDH2*2 Gene Allele," *Pharmacogenetics and Genomics* 17(10) (October 2007): 845–855.

Segal, B., "ADH and ALDH Polymorphisms Among Alaska Natives Entering Treatment for Alcoholism," *Alaska Medicine* 41(1) (January–March 1999): 9–12.

Tipton, K.F., G.T.M. Heneman, and J.M. McCrodden, "Metabolic and Nutritional Aspects of Alcohol," *Biochemical Society Transactions* 11 (1983): 59–61.

Heart Attack (Myocardial Infarction)

Ascherio, A., E.B. Rim, E.L. Giovannucci, et al., "Dietary Fat and Risk of Coronary Heart Disease in Men: Cohort Follow-Up Study in the United States," *British Medical Journal* 313(7049) (13 July 1996): 84–90.

Cumming, R.G., and P. Mitchell, "Medications and Cataract: The Blue Mountains Eye Study," *Ophthalmology* 105(9) (September 1998): 1751–1758.

Desci, T., D. Molnar, and B. Koletzko, "Reduced Plasma Concentrations of Alpha-Tocopherol and Beta-Carotene in Obese Boys," *Journal of Pediatrics* 130 (1997): 653–655.

Einvik, G., T.O. Klemsdal, L. Sandvik, et al., "A Randomized Clinical Trial on n-3 Polyunsaturated Fatty Acids Supplementation and All-Cause Mortality in Elderly Men at High Cardiovascular Risk," *European Journal of Cardiovascular Prevention and Rehabilitation* 17(5) (October 2010): 588–592.

Goldman, I.L., M. Kopelberg, J.E. Debaene, et al., "Antiplatelet Activity in Onion (*Allium cepa*) Is Sulfur Dependent," *Thrombosis and Haemostasis* 76(3) (September 1996): 450–452.

Grandi, N.C., L.P. Breitling, C.Y. Vossen, et al., "Serum Vitamin D and Risk of Secondary Cardiovascular Disease Events in Patients with Stable Coronary Heart Disease," *American Heart Journal* 159(6) (June 2010): 1044–1051.

Guyton, J.R., "Effect of Niacin on Atherosclerotic Cardiovascular Disease," *American Journal of Cardiology* 82(12A) (17 December 1998): 18U–23U; discussion 39U–41U.

Hu, F.B., M.J. Stampfer, J.E. Manson, et al., "Dietary Fat Intake and the Risk of Coronary Heart Disease in Women," *The New England Journal of Medicine* 337(21) (20 November 1997): 1491–1499.

Karppi, J., T.H. Rissanen, K. Nyyssönen, et al., "Effects of Astaxanthin Supplementation on Lipid Peroxidation," *International Journal for Vitamin Nutrition Research* 77(1) (2007): 3–11.

Klipstein-Grobusch, K., J.M. Geleijnse, J.H. Den Breeijen, et al., "Dietary Antioxidants and Risk of Myocardial Infarction in the Elderly: The Rotterdam Study," *American Journal of Clinical Nutrition* 69(2) (February 1999): 261–266.

Klipstein-Grobusch, K., D.E. Grobbee, J.H. Den Breeijen, et al., "Dietary Iron and Risk of Myocardial Infarction in the Rotterdam Study," *American Journal of Epidemiology* 149(5) (1 March 1999): 421–428.

Lemaitre, R.N., D.S. Siscovick, T.E. Raghunathan, et al., "Leisure-Time Physical Activity and the Risk of Primary Cardiac Arrest," *Archives of Internal Medicine* 159 (1999): 686–690.

Muller, J.E., "Circadian Variation and Triggering of Acute Coronary Events," *American Heart Journal* 137(4, Part 2) (April 1999): S1–S8.

O'Keefe, J.H., Jr., J.M. Miles, W.H. Harris, et al., "Improving the Adverse Cardiovascular Prognosis of Type 2 Diabetics," *Mayo Clinic Proceedings* 74(2) (February 1999): 171–180.

Palace, V.P., M.F. Hill, F. Farahmand, et al., "Mobilization of Antioxidant Vitamin Pools and Hemodynamic Function after Myocardial Infarction," *Circulation* 99(1) (5–12 January 1999): 121–126.

Ridker, P.M., J.E. Manson, J.E. Buring, et al., "Homocysteine and Risk of Cardiovascular Disease Among Postmenopausal Women," *Journal of the American Medical Association* 281(19) (19 May 1999): 1817–1821.

Sesso, H.D., J.E. Buring, W.G. Christen, et al., "Vitamin E and C in the Prevention of Cardiovascular Disease in Men: The Physicians' Health Study II Randomized Controlled Trial," *Journal of the American Medical Association* 300(18) (November 2008): 2123–2133.

Tripathi, P., and M.K. Misra, "Therapeutic Role of L-Arginine on Free Radical Scavenging System in Ischemic Heart Diseases," *Indian Journal of Biochemistry and Biophysics* 46(6) (December 2009): 498–502.

Vercellotti, G., "Infectious Agents That Play a Role in Atherosclerosis and Vasculopathies. What Are They? What

Can We Do About Them?" *Canadian Journal of Cardiology* 15 (Supplement B) (April 1999): 13B–15B.

Heat Stress

Squire, D.L., "Heat Illness: Fluid and Electrolyte Issues for Pediatric and Adolescent Athletes," *Pediatric Clinician North America* 37 (1990): 1085–1090.

Hemorrhoids

Perez-Miranda, M., A. Gomez-Cedenilla, T. León-Colombo, et al., "Effect of Fiber Supplements on Internal Bleeding Hemorrhoids," *Hepatogastroenterology* 43(12) (November–December 1996): 1504–1507.

Saggloro, A., et al., "Treatment of Hemorrhoidal Syndrome with Mesoglycan," *Minerva Dietética é Gastroenterlogica* 31 (1985): 311–315.

Wadworth, A.N., and D. Faulds, "Hydroxyethylrutosides: A Review of Its Pharmacology and Therapeutic Efficacy to Venous Insufficiency and Related Disorders," *Drugs* 44 (1992): 1013–1032.

Hepatitis

Bannasch, P., N.I. Khoshkhou, H.J. Hacker, et al., "Synergistic Hepatocarcinogenic Effect of Hepadnaviral Infection and Dietary Aflatoxic B1 in Woodchucks," *Cancer Research* 55(15) (August 1995): 3318–3330.

Bayraktar, Y., F. Sglam, A. Temizer, et al., "The Effect of Interferon and Desferrioxamine on Serum Ferritin and Hepatic Iron Concentrations in Chronic Hepatitis B," *Hepatogastroenterology* 45(240) (November–December 1998): 2322–2327.

Braunwald, J., H. Nonnenmacher, C. Pereira, et al., "Increased Susceptiblity to Mouse Hepatitis Virus Type 3 (MHV3) Infection Induced by a Hypercholsterolaemic Diet with Increased Adsorption of MHV3 to Primary Hepatocyte Cultures," *Reserches virologiques* 142(1) (January–February 1991): 5–15.

Liu, J., E. Manheimer, K. Tsutani, et al., "Medicinal Herbs for Hepatitis C Virus Infection: A Cochrane Hepatobiliary Systematic Review of Randomized Trials," *American Journal of Gastroenterology* 98(3) (March 2003): 538–544.

Melhem, A., M. Stern, O. Shibolet, et al., "Treatment of Chronic Hepatitis C Virus Infection via Antioxidants: Results of a Phase I Clinical Trial," *Journal of Clinical Gastroenterology* 39(8) (September 2005): 737–742.

Murata, A., "Viricidal Activity of Vitamin C. Vitamin C for Prevention and Treatment of Viral Disease," in T. Hasegawa, ed., *Proceedings of the First Intersectional Congress of the International Associated Microbiological Societies* 3 (Tokyo: Tokyo University Press, 1975), pp. 432–442.

Nakaya, Y., K. Okita, K. Suzuki, et al., "BCAA-Enriched Snack Improves Nutritional State of Cirrhosis," *Nutrition* 23(2) (February 2007): 113-120.

Pramooisinsap, C., N. Promvanit, S. Komindr, et al., "Serum Trace Metals in Chronic Viral Hepatitis and Hepatocellular Carcinoma in Thailand," *Journal of Gastroenterology* 29(5) (October 1994): 610–615.

Sumida, Y., K. Kanemasa, K. Fukumoto, et al., "Effects of Dietary Iron Reduction Versus Phlebotomy in Patients with Chronic Hepatitis C: Results from a Randomized, Controlled Trial on 40 Japanese Patients," *Internal Medicine* 46(10) (2007): 637–642.

Torres, M., F. Rodríguez-Serrano, D.J. Rosario, et al., "Does *Silybum marianum* Play a Role in the Treatment of Chronic Hepatitis?" *Puerto Rico Health Sciences Journal* 23(2 supp) (June 2004): 69–74.

Wang, X., "Treatment of 100 Cases of Viral Hepatitis with Compound 370," *Shanghai Journal of Traditional Chinese Medicine* 4:5, cited in *Medicinal Mushrooms: An Exploration of Tradition, Healing, and Culture*, 2d. ed., ed. Christopher Hobbs and Michael Miovic (Botanica Press: Santa Cruz, CA, 1995), p. 241.

Yip, A.Y., W.T. Loo, and L.W. Chow, "*Fructus schisandrae (Wuweizi)* Containing Compound in Modulating Human Lymphatic System—A Phase I Minimization Clinical Trial," *Biomedicine and Pharmacotherapy* 61(9) (October 2007): 588–590.

Hepatitis: ABCs

Feinman, S.V., J.P. Kim, M.A. Blajchman, et al., "Post-Transfusion Hepatitis G (PTH-G)," *Hepatology* 24 (1996): 415A.

Pilot-Matias, T.J., R.J. Carrick, P.F. Coleman, et al., "Expression of the GB Virus C E2 Glycoprotein Using the Semliki Forest Virus Vector System and Its Utility as a Serologic Marker," *Virology* 225 (1996): 282–292.

Polish, L.B., M. Gallagher, H.A. Fields, et al., "Delta Hepatitis: Molecular Biology and Clinical and Epidemiologic Features," *Clinical Microbiology Review* 6 (1993): 211–219.

Herpesvirus Infection

Kurokawa, M., K. Nagasaka, T. Hirabayashi, et al., "Efficacy of Traditional Herbal Medicines in Combination with Acyclovir Against Herpes Simplex Virus Type 1 Infection in Vitro and in Vivo," *Antiviral Research* 27(1–2) (May 1995): 19–37.

Richards, C.M., C. Shimeld, N.A. Williams, et al., "Induction of Mucosal Immunity Against Herpes Simplex Virus Type 1 in the Mouse Protects Against Ocular

Infection and Establishment of Latency," *Journal of Infectious Disease* 77(6) (June 1998): 451–457.

Robertson, A.L., Jr., Y. Katsura, and R.J. Stein, "Viral Genomes and Arterial Disease," *Annals of the New York Academy of Sciences* 748 (17 January 1995): 57–73.

Tangri, K.K., P.K. Seth, S.S. Parmar, and K.P. Bhargava, "Biochemical Study of Anti-Inflammatory and Anti-Arthritic Properties of Glycyrrhetic Acid," *Biochemical Pharmacology* 14(8) (August 1965): 1277–1281.

High Blood Pressure (Hypertension)

Al-Solaiman, Y., A. Jesri, W.K. Mountford, et al., "DASH Lowers Blood Pressure in Obese Hypertensives Beyond Potassium, Magnesium, and Fibre," *Journal of Human Hypertension* 24(4) (April 2010): 237–246.

Belcaro, G., M.R. Cesarone, A. Ricci, et al., "Control of Edema in Hypertensive Subjects Treated with Calcium Antagonist (Nifedipine) or Angiotensin-Converting Enzyme Inhibitors with Pycnogenol," *Clinical and Applied Thrombosis/Hemastasis* 12(4) (October 2006): 440–444.

Clerous, J., R.D. Feldman, and R.J. Petrella, "Lifestyle Modifications to Prevent and Control Hypertension. 4. Recommendations on Physical Exercise Training. Canadian Hypertension Society, Canadian Coalition for High Blood Pressure Prevention and Control, Laboratory Centre for Disease Control at Health Canada, Heart and Stroke Foundation of Canada," *Canadian Medical Association Journal* 160(9) (Supplement) (4 May 1999): S21–S28.

Graudal, N.A., A.M. Galloe, and P. Garred, "The Effect of Reduced Sodium Intake on Blood Pressure, Body Weight, Renin, Aldosterone, Catecholamines, Cholesterol and Triglyercides: A Meta-Analysis," *Ugeskrift für Læger* [*Weekly Journal for Physicians*] 161(17) (26 April 1999): 2526–2530.

Kuroda, S., T. Uzu, T. Fujii, et al., "Role of Insulin Resistance in the Genesis of Sodium Sensitivity in Essential Hypertension," *Journal of Human Hypertension* 13(4) (April 1999): 257–262.

Margolis, K.L., R.M. Ray, L. Van Horn, et al., "Effect of Calcium and Vitamin D Supplementation on Blood Pressure: The Women's Health Initiative Randomized Trial," *Hypertension* 52(2) (November 2008): 847–855.

Morris, R.C., Jr., A. Sebastian, A. Forman, et al., "Normotensive Salt Sensitivity: Effects of Race and Dietary Potassium," *Hypertension* 33(1) (January 1999): 18–23.

Rinkley, T.E., J.F. Lovato, A.M. Arnold, et al., "Effect of *Gingko biloba* on Blood Pressure and Incidence of Hypertension in Elderly Men and Women," *American Journal of Hypertension* 23(5) (May 2010): 528–533.

Rostand, S.G., "Ultraviolet Light May Contribute to Geographic and Racial Blood Pressure Differences," *Hypertension* 20(2, Part 1) (August 1997): 150–156.

Thierry-Palmer, M., K.S. Carlyle, M.D. Williams, et al., "Plasma 25-Hydroxyvitamin D Concentrations Are Inversely Associated with Blood Pressure of Dahl Salt-Sensitive Rats," *Journal of Steroid Biochemistry and Molecular Biology* 66(4) (August 1998): 255–261.

Thomas, M.K., D.M. Lloyd-Jones, R.I. Thadhani, et al., "Hypovitaminosis D in Medical Inpatients," *The New England Journal of Medicine* 338(12) (19 March 1998): 777–783.

Van Der Schaaf, M.R., H.A. Koomans, and J.A. Joles, "Dietary Sucrose Does Not Increase Twenty-Four-Hour Ambulatory Blood Pressure in Patients with Either Essential Hypertension or Polycystic Kidney Disease," *Journal of Hypertension* 17(3) (March 1999): 453–454.

Walker, A.F., G. Marakis, E. Simpson, et al., "Hypotensive Effects of Hawthorn for Patients with Diabetes Taking Prescription Drugs: A Randomized Controlled Trial," *British Journal of General Practice* 56(527) (June 2006): 437–443.

Wang, C., Y. Li, K. Zhu, Y.M. Dong, et al., "Effects of Supplementation with Multivitamin and Mineral on Blood Pressure and C-Reactive Protein in Obese Chinese Women with Increased Cardiovascular Disease Risk," *Asia Pacific Journal of Clinical Nutrition* 18(1) (2009): 121–130.

Wong, N.D., S. Ming, H.Y. Zhou, et al., "A Comparison of Chinese Traditional and Western Medical Approaches for the Treatment of Mild Hypertension," *Yale Journal of Biology and Medicine* 64(1) (January 1991): 79–87.

Zhang, H.Y., S. Reddy, and T.A. Kotchen, "A High Sucrose, High Linoleic Acid Diet Potentiates Hypertension in the Dahl Salt Sensitive Rat," *American Journal of Hypertension* 12(2, Part 1) (February 1999): 183–187.

High Cholesterol

Arsenio, L., P. Bodria, and G. Magnati, "Effectiveness of Long-Term Treatment with Pantethine in Patients with Dyslipidemias," *Clinical Therapy* 8 (1986): 537–545.

Glueck, C.J., M. Tieger, R. Kunkel, et al., "Hypocholesterolemia and Affective Disorders," *American Journal of the Medical Sciences* 308(4) (October 1994): 218–225.

Gordon, R.Y., T. Cooperman, W. Obermeyer, et al., "Marked Variability of Monacolin Levels in Commercial Red Yeast Rice Products: Buyer Beware!" *Archives of Internal Medicine* 170(19) (2010): 1722–1727.

Guyton, J.R., "Effect of Niacin on Atherosclerotic Cardiovascular Disease," *American Journal of Cardiology*

82(12A) (17 December 1998): 18U–23U; discussion 39U–41U.

Kereveur, A., M. Cambillau, and M. Kazatchkine, "Lipoprotein Anomalies in HIV Infections," *Annales de medicine interne* [*Annals of Internal Medicine*] 147(5) (1996): 333–343.

Muldoon, M.F., S.B. Kritchevsky, R.W. Evans, et al., "Serum Total Antioxidant Activity in Relative Hypo- and Hypercholesterolemia," *Free Radical Research* 25(3) (September 1996): 239–245.

Rahbar, A.R., and I. Nabipour, "The Hypolipidemic Effect of *Citrullus colocynthis* on Patients with Hyperlipidemia," *Pakistan Journal of Biological Sciences* 13(24) (December 2010): 1202–1207.

Tam, W.Y., P. Chook, M. Qiao, et al., "The Efficacy and Tolerability of Adjunctive Alternative Herbal Medicine (*Salvia miltiorrhiza* and *Pueraria lobata*) on Vascular Function and Structure in Coronary Patients," *Journal of Alternative and Complementary Medicine* 15(4) (April 2009): 415–421.

HIV/AIDS

Andrieu, J.M., and W. Lu, "Viro-Immunopathogenesis of HIV Disease: Implications for Therapy," *Immunology Today* 16 (1995): 5–7.

Anukam, K.C., E.O. Osazuwa, H.B. Osadolor, et al., "Yogurt Containing Probiotic *Lactobacillus rhamnosus* GR-1 and L. Reuteri RC-14 Helps Resolve Moderate Diarrhea and Increases CD4 Count in HIV/AIDS Patients," *Journal of Clinical Gastroenterology* 42(3) (March 2008): 239–243.

Arora, P.K., E. Fride, J. Petitio, et al., "Morphine-Induced Immune Alterations in Vivo," *Cellular Immunology* 126 (1990): 343–353.

Austin, J., N. Singhai, R. Voigt, et al., "A Community Randomized Controlled Clinical Trial of Mixed Carotenoids and Micronutrient Supplementation of Patients with Acquired Immunodeficiency Syndrome," *European Journal of Clinical Nutrition* 60(11) (November 2006): 1266–1276.

Clark, R.H., G. Feleke, M. Din, et al., "Nutritional Treatment for Acquired Immunodeficiency Virus-Associated Wasting Using Beta-Hydroxy Beta-Methylbutyrate, Glutamine, Arginine: A Randomized Double-Blind, Placebo-Controlled Study," *Journal of Parenteral and Enteral Nutrition* 24(3) (May–June 2000): 133–139.

Huss, R., "Inhibition of Cyclophilin Function in HIV-1 Infection by Cyclosporin A," *Immunology Today* 17 (1996): 259–260.

Kusum, M., V. Kinbuayaem, M. Bunjob, et al., "Preliminary Efficacy and Safety of Oral Suspension SH,

Combination of Five Chinese Medicinal Herbs, in People Living with HIV/AIDS: The Phase I/II Study," *Journal of the Medical Association of Thailand* 87(9) (September 2004): 1065–1070.

Maiman, M., "Management of Cervical Neoplasia in Human Immunodeficiency Virus-Infected Women," *Journal of the National Cancer Institute Monographs* 23 (January 1998): 43–49.

Munro, S., K.L. Thomas, and M. Abu-Shaar, "Molecular Characterization of Peripheral Receptor for Cannabinoids," *Nature* 365 (1993): 61–65.

Rancinan, C., P. Morlat, G. Chene, et al., "IgE Serum Level: A Prognostic Marker for AIDS in HIV-Infected Adults?" *Journal of Allergy and Clinical Immunology* 102(2) (August 1998): 329–330.

Roederer, M., F.J. Staa, M. Anderson, et al., "Disregulation of Leukocyte Glutathione in AIDS," *Annals of the New York Academy of Sciences* 677 (20 March 1993): 113–125.

Stanley, S.K., M.A. Ostrowski, J.S. Justement, et al., "Effect of Immunization with a Common Recall Antigen on Viral Expression in Patients Infected with HIV1," *The New England Journal of Medicine* 334(19) (9 May 1996): 1222–1230.

Tang, A.M., N.M. Graham, R.D. Semba, et al., "Association Between Serum Vitamin A and E Levels and HIV-1 Disease Progression," *AIDS* 11(5) (April 1997): 613–620.

Zinkernagel, R.M., "MHC-Restricted T-Cell Recognition," *Journal of the American Medical Association* 274 (1995): 1069–1071.

Hives

Atkins, F.M., "The Basis of Immediate Hypersensitivity Reactions to Foods and Nutrition," *Nutrition Reviews* 41 (1983): 229–234.

Birkmayer, J.G.D., and W. Beyer, "Biological and Clinical Relevance of Trace Elements," *Ärztliche Laboratorie* [*Doctor's Laboratory*] 36 (1990): 284–287.

Bjarnason, I., P. Williams, P. Smethusrt, et al., "Effect of Non-Steroidal Anti-Inflammatory Drugs and Prostaglandins on the Permeability of the Human Small Intestine," *Gut* 27 (1986): 1292–1297.

Fuglsang, G., G. Madsen, S. Haiken, et al., "Adverse Reactions to Food Additives in Children with Atopic Symptoms," *Allergy* 49(1) (January 1994): 31–37.

Galant, S.P., J. Bullock, and O.I. Frick, "An Immunological Approach to the Diagnosis of Food Sensitivity," *Clinical Allergy* 3 (1973): 363–372.

Hannuksela, M., "Food Allergy and Skin Disease," *Annals of Allergy* 51 (1983): 269–271.

Juhlin, L., "Additives and Chronic Urticaria," *Annals of Allergy* 59 (1987): 119–123.

Lessof, M.H., "Reactions to Food Additives," *Clinical Experiences in Allergy* 25 (Supplement 1) (1995): 27–28.

Lockey, S.D., "Allergic Reactions to F D and C Yellow No. 5, Tartrazine, an Aniline Dye Used as a Coloring and Identifying Agent in Various Steroids," *Annals of Allergy* 17 (1959): 719–721.

Mageri, M., D. Pisarevskaja, R. Scheufele, et al., "Effects of a Pseudoallergen-Free Diet on Chronic Spontaneous Urticaria: A Prospective Trial," *Allergy* 65(1) (January 2010): 78–83.

Merk, G., and G. Goerz, "Analgetika-Intoleranz," *Zeitschrift für Hautkrankheiten* [*Journal for Skin Diseases*] 58 (1983): 535–554.

Meynadier, J., J.J. Guilhou, J. Meyn-Adier, et al., "Chronic Urticaria," *Annals of Dermatology and Venereology* 106(2) (February 1979): 153–158.

Ormerod, A.D., T.M.S. Reid, and R.A. Main, "Penicillin in Milk—Its Importance in Urticaria," *Clinical Allergy* 17 (1987): 229–234.

Panzani, R.C., D. Schiavino, E. Nucera, et al., "Oral Hyposensitization to Nickel Allergy: Preliminary Clinical Results," *International Archives of Allergy and Immunology* 107(1–3) (May–June 1995): 251–254.

Schwartz, H.J., and T.H. Sher, "Anaphylaxis to Penicillin in a Frozen Dinner," *Annals of Allergy* 52 (1984): 342–343.

Steeipane, R.A., H.P. Constatine, and G.A. Steeipane, "Aspirin Intolerance and Recurrent Urticaria in Adults," *Allergy* 35 (1980): 149–154.

Wicher, K., and R.E. Reisman, "Anaphylactic Reaction to Penicillin in a Soft Drink," *Journal of Allergy and Clinical Immunology* 66 (1980): 155–157.

Winkelmann, R.K., "Food Sensitivity and Urticaria or Vasculitis," in *Food Allergy and Intolerance,* ed. Jonathan Brostoff and Stephen J. Challacombe (Philadelphia, PA: W.W. Saunders, 1987), pp. 602–617.

Wraith, D.G., J. Merrett, A. Roth, et al., "Recognition of Food Allergic Patients and Their Allergens by the RAST Technique and Clinical Investigation," *Clinical Allergy* 9 (1969): 25–36.

Hodgkin's Disease

Campbell, A., and T. Jack, "Acute Reactions to Mega Ascorbic Acid Therapy in Malignant Disease," *Scottish Medical Journal* 24 (1979): 151–153.

Kelemen, L.E., S.S. Wang, U. Lim, et al., "Vegetables- and Antioxidant-Related Nutrients, Genetic Susceptibility, and Non-Hodgkin Lymphoma Risk," *Cancer Causes & Control* 19(5) (June 2008): 491-503.

Tavani, A., A. Pregnolato, E. Negri, et al., "Diet and Risk of Lymphoid Neoplasms and Soft Tissue Sarcomas," *Nutrition and Cancer* 27(3) (March 1990): 256–260.

Ward, M.H., J.R. Cerhan, J.S. Colt, et al., "Risk of Non-Hodgkin Lymphoma and Nitrate and Nitrite from Drinking Water and Diet," *Epidemiology* 17(4) (July 2006): 375–382.

Hyperthyroidism

Hidaka, Y., T. Masai, H. Sumizaki, et al., "Onset of Graves' Thyrotoxicosis after an Attack of Allergic Rhinitis," *Thyroid* 6(4) (August 1996): 349–351.

Isselbacher, K.J., E. Braunwald, J. Wilson, eds., *Harrison's Principles of Internal Medicine,* 13th ed. (New York, NY: McGraw-Hill, 1995), pp. 1952–1953.

Mizokami, T., K. Okamura, T. Kohno, et al., "Human T-Lymphotropic Virus Type I-Associated Uveitis in Patients with Graves' Disease Treated with Methylmercaptoimidazole," *Journal of Clinical Endocrinology and Metabolism* 80(6) (June 1995): 1904–1907.

Venditti, P., T. De Leo, and S. Di Meo, "Vitamin E Administration Attenuates the Tri-Iodothyronine-Induced Modification of Heart Electrical Activity in the Rat," *Journal of Experimental Biology* 200 (Part 5) (March 1997): 909–914.

Yanagawa, T., K. Ito, E.L. Kaplan, et al., "Absence of Association Between Human Spumaretrovirus and Graves' Disease," *Thyroid* 5(5) (October 1995): 379–382.

Hypothyroidism

Diekman, T., P.N. Demacker, J.J. Kastelein, et al., "Increased Oxidizability of Low-Density Lipoproteins in Hypothyroidism," *Journal of Clinical Endocrinology and Metabolism* 83(5) (May 1998): 1752–1755.

Isselbacher, K.J., E. Braunwald, J. Wilson, et al., eds. *Harrison's Principles of Internal Medicine,* 13th ed. (New York, NY: McGraw-Hill, 1995), pp. 1952–1953.

Indigestion, Heartburn

Hebbard, G.S., W.M. Sun, J. Dent, et al., "Hyperglycaemia Affects Proximal Gastric Motor and Sensory Function in Normal Subjects," *European Journal of Gastroenterology and Hepatology* 8(3) (March 1996): 211–217.

Katagiri, F., S. Inoue, Y. Sato, et al., "Comparison of the Effects of *Sho-hange-ka-bukuryo-to* and *Nichin-to* on Human Plasma Adrenocorticotropic Hormone and Cortisol Levels with Continual Stress Exposure," *Biological & Pharmaceutical Bulletin* 27(10) (October 2004): 1679–1682.

Khoury, R.M., L. Camacho-Lobato, P.O. Katz, et al., "Influence of Spontaneous Sleep Positions on Nighttime Recumbent Reflux in Patients with Gastroesophageal Reflux Disease," *American Journal of Gastroenterology* 94 (August 1999): 2069–2073.

Suarez, F.L., J.K. Furne, J. Springfield, et al., "Bismuth Subsalicylate Markedly Decreases Hydrogen Sulfide Release in the Human Colon," *Gastroenterology* 114(5) (May 1998): 923–929.

Yamada, K., G. Yagi, and S. Kanaba, "Effectiveness of *Gorei-san* (TJ-17) for Treatment of SSRI-Induced Nausea and Dyspepsia: Preliminary Observations," *Clinical Neuropharmacology* 26(3) (May–June 2003): 112–114.

Infertility in Men

Cormio, L., M. De Siai, F. Lorusso, et al., "Oral L-Citrulline Supplementation Improves Erectile Hardness in Men with Mild Erectile Dysfunction," *Urology* 77(1) (January 2011): 119–122.

de Andrade, E., A.A. de Mesquita, J.A. Claro, et al., "Study of the Efficacy of Korean Red Ginseng in the Treatment of Erectile Dysfunction," *Asian Journal of Andrology* 9(2) (2007): 241–244.

Hunt, C.D., P.E. Johnson, L.O.L. Herbel, et al., "Effects of Dietary Zinc Depletion on Seminal Volume and Zinc Loss, Serum Testosterone Concentrations, and Sperm Morphology in Young Men," *American Journal of Clinical Nutrition* 56 (1992): 148–157.

Keskes-Ammar, L., N. Feki-Chakroun, T. Rebai, et al., "Sperm Oxidative Stress and the Effect of an Oral Vitamin E and Selenium Supplement on Semen Quality in Infertile Men," *Archive of Andrology* 49(2) (March–April 2003): 83–94.

Lau, B.H., and E.W. Lau, "Kyo-Green Improves Sexual Dysfunction in Men and Women," *Medical Science Monitor* 9(2) (February 2003): P112–118.

Mendiola, J., A.M. Torres-Cantero, J.M. Moreno-Grau, et al., "Food Intake and Its Relationship with Semen Quality: A Case-Control Study," *Fertility and Sterility* 91(3) (March 2009): 812–818.

Netter, A., R. Hartoma, and K. Nahoul, "Effect of Zinc Administration on Plasma Testosterone, Dihydrotestosterone and Sperm Count," *Archives of Andrology* 7 (1981): 69–73.

Raymond-Hamet, H., and R. Goutarel, "Are the Stimulant Effects of *Alchornea floribunda* Mueller Arg. in Men Due to Yohimbine?" *Comptes rendus hebdomadaires des seances de l'Academie des Sciences. Serie D: Sciences naturelles* [*Weekly Reports of Sessions of the Academy of Sciences. Series D: Natural Sciences*] 261(16) (18 October 1965): 3223–3224.

Sanderl, B., and B. Fragher, "Treatment of Oligospermia with Vitamin B$_{12}$," *Infertility* 7 (1984): 133–138.

Scott, B.C., J. Butler, B. Halliwell, et al., "Evaluation of the Antioxidant Actions of Ferulic Acid and Catechins," *Free Radical Research Communications* 19(4) (1993): 241–253.

Vitali, G., R. Parente, and C. Melotti, "Carnitine Supplementation in Human Idiopathic Asthenospermia: Clinical Results," *Drugs in Experimental Clinical Research* 21 (1995): 157–159.

Infertility in Women

Anderson, L., S.E. Lewis, and N. McClure, "The Effects of Coital Lubricants on Sperm Motility in Vitro," *Human Reproduction* 13(12) (December 1998): 3351–3356.

Baird, P.A., "Occupational Exposure to Nitrous Oxide—Not a Laughing Matter," *The New England Journal of Medicine* 327(14) (1 October 1992): 1026–1027.

Murray, J.A., "The Widening Spectrum of Celiac Disease," *American Journal of Clinical Nutrition* 69(3) (March 1999): 354–365.

Palomba, S., A. Falbo, F. Giallauria, et al., "Six Weeks of Structured Exercise Training and Hypocaloric Diet Increases the Probability of Ovulation After Clomiphene Citrate in Overweight and Obese Patients with Polycystic Ovary Syndrome: A Randomized Controlled Trial," *Human Reproduction* 25(11) (November 2010): 2783–2791.

Smith, E.M., M. Hammonds-Ehlers, M.K. Clark, et al., "Occupational Exposures and Risk of Female Infertility," *Journal of Occupational and Environmental Medicine* 39(2) (February 1997): 138–147.

Vujkovic, M., J.H. de Vries, J. Lindemans, et al., "The Preconception Mediterranean Dietary Pattern in Couples Undergoing In Vitro Fertilization/Intracytoplasmic Sperm Injection Treatment Increases the Chance of Pregnancy," *Fertility and Sterility* 94(6) (November 2010): 2096–2101.

Influenza

Byleveld, P.M., G.T. Pang, R.L. Clancy, et al., "Fish Oil Feeding Delays Influenza Virus Clearance and Impairs Production of Interferon-Gamma and Virus-Specific Immunoglobulin A in the Lungs of Mice," *Journal of Nutrition* 129(20) (February 1999): 328–335.

Goldberg, A.S., E.C. Mueller, E. Eigen, et al., "Isolation of the Anti-Inflammatory Principles from *Achillea millefolium* (Compositae)," *Journal of Pharmacological Science* 58 (1969): 938–941.

Gorton, H.C., and K. Jarvis, "The Effectiveness of Vitamin C in Preventing and Relieving the Symptoms of Virus-Induced Respiratory Infections," *Journal of Manipulative and Physiological Therapeutics* 22(8) (October 1999): 530–533.

Hamazaki, K., S. Sawazaki, M. Itomura, et al., "No Effect of a Traditional Chinese Medicine, *Hochu-ekki-to*, on Antibody Titer After Influenza Vaccination in Man: A Randomized, Placebo-Controlled Double-Blind Trial," *Phytomedicine* 14(1) (January 2007): 11–14.

Hennte, T., E. Peterhaus, and R. Stocker, "Alterations in Antioxidants Defences in Lung and Liver of Mice Infected with Influenza A Virus," *Journal of General Virology* 73(Part 1) (January 1992): 39–46.

Kimmel, M., D. Keller, S. Farmer, et al., "A Controlled Clinical Trial to Evaluate the Effect of GanedenBC(30) on Immunological Markers," *Methods and Findings in Experimental and Clinical Pharmacology* 32(2) (March 2010): 129–132.

Miyagawa, K., Y. Hayashi, S. Kurihara, et al., "Co-Administration of L-Cystine and L-Theanine Enhances Efficacy of Influenza Vaccination in Elderly Persons: Nutritional Status-Dependent Immunogenicity," *Geriatrics and Gerontology International* 8(4) (December 2008): 243–250.

Urashima, M., T. Segawa, M. Okazaki, et al., "Randomized Trial of Vitamin D Supplementation to Prevent Seasonal Influenza A in Schoolchildren," *American Journal of Clinical Nutrition* 91(5) (May 2010): 1255–1260.

Insect Bites

"Chinese Herbs and Immunity," *Bulletin of the OHAI* 9(8): 395.

Insomnia

Morris, M., H. Steinberg, E.A. Sykes, et al., "Effects of Temporary Withdrawal from Regular Running," *Journal of Psychosomatic Research* 34(5) (1990): 493–500.

Pigeon, W.R., M. Carr, C. Gorman, et al., "Effects of a Tart Cherry Juice Beverage on the Sleep of Older Adults with Insomnia: A Pilot Study," *Journal of Medicinal Food* 13(3) (June 2010): 579–583.

Intermittent Claudication

Berenbarum, F., M. Revel, C. Deshays, et al., "Lumbo-Radicular Pain Caused by Epidural Lipomatosis in the Obese Patient: Recovery after Hypocaloric Diet," *Revue du rhumatisme et des maladies osteo-articulaires* [*Review of Rheumatism and Bone and Joint Disorders*] 59(3) (March 1992): 225–227.

Ducimetiere, P., J.L. Richard, G. Pequignot, et al., "Varicose Veins: A Risk Factor for Atherosclerotic Dis-

ease in Middle-Aged Men?" *International Journal of Epidemiology* 10(4) (December 1981): 329–335.

Khandanpour, N., M.P. Armon, B. Jennings, et al., "Randomized Clinical Trial of Folate Supplementation in Patients with Peripheral Arterial Disease," *British Journal of Surgery* 96(9) (September 2009): 990–998.

Leng, G.C., D.F. Horrobin, F.G. Fowkes, et al., "Plasma Essential Fatty Acids, Cigarette Smoking and Dietary Antioxidants in Peripheral Arterial Disease: A Population-Based Case-Control Study," *Arteriosclerosis and Thrombosis* 14(3) (March 1994): 471–478.

Machlin, L.J., "Use and Safety of Elevated Dosages of Vitamin E in Adults," *International Journal of Vitamin and Nutrition Research* 30 (supplement) (1989): 56–58.

Sommerfield, T., J. Price, and W.R. Hiatt, "Omega-3 Fatty Acids for Intermittent Claudication," *Cochrane Database of Systematic Reviews* 2007, Issue 4. Art. No. CD003833. DOI: 10.1002/14651858.CD003833.pub3.

Iron Overload

Klipstein-Grobusch, K., D.E. Grobbee, J.H. Den Breeijen, et al., "Dietary Iron and Risk of Myocardial Infarction in the Rotterdam Study," *American Journal of Epidemiology* 149(5) (1 March 1999): 421–428.

Milward, E.A., S.K. Baines, M.W. Knuiman, et al., "Noncitrus Fruits as Novel Dietary Environmental Modifiers of Iron Stores in People with or Without HFE Gene Mutations," *Mayo Clinic Proceedings* 83(5) (May 2008): 543–549.

Irritable Bowel Syndrome

Bittner, A.C., R.M. Croffut, M.C. Stranahan, et al., "Prescript-assist Probiotic-Prebiotic Treatment for Irritable Bowel Syndrome: An Open-Label, Partially Controlled, 1-Year Extension of a Previously Published Controlled Clinical Trial," *Clinical Theraeutics* 29(6) (June 2007): 1153–1160.

Brinkhaus, B., C. Hentschel, C. Von Keudell, et al., "Herbal Medicine with Curcuma and Fumitory in the Treatment of Irritable Bowel Snydrome: A Randomized, Placebo-Controlled, Double-Blind Clinical Trial," *Scandanavian Journal of Gastroenterology* 40(8) (August 2005): 936–943.

Dolin, B.J., "Effects of a Proprietary *Bacillus coagulans* Preparation on Symptoms of Diarrhea-Predominant Irritable Bowel Syndrome," *Methods and Findings in Experimental and Clinical Pharmacology* 31(10) (December 2009): 655–659.

Evans, P.R., C. Piesse, Y.T. Bak, et al., "Fructose-Sorbitol Malabsorption and Symptom Provocation in Irritable Bowel Syndrome: Relationship to Enteric Hypersensitivity and Dysmotility," *Scandinavian Journal of Gastroenterology* 33(11) (November 1998): 1158–1163.

King, T.S., M. Elia, and J.O. Hunter, "Abnormal Colonic Fermentation in Irritable Bowel Syndrome," *Lancet* 352(9135) (10 October 1998): 1187–1189.

Leung, W.K., J.C. Wu, S.M. Liang, et al., "Treatment of Diarrhea-Predominant Irritable Bowel Syndrome with Traditional Chinese Herbal Medicine: A Randomized Placebo-Controlled Trial," *American Journal of Gastroenterology* 101(7) (July 2006): 1574–1580.

Kidney Cancer (Renal Cell Carcinoma)

Aune, D., E. De Stefani, A. Ronco, et al., "Legume Intake and the Risk of Cancer: A Multisite Case-Control Study in Uruguay," *Cancer Causes & Control* 20(9) (November 2009): 1605–1615.

De Stefani, E., L. Fierro, P. Correa, et al., "Maté Drinking and Risk of Lung Cancer in Males: A Case-Control Study from Uruguay," *Cancer Epidemiological Biomarkers Preview* 5(7) (July 1996): 515–519.

Frampton, R., S.A. Omond, and J.A. Eisman, "Inhibition of Human Cancer Cell Growth by 1,25-Dihydroxyvitamin D3 Metabolites," *Cancer Research* 43 (1983): 4443–4447.

Galeone, C., C. Pelucchi, L.D. Maso, et al., "Glycemic Index, Glycemic Load and Renal Cell Carcinoma Risk," *Annals of Oncology* 20(11) (November 2009): 1881–1885.

Garland, C.F., F.C. Garland, and E.D. Gorham, "Can Colon Cancer Incidence and Death Rates Be Reduced with Calcium and Vitamin D?" *American Journal of Clinical Nutrition* 54 (1991): 193S–201S.

Lindblad, P., A. Wolk, R. Bergstrom, et al., "Diet and Risk of Renal Cell Cancer: A Population-Based Case-Control Study," *Cancer Epidemiology, Biomarkers, and Prevention* 6(4) (April 1997): 215–223.

Lissoni, P., V. Arosio, E. Mocchegiani, et al., "Zinc Levels in Serum During Subcutaneous Interleukin-2 Immunotherapy of Cancer," *International Journal of Biomarkers* 10(2) (April–June 1995): 124–125.

Lissoni, P., S. Barni, C. Archili, et al., "Endocrine Effects of A 24-Hour Intravenous Infusion of Interleukin-2 in the Immunotherapy of Cancer," *Anticancer Research* 10(3) (May–June 1990): 753–757.

Liu, J.Z., S.G. Chen, B. Zhang, et al., "Effect of *Haishengsu* as an Adjunct Therapy for Patients with Advanced Renal Cell Cancer: A Randomized and Placebo-Controlled Clinical Trial," *Journal of Alternative and Complementary Medicine* 15(10) (October 2009): 1127–1130.

Mellemgaard, A., J.K. McLaughlin, K. Overvad, et al., "Dietary Risk Factors for Renal Cell Carcinoma in Denmark," *European Journal of Cancer* 32A (4) (April 1996): 673–682.

Ravaud, A., and M. Debled, "Present Achievements in the Medical Treatment of Metastatic Renal Cell Carcinoma," *Critical Reviews of Oncology and Hematology* 31(1) (June 1999): 77–87.

Taper, H.S., C. Lemort, and M.B. Roberfroid, "Inhibition Effect of Dietary Inulin and Oligofructose on the Growth of Transplantable Mouse Tumor," *Anticancer Research* 18(6A) (November–December 1998): 4123–4126.

Wolk, A., G. Gridley, S. Niwa, et al., "International Renal Cell Cancer Study. VII. Role of Diet," *International Journal of Cancer* 65(1) (January 1996): 67–73.

Yu, M.C., T.M. Mack, R. Hanisch, et al., "Cigarette Smoking, Obesity, Diuretic Use, and Coffee Consumption as Risk Factors for Renal Cell Carcinoma," *Journal of the National Cancer Institute* 77(2) (August 1986): 351–356.

Kidney Disease

Malyszko, J.S., J. Malyszko, D. Pawlak, et al., "Hemostasis, Platelet Functions, Serotonin and Serum Lipids During Omega-3 Fatty Acid Treatment in Patients with Glomerulonephritis," *Nephron* 80(1) (September 1998): 94–96.

Nakamoto, H., T. Mimura, and N. Honda, "Orally Administered *Juzen-taiho-to*/TJ-48 Ameliorates Erythropoietin (rHuEPO)-Resistant Anemia in Patients on Hemodialysis," *Hemodialysis* (Supplement 9) (October 2008): S9–S14.

Pollock, C.A., L.S. Ibels, F.Y. Zhu, et al., "Protein Intake in Renal Disease," *Journal of the American Society for Nephrology* 8(5) (May 1997): 777–783.

Rahn, K., "Renal Function in Treated and Untreated Hypertension," *Journal of Human Hypertension* 12(9) (September 1998): 599–601.

Trachtman, H., J.C. Chan, W. Chan, et al., "Vitamin E Ameliorates Renal Injury in an Experimental Model of Immunoglobulin A Nephropathy," *Pediatrics Research* 40(4) (October 1996): 620–626.

Yagi, M., S. Kato, T. Nishitoba, et al., "Effects of Chitosan-Coated Dialdehyde Cellulose, a Newly Developed Oral Adsorbent, on Glomerulonephritis Induced by Anti-Thy-1 Antibody in Rats," *Nephron* 78(4) (1998): 433–439.

Kidney Stones

Conte, A., P. Piza, and A. Garcia-Raja, "Urinary Lithogen Risk Test: Usefulness in the Evaluation of Renal

Lithiasis Treatment Using Crystallization Inhibitors (Citrate and Phytate)," *Archivos Españas de Urología* [*Spanish Archives of Urology*] 52(1) (January–February 1999): 94–99.

Garg, A., A. Bonanome, S.M. Grundy, et al., "Effects of Dietary Carbohydrates on Metabolism of Calcium and Other Minerals in Normal Subjects and Patients with Noninsulin-Dependent Diabetes Mellitus," *Journal of Clinical Endocrinology and Metabolism* 70(4) (April 1997): 1007–1013.

Heller, H.J., M.F. Doerner, L.J. Brinkley, et al., "Effect of Dietary Calcium on Stone Forming Propensity," *Journal of Urology* 169(2) (February 2003): 470–477.

Huang, Kee C., and Kee Chang, eds., *The Pharmacology of Chinese Herbs* (Boca Raton, FL: CRC Press, 1992), p. 293.

Hughes, J., and R.W. Norman, "Diet and Calcium Stones," *Canadian Medical Association Journal* 146(2) (15 January 1992): 137–143.

Hunt, C.D., J.L. Herbel, and F.H. Nielsen, "Metabolic Responses of Postmenopausal Women to Supplemental Dietary Boron and Aluminum During Usual and Low Magnesium Intake: Boron, Calcium, and Magnesium Absorption and Retention and Blood Mineral Concentrations," *American Journal of Clinical Nutrition* 65(3) (March 1997): 803–813.

Kleiner, S.M., "Water: An Essential But Overlooked Nutrient," *Journal of the American Dietetic Association* 99(2) (February 1999): 200–206.

Massey, L.K., M. Liebman, and S.A. Kynast-Gales, "Ascorbate Increases Human Oxaluria and Kidney Stone Risk," *Journal of Nutrition* 135(7) (July 2005): 1673–1677.

Mussa, G.C., and M. Martini-Mauri, "Infections of the Urinary Tract in the Pediatric Age: Pathogenesis," *Minerva Pediatrica* 25(38) (3 November 1973): 1681–1716.

Shaw, P., "Idiopathic Hypercalciuria: Its Control with Unprocessed Bran," *British Journal of Urology* 52 (1980): 426–429.

Singh, P.P., R. Kiran, A.K. Pendse, et al., "Ascorbic Acid Is an Abettor in Calcium Urolithiasis: An Experimental Study," *Scanning Microscopy* 7(3) (September 1993): 1041–1047; discussion 1047–1048.

Laryngitis

Damste, P.H., "Voice Changes in Adult Women Caused by Virilizing Agents," *Journal of Speech and Hearing Disorders* 32 (1967): 126.

Gupta, O.P., P.L. Bhatia, and M.K. Agarwalk, "Nasal, Pharyngeal, and Laryngeal Manifestations of Hypothyroidism," *Ear, Nose, and Throat Journal* 56(9) (1977): 10.

Jackson-Menaldi, C.A., A.I. Dzul, et al., "Allergies and Vocal Fold Edema: A Preliminary Report," *Journal of Voice* 13(1) (March 1999): 113–122.

Wallner, L.J., B.J. Hill, and W. Waldrop, "Voice Change Following Adenotonsillectomy," *Laryngosocope* 78 (1968): 1410.

Wendler, J., "Zyklusabhangige Leistungsschwankungen der Stimme und Ihre Beeinflussung Durch Ovulationshemmer," *Folia Phoniatrica* 24 (1972): 259.

Leukemia

Abe, T., "Infantile Leukemia and Soybeans—a Hypothesis," *Leukemia* 13(3) (March 1999): 317–320.

Amir, H., M. Karas, J. Giat, et al., "Lycopene and 1,25-Dihydroxyvitamin D3 Cooperate in the Inhibition of Cell Cycle Progression and Induction of Differentiation in HL-60 Leukemic Cells," *Nutrition and Cancer* 33(1) (1999): 105–112.

Bargetzi, M.J., A. Schonenberger, A. Tichelli, et al., "Celiac Disease Transmitted by Allogeneic Non-T Cell-Depleted Bone Marrow Transplantation," *Bone Marrow Transplantation* 20(7) (October 1997): 607–609.

Campbell, M.J., M.T. Drayson, J. Durham, et al., "Metabolism of 1alpha,25(OH)2D3 and Its 30-epi Analog Integrates Clonal Expansion, Maturation and Apoptosis During HL-60 Cell Differentiation," *Molecular and Cellular Endocrinology* 149(1–2) (25 March 1999): 169–183.

Conney, A.H., Y.R. Lou, J.G. Xie, et al., "Some Perspectives on Dietary Inhibition of Carcinogenesis: Studies with Curcumin and Tea," *Proceedings of the Society for Experimental Biology and Medicine* 216(2) (November 1997): 234–245.

Humer, Richard P., and Jack Challem, *The Natural Health Guide to Beating the Supergerms* (New York, NY: Pocket Books, 1997), p. 248.

Mego, M., R. Koncekova, E. Mikuskova, et al., "Prevention of Febrile Neutropenia in Cancer Patients by Probiotic Strain *Enterococcus faecium* M-74. Phase II Study," *Supportive Care in Cancer* 14(3) (March 2000): 285–290.

Smith, S.J., L.M. Green, M.E. Hayes, et al., "Prostaglandin E2 Regulates Vitamin D Receptor Expression, Vitamin D-24 Hydroxylase Activity and Cell Proliferation in an Adherent Myeloid Leukemia Cell Line (Ad-HL60)," *Prostaglandins and Other Lipid Mediators* 57(2–3) (May 1999): 73–85.

"Smoking Tied to Leukemia Risk," *New York Times*, 23 February 1993.

Yamada, H., "Chemical Characterization and Biological Activity of the Immunologically Active Substances in

Juzen-taiho-to," *Gan to Kagaku Ryoho* [*Japanese Journal of Cancer and Chemotherapy*] 16(4, Part 2–2) (April 1989): 1500–1505.

Liver Cancer

Dashwood, R., T. Negishi, H. Hayatsu, et al., "Chemopreventive Properties of Chlorophylls Towards Aflatoxin B1: A Review of the Antimutagenicity and Anticarcinogenicity Data in Rainbow Trout," *Mutation Research* 399(2) (20 March 1998): 245–253.

Dehmlow, C., J. Erhard, and H. De Groot, "Inhibition of Kupffer Cell Functions as an Explanation for the Hepatoprotective Properties of Silibinin," *Hepatology* 23(4) (April 1996): 749–754.

Griffini, P., O. Fehres, L. Klieverik, et al., "Dietary Omega-3 Polyunsaturated Fatty Acids Promote Colon Carcinoma Metastasis in Rat Liver," *Cancer Research* 58(15) (1 August 1998): 3312–3319.

Ishak, K.G., "Hepatic Neoplasia Associated with Contraceptive and Anabolic Steroids," *Recent Results in Cancer Research* 66 (1979): 73–128.

Lasky, T., and I. Magder, "Hepatocellular Carcinoma P53 G.T. Transversions at Codon 249: The Fingerprint of Aflatoxin Exposure?" *Environmental Health Perspective* 105(4) (April 1997): 392–397.

Mabed, M., L. El-Helw, and S. Shamaa, "Phase II Study of Viscum Fraxini-2 in Patients with Advanced Hepatocellular Carcinoma," *British Journal of Cancer* 90(1) (January 2004): 65–69.

Millis, R.M., C.A. Diya, M.E. Reynolds, et al., "Growth Inhibition of Subcutaneously Transplanted Hepatomas without Cachexia by Alteration of the Dietary Arginine-Methionine Balance," *Nutrition and Cancer* 31(1) (1998): 49–55.

Okuno, M., T. Tanaka, C. Komaki, et al., "Suppressive Effect of Low Amounts of Safflower and Periolla Oils on Diethylnitrosamine-Induced Hepatocarcinogenesis in Male F344 Rats," *Nutrition and Cancer* 30(3) (1998): 186–193.

Taper, H.S., C. Lemort, and M.B. Roberfroid, "Inhibition Effect of Dietary Inulin and Oligofructose on the Growth of Transplantable Mouse Tumor," *Anticancer Research* 18(6A) (November–December 1998): 4123–4126.

Theis, K., "Liver Cancer Marker," *Clinician Reviews* 8(1) (1998): 89.

Yu, M.W., H.H. Hsieh, W.H. Pan, et al., "Vegetable Consumption, Serum Retinol Level, and Risk of Hepatocellular Carcinoma," *Cancer Research* 55(6) (March 1995): 1301–1305.

Yu, S.Y., Y.J. Zhu, and W.J. Li, "Protective Role of Selenium Against Hepatitis B Virus and Primary Liver Cancer in Qidong," *Biological Trace Element Research* 56(1) (January 1997): 117–124.

Zheng, C., G. Feng, and H. Liang, "*Bletilla striata* as a Vascular Embolizing Agent in Interventional Treatment of Primary Hepatic Carcinoma," *Chinese Medical Journal* (Engl) 111(12) (December 1998): 1060–1063.

Lung Cancer

Albanes, D., "Beta-Carotene and Lung Cancer: A Case Study," *American Journal of Clinical Nutrition* 69(6) (June 1999): 1345S–1350S.

Baker, D.L., E.S. Krol, N. Jacobsen, et al., "Reactions of Beta-Carotene with Cigarette Smoke Oxidants. Identification of Carotenoid Oxidation Products and Evaluation of the Prooxidant/Antioxidant Effect," *Chemical Research in Toxicology* 12(6) (June 1999): 535–543.

Begin, M.E., "Selective Killing of Human Cancer Cells by Polyunsaturated Fatty Acids," *Prostaglandins and Leukotrienes in Medicine* 30 (1985): 37–49.

Blumberg, J., and G. Block, "The Alpha-Tocopherol, Beta-Carotene Cancer Prevention Study in Finland," *Nutrition Review* 52(7) (July 1994): 242–245.

Cerchietti, L.C., A.H. Navigente, and M.A. Castro, "Effects of Eicosapentaenoic and Docosahexaenoic n-3 Fatty Acids From Fish Oil and Preferential Cox-2 Inhibition on Systemic Syndromes in Patients with Advanced Lung Cancer," *Nutrition and Cancer* 59(1) (2007): 14–20.

Fujimura, M., K. Kasahara, H. Shirasaki, et al., "Up-Regulation of ICH-1L Protein by Thromboxane A2 Antagonists Enhances Cisplatin-Induced Apoptosis in Non-Small-Cell Lung-Cancer Cell Lines," *Journal of Cancer Research and Clinical Oncology* 125(7) (July 1999): 389–394.

Garcia-Closas, R., A. Agudo, C.A. Gonzalez, et al., "Intake of Specific Carotenoids and Flavonoids and the Risk of Lung Cancer in Women in Barcelona, Spain," *Nutrition and Cancer* 32(3) (1998): 154–158.

Guzey, M., C. Sattler, and H.F. DeLuca, "Combinational Effects of Vitamin D_3 and Retinoic Acid (All Trans and 9 Cis) on Proliferation, Differentiation, and Programmed Cell Death in Two Small Cell Lung Carcinoma Cell Lines," *Biochemical and Biophysical Research Communications* 249(3) (28 August 1998): 735–744.

Isselbacher, K.J., E. Braunwald, J. Wilson, et al., eds., *Harrison's Principles of Internal Medicine,* 13th ed. (New York, NY: McGraw-Hill, 1995), p. 1221.

Jatoi, A., B.D. Daly, G. Kramer, et al., "A Cross-Sectional Study of Vitamin Intake in Postoperative Non-Small

Cell Lung Cancer Patients," *Journal of Surgical Oncology* 68(4) (August 1998): 231–236.

Knekt, P., R. Jarvinene, R. Seppanen, et al., "Dietary Flavonoids and the Risk of Lung Cancer and Other Malignant Neoplasms," *American Journal of Epidemiology* 146(3) (1 August 1997): 223–230.

Knekt, P., J. Marniemi, L. Teppol, et al., "Is Low Selenium Status a Risk Factor for Lung Cancer?" *American Journal of Epidemiology* 148(10) (15 November 1998): 975–982.

Lee, B.W., J.C. Wain, K.T. Kelsey, et al., "Association Between Diet and Lung Cancer Location," *American Journal of Respiratory Critical Care Medicine* 158(4) (October 1998): 1197–1203.

Mendilharsu, M., E. De Stefani, H. Deneo-Pellegrini, et al., "Consumption of Tea and Coffee and the Risk of Lung Cancer in Cigarette-Smoking Men: A Case-Control Study in Uruguay," *Lung Cancer* 19(2) (February 1998): 101–107.

Nyberg, F., V. Agrenius, K. Svartengren, et al., "Dietary Factors and Risk of Lung Cancer in Never-Smokers," *International Journal of Cancer* 78(40) (9 November 1998): 430–436.

Reid, M.E., A.J. Duffield-Lillico, E. Slate, et al., "The Nutritional Prevention of Cancer: 400 mcg Per Day Selenium Treatment," *Nutrition and Cancer* 60(2) (2008): 155–163.

Sinha, R., M. Kulldorff, J. Curtin, et al., "Fried, Well-Done Red Meat and Risk of Lung Cancer in Women (United States)," *Cancer Causes and Control* 9(6) (December 1998): 621–630.

van der Meij, B.S., J.A. Langius, E.F. Smit, et al., "Oral Nutritional Supplements Containing (n-3) Polyunsaturated Fatty Acids Affect the Nutritional Status of Patients with Stage III Non-Small Cell Lung Cancer During Multimodality Treatment," *Journal of Nutrition* 140(10) (October 2010): 1774–1780.

Van Rensburg, C.E., G. Joone, and R. Anderson, "Alpha-Tocopherol Antagonizes the Multidrug-Reistance-Reversal Activity of Cyclosporin A, Verapamil, FG120918, Clofazimine and B69," *Cancer Letters* 127[1–2] (May 1998): 107–112.

Zheng, G.Q., P.M. Kenney, J. Zhang, et al., "Inhibition of Benzo-[a]pyrene-Induced Tumorigenesis by Myristicin, a Volatile Aroma Constituent of Parsley Leaf Oil," *Carcinogenesis* 13(10) (October 1992): 1921–1923.

Lupus

Clark, W.F., C. Kortas, A.P. Heidenheim, et al., "Flaxseed in Lupus Nephritis: A Two-Year Nonplacebo-Controlled Crossover Study," *Journal of the American College of Nutrition* 20(2) (supplement) (April 2001): 143–148.

Comstock, G.W., A.E. Burke, S.C. Hoffman, et al., "Serum Concentrations of Alpha Tocopherol, Beta Carotene, and Retinol Preceding the Diagnosis of Rheumatoid Arthritis and Systemic Lupus Erythematosus," *Annals of Rheumatological Disease* 56(5) (May 1997): 323–325.

Kipen, Y., E.M. Briganti, B.J. Strauss, et al., "Three-Year Follow-Up of Body Composition Changes in Pre-Menopausal Women with Systemic Lupus Erythematosus," *Rheumatology* (Oxford) 38(1) (January 1999): 59–65.

Lappé, Marc, *Evolutionary Medicine: Rethinking the Origins of Disease* (San Francisco, CA: Sierra Club Books, 1994), pp. 141–147.

Serban, M.G., E. Balanescu, and V. Nita, "Lipid Peroxidase and Erythrocyte Redox System in Systemic Vasculitides Treated with Corticoids: Effect of Vitamin E Administration," *Romanian Journal of Internal Medicine* 32(4) (October–December 1994): 283–289.

Tam, L.S., E.K. Li, V.Y. Leung, et al., "Effects of Vitamin C and E on Oxidative Stress Markers and Endothelial Function in Patients with Systemic Lupus Erythematosus: A Double Blind, Placebo Controlled Pilot Study," *Journal of Rheumatology* 32(2) (February 2005): 275–282.

Wright, S.A., F.M. O'Prey, M.T. McHenry, et al., "A Randomized Interventional Trial of Omega-3-Polyunsaturated Fatty Acids on Endothelial Function and Disease Activity in Systemic Lupus Erythematosus," *Annals of Rheumatic Diseases* 67(6) (June 2008): 841–848.

Lyme Disease

Cantorna, M.T., and C.E. Hayes, "Vitamin A Deficiency Exacerbates Murine Lyme Arthritis," *Journal of Infectious Disease* 174(4) (October 1996): 747–751.

Cantorna, M.T., C.E. Hayes, and H.F. DeLuca, "1,25-Dihydroxycholecalciferol Inhibits the Progression of Arthritis in Murine Models of Human Arthritis," *Journal of Nutrition* 128(1) (January 1998): 68–72.

Fokina, G.I., V.M. Roikhel, M.P. Frolova, et al., "The Antiviral Action of Medicinal Plant Extracts in Experimental Tick-Borne Encephalitis," *Voprosy Virusologii* [*Questions in Virology*] 38(4) (July–August 1993): 170–173.

Lymphedema

Casley-Smith, J.R., "Treatment of Lymphedema by Complex Physical Therapy, with and without Oral and Topical Benzopyrones: What Should Therapists and Patients Expect?" *Lymphology* 29(2) (June 1996): 76–82.

Korpan, M.I., and V. Fialka, "Wobenzym and Diuretic Therapy in Lymphedema after Breast Surgery," *Wiener Medizinischer Wochenschrift* [*Vienna Medicine Weekly*] 146(4) (1996): 67–72, 74.

Loprinzi, C.L., J.W. Kugler, J.A. Soan, et al., "Lack of Effect of Coumarin in Women with Lymphedema after Treatment for Breast Cancer," *The New England Journal of Medicine* 340(5) (4 February 1999): 346–350.

Shaw, C., P. Mortimer, and P.A. Judd, "Randomized Controlled Trial Comparing a Low-Fat Diet with a Weight-Reduction Diet in Breast Cancer–Related Lymphedema," *Cancer* 109(10) (May 2007): 1949–1956.

Shaw, C., P. Mortimer, and P.A. Judd, "A Randomized Controlled Trial of Weight Reduction as a Treatment for Breast Cancer–Related Lymphedema," *Cancer* 110(8) (October 2007): 1868–1874.

Soria, P., A. Cuesta, H. Romero, et al., "Dietary Treatment of Lymphedema by Restriction of Long-Chain Triglycerides," *Angiology* 45(8) (August 1994): 703–707.

Swirsky, Joan, and Diane Sackett Nannery, *Coping with Lymphedema* (Garden City Park, NY: Avery Publishing Group, 1998), p. 22.

Yasuhara, H., H. Shigematsu, and T. Muto, "A Study of the Advantages of Elastic Stockings for Leg Lymphedema," *International Angiology* 15(3) (September 1996): 272–277.

Macular Degeneration

Christen, W.G., U.A. Ajani, R.J. Glynn, et al., "Prospective Cohort Study of Antioxidant Vitamin Supplement Use and the Risk of Age-Related Maculopathy," *American Journal of Epidemiology* 149(5) (1 March 1999): 476–484.

Darzins, P., P. Mitchell, and R.G. Heller, "Sun Exposure and Age-Related Macular Degeneration. An Australian Case-Control Study," *Ophthalmology* 104(5) (May 1997): 770–776.

Hammond, B.R., Jr., E.J. Johnson, R.M. Russell, et al., "Dietary Modification of Human Macular Pigment Density," *Investigations in Ophthalmologic and Visual Science* 38(9) (August 1997): 1795–1801.

Johnson, E.J., H.Y. Chung, S.M. Caldarella, et al., "The Influence of Supplemental Lutein and Docosahexaenoic Acid on Serum, Lipoproteins, and Macular Pigmentation," *American Journal of Clinical Nutrition* 87(5) (May 2008): 1521–1529.

Mitchell, P., W. Smith, and J.J. Wang, "Iris Color, Skin Sun Sensitivity, and Age-Related Maculopathy: The Blue Mountains Eye Study," *Ophthalmology* 195(8) (August 1998): 1359–1363.

Miyamoto, H., Y. Ogura, and Y. Honda, "Hyperbaric Oxygen Treatment for Macular Edema After Retinal Vein Occlusion—Fluorescein Angiographic Findings and Visual Prognosis," *Nippon Ganka Gakkai Zasshi* [*Japanese Journal of Ophthalmology*] 99(2) (February 1995): 220–225.

Querques, G., P. Benlian, B. Chanu, et al., "Nutritional AMD Treatment Phase I (NAT-1): Feasibility of Oral DHA Supplementation in Age-Related Macular Degeneration," *European Journal of Ophthalmology* 19(1) (January–February 2009): 100–106.

Snodderly, D.M., "Evidence for Protection Against Age-Related Macular Degeneration by Carotenoids and Antioxidant Vitamins," *American Journal of Clinical Nutrition* 62(6) (Supplement) (December 1995): 1448S–1461S.

Sommerburg, O., J.E. Keunen, A.C. Brid, et al., "Fruits and Vegetables That Are Sources for Lutein and Zeaxanthin: The Macular Pigment in Human Eyes," *British Journal of Ophthalmology* 82(8) (August 1998): 907–910.

Tobe, T., K. Takahashi, H. Ohkuma, et al., "The Effect of Interferon-Beta on Experimental Choroidal Neovascularization," *Nippon Ganka Gakkai Zasshi* [*Japanese Journal of Ophthalmology*] 99(5) (May 1995): 571–581.

Young, R.W., "Pathophysiology of Age-Related Macular Degeneration," *Survey of Ophthalmology* 31 (1987): 291–306.

Mastitis

Bodley, V., and D. Powers, "Long-Term Treatment of a Breastfeeding Mother with Fluconazole-Resolved Nipple Pain Caused by Yeast: A Case Study," *Journal of Human Lactation* 13(4) (December 1997): 307–311.

Hunfeld, K.P., and R. Bassler, "Lymphocytic Mastitis and Fibrosis of the Breast in Long-standing Insulin-Dependent Diabetics: A Histopathologic Study on Diabetic Mastopathy and Report of Ten Cases," *General Diagnosis and Pathology* 143(1) (July 1997): 49–58.

Takeuchi, S., K. Ishiguro, M. Ikegami, et al., "Production of Toxic Shock Syndrome Toxin by Staphylococcus Aureus Isolated from Mastitic Cow's Milk and Farm Bulk Milk," *Veterinary Microbiology* 59(4) (January 1998): 251–258.

Measles

Alm, J.S., J. Swartz, G. Lilja, et al., "Atopy in Children of Families with an Anthroposophic Lifestyle," *Lancet* 353(9163) (1 May 1999): 1485–1488.

Burney, P.G.J., S. Chinn, and R.J. Rona, "Has the Prevalence of Asthma Increased in Children? Evidence from the National Study of Health and Growth, 1973–1986," *British Medical Journal* 300 (1990): 1306–1310.

Christensen, M., T. Ronne, and A.H. Christiansen, "MMR-Vaccination of Children Allergic to Eggs," *Ugeskrift Læger* [*Weekly Journal for Physicians*] 161(9) (1 March 1999): 1270–1272.

Christian, P., and K.P. West, Jr., "Interactions Between Zinc and Vitamin A: An Update," *American Journal of Clinical Nutrition* 68 (1998): 435S–441S.

Paunio, M., H. Peltola, M. Valle, et al., "Explosive School-Based Measles Outbreak: Intense Exposure May Have Resulted in High Risk, Even Among Revaccinees," *American Journal of Epidemiology* 148(11) (1 December 1998): 1103–1110.

Shaheen, S.O., P. Aaby, A.J. Hall, et al., "Measles and Atopy in Guinea-Bisseau," *Lancet* 347 (1996): 1792–1796.

Solon, F.S., B.M. Popkin, T.L. Fernandez, et al., "Vitamin A Deficiency in the Philippines: A Study of Xerophthalmia in Cebu," *American Journal of Clinical Nutrition* 31(2) (February 1978): 360–368.

Usonis,V., V. Bakasenas, A. Kaufhold, et al., "Reactogenicity and Immunogenicity of a New Live Attenuated Combined Measles, Mumps and Rubella Vaccine in Healthy Children," *Pediatric Infectious Disease Journal* 18(1) (January 1999): 42–48.

Melanoma

Abdallah, R.M., J.R. Starkey, and G.G. Meadows, "Dietary Restriction of Tyrosine and Phenylalanine: Inhibition of Metastasis of Three Rodent Tumors," *Journal of the National Cancer Institute* 78(4) (April 1987): 759–769.

Ainsleigh, H.G., "Beneficial Effects of Sun Exposure on Cancer Mortality," *Preventive Medicine* 22(1) (January 1993): 132–140.

Braun, M.M., and M.A. Tucker, "A Role for Photoproducts of Vitamin D in the Etiology of Cutaneous Melanoma?" *Medical Hypotheses* 48(4) (April 1997): 351–354.

Danielsson, C., K. Fehsel, P. Polly, et al., "Differential Apoptotic Response of Human Melanoma Cells to 1 Alpha, 25-Dihydroxyvitamin D3 and Its Analogues," *Cell Death and Differentiation* 5(11) (November 1998): 946–952.

Danielsson, C., H. Torma, A. Vahlquist, et al., "Positive and Negative Interaction of 1,25-Dihydroxyvitamin D3 and the Retinoid CD437 in the Induction of Human Melanoma Cell Apoptosis," *International Journal of Cancer* 81(3) (5 May 1999): 467–470.

Reich, R., L. Royce, and G.R. Martin, "Eicosapentaenoic Acid Reduces the Invasive and Metastatic Activities of Malignant Tumor Cells," *Biochemical Biophysical Research Communications* 160(2) (28 April 1989): 559–564.

Rose, M.L., J. Madren, H. Bunzendahl, et al., "Dietary Glycine Inhibits the Growth of B16 Melanoma Tumors in Mice," *Carcinogenesis* 20(5) (May 1999): 793–798.

Veierod, M.B., D.S. Thelle, and P. Laake, "Diet and Risk of Cutaneous Malignant Melanoma: A Prospective Study

of 50,757 Norwegian Men and Women," *Internal Journal of Cancer* 71(4) (May 1997): 600–604.

Yan, L., J.A. Yee, D. Li, et al., "Dietary Supplementation of Selenomethionine Reduces Metastasis of Melanoma Cells in Mice," *Anticancer Research* 12(2A) (March–April 1999): 1337–1342.

Memory Problems

Bernstein, G.A., M.E. Carroll, N.W. Dean, et al., "Caffeine Withdrawal in Normal School-Age Children," *Journal of the American Academy of Child and Adolescent Psychiatry* 37(8) (August 1998): 858–865.

Deijen, J.B., C.J. Wientjes, H.F. Vullinghs, et al., "Tyrosine Improves Cognitive Performance and Reduces Blood Pressure in Cadets after One Week of a Combat Training Course," *Brain Research Bulletin* 48(2) (15 January 1999): 203–209.

Dodge, H.H., T. Zitzelberger, B.S. Oken, et al., "A Randomized Placebo-Controlled Trial of *Gingko biloba* for the Prevention of Cognitive Decline," *Neurology* 70 (19) (2008): 1809–1817.

Easton, C.J., and L.O. Bauer, "Beneficial Effects of Thiamine on Recognition Memory and P300 in Abstinent Cocaine-Dependent Patients," *Psychiatry Research* 70(3) (30 May 1997): 165–174.

Grealy, M.A., D.A. Johnson, and S.K. Rushton, "Improving Cognitive Function after Brain Injury: The Use of Exercise and Virtual Reality," *Archives of Physical Medicine and Rehabilitation* 80(6) (June 1999): 661–667.

Kalmijn, S., E.J. Feskens, L.J. Launer, et al., "Polyunsaturated Fatty Acids, Antioxidants, and Cognitive Function in Very Old Men," *American Journal of Epidemiology* 145(1) (1 January 1997): 33–41.

Kenealy, P.M., "Mood-State-Dependent Retrieval: The Effects of Induced Mood on Memory Reconsidered," *Quarterly Journal of Experimental Psychology* 50(2) (May 1997): 290–317.

Kennedy, D.O., C.F. Haskell, B. Robertson, et al., "Improved Cognitive Performance and Mental Fatigue Following a Multi-Vitamin and Mineral Supplement with Added Guaraná (*Paullinia cupana*)," *Appetite* 50(2–3) (March–May 2008): 506–513.

Ng, T.P., P.C. Chiam, T. Lee, et al., "Curry Consumption and Cognitive Function in the Elderly," *American Journal of Epidemiology* 164(9) (July 2006): 898–906.

Nielsen, F.H., "The Justification for Providing Dietary Guidance for the Nutritional Intake of Boron," *Biological Trace Element Research* 66(1–3) (Winter 1998): 319–330.

Perkins, A.J., H.C. Hendrie, C.M. Callahan, et al., "Association of Antioxidants with Memory in a Multiethnic Elderly Sample Using the Third National Health and

Nutrition Examination Survey," *American Journal of Epidemiology* 150(1) (1 July 1999): 37–44.

Perrig, W.J., P. Perrig, and H.B. Sthaelin, "The Relation Between Antioxidants and Memory Performance in the Old and Very Old," *Journal of the American Geriatric Society* 45(6) (June 1997): 718–724.

Solfrizzi, V., F. Panza, F. Torres, et al., "High Monounsaturated Fatty Acids Intake Protects Against Age-Related Cognitive Decline," *Neurology* 52(8) (12 May 1999): 1563–1569.

Verger, P., D. Lagarde, D. Batejat, et al., "Influence of the Composition of a Meal Taken after Physical Exercise on Mood, Vigilance, Performance," *Physiology of Behavior* 64(3) (1 June 1998): 317–322.

Westrick, E.R., A.P. Shapiro, P.E. Nathan, et al., "Dietary Tryptophan Reverses Alcohol-Induced Impairment of Facial Recognition But Not Verbal Recall," *Alcoholism in Clinical and Experimental Research* 12(4) (August 1988): 531–533.

Ménière's Disease

Brookler, K.H., and M.B. Glenn, "Ménière's Syndrome: An Approach to Therapy," *Ear, Nose, and Throat Journal* 74(8) (August 1995): 534–538, 540, 542.

Hanner, P., H. Rask-Andersen, S. Lange, et al., "Antisecretory Factor-Inducing Therapy Improves the Clinical Outcome in Patients with Ménière's Disease," *Acta Otolaryngologica* 130(2) (February 2010): 223–227.

López-Gónzales, M.A., J.M. Guerrero, B. Sánchez, et al., "Melatonin Induces Hyporeactivity Caused by Type II Collagen in Peripheral Blood Lymphocytes from Patients with Autoimmune Hearing Losses," *Neuroscience Letters* 239(1) (December 1997): 1–4.

Mangabeira Albernaz, P.L., and Y. Fukuda, "Glucose, Insulin, and Inner Ear Pathology," *Acta Otolaryngolica* (Stockholm) 97(5–6) (May–June 1984): 496–501.

Rosingh, H.J., H.P. Wit, and F.W. Albers, "Perilymphatic Pressure Dynamics Following Posture Change in Patients with Ménière's Disease and in Normal Hearing Subjects," *Acta Otolaryngolica* (Stockholm) 118(1) (January 1998): 1–5.

Silverstein, H., J.E. Isaacson, M.J. Olds, et al., "Dexamethasone Inner Ear Perfusion for the Treatment of Ménière's Disease: A Prospective, Randomized, Double-Blind, Crossover Trial," *American Journal of Otology* 19(2) (March 1998): 196–201.

Menopause-Related Problems

Ishihara, M., Y. Ito, T. Nakakita, et al., "Clinical Effect of Gamma-Oryzanol on Climacteric Disturbance and Serum Lipid Peroxides," *Nippon Sanka Fujinka Gakkai Zasshi* 34(20) (February 1982): 243–251.

Qian, L.Q., B. Wang, J.Y. Niu, et al., "Assessment of the Clinical Effect of Chinese Medicine Therapy Combined with Psychological Intervention for Treatment of Patients of Peri-Menopausal Syndrome Complicated by Hyperlipidemia," *Chinese Journal of Integrative Medicine* 16(2) (April 2010): 124–130.

Qu, F., X. Cai, Y. Gu, et al., "Chinese Medicinal Herbs in Relieving Perimenopausal Depression: A Randomized, Controlled Trial," *Journal of Alternative and Complementary Medicine* 15(1) (January 2009): 93–100.

Reed, S.D., K.M. Newton, A.Z. LaCroix, et al., "Vaginal, Endometrial, and Reproductive Hormone Findings: Randomized, Placebo-Controlled Trial of Black Cohosh, Multibotanical Herbs, and Dietary Soy for Vasomotor Symptoms: The Herbal Alternatives For Menopause (HALT) Study," *Menopause* 15(1) (January–February 2008): 51–58.

van Die, M.D., K.M. Bone, H.G. Burger, et al., "Effects of a Combination of *Hypericum perforatum* and *Vitex agnus-castus* on PMS-like Symptoms in Late-Perimenopausal Women: Findings from a Subpopulation Analysis," *Journal of Alternative and Complementary Medicine* 15(9) (September 2009): 1045–1048.

Menstrual Problems

Abdul-Razzak, K.K., N.M. Ayoub, A.A. Abu-Taleb, et al., "Influence of Dietary Intake of Dairy Products on Dysmenorrhea," *Journal of Obstetrics and Gynaecology Research* 36(2) (April 2010): 377–383.

Harel, Z., F.M. Biro, R.K. Kottenhahn, et al., "Supplementation with Omega-3 Polyunsaturated Fatty Acids in the Management of Dysmenorrhea in Adolescents," *American Journal of Obstetrics and Gynecology* 174(4) (April 1996): 1335–1338.

Kopp-Woodroffe, S.A., M.M. Manore, C.A. Dueck, et al., "Energy and Nutrient Status of Amenorrheic Athletes Participating in a Diet and Exercise Training Intervention Program," *International Journal of Sport Nutrition* 9(1) (March 1999): 70–88.

Migraine

Baischer, W., "Psychological Aspects as Predicting Factors for the Indication of Acupuncture in Migraine Patients," *Wienerischer Klinischer Wochenschrift* 105(7) (1993): 200–203.

Diener, H.C., V. Pfaffenrath, J. Schnitker, et al., "Efficacy and Safety of 6.25 mg t.i.d. Feverfew CO2-Extract (MIG-99) in Migraine Prevention—A Randomized, Double-Blind, Multicentre, Placebo-Controlled Study," *Cephalalgia* 25(11) (November 2005): 1031–1041.

Facchinetti, F., G. Sances, P. Borella, et al., "Magnesium Prophylaxis of Menstrual Migraine: Effects on Intracellular Magnesium," *Headache* 31 (1991): 298–301.

Harel, Z., G. Gascon, S. Riggs, et al., "Supplementation with Omega-3 Polyunsaturated Fatty Acids in the Management of Recurrent Migraines in Adolescents," *Journal of Adolescent Health* 31(2) (August 2002): 154–161.

Hershey, A.D., S.W. Powers, A.L. Vockell, et al., "Coenzyme Q_{10} Deficiency and Response to Supplementation in Pediatric and Adolescent Migraine," *Headache* 47(1) (January 2007): 73–80.

Launso, L., E. Brendstrup, and S. Arnberg, "An Exploratory Study of Reflexological Treatment for Headache," *Alternative Therapies in Health and Medicine* 5(3) (May 1999): 57–65.

Leíra, R., and R. Rodríguez, "Diet and Migraine," *Revista Neurolgica* 24(129) (May 1996): 534–538.

MacGregor, E.A., and J. Guillebaud, "Combined Oral Contraceptives, Migraine and Ischaemic Stroke," *British Journal of Family Planning* 24(2) (July 1998): 55–60.

Marcus, D.A., L. Scharff, D. Turk, et al., "A Double-Blind Provocative Study of Chocolate as a Trigger of Headache," *Cephalagia* 17(8) (December 1997): 855–862.

Molaie, M., "Serotonin Syndrome Presenting with Migrainelike Stroke," *Headache* 37(8) (September 1997): 519–521.

Nelson-Piercy, C., and M. De Swiet, "Diagnosis and Management of Migraine. Low Dose Aspirin May Be Used for Prophylaxis," *British Medical Journal* 313(7058) (14 September 1996): 691–692.

Ostergaard, J.R., and M. Kraft, "Benign Coital Headache," *Cephalalgia,* 12(6) (December 1992): 353–355.

Parker, G.B., H. Tupling, and D.S. Pryor, "A Controlled Trial of Cervical Manipulation of Migraine," *Australia and New Zealand Journal of Medicine* 8(6) (December 1978): 589–593.

Pittler, M.H., and E. Ernst, "Feverfew for Preventing Migraine," *Cochrane Database of Systematic Reviews* 2004, Issue 1. Art. No.: CD002286. DOI: 10.1002/14651858.CD002286.pub2.

Sartory, G., B. Müller, J. Metsch, et al., "A Comparison of Psychological and Pharmacological Treatment of Pediatric Migraine," *Behavior Research and Therapy* 36(12) (December 1998): 1155–1170.

Schoenen, J., J. Jacquy, and M. Lenaerts, "Effectiveness of High-Dose Riboflavin in Migraine Prophylaxis: A Randomized Trial," *Neurology* 50(2) (February 1998): 466–470.

Schwartz, C.E., "A Surfeit of Serotonin: Sumatriptan and Serotonergic Antidepressants," *Archives of Internal Medicine* 1141 (24 May 1999): 159.

Mononucleosis

Enger, S.M., R.K. Ross, B. Henderson, et al., "Breastfeeding History, Pregnancy Experience and Risk of Breast Cancer," *British Journal of Cancer* 76(1) (1997): 118–123.

Morning Sickness

Rickinson, A., "The Role of Herpesviruses in Immune Deficiency-Associated Lymphomas," *Acquired Immune Deficiency Syndromes and Human Retrovirology* (14)4 (1997): A15.

Seto, A., T. Einarson, and G. Koren, "Pregnancy Outcome Following First Trimester Exposure to Antihistamines: Meta-Analysis," *American Journal of Perinatology* 14(3) (March 1997): 119–124.

van Stuijvenberg, M.E., I. Schabort, D. Labadarios, et al., "The Nutritional Status and Treatment of Patients with Hyperemesis Gravidarum," *American Journal of Ostetrics and Gynecology* 172(5) (May 1995): 1585–1591.

Motion Sickness

Howarth, P.A., and M. Finch, "The Nauseogenicity of Two Methods of Navigating within a Virtual Environment," *Applied Ergonomics* 30(1) (February 1999): 39–45.

Kolansinski, E.M., and R.D. Gilson, "Ataxia Following Exposure to a Virtual Environment," *Aviation, Space, and Environmental Medicine* 70 (3, Part 3) (March 1999): 264–269.

Murray, J.B., "Psychophysiological Aspects of Motion Sickness," *Perceptual and Motor Skills* 85(3, Part 2) (December 1997): 1163–1167.

Sharma, K., et al., "Prevalence and Correlates of Susceptibility to Motion Sickness," *Acta Geneticae Medicae et Gemellologie* (Rome) 46(2) (1997): 105–121.

Multiple Sclerosis

Cullen, C.F., and R.L. Swank, "Intravascular Aggregation and Adhesiveness of the Blood Elements Associated with Alimentary Lipemia and Injection of Large Molecular Substances: Effect on Blood-Brain Barrier," *Circulation* 9 (1954): 335–346.

Haeren, A.F., W.W. Tourtellotte, K.A. Richard, et al., "A Study of the Blood Cerebrospinal Fluid-Brain Barrier in Multiple Sclerosis," *Neurology* 14 (1964): 345–351.

Hayes, C.E., M.T. Cantorna, and H.F. DeLuca, "Vitamin D and Multiple Sclerosis," *Proceedings of the Society for Experimental Biology and Medicine* 216(1) (October 1997): 21–27.

Santiago, E., L.A. Perez-Mediavilla, and N. Lopez-Moratalla,

"The Role of Nitric Oxide in the Pathogenesis of Multiple Sclerosis," *Journal of Physiological Biochemistry* 54(4) (December 1998): 229–237.

Swank, R.L., and A. Grimsgaard, "Multiple Sclerosis: The Lipid Relationship," *American Journal of Clinical Nutrition* 48 (1988): 1387–3193.

Mumps

Alm, J.S., J. Swartz, G. Lilja, et al., "Atopy in Children of Families with an Anthroposophic Lifestyle," *Lancet* 353(9163) (1 May 1999): 1485–1488.

Christensen, M., T. Ronne, and A.H. Christiansen, "MMR-Vaccination of Children Allergic to Eggs," *Ugeskrift for Læger* [*Weekly Journal for Physicians*] 161(9) (1 March 1999): 1270–1272.

Isselbacher, K.J., E. Braunwald, J. Wilson, et al., eds., *Harrison's Principles of Internal Medicine*, 13th ed. (New York, NY: McGraw-Hill, 1995), p. 830.

Ruther, U., S. Stilz, E. Rohl, et al., "Successful Interferon-Alpha 2: A Therapy for a Patient with Acute Mumps Orchitis," *European Urologist* 27(2) (1995): 174–176.

Usonis, V., V. Bakasenas, A. Kaufhold, et al., "Reactogenicity and Immunogenicity of a New Live Attenuated Combined Measles, Mumps and Rubella Vaccine in Healthy Children," *Pediatric Infectious Disease Journal* 18(1) (January 1999): 42–48.

Muscles, Sore

Eston, R., and D. Peters, "Effects of Cold Water Immersion on the Symptoms of Exercise-Induced Muscle Damage," *Journal of Sports Science* 17(3) (March 1999): 231–238.

Slauterbeck, J., C. Clevenger, W. Lundberg, et al., "Estrogen Level Alters the Failure Load of the Rabbit Anterior Cruciate Ligament," *Journal of Orthopedic Research* 17(3) (May 1999): 405–408.

Myasthenia Gravis

Dong, S.T., V.T. Nguyen, et al., "Acupuncture Anesthesia in Thymectomy on Myasthenia Gravis Patients," *Acupuncture and Electrotherapy Research* 13(1) (1988): 25–30.

Kaeser, H.E., "Drug-Induced Myasthenic Syndromes," *Acta Neurological Scandinavica* 100 (Supplement) (1984): 39–47.

Liang, H., Y. Zhang, and B. Geng, "The Effect of Astragalus Polysaccharides (APS) on Cell Mediated Immunity (CMI) in Burned Mice," *Chung-Hua Cheng Hsing Shao Shang Wai Ko Tsa Chih* 10(2) (March 1994): 138–141.

Tu, L.H., D.R. Huang, R.Q. Zhang, et al., "Regulatory Action of Astragalus Saponins and Buzhong Yiqi Compound on Synthesis of Nicotinic Acetylcholine Receptor Antibody in Vitro for Myasthenia Gravis," *Chinese Medical Journal* 107(4) (April 1994): 300–303.

Nails, Infected

Buck, D.S., D.M. Nidorf, and J.G. Addino, "Comparison of Two Topical Preparations for the Treatment of Onychomycosis: *Melaleuca alternifolia* (Tea Tree) Oil and Clotrimazole," *Journal of Family Practice* 38(6) (June 1994): 601–605.

Gupta, A.K., R.G. Sibbald, C.W. Lynde, et al., "Onychomycosis in Children: Prevalence and Treatment Strategies," *Journal of the American Academy of Dermatology* 36 (1997): 395.

Kemna, M.E., and E.E. Elewski, "A U.S. Epidemiologic Survey of Superficial Fungal Diseases," *Journal of the American Academy of Dermatology* 35 (1996): 359.

Williams, H.C., R. Buffham, and A. Du Vivier, "Successful Use of Topical Vitamin E Solution in the Treatment of Nail Changes in Yellow Nail Syndrome," *Archives of Dermatology* 127 (1991): 1023–1028.

Nausea

Murray, Michael T., *Encyclopedia of Nutritional Supplements* (Rocklin, CA: Prima Press, 1998), p. 203.

Osteoarthritis

Berger, R., and H. Nowak, "A New Medical Approach to the Treatment of Osteoarthritis: Report of an Open Phase IV Study with Ademethionine (Gumbaral)," *American Journal of Medicine* 83(5a) (20 November 1987): 8408.

Dingle, J.T., "Cartilage Maintenance in Osteoarthritis: Interaction of Cytokines, NSAIDs, and Prostaglandins in Articular Cartilage Damage and Repair," *Journal of Rheumatology* 28 (Supplement) (March 1991): 30–37.

Fassbender, H., "Role of Chondrocyte in the Development of Osteroarthritis," *American Journal of Medicine* 83(5a) (20 November 1987): 17–24.

Hurley, M.V., "The Role of Muscle Weakness in the Pathogenesis of Osteoarthritis," *Rheumatological Disease Clinician in North America* 25(2) (May 1999): 283–298.

Jacquet, A., P.O. Girodet, and A. Pariente, "Phytalgic, a Food Supplement, vs. Placebo in Patients with Osteoarthritis of the Knee or Hip: A Randomised Double-Blind Placebo-Controlled Clinical Trial," *Arthritis Research & Therapy* 11(6) (2009): R192.

Kerrigan, D.C., M.K. Todd, and P.O. Riley, "Knee Osteoarthritis and High-Heeled Shoes," *Lancet* 351(9113) (9 May 1998): 1399–1401.

Kim, L.S., L.J. Axelrod, P. Howard, et al., "Efficacy of Methylsulfonylmethane (MSM) in Osteoarthritis Pain of the Knee: A Pilot Clinical Trial," *Osteoarthritis and Cartilage* 14(3) (March 2006): 286–294.

Leffler, C.T., A.F. Philippi, S.G. Leffler, et al., "Glucosamine, Chondroitin, and Manganese Ascorbate for Degenerative Joint Disease of the Knee or Low Back: A Randomized, Double-Blind, Placebo-Controlled Pilot Study," *Military Medicine* 164(2) (February 1999): 85–91.

Lopes, V.A., "Double-Blind Clinical Evaluation of the Relative Efficacy of Ibuprofen and Glucosamine Sulphate in the Management of Osteoarthrosis of the Knee in Out-Patients," *Current Medical Research and Opinion* 8(3) (1982): 145–149.

Manicourt, D.H., A. Druetz-Van Egeren, L. Haazen, et al., "Effects of Tenoxicam and Aspirin on the Metabolism of Proteglycans and Hyaluronan in Normal and Osteoarthritic Human Articular Cartilage," *British Journal of Pharmacology* 113(4) (December 1994): 1113–1120.

McAlindon, T.E., D.T. Felson, Y. Zhang, et al., "Relation of Dietary Intake and Serum Levels of Vitamin D to Progression of Osteoarthritis of the Knee Among Participants in the Framingham Study," *Annals of Internal Medicine* 125(5) (1 September 1996): 353–359.

Roberts, N.B., J.D. Holding, H.P. Walsh, et al., "Serial Changes in Serum Vitamin K1, Triglyceride, Cholesterol, Osteocalcin and 25-Hydroxyvitamin D3 in Patients after Hip Replacement for Fractured Neck of Femur or Osteoarthritis," *European Journal of Clinical Investigation* 26(1) (January 1996): 24–29.

Sawitzke, A.D., H. Shi, M.F. Finco, et al., "The Effect of Glucosamine and/or Chondroitin Sulfate on the Progression of Knee Osteoarthritis: A Report from the Glucosamine/Chondroitin Arthritis Intervention Trial," *Arthritis and Rheumatism* 58(10) (October 2008).

Summers, M.N., W.E. Haley, J.D. Reveille, et al., "Radiographic Assessment and Psychologic Variables as Predictors of Pain and Functional Impairment in Osteoarthritis of the Knee or Hip," *Arthritis and Rheumatology* 31(2) (February 1988): 204–209.

Toda, Y., T. Today, S. Takemura, et al., "Change in Body Fat, But Not Body Weight or Metabolic Correlates of Obesity, Is Related to Symptomatic Relief of Obese Patients with Knee Osteoarthritis after a Weight Control Program," *Journal of Rheumatology* 25(11) (November 1998): 2181–2186.

Van Baar, M.E., J. Dekker, R.A. Ootsendorp, et al., "The Effectiveness of Exercise Therapy in Patients with Osteoarthritis of the Hip or Knee: A Randomized Clinical Trial," *Journal of Rheumatology* 25(12) (December 1998): 2432–2349.

Wluka, A.E., S. Stuckey, C. Brand, et al., "Supplementary

Vitamin E Does Not Affect the Loss of Cartilage Volume in Knee Osteoarthritis: A 2 year Double Blind Randomized Placebo Controlled Study," *Journal of Rheumatology* 29(12) (December 2002): 2585–2591.

Osteoporosis

Cao, J.J., L.K. Johnson, and J.R. Hunt, "A Diet High in Meat Protein and Potential Renal Acid Load Increase Fractional Calcium Absorption and Urinary Calcium Excretion, Without Effecting Markers of Bone Resorption or Formation in Postmenopausal Women," *Journal of Nutrition* 141(3) (March 2011): 391–397.

Feskanich, D., P. Weber, W.C. Willett, et al., "Vitamin K Intake and Hip Fractures in Women: A Prospective Study," *American Journal of Clinical Nutrition* 69(1) (January 1999): 74–79.

Gambacciani, M., M. Ciaponi, B. Cappaglis, et al., "Effects of Combined Low Dose of the Isoflavone Derivative Ipriflavone and Estrogen Replacement on Bone Mineral Density and Metabolism in Postmenopausal Women," *Maturitas* 28(1) (September 1997): 75–81.

Henderson, N.K., C.P. White, and J.A. Eisman, "The Roles of Exercise and Fall Risk Reduction in the Prevention of Osteoporosis," *Endocrinology and Metabolism Clinician in North America* 27(21) (June 1998): 369–387.

Li, Z., H. Karp, A. Zerlin, et al., "Absorption of Silicon from Artesian Aquifer Water and Its Impact on Bone Health in Postmenopausal Women: A 12 Week Pilot Study," *Nutrition Journal* 9 (October 2010): 44.

Melhus, H., K. Michaelsson, A. Kindmark, et al., "Excessive Dietary Intake of Vitamin A Is Associated with Reduced Bone Mineral Density and Increased Risk for Hip Fracture," *Annals of Internal Medicine* 129(10) (15 November 1998): 770–778.

Moschonis, G., I. Kasaroli, and G.P. Lyritis, "The Effects of a 30-Month Dietary Intervention on Bone Mineral Density: The Postmenopausal Health Study," *British Journal of Nutrition* 104(1) (July 2010): 100–107.

Munger, R.G., J.R. Cerhan, and B.C. Chiu, "Prospective Study of Dietary Protein Intake and Risk of Hip Fracture in Postmenopausal Women," *American Journal of Clinical Nutrition* 69(1) (January 1999): 147–152.

Murkies, A.L., G. Wilcox, and S.R. Davis, "Clinical Review 92: Phytoestrogens," *Journal of Clinical Endocrinology and Metabolism* 83(2) (February 1998): 297–303.

Shedd-Wise, K.M., D.L. Alekel, H. Hofmann, et al., "The Soy Isoflavones for Reducing Bone Loss Study: 3-year Effects on pQCT Bone Mineral Density and Strength Measures in Postmenopausal Women," *Journal of Clinical Densitometry* 14(1) (January–March 2011): 47–57.

Silverman, N.E., B.J. Nicklas, and A.S. Ryan, "Addition of Aerobic Exercise to a Weight Loss Program Increases BMD, with an Associated Reduction in Inflammation in Overweight Postmenopausal Women," *Calcified Tissue International* 84(4) (April 2009): 257–265.

Thomas, M.K., D.M. Lloyd-Jones, R.I. Thadhani, et al., "Hypovitaminosis D in Medical Inpatients," *The New England Journal of Medicine* 338(12) (19 March 1998): 777–783.

Ovarian Cancer

Gersshenson, D.M., M.F. Mitchell, N. Atkinson, et al., "The Effect of Prolonged Cisplatin-Based Chemotherapy on Progression-Free Survival in Patients with Optimal Epithelial Ovarian Cancer: 'Maintenance' Therapy Reconsidered," *Gynecologic Oncology* 47(1) (1992): 7–13.

Helzlhouser, K.J., A.J. Alberg, E.P. Norkus, et al., "Prospective Study of Serum Micronutrients and Ovarian Cancer," *Journal of the National Cancer Institute* 88(1) (3 January 1996): 32–37.

Isselbacher, K.J., E. Braunwald, J. Wilson, et al., eds., *Harrison's Principles of Internal Medicine*, 13th ed. (New York, NY: McGraw-Hill, 1995), pp. 1853–1854.

Kushi, L.H., P.J. Mink, A.R. Folsom, et al., "Prospective Study of Diet and Ovarian Cancer," *American Journal of Epidemiology* 149(1) (1 January 1999): 21–31.

La Vecchia, C., E. Negri, S. Franceschi, et al., "Alcohol and Epithelial Ovarian Cancer," *Journal of Clinical Epidemiology* 45(9) (September 1992): 1025–1030.

McGuire, W.P., W.J. Hoskins, M.F. Brady, et al., "Cyclophosphamide and Cisplatin Compared with Paclitaxel and Cisplatin in Patients with Stage II and Stage IV Ovarian Cancer," *The New England Journal of Medicine* 334(1) (1996): 1–6.

Pan, S.Y., A.M. Ugnat, Y. Mao, et al., "A Case-Control Study of Diet and the Risk of Ovarian Cancer," *Cancer Epidemiology, Biomarkers and Prevention* 13(9) (September 2004): 1521–1527.

Risch, H.A., M. Jain, L.D. Marrett, et al., "Dietary Fat Intake and Risk of Epithelial Ovarian Cancer," *Journal of the National Cancer Institute* 86(18) (21 September 1994): 1409–1415.

Rossi, M., E. Negri, P. Lagiou, et al., "Flavonoids and Ovarian Cancer Risk: A Case-Control Study in Italy," *International Journal of Cancer* 123(4) (August 2008): 895–898.

Shen, F., and G. Weber, "Synergistic Action of Quercetin and Genistein in Human Ovarian Carcinoma Cells," *Oncology Research* 9(11–12) (1997): 597–602.

Sieja, K., "Selenium Deficiency in Women with Ovarian Cancer Undergoing Chemotherapy and the Influence of Supplementation with This Supplement on Biochemical Parameters," *Pharmazie* 53(7) (July 1998): 473–476.

Tessitore, L., M. Chara, E. Sesca, et al., "Fasting During Promotion, But Not During Initiation, Enhances the Growth of Methylnitrosourea-Induced Mammary Tumors," *Carcinogensis* 18(8) (August 1997): 1679–1681.

Ovarian Cyst

Huber-Buchholz, M.M., D.G. Carey, and R.J. Norman, "Restoration of Reproductive Potential by Lifestyle Modification in Obese Polycystic Ovary Syndrome: Role of Insulin Sensitivity and Luteinizing Hormone," *Journal of Clinical Endocrinology and Metabolism* 84(4) (April 1999): 1470–1474.

Hudson, T., and A. Lewin, "Naturopathic Specific Condition Review: Ovarian Cysts," *Protocol Journal of Botanical Medicine* 1(4) (Spring 1996): 32.

Mohammed, H.O., M.E. White, C.L. Guard, et al., "A Case-Controlled Study of the Association Between Blood Selenium and Cystic Ovaries in Lactating Dairy Cattle," *Journal of Dairy Science* 74(7) (July 1999): 2180–2185.

Tarquini, R., V. Bruni, F. Perfetto, et al., "Hypermelatoninemia in Women with Polycystic Ovarian Syndrome," *European Journal of Contraception and Reproductive Health Care* 1(4) (December 1996): 349–350.

Overweight

Blackburn, G.L., "Benefits of Weight Loss in the Treatment of Obesity," *American Journal of Clinical Nutrition* 69(3) (March 1999): 347–349.

Foster, G.D., T.A. Wadden, R.M. Swain, et al., "Changes in Resting Energy Expenditure After Weight Loss in Obese African American and White Women," *American Journal of Clinical Nutrition* 69(1) (January 1999): 13–17.

Gilbert, J.A., D.R. Joanisse, J.P. Chaput, et al., "Milk Supplementation Facilitates Appetite Control in Obese Women During Weight Loss: A Randomised, Single-Blind, Placebo-Controlled Trial," *British Journal of Nutrition* 105(1) (January 2011): 133–143.

Rogers, P.J., and J.E. Blundell, "Separating the Actions of Sweetness and Calories: Effects of Saccharin and Carbohydrates on Hunger and Food Intake on Human Subjects," *Physiology and Behavior* 45 (1989): 1093–1099.

Rogers, P.J., P. Keedwell, and J.E. Blundell, "Further Analysis of the Short-Term Inhibition of Food Intake in Humans by the Dipeptide L-Aspartyl-L-Phenylalanine Methyl Ester (Aspartame)," *Physiology and Behavior* 49 (1991): 739–743.

Rolls, B.J., E.A. Bell, V.H. Castellanos, et al., "Energy Density But Not Fat Content of Foods Affected Energy Intake in Lean and Obese Women," *American Journal of Clinical Nutrition* 69(5) (May 1999): 863–871.

Rolls, B.J., P.A. Pirraglia, M.B. Jones, et al., "Effects of Olestra, a Noncaloric Fat Substitute, on Daily Energy and Fat Intakes in Lean Men," *American Journal of Clinical Nutrition* 56 (1992): 84–92.

Soenen, S., G. Plasqui, A.J. Smeets, et al., "Protein Intake Induced an Increase in Exercise Stimulated Fat Oxidation During Stable Body Weight," *Physiology and Behavior* 101(5) (December 2010): 770–774.

Wyatt, H.R., G.K. Grunwald, H.M. Seagle, et al., "Resting Energy Expenditure in Reduced-Obese Subjects in the National Weight Control Registry," *American Journal of Clinical Nutrition* 69(6) (June 1999): 1189–1193.

Pain, Chronic

Lee, S.W., M.L. Liong, K.H. Yuen, et al., "Acupuncture Versus Sham Acupuncture for Chronic Prostatitis/Chronic Pelvic Pain," *Amercian Journal of Medicine* 121(1) (January 2008): e1–7.

Shir, Y., A. Ratner, S.N. Raja, et al., "Neuropathic Pain Following Partial Nerve Injury in Rats Is Suppressed by Dietary Soy," *Neuroscience Letters* 240(2) (9 January 1998): 73–76.

Parasitic Infection

Vogel, H.C.A., *The Nature Doctor* (New Canaan, CT: Keats Publishing, 1991), p. 446.

Parkinson's Disease

Anderson, C., H. Checkoway, G.M. Franklin, et al., "Dietary Factors in Parkinson's Disease: The Role of Food Groups and Specific Foods," *Movement Disorders* 14(1) (January 1999): 21–27.

Chung, W., R. Poppen, and D.A. Lundervold, "Behavioral Relaxation Training for Tremor Disorders in Older Adults," *Biofeedback and Self Regulation* 20(2) (June 1995): 123–125.

da Silva, T.M., R.P. Munhoz, C. Alvarez, et al., "Depression in Parkinson's Disease: A Double-Blind, Randomized, Placebo-Controlled Pilot Study of Omega-3 Fatty Acid Supplementation," *Journal of Affective Disorders* 111(2–3) (December 2008): 351–359.

de Lau, L.M., P.J. Koudstaal, J.C. Witteman, et al., "Dietary Folate, Vitamin B_{12}, and Vitamin B_6 and the Risk of Parkinson Disease," *Neurology* 67(3) (July 2006): 315–318.

Foy, C.J., A.P. Passmore, M.D. Vahidassr, et al., "Plasma Chain-Breaking Antioxidants in Alzheimer's Disease, Vascular Dementia and Parkinson's Disease," *Quarterly Journal of Medicine* 92(1) (January 1999): 39–45.

Kao, H.J., W.H. Chen, and J.S. Liu, "Rapid Progression of Parkinsonism Associated with an Increase of Blood Manganese," *Kaohsiung I Hsueh Ko Hsueh Tsa Chih* [*Kaohsiung Journal of Medical Sciences*] 15(5) (May 1999): 297–301.

Karstaedt, P.J., J.H. Pincus, and S.S. Coughlin, "Standard and Controlled Release Levodopa/Carbidopa in Patients with Fluctuating Parkinson's Disease on a Protein Redistribution Diet: A Preliminary Report," *Archives of Neurology* 48(4) (April 1991): 402–405.

Montgomery, E.B., "Heavy Metals and the Etiology of Parkinson's Disease and Other Movement Disorders," *Toxicology* 97(1–3) (31 March 1995): 3–9.

Takacs, M., J. Vamos, Q. Papp, et al., "In Vitro Interaction of Selegiline, Riboflavin and Light: Sensitized Photodegradation of Drugs. I," *Acta Pharmacologica Hungarica* 69(3) (June 1999): 103–107.

Pelvic Inflammatory Disease

Isselbacher, K.J., E. Braunwald, J. Wilson, et al., eds., *Harrison's Principles of Internal Medicine*, 13th ed. (New York, NY: McGraw-Hill, 1995), p. 544.

Landers, D.V., K.K. Holmes, D.A. Eschenbach, et al., "Combination Antimicrobial Therapy in Treatment of Acute Pelvic Inflammatory Disease," *American Journal of Obstetrics and Gynecology* 164 (1991): 849.

Omura, Y., and S.L. Beckman, "Role of Mercury (Hg) in Resistant Infections and Effective Treatment of *Chlamydia trachomatis* and Herpes Family Viral Infections (and Potential Treatment for Cancer) by Removing Localized Hg Deposits with Chinese Parsley and Delivering Effective Antibiotics Using Various Drug Uptake Enhancement Methods," *Acupuncture and Electrotherapy Research* 20(3–4) (August 1995): 195–229.

Peptic Ulcer

Cheney, G., "Anti–Peptic Ulcer Dietary Factor," *Journal of the American Dietetic Association* 26 (1950): 668–672.

Elmstahl, S., U. Svensson, and G. Berglund, "Fermented Milk Products Are Associated to Ulcer Disease. Results from a Cross-Sectional Population Study," *European Journal of Clinical Nutrition* 52(9) (September 1998): 668–674.

Kang, J.Y., K.G. Yeoh, H.P. Chia, et al., "Chili—Protective Factor Against Peptic Ulcer?" *Digestive Diseases and Sciences* 40(3) (March 1995): 576–579.

Magistretti, M.J., M. Conti, and A. Cristoni, "Antiulcer Activity of an Anthocyanidin from *Vaccinium myrtillus*," *Arzneimittel-forschung* [*Medication Research*] 38(5) (May 1988): 686–690.

Murray, F.E., J. Ennis, J.R. Lennon, et al., "Management of Reflux Oesophagitis: Role of Weight Loss and Cimetidine," *Irish Journal of Medical Science* 160(1) (January 1991): 2–4.

Sharma, D., "Dry Meals—Physiological Approach to Management of Duodenal Ulcer," *Tropical Gastroenterology* 18(3) (July–September 1997).

Wada, T., Y. Aiba, K. Shimizu, et al., "The Therapeutic Effect of Bovine Lactoferrin in the Host Infected with *Helicobacter pylori*," *Scandinavian Journal of Gastroenterology* 34(3) (March 1999): 238–243.

Yeoh, K.G., J.Y. Kang, L. Yap, et al., "Chili Protects Against Aspirin-Induced Gastroduodenal Mucosal Injury in Humans," *Digestive Diseases and Sciences* 40(3) (March 1995): 580–583.

Periodontal Disease

Kweider, M., G.D. Lowe, G.D. Murray, et al., "Dental Disease, Fibrinogen and White Cell Count: Links with Myocardial Infarction?" *Scottish Medical Journal* 38(3) (June 1993): 73–74.

Morrison, H.I., L.F. Ellison, and G.W. Taylor, "Periodontal Disease and Risk of Fatal Coronary Heart and Cerebrovascular Diseases," *Journal of Cardiovascular Risk* 6(1) (February 1999): 7–11.

O'Hehir, S., " 'Dry Brushing' Beats Dental Plaque," *Prevention* 49(9) (September 1997): 45.

Weiss, E.I., R. Lev-Dor, Y. Kashamn, et al., "Inhibiting Interspecies Coaggregation of Plaque Bacteria with a Cranberry Juice Constituent," *Journal of the American Dental Association* 129(12) (December 1998): 1719–1723.

Premenstrual Syndrome (PMS)

Chocano-Bedoya, P.O., J.E. Manson, S.E. Hankinson, et al., "Dietary B Vitamin Intake and the Incident of Premenstrual Syndrome," *The American Journal of Clinical Nutrition* 93 (5) (May 2011): 1080–1086. Epub 2311, February 23.

Christie, S., A.F. Walker, S.M. Hicks, et al., "Flavonoid Supplement Improves Leg Health and Reduces Fluid Retention in Pre-Menopausal Women in a Double-Blind, Placebo-Controlled Study," *Phytomedicine* 11(1) (January 2004): 11–17.

Jones, D.Y., "Influence of Dietary Fat on Self-Reported Menstrual Symptoms," *Physiology and Behavior* 40(4) (1987): 483–487.

Muneyvirci-Delale, O., V.L. Nacharaju, B.M. Altura, et al., "Sex Steroid Hormones Modulate Serum Ionized Magnesium and Calcium Levels Throughout the Menstrual Cycle in Women," *Fertility and Sterility* 69(5) (May 1998): 958–962.

Murakami, K., S. Sasaki, Y. Takahashi, et al., "Dietary Glycemic Index Is Associated with Decreased Premenstrual Symptoms in Young Japanese Women," *Nutrition* 24(6) (June 2008): 554–561.

Olso, B.R., M.R. Forman, E. Lanza, et al., "Relation Between Sodium Balance and Menstrual Cycle Symptoms in Normal Women," *Annals of Internal Medicine* 125 (1 October 1996): 564–567.

Peiffer, A., B. Lapointe, and N. Barden, "Hormonal Regulation of Type II Glucocorticoid Receptor Messenger Ribonucleic Acid in Rat Brain," *Endocrinology* 129 (1991): 2166–2174.

Ramno, S., R. Judge, J. Dillon, et al., "The Role of Fluoxetine in the Treatment of Premenstrual Dysphoric Disorder," *Clinical Therapy* 21(4) (April 1999): 615–633; discussion, 613.

Tarasuk, V., and G.H. Beaton, "Menstrual-Cycle Patterns in Energy and Macronutrient Intake," *American Journal of Clinical Nutrition* 53 (1991): 442–447.

Thys-Jacobs, S., "Vitamin D and Calcium in Menstrual Migraine," *Headache* 34(9) (October 1994): 544–546.

Wyatt, K.M., P.W. Dimmock, P.W. Jones, et al., "Efficacy of Vitamin B_6 in the Treatment of Premenstrual Syndrome: Systematic Review," *British Medical Journal* 318(7195) (22 May 1999): 1375–1381.

Prostate Cancer

Adlercreutz, H., H. Markkanen, and S. Watanabe, "Plasma Concentrations of Phyto-Estrogens in Japanese Men," *Lancet* 342(8881) (13 November 1993): 1209–1210.

Adlercreutz, H., Y. Mousavi, J. Clark, et al., "Dietary Phytoestrogens and Cancer: In Vitro and in Vivo Studies," *Journal of Steroid Biochemistry and Molecular Biology* 41(3–8) (1992): 331–337.

Ansari, M.S., and N.P. Sgupta, "A Comparison of Lycopene and Orchidectomy vs. Orchidectomy Alone in the Management of Advanced Prostate Cancer," *British Journal of Urology International* (92) (2003): 375–378.

Bairati, I., F. Meyer, V. Frader, et al., "Dietary Fat and Advanced Prostate Cancer," *Journal of Urology* 159(4) (April 1998): 1271–1275.

Campbell, M.J., S. Park, M.R. Uskokovic, et al., "Synergistic Inhibition of Prostate Cancer Cell Lines by a 19-Nor-Hexafluoride Vitamin D_3 Analogue and Anti-Activator Protein 1 Retinoid," *British Journal of Cancer* 79(1) (January 1999): 101–107.

Catalona, W.J., D.S. Smith, T.L. Ratliff, et al., "Measurement of Prostate-Specific Antigen in Serum as a Screening Test for Prostate Cancer," *The New England Journal of Medicine* 324(17) (1991): 1156–1161.

Gann, P.H., J. Ma, E. Giovannucci, et al., "Lower Prostate Cancer Risk in Men with Elevated Plasma Lycopene Levels: Results of a Prospective Analysis," *Cancer Research* 59(6) (15 March 1999): 1225–1230.

Gartner, C., W. Stahl, and H. Sies, "Lycopene Is More Bioavailable from Tomato Paste Than from Fresh Tomatoes," *American Journal of Clinical Nutrition* 66 (1997): 116–122.

Giovannucci, E., "Tomatoes, Tomato-Based Products, Lycopene, and Cancer: Review of the Epidemiologic Literature," *Journal of the National Cancer Institute* 91(4) (17 February 1999): 317–331.

Hayes, R.B., R.G. Ziegler, G. Gridley, et al., "Dietary Factors and Risks for Prostate Cancer Among Blacks and Whites in the United States," *Cancer Epidemiology and Biomarkers Preview* 8(1) (January 1999): 25–34.

Kristal, A.R., K.B. Arnold, M.L. Neuhouser, et al., "Diet, Supplement Use, and Prostate Cancer Risk: Results from the Prostate Cancer Prevention Trial," *American Journal of Epidemiology* 172(5) (September 2010): 566–577.

Lippman, S.M., E.A. Klein, P.J. Goodman, et al., "Effect of Selenium and Vitamin E on Risk of Prostate Cancer and Other Cancers: The Selenium and Vitamin E Cancer Prevention Trial (SELECT)," *Journal of the American Medical Association* 301(1) (January 2009): 39–51.

Matzkin, H., P. Eber, B. Todd, et al., "Prognostic Significance of Changes in Prostate-Specific Markers After Endocrine Treatment of Stage D2 Prostatic Cancer," *Cancer* 70(9) (1992): 2302–2309.

Onozawa, M., K. Fukuda, M. Ohtani, et al., "Effects of Soybean Isoflavones on Cell Growth and Apoptosis of the Human Prostatic Cancer Cell Line LNCaP," *Japanese Journal of Clinical Oncology* 28(6) (June 1998): 360–363.

Pastori, M., H. Pfander, D. Bocobnoinik, et al., "Lycopene in Association with Alpha-Tocopherol Inhibits at Physiological Concentrations Proliferation of Prostate Carcinoma Cells," *Biochemistry and Biophysics Research Communications* 250(3) (29 September 1998): 582–585.

Rose, D.P., "Dietary Fatty Acids and Prevention of Hormone-Responsive Cancer," *Proceedings of the Society for Experimental Biology and Medicine* 216(2) (November 1997): 224–233.

Shamsuddin, A.M., and G.Y. Yang, "Inositol Hexaphosphate Inhibits Growth and Includes Differentiation of PC-3 Human Prostate Cancer Cells," *Carcinogenesis* 16(8) (August 1995): 1976–1979.

Strom, S.S., Y. Yamamura, C.M. Duphorne, et al., "Phytoestrogen Intake and Prostate Cancer: A Case-Control Study Using a New Database," *Nutrition and Cancer* 33(1) (1999): 20–25.

Vidlar, A., J. Vostalova, J. Ultrichova, et al., "The Safety and Efficacy of a Silymarin and Selenium Combination in Men After Radical Prostatectomy—A Six Month Placebo-Controlled Double-Blind Clinical Trial," *Biomedical Papers of the Medical Faculty of the University Palacky*, (Olomouc, Czech Republic) 154(3) (September 2010): 239–244.

Yoshizawa, K., W.C. Willett, S.J. Morris, et al., "Study of Prediagnostic Selenium Level in Toenails and the Risk of Advanced Prostate Cancer," *Journal of the National Cancer Institute* 90(16) (19 August 1998): 1219–1224.

Zentner, P.G., L.K. Pao, M.C. Benson, et al., "Prostate-Specific Antigen Density: A New Prognostic Indicator for Prostate Cancer," *International Journal of Radiation, Oncology Biology, and Physics* 27(1) (1993): 47–58.

Prostatitis

Ofek, I., J. Goldhar, D. Zafrini, et al., "Anti-*Escherichia coli* Adhesion Activity of Cranberry and Blueberry Juices," *The New England Journal of Medicine* 327 (1991): 1599.

Psoriasis

Bazex, A., "Diet without Gluten and Psoriasis," *Annals of Dermatology Symposia* 103 (1976): 648.

Boer, J., J. Hermans, A. Schothorst, et al., "Comparison of Phototherapy (UV-B) and Photochemotherapy (PUVA) for Clearing and Maintenance Therapy of Psoriasis," *Archives of Dermatology* 120 (1984): 52–57.

Collier, P.M., A. Ursell, K. Zaremba, et al., "Effect of Regular Consumption of Oily Fish Compared with White Fish on Chronic Plaque Psoriasis," *European Journal of Clinical Nutrition* 47(4) (April 1993): 251–254.

Danno, K., and N. Sugie, "Combination Therapy with Low-Dose Etretinate and Eicosapentanoic Acid for Psoriasis Vulgaris," *Journal of Dermatology* 25(11) (November 1998): 703–705.

Douglass, J.M., "Psoriasis and Diet," *California Medicine* 133 (1980): 450.

Fratino, P., C. Pelfini, A. Jucci, et al., "Glucose and Insulin in Psoriasis: The Role of Obesity and Genetic History," *Panminerva Medica* 21 (1979): 167.

Gisondi, P., M. Del Giglio, V. Di Francesco, et al., "Weight Loss Improves the Response of Obese Patients with Moderate-to-Severe Chronic Plaque Psoriasis to Low-Dose Cyclosporine Therapy: A Randomized, Controlled, Investigator-Blinded Clinical Trial," *American*

Journal of Clinical Nutrition 88(5) (November 2008): 1242–1247.

Kragballe, K., and M.D. Herlin, "Benoxaphren Improves Psoriasis," *Archives of Dermatology* 119 (1983): 548–552.

Misery, L., "Skin, Immunity and the Nervous System," *British Journal of Dermatology* 137(6) (December 1997): 843–850.

Monk, B.E., and S.M. Neill, "Alcohol Consumption and Psoriasis," *Dermatologica* 173 (1986): 57–60.

Proctor, M., D.I. Wilkinson, E.K. Orenberg, et al., "Lowered Cutaneous and Urinary Levels of Polyamines with Clinical Improvement in Treated Psoriasis," *Archives of Dermatology* 15(8) (August 1979): 945–949.

Prystowsky, J.H., A. Orologa, and S. Taylor, "Update on Nutrition and Psoriasis," *International Journal of Dermatology* 32(8) (August 1993): 582–586.

Scholzen, T., C.A. Armstrong, N.W. Bunnett, et al., "Neuropeptides in the Skin: Interactions Between the Neuroendocrine and the Skin Immune Systems," *Experimental Dermatology* 7(2–3) (April 1998): 81–96.

Seveille, R.H., "Psoriasis and Stress," *British Journal of Dermatology* 97 (1977): 297.

Thurmon, F.M., "The Treatment of Psoriasis with a Sarsaparilla Compound," *The New England Journal of Medicine* 227 (1942): 128–133.

Van Ruissen, F., M. Le, J.M. Carroll, et al., "Differential Effects of Detergents on Keratinocyte Gene Expression," *Journal of Investigational Dermatology* 110(4) (April 1998): 358–363.

Radiation Therapy Side Effects

Clemens, M.R., C.I. Müller-Ladner, and K.F. Gey, "Vitamins During High Dose Chemo- and Radiotherapy," *Zeitschrift für Ernährungswissenschaft* [*Journal for Nutritional Science*] 31(2) (June 1992): 110–120.

Hartmann, A., M. Vormstein, T. Schnabel, et al., "An Absent Correlation Between Antioxidant Blood Concentrations and the Remission Response of Preoperatively Treated Breast Carcinomas," *Strahlentherapie und Onkologie* [*Radiation Therapy and Oncology*] 72(8) (August 1996): 434–438.

Kaya, H., N. Delibas, M. Sertester, et al., "The Effect of Melatonin on Lipid Perioxidation During Radiotherapy in Female Rats," *Strahlentherapie und Onkologie* [*Radiation Therapy and Oncology*] 175(6) (June 1999): 285–288.

Redlich, C.A., S. Rockwell, J.S. Chung, et al., "Vitamin A Inhibits Radiation-Induced Pneumonitis in Rats," *Journal of Nutrition* 128(10) (October 1998): 1661–1664.

Restless Legs Syndrome

Lavigne, G.J., and J.Y. Montplaisir, "Restless Legs Syndrome and Sleep Bruxism: Prevalance and Association Among Canadians," *Sleep* 17 (1994): 739.

Ondo, W., and J. Jankovic, "Restless Legs Syndrome: Clinicoetiologic Correlates," *Neurology* 47 (1996): 1435.

Picchietti, D., "Growing Pains: RLS in Children," in V. Wilson, A. Walters, eds., *Sleep Thief: Restless Legs Syndrome* (Orange Park, FL: Galaxy Books, 1996), p. 82–93.

Rheumatoid Arthritis

Bálint, G., A. Apáthy, M. Gaál, et al., "Effect of Avemar—A Fermented Wheat Germ Extract—On Rheumatoid Arthritis. Preliminary Data," *Clinical and Experimental Rheumatology* 24(3) (May–June 2006): 325–328.

Berbert, A.A., C.R. Kondo, C.L. Almendra, et al., "Supplementation of Fish Oil and Olive Oil in Patients with Rheumatoid Arthritis," *Nutrition* 21(2) (February 2005): 131–136.

Fleischer, B., R. Gerardy-Schahn, B. Metzroth, et al., "An Evolutionary Conserved Mechanism to T Cell Activation by Microbial Toxins," *Journal of Immunology* 146(1) (January 1991): 11–17.

Jenkins, R., P. Rooney, D. Jones, et al., "Increased Intestinal Permeability in Patients with Rheumatoid Arthritis: A Side Effect of Oral Nonsteroidal Anti-Inflammatory Drug Use," *Gastroenterology* 96 (1989): 647–655.

Lappé, Marc, *Evolutionary Medicine: Rethinking the Origins of Disease* (San Francisco, CA: Sierra Club Books, 1994), p. 137.

Shapiro, J.A., T.D. Koepsell, L.F. Voigt, et al., "Diet and Rheumatoid Arthritis in Women: A Possible Protective Effect of Fish Consumption," *Epidemiology* 7(3) (May 1996): 256–263.

Tao, X., J.J. Cush, M. Garret, et al., "A Phase I Study of Ethyl Acetate Extract of the Chinese Antirheumatic Herb *Tripterygium wilfordii hook* F in Rheumatoid Arthritis," *Journal of Rheumatology* 28(10) (October 2001): 2160–2167.

Warnock, M., D. McBean, A. Suter, et al., "Effectiveness and Safety of Devil's Claw Tablets in Patients with General Rheumatic Disorders," *Phytotherapy Research* 21(12) (December 2007): 1228–1233.

Zaphiropoulos, G.C., "Rheumatoid Arthritis and the Gut," *British Journal of Rheumatology* 25 (1986): 138–140.

Seizure Disorders

De Vivo, D.C., T.P. Bohan, D.L. Coulter, et al., "L-Carnitine Supplementation in Childhood Epilepsy: Current

Perspectives," *Epilepsia* 39(11) (November 1998): 1216–1225.

DeGiorgio, C.M., P. Miller, S. Meymandi, et al., "n-3 Fatty Acids (Fish Oil) for Epilepsy, Cardiac Risk Factors, and the Risk of SUDEP: Clues from a Pilot, Double-Blind, Exploratory Study," *Epilepsy & Behavior* 13(4) (November 2008): 681–684.

Hardman, J.G., L.E. Limbird, P.B. Molinoff, et al., *Goodman and Gilman's the Pharmacological Basis of Therapeutics* (New York, NY: McGraw-Hill, 1996), p. 461.

Kossoff, E.H., J.L. Bosarge, M.J. Miranda, et al., "Will Seizure Control Improve by Switching from the Modified Atkins Diet to the Traditional Ketogenic Diet?" *Epilepsia* 51(12) (December 2010): 2496–2499.

Morrell, M.J., "Guidelines for the Care of Women with Epilepsy," *Neurology* 51(5) (Supplement 4) (November 1998): S21–S27.

Muzykewicz, D.A., D.A. Lyczkowski, N. Memon, et al., "Efficacy, Safety, and Tolerability of the Low Glycemic Index Treatment in Pediatric Epilepsy," *Epilepsia* 50(5) (February 2009): 1118–1126.

Nagatomo, I., Y. Akasaki, M. Uchida, et al., "Influence of Dietary Zinc on Convulsive Seizures and Hippocampal NADPH Diaphorase-Positive Neurons in Seizure Susceptible EL Mouse," *Brain Research* 789(2) (13 April 1998): 213–220.

Sapolsky, R.M., "Potential Behavioral Modification of Glucocorticoid Damage to the Hippocampus," *Behavioral Brain Research* 57(2) (30 November 1998): 175–182.

Sex Drive, Diminished

Arreola, F., R. Paniagua, J. Herrera, et al., "Low Plasma Zinc and Androgen in Insulin-Dependent Diabetes Mellitus," *Archives of Andrology* 16(2) (1986): 151–154.

Gray, A., H.A. Feldman, J.B. McKinley, et al., "Age, Disease, and Changing Sex Hormone Levels in Middle-Aged Men: Results of the Massachusetts Male Aging Study," *Journal of Endocrinology and Metabolism* 73(5) (November 1991): 1016–1025.

Green, J., A. Denhan, J. Ingram, et al., "Treatment of Menopausal Symptoms by Qualified Herbal Practitioners: A Prospective, Randomized, Controlled Trial," *Family Practice* (2007). DOI: 10.1093/fampra/cmm048.

Lucà-Moretti, M., A. Grandi, E. Lucà, et al., "Master Amino Acid Pattern as Substitute for Dietary Proteins During a Weight-Loss Diet to Achieve the Body's Nitrogen Balance Equilibrium with Essentially No Calories," *Advances Therapy* 20(5) (September–October 2003): 282–291.

Ziegenfuss, T., and L. Lamber, "Comparison of Androstenedione and 4-Androstenediol and Testosterone

Levels," cited in Joshua Shackman, Greg Ptacek, and Karlis C. Ullis, *Super "T": The Complete Guide to Creating an Effective, Safe, and Natural Testosterone Enhancement Program for Men and Women* (New York, NY: Fireside Books, 1999), p. 256.

Sinusitis

Khoury, R.M., L. Camacho-Lobato, P.O. Katz, et al., "Influence of Spontaneous Sleep Positions on Nighttime Recumbent Reflux in Patients with Gastroesophageal Reflux Disease," *American Journal of Gastroenterology* 94 (August 1999): 2069–2073.

Laino, C., "*H. Pylori* Implicated in Allergies," *Medical Tribune*, 24 March 1994, p. 1.

Ulualp, S.O., R.J. Toohill, R. Hoffmann, et al., "Possible Relationship of Gastroesophagopharyngeal Acid Reflux with Pathogenesis of Chronic Sinusitis," *American Journal of Rhinology* 13(3) (May–June 1999): 197–202.

Westerveld, G.J., I. Dekker, H.P. Voss, et al., "Antioxidant Levels in the Nasal Mucosa of Patients with Chronic Sinusitis and Healthy Controls," *Archives of Otolaryngology* 123 (1997): 201–204.

Skin Cancer

Clark, L.C., G.F. Combs, Jr., B.W. Turnbull, et al., "Effects of Selenium Supplementation for Cancer Prevention in Patients with Carcinoma of the Skin: A Randomized Controlled Trial. Nutritional Prevention of Cancer Study Group," *Journal of the American Medical Association* 276(24) (25 December 1996): 1957–1963.

Huang, M.T., W. Ma, P. Yen, et al., "Inhibitory Effects of Topical Application of Low Doses of Curcumin on 12-O-Tetradecanoylphorbol-13-Acetate-Induced Tumor Promotion and Oxidized DNA Bases in Mouse Epidermis," *Carcinogenesis* 18(1) (January 1997): 83–88.

Ishizaki, C., T. Oguro, T. Yoshida, et al., "Enhancing Effect of Ultraviolet A on Ornithine Decarboxylase Induction and Dermatitis Evoked by 12-O-Tetradecanoylphorbol-13-Acetate and Its Inhibition by Curcumin in Mouse Skin," *Dermatology* 193(4) (1996): 311–317.

Kahn, H.S., L.M. Tatham, A.V. Patel, et al., "Increased Cancer Mortality Following a History of Nonmelanoma Skin Cancer," *Journal of the American Medical Association* 280(10) (9 September 1998): 910–912.

Namba, T., K. Sekiya, A. Toshinal, et al., "Study on Baths with Crude Drug. II.: The Effects of *Coptidis rhizoma* Extracts as Skin Permeation Enhancer," *Yakugaku Zasshi* [*Journal of the Pharmaceutical Society of Japan*] 115(8) (August 1995): 618–625.

Yasukawa, K., Y. Ikeya, H. Mitsuhashi, et al., "Gomisin A Inhibits Tumor Promotion by 12-O-Tetradecanoylphorbol-13-Acetate in Two-stage Carcinogenesis in Mouse Skin," *Oncology* 49(1) (1992): 68–71.

Stomach Cancer

Akimoto, M., T. Nishihira, and M. Kasai, "Modulation of the Antitumor Effect of BRM Under Various Nutritional or Endocrine Conditions," *Gan to Kagaku Ryoho* [*Japanese Journal of Cancer and Chemotherapy*] 13(4, Part 2) (April 1986): 1270–1276.

Fernandez, E., L. Chatenoud, C. La Vecchia, et al., "Fish Consumption and Cancer Risk," *American Journal of Clinical Nutrition* 70(1) (July 1999): 85–90.

Huang, Kee C., and Kee Chang, eds., *The Pharmacology of Chinese Herbs* (Boca Raton, FL: CRC Press, 1992), p. 39.

Knekt, P., A. Aromaa, J. Maatela, et al., "Serum Vitamin E, Serum Selenium, and the Risk of Gastrointestinal Cancer," *International Journal of Cancer* 42 (1988): 846–850.

Linder, Maria C., ed., *Nutritional Biochemistry and Metabolism,* 2d. ed. (New York, NY: Elsevier Science Publishing Co., 1991), pp. 499, 512.

Moss, Ralph W., *Cancer Therapy* (Brooklyn, NY: Equinox Press, 1996), p. 234.

Yin, G.Y., X.F. He, and Y.F. Yin, "Study on Mitochondrial Ultrastructure, Trace Elements and Correlative Factors of Gastric Mucosa in Patients with Spleen Deficiency Syndrome," *Chung-Kuo Chung Hsi I Chieh Ho Tsa Chih* [*Chinese Journal of Modern Developments in Traditional Medicine*] 15(12) (December 1995): 719–723.

Zhang, L., L.W. Yang, and L.J. Yang, "Relation Between *Helicobacter pylori* and Pathogenesis of Chronic Atrophic Gastritis and the Research of Its Prevention and Treatment," *Chung-Kuo Chung Hsi I Chieh Ho Tsa Chih* [*Chinese Journal of Modern Developments in Traditional Medicine*] 12(9) (September 1992): 515–516, 521–523.

Zheng, G.Q., P.M. Kenney, J. Zhang, et al., "Chemoprevention of Benzo[a]pyrene-Induced Forestomach Cancer in Mice by Natural Phthalides from Celery Seed Oil," *Nutrition and Cancer* 19(1) (1993): 77–86.

Strep Throat

Badgett, J.T., and L.K. Hersterberg, "Management of Group A Streptococcus Pharyngitis with a Second-Generation Rapid Strep Screen: Strep A O1A," *Microbial Drug Resistance* 2 (1996): 371–376.

Bensky, Dan, and Andrew Gamble, compilers, *Chinese Herbal Medicine: Materia Medica,* rev. ed. (Seattle, WA: Eastland Press, 1993), p. 76.

Brook, I., "Treatment of Group A Streptococcal Pharyngotonsillitis," *Journal of the American Medical Association* 247 (1982): 2496.

McIsaac, W.J., V. Goel, P.M. Slaughter, et al., "Reconsidering Sore Throats. Part 1: Problems with Current Clinical Practice," *Canadian Family Physician* 43 (1997): 485–493.

McIsaac, W.J., V. Goel, P.M. Slaughter, et al., "Reconsidering Sore Throats. Part 2: Alternative Approach and Practical Office Tool," *Canadian Family Physician* 43 (1997): 495–500.

Rinehart, J.F., "Studies Relating Vitamin C Deficiency to Rheumatic Fever and Rheumatoid Arthritis: Experimental, Clinical, and General Considerations. I: Rheumatic Fever," *Annals of Internal Medicine* 9 (1935): 586–599.

Rinehart, J.F., "Studies Relating Vitamin C Deficiency to Rheumatic Fever and Rheumatoid Arthritis: Experimental, Clinical, and General Consideration. II. Rheumatoid (Atrophic) Arthritis," *Annals of Internal Medicine* 9 (1935): 671–689.

Stroke

Agnarsson, U., G. Thorgeirsson, H. Sigvaldason, et al., "Effects of Leisure-Time Physical Activity and Ventilatory Function on Risk for Stroke in Men: The Reykjavik Study," *Annals of Internal Medicine* 130 (15 June 1999): 987–990.

Almeida, O.P., K. Marsh, and H. Alfonso, "B-Vitamins Reduce the Long-Term Risk for Depression After Stroke: The VITATOPS-DEP Trial," *Annals of Neurology* 68(4) (October 2010): 503–510.

Garbagnati, F., G. Cairella, A. De Martino, et al., "Is Antioxidant and n-3 Supplementation Able to Improve Functional Status in Poststroke Patients? Results from the Nutristroke Trial," *Cerebrovascular Diseases* 27(4) (2009): 375–383.

Mcintosh, T.K., M. Juhler, and T. Wieloch, "Novel Pharmacologic Strategies in the Treatment of Experimental Traumatic Brain Injury: 1998," *Journal of Neurotrauma* 15(10) (October 1998): 731–769.

Morrison, H.I., L.F. Ellison, and G.W. Taylor, "Periodontal Disease and Risk of Fatal Coronary Heart and Cerebrovascular Diseases," *Journal of Cardiovascular Risk* 6(1) (February 1999): 7–11.

Robinson, K., K. Arheart, H. Refsum, et al., "Low Circulating Folate and Vitamin B₆ Concentrations: Risk Factors for Stroke, Peripheral Vascular Disease, and Coronary Artery Disease. European COMAC Group," *Circulation* 97(5)(10 February 1998): 437–443.

Tanne, D., S. Yaari, and U. Goldbourt, "High-Density Lipoprotein Cholesterol and Risk of Ischemic Stroke

Mortality: A 21-Year Follow-Up of 8586 Men from the Israeli Ischemic Heart Disease Study," *Stroke* 28 (January 1997): 83–87.

Van Der Worp, H.B., P.R. Bar, L.J. Kappelle, et al., "Dietary Vitamin E Levels Affect Outcome of Permanent Focal Cerebral Ischemia in Rats," *Stroke* 29 (1998): 1002–1006.

Sweating, Excessive

Blanco, C., and F.R. Schneier, "Current and New Approaches to Social Phobia," *Medscape Mental Health* 2(4) (1997): 1–10.

Goh, C.L., and K. Yoyong, "A Comparison of Topical Tannic Acid Versus Iontophoresis in the Medical Treatment of Palmar Hyperhidrosis," *Singapore Medical Journal* 37(5) (October 1996): 466–468.

Syphilis

Cardin De Stefani, E., and C. Costa, "Tryptophan Metabolism in Syphilis Infections," *Bolletina de la Societa Italiana de la Biologia Spermimentale* 60(8) (31 August 1984): 1541–1547.

Tendinitis

Saveriano, G., P. Lioretti, F. Maiolo, et al., "Our Experience in the Use of a New Objective Pain Measuring System in Rheumarthropatic Subjects Treated with Transcutaneous Electroanalgesia and Ultrasound," *Minerva Medica* 77 (1986): 745–752.

Tinnitus

Grossi, M.G., G. Belcaro, M.R. Cesarone, et al., "Improvement in Cochlear Flow with Pycnogenol in Patients with Tinnitus: A Pilot Evaluation," *Panminerva Medica* 52(2 supplement 1) (2010): 63–68.

Toothache

Koba, K., Y. Kimura, K. Matsumoto, et al., "Post-Operative Symptoms and Healing After Endodontic Treatment of Infected Teeth Using Pulsed Nd:YAG Laser," *Endodontics and Dental Traumatology* 15(2) (April 1999): 68–72.

Pihistrom, B.L., K.M. Hargreaves, O.J. Bouwsma, et al., "Pain After Periodontal Scaling and Root Planing," *Journal of the American Dental Association* 130(6) (June 1999): 801–807.

Tidwell, E., B. Huston, N. Burkhart, et al., "Herpes Zoster of the Trigeminal Nerve Third Branch: A Case Report and Review of the Literature," *International Endodontics Journal* 32(1) (January 1999): 61–66.

Tripp, D.A., N.R. Neish, and M.J. Sullivan, "What Hurts During Dental Hygiene Treatment," *Journal of Dental Hygiene* 72(4) (Fall 1998): 25–30.

Tuberculosis

Dhople, A.M., M.A. Ibanez, and T.C. Poirier, "Role of Iron in the Pathogenesis of *Mycobacterium avium* Infection in Mice," *Microbios* 87(351) (1996): 77–87.

Isselbacher, K.J., E. Braunwald, J. Wilson, et al., eds., *Harrison's Principles of Internal Medicine,* 13th ed. (New York, NY: McGraw-Hill, 1995), p. 710.

Onodera, H., Y. Kasamatsu, S. Tsujimoto, et al., "A Case of Pulmonary Tuberculosis Complicated with Drug Toxicosis—Value of Shosaikoto and Hochuekito as Anti-Allergic Agents," *Kekkaku* 68(1) (January 1993): 23–29.

Paton, N.I., Y.K. Chua, A. Earnest, et al., "Randomized Controlled Trial of Nutritional Supplementation in Patients with Newly Diagnosed Tuberculosis and Wasting," *American Journal of Clinical Nutrition* 80(2) (August 2004): 460–465.

Range, N., A.B. Andersen, P. Magnussen, et al., "The Effect of Micronutrient Supplementation on Treatment Outcome in Patients with Pulmonary Tuberculosis: A Randomzied Controlled Trial in Mwanza, Tanzania," *Tropical Medicine & International Health* 10(9) (September 2005): 826–832.

Rockett, K.A., R. Brookes, I. Udalova, et al., "1,25-Dihydroxyvitamin D3 Induces Nitric Oxide Synthase and Suppresses Growth of Mycobacterium Tuberculosis in a Human Macrophage-Like Cell Line," *Infection and Immunity* 66(11) (November 1998): 5314–5321.

Vaginosis

Goldenberg, R.L., E. Thorn, A.H. Moawad, et al., "The Preterm Prediction Study: Fetal Fibronectin, Bacterial Vaginosis, and Peripartum Infection. NICHD Maternal Fetal Medicine Units Network," *Obstetrics and Gynecology* 87(5, Part 1) (1996): 656–660.

Marrazzo, J.M., R.L. Cook, H.C. Wiesenfeld, et al., "Women's Satisfaction with an Intravaginal *Lactobacillus* Capsule for the Treatment of Bacterial Vaginosis," *Journal of Women's Health* 15(9) (November 2006): 1053–1060.

Varicose Veins

Diehm, C., H.J. Trampisch, S. Lange, et al., "Comparison of Leg Compression Stocking and Oral Horse-Chestnut Seed Extract Therapy in Patients with Chronic Venous Insufficiency," *Lancet* 347(8997) (3 February 1996): 292–294.

Ducimetiere, P., J.L. Richard, G. Pequignot, et al., "Varicose Veins: A Risk for Atherosclerotic Disease in Middle-Aged Men?" *International Journal of Epidemiology* 10(4) (December 1981): 329–335.

Iannuzzi, A., S. Panico, A.V. Ciardulio, et al., "Varicose Veins of the Lower Limbs and Venous Capacitance in

Postmenopausal Women: Relationship with Obesity," *Journal of Vascular Surgery* 36(5) (November 2002): 965–968.

Pittler, M.H., and E. Ernst, "Horse Chestnut Seed Extract for Chronic Venous Insufficiency," Cochrane Database of Systematic Reviews 2006, Issue 1. Art. No.: CD003230. DOI: 10.1002/14651858.CD003230.pub3.

Vitiligo

Schallreuter, K.U., J.M. Wood, K.R. Lemke, et al., "Treatment of Vitiligo with a Topical Application of Pseudocatalase and Calcium in Combination with Short-Term UVB Exposure: A Case Study on 33 Patients," *Dermatology* 190(3) (1995): 223–229.

Schulpis, C.H., C. Antoniou, T. Michas, et al., "Phenylalanine Plus Ultraviolet Light: Preliminary Report of a Promising Treatment for Childhood Vitiligo," *Pediatric Dermatology* 6 (1989): 332–335.

Siddiqui, A.H., L.M. Stolk, R. Bhaggoe, et al., "L-Phenylalanine and UVA Radiation in the Treatment of Vitiligo," *Dermatology* 188 (1994): 215–218.

Warts

Bairati, I., K.J. Sherman, B. McKnight, et al., "Diet and Genital Warts: A Case-Control Study," *Sexually Transmitted Diseases* 21(3) (May–June 1994): 149–154.

Ewin, D.M., "Hypnotherapy for Warts (Verruca Vulgaris): 41 Consecutive Cases with 33 Cures," *American Journal of Clinical Hypnosis* 35(1) (July 1992): 1–10.

Schneider, A., A. Morabia, U. Papendick, et al., "Pork Intake and Human Papillomavirus-Related Disease," *Nutrition and Cancer* 13(4) (1990): 209–211.

Wrinkles

Contet-Audonneau, J.L., C. Jeanmaire, and G. Pauly, "A Histological Study of Human Wrinkle Structures: Comparison Between Sun-Exposed Areas of the Face, with or without Wrinkles, and Sun-Protected Areas," *British Journal of Dermatology* 140(6) (June 1999): 1038–1047.

Ernster, V.L., D. Grady, R. Miike, et al., "Facial Wrinkling in Men and Women, by Smoking Status," *American Journal of Public Health* 85(1) (January 1995): 78–82.

Hoppe, U., J. Bergemann, W. Diembeck, et al., "Coenzyme Q_{10}, a Cutaneous Antioxidant and Energizer," *Biofactors* 9(2–4) (1999): 371–378.

Schmidt, J.B., M. Binder, G. Demschik, et al., "Treatment of Skin Aging with Topical Estrogens," *International Journal of Dermatology* 35(9) (September 1996): 669–674.

Yeast Infection (Yeast Vaginitis)

Buslau, M., I. Menzel, and H. Holzmann, "Fungal Flora of Human Faeces in Psoriasis and Atopic Dermatitis," *Mycoses* 33(2) (February 1990): 90–94.

Kennedy, M.J., and P.A. Volz, "Ecology of *Candida albicans* Gut Colonization: Inhibition of Candida Adhesion, Colonization, and Dissemination from the Gastrointestinal Tract by Bacterial Antagonism," *Infection and Immunity* 49(3) (September 1985): 654–663.

Larmas, M.M., K.K. Makinene, and A. Scheinin, "Turku Sugar Studies. III. An Intermediate Report on the Effect of Sucrose, Fructose and Xylitol Diets on the Numbers of Salivary Lactobacilli, Candida, and Streptococci," *Acta Odontologica Scandinavica* 32 (1974): 423–433.

Senff, H., C. Bothe, J. Busacker, et al., "Studies on the Yeast Flora in Patients Suffering from Psoriasis Capillitii or Seborrhoic Dermatitis of the Scalp," *Mycoses* 33(1) (January 1990): 29–32.

Weig, M., E. Werner, M. Frosch, et al., "Limited Effect of Refined Carbohydrate Dietary Supplementation on Colonization of the Gastrointestinal Tract of Healthy Subjects by *Candida albicans*," *American Journal of Clinical Nutrition* 69(6) (June 1999): 1170–1173.

PART THREE: TECHNIQUES OF HERBAL HEALING

Acupuncture

National Institutes of Health, Consensus Paper Group 107, *Acupuncture* (5 November 1997).

Shi, R., G. Ji, L. Zhao, et al., "Effects of Electroacupuncture and Twirling Reinforcing-Reducing Manipulations on Volume of Microcirculatory Blood Flow in Cerebral Pia Mater," *Journal of Traditional Chinese Medicine* 18(3) (September 1998): 220–224.

Timofeev, M.F., "Effects of Acupuncture and an Agonist of Opiate Receptors on Heroin Dependent Patients," *American Journal of Chinese Medicine* 27(2) (1999): 143–148.

Toriizuka, K., M. Okumura, K. Iijima, et al., "Acupuncture Inhibits the Decrease in Brain Catecholamine Contents and the Impairment of Passive Avoidance Task in Ovariectomized Mice," *Acupuncture and Electrotherapy Research* 24(1) (1999): 45–57.

Yamashita, H., H. Tsukayama, Y. Tanno, et al., "Adverse Events Related to Acupuncture," *Journal of the American Medical Association* 280(18) (11 November 1998): 1563–1564.

Aromatherapy

Diego, M.A., N.A. Jones, T. Field, et al., "Aromatherapy Positively Affects Mood, EEG Patterns of Alertness and Math Computations," *International Journal of Neuroscience* 96(3–4) (December 1998): 217–224.

Fujiwara, R., T. Komori, Y. Noda, et al., "Effects of a Long-Term Inhalation of Fragrances on the Stress-Induced Immunosuppression in Mice," *Neuroimmunomodulation* 5(6) (November/December 1998): 318–322.

Hay, I.C., M. Jamieson, and A.D. Ormerod, "Randomized Trial of Aromatherapy: Successful Treatment for Alopecia Areata," *Archives of Dermatology* 134(11) (November 1998): 1349–1352.

Hu, P.H., Y.C. Peng, Y.T. Lin, et al., "Aromatherapy for Reducing Colonoscopy Related Procedural Anxiety and Physiological Parameters: A Randomized Controlled Study," *Hepatogastroenterology* 57(102–103) (September–October 2010): 1082–1086.

Kiecolt-Glaser, J.K., J.E. Graham, W.B. Malarkey, et al., "Olfactory Influences on Mood and Autonomic, Endocrine, and Immune Funtion," *Psychoneuroendocrinology* 33(3) (2008): 328–339.

Kilstoff, K., and L. Chenoweth, "New Approaches to Health and Well-Being for Dementia Day-Care Clients, Family Carers and Day-Care Staff," *International Journal of Nursing Practice* 4(2) (June 1998): 70–83.

Oz, M.C., E.J. Lemole, L.L. Oz, et al., "Treating CAD with Cardiac Surgery Combined with Complementary Therapy," *Medscape Women's Health* 1(10) (October 1996): 7.

Romine, I.J., A.M. Bush, and C.R. Geist, "Lavender Aromatherapy in Recovery from Exercise," *Perceptual and Motor Skills* 88(3, Part 1) (June 1999): 756–758.

Sayette, M.A., and D.J. Parrott, "Effects of Olfactory Stimuli on Urge Reduction in Smokers," *Experimental and Clinical Psychopharmacology* 7(2) (May 1999): 151–159.

Compresses

Arora, S., M. Vatsa, and V. Dadhwal, "A Comparison of Cabbage Leaves vs. Hot and Cold Compresses in the Treatment of Breast Engorgement," *Indian Journal of Community Medicine* 33(3) (July 2008): 160–162.

Rana, M., N.C. Gellrich, A. Ghassemi, et al., "Three-Dimensional Evaluation of Postoperative Swelling After Third Molar Surgery Using 2 Different Cooling Therapy Methods: A Randomized Observer-Blind Propsective Study," *Journal of Oral and Maxillofactory Surgery* 14 (April 2011).

Douches

Hassan, S., A. Chatwani, H. Brovender, et al., "Douching for Perceived Vaginal Odor with No Infectious Cause of Vaginitis: A Randomized Controlled Trial," *Journal of Lower Genital Tract Disease* 15(2) (April 2011): 128–133.

Onderdonk, A.B., M.L. Delaney, P.L. Hinkson, et al., "Quantitative and Qualitative Effects of Douche Preparations on Vaginal Microflora," *Obstetrics and Gynecology* 80 (3, Part 1) (September 1992): 333–338.

Rosenberg, M.J., and R.S. Phillips, "Does Douching Promote Ascending Infection?" *Journal of Reproductive Medicine* 37(11) (November 1992): 930–938.

Scholes, D., A. Stergachis, L.E. Ichikawa, et al., "Vaginal Douching as a Risk Factor for Cervical Chlamydia Trachomatis Infection," *Obstetrics and Gynecology* 91(6) (June 1998): 993–997.

Estrogen-Reducing Diet

Adlercreutz, H., "Diet, Breast Cancer and Sex Hormone Metabolism," *Annals of the New York Academy of Sciences* 595 (1990): 281.

Begin, M.E., U.N. Das, G. Ells, et al., "Selective Killing of Human Cancer Cells by Polyunsaturated Fatty Acids," *Prostaglandins and Leukotrienes in Medicine* 30 (1987): 37–49.

De Waard, F., J. Poortman, M. De Pedro-Alvarez, et al., "Weight Reduction and Oestrogen Excretion in Obese Post-Menopausal Women," *Maturitas* 4 (1982): 155.

Longcope, C., S. Gorbach, B. Goldin, et al., "The Effect of a Low-Fat Diet on Estrogen Metabolism," *Journal of Clinical Endocrinology and Metabolism* 46 (1987): 146.

Rose, D.P., M. Lubin, and J.M. Connolly, "Effects of Diet Supplementation with Wheat Bran on Serum Estrogen Levels in the Follicular and Luteal Phases of the Menstrual Cycle," *Nutrition* 13(6) (June 1997): 535–539.

Tegelman, R., P. Lindeskog, K. Carlström, et al., "Peripheral Hormone Levels in Healthy Subjects During Fasting," *Acta Endocronilogica* (Denmark) 133 (1986): 457.

Kegel Exercises

Aslan, E., N. Komurcu, N.K. Beji, et al., "Bladder Training and Kegel Exercises for Women with Urinary Complaints Living in a Rest Home," *Gerontology* 54(4) (2008): 224–231.

McKenna, P.H., C.D. Herndon, S. Connery, et al., "Pelvic Floor Muscle Retraining for Pediatric Voiding Dysfunction Using Interactive Computer Games," *Journal of Urology* 162(3, Part 2) (September 1999): 1056–1063.

Payne, C.K., "Biofeedback for Community-Dwelling Individuals with Urinary Incontinence," *Urology* 51(2A) (Supplement) (February 1998): 35–39.

Vasconcelos, M., E. Lima, L. Caiafa, et al., "Voiding Dysfunction in Children. Pelvic-floor Exercises or Biofeedback Therapy: A Randomized Study," *Pediatric Nephrology* 21(12) (December 2006): 1858–1864.

Massage

McClurg, D., and A. Lowe-Strong, "Does Abdominal Massage Relieve Constipation?" *Nursing Times* 107(12) (April–May 2011): 20–22.

McIntosh, G., and H. Hall, "Low Back Pain (Acute)," *Clinical Evidence* (Online) (9) (May 2011): 1102.

Ointments

Eshghi, F., S.J. Hosseinimehr, N. Rahmani, et al., "Effects of Aloe Vera Cream on Posthemorrhoidectomy Pain and Wound Healing: Results of a Randomized, Blind, Placebo-Controlled Study," *Journal of Alternative and Complementary Medicine* 16(6) (June 2010): 647–650.

Pawar, P.L., and B.M. Nabar, "Effect of Plant Extracts Formulated in Different Ointment Bases on MDR Strains," *Indian Journal of Pharmaceutical Sciences* 72(3) (May 2010): 397–401.

Plasters

Bensky, Dan, and Andrew Gamble, compilers, *Chinese Herbal Medicine: Materia Medica,* rev. ed. (Seattle, WA: Eastland Press, 1993), p. 304.

Huang, Kee C., and Kee Chang, eds., *The Pharmacology of Chinese Herbs* (Boca Raton, FL: CRC Press, 1992), p. 197.

Tian, L., S. Yuan, E. Ba, et al., "Composite Acupuncture Treatment of Mental Retardation in Children," *Journal of Traditional Chinese Medicine* 15(1) (March 1995): 34–37.

Poultices

Akbulut, S., H. Semur, O. Kose, et al., "Phytocontact Dermatitis Due to *Ranunculus arvensis* Mimicking Burn Injury: Report of Three Cases and Literature Review," *International Journal of Emergency Medicine* 21 (February 2011): 4–7.

Fröhlich, H.H., and W. Müller-Limmroth, "Physical Investigations into the Thermotherapeutic Action of the Kneipp Hay Flower Sack," *Münchener Medizinisher Wochenschrift* [*Munich Medical Weekly*] 117(11) (14 March 1975): 443–448.

Relaxation Techniques

Davy, K.P., P.P. Jones, and D.R. Seals, "Influence of Age on the Sympathetic Neural Adjustments to Alterations in Systemic Oxygen Levels in Humans," *American Journal of Physiology* 273 (2, Part 2) (August 1997): R690–695.

Dusek, J.A., P.L. Hibberd, B. Buczynski, et al., "Stress Management Versus Lifestyle Modification on Systolic Hypertension and Medication Elimination: A Randomized Trial," *Journal of Alternative and Complementary Medicine* 14(2) (March 2008): 129–136.

Janke, J., "The Effect of Relaxation Therapy on Preterm Labor Outcomes," *Journal of Obstetrics, Gynecology, and Neonatal Nursing* 28(3) (May–June 1999): 255–263.

Kroner-Herwig, B., U. Mohn, and R. Pothmann, "Comparison of Biofeedback and Relaxation in the Treatment of Pediatric Headache and the Influence of Parent Involvement on Outcome," *Applied Psychophysiology and Biofeedback* 23(3) (September 1998): 143–157.

Mahajan, A.S, K.S. Reddy, and U. Sachdeva, "Lipid Profile of Coronary Risk Subjects Following Yogic Lifestyle Intervention," *Indian Heart Journal* 51(1) (January–February 1999): 37–40.

Malathi, A., and A. Damodaran, "Stress Due to Exams in Medical Students—Role of Yoga," *Indian Journal of Physiology and Pharmacology* 43(2) (April 1999): 218–224.

Manjunath, N.K., and S. Telles, "Factors Influencing Changes in Tweezer Dexterity Scores Following Yoga Training," *Indian Journal of Physiology and Pharmacology* 43(2) (April 1999): 225–229.

Naga Venkatesha Murthy, P.J., N. Janakiramaiah, B.N. Gangadhar, et al., "P300 Amplitude and Antidepressant Response to Sudarshan Kriya Yoga (SKY)," *Journal of Affective Disorders* 50(1) (July 1998): 45–48.

Stachenfeld, N.S, G.W. Mack, L. DiPietro, et al., "Regulation of Blood Volume During Training in Post-Menopausal Women," *Medical Science in Sports and Exercise* 30(1) (January 1998): 92–98.

Twohig, M.P., S.C. Hayes, J.C. Plumb, et al., "A Randomized Clinical Trial of Acceptance and Commitment Therapy Versus Progressive Relaxation Training for Obsessive-Compulsive Disorder," *Journal of Consultanting and Clinical Psychology* 78(5) (October 2010): 705–716.

Sitz bath

Jensen, S.L., "Treatment of First Episodes of Acute Anal Fissure: Prospective Randomised Study of Lignocaine Ointment Versus Hydrocortisone Ointment or Warm Sitz Baths Plus Bran," *British Medical Journal* (Clinical Research Edition) 292(6529) (May 1986): 1167–1169.

Appendix A: Glossary

ACLE. Acute cutaneous lupus erythematosus.

ACTH. *See* adrenocorticotropic hormone (ACTH).

actinic keratosis. Abnormal skin growth stimulated by ultraviolet radiation from sunlight; may lead to a type of cancer called basal cell carcinoma.

acute illness. An illness that may cause severe symptoms but is of limited duration. Term is also sometimes used to mean "severe."

Addison's disease. A disease caused by failure of the adrenal glands, marked by lack of appetite, weakness, digestive problems, and darkening of the skin.

adrenaline. *See* epinephrine.

adrenocorticotropic hormone (ACTH). A hormone that stimulates the secretion of epinephrine (adrenaline) as part of the body's response to stress.

aldose reductase. An enzyme that converts glucose into sorbitol, a step that could lead to the formation of diabetic cataracts.

allergen. A normally harmless substance, such as pollen, that provokes an immune response.

allergy. An immune response to an allergen, such as hay fever developing in response to grass pollen.

alopecia. Medical term for hair loss.

amino acid. One of the twenty-two nitrogen-bearing substances that the body uses to create proteins.

analgesic. An agent that reduces pain.

anaphylactic shock. A severe allergic reaction that can occur within seconds of contact with the allergen, marked by very low blood pressure and breathing difficulties.

anemia. A condition in which the bloodstream cannot carry enough oxygen to meet the needs of the body's tissues.

angina. A spasmodic, choking, or suffocating pain caused by a reduction in the heart muscle's supply of oxygen.

angiogenesis. The development of blood vessels that provide oxygen and nutrients to a tissue, healthy or malignant.

antibiotic. An agent that acts against bacteria.

antibody. A protein, created by the immune system, designed to react to a specific microorganism or other foreign matter.

antigen. A foreign substance that triggers the body to produce antibodies.

antihistamine. An agent that opposes the action of histamine. (*See* histamine.)

antioxidant. Substance that protects cells against the effects of free radicals. Free radicals can damage cells, and may play a role in heart disease, cancer, and other diseases. Some antioxidants are beta-carotene, lutein, lycopene, selenium, and vitamins A, C, and E.

aromatase. An enzyme involved in regulating sex hormone balances.

arrhythmia. Any deviation from the heartbeat's normal rhythm.

arteriosclerosis. A stiffening and thickening of the walls of arteries caused by cholesterol or calcium deposits.

artery. A blood vessel that carries blood away from the heart and toward the rest of the body's tissues.

ascites. The accumulation of fluid in the abdominal cavity, usually caused by liver disease.

astringent. An agent that causes contraction, especially after being applied to the skin.

atherosclerosis. A common form of arteriosclerosis in which fatty deposits form within the inner linings of arteries.

autoimmune disease. A condition in which the immune system attacks the body's own tissues. Examples include lupus, multiple sclerosis, and rheumatoid arthritis.

ayurvedic medicine. Also called ayurveda, it is one of the world's oldest medical systems. It originated in India and has evolved there over thousands of years. Ayurvedic medicine utilizes diet, detoxification, and purification techniques, herbal and mineral remedies, yoga, breathing exercises, meditation, and massage therapy as holistic healing methods.

B cell. An immune-system cell that creates antibodies. (*See* antibody.)

bacteria. Single-celled microbes. Some bacteria can cause disease, while others, known as "friendly" bacteria, help the body by aiding digestion and protecting against harmful organisms.

basic fibroblast growth factor (bFGF). A hormone that stimulates the growth of blood vessels.

benign. Pertaining to cells or tumors that are not cancerous.

bFGF. Basic fibroblast growth factor.

bile. A yellowish secretion, created in the liver, that is released into the small intestine to aid in fat digestion.

biopsy. Removal of tissue for diagnostic purposes.

blood-brain barrier. A protective feature, involving capillary walls and other cells, that permits the entry of only certain substances into the brain.

blood lipids. Lipids (fats) are needed by the body to build cell membranes, make certain hormones, and store energy. Cholesterol and triglycerides are the main types of lipids measured in routine blood tests.

candidiasis. Infection with the yeast *Candida*, especially *Candida albicans*.

capillaries. Tiny blood vessels that link arteries with veins, and through which nutrients and wastes pass to and from the body's cells.

carcinoma. A cancer that arises from the cells, called epithelial cells, that line the body inside and out.

cardiac. Pertaining to the heart. Also, pertaining to the stomach area adjacent to the esophagus.

cell line study. A study performed in a laboratory on human or animal cells from a specific part of the body such as liver cells. Many drugs and herbs are tested in this manner before being tested in a clinical study. This way a scientist will get some idea of how the drug or herb will perform in the human body.

cervical dysplasia. Abnormal cell growth on the cervix that may lead to cervical cancer.

chemotherapy. The use of drugs to treat disease, especially drug therapy for cancer.

cholagogue. A substance that stimulates the production of bile.

cholecystitis. Inflammation of the gallbladder.

cholesterol. A waxy substance used by the body for a number of purposes, including the creation of cell membranes and hormones. Most, approximately 85 percent, of the body's cholesterol supply is made in the liver, with the rest being obtained from food.

chronic illness. An illness that recurs or persists for an extended period of time.

chyme. Undigested food in the stomach.

cirrhosis. Liver disease marked by the development of scar tissue and nodules, which eventually leads to loss of liver function.

climacteric. A period of transition from fertility to menopause in which production of estrogen, the main female hormone, diminishes. Also called perimenopause.

collagen. A gelatinous protein found in connective tissue.

complication. A secondary problem that arises as the result of the initial illness, and that tends to make recovery longer and/or more difficult.

compress. A cloth used to apply heat, cold, or drugs to the body's surface.

constipation. A condition in which bowel movements are infrequent or difficult.

cortisol. A hormone produced in response to stress.

costochondritis. Inflammation of the cartilage attached to a rib.

Crohn's disease. A chronic inflammatory disease that leads to ulceration, anywhere from the mouth to the anus.

cystitis. Inflammation of the bladder.

decoction. Liquid medicine made with boiled extracts of water-soluble substances.

dehydroepiandrosterone (DHEA). One of the most abundant hormones in the bloodstream. It is converted by the body into sex hormones.

dementia. A breakdown of mental function, marked by personality changes and decline in the ability to speak, remember, think, and/or orient oneself to the outside world.

dermatitis. Inflammation of the skin.

DGL. Deglycyrrhizinated licorice.

DHEA. *See* dehydroepiandrosterone.

diarrhea. A condition in which bowel movements are more frequent or contain more fluid than normal.

diastolic pressure. The blood pressure exerted between heartbeats.

differentiation. Process of the life of a cell. All cells develop and mature to be able to have a distinct useful function in the body.

diuretic. An agent that increases urine output.

dopamine. A substance created by the body that serves as a neurotransmitter. (*See* neurotransmitter.)

duodenal. Pertaining to the first portion of the intestine just after the stomach.

dysentery. Inflammation of the large intestine marked by bloody diarrhea and cramps.

dysmenorrhea. Difficult or painful menstruation.

EBV. *See* Epstein-Barr virus.

edema. Swelling caused by fluid retention.

EFA. *See* essential fatty acid.

ejection fraction. Amount of blood pumped by the heart into circulation with each heartbeat.

electrolyte. A substance, such as calcium and other minerals, that can conduct electrical impulses when dissolved in body fluids. Usually associated with maintenance of the body's fluid balance.

enzyme p450. A liver enzyme necessary for the activation of many chemicals, including some cancer treatment drugs. Inappropriate p450 activity can lead to the development of toxins that damage liver tissue.

epididymitis. Inflammation of the ducts through which sperm leave the testes.

epinephrine. A stimulant hormone that increases the rate and force of the heartbeat, quickens the breathing, causes the liver to break down its energy stores for immediate use, and serves as a neurotransmitter. (*See* neurotransmitter.) Also known as adrenaline.

Epstein-Barr virus (EBV). A virus responsible for infectious mononucleosis (a disease marked by fatigue, sore throat, and swollen glands) and linked to a number of other disorders.

essential fatty acid (EFA). A fatty acid that is required by the body, but which the body cannot create itself. There are two types of EFAs, omega-3s and omega-6s, which must be obtained from food.

essential oil. A volatile substance responsible for the odor or taste of a plant.

estradiol. The most active form of estrogen in the body.

estrogen. The main female hormone, important to both the menstrual cycle and to the development of secondary sex characteristics such as breast growth.

expectorant. An agent that promotes the elimination of mucus from the respiratory tract.

extract (herbal). Liquid extracts are made of active herbal ingredients dissolved in a liquid (usually water, alcohol, or glycerol). Liquid extracts are more concentrated than tinctures and are typically a 1:1 concentration.

exudate. Fluid expelled through the skin.

fibrin. A protein-based substance that forms strands on which new blood vessels may grow.

flatulence. The presence of an abnormally large amount of gas in the stomach and intestines.

flavonoid. Any of a large group of crystalline compounds found in plants. Although not technically vitamins, flavonoids are labeled as vitamin P. They enhance vitamin C's functions by protecting it from oxidation and improving how vitamin C is absorbed.

follicle-stimulating hormone (FSH). A hormone that allows eggs to "mature" within the ovary.

free radical. An unstable molecule produced during the body's use of oxygen. Such a molecule can damage tissues.

free-radical scavenger. A substance that eliminates free radicals.

frostbite. Localized tissue destruction resulting from exposure to extreme cold.

FSH. *See* follicle-stimulating hormone.

gallstone. A hard, crystal-like structure found in the gallbladder or a bile duct, composed chiefly of cholesterol.

gastric. Pertaining to the stomach.

gastritis. Inflammation of the stomach lining.

gene p53. A gene that stops the multiplication of defective cells.

German Commission E Monographs. In 1978 the German government established an expert committee, the Commission E, to evaluate the safety and efficacy of over 300 herbs and herb combinations sold in Germany. The results were published as official monographs that give the approved uses, contraindications, side effects, dosage, drug interactions, and other therapeutic information essential for the responsible use of herbs and phytomedicines. It has since been translated into English.

gingivitis. Inflammation of the gums.

glomerulonephritis. Inflammation of that portion of the kidney, the glomerulus, which filters wastes from the blood.

glucose. A simple sugar that is one of the body's primary sources of energy.

gluten-free. A gluten-free diet is a diet that excludes foods containing gluten. Gluten is a protein found in wheat (including kamut and spelt), barley, rye, malts, and triticale.

good manufacturing practices (GMP). FDA rules that ensure that all supplements, including herbs, are manufactured in a uniform way and that what appears on the label is what is in the product. This helps to assure safety.

hemorrhage. Abnormal or profuse bleeding.

hepatitis. Inflammation of the liver, usually caused by a virus but sometimes caused by other agents, such as toxins.

hepatotoxic. Poisoning the liver.

herpes. A family of viruses responsible for a number of different disorders, including chickenpox, cold sores, genital herpes, ocular keratitis, and shingles.

histamine. A chemical, produced by the body in response to an allergen, that can cause breathing difficulties and low blood pressure.

HIV. Human immunodeficiency virus.

homeopathy. A whole medical system that was developed in Germany more than 200 years ago. Homeopathy seeks to stimulate the body's ability to heal itself by giving very small doses of highly diluted substances.

hormone. A chemical messenger that regulates bodily functions.

HPV. *See* human papillomavirus.

human papillomavirus (HPV). A virus that causes genital warts and could be a cause of cervical cancer.

hypertension. High blood pressure.

hypertrophy. A general increase in the bulk of a tissue or organ that is not due to a tumor.

hypoglycemia. Low blood sugar.

hypotension. Low blood pressure.

immunity. The ability to resist infection or illness.

immunostimulant. Increasing the ability of the immune system to fight infection.

immunosuppressant. Decreasing the ability of the immune system to fight infection.

immunotherapy. The use of immune-strengthening techniques to fight illness.

incontinence. The inability to hold urine or stool for voluntary excretion.

infection. Invasion of the body by harmful microorganisms such as bacteria, fungi, or viruses.

inflammation. The body's response to irritation or injury, generally involving redness, swelling, and warmth.

insomnia. The inability to sleep.

insulin. A hormone that enables the transport of sugar or fatty acids into most of the body's cells.

insulin resistance. *See* type 2 diabetes.

insulinlike growth factor I. A hormone secreted by the liver in response to growth hormone that regulates normal physiology.

intercostal. Pertaining to the spaces between the ribs.

interferon. Any of a family of protein compounds that slow the course of viral infection.

interleukin. Any of a family of proteins that stimulate the immune system, including to produce B cells and T cells. (*See* B cell, T cell.)

intermittent claudication. A condition caused by interrupted blood supply to the muscles, chiefly the calf muscles. It is marked by attacks of lameness and pain.

intramuscular. Refers to injections given into muscle tissue.

isoflavones. A class of phytochemicals that have weak estrogen-like effects; their use should be discussed with a doctor in patients with estrogen-based cancers such as breast cancer or those at risk for them. They have been shown to offer mild protection for the bones and heart.

jaundice. A yellowish staining of the skin, eyes, and mucous membranes, caused by too much bile pigment (bilirubin) in the blood.

keratitis. Inflammation of the cornea.

ketoacidosis. Acidification of the blood, generally caused by diabetes.

LAK cell. *See* lymphokine-activated killer cell.

laxative. An agent that loosens the bowels.

leaky gut syndrome. A condition in which the intestinal walls allow relatively large food particles or bacteria to pass into the bloodstream.

leukocyte. *See* white blood cell.

leukopenia. Low white blood cell count.

LH. *See* luteinizing hormone.

lipid peroxides. Harmful substances that break down fats.

lipoprotein. A molecule that combines protein and fat, which allows fatty substances to be transported through the watery bloodstream.

luteinizing hormone (LH). A hormone that stimulates the release of eggs from the ovary.

lymph node. One of a number of organs that filter foreign material from lymph, a clear fluid that circulates within the body's tissues. Lymph nodes also create lymphocytes. (*See* lymphocytes.)

lymphocyte. Any of a group of white blood cells with specialized immune functions, such as B cells and T cells. (*See* B cell, T cell.)

lymphokine-activated killer (LAK) cell. A hormonally activated immune cell that uses chemicals to destroy tumor cells.

macrophage. A "germ-eating" immune-system cell.

malignant. Pertaining to cells that are cancerous.

melatonin. An antioxidant hormone that protects damaged cells; also involved in the sleep-wake cycle.

menopause. The termination of menstruation, caused by decreases in the levels of estrogen and progesterone.

menorrhagia. Abnormally heavy menstrual periods.

metastatic. Pertaining to cancer that has spread from the site where it first developed.

mucous membrane. Any of the membranes that line those moist parts of the body in contact with air, such as the anus, mouth, nasal passages, and vagina.

myasthenia gravis. A condition in which the immune system attacks the connection between nerves and muscles, especially the muscles around the eyes and the lungs.

myeloma. A tumor composed of the blood-producing cells in the bone marrow.

myoma. A benign growth composed of muscle tissue.

natural killer (NK) cell. An immune-system cell, activated by antibodies, that secretes chemicals to destroy cancer cells and infectious microbes.

neuralgia. Severe, throbbing, or stabbing pain along the course of a nerve.

neuropathy. Damage to nerve tissue.

neurotransmitter. A substance that relays impulses from one nerve cell to another.

neutraceutical. Naturally occurring food chemical used to benefit health when extracted and isolated and taken as a supplement.

NK cell. *See* natural killer cell.

norepinephrine. A stimulant hormone produced in response to low blood pressure and physical stress. Also serves as a neurotransmitter. (*See* neurotransmitter.)

onset of action. Time required for a drug or herb to take effect.

orchitis. Inflammation of the testes.

orifice. A term for a body opening and, in Oriental medicine, any of the sense organs in the head.

osteomyelitis. Inflammation of the bone.

osteoporosis. A thinning and weakening of the bones, caused by the loss of minerals from bone tissue.

PAF. *See* platelet-activating factor.

parasite. An organism that lives on or in, and obtains nourishment from, another organism.

pathogen. A disease-causing entity.

peritoneum. The membrane lining the abdominal cavity.

pernicious anemia. Anemia caused by vitamin B_{12} deficiency, marked by red blood cells that are very large.

pharyngitis. Inflammation of the pharynx, the upper portion of the digestive tube from the esophagus to the mouth and nasal cavities.

pinnate. Pin shaped.

placebo. An inactive substance used in research to provide a basis for comparison with an active substance.

plaque. A deposit of undesired material on tissue, such as the buildup of plaque in arteries that leads to atherosclerosis.

plasmin. A substance that breaks up clots.

platelet-activating factor (PAF). A substance that causes red blood cells to clump together. This starts a process that could lead to allergic and asthmatic reactions.

PMS. *See* premenstrual syndrome.

polycystic ovarian disease. A condition in which the ovaries contain many cysts, and high levels of male hormones are present.

poultice. A soft mush prepared by wetting powders or other absorbent substances with oils or water. The mush is then placed in a cloth and applied to the skin.

premenstrual syndrome (PMS). Term for a variety of symptoms that may be experienced a week or two before the start of menstruation, including acne, backache, breast tenderness, irritability, mood swings, and water retention.

progesterone. A female sex hormone that acts in concert with estrogen to control the menstrual cycle.

prolactin. A hormone that starts and maintains milk flow.

prolapse. The sinking or falling of an organ or other body part, especially at its orifice.

prostaglandin. Any of a class of proteins present in many tissues. These substances regulate bodily processes such as blood pressure, inflammation reaction, and smooth-muscle contraction in the windpipe, intestines, and uterus.

pulmonary. Pertaining to the lungs.

purgative. An agent that empties the bowels by encouraging defecation.

purpura. Purple discoloration of the skin, caused by bleeding.

radiation therapy. The use of radiation to treat disease, especially when used to treat cancer.

randomized study. A study in which people are allocated at random (by chance alone) to receive one of several clinical interventions. One of these interventions is the standard of comparison or control. The control may be a standard practice, a placebo ("sugar pill"), or no intervention at all.

receptor site. A site on a cell that accepts a specific substance, such as an estrogen receptor site on a breast cell.

red blood cell. A cell that contains hemoglobin, a substance that carries oxygen through the bloodstream.

reflux. Upward flow of substances that should normally flow downward, such as stomach acid backing up into the esophagus.

remission. The reduction or reversal of symptoms in chronic disease, such as cancer or multiple sclerosis.

renal. Pertaining to the kidneys.

restenosis. Closure of arteries after angioplasty.

reverse transcriptase. An enzyme that allows HIV and similar viruses to insert their genetic information into the DNA of a human cell, causing the cell to produce more viruses.

Reye's syndrome. A condition that can follow viral infection. It involves brain inflammation and fatty-tissue invasion of the internal organs. In children it can be caused by aspirin intake.

rhinovirus. A family of viruses that cause colds.

sarcoma. A cancer of the connective tissue.

sedative. An agent that quiets nervous excitement.

serotonin. A hormone that influences a number of bodily functions, including digestion, respiration, and blood pressure maintenance. Also serves as a neurotransmitter. (*See* neurotransmitter.)

shingles. An infection with the herpes varicella-zoster virus, marked by painful blisters that follow the course of a nerve.

sign. An indication of disease that is not necessarily noticeable to the patient, but that is noticeable to the examiner.

Sjögren's syndrome. A condition in which the immune system attacks the body's moisture-producing glands. It is marked by dryness of the eyes and mouth.

sleep latency. Time required to fall asleep.

spasm. Involuntary contraction of one or more muscle groups.

sperm motility. A sperm cell's ability to move through the female reproductive tract.

spermatorrhea. Any condition involving the involuntary release of sperm.

stomatitis. Inflammation of the mouth.

symptom. An indication of disease that is noticeable to the patient.

systolic pressure. The blood pressure exerted during heartbeats.

T cell. Any of a group of immune-system cells. Helper T cells coordinate the immune response against infectious microbes and cancerous cells, enabling the body to defend itself, while suppressor T cells suppress the immune response, preventing the immune system from attacking the body itself.

tachycardia. Excessively rapid heart rate.

tachyphylaxis. A condition without addiction but in which larger and larger doses of a drug or herb must be taken to get the same effect.

tea. An infusion made by simmering plant material in water.

testosterone. The main male hormone, important to proper sexual function, fertility, and the development of such secondary sex characteristics as facial hair.

therapeutic range. Range from lowest effective dosage to greatest nontoxic dosage of an herb or medication.

thrush. An infection by the fungus *Candida albicans* of the mouth and throat, as shown by white spots on the tongue and insides of the cheeks.

TIA. *See* transient ischemic attack.

tincture. An alcohol solution prepared from herbal materials.

tinnitus. A ringing or roaring in the ear in the absence of any actual sound.

TNF. *See* tumor necrosis factor.

tonic. An agent designed to restore enfeebled function and to promote vigor and a sense of well-being.

tonifying. Promoting vigor in an organ system.

topical. Pertaining to the surface of the body.

toxin. A poison that impairs bodily health; in Oriental medicine, pathogenic energy.

transient ischemic attack (TIA). A brief (lasting anywhere from several minutes to two hours) disruption in brain function caused by a temporary interruption in the brain's oxygen supply. It may produce momentary dizziness or any of the symptoms associated with a stroke, such as slurred speech, paralysis, or vision problems.

trigeminal. Pertaining to the nerves that enable facial sensation and movement.

triglycerides. The primary form in which fat is both found in food and stored in the body.

tumor necrosis factor (TNF). A substance produced by the immune system that can kill cancer cells.

type 1 diabetes. A form of diabetes in which the body cannot produce enough insulin to meet its needs. It used to be called insulin-dependent or juvenile-onset diabetes.

type 2 diabetes. A form of diabetes in which the body produces enough insulin, or sometimes too much, but cannot use that insulin properly (insulin resistance). It used to be called non-insulin-dependent or adult-onset diabetes.

ulcer. A lesion on the skin or a mucous membrane.

uveitis. Inflammation of the uveal tract, the vascular system of the eye.

vascular. Pertaining to the blood vessels.

vein. A blood vessel that carries blood away from the body's tissues and toward the heart.

vertigo. Faintness, dizziness, or inability to maintain one's balance.

viral load. Measurement of the total number of viruses in circulation.

virus. Any of a group of tiny disease-causing entities with very simple structures. They cannot reproduce on their own, and so must take over cells within the host organism to do so.

vitiligo. Appearance of nonpigmented patches on otherwise normal skin.

volatile oils. Easily evaporated taste- and aroma-imparting compounds found in plants.

white blood cell. An immune-system cell that destroys invading organisms along with infected or damaged cells. Also known as a leukocyte.

yeast. Any of a group of single-celled fungi. Some yeasts, such as *Candida albicans*, can cause infection.

Appendix B: Resources

This appendix provides information on where to find herbal services and products. Product names and their distributors change frequently. Some of the sources and addresses here may have changed since they were listed in this book. For up-to-date product and vendor listings for the herbs listed in this book, look online for the manufacturers or herbal organizations that we list in the appendices. Also, many big box stores (such as Walmart) and pharmacies sell a wide range of herbal products.

HERBAL AND OTHER ALTERNATIVE HEALTH SERVICES

Acupressure Institute
1533 Shattuck Avenue
Berkeley, CA 94709
800-442-2232
510-845-1059
www.acupressureinstitute.com

American Association of Acupuncture and Oriental Medicine (AAAOM)
P.O. Box 96503 PMB 93504
Washington, DC 20090-6503
866-455-7999
www.aaaomonline.org
Maintains a list of over 10,000 licensed professionals who provide traditional Chinese herbal formulas, acupuncture, and tui nei massage.

American Association of Naturopathic Physicians
4435 Wisconsin Avenue, NW, Suite 403
Washington, DC 20016
866-538-2267
202-237-8150
www.naturopathic.org
Naturopathic physicians are extensively trained in the use of herbs and nutrition in the treatment of disease. The American Association of Naturopathic Physicians provides referrals to a nationwide network of licensed practitioners.

American Botanical Council
6200 Manor Road
Austin, TX 78723
512-926-4900
www.herbalgram.org
The American Botanical Council provides specialized publications and current information about developments in herbal medicine through its publication, Herbalgram.

American Chiropractic Association
1701 Clarendon Boulevard
Arlington, VA 22209
703-276-8800
www.acatoday.org

American Herb Association
P.O. Box 1673
Nevada City, CA 95959
530-265-9552
www.ahaherb.com
Provides information about herbs and herbal products.

American Herbal Pharmacopoeia
P.O. Box 66809
Scotts Valley, CA 95067
831-461-6318
Fax: 831-475-6219
www.herbal-ahp.org

American Herbal Products Association
8630 Fenton Street, Suite 918
Silver Spring, MD 20910
301-588-1171
www.ahpa.org

American Holistic Medical Association
23366 Commerce Park, Suite 101B
Beachwood, OH 44122
216-292-6644
Fax: 216-292-6688
www.holisticmedicine.org

American Institute of Holistic Theology
2112 Eleventh Avenue South, Suite 520
Birmingham, AL 35205-2841
800-650-4325
www.aiht.edu
Provides instruction in a variety of natural approaches to health care and maintenance.

American Massage Therapy Association
500 Davis Street
Evanston, IL 60201
877-905-0577
847-864-0123
Fax: 847-864-5196
www.amtamassage.org
Can assist you in locating a qualified massage therapist in your area.

American Reflexology Certification Board
P.O. Box 141553
Grand Rapids, MI 49514
303-933-6921
Fax: 303-904-0460
www.arcb.net
Can provide information on programs for learning this technique.

Association for Applied Psychophysiology and Biofeedback
10200 West 44th Avenue, Suite 304
Wheat Ridge, CO 80033
800-477-8892
303-422-8436
www.aapb.org
Provides information about behavior modification by biofeedback.

Charlie Foundation to Help Cure Pediatric Epilepsy
1223 Wilshire Blv., Box 815
Santa Monica, CA 90403
310-393-2347
www.charliefoundation.org
Offers information on curing pediatric epilepsy through the ketogenic diet.

Homeopathic Academy of Naturopathic Physicians
1607 Siskiyou Boulevard
Ashland, OR 97520
541-840-2422
Fax: 815-301-6595
www.hanp.net

International Academy of Compounding Pharmacists (IACP)
4638 Riverstone Boulevard
Missouri City, TX 77459
800-927-4227
281-933-8400
Fax: 281-495-0602
www.iacprx.org
Can help you to find a compounding pharmacist in your area.

National Association for Holistic Aromatherapy
P.O. Box 1868
Banner Elk, NC 28604
828-898-6161
www.naha.org
Provides information on aromatherapy.

National Ayurvedic Medical Association
620 Cabrillo Avenue
Santa Cruz, CA 95065
800-669-8914
505-323-2838
www.ayurveda-nama.org

National Center for Complimentary and Alternative Medicine (NCCAM)
National Institutes of Health
9000 Rockville Pike
Bethesda, MD 20892
www.nccam.nih.gov
Provides information on complementary and alternative medicine and clinical trials for supplements.

National Certification Commission for Acupuncture and Oriental Medicine (NCCAOM)
76 South Laura Street, Suite 1290
Jacksonville, FL 32202
904-598-1005
www.nccaom.org

National Vitiligo Foundation
P.O. Box 23226
Cincinnati, OH 45223
513-541-3903
www.nvfi.org

Natural Healing Institute
543 Encinitas Boulevard, Suites 105–108
Encinitas, CA 92024-2930
760-943-8485
www.naturalhealinginst.com
Offers license and certificate programs in naturopathic medicine, holistic health, nutrition, herbology, and massage.

Rolf Institute of Structural Integration
5055 Chaparral Court, Suite 103
Boulder, CO 80301
800-530-8875
303-449-5903
www.rolf.org
Provides information on the Rolfing method of massage.

United States Pharmacopeia
12601 Twinbrook Parkway
Rockville, MD 20852-1790
800-227-8772
301-881-0666
www.usp.org/aboutusp/contactus.html

MARKETERS OF HERBAL PRODUCTS

AkPharma, Inc.
P.O. Box 111
Pleasantville, NJ 08232
800-994-4711
609-645-5100
www.akpharma.com
Beano, Lactaid.

Allovedic Remedies
American Formulary, Inc.
140 Ethel Road West, Suite S-T
Piscataway, NJ 08854
732-985-9899
www.americanformulary.com
Herbal dietary supplements.

Ayush Herbs Inc.
2239 152nd Avenue NE
Redmond, WA 98052
800-925-1371
425-637-1400
Fax: 425-451-2670
www.ayush.com
Ayurvedic herbal extracts and finished products.

The Backstore
VitalityWeb.com, Inc.
13820 Stowe Drive
San Diego (Poway), CA 92064-8800
800-796-9656
858-218-1320
www.thebackstore.com
Home TENS units.

BioHerb, Inc.
Saintech International, Inc.
1584 Kensington Road
San Marino, CA 91108
800-978-8323
Fax: 626-449-4515
www.bioherbusa.com

Blue Light, Inc.
530 West State Street
Ithaca, NY 14850
888-258-3548
Fax: 888-666-9888
www.treasureofeast.com
Freeze-dried herbal concentrates

Body Dynamics, Inc.
2034 Statler Drive
Carrollton, TX 75007
972-245-5500
Fax: 972-245-5522
www.bodydynamics.com
Herbal, vitamin, and skin-care formulas.

Botanical Laboratories, Inc.
1441 West Smith Road
Ferndale, WA 98248
800-232-4005
360-384-5656
www.botlab.com

Brion Herbs Corporation
9200 Jeronimo Road
Irvine, CA 92618
800-333-4372
949-587-1238
Fax: 800-557-1260
www.brionherbs.com

Cayenne Company, Inc.
2235 East 38th Street
Minneapolis, MN 55407-3083
800-229-3663
612-724-5266
www.cayennecompany.com
Cayenne products, including Heart Food Caps, Power Caps, Power Plus.

CC Pollen Company
3627 East Indian School Road, Suite 209
Phoenix, AZ 85018
800-875-0096
602-957-0096
www.ccpollen.com
Bee products: Aller Bee-Gone, bee pollen, bee propolis, royal jelly products.

Cellulite USA
www.celluliteusa.com
Provides information about Endermologie and assists in locating practitioners.

Country Life
180 Vanderbilt Motor Parkway
Hauppauge, NY 11788
800-645-5768
www.country-life.com
Herbal products, vitamin and mineral supplements, and amino acids made from natural raw materials.

Crane Herb Company (sells to licensed practitioners only)
745 Falmouth Road
Mashpee, MA 02649
Fax: 508-539-1700
www.craneherb.com
Herbs, formulas.

Cyvex Nutrition
1851 Kaiser Avenue
Irvine, CA 92614
949-622-9030
Fax: 949-622-9033
www.cyvex.com
Bulk nutraceutical ingredients: BioVin grapeseed extract, BioVinca, Vinpocetine.

East Earth Trade Winds
P.O. Box 493151
Redding, CA 96049-3151
800-258-6878 (orders)
530-226-6161 (information)
Fax: 800-258-6878
http://eastearthtrade.com
Herbs, ready-made formula teas, patent medicines.

Eclectic Institute
36350 Southeast Industrial Way
Sandy, OR 97055
800-332-4372
www.eclecticherb.com
Freeze-dried botanicals, organic herbs, herbal extracts, nutritional supplements.

EcoNugenics, Inc.
2208 Northpoint Parkway
Santa Rosa, CA 95407
800-308-5518
707-521-3370
www.econugenics.com
Padma Basic and other herbal supplements.

Emerson Ecologies
7 Commerce Drive
Bedford, NH 03110
800-654-4432
www.emersonecologies.com

Energique, Inc.
201 Apple Boulevard
Woodbine, IA 51579
800-869-8078
Fax: 800-503-2588
www.energiqueherbal.com
Liquefied herbal extracts, available on a private-label basis.

Essiac Canada International
3551 St. Charles
No. 241
Kirkland, Quebec
Canada H9H 3C4
888-900-2299
Fax: 514-695-2287
www.essiac-canada-intl.com

FoodScience of Vermont
20 New England Drive
Essex Junction, VT 0545
800-874-9444
Fax: 802-878-0549
www.foodscienceofvermont.com
Aangamik DMG, multivitamins, herbals (liquids, capsules, tablets), supplements for seniors.

Fountain of Youth Technologies
P.O. Box 608
Millersport, OH 43046
800-939-4296
www.foytech.com
Doctor's Growth Hormone.

Gaia Herbs, Inc.
101 Gaia Herbs Drive
Brevard, NC 28712
800-831-7780
www.gaiaherbs.com
Liquid herbal extracts and gel caps, saw palmetto.

Garden of Life
5500 Village Boulevard, Suite 202
West Palm Beach, FL 33407
866-465-0051
www.gardenoflife.com

Ginco International
725 Cochran Street, Unit C
Simi Valley, CA 93065
800-284-2598
805-520-2592
www.gincointernational.com
Herbal supplements, Acu-Life Massage sandals, royal jelly, bee pollen.

Golden Flower Chinese Herbs
2724 Vassar Place NE
Albuquerque, NM 87107
800-729-8509
505-837-2040
Fax: 866-298-7541; 505-837-2052
www.gfcherbs.com

Health From The Sun
1 Clock Tower Place, Suite 100
Maynard, MA 01754
800-447-2249
www.healthfromthesun.com

Herb Pharm
P.O. Box 116
Williams, Oregon 97544
800-545-7392
541-846-6262
www.herb-pharm.com

The Herbal Apothecary
P.O. Box 598
Graton, CA 95444
707-829-4704
http://herbalapothecaryonline.com

HerbaSway
101 N. Plains Industrial Road
Wallingford, CT 06492-4048
800-672-7322
www.herbasway.com
Liquid herbal concentrates.

Herbs, Etc.
1345 Cerrillos Road
Santa Fe, NM 87505
888-694-3727
505-982-1265
www.herbsetc.com
Alcohol-free herbal extracts, including Deep Health, Deep Sleep, Lung Tonic, Singer's Saving Grace.

Herbs for Kids
1441 West Smith Road
Ferndale, WA 98248-5935
800-258-4463
www.herbsforkids.com
Alcohol-free organic herbal extracts.

Himalaya Herbal Healthcare
10440 Westoffice Drive
Houston, TX 77042
800-869-4640
713-863-1622
www.himalayausa.com
GastriCare, GlucoCare, HeartCare, ImmunoCare, JointCare, LaxaCare, LeanCare, LiverCare, MindCare, ProstaCare, StressCare, UriCare, VeinCare, VigorCare.

Hyland's, Inc.
210 West 131st Street
Los Angeles, CA 90061
800-624-9659
310-768-0700
www.hylands.com
Homeopathic products, Calms Forte tablets, Nerve Tonic.

Irwin Naturals
5310 Beethoven Street
Los Angeles, CA 90066
800-297-3273
310-306-3636
www.irwinnaturals.com

Jarrow Formulas
1824 South Roberson Boulevard
Los Angeles, CA 90035
310-204-6936
www.jarrow.com

JHS Natural Products
P.O. Box 23936
Eugene, OR 97402
888-330-4691
541-344-1396
Fax: 541-344-3107
www.jhsnp.com
PSK.

KPC Herbs, Inc.
16 Goddard
Irvine, CA 92618
800-572-8188 (orders)
949-727-4000
Fax: 949-727-3577
www.kpc.com
KPC herbal formulas for southern California and southwestern states.

Lactaid
McNeill Consumer Products Company
7050 Camp Hill Road
Fort Washington, PA 19034-2299
800-522-8243
215-233-7000
www.lactaid.com
Lactaid.

Lalilab, Inc.
1415 Hamlin Road
Durham, NC 27704
800-639-3436
919-620-6767
Fax: 919-620-9575
www.lalilab.com
Botanical extracts.

LaneLabs-USA, Inc.
3 North Street
Waldwick, NJ 07463
201-661-6000
Fax: 201-661-6001
www.lanelabs.com

Lily of the Desert
1887 Geesling Road
Denton, TX 76208
800-229-5459
940-566-9914
Fax: 940-566-9915
www.lilyofthedesert.com
Aloe vera products.

Long Life Teas (*See* Country Life)

Mushroom Wisdom, Inc.
1 Madison Street, Suite F6
East Rutherford, NJ 07073
800-747-7418
973-470-0010 (international)
www.maitake.com
Grifron Maitake caplets, Grifron Maitake D-fraction, Mai Green Tea, Prost-Mate.

Maypro Industries
2975 Westchester Avenue
Purchase, NY 10577
914-251-0701
www.maypro.com

Mayway Trading Corporation
1338 Mandela Parkway
Oakland, CA 94607
510-208-3113
510-208-3069
www.mayway.com
Only sells its products to health-care practitioners, health-related businesses, and students of traditional Chinese medicine.

MedicAlert
MedicAlert Foundation
2323 Colorado Avenue
Turlock, CA 95382
888-633-4298
www.medicalert.org
Provides bracelets that warn about serious chronic medical conditions such as severe allergies, diabetes, and epilepsy.

Metagenics
100 Avenue La Pata
San Clemente, CA 92673
800-692-9400
949-366-0818
www.metagenics.com
UltraBalance products.

Michael's Naturopathic Programs
6003 Randolf Blvd.
San Antonio, TX 78233
800-845-2730
www.michaelshealth.com
Herbal product manufacturer and distributor.

NatraBio
A Division of Nutraceutical International Corporation
P.O. Box 5935
Bellingham, WA 98227-5935
800-260-5514
360-384-5656
www.natrabio.com
Homeopathic remedies: Adrenal Support; Acne Relief; Allergy Relief formulas.

Naturade, Inc.
A division of NNC LLC
1 City West Boulevard, Suite 1440
Orange, CA 92868
800-421-1830
Fax: 714-935-9837
www.naturade.com

Natural-Immunogenics Corporation
3265 West McNab Road
Pompano Beach, FL 33069
888-328-8840
Fax: 954-979-0838
www.natural-immunogenics.com
Sovereign Silver 10ppm colloidal silver.

Nature's Answer
85 Commerce Drive
Hauppauge, NY 11788
800-439-2324
631-231-7492
www.naturesanswer.com

Nature's Best, Inc.
195 Engineers Road
Hauppauge, NY 11788
800-345-2378
631-232-3355
www.naturesbest.com

Nature's Plus
548 Broadhollow Road
Melville, NY 11747
800-645-9500
www.naturesplus.com
Herbal products.

Nature's Way Products, Inc.
Customer Service Department
3051 West Maple Loop Dr., Suite 125
Lehi, UT 84043
800-962-8873
www.naturesway.com
Herbal supplements.

Nordic Naturals
111 Jennings Drive
Watsonville, CA 95076
800-662-2544
Fax: 831-724-6200
www.nordicnaturals.com
Essential fatty acids; Children's DHA; EPA; Ultimate Omega.

North American Herb and Spice
P.O. Box 4885
Buffalo Grove, IL 60089
800-243-5242
847-473-4700
www.oreganol.com
Oreganol P73, Oregamax, oil of rosemary.

North American Medicinal Mushroom Extracts
Box 1780
Gibsons, BC
Canada, V0N 1V0
604-886-7799
www.nammex.com
Cordyceps, maitake, reishi, shiitake.

Nuherbs
3820 Penniman Avenue
Oakland, CA 94619-1759
800-233-4307
510-534-4372
Fax: 510-534-4384
www.nuherbs.com
Chinese patent medicines. Only sells its products to health-care practitioners.

Nutraceutical Corporation
1400 Kearns Boulevard
Park City, UT 84060
800-669-8877
www.nutraceutical.com
Bioallers, Herbs for Kids, KAL, Natrabio, Nature's Life, Natural Balance brands, Solray, Zand products, including L-5-HTP, Kidney Blend SP-6, Heart Blend SP-8, Nerve Blend SP-14.

Optimum Nutrition, Inc.
600 North Commerce Street
Aurora, IL 60504
630-236-0097
www.optimumnutrition.com
Herbs, sports drinks, protein powders.

Phapros/Argomed
Denpasar Raya Kav D3
Mega Kuningan
South Jakarta, DKI Jakarta, 12950
Indonesia
62-21-5276263
Fax: 62-21-5209381
www.ptphapros.fuzing.com
Food supplements, herbal medicines.

Pines International, Inc.
1992 East 1400 Road
Lawrence, KS 66044
800-697-4637
Fax: 785-841-1252
www.wheatgrass.com
Wheatgrass, barley grass, alfalfa, beet-juice powder, and green-foods supplements.

Planetary Herbals
P.O. Box 1760
Soquel, CA 95073
800-606-6226
831-438-1700
www.planetaryherbals.com
Horse chestnut cream, triphala. Chinese herbs and ayurvedic preparations.

Prince of Peace Enterprises, Inc.
3536 Arden Road
Hayward, CA 94545
510-887-1899
Fax: 510-887-1799
www.popus.com
Ginseng, nutritional supplements.

Puritan's Pride
1233 Montauk Highway
Oakdale, NY 11769-9001
800-645-1030
www.puritan.com
Vitamin, mineral, and herbal supplements.

Qualiherb Online
116 Pleasant Street, Suite 328
Easthampton, MA 01027
413-282-1001
Fax: 413-282-1099
www.qualiherb.net
Chinese herbs. Only sells its products to health-care practitioners.

Raintree Nutrition, Inc.
3579 Hwy 50 East, Suite 222
Carson City, NV 89701
www.rain-tree.com
Herbal combination formulas.

Rich Nature Labs, Inc.
9700 Harbour Place, Suite 128
Mukilteo, WA 98275
888-708-8127
Fax: 425-493-1803
www.richnature.com
Herbal remedies, formulas, and raw materials.

Solaray. *See* **Nutraceutical Corporation.**

Solgar, Inc.
500 Willow Tree Road
Leonia, NJ 07605
201-944-2311
Fax: 201-944-7351
www.solgar.com

Source Naturals
23 Janis Way
Scotts Valley, CA 95066
800-815-2333
831-438-1144
Fax: 831-438-7410
www.sourcenaturals.com
Herbs.

Spring Wind Herbs Company
2325 Fourth Street, Suite 6
Berkeley, CA 94710
800-588-4883 (orders)
510-849-1820 (information)
Fax: 510-849-4886
www.springwind.com

Sundown Naturals
110 Orville Drive
Bohemia, NY 11716
888-848-2435
www.sundownnaturals.com

Superior Trading Company
835 Washington Street
San Francisco, CA 94108
415-495-7988
Fax: 415-495-7990
www.superiortrading.com
Ginseng products.

Taiyo International
5960 Golden Hills Drive
Minneapolis, MN 55416
763-398-3003
Fax: 763-398-3007
www.taiyointernational.com
Green tea extracts.

Traditional Medicinals
4515 Ross Road
Sebastopol, CA 95472
800-543-4372
www.traditionalmedicinals.com
Medicinal herbal teas.

Trillium Herbal Company, Inc.
185 East Walnut Street
Sturgeon Bay, WI 54235
920-746-5207
Fax: 920-746-7649
www.trilliumherbal.com
Organic Body ayurvedic aromatherapy blends.

Twinlab Corporation
600 East Quality Drive
American Fork, UT 84003
800-645-5626
www.twinlab.com

Uptown Health Foods
130-22529 Lougheed Highway
Maple Ridge, BC
Canada, V2X OL4
877-467-3698
604-467-5587
www.uptownhealth.com
Herbs.

Växa International
600 North Westshore Boulevard, Suite 800
Tampa, FL 33609
877-622-8292
813-870-2904
Fax: 888-734-4154
www.vaxa.com
Herbs and herbal formulas.

Wakunaga of America
23501 Madero
Mission Viejo, CA 92691
800-421-2998
949-855-2776
www.kyolic.com
Ginko-Go, Kyolic aged garlic extract.

ZAND Herbal Formulas
A Division of Nutraceutical International Corporation
P.O. Box 5935
Bellingham, WA 98227-5935
800-241-0859
www.zand.com

Index

Page numbers in italics refer to illustrations, sidebars, and table heads.

abrasions. *See* cuts, scrapes, and abrasions
acerola, 14–15
acne, 188–90
  aloe and, 18
  arjuna and, 24
  guggul and, 82–83
  lavender and, 93
acorus, 15–16
acupuncture, 489–90
adaptogen, 21, 27, 127, 132
ADD/ADHD, 212–14
  American ginseng and, 21
  avena and, 30
  brahmi and, 36
  chamomile and, 46
  hawthorn and, 84
  oligomeric proanthocyanidins (OPCs) and, 106
  scutellaria and, 129
addiction
  passionflower and, 111
adrenocorticotropic hormone (ACTH), 46, 467
advanced breathing exercises, 497
aescin, 87
aging
  acerola and, 14
agrimony, 16–17
AIDS. *See* HIV/AIDS
alcoholism, 190–91
  kudzu and, 92
  milk thistle and, 100
  reishi and, 122
alfalfa, 17–18
allergic rhinitis. *See under* allergies, respiratory
allergies, 191–96
  bupleurum and, 38
  chamomile and, 46
  chen-pi and, 48
  eucalyptus and, 65
  food, 191–93
  oligomeric proanthocyanidins (OPCs) and, 106
  pollen and, 114
  quercetin and, 119
  respiratory, 193–96
  scutellaria and, 129
aloe, 18–20
alopecia. *See* hair loss
alternative medicine, 5
Alzheimer's disease, 196–98
  ashwagandha and, 27
  brahmi and, 36
  ginkgo biloba and, 74–75
  hawthorn and, 83
  lemon balm and, 94
  oligomeric proanthocyanidins (OPCs) and, 106
  rosemary and, 123–24
amebiasis. *See under* parasitic infection
American ginseng, 20–22
American Herbal Pharmacopeia, 6
andiroba, 22
andrographis, 22–23
anemia, 198–200
angelica, 23
angina, 200–202
  acerola and, 14
  angelica and, 23

arjuna and, 24
astragalus and, 28–29
hawthorn and, 83–84
khella and, 91
anise, 23–24
ankles, swollen, 202–3
  gotu kola and, 80
  horse chestnut and, 87
  oligomeric proanthocyanidins (OPCs) and, 106–7
anthocyanosides, 31–32
anxiety disorder, 203–5
  brahmi and, 36
  California poppy and, 42
  chamomile and, 46
  corydalis and, 56
  ginseng and, 77
  hawthorn and, 84
  kava kava and, 90
  lavender and, 94
  lemon balm and, 94–95
  passionflower and, 111
  scutellaria and, 129
arjuna, 24–25
arnica, 25–26
aromatherapy, 490–91
arrhythmia, cardiac. *See under* congestive
    heart failure
artemisia, 26, *26*
arteriosclerosis. *See* atherosclerosis
arthritis
  andiroba and, 22
  ashwagandha and, 27
  birch and, 33
  boswellia and, 35–36
  burdock and, 39
  cat's claw and, 43
  cayenne and, 45
  chaparral and, 48
  copaiba and, 53–54
  devil's claw and, 59
  ginger and, 73
  osha and, 109
  See also gout; osteoarthritis; rheumatoid
    arthritis
asafoetida, 26–27
ashwagandha, 27–28
asthma, 205–9
  coleus and, 51
  elderberry and, 63
  fennel seed and, 67
  green tea and, 81
  khella and, 91
  quercetin and, 119
astragalus, 28–30
Astragalus Decoction to Construct the Middle, 160
atherosclerosis, 209–11
  alfalfa and, 17
  andrographis and, 22
  astragalus and, 28–29
  dong quai and, 60
  ginger and, 73
  green tea and, 81
  hawthorn and, 84
  khella and, 91
  polysaccharide kureha and, 115

quercetin and, 119
scutellaria and, 129
snow fungus and, 135
athlete's foot, 211–12
attention deficit disorder/attention deficit
    hyperactivity disorder. *See* ADD/ADHD
Augmented Rambling Powder, 160–61
autoimmune disorders
  ashwagandha and, 27
avena, 30
ayurveda, 49
  herbal formulas, 181–84

Bacteriodes, 466
bad breath. *See* halitosis
baldness. *See* hair loss
ballistic stretching, 497
barberry, 30–31
basal cell carcinoma. *See under* skin cancer
bed-wetting, 215–16
  agrimony and, 16
belching. *See under* indigestion
Bell's palsy, 216–17
beneficial herbs
  acne, *188*
  ADD/ADHD, *213*
  AIDS, *350*
  alcoholism, *191*
  allergies, *192*
  Alzheimer's disease, *197*
  anemia, *199*
  angina, *201*
  ankles, swollen, *202*
  anxiety disorder, *203*
  asthma, *206*
  atherosclerosis, *210*
  athlete's foot, *212*
  bed-wetting, *215*
  Bell's palsy, *217*
  benign prostatic hypertrophy, *218*
  bladder cancer, *220*
  bladder infection, *222*
  boil, *224*
  bone cancer, *225*
  breast cancer, *227*
  bronchitis and pneumonia, *231*
  bruising, *233*
  burns, *234*
  bursitis, *235*
  cancer, *237–45*
  canker sores, *246*
  carpal tunnel syndrome, *247*
  cataracts, *249*
  celiac disease, *251*
  cellulite, *252*
  cervical cancer, *253*
  chronic fatigue syndrome, *255*
  cirrhosis of the liver, *258*
  colic, *259*
  colorectal cancer, *261*
  common cold, *263*
  congestive heart failure, *265*
  constipation, *268*
  cough, *270*
  Crohn's disease, *272*

cuts, scrapes, and abrasions, 274
dandruff, 275
depression, 277
diabetes, 281
diabetic retinopathy, 284
diaper rash, 286
diarrhea, 287
dry mouth, 289
ear infection, 291
eczema, 293
emphysema, 295
endometrial cancer, 296
endometriosis, 298
erectile dysfunction, 300
eye problems, 302–5
fibrocystic breasts, 306
fibromyalgia syndrome, 309
food poisoning, 311
fracture, 313
gallstones, 315
gastritis, 317
glaucoma, 319
gonorrhea and chlamydia, 321
gout, 323
hair loss, 324
halitosis, 325
hangover, 327
headache, 328
heart attack, 330
heat stress, 333
hemorrhoids, 334
hepatitis, 337
herpesvirus infection, 339
hiccups, 361
high blood pressure, 341
high cholesterol, 344
HIV/AIDS, 347
hives, 352
Hodgkin's lymphoma, 354
hyperthyroidism, 355
hypothyroidism, 357
indigestion, 358–60
infertility, 362–63
influenza, 365
insect bites, 367
insomnia, 368
intermittent claudication, 370
iron overload, 371
irritable bowel syndrome, 372
kidney cancer, 374
kidney disease, 376
kidney stones, 377
laryngitis, 379
leukemia, 381
liver cancer, 383
lung cancer, 385
lupus, 387
Lyme disease, 389
lymphedema, 391
macular degeneration, 392
mastitis, 393
measles, 394
memory problems, 396
Ménière's disease, 398
menopause-related problems, 399
menstrual problems, 402
migraine, 404
mononucleosis, 406
morning sickness, 407
motion sickness, 408
multiple sclerosis, 409
mumps, 411
muscles, sore, 412
myasthenia gravis, 413
nails, infected, 414
nausea, 415

nosebleed, 416
osteoarthritis, 418
osteoporosis, 420
ovarian cancer, 423
ovarian cyst, 424
overweight, 426
pain, chronic, 428
parasitic infection, 431
Parkinson's disease, 433
pelvic inflammatory disease, 434
peptic ulcer, 435
periodontal disease, 438
premenstrual syndrome, 440
prostate cancer, 442
prostatitis, 445
psoriasis, 447
respiratory allergies, 194
restless legs syndrome, 449
rheumatoid arthritis, 451
ringworm, 453
seizure disorders, 454
sex drive, diminished, 456
shin splints, 458
sinusitis, 458
skin cancer, 460, 462
sprains and strains, 463
stomach cancer, 464
strep throat, 466
stress, 467
stroke, 469
sweating, excessive, 471
syphilis, 472
tinnitus, 474
toothache, 475
tuberculosis, 476
uterine fibroids, 308
vaginosis, 478
varicose veins, 479
vitiligo, 481
vomiting, 482
warts, 483
wrinkles, 484
yeast infection, 486
benign prostatic hypertrophy (BPH), 217–19
    papain and, 110
    pollen and, 114
    pygeum and, 118–19
    saw palmetto and, 126–27
berberine, 79
Bifidobacterium bifidus, 71, 466, 472
bilberry, 31–32
biofeedback, 496
Biota Seed Pill to Nourish the Heart, 161
birch, 32–33
bite, insect. *See* insect bites
bitter melon, 33
bitter orange, 33–34
black cohosh, 34–35
black tea, 81
bladder cancer, 219–21
    red wine catechins and, 121
bladder infection, 221–23
    agrimony and, 16
    artemisia and, 26
    barberry and, 30–31
    dandelion and, 58
bleeding
    agrimony and, 16
bleeding gums. *See under* periodontal disease
bloating. *See under* indigestion; premenstrual
        syndrome
blood cholesterol levels, 83–84
blood pressure problems. *See* high blood pressure
bloodshot eyes. *See under* eye problems
blood sugar levels, 47, 64, 66, 68, 71, 74, 78, 117
blurred vision. *See under* eye problems

boils, 223–24
    burdock and, 39
    schizonepeta and, 128
bone, broken. *See* fracture
bone cancer, 225–26
    bupleurum and, 38
boswellia, 35–36
bowel diseases
    calendula and, 41
    cat's claw and, 43
bowel retraining, 491–92
brahmi, 36–37
breast cancer, 226–30
    green tea and, 81
    red wine catechins and, 121
breast-feeding-related problems. *See* mastitis
breast infection. *See* mastitis
breast pain. *See under* fibrocystic breasts; mastitis;
        premenstrual syndrome
breathing techniques, 496–97
bromelain, 37–38
bronchitis and pneumonia, 230–32
    acerola and, 14
    coltsfoot and, 52
    elderberry and, 63
    elecampane and, 64
    eucalyptus and, 65
    fennel seed and, 67
    horehound and, 86
    horsetail and, 88
    mullein and, 104
    osha and, 109
    reishi and, 122
bruising, 232–33
    horse chestnut and, 87
    papain and, 110
bupleurum, 38
Bupleurum and Cinnamon Twig Decoction, 161–62
Bupleurum Plus Dragon Bone and Oyster Shell
        Decoction, 162
burdock, 38–39
burns, 233–34
    aloe and, 18
    lavender and, 94
    raspberry leaf and, 120
bursitis, 234–36
butcher's broom, 39–40

caffeine, 82
cajueiro, 40
calendula, 40–42
California poppy, 42
cancer, 236–45
    acerola and, 14
    alfalfa and, 17
    aloe and, 18–19
    American ginseng and, 21
    andrographis and, 22
    ashwagandha and, 28
    astragalus and, 29
    bitter melon and, 33
    bromelain and, 37
    burdock and, 39
    cat's claw and, 43–44
    cordyceps and, 55
    garlic and, 70–71
    ginkgo biloba and, 75
    ginseng and, 77–78
    goldenseal and, 79
    green tea and, 81
    jambul and, 89
    kelp and, 91
    kudzu and, 92–93
    licorice and, 95–96
    maitake and, 98
    milk thistle and, 100–101

cancer (*cont.*)
  mistletoe and, 102
  morinda and, 102–3
  oligomeric proanthocyanidins (OPCs)
    and, 106
  papain and, 110
  pau d'arco and, 112
  polysaccharide kureha and, 115
  quercetin and, 119
  reishi and, 122
  rosemary and, 124
  schisandra and, 127
  scutellaria and, 129
  shiitake and, 131
  Siberian ginseng and, 132–33
  side effects of treatment, 237–44
  slippery elm and, 134
  snow fungus and, 135
  warning signs, 236
  See also individual cancers
Candida albicans, 61, 108
candidiasis. *See* yeast infection
canker sores, 246–47
  myrrh and, 105
  quercetin and, 120
capsaicin, 45
capsules, 10–11
carboplatin, *237–38*
cardamom, 42
cardiac arrhythmia. *See under* congestive
    heart failure
cardiomyopathy
  schisandra and, 128
cardiovascular disease. *See* angina; atherosclerosis;
    congestive heart failure; heart attack; stroke
cardiovascular system, *xvii*
carpal tunnel syndrome, 247–48
  arnica and, 25
  ashwagandha and, 27
  chaparral and, 48
  corn silk and, 55
  devil's claw and, 59
catalogs, 12
cataracts, 248–50
  bilberry and, 31
  corydalis and, 56
  ginkgo biloba and, 75
  quercetin and, 120
catnip, 43
cat's claw, 43–44
catuaba, 44
cayenne, 44–46
celiac disease, 250–52
cellulite, 252
  kelp and, 91
cervical cancer, 252–54
Chagas'disease. *See under* parasitic infection
chamomile, 46–47
chanca piedra, 47
chancre, 471–72
chaparral, 47–48
chemoresistance, 119
chemotherapy side effects. *See under* cancer
chen-pi, 48
chicken pox. *See under* herpesvirus
    infection
Chinese senega root, 48–49
chiretta, 49
chlamydia. *See* gonorrhea and chlamydia
cholesterol problems. *See* high cholesterol
chronic fatigue syndrome (CFS), 255–57
  echinacea and, 61
  ginseng and, 78
  licorice and, 96
  shiitake and, 131–32
  Siberian ginseng and, 133

cinnamon, 49–50
circulatory problems
  prickly ash and, 115–16
  rosemary and, 124
  See also congestive heart failure; high blood
    pressure; intermittent claudication
cirrhosis of the liver, 257–59
  milk thistle and, 100
  reishi and, 122
cisplatin, *237–38*
Clostridium, 81
clove, 50
cochlear damage
  astragalus and, 29
Cochrane Collaboration, 62
codonopsis, 50–51
cofactors, 83
cognition
  ginkgo biloba and, 74–75
  ginseng and, 78
  gotu kola and, 80
coix, 51
cold. *See* common cold
cold sores. *See under* herpesvirus infection
coleus, 51–52
colic, 259–60
  anise and, 24
  asafoetida and, 27
colorectal cancer, 260–62
  green tea and, 81
coltsfoot, 52
comfrey, 52–53
common cold, 262–64
  acerola and, 15
  American ginseng and, 21
  andrographis and, 22–23
  astragalus and, 29
  cat's claw and, 44
  echinacea and, 61–62
  eucalyptus and, 65
  horehound and, 86
  osha and, 109
Complete German Commission E Monographs,
    xvii, 4, 6
compounding pharmacies, 12–13
compresses, 492
congestion
  myrrh and, 105
congestive heart failure, 264–67
  arjuna and, 24
  astragalus and, 28–29
  cordyceps and, 55
  guggul and, 83
  hawthorn and, 83–84
  motherwort and, 103
conjunctivitis
  calendula and, 41
  eyebright and, 66
  See also eye problems
constipation, 267–69
  aloe and, 19
  artemisia and, 26
  dandelion and, 58
  kelp and, 91
  psyllium and, 117–18
conventional medicine, 5–6
copaiba, 53–54
coptis, 54
Coptis Decoction to Relieve Toxicity, 163
cordyceps, 54–55
corn silk, 55
coronary artery disease (CAD)
  red wine catechins and, 121
corydalis, 55–56
couch grass, 56
cough, 269–71

cayenne and, 45
coltsfoot and, 52
echinacea and, 61–62
eucalyptus and, 65
fennel seed and, 67
fritillaria and, 70
marshmallow root and, 98
mullein and, 104
creams. *See* ointments
Crohn's disease, 271–73
  boswellia and, 36
  bromelain and, 37
  slippery elm and, 134
croup. *See under* cough
cuts, scrapes, and abrasions, 274–75
  barberry and, 30–31
  chamomile and, 46
  eucalyptus and, 66
  gotu kola and, 80
  mullein and, 104
  myrrh and, 105
  oligomeric proanthocyanidins (OPCs)
    and, 106–7
  sangre de drago and, 124–25
cyclophosphamide, *238–39*
cystitis. *See* bladder infection
cytomegalovirus
  licorice and, 96

damiana, 56–57
dandelion, 58–59
dandruff, 275–76
  burdock and, 39
dan shen, 57–58
deafness, sudden
  ginkgo biloba and, 76
deep-breathing, 497
depression, 276–79
  damiana and, 57
  ginkgo biloba and, 76
  kava kava and, 90
  lavender and, 94
  schisandra and, 128
dermatitis. *See* eczema; hives
devil's claw, 59
diabetes, 279–84
  agrimony and, 16
  American ginseng and, 21
  ashwagandha and, 28
  astragalus and, 29
  bilberry and, 31–32
  bitter melon and, 33
  bromelain and, 37
  cajueiro and, 40
  chanca piedra and, 47
  chiretta and, 49
  coptis and, 54
  fenugreek and, 68
  garlic and, 71
  ginseng and, 78
  green tea and, 81–82
  jambul and, 89
  milk thistle and, 101
  psyllium and, 118
  risk factors, 279
  scutellaria and, 129
diabetic neuropathy
  cayenne and, 45
diabetic retinopathy, 284–85
  arnica and, 25
  hawthorn and, 84
  jambul and, 89
  oligomeric proanthocyanidins (OPCs) and, 106
  quercetin and, 120
diaper rash, 285–86
  licorice and, 96

diarrhea, 286–88
  agrimony and, 16
  andrographis and, 23
  artemisia and, 26
  barberry and, 31
  chen-pi and, 48
  mullein and, 104
  Oregon grape root and, 109
  psyllium and, 117–18
  raspberry leaf and, 120
  sangre de drago and, 125
digestive system, xx
dioscorea. See wild yam
diseases/disorders. See individual medical
    conditions
Doctrine of Signatures, 66
dong quai, 59–61
Dong Quai and Peony Powder, 164
double-blind tests, 3
douches, 492
doxorubicin, 239
drug withdrawal
  acorus and, 16
dry mouth, 288–90
dyspepsia. See indigestion

ear infection, 290–92
  echinacea and, 62
  garlic and, 71
  mullein and, 104
echinacea, 61–63
eczema, 292–94
  avena and, 30
  burdock and, 39
  coleus and, 51
  copaiba and, 53–54
  quercetin and, 120
  rosemary and, 124
  sangre de drago and, 124–25
  sarsaparilla and, 125
edema. See ankles, swollen; lymphedema. See also
    under premenstrual syndrome
Egyptian medicine, 11
Eight-Ingredient Pill with Rehmannia, 164–65
elderberry, 63
elecampane, 63–64
emphysema, 295–96
  horsetail and, 88
  quercetin and, 119
endocrine system, xix
endometrial cancer, 296–97
  chamomile and, 46
endometriosis, 297–99
  alfalfa and, 17
  green tea and, 81
enlarged prostate. See benign prostatic hypertrophy;
    prostate cancer; prostatitis
enteric coating, 11, 59
enuresis. See bed-wetting
ephedra, 64, 187
Ephedra, Asiasarum, and Prepared
    Aconite Decoction, 165
Ephedra Decoction, 165
epilepsy. See seizure disorders
epimedium, 64–65
erectile dysfunction, 299–301
  catuaba and, 44
  damiana and, 57
  ginkgo biloba and, 75
  ginseng and, 78
  iporuru and, 88–89
  muira puama and, 104
Escherichia coli, 44
espinheira santa, 65
essential oils, 11, 490–91
Essiac tea, 165–66

estrogen-reducing diet, 492–93
estrogen-replacement therapy (ERT), 34, 93, 151, 400
eucalyptus, 65–66
exercise, 497
extracts, 11, 13
eyebright, 66–67
eye problems, 301–5
  bags beneath eyes, 301
  barberry and, 30–31
  bloodshot eyes, 301–2
  blurred vision, 302–3
  conjunctivitis (pinkeye), 303–5
  eyebright and, 66
  floaters, 305

fatigue
  schisandra and, 128
fennel seed, 67
fenugreek, 67–68
fever
  andrographis and, 22–23
fever blisters. See under herpesvirus infection
feverfew, 68–69
fibrocystic breasts, 305–7
  green tea and, 81
fibroids, uterine, 307–9
  black cohosh and, 34
  cinnamon and, 49
  dan shen and, 57
fibromyalgia syndrome, 309–10
Five-Accumulation Powder, 166
Five-Ingredient Powder with Poria, 167
flatulence. See under indigestion
flavonoids, 107
floaters. See under eye problems
flu. See influenza
foam cells, 119
food allergies. See under allergies
Food and Drug Administration, U.S. (FDA), 4, 8, 102
food poisoning, 310–13
  clove and, 50
  green tea and, 81
  slippery elm and, 134
foot baths, 493
forskolin, 51–52
Four-Gentlemen Decoction, 167–68
Four-Substance Decoction, 168
fracture, 313–14
  arnica and, 25
free radicals, 89
friendly bacteria, 38
Frigid Extremities Decoction, 168
Frigid Extremities Powder, 169
fritillaria, 69–70
fungal infection
  alfalfa and, 17
  eucalyptus and, 65
  See also athlete's foot; ringworm; yeast infection

gallbladder problems
  andrographis and, 23
gallstones, 314–16
  barberry and, 31
  dandelion and, 58
  gentian and, 72
  peppermint and, 113
  prickly ash and, 115–16
Gardnerella, 477
garlic, 70–72
gas. See under indigestion
gastric ulcers
  bromelain and, 37
gastritis, 316–18
  barberry and, 31
  calendula and, 41
  espinheira and, 65

licorice and, 96
  Oregon grape root and, 109
Gastrodia and Uncaria Decoction, 169
gastroenteritis. See under food poisoning
gastrointestinal tract ailments
  astragalus and, 29
Generally Recognized as Safe (GRAS) list, 48
genital warts
  green tea and, 82
gentian, 72
Gentiana Longdancao Decoction to Drain the Liver,
    169–70
German Commission E, 8–9
giardiasis. See under parasitic infection
ginger, 72–74
gingivitis
  myrrh and, 105
  See also periodontal disease
ginkgo biloba, 11, 74–77, 196
ginseng, 77–79. See also American ginseng; Siberian
    ginseng
Ginseng Decoction to Nourish the Nutritive Chi,
    170–71
glaucoma, 318–20
  acerola and, 15
  coleus and, 51–52
  ginkgo biloba and, 75
glomerulonephritis. See under kidney disease
glucose, 74, 117
goldenseal, 62, 79–80
gonorrhea and chlamydia, 320–22
  scutellaria and, 129–30
good manufacturing practices (GMPs), 8
gotu kola, 80–81
gout, 322–23
  burdock and, 39
  devil's claw and, 59
  green tea and, 82
granules, 11
Graves' disease. See under hyperthyroidism
green tea, 81–82
guggul, 82–83
gum disease. See under periodontal disease
gums, bleeding. See under periodontal disease

hair loss, 323–25
halitosis, 325–26
  anise and, 24
hand baths, 493
hangover, 326–27
  ginseng and, 78
  scutellaria and, 130
hawthorn, 83–84
hay fever. See respiratory allergies under allergies
headache, 327–29
  clove and, 50
  codonopsis and, 50
  eucalyptus and, 66
  lavender and, 93–94
  peppermint and, 113
  scutellaria and, 129
health food stores, 12
heart attack, 329–32
  andrographis and, 22
  arjuna and, 24
  astragalus and, 28–29
  dong quai and, 60
  garlic and, 71
  ginkgo biloba and, 75–76
  hawthorn and, 84
  scutellaria and, 129
heartburn. See under indigestion
heart disease
  bilberry and, 32
  coleus and, 52
  dan shen and, 57

heart disease (cont.)
  fenugreek and, 68
  goldenseal and, 79–80
  kudzu and, 93
  oligomeric proanthocyanidins (OPCs) and, 106
  olive leaf and, 108
  psyllium and, 118
  Siberian ginseng and, 133
  See also angina; congestive heart failure; heart attack
heart failure. See congestive heart failure
heat stress, 332–33
Helicobacter pylori, 31
hemochromatosis. See iron overload
hemorrhoids, 333–35
  aloe and, 19
  butcher's broom and, 39
  dandelion and, 58
  horse chestnut and, 87
  mullein and, 104
  psyllium and, 117–18
hepatitis, 335–38
  ABCs of, 336
  andrographis and, 23
  dan shen and, 57
  licorice and, 96
  milk thistle and, 100
  schisandra and, 127–28
herbal formulas, 159
  acne, 189
  ADD/ADHD, 213
  AIDS, 351
  alcoholism, 191
  allergies, 192
  Alzheimer's disease, 198
  anemia, 199
  angina, 201
  anxiety disorder, 204
  Arrest Wheezing Decoction, 160
  asthma, 207
  Astragalus Decoction to Construct the Middle, 160
  atherosclerosis, 211
  Augmented Rambling Powder, 160–61
  bed-wetting, 215
  Bell's palsy, 217
  benign prostatic hypertrophy, 218
  Biota Seed Pill to Nourish the Heart, 161
  bladder cancer, 220
  boil, 224
  bone cancer, 226
  breast cancer, 228
  bronchitis and pneumonia, 232
  Bupleurum and Cinnamon Twig Decoction, 161–62
  Bupleurum Plus Dragon Bone and Oyster Shell Decoction, 162
  Calm the Stomach Powder, 162
  cancer, 237–45
  cataracts, 249
  cervical cancer, 253
  chronic fatigue syndrome, 256
  Cinnamon Twig and Poria Pill, 162–63
  colorectal cancer, 261
  constipation, 268
  Coptis Decoction to Relieve Toxicity, 163
  cough, 271
  Crohn's disease, 272
  depression, 277
  diabetes, 282
  diabetic retinopathy, 284
  diarrhea, 287
  Dong Quai and Peony Powder, 164
  dry mouth, 289
  ear infection, 291
  eczema, 293
  Eight-Ingredient Pill with Rehmannia, 164–65

endometrial cancer, 297
endometriosis, 298
Ephedra, Asiasarum, and Prepared Aconite Decoction, 165
Ephedra Decoction, 165
Essiac tea, 165–66
eye problems, 302–4
fibrocystic breasts, 306
Five-Accumulation Powder, 166
Five-Ingredient Powder with Poria, 167
food poisoning, 312
Four-Gentlemen Decoction, 167–68
Four-Substance Decoction, 168
Frigid Extremities Decoction, 168
Frigid Extremities Powder, 169
gallstones, 316
gastritis, 317
Gastrodia and Uncaria Decoction, 169
Gentiana Longdancao Decoction to Drain the Liver, 169–70
Ginseng Decoction to Nourish the Nutritive Chi, 170–71
glaucoma, 319
gonorrhea and chlamydia, 321
hair loss, 324
headache, 328
heart attack, 330
heat stress, 333
hepatitis, 337
herpesvirus infection, 340
high blood pressure, 342
high cholesterol, 345
HIV/AIDS, 348
hives, 352
Hochu-Ekki-To, 171
Hodgkin's lymphoma, 354
Honey-Fried Licorice Decoction, 171–72
Hoxsey Formula, 172
hyperthyroidism, 356
hypothyroidism, 357
infertility, 362, 364
insomnia, 369
irritable bowel syndrome, 373
kidney cancer, 375
Kidney Chi Pill from the Golden Cabinet, 172–73
kidney disease, 376
kidney stones, 378
Kudzu Decoction, 173
laryngitis, 380
Ledebouriella Decoction that Sagely Unblocks, 173–74
leukemia, 381
Licorice, Wheat, and Jujube Decoction, 174
liver cancer, 383
lung cancer, 386
lupus, 388
Major Bupleurum Decoction, 174–75
Major Construct the Middle Decoction, 175
measles, 394
memory problems, 396
Ménière's disease, 398
menopause-related problems, 400
menstrual problems, 402
migraine, 404
Minor Bluegreen Dragon Decoction, 175
Minor Bupleurum Decoction, 175–76
multiple sclerosis, 409
mumps, 411
myasthenia gravis, 413
nosebleed, 417
Ophiopogonis Decoction, 176
osteoarthritis, 419
osteoporosis, 420
ovarian cancer, 423
ovarian cyst, 425
overweight, 426

Oyster Shell Powder, 176–77
pain, chronic, 428
parasitic infection, 432
pelvic inflammatory disease, 434
Peony and Licorice Decoction, 177
peptic ulcer, 436
periodontal disease, 438
Pill for Deafness That is Kind to the Left Kidney, 177
Pinellia and Magnolia Bark Decoction, 177–78
Pinellia Decoction to Drain the Epigastrium, 178
Polyporus Decoction, 178
premenstrual syndrome, 441
prostate cancer, 443
prostatitis, 446
psoriasis, 448
respiratory allergies, 195
restless legs syndrome, 449
rheumatoid arthritis, 451
Robert's Formula, 178–79
Sairei-to, 179
seizure disorders, 454
Seven-Treasure Pill for Beautiful Whiskers, 179–80
Shih Qua Da Bu Tang, 180
Six-Ingredient Pill with Rehmannia, 180–81
skin cancer, 460, 462
stomach cancer, 464
strep throat, 466
stress, 468
stroke, 469
sweating, excessive, 471
tinnitus, 474
triphala, 181
True Man's Decoction to Nourish the Organs, 181
True Warrior Decoction, 181–82
tuberculosis, 477
uterine fibroids, 308
Vacha Rasayanas, 182
vitiligo, 481
vomiting, 482
Warm the Gallbladder Decoction, 182–83
Warm the Menses Decoction, 183
White Tiger Decoction, 183
yeast infection, 486
Yogaraj Guggulu, 183–84
herbalism, 3
herbs, 3
  buying, 12–13
  forms of, 10–12
  potentially dangerous, 8–9
  standardization, 13
  top reasons for taking, 9–10
  treatment rules, 5–9
  See also beneficial herbs; herbal formulas; individual herbs; techniques
herb shops, 12
herpes simplex
  aloe and, 19
herpesvirus infection, 338–41
  acerola and, 15
  clove and, 50
  echinacea and, 62
  lemon balm and, 95
  papain and, 110
  prunella and, 116
herpes zoster. See under herpesvirus infection
hiccups. See under indigestion
high blood pressure, 341–44
  American ginseng and, 21
  angelica and, 23
  chanca piedra and, 47
  coleus and, 52
  corn silk and, 55
  dong quai and, 60
  ginseng and, 78
  hawthorn and, 84

olive leaf and, 108
reishi and, 122
scutellaria and, 129
high cholesterol, 344–46
ginger and, 73
green tea and, 81
guggul and, 83
hawthorn and, 84
ho she wu and, 84
scutellaria and, 129
shiitake and, 132
snow fungus and, 135
high-density lipoprotein (HDL), 68
high-protein diet, 422
HIV/AIDS, 346–49
cat's claw and, 44
catuaba and, 44
licorice and, 96
maitake and, 98
olive leaf and, 108
prunella and, 116
rooibos and, 123
shiitake and, 132
hives, 351–53
quercetin and, 119
Hochu-Ekki-To, 171
Hodgkin's lymphoma, 353–55
hoelen, 85
homeopathy, 10, 25
Honey-Fried Licorice Decoction, 171–72
hops, 85–86
horehound, 86–87
hormone replacement therapy (HRT), 97
horse chestnut, 87
horsetail, 87–88
ho she wu, 84–85
hot flashes. See under menopause-related
problems
Hoxsey Formula, 172
human immunodeficiency virus.
See HIV/AIDS
hyperactivity. See ADD/ADHD
hyperlipidemia
myrrh and, 105
hypertension. See high blood pressure
hyperthyroidism, 355–56
motherwort and, 103
hypothyroidism, 356–58

immune system, 20
barberry and, 31
garlic and, 71
indigestion, 358–60
belching, 358, 358–59
bitter orange and, 34
bloating and flatulence, 359, 359–60
cardamom and, 42
chen-pi and, 48
cinnamon and, 49
dandelion and, 58
fennel seed and, 67
gentian and, 72
ginger and, 73
goldenseal and, 79
heartburn, 360, 360
hops and, 85
horehound and, 86
lavender and, 94
peppermint and, 113
rosemary and, 124
infertility, 361–64
American ginseng and, 21
astragalus and, 29
black cohosh and, 34
dong quai and, 60
ginseng and, 78

iporuru and, 88–89
in men, 361–63, 362
in women, 363–64, 363–64
inflammation
boswellia and, 36
calendula and, 41
comfrey and, 53
influenza, 364–66
acerola and, 15
American ginseng and, 21
andrographis and, 22–23
anise and, 24
catnip and, 43
echinacea and, 61–62
elderberry and, 63
fritillaria and, 70
mullein and, 104
osha and, 109
scutellaria and, 130
injuries. See bruising; burns; cuts, scrapes, and
abrasions; fracture; muscles, sore; shin
splints; sprains
insect bites, 366–67
asafoetida and, 27
eucalyptus and, 66
sangre de drago and, 124–25
insomnia, 368–70
catnip and, 43
chamomile and, 46
corydalis and, 56
hops and, 85–86
kava kava and, 90
lavender and, 94
lemon balm and, 95
rooibos and, 123
schisandra and, 128
insulin resistance, 101
intermittent claudication, 370–71
ginkgo biloba and, 75–76
Internet, 12
inula. See elecampane
iodine, 91
iporuru, 88–89
iron overload, 371
irritable bowel syndrome (IBS), 371–74
asafoetida and, 27
brahmi and, 36
chamomile and, 46
lemon balm and, 95
peppermint and, 113
psyllium and, 117–18
rosemary and, 124
slippery elm and, 134
isoflavones, 93

jambul, 89

kava kava, 89–90
Kegel exercises, 493–94
kelp, 90–91
khella, 91–92
kidney cancer, 374–75
Kidney Chi Pill from the Golden Cabinet,
172–73
kidney disease, 375–77
cordyceps and, 55
couch grass and, 56
hoelen and, 85
kidney stones, 47, 377–79
barberry and, 31
chanca piedra and, 47
khella and, 91
knee joint inflammation:
arnica and, 25
kudzu, 92–93
Kudzu Decoction, 173

Lactobacillus acidophilus, 71, 466, 472, 477, 492–93
laryngitis, 379–81
coltsfoot and, 52
fritillaria and, 70
marshmallow root and, 98
lavender, 93–94
laxatives, bulk-forming, 117
leaky gut, 450
Ledebouriella Decoction that Sagely Unblocks,
173–74
lemon balm, 94–95
lentinan. See shiitake
leukemia, 381–82
dong quai and, 60
red wine catechins and, 121
leukoderma. See vitiligo
licorice, 95–97
Licorice, Wheat, and Jujube Decoction, 174
Listeria, 113
liver cancer, 383–85
cinnamon and, 49–50
liver disease
agrimony and, 16
andrographis and, 23
artemisia and, 26
astragalus and, 29
barberry and, 31
burdock and, 39
dandelion and, 58
green tea and, 82
Oregon grape root and, 109
schisandra and, 127–28
See also cirrhosis of the liver; hepatitis; liver cancer
low blood sugar, 40, 57
low-density lipoprotein (LDL), 32
low-protein diet, 376
lozenges, 11
lung cancer, 385–87
cordyceps and, 55
lupus, 387–89
codonopsis and, 51
Lyme disease, 389–90
lymphedema, 390–91
horse chestnut and, 87
oligomeric proanthocyanidins (OPCs) and, 106–7

macular degeneration, 391–93
ginkgo biloba and, 75
oligomeric proanthocyanidins (OPCs) and, 106
quercetin and, 120
maitake, 97–98
Major Bupleurum Decoction, 174–75
Major Construct the Middle Decoction, 175
malaria. See under parasitic infection
marrubiin, 86
marshmallow root, 98–99
massage, 494
mastitis, 393–94
schizonepeta and, 128
maté, 99
measles, 394–95
medical conditions, 187
acne, 188–90
ADD/ADHD, 212–14
AIDS, 349–51
alcoholism, 190–91
allergies, 191–96
Alzheimer's disease, 196–98
anemia, 198–200
angina, 200–202
ankles, swollen, 202–3
anxiety disorder, 203–5
asthma, 205–9
atherosclerosis, 209–11
athlete's foot, 211–12
bed-wetting, 215–16

medical conditions (cont.)
  Bell's palsy, 216–17
  benign prostatic hypertrophy, 217–19
  bladder cancer, 219–21
  bladder infection, 221–23
  boil, 223–24
  bone cancer, 225–26
  breast cancer, 226–30
  bronchitis and pneumonia, 230–32
  bruising, 232–33
  burns, 233–34
  bursitis, 234–36
  cancer, 236–45
  canker sores, 246–47
  carpal tunnel syndrome, 247–48
  cataracts, 248–50
  celiac disease, 250–52
  cellulite, 252
  cervical cancer, 252–54
  chronic fatigue syndrome, 255–57
  cirrhosis of the liver, 257–59
  colic, 259–60
  colorectal cancer, 260–62
  common cold, 262–64
  congestive heart failure, 264–67
  constipation, 267–69
  cough, 269–71
  Crohn's disease, 271–73
  cuts, scrapes, and abrasions, 274–75
  dandruff, 275–76
  depression, 276–79
  diabetes, 279–84
  diabetic retinopathy, 284–85
  diaper rash, 285–86
  diarrhea, 286–88
  dry mouth, 288–90
  ear infection, 290–92
  eczema, 292–94
  emphysema, 295–96
  endometrial cancer, 296–97
  endometriosis, 297–99
  erectile dysfunction, 299–301
  eye problems, 301–5
  fibrocystic breasts, 305–7
  fibroids, uterine, 307–9
  fibromyalgia syndrome, 309–10
  food poisoning, 310–13
  fracture, 313–14
  gallstones, 314–16
  gastritis, 316–18
  glaucoma, 318–20
  gonorrhea and chlamydia, 320–22
  gout, 322–23
  hair loss, 323–25
  halitosis, 325–26
  hangover, 326–27
  headache, 327–29
  heart attack, 329–32
  heat stress, 332–33
  hemorrhoids, 333–35
  hepatitis, 335–38
  herpesvirus infection, 338–41
  high blood pressure, 341–44
  high cholesterol, 344–46
  HIV/AIDS, 346–49
  hives, 351–53
  Hodgkin's lymphoma, 353–55
  hyperthyroidism, 355–56
  hypothyroidism, 356–58
  indigestion, 358–60
  infertility, 361–64
  influenza, 364–66
  insect bites, 366–67
  insomnia, 368–70
  intermittent claudication, 370–71
  iron overload, 371

  irritable bowel syndrome, 371–74
  kidney cancer, 374–75
  kidney disease, 375–77
  kidney stones, 377–79
  laryngitis, 379–81
  leukemia, 381–82
  liver cancer, 383–85
  lung cancer, 385–87
  lupus, 387–89
  Lyme disease, 389–90
  lymphedema, 390–91
  macular degeneration, 391–93
  mastitis, 393–94
  measles, 394–95
  memory problems, 395–97
  Ménière's disease, 397–99
  menopause-related problems, 399–401
  menstrual problems, 401–3
  migraine, 403–6
  mononucleosis, 406–7
  morning sickness, 407
  motion sickness, 407–8
  multiple sclerosis, 409–10
  mumps, 410–12
  muscles, sore, 412
  myasthenia gravis, 412–13
  nails, infected, 413–15
  nausea, 415–16
  nosebleed, 416–17
  osteoarthritis, 417–20
  osteoporosis, 420–22
  ovarian cancer, 422–24
  ovarian cyst, 424–25
  overweight, 425–27
  pain, chronic, 427–29
  parasitic infection, 429–32
  Parkinson's disease, 432–33
  pelvic inflammatory disease, 433–35
  peptic ulcer, 435–37
  periodontal disease, 437–39
  premenstrual syndrome, 439–42
  prostate cancer, 442–45
  prostatitis, 445–46
  psoriasis, 446–48
  restless legs syndrome, 448–50
  rheumatoid arthritis, 450–52
  ringworm, 452–53
  seizure disorders, 453–55
  sex drive, diminished, 455–57
  shin splints, 457–58
  sinusitis, 458–59
  skin cancer, 460–63
  sprains and strains, 463–64
  stomach cancer, 464–65
  strep throat, 465–66
  stress, 467–68
  stroke, 468–70
  sweating, excessive, 470–71
  syphilis, 471–72
  tendinitis, 472–73
  tinnitus, 473–74
  toothache, 474–76
  tuberculosis, 476–77
  vaginosis, 477–78
  varicose veins, 478–80
  vitiligo, 480–81
  vomiting, 481–82
  warts, 482–84
  wrinkles, 484–85
  yeast infection, 485–86
medicinal spirits (essences), 11
meditation, 497–98
melanoma. See under skin cancer
memory problems, 395–97
  ashwagandha and, 27
  brahmi and, 36

  ginkgo biloba and, 74–75
  hawthorn and, 83
  rosemary and, 123–24
men
  breast cancer in, 226
  infertility in, 361–63, 362
Ménière's disease, 397–99
menopause-related problems, 399–401
  alfalfa and, 17
  avena and, 30
  black cohosh and, 34–35
  damiana and, 57
  dong quai and, 60
  ginseng and, 78
  hops and, 86
  kudzu and, 93
menstrual cramps. See under menstrual problems;
    premenstrual syndrome
menstrual problems, 401–3
  cinnamon and, 49
  dan shen and, 57
  dong quai and, 60
  kelp and, 91
  morinda and, 103
  rosemary and, 124
  shepherd's purse and, 130
methotrexate, 240
migraine, 403–6
  dong quai and, 60
  feverfew and, 69
milk thistle, 99–101
Minor Bluegreen Dragon Decoction, 175
Minor Bupleurum Decoction, 175–76
mistletoe, 101–2
mitomycin, 241
monoamine oxidase (MAO) inhibitors, 48
mononucleosis, 406–7
morinda, 102–3
morning sickness, 407
  chamomile and, 46
  ginger and, 73
motherwort, 103
motion sickness, 407–8
  ginger and, 73
mouth and gum problems. See canker sores; dry
    mouth; halitosis; periodontal disease
muira puama, 104
mullein, 104–5
multiple myeloma. See under bone cancer
multiple sclerosis, 409–10
  ginkgo biloba and, 76
mumps, 410–12
muscle injury. See muscles, sore; sprains and strains
muscles, sore, 412
  arnica and, 25
  birch and, 33
  cayenne and, 45
  papain and, 110
  rosemary and, 124
mushroom. See maitake; reishi; shiitake
myasthenia gravis, 412–13
myocardial infarction. See heart attack
myrrh, 105

nails, infected, 413–15
  barberry and, 30–31
  coix and, 51
  scutellaria and, 129–30
National Center for Complementary and
    Alternative Medicine (NCCAM), 3
National Formulary, 6
Native Americans, 20, 155
nausea, 415–16
  chen-pi and, 48
  chiretta and, 49
  ginger and, 73

nephritis. *See under* kidney disease
nervousness
  asafoetida and, 27
  avena and, 30
  damiana and, 57
  See also anxiety disorder; stress
nervous system, *xix*
nightmares
  ho she wu and, 85
night vision problems
  bilberry and, 32
noni. *See* morinda
nosebleed, 416–17
  alfalfa and, 18
  oligomeric proanthocyanidins (OPCs)
    and, 106–7
  shepherd's purse and, 130

obesity. *See* overweight
Office of Dietary Supplements (ODS), 3
ointments, 494–95
oligomeric proanthocyanidins (OPCs), 105–7
olive leaf, 108
onset of action, 6
Ophiopogonis Decoction, 176
Oregon grape root, 108–9
osha, 109–10
osteoarthritis, 417–20
  bromelain and, 37
osteoporosis, 420–22
  alfalfa and, 18
  epimedium and, 64
osteosarcoma. *See under* bone cancer
ovarian cancer, 422–24
ovarian cyst, 424–25
  dong quai and, 60
over-the-counter (OTC) drugs, 9, 159
overweight, 425–27
  bitter orange and, 34
  cayenne and, 45
  coleus and, 52
  dandelion and, 58
Oyster Shell Powder, 176–77

pain, chronic, 427–29
  arnica and, 25
  comfrey and, 53
  ginger and, 73
panic attack. *See under* anxiety disorder
papain, 110
parasitic infection, 429–32
  artemisia and, 26
  barberry and, 30–31
  cajueiro and, 40
  most common, *430–31*
  ginger and, 73–74
  pau d'arco and, 112
  prickly ash and, 116
Parkinson's disease, 432–33
  acerola and, 15
  brahmi and, 36
  ginkgo biloba and, 74–75
passionflower, 110–11
patent protection, 10
pau d'arco, 111–12
pelvic inflammatory disease (PID), 433–35
Peony and Licorice Decoction, 177
peppermint, 112–14
peptic ulcer, 435–37
  barberry and, 31
  bilberry and, 32
  chamomile and, 46
  chen-pi and, 48
  cinnamon and, 50
  clove and, 50
  codonopsis and, 51

garlic and, 71
  licorice and, 96
periodontal disease, 437–39
  clove and, 50
  goldenseal and, 80
  gotu kola and, 80–81
  green tea and, 82
  scutellaria and, 130
pharmacopeias, 6
phobia. *See under* anxiety disorder
PDR for Herbal Medicines, xvii, 4, 6
Pill for Deafness That is Kind to the Left Kidney, 177
Pinellia and Magnolia Bark Decoction, 177–78
Pinellia Decoction to Drain the Epigastrium, 178
pinkeye. *See* conjunctivitis *under* eye problems
pinworms. *See under* parasitic infection
plant juices, 12
plants, 3
plasters, 495
PMS. *See* premenstrual syndrome
pneumonia. *See* bronchitis and pneumonia
poisoning. *See* food poisoning
pollen, 114
Polyporus Decoction, 178
polysaccharide kureha (PSK), 114–15
poppy. *See* California poppy
poultices, 495–96
premenstrual syndrome (PMS), 439–42
  black cohosh and, 34–35
  bromelain and, 37
  chamomile and, 46
  corn silk and, 55
  dandelion and, 58
  dong quai and, 60
  motherwort and, 103
  raspberry leaf and, 120–21
prickly ash, 115–16
progressive relaxation, 498
prostate, enlarged. *See* benign prostatic
    hypertrophy; prostate cancer; prostatitis
prostate cancer, 442–45
  pygeum and, 118–19
  red wine catechins and, 121
  saw palmetto and, 126–27
prostate-specific antigen (PSA), 101, 119, 442, 444
prostatitis, 445–46
  catuaba and, 44
  pollen and, 114
  quercetin and, 120
prunella, 116
Pseudomonas, 494
psoralea, 116–17
psoriasis, 446–48
  aloe and, 19
  milk thistle and, 101
  Oregon grape root and, 109
  psoralea and, 117
  sarsaparilla and, 125
psyllium, 117–18
Pycnogenol, 106–7
pygeum, 118–19
pyorrhea. *See under* periodontal disease

quercetin, 119–20

radiation exposure:
  aloe and, 19
radiation therapy. *See under* cancer
rash. *See* diaper rash
raspberry leaf, 120–21
red wine catechins, 121–22
reishi, 122–23
relaxation techniques, 496–98
renal cell carcinoma. *See* kidney cancer
reproductive tract
  barberry and, 30–31

respiratory allergies, 193–96
  licorice and, 96–97
  scutellaria and, 129
respiratory tract, *xx*
restless legs syndrome, 448–50
  corydalis and, 56
  schisandra and, 128
resveratrol. *See* red wine catechins
retail stores, 12
retinopathy. *See* diabetic retinopathy
rheumatism
  andiroba and, 22
  birch and, 33
  rosemary and, 124
rheumatoid arthritis, 450–52
  bromelain and, 37
  feverfew and, 69
RIMS system, 472–73
ringworm, 452–53
Robert's Formula, 178–79
rooibos, 123
rosemary, 123–24

Sairei-to, 179
Salmonella, 113
sangre de drago, 124–25
sarsaparilla, 125–26
saw palmetto, 126–27
scarring
  gotu kola and, 80
schisandra, 127–28
schistosomiasis. *See under* parasitic infection
schizonepeta, 128
schizophrenia
  ginkgo biloba and, 76
sciatica
  burdock and, 39
scrapes. *See* cuts, scrapes, and abrasions
scutellaria, 128–30
seasonal affective disorder (SAD), 76
  ginkgo biloba and, 76
secretagogue, 23
seizure disorders, 453–55
  acorus and, 16
  Chinese senega root and, 49
Seven-Treasure Pill for Beautiful Whiskers, 179–80
severe acute respiratory syndrome (SARS)
  licorice and, 96
sex-drive, diminished, 455–57
  ashwagandha and, 28
  avena and, 30
  damiana and, 57
  ginkgo biloba and, 75
  ginseng and, 78
  kava kava and, 90
  muira puama and, 104
sexual dysfunction
  cayenne and, 45
  epimedium and, 64
sexually transmitted diseases. *See* gonorrhea and
    chlamydia; HIV/AIDS; syphilis
shepherd's purse, 130–31
Shih Qua Da Bu Tang, 180
shiitake, 131–32
shingles. *See under* herpesvirus infection
shin splints, 457–58
Siberian ginseng, 132–34
silymarin. *See* milk thistle
sinusitis, 458–59
  anise and, 24
  barberry and, 30–31
  elderberry and, 63
  horehound and, 86
  osha and, 109
sitz baths, 498–99
Six-Ingredient Pill with Rehmannia, 180–81

Sjögren's syndrome. *See under* dry mouth
skin cancer, 460–63
  schisandra and, 128
skin elasticity
  kelp and, 91
skin problems
  agrimony and, 16
  andiroba and, 22
  barberry and, 30–31
  birch and, 33
  calendula and, 41
  comfrey and, 53
  licorice and, 96
skin washes, 499
sleep problems. *See* insomnia; restless
    legs syndrome
slippery elm, 133–35
snow fungus, 135
sore muscles. *See* muscles, sore
sore throat
  mullein and, 104
  raspberry leaf and, 121
soy isoflavone concentrate, 135–38
soy lecithin, 138–39
sprains and strains, 463–64
  papain and, 110
St. John's wort, 77, 139–42
stamina
  ginseng and, 78
standardization, 13
Staphylococcus aureus, 32, 41, 466
static stretching, 497
steam inhalations, 499
steroid drugs, *241–42*
stinging nettle, 142–43
stomach ailments
  cayenne and, 45
  marshmallow root and, 99
stomach cancer, 464–65
strep throat, 465–66
  myrrh and, 105
Streptococcus, 82, 465
stress, 467–68
  American ginseng and, 21
  ashwagandha and, 28
  brahmi and, 36
  California poppy and, 42
  chamomile and, 46
  ginseng and, 78
  kava kava and, 90
  lemon balm and, 94–95
  peppermint and, 113
  reishi and, 122
  schisandra and, 128
  scutellaria and, 129
stroke, 76, 468–70
  ginkgo biloba and, 75–76
  hawthorn and, 84
structural tissues, *xviii*
surgery
  papain and, 110
sweating, excessive, 470–71
  schisandra and, 128
swelling
  butcher's broom and, 39
swimmer's itch. *See under* parasitic infection
symptoms, emergencies, 5–6
syphilis, 471–72
syrups, 12, 499

tablets, 12
T cells, 98, 115–16, 347, 349, 450

teas, 12, 499–500
tea tree, 143–44
techniques
  acupuncture, 489–90
  aromatherapy, 490–91
  bowel retraining, 491–92
  compresses, 492
  douches, 492
  estrogen-reducing diet, 492–93
  exercise, 497
  foot baths, 493
  hand baths, 493
  Kegel exercises, 493–94
  massage, 494
  meditation, 497–98
  ointments, 494–95
  plasters, 495
  poultices, 495–96
  relaxation, 496–98
  sitz baths, 498–99
  skin washes, 499
  steam inhalations, 499
  syrups, 499
  teas, 499–500
  tinctures, 500
tendinitis, 472–73
  devil's claw and, 59
  oligomeric proanthocyanidins (OPCs) and, 106–7
therapeutic range, 6
thiotepa, *242*
throat infection
  barberry and, 30–31
thyme, 144–45
tilden flower, 145
tinctures, 12, 500
tinnitus, 76, 473–74
  cordyceps and, 55
  ginkgo biloba and, 76
tolu balsam, 145–46
toothache, 474–76
  clove and, 50
traditional Chinese medicine (TCM), 7
  herbal formulas, 160–83
  See also individual disorders; medical conditions
transcutaneous electrical nerve stimulation
    (TENS), 473
treatments. *See* techniques
trichomoniasis. *See under* parasitic infection
triglycerides, 84
triphala, 181
True Man's Decoction to Nourish
    the Organs, 181
True Warrior Decoction, 181–82
tuberculosis, 476–77
turmeric, 146–47

ulcerative colitis
  aloe and, 19
  boswellia and, 36
  psyllium and, 117–18
ulcers
  alfalfa and, 18
  aloe and, 19
United States Pharmacopeia (USP), 6
upper respiratory infection
  echinacea and, 61–62
urinary incontinence
  cardamom and, 42
urinary tract, *xix*
urinary tract infections (UTIs), 47, 54
  coptis and, 54
  sarsaparilla and, 125

uva ursi, 147–48
UV light damage:
  aloe and, 19

Vacha Rasayanas, 182
vaginitis
  sangre de drago and, 125
vaginosis, 477–78
valerian, 148–50
varicose veins, 40, 478–80
  butcher's broom and, 39–40
  gotu kola and, 80
  horse chestnut and, 87
  oligomeric proanthocyanidins (OPCs)
    and, 106–7
varuna, 150
venous insufficiency:
  bilberry and, 32
  horse chestnut and, 87
vincristine, *242*
viral infection
  scutellaria and, 130
  Siberian ginseng and, 133
vision, blurred. *See under* eye
    problems
visualization, 498
vitamin C, 14–15
vitamin deficiency
  aloe and, 19
vitamin K, 82
vitamin K deficiency, 18
vitex, 150–51
vitiligo, 480–81
  khella and, 91–92
  psoralea and, 117
vomiting, 481–82
  codonopsis and, 51
  ginger and, 73
  scutellaria and, 130

walnut leaf, 151–52
Warm the Gallbladder Decoction,
    182–83
Warm the Menses Decoction, 183
warts, 482–84
weight loss
  green tea and, 82
  maté and, 99
weight problems. *See* overweight
White Tiger Decoction, 183
wild angelica, 152
wild yam, 152–53
willow bark, 153–54
wintergreen, 154–55
witch hazel, 155–56
women
  infertility in, 363–64, *363–64*
wounds. *See* burns; cuts, scrapes, and
    abrasions
wrinkles, 484–85
  acerola and, 15
  green tea and, 82
  quercetin and, 120

yarrow, 156–57
yeast infection, 485–86
  echinacea and, 61
  olive leaf and, 108
  pau d'arco and, 112
yoga, 498
Yogaraj Guggulu, 183–84
yohimbe, 157–58

ABOUT THE AUTHOR

Phyllis Balch was a certified nutritional consultant who received her certification from the American Association of Nutritional Consultants, and was a leading nutritional counselor for more than two decades. She came to the field as a result of experiencing directly the benefits of using diet and nutrition as remedies for sickness.

In the 1970s, Balch and her children suffered from a number of undiagnosed (or misdiagnosed) illnesses, and although they had expert medical knowledge very close at hand, their lives continued to be disrupted by these maladies. Balch felt there was something missing in the typical medical approach, which treated the symptoms rather than the cause of illness. Her introduction to the relationship between nutrition and well-being was through Paavo Airola, a well-known naturopath and writer. Balch then pursued her own intensive research into the science of nutrition, and by making radical changes in diet was able to transform her own health and the health of her children.

Convinced that nutrition was, in many cases, the answer to regaining and maintaining health, Balch opened a health food store called Good Things Naturally. In 1983, she published *Nutritional Outline for the Professional and the Wise Man*—now known as *Prescription for Nutritional Healing*—to share her knowledge with a broader audience. Through its five editions, this book has had millions of readers in many countries, and it has been translated into seven foreign languages.

During her lifetime, Balch continually shared her knowledge with others and persuaded many traditionally schooled medical practitioners to incorporate nutritional healing methods of restoring health into their practice. She was highly sought after as a visiting lecturer and appeared on television and radio programs throughout North America. Balch, who lived in Fort Myers, Florida, and Greenfield, Indiana, died in December 2004 while working on the fourth edition of *Prescription for Nutritional Healing*.

ABOUT STACEY BELL, DSC

In addition to revising the second edition of *Prescription for Herbal Healing* and the fifth edition of *Prescription for Nutritional Healing*, Stacey Bell has been a registered dietitian for thirty-five years, and has worked in that capacity and conducted clinical research studies for twenty years. She received a doctorate in nutrition from Boston University, with honors, in 1994. For her dissertation, she evaluated the effect of supplemental fish oil on immune function in patients with HIV infection and AIDS. Bell was on the faculty at Harvard Medical School in Boston, and has published more than seventy peer-reviewed scientific articles. Her research interests include obesity, diabetes, cancer, AIDS, burn patients, critical illness, and dietary supplements. A frequent lecturer around the world on many topics related to nutrition, she serves on the board of a nonprofit agency, Kids Can Cook, which offers basic cooking instruction and nutrition education to Boston middle-school-aged children.

THE #1 BESTSELLING NATURAL HEALTH SERIES

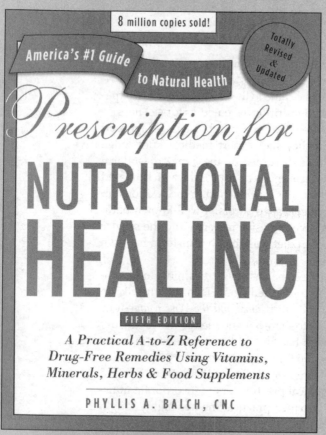

8 million copies sold!

America's #1 Guide to Natural Health

Totally Revised & Updated

Prescription for
NUTRITIONAL HEALING

FIFTH EDITION

A Practical A-to-Z Reference to
Drug-Free Remedies Using Vitamins,
Minerals, Herbs & Food Supplements

PHYLLIS A. BALCH, CNC

ISBN 978-1-58333-400-3

America's #1 Guide to Herbal Healing

MORE THAN 300,000 COPIES SOLD!

Prescription for
HERBAL HEALING

2ND EDITION

TOTALLY REVISED & UPDATED

*An Easy-to-Use A-to-Z
Reference to Hundreds of
Common Disorders and Their
Herbal Remedies*

PHYLLIS A. BALCH, CNC
Revised and updated by Stacey Bell, DSC
bestselling author of *Prescription for Nutritional Healing*, 5th Edition
(more than 8 million copies sold)

ISBN 978-1-58333-452-2

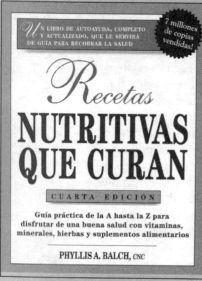

UN LIBRO DE AUTOAYUDA, COMPLETO
Y ACTUALIZADO, QUE LE SERVIRÁ
DE GUÍA PARA RECOBRAR LA SALUD

7 millones de copias vendidas!

Recetas
NUTRITIVAS QUE CURAN

CUARTA EDICIÓN

Guía práctica de la A hasta la Z para
disfrutar de una buena salud con vitaminas,
minerales, hierbas y suplementos alimentarios

PHYLLIS A. BALCH, CNC

ISBN 978-1-58333-352-5

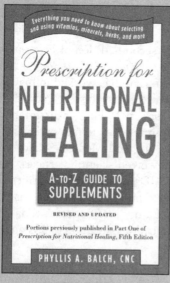

Everything you need to know about selecting
and using vitamins, minerals, herbs, and more

Prescription for
NUTRITIONAL HEALING

A-TO-Z GUIDE TO SUPPLEMENTS

REVISED AND UPDATED

Portions previously published in Part One of
Prescription for Nutritional Healing, Fifth Edition

PHYLLIS A. BALCH, CNC

ISBN 978-1-58333-412-6

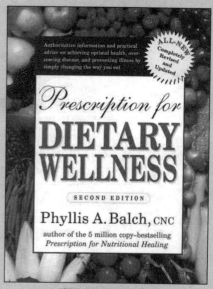

Authoritative information and practical
advice on achieving optimal health, overcoming disease, and preventing illness by
simply changing the way you eat

ALL-NEW
Completely Revised and Updated

Prescription for
DIETARY WELLNESS

SECOND EDITION

Phyllis A. Balch, CNC

author of the 5 million copy-bestselling
Prescription for Nutritional Healing

ISBN 978-1-58333-147-7

Natural remedies that work